OPTOMETRY

To my children, Benjamin, Simon and Daniel
Rosenfield, from whom I learn something new
every day.
Mark Rosenfield

To my daughter, Isla, with all my hopes, dreams and love.
Nicola Logan

For Elsevier:

Commissioning Editor: *Robert Edwards/Russell Gabbedy*
Development Editor: *Nicola Lally*
Project Manager: *Christine Johnston*
Designer: *Stewart Larking*
Illustration Manager: *Merlyn Harvey*
Illustrator: *Cactus*

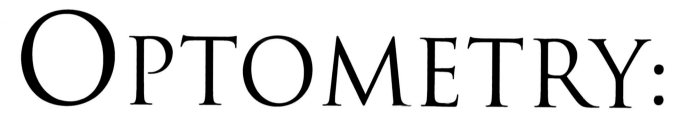

OPTOMETRY:
Science, Techniques AND Clinical Management

SECOND EDITION

Edited by

MARK ROSENFIELD, MCOPTOM, PHD, FAAO

SUNY College of Optometry, New York, USA

NICOLA LOGAN, MCOPTOM, PHD

School of Life and Health Sciences, Aston University, Birmingham, UK

Contributing Editor

KEITH EDWARDS, FCOPTOM, DIPCLP, FAAO

Bausch & Lomb, New York, USA

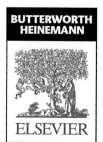

Edinburgh London New York Oxford Philadelphia St Louis Sydney Toronto 2009

BUTTERWORTH
HEINEMANN
ELSEVIER

First edition 1988
Second edition 2009

ISBN 978 0 7506 8778 2

British Library Cataloguing in Publication Data
A catalogue record for this book is available from the British Library

Library of Congress Cataloging in Publication Data
A catalog record for this book is available from the Library of Congress

Notice

Knowledge and best practice in this field are constantly changing. As new research and experience broaden our knowledge, changes in practice, treatment and drug therapy may become necessary or appropriate. Readers are advised to check the most current information provided (i) on procedures featured or (ii) by the manufacturer of each product to be administered, to verify the recommended dose or formula, the method and duration of administration, and contraindications. It is the responsibility of the practitioner, relying on their own experience and knowledge of the patient, to make diagnoses, to determine dosages and the best treatment for each individual patient, and to take all appropriate safety precautions. To the fullest extent of the law, neither the Publisher nor the Editors assumes any liability for any injury and/or damage to persons or property arising out of or related to any use of the material contained in this book.

The Publisher

Transferred to Digital Printing, 2014

Printed in the United States of America

Contents

PART 3 Management

Foreword

Optometry can trace its origins back to 1611 when Johannes Kepler wrote his *Dioptrice* concerning the mathematics of lenses, prisms and mirrors, as well as describing how the image is formed in the eye. In 1623, Daza de Valdes published the first treatise on the use and fitting of spectacles. Over the next centuries, optical instruments including telescopes and special lenses (e.g. achromatic lenses) appeared. By the end of the 19th century, opticians were performing ocular refractions based on prior scientific discoveries in optics and particularly the explanations of the refractive errors by Donders in 1864 in his classic textbook: '*Anomalies of Refraction and Accommodation of the Eye*'. By this time, Thomas Young had discovered astigmatism (in 1801) and described a famous experiment which demonstrated the role of the crystalline lens in accommodation. Other landmark contributions included the law of refraction (Snell, 1621), the sphero-cylindrical lens (Airy, 1825), optotypes (Snellen, 1862), and optical instruments to examine the eye, such as the ophthalmoscope (Helmholtz. 1851), ophthalmometer (Ramsden, 1795) and the first subjective instrument to measure accommodation (Porterfield, 1759) which was improved subsequently by Badal (1876). The dioptre, which became the standard optical unit, was first introduced by Monoyer in 1875.

The distinguished heritage of optometry comes from these classical optical and physical concepts, and many university departments or schools of optometry, such as those in Berkeley, Cardiff, London, Manchester and Sydney originated as a division of their respective physics departments. The emphasis of the optometry course was in the physical sciences and that is partly the reason why in the UK the appellation 'ophthalmic optics' was used until relatively recently. Today, the emphasis of the curriculum has shifted toward the biological sciences as optometry has become involved in health care delivery as a primary care profession. Many optometrists now participate in the treatment and management of ocular disease including diabetes and glaucoma. These developments have been facilitated by legislation in several countries including Australia, USA and the UK allowing optometrists to use diagnostic and therapeutic drugs for the management of abnormal ocular conditions. Other recent developments including the introduction of contact lens materials which are more compatible with the eye (e.g. silicone hydrogels), procedures to examine both the eye and vision using electronic and computer technology (e.g. short-wave perimetry, optical coherence tomography), better understanding of the optics of the eye (e.g. wavefront refraction) and knowledge of the complex neurology of the visual system have all contributed to contemporary optometric examination and management techniques.

Optometry: Science, Techniques and Clinical Management expertly reflects the present wide breadth of the scope and practice of optometry including eye and vision care for adults, children and the elderly, low vision, eye protection, contact lenses, as well as communication skills with patients. Each chapter represents an enlightened synthesis of the various aspects of modern optometry, although not in the detailed fashion of a textbook devoted to a given aspect (e.g. binocular vision, ophthalmic drugs). The chapters are written with up-to-date, evidenced-based information of the various examination procedures and management. There are some variations of style as one might expect in a multi-authored book, but it is to the credit of the editors that the overall presentation and flow of the text has attained uniformity without significant redundancy. Within the book, one will find the scientific foundation and basic clinical knowledge needed to understand and apply to the practice of optometry. The scope and quality of this book admirably reflects the maturity of optometry, a profession which has become utterly professional, independent and socially responsible.

The editors, Drs Mark Rosenfield and Nicola Logan are both well-known optometric scientists. They have gathered a group of eminent co-authors from various countries, each an expert in their own field. It is an enormous and arduous task to edit a book written by so many authors, as one becomes involved in a string of administrative tasks to gather the manuscripts. The whole process always proceeds at the speed of the slowest, who sometimes holds up the book for long periods of time. But they have succeeded brilliantly.

Michel Millodot, OD, FCOptom, PhD, DOSc (Hon), FAAO
Honorary Professor, School of Optometry and Vision Sciences, Cardiff University, UK;
Professor Emeritus, The Hong Kong Polytechnic University, Hong Kong

Preface

This book is the successor to *Optometry*, edited by Keith Edwards and Richard Llewellyn, which was published in 1988. In the preface to that work, the editors wrote that 'no single volume fulfilled the perceived need or covered the theoretical background to the visual and perceptive processes together with the techniques for the practical investigation and subsequent management of the normal and abnormal'. While the goal of this new work remains to meet that need, some 20 years later the scope and practice of optometry has changed dramatically. New techniques and procedures have been incorporated into everyday patient care, some of which were not even invented at the time the last edition was written. Now the practitioner can access sophisticated techniques for imaging the eye using procedures such as optical coherence tomography, test visual performance with function-specific perimeters, administer modern therapeutic pharmaceutical agents for a wide range of ophthalmic conditions and prescribe contact lenses manufactured using materials that seek to maintain the natural physiology of the cornea. In addition to these dramatic technological advancements, the patient base is also changing. As life expectancy rises, the number of patients over 70 years of age has increased significantly, with a concurrent expansion in the need for eye care services in this age group. At the same time, the younger members of the population are also in need of both routine and advanced care. Optometry has a responsibility to provide high-quality primary eye care to all members of society.

With the rapidly expanding scope of practice of optometry, one might ask how a single volume can cover all aspects of this growing profession. The simple answer is it cannot, particularly since many of the topics covered by a single chapter in this volume have entire textbooks devoted to them, such as contact lenses, visual fields or binocular vision. Nevertheless, the goal of this book is to provide the reader with an introduction to each area. Hopefully, this will whet the appetite and motivate them to move on to more advanced sources of information, such as specialist texts and journal articles. However, it is hoped that this integrated approach will appeal to both students new to the field of optometry and established practitioners seeking to update their knowledge.

The book is divided into three sections, namely science, techniques and clinical management. The first section reviews the anatomy, physiology and psychology of vision, examines visual performance and development and discusses ocular disease and the pharmacological interventions available to treat abnormal ocular conditions. In the second section, techniques for assessing the status and function of the eye are described together with the correction of refractive error using spectacles and contact lenses or by alternative means such as temporary or permanent anatomical changes. The final section discusses patient management, communication and legal aspects of optometry, and reviews the needs of special populations such as children, the elderly, low vision and special needs groups.

To reflect the international spectrum of optometry, we have included contributions from 40 authors based on four different continents. Currently, the breadth and type of practice varies markedly from one country to another, and we have tried to select internationally renowned authors who can provide a flavour of the way they practise in their particular location, even if some of the procedures or techniques may be more relevant to one particular region of the world than another. With the development of readily accessible and instantaneous global communication, geographic boundaries may become increasing irrelevant, and it is likely that optometry, like many other professions and political entities, will become more equitable in scope of practice. It is to be hoped that this volume can make a contribution to the 'globalisation' of our profession so that high-quality primary eye care can be provided to everyone around the world.

Finally, we thank the contributors to this volume. It has been a pleasure to work with such an outstanding group of people, and we apologize for all the nagging e-mails that production of a work such as this necessitates. Their willingness to pass on their expertise to both present and future practitioners is a tribute to their generosity and wisdom, and bodes well for the future of this expanding profession.

Mark Rosenfield
Nicola Logan

Contributors

David A Atchison MSc (Optom), PhD, DSc, FAAO, FOSA, CertEd (Higher Ed)
Institute of Health and Biomedical Innovation, Queensland University of Technology, Brisbane, Australia

Gary E Baker PhD
Department of Optometry and Visual Science, City University, London, UK

Sherry J Bass OD, MS, FAAO
SUNY College of Optometry, New York, USA

Christopher Bentley MCOptom, FRCOphth
Central Middlesex Hospital, London, UK

Susan Blakeney FCOptom, PhD, LLM, LLB
The College of Optometrists, London, UK

W Neil Charman FCOptom (Hon), PhD, DSc, FOptSocAm
Department of Optometry and Neuroscience, University of Manchester, Manchester, UK

Kent M Daum OD, PhD
Illinois College of Optometry, Chicago, USA

Leon N Davies MCOptom, PhD, FAAO, FHEA
School of Life and Health Sciences, Aston University, Birmingham, UK

Michael J Doughty PhD
Department of Vision Sciences, Glasgow Caledonian University, Glasgow, UK

Kathryn Dumbleton MCOptom, MSc, FAAO (DipCL), FBCLA
Centre for Contact Lens Research, School of Optometry, University of Waterloo, Waterloo, Canada

Keith Edwards FCOptom, DipCLP, FAAO
Bausch & Lomb, New York, USA

Bruce J W Evans FCOptom, PhD, DipCLP, DipOrth, FAAO, FBCLA
Institute of Optometry, London, UK; Optometry and Visual Science, City University, London, UK

John G Flanagan MCOptom, PhD, FAAO
School of Optometry, University of Waterloo, Waterloo, Canada; Department of Ophthalmology and Vision Sciences, University of Toronto, Toronto, Canada

James M Gilchrist FCOptom, PhD
Bradford School of Optometry and Vision Science, University of Bradford, Bradford, UK

Bernard Gilmartin FCOptom, PhD, FAAO
School of Life and Health Sciences, Aston University, Birmingham, UK

Graham Hopkins BPharm, PhD, MRPharmS
Community Pharmacist, Cheltenham, UK

Lyndon Jones FCOptom, PhD, DipCLP, DipOrth, FAAO (DipCL)
Centre for Contact Lens Research, School of Optometry, University of Waterloo, Waterloo, Canada

Carly S Y Lam MCOptom, PhD, FAAO
School of Optometry, The Hong Kong Polytechnic University, Hong Kong

Marc Lay BS
SUNY College of Optometry, New York, USA

Susan J Leat FCOptom, PhD, FAAO
School of Optometry, University of Waterloo, Waterloo, Canada

Nicola Logan MCOptom, PhD
School of Life and Health Sciences, Aston University, Birmingham, UK

Jan Lovie-Kitchin MSc (Optom), PhD, FAAO
School of Optometry, Queensland University of Technology, Brisbane, Australia

Shabbir Mohamed MBChB (Hons), MRCOphth, FRCSEd
University Hospital Birmingham, NHS Foundation Trust, Birmingham, UK

Shehzad A Naroo MCOptom, PhD, FIACLE, FAAO, FBCLA
School of Life and Health Sciences, Aston University, Birmingham, UK

Rachel North FCOptom, PhD
School of Optometry and Vision Sciences, Cardiff University, Cardiff, UK

Catherine Pace Watson OD
SUNY College of Optometry, New York, USA

Joan K Portello OD, MPH, MS, FAAO
SUNY College of Optometry, New York, USA

Christine Purslow MCOptom, PhD, FBCLA, FIACLE
School of Optometry and Vision Sciences, Cardiff University, Cardiff, UK

Mark Rosenfield MCOptom, PhD, FAAO
SUNY College of Optometry, New York, USA

Bruce P Rosenthal OD, FAAO
Low Vision Programs, Lighthouse International; SUNY College of Optometry, New York, USA; Low Vision Service, Mt Sinai Hospital, New York, USA

Ranjit Sandhu MRCOphth
Central Middlesex Hospital, London, UK

Kathryn J Saunders MCOptom, PhD
School of Biomedical Sciences, University of Ulster, Coleraine, UK

Sunil Shah MBBS, FRCOphth, FRCS (Ed), FBCLA
Midland Eye Institute, Solihull, UK; School of Life and Health Sciences, Aston University, Birmingham, UK; School of Biomedical Sciences, University of Ulster, Coleraine, UK

Jerome Sherman OD, FAAO
SUNY College of Optometry, New York, USA

Glyn Walsh FCOptom, PhD
Department of Vision Sciences, Glasgow Caledonian University, Glasgow, UK

Carol Westall PhD
Ophthalmology and Vision Science, University of Toronto and The Hospital for Sick Children, Toronto, Canada

Elizabeth Wickware BS
SUNY College of Optometry, New York, USA

CHAPTER **1**

Forming an optical image: the optical elements of the eye

W Neil Charman

Introduction

The role of any sensory system is to gather such information about the environment as is appropriate to an animal's needs. This information can then be used by the animal to make decisions about such basic activities as feeding, navigation, sex and avoidance of predators. The information acquired might be conveyed over considerable distances in the form of sound, smell, or electric or magnetic fields. Alternatively, it might involve closer contact through, for example, touch or taste. Sensory systems based on the detection of electromagnetic radiation ('light') have the obvious advantage of providing line-of-sight data over substantial distances, hence allowing maximal time for decisions to be made about the appropriate behavioural response. Unlike systems based on sound or smell, these visual systems are unaffected by wind speed and direction but they do demand either a source of light, to be reflected by the environment, or that objects within the environment themselves emit radiation. Most vertebrates and invertebrates depend upon passively reflected light as the basis of their visual systems, although the pit organs of some snakes have developed to detect the thermal infrared radiation which is actively emitted by some prey animals, and the light emitted by many deep-sea creatures plays an important role in their activities. In this chapter we will be concerned with how the human eye is constructed to use electromagnetic radiation to form an image of the outside world on the light-sensitive retina for subsequent processing by the neural system.

The various stages of our visual system developed collectively to gather optical radiation from different directions in the environment and to process the information contained to ultimately generate the final perceived representation of the individual's surroundings. Ideally, this final percept might include information on the spatial, motion, depth, colour and other aspects of the environment. This data extraction should occur over as wide a range of illumination levels as possible. In practice, the reduced photon flux available at lower light levels has forced the evolution of a flexible visual system in which, as the illumination level falls, some sacrifices are made in the amount of detailed information that can be acquired, in order to retain sensitivity to light combined with a reasonable temporal response.

In the evolutionary past, the only widely available electromagnetic radiation available for the development of a sensory system based on its detection was direct and reflected sunlight (**Fig. 1.1**). Although in space the solar spectrum corresponds fairly closely to that of a black body at a temperature of 5760 K, at the earth's surface such radiation has an abrupt shortwave cutoff at about 280 nm, set by ozone absorption in the upper atmosphere. Its peak spectral irradiance occurs over a band from about 400 to 800 nm. A series of absorption bands caused mainly by water vapour reduce irradiance in the near infrared. The exact spectrum varies with such factors as the solar zenith angle, cloud cover and viewing direction. From the evolutionary point of view, then, this spectrum and its variations not only set a limit to the maximum photon energy available to initiate photochemical events within the eye but also necessarily influenced the evolution

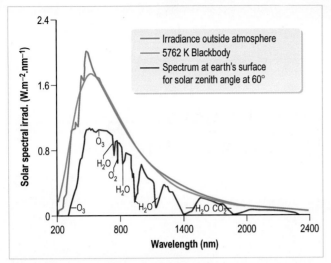

Figure 1.1 The solar irradiance spectrum. The solar spectrum as incident from outside the atmosphere (*green*) is modified by atmospheric absorption during its passage to the earth's surface. For comparison, the spectrum for a 5762 K black body is also shown (blue). The red curve gives the solar spectrum at the earth's surface when the solar zenith angle is 60°. The 'visible' region of the spectrum extends from about 400 to 700 nm. (After Mecherikunne et al 1983.)

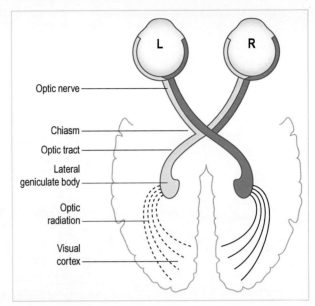

Figure 1.2 Schematic diagram showing the visual pathways, viewed from above the head.

of the overall spectral sensitivity and potential for colour vision of terrestrial animals: the spectrum available to aquatic species was modified by absorption characteristics of the relevant depth of water. Further, if we assume that the human visual system developed to provide useful information over illuminances between the 150 000 lux of bright sunlight and the 0.0001 lux of the overcast night sky, we can see that it needed an enormous dynamic range. One consequence of the need to respond over a range of up to 10 $\log_{10}$ units of illuminance is that our visual system is rather poor at judging absolute levels of light and is primarily concerned with contrasts, that is, the relative luminances in different parts of a scene. Other species, with different needs and environments, have developed quite different visual systems (e.g. Duke-Elder 1958; Lythgoe 1979; Cronly-Dillon & Gregory, 1991).

It will be helpful to start this brief review of the optical part of the visual system and its properties by reminding ourselves of the basic overall form of the visual pathways (**Fig. 1.2**). Twin optical images are first formed on the light-sensitive retinas of the two eyes. Each eye must be directed so that the image of the object of interest falls on the central fovea, this being achieved with the aid of appropriate head turns together with the extraocular muscles which move the eyes within their orbits. Due to the lateral separation of the eyes, each receives a slightly different view of the world, giving the possibility of stereoscopic vision.

At the retina the optical images are encoded in the form of spatially and temporally related neural activity that is transmitted via the optic nerves and chiasma through the lateral geniculate nuclei (LGNs) to the primary visual cortex at the back of the brain. The nasal halves of the fibres within each optic nerve cross at the chiasma (decussate), so that those from the same half of the visual field of both eyes arrive at the same side of the brain. Thus the left side of the visual field is represented at the right side of the cortex

and the right half on the left side. Other pathways (not shown) link to other areas of the brain. Signal processing at the retina, LGNs and cortex enhances the extraction of specific types of spatial and temporal information from the incoming light signal (see Ch. 2).

Although, in this and the next chapter, it will be convenient to take these various stages in sequence, it must be remembered that the whole system evolved collectively, so that the characteristics of each element developed in relation to the abilities and demands of other elements.

Over the years in which the structure and function of the visual system have been studied, an enormous, and still growing, volume of information has been accumulated, admirably summarized by a variety of authors (e.g. Davson 1990; Pipe & Rapley 1997; Bron et al 1997; Forrester et al 2002; Kaufman & Alm 2003). Valuable discussions of the characteristics of the anterior eye in relation to contact lens wear have been given by several authors (e.g. Lawrenson 2002). The present chapter can only serve as an introduction to the more important results on the optical components of the eye itself.

The eyeball and its neighbouring structures

Each eyeball or globe lies within its orbit (**Fig. 1.3**). Viewed from the outside, the larger opaque portion, the sclera, approximates to a sphere about 25 mm in diameter. The anterior transparent portion, the cornea, has a smaller radius of curvature of about 7.8 mm. These two regions are linked by a transition zone, the limbus or corneoscleral junction, where two connective tissue sacs merge. One of these, Tenon's capsule, surrounds the globe and the other, the conjunctiva, links the globe to the eyelids. The palpebral conjunctiva lines the inner surfaces of the lids: the conjunctiva then continues posteriorly via the upper and lower fornices to cover the anterior globe as the bulbar conjunctiva,

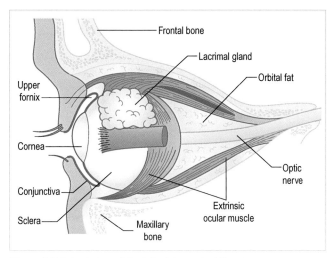

Figure 1.3 Lateral view of the left globe and orbit.

ending at the limbus. Nerves, blood vessels and the tendons of the extraocular muscles penetrate Tenon's capsule, which is continuous with the tissue sheaths of these.

The globe is supported by the fat that lies between it and the periosteum lining the orbital walls and by the extraocular muscle sheaths. The lacrimal gland lies on the upper temporal side of the globe and is responsible for producing the bulk of the tears.

Anterior to the globe the eyelids, through their reflex closure, form a protective external barrier against injury from excessive light or mechanical trauma. Their action during blinking (typical rate around 12 blinks/min) removes debris from the cornea, and spreads the tear film across the corneal surface. Tears collect at the inner canthal angle (i.e. the nasal junction of the upper and lower lids) and, under the action of blinking, drain into the neighbouring punctae (about 0.25 mm in diameter) of the upper and lower lids, to flow through the canaliculi (about 10 mm long and 0.5 mm in diameter) into the lacrimal sac and thence to the nasolacrimal duct. The lids also contain the meibomian glands

(about 30–40 opening on the margin of the upper lid and slightly fewer, 20–40, on the lower), which secrete the lipids for the tear layer.

The globe itself (**Fig. 1.4**) is made up of three basic concentric layers or coats, also sometimes known as tunics. Proceeding inwards from the outside of the eye, these are successively the outer fibrous (corneoscleral) coat, the vascular uvea (choroid, ciliary body and iris), much of which is nutritive in function, and the neural layer (retina) where the optical image is received and converted to neural activity (see Ch. 2). The outer fibrous coat provides a tough protective envelope for the other ocular structures, together with structural support for the intraocular contents and for the attachments of the extraocular muscles. The iris contains the pupil, which has several important optical roles. The crystalline lens is suspended from the ciliary body or muscle by the zonular fibres (which collectively make up the zonule of Zinn) so that, in the young eye, changes in shape of the ciliary body vary the tension of the zonule and alter the shape of the lens to allow accommodation or focusing on objects at different distances. The choroid offers support and nourishment to the neural retina. Together, the three coats enclose the optical media of the eye: the aqueous, the lens and the vitreous.

The dioptric apparatus

General characteristics

The first stage of vision is the formation of an optical image on the retina. Information lost at this stage cannot be retrieved by later stages of the visual system and, indeed, the major cause of poor vision remains the defocus blur of the retinal image caused by uncorrected refractive error. Since the retinal receptors can only respond over a limited range of wavelengths, it is important that the optical media of the eye – tear film, cornea, aqueous, lens and vitreous – have good transmittance within this wavelength range. Moreover, they are required to produce a retinal image with a quality compatible with the spatial resolution of the neural retina. As the smallest foveal receptors measure about

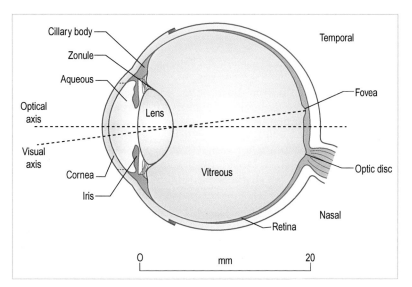

Figure 1.4 Schematic horizontal section of the eye. The bar gives the approximate scale. The angle between the visual and optical axes is angle alpha (α).

2 μm in diameter (see Ch. 2) and subtend about 0.4 min arc at the posterior nodal point of the eye, this demands that the optical resolution of the eye be of a similar order. Recalling that the limit set by diffraction to the optical resolution of the eye is about 1.22 λ/D radians, where λ is the wavelength and D the pupil diameter, the diffraction-limited resolution of an eye with the typical photopic pupil diameter of 4 mm would be around 0.6 min arc. Thus, the optical system of the eye needs to be both transparent at solar wavelengths and, at least at the fovea, of remarkably good optical quality. No other body structure is transparent over distances of 25 mm and, as we shall see, almost all the structures anterior to the retina through which light has to pass are avascular.

The basic layout of the eye is illustrated in **Figure 1.4**. Its optical properties have been modelled with various degrees of sophistication by numerous authors (Atchison & Smith 2000; Rabbetts 2007). **Figure 1.5** shows some common paraxial models of the unaccommodated eye. The most complex model has dimensions, curvatures and refractive indices which approximate to those of typical real eyes. The three models are progressively simpler in their optics, the main difference being that they have different numbers of optical surfaces: their major optical parameters are listed in **Table 1.1**. The single-surface, reduced eye is adequate for many calculations in visual optics on the effects of corrective lenses in ametropia (e.g. Rabbetts 2007). In practice, the dimensional parameters of individual, normal, adult eyes show spreads of at least ±10% about the 'typical' values of the models. For example, radii of curvature for the anterior cornea may lie between about 7.0 and 8.8 mm and axial lengths between 20 and 28 mm. It has been found that the distributions of the values of individual parameters across the population are approximately normal but that correlation between the individual parameters for any single eye results in the distribution of refractive error showing a strong peak near emmetropia, rather than being a normal distribution. The development of refractive error is discussed in a later chapter (Ch. 11). We now consider the actual optical structures in more detail.

The tear film

The first optical element is the tear film (see Korb et al 2002 for an extensive review). Its quality is of major importance, as there is a large change in refractive index over its anterior boundary, giving a surface power of around 43 D, and it must provide a smooth optical surface. It also plays a role in metabolic support, particularly in providing oxygen to the avascular cornea, protection against microbial colonization, and lubrication to allow the lids to move smoothly across the anterior eye. The tear film is, of course, a dynamic structure due to evaporation, tear loss through the punctae, absorption by the conjunctiva, and tear flow, and it is important that its smoothness be maintained during the period between blinks.

In the past, the tear film was usually described as having a trilaminar structure: a superficial lipid or oily layer around 0.1 μm thick; an aqueous layer around 7 μm thick; and, in contact with the corneal epithelium, a mucus layer around 0.02–0.05 μm thick. Current ideas favour a more complex structure, with a gradient of mucin continuing into the aqueous layer, but debate continues on the true thicknesses of its components, particularly that of the aqueous layer. The majority of the lipid layer, which among other functions plays the important role of reducing evaporation of the underlying aqueous layer, originates in the meibomian glands on the lid margins. The aqueous phase, which contains dissolved ions and proteins, comes from the main lacrimal gland, with some contributions from the accessory glands of Krause and Wolfring in the conjunctiva. Most of the mucin originates in the goblet cells of the conjunctiva. Amongst other roles, such as protecting the epithelium against local drying effects, the mucous layer effectively forms a self-healing barrier against bacterial infiltration.

The normal rate of tear production is between 1 and 2 μL/min, equivalent to a turnover of around 16% per minute in normal subjects. In the normal eye, the interval between blinks is typically around 5 seconds. This is much shorter than the time taken for the film to start to break up when the eye is deliberately kept open after a blink (typically around 30 seconds, depending upon how break-up is assessed, see Ch. 17).

The cornea

Looked at from the front, the cornea measures about 12 mm in the horizontal meridian and 11 mm in the vertical meridian, so that its surface constitutes around 6% of the area of the globe. It is thinner at its centre (around 0.52 mm) than at its periphery (around 0.67 mm). While the tear film is important in providing a locally smooth anterior surface to the eye, the shape of this surface is determined by the contour of the underlying cornea. This typically approximates to a conicoid of the form $x^2 + y^2 + pz^2 = 2r_0z$, where x and y are Cartesian coordinates perpendicular to the axis of symmetry, z; r_0 is the radius of curvature at the corneal apex; and p is an asphericity parameter or shape factor. Values of p<0 represent hyperboloids, p = 0 paraboloids, 0<p<1 flattening (prolate) ellipsoids, p = 1 spheres and p>1 steepening

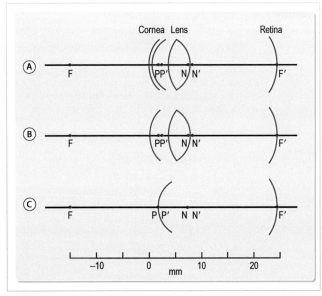

Figure 1.5 Typical paraxial optical models of the unaccommodated, emmetropic eye, showing the positions of the cardinal points in relation to the various surfaces. P, P′ are the principal points, F, F′ the focal points and N, N′ the nodal points. The parameters of these eyes are listed in **Table 1.1**.

Table 1.1 Parameters of some paraxial models of the relaxed, emmetropic human eye.

		Schematic eye	Simplified schematic eye	Reduced eye
Surface radii	Anterior cornea	7.80	7.80	5.55
	Posterior cornea	6.50		
	Anterior lens	10.20	10.00	
	Posterior lens	−6.00	−6.00	
Distances from anterior cornea	Posterior cornea	0.55		
	Anterior lens	3.60	3.60	
	Posterior lens	7.60	7.20	
	Retina	24.20	23.90	22.22
Refractive indices	Cornea	1.3371		
	Aqueous humour	1.3374	1.333	1.333
	Lens	1.4200	1.416	
	Vitreous humour	1.3360	1.333	

Dimensions are in millimetres.
The schematic eye is that suggested by Le Grand and el Hage; the other two models are due to Emsley.
(After Charman 1991.)

(oblate) ellipsoids. The same conicoid equation is sometimes written in terms of either an alternative asphericity factor Q, or the eccentricity e of the conic section, where $p = 1 + Q = 1 − e^2$. Studies (Kiely et al 1982; Guillon et al 1986) suggest that the mean p value and its standard deviation are around 0.8±0.15. The mean corresponds to a prolate ellipsoid with flattening in the periphery although individual eyes may vary substantially from this value (range 0.2<p<1.5) (**Fig. 1.6**). The flattening of the cornea in its periphery helps to reduce ocular spherical aberration and is of obvious importance in relation to the fit of rigid contact lenses. With r_0 around 7.8 mm, the tear film and cornea typically provide about two-thirds of the overall optical power of the eye.

When viewed in transverse section, the cornea consists of five layers of varying thicknesses (**Fig. 1.7A**). Moving from the anterior to the posterior surface these are: the epithelium (50 μm thick); the basal lamina (between 0.5 and 1.0 μm)

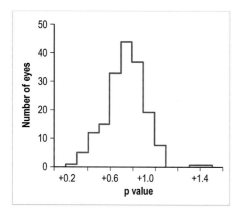

Figure 1.6 Histogram showing the distribution of values for the corneal asphericity parameter or shape factor p in a sample of 176 eyes. (After Kiely et al 1982.)

and Bowman's layer (8–14 μm); the stroma (about 450 μm); Descemet's membrane (10–12 μm); and the endothelium (5 μm).

The stratified, squamous, non-keratinized epithelium consists mainly of 5–6 layers of cells, these being a single row of columnar basal cells, 2–3 rows of wing cells and a further 2–3 layers of flattened, superficial (squamous) cells. The epithelium forms a permeability barrier to small molecules, water and ions, as well as to pathogens. Mitosis in the basal layer produces new cells which move up into the wing-cell layer. In turn, the wing cells move into the superficial layers. At the anterior surface of the superficial cells small finger- and ridge-like projections (microvilli and microplicae) protrude into the tear film and are thought to be of importance in relation to the spreading and attachment of the tear film. The surface cells are eventually lost to the tears, to be replaced by new cells from beneath, the normal turnover time of the epithelial cells being about a week. If the epithelium is damaged to the level of the basement membrane, the basal cells spread out to cover the damaged area: after a few hours of initial inhibition, cell growth recommences so that the epithelium is restored to its normal thickness in a few days. The integrity of the limbus is important to the regeneration process. The ability of the epithelium to recover after trauma is one of the factors that make possible excimer laser refractive surgical techniques, such as photorefractive keratectomy, which involve removing the central area of the epithelium.

The acellular Bowman's layer consists of a randomly oriented array of fine collagen fibrils with diameters around 25 nm. Interestingly, it is not present in the cornea of most mammals and its removal over the central cornea in photorefractive keratectomy does not appear to affect corneal integrity.

The bulk of the corneal thickness is provided by the stroma, consisting of ribbons or layers (lamellae) of collagen fibrils in a matrix of proteoglycans with fibroblasts

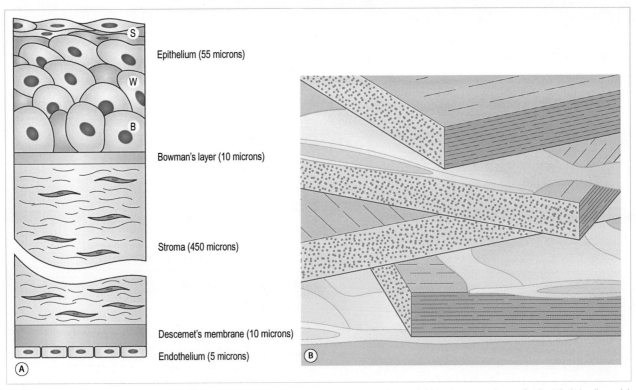

Epithelium (55 microns)

Bowman's layer (10 microns)

Stroma (450 microns)

Descemet's membrane (10 microns)

Endothelium (5 microns)

Figure 1.7 Schematic diagrams showing **(A)** section of the layers of the cornea (not to scale). Typical basal, wing and superficial epithelial cells are labelled B, W and S, respectively. **(B)** Arrangement of collagen fibrils in adjacent laminae, together with keratocytes: each lamella is about 2 microns thick and the flattened keratocytes lie between neighbouring lamellae.

(keratocytes) spread between the layers. There are about 200 lamellae, each around 2 µm thick and 10–260 µm wide: they extend right across the cornea, from limbus to limbus. Within each lamella the collagen fibrils, each around 31 nm in diameter, are oriented parallel to one another and the interfibrillar spacing is almost constant at about 55 nm. Fibrils of neighbouring lamellae make large angles (almost 90 degrees) with each other, giving the overall cornea considerable mechanical strength. The keratocytes, which are stellate cells flattened in the plane of the cornea and lie between the lamellae, maintain the corneal collagen and proteoglycans (**Fig. 1.7B**).

Descemet's membrane acts as the basement membrane for the endothelium and is composed of fine collagen fibrils. Its thickness increases after birth from an initial value of about 4 µm to adult values of around 10 µm. Finally, the endothelium consists of a single layer of squamous cells which, when viewed from a direction perpendicular to the corneal surface, appears as a polygonal (typically hexagonal), quasi-regular mosaic. At birth, the cell density is about 4500 cells/mm^2 but as, unlike the situation in the epithelium, there is a limited capacity for mitosis, the cell density decreases with age. Studies suggest, however, that functional normality is still maintained when the cell density falls to 1000 cells/mm^2.

The cornea is richly innervated, receiving its mainly sensory nerve supply from the nasociliary branch of the trigeminal nerve. Most of the 50–80 nerve trunks enter the cornea at mid-stromal level. Their starting direction is radial. Although initially the trunks contain a mixture of myelinated and unmyelinated fibres, myelin is soon lost. The fibres run anteriorly and progressively divide to form the subepithelial nerve plexus. Fibres from this plexus then penetrate Bowman's layer and form a quasi-regular meshwork at the basal cell layer. Small branches extend towards the more superficial epithelial layers. It is of interest that nerves from any particular point in the corneal periphery branch out to serve multiple points on the cornea, so that there is no correspondence between an individual nerve trunk and any particular region of the cornea: thus corneal touch or pain is not experienced as a localized sensation.

A key question is why the corneal stroma is transparent whereas the sclera, which is comprised of broadly similar material, is not. Maurice (1957) suggested that the explanation lay primarily in the uniformity in diameter and regularity in spacing of the fibrils comprising the corneal lamellae. He proposed that this arrangement led to strong constructive interference in the forward direction of the light waves diffracted by each fibril and hence forward propagation of the light. In contrast, the scleral fibrils lack such characteristics, being on average both larger and more variable in diameter (105±37 nm in the limbal area of sclera): thus there are no systematic phase differences between the diffracted waves and light is strongly scattered in all directions, to give the sclera its 'white' appearance. Although Maurice's concept of a completely regular lattice has been modified by later authors, it remains of prime importance.

Maintenance of the spacing of the corneal fibrils demands control of corneal hydration. When the cornea swells, the disruption associated with the changed fibrillary spacing causes an increase in scattering and a loss in transparency. In practice, it appears that excess water results in clumping of fibrils in some stromal regions, with other regions having no fibrils. The corneal endothelium plays a vital role in maintaining hydration at the appropriate level of 78±5% (Hodson 1997). The endothelium acts both as a barrier, through tight junctions between neighbouring cells, and a metabolically driven pump which ensures the interchange of appropriate ions and small molecules between the aqueous and the stroma.

To maintain its integrity and function, the cornea needs to be supplied with oxygen and essential metabolites such as glucose, vitamins and amino acids. Since the optical requirement of transparency has led to an avascular structure, these metabolic needs must be met from other sources. Under open-eye conditions, oxygen comes largely from the atmosphere after diffusion across the tear film, with the tears being saturated with oxygen. Contact lenses may interfere with this process (and with the normal egress of carbon dioxide from the cornea) and, as a result, enormous efforts have been made over the years to improve the oxygen transmissibility of contact lens materials. During eye closure, the oxygen level in the tears is in equilibrium with that of the palpebral vasculature. The aqueous appears to be the primary source of glucose and amino acids for the cornea, rather than the tears and perilimbal vasculature.

The aqueous humour

The non-cellular aqueous has the twin roles of providing a clear optical medium and a supply of metabolites for the neighbouring ocular structures. Like the vitreous, it contains about 99% water. Its density and viscosity are essentially the same as those of water. Unlike the vitreous, it is continuously renewed. The total volume is about 340 μL, with about 270 μL in the anterior chamber and 70 μL in the posterior chamber, although the volume of the anterior chamber decreases with age and tends to be smaller in hyperopic eyes. The aqueous originates in the ciliary body and carries fluid and metabolites, such as glucose and amino acids, that have diffused from the capillaries of the ciliary processes: there are about of these 70 processes, forming ridges each about 1 mm high, 2 mm long and 0.5 mm wide, arranged radially on the rear part of the ciliary body and collectively forming the pars plicata. The aqueous circulates from the posterior chamber, through the pupil, and into the anterior chamber. Most of it finally passes through the trabecular meshwork and is removed from the eye via the canal of Schlemm, a narrow tube which follows an annular course some 30 mm long circumferential to the borders of the anterior chamber, to the episcleral venous network (**Fig. 1.8**), although some aqueous is removed by other routes. The rate of replacement of aqueous is about 1% of its volume (i.e. 2–3 μL) per minute.

During its passage through the posterior and anterior chambers the aqueous provides metabolites to the avascular lens and cornea and carries away their waste products. Circulation also helps to maintain optical clarity. The aqueous humour provides positive pressure to give shape to the globe and maintain contact between the neural layers of the retina and the pigment epithelium. In combination with the pressure from the vascular system, it largely controls the intraocular pressure (IOP), which, when measured by applanation tonometry, has an average value of around 15–16 mmHg, with higher readings being obtained in the

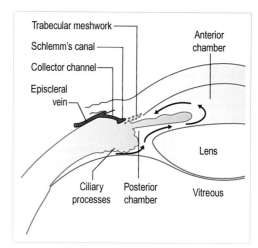

Figure 1.8 Bulk flow of aqueous humour.

early morning and lower in the evening. If the circulation of the aqueous is impeded, intraocular pressure will change, leading to a variety of clinical problems (see Ch. 24).

The crystalline lens

The biconvex crystalline lens, which in its unaccommodated state has a smaller radius of curvature in its posterior surface (see **Table 1.1**), is basically composed of 65% water and 35% protein. It is completely enclosed within its transparent, elastic capsule, a thickened, smooth, basement membrane. This varies in thickness across its area: the anterior portion is thicker than the posterior portion (thicknesses at the anterior and posterior poles are about 3 and 16 μm, respectively) and both portions are thicker towards the equator, where the zonular fibres are attached (**Fig. 1.9**). When not affected by forces from the supporting zonular fibres the elastic forces from the capsule mould the young, excised lens into a more convex, optically more powerful, accommodated shape. At the anterior surface of the lens, below the capsule, lies a single layer of cuboidal epithelial cells: these are about 6 μm high and 15 μm wide near the lens axis but become progressively longer towards the lens equator. At and near the lens equator,

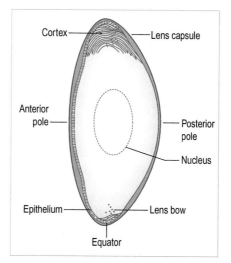

Figure 1.9 The lens in section. The thicknesses of the capsule and the epithelium have been exaggerated for clarity.

the cells undergo mitotic division throughout life. The new cells produce processes which pass anteriorly between the epithelium and the rest of the lens and posteriorly along the inner surface of the capsule to become new lens fibres. Thus, the outer layers of the lens (the cortex) are composed of younger fibres, whereas the inner regions (the nucleus) contain older fibres. The lens fibres are flattened hexagons in section and are linked to their neighbours by 'ball and socket' and other junctions along their lengths, so that the lens acts as a single body during the shape changes accompanying accommodation, no sliding of the fibres with respect to one another being possible.

Due to the continuous addition of new fibres, lens thickness increases from about 3.5 to 5.0 mm between birth and 80 years, while the weight increase from 65 to 270 mg. Lens growth additionally affects the surface curvatures (the anterior surface becomes steeper with age while the posterior surface does not) and reduces the depth of the anterior chamber as the position of the posterior pole of the lens changes little throughout life. Finally, it affects the refractive index distribution of the lens, since the nuclear regions are older and more compressed than the outer cortical regions, giving a higher refractive index in the nucleus (around 1.41) than in the cortex (about 1.36). The exact nature of the refractive index distribution, and its change with age, is still uncertain but it contributes significantly to both the power and the aberrations of the lens.

The lens is supported from its equatorial region by a complex arrangement of mainly radially directed zonular fibres (the zonule of Zinn) anchored to the lens capsule up to around 2 mm from the equator anteriorly and 1 mm posteriorly. Each 'fibre', with a diameter of around 5–35 μm, is actually a bundle of smaller fibres, themselves composed of 8–12 nm collagen fibrils. The other ends of the zonular fibres arise from the pars plana ciliary epithelium, so that shape changes in the ciliary body or muscle alter the tension in the fibres and hence affect the shape of the elastic capsule and lens.

The modest metabolic requirements of the lens have to be satisfied by metabolites which have diffused through the capsule from the aqueous and vitreous, with waste products moving in the reverse direction.

The vitreous body

The bulk of the optical path to the retina is provided by the transparent, jelly-like vitreous body. In the young eye this has a consistency somewhat firmer than uncooked egg white. The vitreous approximates to a sphere with an anterior depression (the patellar or hyaloid fossa) to accommodate the rear surface of the lens. Running axially back through the vitreous from the posterior pole of the lens to the optic disc is the fluid-filled Cloquet's canal, 1–2 mm wide, which marks the path of the fetal hyaloid artery. The vitreous consists of a network of collagen filaments (about 15–20 nm in diameter) in a fluid matrix which has a very similar composition to the aqueous. The more liquid central vitreous is surrounded by a cortical zone where the collagen fibres are more densely arranged, a similar condensation of fibrils constituting the walls of Cloquet's canal. The vitreous is essentially acellular but isolated cells may occur and larger numbers may be seen in some pathologies. It is attached to other ocular structures at various points, particularly to the

retina around the optic disc, and to the posterior lens capsule and the peripheral retina and pars plana via the vitreous base, a 3–4 mm wide annular band. The vitreous tends to become more liquid with age. It is usually considered that the vitreous is optically homogeneous but it may be that variations in its local composition contribute to irregular ocular aberration and scattering.

The pupil

The final optical component of the eye is the pupil, whose margin rests on the anterior lens. The pupil acts as the aperture stop of the system. Its diameter therefore plays an important role in relation to the quantity of light reaching the retina, ocular depth-of-focus, diffractive effects and optical aberrations. The main factors affecting its diameter are the light and the near reflexes, with neural pathways involving autonomic parasympathetic (constriction) and sympathetic (dilation) mechanisms, acting on the sphincter and dilator pupillae muscles, respectively. Pupil diameter is also affected by a variety of other factors, including emotional state, pain and drugs, and tends to decrease with age.

Figure 1.10 shows typical data for the pupil diameter of young adult observers as a function of scene luminance. Note that even when the ambient light level changes by about eight orders of magnitude the pupil diameter changes by less than a factor of four, so its area changes by $<16\times$. Thus, the changes in pupil area are by no means great enough to maintain constant retinal illuminance under changing lighting conditions. (Retinal illuminance is generally specified in trolands, where an illuminance of 1 troland corresponds to that produced by a field of luminance 1 cd/m^2 seen through a pupil of area 1 mm^2.)

The optical performance of the eye

Transmittance

The cumulative effect of the spectral transmittances of the elements of the eye is illustrated in **Figure 1.11**. What is plotted is the cumulative transmittance up to the rear

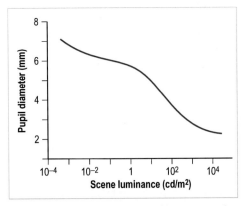

Figure 1.10 Ocular entrance pupil diameter as a function of scene luminance for young observers. Pupil diameter is influenced by a variety of other factors, so the values given can only be considered as being typical. For comparison with later chapters, the photopic region, where cone vision dominates, extends down to about 3 cd/m^2 and the scotopic region, where only rods are operative, up to about 10^{-3} cd/m^2. Between these two regions lies the transitional mesopic range, where both types of retinal receptor contribute to vision.

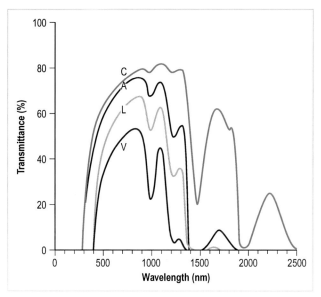

Figure 1.11 Cumulative spectral transmittances at the posterior surfaces of the ocular structures in the young adult eye. Transmittances up to the posterior cornea, aqueous, lens and vitreous are labelled C, A, L and V, respectively. (After Boettner and Wolter 1962.)

surface of each ocular component. It can be seen that the cornea provides the first line of defence against energetic ultraviolet photons which could potentially harm the retina, although too much ultraviolet light can damage the cells of the corneal epithelium and result in photokeratitis (snow blindness, arc eye, welder's flash). It is evident that the lens provides a second major cutoff at the blue-violet end of the spectrum, which additionally helps to protect the retina against damage from higher-energy photons (the 'blue light hazard'). Blue-absorbing macular pigment extending over the central 5 degrees of the retina further protects the central fovea from damage. The media continue to transmit (and form an optical image) at infrared wavelengths (at least up to 1300 nm) to which the retina is not sensitive, a characteristic which is made use of in several types of optometric instruments, such as many autorefractors. With age, the transmittance of the lens decreases, particularly at the blue end of the spectrum, even when no cataract is present.

Foveal image quality

As in any optical system, the quality of the ocular image is affected by a number of factors, several of which are functions of the pupil diameter. Assuming that focus errors due to errors of refraction or accommodation are absent, the main factors are diffraction, monochromatic and chromatic aberrations and scattering in the ocular media. It might be thought that, ideally, the fovea should lie on the optical axis of the eye, where aberrations would be expected to have their smallest values. This would correspond to the position of the second focal point of an emmetropic eye. In practice, this focal point usually lies between the fovea and the optic disc (see **Fig. 1.4**) as well as being displaced slightly upwards. The resultant angle between the visual and optical axes is termed angle alpha (α) and it typically has components of about 3–5 degrees in the horizontal direction and 2 degrees in the vertical direction.

As noted earlier, due to the finite wavelength of light, in the absence of aberration the image of a point in monochromatic light appears as an Airy diffraction pattern, and consequently the image of any object (which can be considered as being equivalent to an array of points) is slightly blurred. The dimensions of the Airy pattern are usually specified in terms of the radius of its first dark ring ($1.22\lambda/D$ radians, where λ is the wavelength and D the pupil diameter in the same units). Thus the blur due to diffraction decreases as the pupil diameter increases and the wavelength reduces. In the absence of aberration, an eye working at visible wavelengths (e.g. 500 nm) would be expected to have less diffractive blur and hence better optical resolution than one working in the near infrared (e.g. 1000 nm).

In contrast to the influence of diffraction, in most eyes the image-degrading effects of monochromatic aberration tend to increase as the pupil diameter increases. Although, at the fovea, aberrations are small enough to have little effect when the pupil is less than 3 mm in diameter, thereafter their impact usually increases steadily. While the majority of young eyes suffer from small amounts of positive (under-corrected) spherical aberration, there are wide inter-subject variations and most eyes also suffer idiosyncratically from a complex mixture of aberrations due to such factors as the individual tilts and asymmetries of the ocular surfaces. There is a tendency for lens aberrations to at least partially compensate for those of the cornea. Interestingly, if the individual axial aberrations are averaged across a large population, the average of most is close to zero, although individual values vary about this mean (Porter et al 2001; Thibos et al 2002). Thus it appears as though the normal growth processes aim to produce an essentially aberration-free eye: however, small idiosyncratic asymmetries about this state are tolerated, leading to the inter-subject variations in aberration observed. It is important to stress that the blur caused by these aberrations is quite modest and if we approximate it to the effects of blur due to spherical defocus, the equivalent defocus rarely exceeds 0.25 D.

Chromatic aberration, caused by variation in the refractive indices of the optical media of the eye with wavelength, i.e. dispersion, also affects the foveal image. The major effect is longitudinal chromatic aberration, the eye being relatively myopic at the blue end of the spectrum and relatively hyperopic in the red (**Fig. 1.12**). This aberration varies very little between individual subjects and is made use of in the duochrome test in refraction (Ch. 14). Although the dioptric difference in refraction across the spectrum is quite large, its effects are not usually noticed, mainly because the relative luminous efficiency of the eye is much reduced at the ends of the visible spectrum. There is also a little transverse chromatic aberration at the fovea (approximately a minute of arc) since, as noted earlier, the fovea lies a few degrees away from the optic axis of the eye (angle alpha).

Scattering occurs because none of the optical media of the eye is perfectly transparent. Indeed, it would not be possible to visualize corneal sections with the slit-lamp microscope without the back-scattered light from the cornea. It is forward-scattered light which tends to degrade the contrast of the retinal image. Such light is usually weak enough to have little effect in young, healthy eyes but lenticular scattering tends to increase with age and, for older people, creates real problems with glare in such situations as night driving.

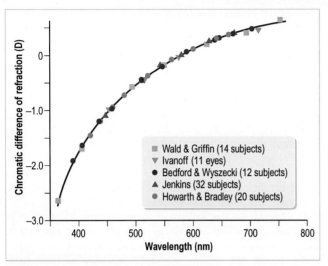

Figure 1.12 Longitudinal chromatic aberration of the eye as found by the authors indicated. (After Charman 1991.)

The overall image quality can be summarized in a number of ways. Perhaps the most convenient are the line-spread function (LSF) and the modulation transfer function (MTF). The LSF is simply the distribution of light (in our case, the retinal illuminance) in the image of a line, as measured in a direction perpendicular to its length. The MTF is a plot of the way in which an optical system degrades the modulation or contrast in the image of a sinusoidal grating (i.e. the modulation transfer) as a function of the spatial frequency of the grating. By spatial frequency we mean the reciprocal of the period of the grating (where the period is the angular width of one cycle, comprising one bright and one dark bar). Gratings of low spatial frequency have broad bars and those of high spatial frequency have narrow bars. In a visual context, spatial frequency is usually measured in cycles per degree. If I_{max} and I_{min} are the maxima and minima of the grating, then the modulation is $(I_{max}-I_{min})/(I_{max}+I_{min})$. The modulation transfer at any spatial frequency is then given by M_I/M_O, where M_I is the modulation of the image and M_O the modulation of the object grating (**Fig. 1.13**). If the image of a point (the point-spread function) is asymmetric, due to such aberrations as coma, the LSF and MTF will vary with orientation. Moreover, the peaks of the image of the sinewave grating will in general be displaced slightly from the expected position, creating a phase shift which varies with spatial frequency. The plot of this phase shift as a function of spatial frequency is called the phase transfer function (PTF). As will be discussed later, the concept of the MTF ties in well with the psychophysically measured contrast sensitivity function, in which the sensitivity (reciprocal of the modulation of the just detectable sinewave grating) is plotted as a function of the spatial frequency of the grating (see Ch. 12).

Figure 1.14 shows experimental measurements of the profiles of the foveal LSF as a function of pupil diameter for an eye which has been corrected for any sphero-cylindrical error. The measured profiles are compared with those expected for a theoretical eye affected only by diffraction, where the line images get narrower as the pupil diameter increases. It can be seen that with small pupils the aberrations have little effect but that, for pupil diameters greater than 3 mm, the measured image is substantially broadened by aberration. The best compromise between diffraction and aberration, yielding the narrowest line image, occurs when the pupil diameter is around 2–3 mm.

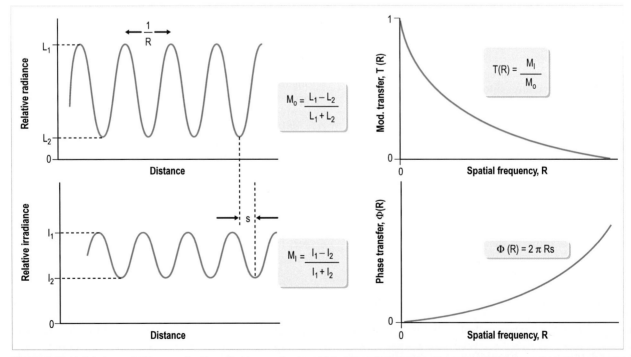

Figure 1.13 Modulation and phase transfer. The retinal image of a sinusoidal grating of modulation M_O and spatial frequency R has the reduced modulation M_I, and may also suffer a phase shift φ (R) = 2πRs. Plots of the modulation transfer T(R) = M_I/M_O, and phase shift φ (R) as a function of R comprise the modulation transfer function (MTF) and phase transfer function (PTF) of the eye for the pupil diameter and other imaging conditions in use.

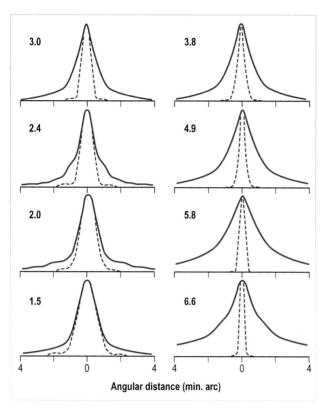

Figure 1.14 Typical measurements of the foveal line-spread function (LSF) in white light (*continuous curves*), compared with the theoretical results for an aberration-free eye (*dashed curves*). Each pair of curves is labelled with the corresponding pupil diameter (mm). (After Campbell & Gubisch 1966.)

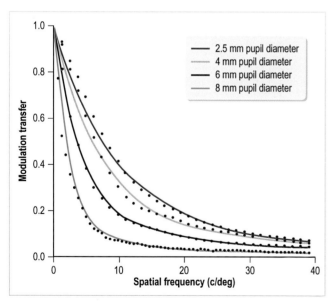

Figure 1.15 Typical measurements of the ocular MTF for different pupil diameters. Monochromatic light of wavelength 633 nm has been used. (After Artal and Navarro 1994.)

The corresponding pupil dependence of the modulation transfer function is shown in **Figure 1.15**, the data in this case having been obtained in monochromatic light. Evidently, as the pupil size is increased above about 2.5 mm the MTF tends to degrade, meaning that the retinal image of a grating of any spatial frequency has progressively lower

contrast, making it harder for the neural system to detect. Although it might appear worrying that the optical performance is poor when the pupil diameter is large, it must be remembered that, under natural conditions, large pupils are normally only found when light levels are low, and neural resolution is also poor.

Effects of defocus on the foveal image: ocular depth-of-focus and field

We have so far assumed that the eye is optimally focused. In practice, this is not necessarily the case. As the eye moves away from the correct position of focus, due either to uncorrected refractive error or to an incorrect accommodative response, the defocus blur steadily increases (**Fig. 1.16B**). As can be appreciated from **Figure 1.16A**, the amount of defocus blur increases with the pupil diameter.

If we use a simple geometrical optics approximation, in angular terms the blur circle diameter, β, is given by β ≈ 3.44.△F.D min arc, where △F is the dioptric error of focus and D is the pupil diameter in millimetres, although diffraction and aberration make this formula inapplicable near the correct focus. Evidently, if the pupil diameter is reduced, blur also reduces and for any given error of focus the retinal image becomes clearer. This is why uncorrected myopes often narrow their palpebral aperture in an attempt to improve distance vision or why the near vision of presbyopes is improved by using higher levels of lighting, which contract the pupil and reduce the diameter of the retinal blur circles: it is also the basis of the clinical pinhole test to determine whether reduced vision is due to a refractive error.

The dioptric depth-of-field is the vergence (reciprocal of object distance) range over which an object can be moved without any blur being detected. The depth-of-focus is the numerically equal dioptric range in the image space. Both quantities can, of course, also be expressed in terms of

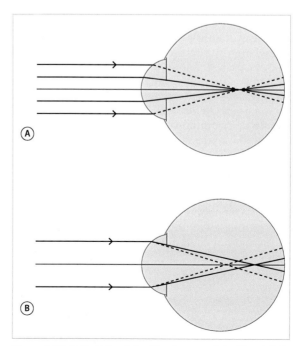

Figure 1.16 Retinal blur circles. The diameter of the blur circle increases with **(A)** the pupil diameter and **(B)** the dioptric error of focus.

object and image distances. Actual values depend upon a variety of factors, including the individual, the pupil diameter, the lighting conditions and the test object used (see, e.g., Charman 1991).

Although our blur circle formula is very approximate, we find that if D takes the typical photopic value of 3 mm, $\beta \approx 10.\triangle F$ min arc, so that a focus error of 0.2 D would produce a blur circle of 2 min arc in diameter. This is the separation of the limb centres in the bars of a 6/6 (20/20) Snellen E, suggesting that 0.2 D might be a rough theoretical estimate of the tolerable error of focus. In practice, the precision attained by most methods of refraction is around ± 0.25 D and we can usually move objects over at least a ± 0.25 D vergence range without detecting any obvious image blur: the range over which an object can be moved before people judge the blur to be troublesome is substantially greater (at least ± 0.50 D, see, e.g., Atchison et al 2005; Ciuffreda et al 2006). This has obvious relevance to such clinical questions as the change in refractive error required to necessitate a new spectacle correction.

Accommodation

We have so far assumed that the optics of the eye are static. In fact, the younger eye can change the power of its lens, and hence of the whole eye, to view near objects clearly. This process is called accommodation. In the unaccommodated eye, the relaxed ciliary muscle and the elastic choroid maintain tensional forces in the zonule. These are transmitted to the lens through its capsule and result in the lens (particularly its anterior surface) taking a less powerful, flatter form appropriate to distance vision. For near vision, the contracted ciliary muscle changes its shape in such a way as to reduce the tension in the zonular fibres. As a result, the elastic lens and capsule can progressively take up their unconstrained, natural, more powerful form, with the anterior surface steepening markedly. These changes are illustrated in **Figure 1.17**.

Unfortunately, the efficiency of this process declines with age, from at least the early teens. The clinical measurement of accommodation is discussed in Chapter 15. Usually the range of power change that the eye is capable of, or amplitude of accommodation, has diminished to zero by the age of around 50 years of age, with the symptoms of presbyopia appearing some years before that. Under clinical conditions, the amplitude of accommodation is usually measured subjectively, when the actual change in ocular power is supplemented by the subjective depth-of-focus of the eye. This means that, even when true changes in lens power have ceased, a non-zero subjective amplitude of accommodation (around 1 D) is still found (**Fig. 1.18**). Debate still continues on the factors responsible for the progressive accommodative loss but there is no doubt that the changing form and mechanical characteristics of the lens play major roles.

If we examine the performance of the accommodation system in more detail, the following important points emerge:

1. Under good lighting conditions when retinal cones are active (photopic vision) accommodation is quite accurate, provided that the object of interest lies within the amplitude of accommodation. It is usual, however, to find slight over-accommodation ('lead') for distant

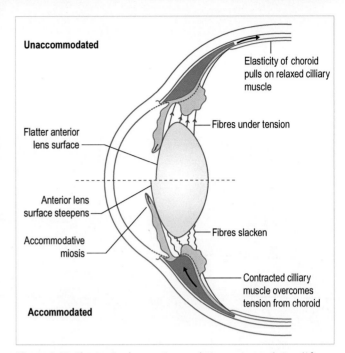

Figure 1.17 Changes in the anterior eye during accommodation. (After Pipe & Rapley 1997.)

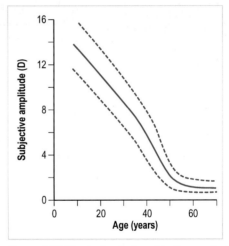

Figure 1.18 The decline in the subjective amplitude of accommodation with age. The continuous curve represents the mean and the dashed curves the limits of the distribution for normal subjects. It is assumed that any refractive error is corrected so that the far point of the eye lies at infinity. The dioptric amplitude is then the reciprocal of the shortest distance (in metres) at which an object can be seen without detectable blur. An amplitude of, say, 5 D thus means that the shortest distance at which an object can be seen clearly lies at 0.2 m from the eye.

objects and slight under-accommodation ('lag') for near objects, even though all of these lie within the normal amplitude of accommodation. As, however, the light level is reduced and the rods of the retina become more active the accuracy reduces and leads and lags in accommodation increase in magnitude. Finally, when the light level is too low for cones to function effectively (scotopic vision, when only rod receptors are active) the accommodation system ceases to function and the eye remains at a slightly myopic tonic level (some times called the dark focus), typically around −1 D.

2. Under good lighting conditions when the distance of the object of regard is changed, there is a reaction time (latency) of about one-third of a second before the power of the lens starts to change. The actual response change usually takes 0.5 secs or more to complete (response time).

3. Even though observation may be monocular, accommodation causes the eyes to converge (accommodative convergence), while convergence causes some accommodation (convergence accommodation). Additionally, in most cases accommodation on a near object causes the pupil to constrict (accommodative miosis).

Off-axis image quality

Although foveal imagery is of importance for tasks demanding the highest spatial resolution, in solid-angle terms the peripheral field is much more important. Generally speaking, objects of interest will be detected in peripheral vision and then head or eye turns will bring their images onto the fovea for detailed inspection. In fact, the eye is a system with a remarkably wide field, the absolute monocular field being roughly 100, 70, 70 and 80 degrees in the temporal, nasal, superior and inferior directions, respectively.

What is image quality like in the peripheral field? For most eyes, the dominant factor governing image blur is what approximates to oblique astigmatism, with a point object being imaged as two longitudinally separated focal lines oriented either along the meridian in which the off-axis point lies, or perpendicular to it (the radial and tangential line foci, respectively). The amount of astigmatism increases with the field angle (**Fig. 1.19**). Note that if we wish to make an accurate determination of the axial refractive error, for example by retinoscopy (see Ch. 13), we must be careful to be as close to the visual axis as possible; otherwise the results will be contaminated by the eye's oblique astigmatism. In most eyes, the two astigmatic image fields lie on either side of the retinal surface, so that the circle of least

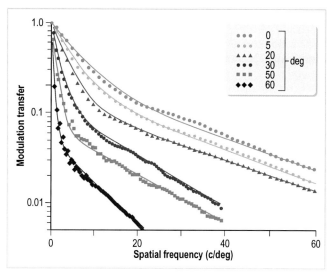

Figure 1.20 Ocular modulation transfer functions for a 4 mm pupil at the different field angles indicated. (After Navarro et al 1993.)

confusion lies close to the retina. There are, however, considerable inter-subject differences.

Clearly, the increasing amounts of oblique astigmatism in the peripheral field have a degrading effect on image quality. The nature of the point image will depend upon where the retina lies with respect to the astigmatic foci and, in general, the image will lack circular symmetry. **Figure 1.20** shows the MTF for a fixed 4 mm pupil at several field angles, where the focus corresponds to that producing the most symmetrical point image: the MTFs have been averaged over all orientations. The important feature is that the retinal image quality reduces as we move away from the visual axis. However, as will be discussed later (Ch. 2), the resolution abilities of the neural retina also decline with field angle, and visual acuity in the periphery is usually limited by neural, rather than optical, factors.

Eye movements

It is clear that, since both optical and neural performance are optimal on the visual axis, a system is needed to rapidly direct the eyes so that the images of interest fall on the fovea of each eye (gaze shifting leading to fixation). A scene is explored through a series of such fixational movements (or saccades) to different points across the visual field. Moreover, the system must be capable of maintaining the images on the two foveas both when the object is fixed and, ideally, when it is moving (gaze holding). These functions are achieved by combined eye and head movements. For these to interact satisfactorily to achieve the desired aim, the eye movement system needs to receive information about the head position. This is derived from the vestibular system or labyrinth of the inner ear, which signals rotational and translational movements of the head. The compensatory vestibulo-ocular responses take place automatically (i.e. they are reflex responses) whereas the fixational changes required to foveate a new object of interest are voluntary responses (e.g. Carpenter 1991; Leigh & Zee 1991).

Each eye is moved in its orbit by the action of six extrinsic or extra-ocular muscles: the medial and lateral recti, the superior and inferior recti, and the superior and inferior

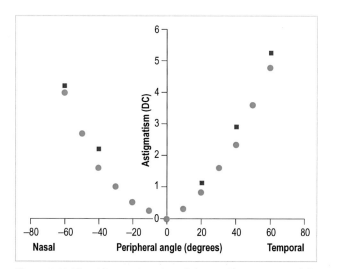

Figure 1.19 The oblique astigmatism of the eye. The experimental data shown come from the work of Lotmar and Lotmar (1974) (blue circles) and Millodot (1981) (red squares). Note that, due to angle α, the points are not quite symmetrical about the visual axis.

obliques. The details and actions of these muscles will be discussed in a later chapter (Ch. 16) but we note here that their action rotates each eye about a 'centre of rotation' lying approximately 13.5 mm behind the cornea. Strictly, however, there is no unique centre for all the different possible rotations: for example, the 'centre of rotation' for vertical movements lies some 2 mm anterior to that for horizontal movements.

Although the two eyes can scan a field extending about 45 degrees in all directions from the straight-ahead or primary position, in practice eye movements rarely exceed about 20 degrees, fixation on more peripheral objects being achieved by combined head and eye rotation. This has obvious implications for the design of progressive addition spectacle lenses.

If the angle between the two visual axes does not change during a movement, the latter is described as a version (or conjugate) movement. However, the lateral separation of the eyes in the head implies the need for an additional class of movements to cope with the differing convergence requirements of objects at various distances. Those movements, which involve a change in the angle between the visual axes, are called vergence (or dysjunctive) movements. Fixational changes may in general involve both types of movement, which appear to be under independent neurological control (Rashbass & Westheimer 1961).

As examples of the speed of versional eye movements, **Figure 1.21** shows the time course of saccades to new fixation points located at progressively greater angles from the original point of fixation. It can be seen that the movements are extremely rapid, reaching more than 700 deg/sec, depending upon the amplitude of the saccade: the saccade latency is about 200 msec. Interestingly, it appears that during the saccade, when the image is moving rapidly across the retina, vision is largely (although not completely) suppressed. This saccadic suppression (or perhaps more properly attenuation) results in, for example, the retinal thresholds for brief flashes of light being elevated, the elevation commencing some 30–40 msec before the actual saccadic movement starts. The subject is usually unaware of this temporary impairment of vision and the exact mechanism responsible remains controversial.

A question of considerable importance to the achievement of good visual acuity is the stability with which fixation can be held on the object of interest. In practice, it is found that a variety of small-amplitude eye movements always occur. These miniature eye movements can be broken down into three components: tremor, drift and microsaccades. The frequency spectrum of tremor falls essentially monotonically with frequency above approximately 10 Hz, extending up to approximately 200 Hz. The amplitude is small, probably less that 0.5 min arc, corresponding roughly to the effective angular subtense of a foveal cone at the nodal point of the eye. Drift movements are larger and slower, with amplitudes of 2–5 min arc and velocities around 4 min/sec. The fixation errors brought about by these slow drifts (which are usually disassociated in the two eyes) are corrected by rapid microsaccades which are correlated in the two eyes. The overall stability of fixation is illustrated in **Figure 1.22**, from which it can be seen that, for most of the time, the point of regard lies within a few minutes of arc from the target.

Stereopsis

It is clear that, because the eyes are laterally separated in the head, each receives a slightly different view of the environment. The resultant disparities between the two retinal images can be used by the visual system to estimate the relative distances of objects, although absolute distance judgement is usually much more dependent on monocular cues such as perspective and size constancy.

Although much of the mechanism of stereopsis depends on the neural system, in particular the existence of binocularly driven neurones, it will be useful at this stage to consider the geometry involved (**Fig. 1.23A**). Suppose we have two points, A and B, lying at distances l and $l + \delta l$ from the observer. The angular separations of the objects at the nodal points of the left and right eyes are θ_L and θ_R. Then the difference, $\delta\theta$, between these angles, or disparity, is:

$$\delta\theta = \theta_R - \theta_L = \alpha_1 - \alpha_2$$

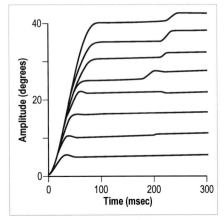

Figure 1.21 Time course of saccades of different amplitudes. The traces have been superimposed so that the beginnings of each saccade occur at time zero. In fact, each is preceded by a latency or reaction time of about 200 msec. (After Robinson 1964.)

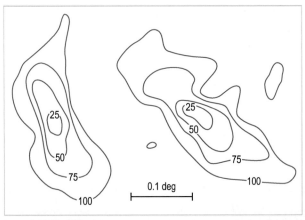

Figure 1.22 Stability of fixation for two subjects. The contours define areas within which the point of fixation was found for 25, 50, 75 and 100% of the time. (After Bennet-Clark 1964.)

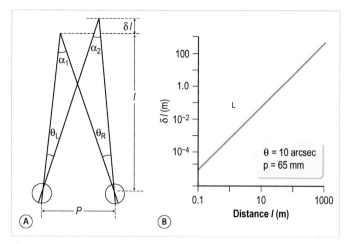

Figure 1.23 (A) Geometry of stereopsis. **(B)** Theoretical just-discriminable change in distance as a function of the object distance for $p = 65$ mm, $\delta\theta = 10$ sec arc (see text).

Approximating all angles as being small (i.e. $l \gg p$, δl) we find that the angular disparity is:

$$\delta\theta = (p/l) - \left(p/(l + \delta\,l)\right) \approx p\delta l/l^2$$

or

$$\delta l \approx \delta\theta.l^2/p$$

where p is interpupillary distance. Evidently our ability to detect that the two points are at different distances depends on the minimum value of $\delta\theta$ that can be detected. As will be discussed in a later chapter (Ch. 16), although just-detectable disparity $\delta\theta$ varies somewhat with such parameters as target distance and the nature of the task, under favourable circumstances it can be around 10 sec arc (i.e. 0.17 min arc). **Figure 1.23B** plots the just-discriminable difference in depth δl as a function of the distance l on the assumptions of this value for $\delta\theta$ and a value of 65 mm for p (the normal range of p is 50–76 mm). In practice, stereopsis is useful up to a distance of a few hundred metres.

Summary

Under normal, photopic, daylight conditions, when the pupil diameter is around 3 mm, the optical system of the eye is capable of delivering a near diffraction-limited optical image to the fovea of the retina, over a wavelength range from about 400 to 1200 nm. As the light level falls to the mesopic and scotopic levels and the pupil dilates, the quality of the foveal image deteriorates. Away from the visual axis, image quality is dominated by increasing amounts of oblique astigmatism. The next chapter will discuss ways in which the neural retina and brain make use of these optical capabilities.

References

Artal P, Navarro R 1994 Monochromatic modulation transfer function of the human eye for different pupil diameters: an analytical expression. Journal of the Optical Society of America A 11:246–249

Atchison D A, Smith, G 2000 Optics of the human eye. Butterworth-Heinemann, Oxford

Atchison D A, Fisher S W, Pedersen C A, Ridall P G 2005 Noticeable, troublesome and objectionable limits of blur. Vision Research 45:1967–1974

Bennet-Clark H C 1964 The oculomotor response to small target displacements. Optica Acta 11:301–314

Boettner E A, Wolter J R 1962 Transmission of the ocular media. Investigative Opthalmology 1:776–783

Bron A J, Tripathi R C, Tripathi B J 1997 Wolff's anatomy of the eye and orbit, 8th edn. Chapman & Hall Medical, London

Campbell F W, Gubisch R W 1966 Optical quality of the eye. Journal of Physiology (London) 186:558–578

Carpenter R H S (ed.) 1991 Vision and visual dysfunction, vol 8: Eye Movements. Macmillan, Basingstoke

Charman W N 1991 Optics of the human eye. In: Charman W N Vision and visual dysfunction, vol.1: Visual optics and instrumentation. Macmillan, Basingstoke, pp 1–26

Ciuffreda K J, Selenov A, Wang B et al 2006 'Bothersome blur': a functional unit of blur perception. Vision Research 46:895–901

Cronly-Dillon F R, Gregory R L 1991 Vision and visual dysfunction, vol 2: Evolution of the eye and visual system. McMillan, Basingstoke

Davson H 1990 Physiology of the eye, 5th edn. Macmillan, Basingstoke

Duke-Elder S 1958 System of ophthalmology, vol 1: The eye in evolution. Kimpton, London

Forrester J V, Dick A D, McMenamin P et al 2002 The eye: basic sciences in practice, 2nd edn. WB Saunders, London

Guillon M, Lydon D P M 1986 Corneal topography: a clinical model. Ophthalmology and Physiological Optics 6:47–56

Hodson S A 1997 Corneal stromal swelling. Progress in Retinal and Eye Research 16:99–116

Kaufman P L, Alm A 2003 Adler's physiology of the eye: clinical applications, 10th edn. Mosby Year Book, St Louis

Kiely P M, Smith G, Carney L G 1982 The mean shape of the human cornea. Optica Acta 29:1027–1040

Korb D R, Craig J, Doughty M et al 2002 The tear film: structure, function and clinical examination. Butterworth-Heinemann, London

Lawrenson J G 2002 The anterior eye. In: Efron N Contact lens practice. Butterworth-Heinemann, Oxford, pp 11–35

Leigh R J, Zee D S 1991 The neurology of eye movements, 2nd edn. Davis, Philadelphia

Lotmar W, Lotmar T 1974 Peripheral astigmatism in the human eye: experimental data and theoretical model predictions. Journal of the Optical Society of America 64:510–513

Lythgoe J N 1979 The ecology of vision. Clarendon, Oxford

Maurice D M 1957 The structure and transparency of the cornea. Journal of Physiology (London) 136:263–286

Mecherikunne A T, Gatlin J A, Richmond J C 1983 Data on total and spectral solar irradiance. Applied Optics 22:1354–1359

Millodot M 1981 Effect of ametropia on peripheral refraction. American Journal of Optometry and Physiological Optics 58:691–695

Navarro R, Artal P, Williams D R 1993 Modulation transfer of the eye as a function of retinal eccentricity. Journal of the Optical Society of America A 10:201–212

Pipe D M, Rapley L 1997 Ocular anatomy and histology, 2nd edn. ABDO, London

Porter J, Guirao A, Cox I G et al 2001 Monochromatic aberrations of the human eye in a large population. Journal of the Optical Society of America A 18:1793–1803

Rabbetts R B 2007 In: Bennett & Rabbetts clinical visual optics, 4th edition. Butterworth-Heinemann Elsevier, Oxford

Rashbass C, Westheimer G 1961 Independence of conjunctive and disjunctive eye movements. Journal of Physiology (London) 159:361–364

Robinson D A 1964 The mechanics of human saccadic eye movements. Journal of Physiology (London) 174:245–264

Thibos L N, Hong X, Bradley A et al 2002 Statistical variation of aberration structure in a normal population of healthy eyes. Journal of the Optical Society of America A 19:2329–2348

CHAPTER 2

Anatomy of vision

Gary E Baker

Introduction

The neural infrastructure of visual processing is spread widely throughout the central nervous system. There are over 30 separate cortical areas implicated as substrates for the various functional attributes of vision but the majority of the visual input to these areas passes initially from the retina via the lateral geniculate nucleus to the striate cortex.

The aim of this chapter is to provide an overview of the structural organization of these initial elements of the visual pathways that provide the raw visual data for the various widespread cortical divisions. In addition, the aim is to provide an introduction to other subcortical pathways involved in visual processes as well as a basis for comprehending the consequences for visual field representation of damage to the initial parts of the visual pathway (see Ch. 20).

Retina

The retina is the eye's innermost coat, lining the posterior two-thirds of the internal surface. It is a thin, mostly transparent layer of tissue that extends forward from the optic disc to its anterior limit, the ora serrata, where it is continuous with the epithelial layers of the ciliary body.

The visual system's photosensitive components are located in the retina. However, the retina represents more than a mere phototransduction apparatus, as its origin as an outpouching of the brain belies. Its cytoarchitecture underlies sophisticated post-receptor processing of the response of the photosensitive cells (for comprehensive reviews see Masland 2001; Sterling & Demb 2004; Wässle 2004).

The retina originates as two primordial layers of invaginating epithelium. An outer layer, identified as the retinal pigment epithelium, and an inner layer that ultimately becomes the multilaminar neural retina. This layered organization of the retina and its nomenclature are described in **Figure 2.1A**.

The histological appearance of the retinal layers shows the distribution of the various cell bodies and processes but fails to reveal their organization as a number of morphologically and physiologically distinct cell types that are organized into vertical (through the layers) and lateral (within layers) paths of cellular interactions. The outermost laminae, adjacent to the pigment layer (retinal pigment epithelium, RPE), are where the majority of photosensitive cells are located. These photoreceptors, the rods and cones, represent the site where the transduction of light energy into the bioelectrical activity essential for vision is accomplished. Within the vertical path through the retina, information flow passes predominantly from the photoreceptors via the second-order neurons, the bipolar cells, to the third-order neurons, the ganglion cells, and thence from the retina to cellular targets centrally in the brain. At successive stages of this vertical path, cellular responses are influenced by lateral interactions, firstly with horizontal cells at the level of the photoreceptors and later by amacrine cells in the inner retina at the level of the ganglion cells. These separate paths are indicated schematically in **Figure 2.1A**.

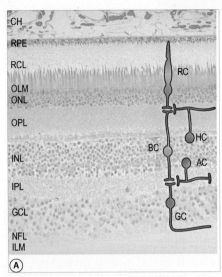

(A)

Figure 2.1A Transverse section through the mid-peripheral retina and choroid (CH) of a macaque retina stained with toluidine blue. Scale bar: 50 μm. The labels on the left side indicate the conventional nomenclature for the individual layers. RPE, retinal pigment epithelium; RCL, rod and cone layer; OLM, outer limiting membrane; ONL, outer nuclear layer; OPL, outer plexiform layer; INL, inner nuclear layer; IPL, inner plexiform layer; GCL, ganglion cell layer; NFL, nerve fibre layer; ILM, inner limiting membrane. The right side of the section is overlaid with diagrammatic representations of the vertical (blue) and horizontal (red) paths of cellular interaction within the retina. RC, receptor cell; BC, bipolar cell; GC, ganglion cell; HC, horizontal cell; AC, amacrine cell.

Foveal specialization

Prior to considering the cellular relationships in the retina, it is important to emphasize that its organization is not homogeneous. At the centre of the retina on the visual axis is a region of approximately 5 mm in diameter known as the macula lutea (yellow spot), so called as a consequence of the xanthophyll derivates found within the retinal cells of the region, which impart a yellowish hue. At the centre of this macular region is a depression or pit, the fovea, with a diameter of approximately 1.5 mm. Peripheral to the fovea are the parafoveal and perifoveal regions, while at the foveal centre is the foveola.

The cellular organization is adapted in the fovea to allow the finest level of visual resolution in the roughly central 5 degrees of visual angle. Specific mention will be made of the consequences of the adaptation of the central retina for the organization of the visual pathways in the relevant sections below. Microscopically, however, the most obvious modification of this retinal region is the reduced thickness (**Fig. 2.1B**). Consequently, the path of light to the photoreceptors is comparatively unobstructed by overlying tissue, a factor that is further enhanced by the absence of the vasculature from the foveal centre.

Pigment epithelium

This, the outermost layer of the retina, is a single-cell-thick layer of tessellating, polygonal and relatively cuboidal epithelium (**Fig. 2.1A**: RPE; **Fig. 2.2A**). It is continuous rostrally with the outer, pigmented epithelial layer of the ciliary body. The basal surface of these cells provides the inner basal lamina component of Bruch's membrane, which separates the pigment epithelium from the adjacent choriocapillaris, the vascular supply that provides for the outer retina including the photoreceptors. Gap junctions, anchoring

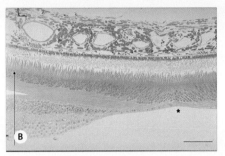

(B)

Figure 2.1B Transverse section through the foveal region stained with toluidine blue. Scale bar: 50 μm. The centre of the fovea, the foveola, is indicated by the asterisk towards the right-hand edge of the micrograph. The left-hand edge is the parafoveal margin and the layer designations defined in **Figure 2.1A** apply there. The foveola is characterized by the virtual absence of the retinal layers vitreal to the outer nuclear layer. The arrow indicates the direction of the light path towards the photoreceptors. Clearly, peripheral to the foveal region, light must pass through the layered array of cells and processes that comprise the retina. However, at the fovea, on which the image is normally fixated, the obstruction is minimal.

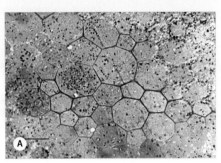

(A)

Figure 2.2A A tangential section through human pigment epithelial cells. Scale bar: 25 μm. The tight junctions between the cells enhance the outline of the cells. There is a large size and shape difference, varying from pentagonal to octagonal. The specimen was taken from a 70-year-old; in younger individuals, there is less variation, with the hexagonal form dominating.

junctions and occluding junctions are found between pigment epithelial cells, the latter towards the apical surface and forming a part of the blood–retina barrier. The apical surface of each of these cells is intimately associated with the rods and cones (**Fig. 2.2B**), and this relationship, which can be disrupted by retinal detachment, is critical for sustaining the photosensitive properties of the rods and cones. The pigment within the cells of this layer is melanin, which is packaged in melanosomes distributed mainly towards the apical (inner) surface of the cells. Melanin will absorb light that passes through the retina and therefore acts to prevent light scatter, thereby reducing image degradation.

Photoreceptor cells

Retinal distribution

Rod photoreceptors are adapted to perform best in scotopic conditions whereas cones are specialized for brighter, photopic, circumstances. They contain different light-sensitive photopigments. There is one basic rod type but cone photoreceptors comprise three major types that differ with respect to their wavelength specificities and are thus subdivided into red, green and blue cone types, also known respectively as L (long-wavelength sensitive), M (mid-wavelength sensitive) and S (short-wavelength sensitive) cones.

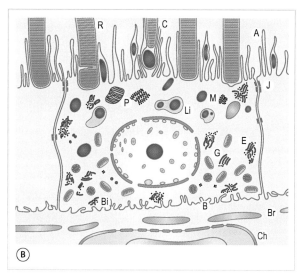

Figure 2.2B Schematic diagram of a retinal pigment epithelial cell. A, apical processes; B, basement membrane; Bi, basal infoldings; E, endoplasmic reticulum; G, Golgi complex; J, tight junction; Li, lipofuscin granule; M, melanosome; P, phagosome; Br, Bruch's membrane; Ch, choriocapillaris; R and C, outer segment tips of rod and cone photoreceptors.

Rods comprise the largest proportion of receptors. Classical accounts describe rods amounting to 120 million/eye while cones total roughly 6 million/eye (Østerberg 1935). However, a recent study utilizing a more appropriate sampling procedure estimates the (mean) rod population at approximately 90 million and that for the cone population at about 4.5 million for each eye, although there appears to be a great deal of individual variability (Curcio et al 1990).

The far greater number of rods implies a much greater density of this photoreceptor but there is important regional specialization in photoreceptor density across the retina. Rods are present at higher density except in the macular region and at the extreme peripheral margin, where cones dominate (Williams 1991). Rods are virtually absent from the centre of the foveal pit (foveola) and are at their highest density at the perifoveal border, especially at its superior aspect (Curcio et al 1990).

The three cone types are not present in equal numbers. It has been estimated that there are roughly 2.9 million red cones, 1.4 green cones and 0.2 million blue cones (Oyster 1999). In addition to their unequal numbers, the different cone types are also distributed differently across the retina; the presence of only red and green cones at the foveola means that we are normally tritanopic in the central fovea (Curcio et al 1991).

Morphology

Both photoreceptor cell types have an outer segment, which is the photosensitive compartment of the cell, joined to an inner segment by a narrow stalk containing a modified cilium. For rods, an outer fibre extends from the inner segment to the cell body region whereas, in general, cone inner segments are immediately adjacent to the cell body. An inner fibre (or axon) projects from the cell body of both receptor types with terminal end feet including synaptic regions that are specialized for each cell type (**Fig. 2.3A**).

Outer segment

The outer segments of rods are of a relatively long, tubular form while those of cones, at least outside the foveal region,

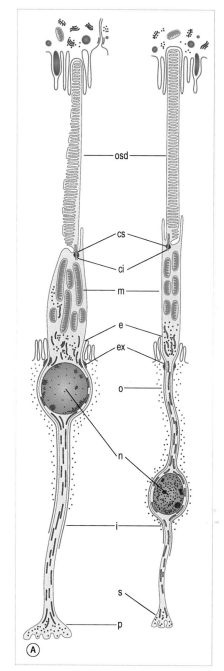

Figure 2.3A Schematic diagrams of a cone (*left*) and rod (*right*). osd, outer segment discs; cs, connecting stalk; ci, cilium; m, myoid; e, ellipsoid; ex, location of outer limiting membrane; o, outer fibre; n, nucleus; i, inner fibre; s, spherule; p, pedicle.

are shorter and conical. Within the fovea, the distinction is not so easily made between rods and cones, with both receptor types having similar cylindrical morphology in this region.

Each outer segment comprises a stack of membranous sacs or discs which incorporate the visual pigment molecules that are the basis of photosensitivity. In rods, these discs can be considered an intracellular organelle in that, except at the base of the outer segment where the discs are produced, they are distinct intracellular compartments separate from the cell membrane (**Fig. 2.3B**). In cones, by

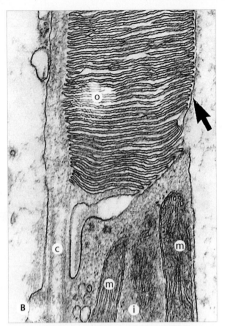

Figure 2.3B Rod photoreceptor of a rhesus monkey at the junction between inner and outer segments. i, inner segment; o, outer segment; c, cilium within connecting stalk; m, mitochondrion. A few discs adjacent to the cilium are continuous with the plasma membrane where they are formed but the remainder are detached from the plasma membrane and are free-floating within the outer segment (*arrow*).

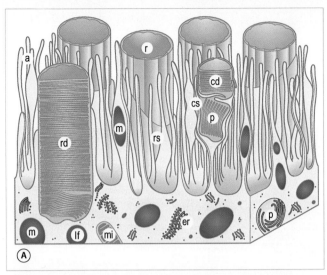

Figure 2.4A Schematic representation of the relationship between rods, cones and pigment epithelial cells. Most of the apical processes of the pigment epithelial cells are fine and finger-like while others form a sheath investment. a, apical process; cd, cone outer segment discs; cs, cone sheath; er, rough endoplasmic reticulum; gl, Golgi complex; lf, lipofuscin granule; m, melanosomes; m', mitochondrion; p, phagosomes – one of them about to enter the body of the pigment epithelial cell; r, rod; rd, rod outer segment discs; rs, rod sheath.

contrast, the discs are produced by a similar infolding of the plasma membrane at the base, but this organization is retained throughout the entire extent of the outer segment so that the disc's internal face is, in the main, part of the massively increased extracellular surface of the cell membrane.

The discs are not static or permanent. In macaque rods, they are removed or shed from the outer segment tips and renewed by continued production at the outer segment base (Young 1971). This cycle of disc shedding and renewal has been shown to be under circadian regulation in various non-primate species with the different photoreceptor types expressing distinct phases. In cone outer segments the discs are shed at the end of the day, while in rods the outer segment tips slough off during the transition from dark to light at the end of the night. The tips of the photoreceptor outer segments are enveloped by processes arising from the apical surfaces of the adjacent pigment epithelial cells (**Figs 2.2B** and **2.4A**). As the outer segment discs are shed, they are phagocytosed in groups of about 10 to 20, or more, by these cells (**Figs 2.4A** and **2.4B**) (Young & Bok 1969).

The extracellular region between the pigment epithelial cell processes and the photoreceptor outer segments, the so-called subretinal space, is occupied by the interphotoreceptor matrix. This is a mixture of proteins and glycosaminoglycans that may possess adhesive properties acting to preserve the close apposition of the adjacent cell layers (Chu & Grunwald 1990). In addition, at least one particular constituent, interstitial retinoid-binding protein, has an important role in transferring molecules essential in the phototransduction regeneration process, to and from the retinal pigment epithelial cells (Bok 1990).

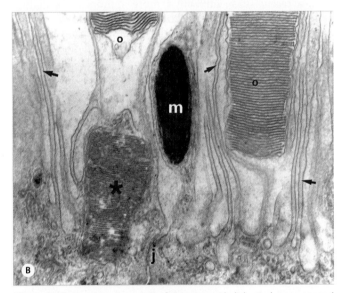

Figure 2.4B Electron micrograph of pigment epithelial apical processes and adjacent receptor outer segments of rhesus monkey. The apical processes, some of which are indicated by arrows, surround the tips of the outer segments. A group of approximately 50 outer segment discs from one of the receptor outer segments (*), in the process of sloughing off, has detached and is partly buried within the epithelial cell preliminary to the formation of a phagosome. m, melanosome; o, outer segment tips.

Inner segment

The inner segment is generally larger in cones than rods outside the foveal region but of roughly equal size in the fovea. It is subdivided into two regions: the region closer to the outer segment is known as the ellipsoid, the other as the myoid (see **Fig. 2.3A**). The ellipsoid houses a large concentration of mitochondria and thus represents the powerhouse of the cell, while the myoid, occupied by endoplasmic reticulum and Golgi apparatus, is a region specialized for the protein production and packaging necessary for the renewal of discs at the base of the outer segment (Steinberg et al 1980) as well as the photopigment components embedded in those membranes (Bok 1985).

Just as the outer segments of photoreceptor cells are separated from each other by enveloping processes of the apical surface of the pigment epithelial cells, the inner segments of adjacent photoreceptors are similarly separated, but by processes of Müller cells. These are large glial, or supporting, cells that extend throughout the entire depth of the retina (**Fig. 2.5**). They form specialized tight junctions (maculae adherens) with the inner segments at their bases as well as with other Müller cell processes, forming a histologically defined retinal layer, the external (outer) limiting membrane, which is the inner border of the subretinal space (**Figs 2.1A and 2.6**).

An outer fibre connects the inner segment to the cell body of the photoreceptor. This fibre is of almost negligible length in cones outside the foveal region, but in the foveola the cone cell body is displaced along the outer fibre. Outside the foveal region, the different lengths of their outer fibres result in the cell bodies of cones and rods, and the nuclei they include; being largely segregated in the outer nuclear layer, the cone cell bodies lying adjacent to the outer limiting membrane separate from several rows of rod nuclei (**Fig. 2.6**). An inner fibre, or axon, extends from the cell body region to terminate in a synaptic end foot. At the fovea, these axons belong predominantly to cones and are particularly evident as Henle's fibre layer (**Fig. 2.6**).

The axon terminal regions are morphologically specialized according to the photoreceptor cell type. Rod terminals, or spherules, are relatively spherical while the different cone types each have larger, flattened terminals known as pedicles (see **Figs 2.3A and 2.6**). These can have small, laterally extending processes which are frequently in gap junction contact with other cone pedicles (Hornstein et al 2004) as well as with rod spherules (Haverkamp et al 2000).

The spherules and pedicles are located within the outer plexiform layer (see **Fig. 2.1A**). As found for their cell bodies in the outer nuclear layer, the different synaptic terminals are partitioned within this layer; rod spherules form several sublaminae towards the border with the outer nuclear layer, while the cone pedicles are distributed further towards the inner margin of the outer plexiform layer.

Invaginations within the photoreceptor terminal regions represent specialized regions for synaptic interaction with other retinal neurons. A flat plate, the 'synaptic ribbon', is found in the photoreceptor component of this specialized region, oriented orthogonally to an electron-dense region of presynaptic membrane and a synaptic ridge (**Fig. 2.7A**). Synaptic vesicles are associated with both sides of the ribbon and the function of the ribbon may be for rapid channelling of synaptic vesicles to their docking sites at the presynaptic membrane (Rao-Mirotznik et al 1995).

Rod spherules generally possess a single invagination (**Fig. 2.7A**) whereas there may be up to 50 invaginations found in the more complex and larger, flattened pedicle terminals (**Fig. 2.7B**) (Chun et al 1996). At these synaptic specializations, contacts are made with bipolar cell dendrites and the processes of horizontal cells. In each cone

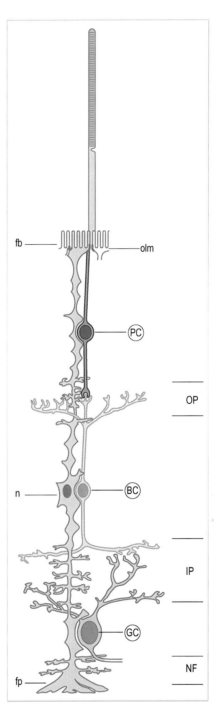

Figure 2.5 Schematic representation of a Müller cell. The soma (n) lies in the inner nuclear layer and its processes form numerous fine branches penetrating the neuropil of the two plexiform layers and the nerve fibre layer. Müller cells terminate in the outer retina in the form of microvilli-like fibre processes (fb) which penetrate the outer limiting membrane (olm) and surround the photoreceptor inner segments. At their inner retinal limit, Müller cells broaden to form footplates (fp) at the inner limiting membrane. OP, outer plexiform layer; IP, inner plexiform layer; NF, nerve fibre layer

invagination, a central bipolar cell dendrite is flanked by two horizontal cell processes found deeper within the invagination, forming an arrangement known as a triad (**Fig. 2.7C**). The term triad implies only three components but the number of processes, especially within the invaginations of rod spherules, can exceed this number.

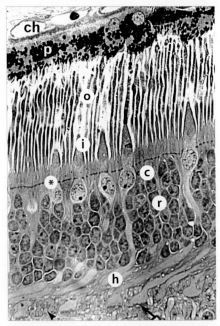

Figure 2.6 Human retina showing the larger, oval cell bodies of the cones (c) with lighter nuclei lying adjacent to the outer limiting membrane (*). They are clearly distinguishable from the smaller, rod cell bodies (r) with more densely staining nuclei, which are more densely packed and form several layers at this retinal location. Cone and rod inner fibres (h) terminate respectively in pedicles (*arrow*) and spherules (*arrowhead*). ch, choriocapillaris; p, retinal pigment epithelium; i, inner segment; o, outer segment.

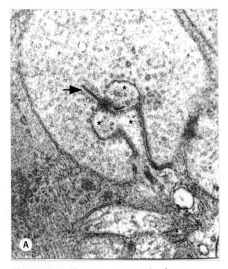

Figure 2.7A Electron micrograph of a transverse section through a rod spherule showing three distinct invaginating profiles (*) and a synaptic ribbon (*arrow*).

Not all synaptic contacts are confined within invaginations of the terminals. Cone pedicles and bipolar cell dendrites also make flat contacts (**Fig. 2.7C**), although there appear to be no flat contacts on spherules. These superficial synapses resemble conventional synapses with presynaptic intramembranous particles and postsynaptic densities, but are virtually devoid of closely adjacent vesicles, suggesting a synaptic mechanism distinct from that at the invaginating ribbon synapses. Nevertheless, both types of synaptic specialization represent an initial

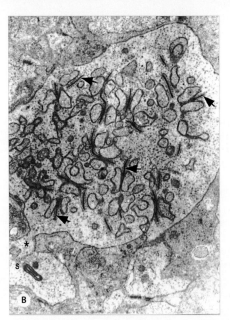

Figure 2.7B Electron micrograph of a cone pedicle sectioned parallel and close to its base, showing approximately 25 synaptic ribbons (*some indicated by arrows*) each with aligned vesicles. In the bottom left-hand corner, a pedicle process (*) appears to be contacting a rod spherule (s).

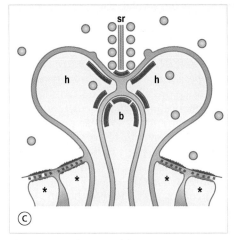

Figure 2.7C Schematic of the synaptic arrangements at a cone pedicle. Two horizontal cell dendrites (h) and one dendrite from a bipolar cell (b) invaginate the base of the pedicle, forming a triad. The ridge of the invaginations is directly opposite the synaptic ribbon (sr) of the pedicle. Synaptic vesicles align either side of the ribbon and the density is located at the base of the ribbon adjacent to the presynaptic membrane. In addition to the invaginating processes, the location of flat bipolar contacts with the pedicle are indicated (*).

locus in the visual pathway for an influence of lateral information transmission on the vertical path of information transmission through the retina.

Postreceptor organization

Vertical interactions

Information passes from the photoreceptors to the second-order neurons, the bipolar cells, at the cone pedicles and rod spherules in the outer plexiform layer. Subsequently,

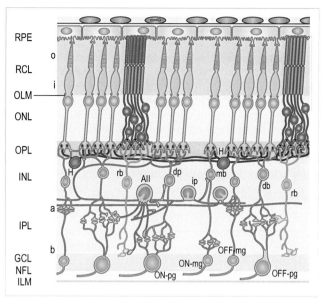

Figure 2.8 A schematic showing the morphological variety of retinal neurons and their connectivities in the context of the histologically defined layers. A number of specific cell types are highlighted: see text for details. Laminar conventions: RPE, retinal pigment epithelium; RCL, rod and cone layer (o, outer segment; i, inner segment); OLM, outer limiting membrane; ONL, outer nuclear layer; OPL, outer plexiform layer; INL, inner nuclear layer; IPL, inner plexiform layer (a, sublamina a/OFF layer; b, sublamina b/ON layer); GCL, ganglion cell layer; NFL, nerve fibre layer; ILM, inner limiting membrane. Cell types: AII, AII amacrine cell; H, horizontal cell; mb, midget bipolar; db, diffuse bipolar; rb, rod bipolar; ip, interplexiform cell; ON-pg, ON-type parasol ganglion cell; OFF-pg, OFF-type parasol ganglion cell; ON-mg, ON-type midget ganglion cell; OFF-mg, OFF-type midget ganglion cell.

with one significant exception that will be addressed further below, information passes from bipolar cells directly to the third-order neurons, the ganglion cells, at the inner plexiform layer (**Fig. 2.8**). This vertical route will be discussed before directing attention to the horizontal and amacrine cell populations that comprise the lateral pathways for information flow in the retina.

Bipolar cells

In the pathway from photoreceptors to bipolar cell to ganglion cell, glutamate is the neurotransmitter at the respective synapses. Nevertheless, the distribution of different post-synaptic glutamate receptors determines that at the photoreceptor–bipolar cell synapse the visual signal is channelled into distinct ON and OFF pathways, this terminology reflecting the response of a cell's receptive field centre to either increasing or decreasing increments in luminance (Werblin and Dowling 1969).

Throughout the retina the connections within the ON and OFF pathways remain largely segregated. At the pedicles, cone ON bipolar cells make contacts within the invaginating synapses of the pedicles, while cone OFF bipolar cells make contacts mainly at the superficial synapses of pedicles (see **Fig. 2.7C**) (Wässle 2004).

Of the estimated 25 million bipolar cells in the human retina (Oyster 1999), Kolb et al (1992) defined nine distinct types of bipolar cell, one type specifically a rod bipolar cell and the remaining eight associated with cones. Their classification of cone bipolar cells, based on

morphology and connectivity, describes various diffuse bipolar cells, flat and invaginating midget bipolar cells, and cone-specific bipolar cell types. It is now generally considered that all mammalian species have a dozen bipolar cell types, all probably having ON and OFF subtypes (Nelson and Kolb 2003).

Most of the cone bipolars are diffuse and may contact between 5 and 20 cones. The so-called midget bipolar cell pathway (named because of the ultimate connections to midget ganglion cells) is, however, characterized by a much lower ratio, especially in the central retina, where cone bipolar cells outnumber cone photoreceptors and where there is at least a one-to-one relationship (**Fig. 2.8**). Given the different wavelength specificities of distinct cone types, the cone pathway in the central retina is therefore adapted for high-resolution spatial detail and colour. In the perifoveal and further peripheral retina a greater number of cones contact each midget bipolar cell, except in the case of the blue cone bipolar, which contacts only one or two blue cones (Kouyama & Marshak 1992).

The solitary rod bipolar cell type is an ON bipolar cell and the number of rods connected to a bipolar cell is greater than the cone bipolar cell ratio (**Fig. 2.8**). Each rod bipolar cell contacts from 20 to 80 rod spherules, lower numbers being characteristic of the rod bipolar cells in the central retina, with higher numbers peripherally. The rod pathway is therefore a convergent pathway. The implication of this arrangement is that, unlike the cone pathways in the central retina, the rod pathway pools inputs from many receptors, diminishing the amount of information relating to detailed spatial form but enhancing the probability of light detection, and consequently underlying the rod system's role in scotopic conditions.

Bipolar cell processes maintain the segregation of ON and OFF subtypes, making their synapses within specific sublaminae of the inner plexiform layer. OFF and ON cone bipolar synapses are segregated, respectively, to sublaminae a and b (**Fig. 2.8**). The bipolar terminal, like the photoreceptor terminal, possesses a specialized ribbon synapse. In this case, commonly there are two postsynaptic elements comprising a dyad, one being a ganglion cell dendrite, the other an amacrine cell process.

Ganglion cells

The retinal output is carried ultimately by the ganglion cells. Unlike most other retinal neurons, ganglion cells generate action potentials, other cell types generally operating via local, graded potentials. Various classifications have been reported, some based on morphological features such as cell body size and characteristics of their dendritic arborization, while other schemes have emphasized the physiological properties of different ganglion cell types. The focus here is on the former, which represent a less ambiguous, definitive description. Further, studies of the macaque retina will also be central (e.g. Leventhal et al 1981; Perry et al 1984; Rodieck 1988; Rodieck & Watanabe 1993).

The median number of ganglion cells in the human retina has been given as 1.12 million (Curcio & Allen 1990) and 18 different types have been described within this population (Kolb et al 1992). The cell bodies of these neurons are located in the ganglion cell layer of the retina, varying in density from the macular region, where, outside the foveola, they can be up to about 10 cells thick, decreasing to one cell thick at the peripheral margin.

Particular morphological types with different patterns of dendritic branching within the inner plexiform layer were initially described by Cajal (in Polyak 1941). Given the likelihood that the distinct branching patterns indicate inputs from different bipolar and/or amacrine cell populations, the clear implication is that the distinct cell types also exhibit different physiological, and consequently functional, properties.

On the basis of their dendritic morphology, Polyak (1941) distinguished parasol and midget ganglion cell types. The midget cell population represents by far the largest ganglion cell type, at about 80% of the total, while parasol ganglion cells make up 10% of the total, both types being distributed across the retina (Perry et al 1984). The midget cell type, as the name implies, possesses a small cell body and fairly compact dendritic tree, but can be further classified as two subtypes on the basis of distinct levels of dendritic stratification in the outer and inner sublaminae of the inner plexiform layers. The parasol cell population has a larger cell body and a larger dendritic expanse than the midget cells at any location on the retina and can also be subtyped on the basis of dendritic stratification: in this case to two different sublaminae within the central zone of the inner plexiform layer (**Fig. 2.8**) (Watanabe & Rodieck 1989). These different levels of dendritic stratification reflect the continued segregation of ON and OFF pathways through the retina, ON cone bipolars making synapses with ON midget or parasol ganglion cells, and OFF cone bipolars with OFF ganglion cells (Kolb & Dekorver 1991; Dacey & Lee 1994). Cone bipolars are therefore intermediates in a direct path from cone photoreceptors to the ganglion cell output from the retina.

However, the rod pathway to ganglion cells is organized differently; rod bipolar cells receive their input from rod photoreceptors and their processes arborize in the inner, ON sublamina of the inner plexiform layer. Here, rather than synapse directly with ganglion cells, the rod bipolar cells connect to the processes of AII type of amacrine cell (**Fig. 2.8**), which pool the inputs from a number of rod bipolars. The rod pathway then joins the cone pathway via gap junctions with the processes of ON cone bipolar cells and GABAergic synapses with OFF cone bipolar cells. These then connect respectively to ON and OFF ganglion cells (DeVries & Baylor 1995).

It seems likely that this is not the only route via which the rod signal influences the cone pathways. The human electroretinogram suggests there may be two rod pathways, a slow path and a faster path. The slow path may reflect the rod bipolar to AII amacrine circuitry, whereas the fast path could be the direct entry of the rod signal into the cone path at the outer retina (Stockman et al 1995). The lateral gap junction connections found between rod spherules and cone pedicles could represent the route for rod responses in cone photoreceptors (Schneeweis & Schnapf 1995).

Midget ganglion cells in the central retina receive their input from bipolar cells which themselves receive input from a single cone (Kolb et al 1992; Dacey 1993a; Calkins et al 1994; Kolb & Marshak 2003). This midget system seems to represent a 'private-line' arrangement in its path to the brain, conveying information relating to specific wavelengths with high acuity. In contrast, parasol cells receive inputs from a number of diffuse bipolars, which receive their input from several photoreceptors (Jacoby et al 2000). These different circuitries imply that the midget and parasol systems differ in their functional properties. This is supported by the observations that the parasol input is divided, with approximately 20% from bipolar cells and 80% from various amacrine cells (Martin & Grünert 2003), while midget cell input appears to be split 50:50 between bipolar and amacrine cell input (Kolb et al 1992). As will be discussed below, these two types of ganglion cell, which together represent 90% of ganglion cells, send their axons to the primary thalamic relay, thus conveying their signal to the primary visual cortex, and represent the neural substrate of the majority of the 'dimensions' of vision.

The remaining 10% of the ganglion cell population comprises a relatively large number of different types, distinguished mainly by their dendritic morphology (e.g. Kolb et al 1992; Peterson & Dacey 2000; Telkes et al 2000). Within this population, the small-field bistratified ganglion cells have received particular attention because these cells, like the midget and parasol types, send their axons to the main retinorecipient thalamic relay nucleus. This cell type, with a dendritic expanse slightly greater than parasol cells, has been described in both monkey and human retina (Dacey 1993b) and appears to correspond to the blue-ON ganglion cell type (Dacey & Lee 1994).

One final type of ganglion cell must be given particular mention. This type, in which the dendritic tree gives the cell its description as a widefield diffuse ganglion cell, is of interest because it is intrinsically photosensitive, and thus represents an inner retinal photoreceptor. There are only about 3000 of these cells in the primate retina (<0.5% of total ganglion cells), with a dendritic tree spread among the largest found, and they express a melanopsin photopigment (Dacey et al 2005). In rodents, these cells have been considered the irradiance-dependent retinal substrate for the pupillary light reflex and for entraining circadian rhythms (Hattar et al 2002). Recent evidence also suggests an involvement of these cells in the primate pupillary light reflex (Gamlin et al 2007), but it is questionable whether the central projections from these cells can be considered a parallel, 'non-image forming' pathway, distinct from those originating at rods and cones (Dacey et al 2005).

Lateral interactions

Horizontal cells

There are at least two types of horizontal cell in the primate retina, H1 and H2, which represent lateral influences on retinal transmission in the outer retina (**Fig. 2.8**). Both types have a maximum density at the foveal margin, but the H2 population is outnumbered by twice the number of H1 cells in the peripheral retina and fourfold at their respective peaks (Wässle et al 2000). Their connections at the cone and rod ribbon synapses provide feedback to rods and cones as well as bipolar cells, with the likely outcome that the presence of a local signal is enhanced relative to more distant inputs. The H1 group has been considered by some to be heterogeneous, including an H3 subdivision (Kolb et al 1992).

The H1 cell type has a long axon terminating in a clustered arborization while the H2 type has a sparse spread of arbors at the ends of its axon (Boycott & Kolb 1973). Within each population the cells are coupled to each other via gap junctions (Dacey et al 1996). However, the two types differ in their photoreceptor connections. The dendritic field of the H1 type contacts red and green cones, whereas the axon terminals connect to rods as the lateral components of the triad in rod terminals. In contrast, the H2 type of horizontal cell connects in particular to blue cone pedicles (Boycott & Kolb, 1973; Ahnelt & Kolb 1994a, b; Dacey et al 1996). The axon, rather than providing a basis for integrating the signals from the dendritic and axonal extremes, has the effect of electronically isolating the dendritic and axonal fields, so these two subsets of horizontal cells can be viewed as primarily processing either blue or red and green signals.

Amacrine cells

Amacrine cells are the substrate for lateral influences in the inner retina (**Fig. 2.8**). A large proportion of synapses on ganglion cells are from amacrine cells (Calkins et al 1994; Jacoby et al 1996), which also input onto the terminal processes of bipolar cells.

Most primate amacrines use either GABA or glycine as a neurotransmitter and may be categorized accordingly (Kalloniatis et al 1996). The majority appear to be glycinergic (Crooks & Kolb 1992; Koontz et al 1993) but the proportion of GABAergic amacrine synapses (80–90%) is much greater (Koontz & Hendrickson 1990), possibly reflecting a greater density of dendritic ramification by GABAergic amacrine cells. Nevertheless, regardless of their relative synaptic distributions, the inhibitory properties of both GABA and glycine appear to result in an amacrine cell circuitry that generally provides negative feedback on to bipolar cell terminals and inhibitory feedforward on to ganglion cells.

There are approximately 25 types of amacrine cell in the primate retina and they are the most morphologically variable retinal cell group (Mariani 1990; Kolb et al 1992). On the basis of their dendritic spread they can be classified into narrow/small-, medium-, or wide/large-field amacrine cells. Most amacrine cell bodies are located in the inner nuclear layer (**Fig. 2.8**), but they may also be found in the inner plexiform layer and in the ganglion cell layer. In the latter case they are often referred to as displaced amacrine cells, and in the peripheral retina they may even outnumber the ganglion cell population in that layer (Curcio & Allen 1990).

Although the vast majority of bipolar and ganglion cells stratify in either the ON or OFF sublaminae of the inner plexiform layer, roughly half of the amacrine cell population appear to have dendrites that arborize in both the ON and OFF sublaminae (Kolb et al 1992). Such bilaminar stratification is characteristic of the AII amacrine cell type, which was discussed above in relation to the vertical retinal pathway for the rod signal (**Fig. 2.8**). This small-field, glycinergic amacrine cell type also contains the calcium-binding protein calretinin, and their peak density is approximately 5000 cells/mm^2 in the perifoveal retina (Wässle et al 1995).

Many amacrine cells co-localize GABA or glycine with another neurotransmitter. A well-characterized example is the starburst amacrine cell, a medium-field type which also contains acetylcholine (Rodieck 1989; Rodieck & Marshak 1992). They also comprise ON and OFF subtypes. The cell bodies of the OFF-type cells are found in the innermost division of the inner nuclear layer and, as might be expected,

their dendrites ramify in the outer, sublamina a, of the inner plexiform layer. The ON-type are included in the displaced amacrine cell group, their cell bodies located in the ganglion cell layer and their dendritic tree arborizes in the inner, sublamina b, of the inner plexiform layer (Rodieck & Marshak 1992).

In Cajal's original descriptions, amacrine cells were named as such because of their apparent lack of an axon (amacrine = axon-less). However, more recently, multiple axonal processes have been identified in a variety of large-field amacrine cells. One of these is the GABAergic, AI amacrine cell, which can, in the central retina, have a dense dendritic tree of about 0.5 mm in diameter but a polyaxonal arborization that can extend to, and maybe even beyond, 4.5 mm. In addition, unlike retinal neurons in the outer retina, these amacrine cells generate action potentials (Stafford & Dacey 1997).

Axon-like processes are also found in a dopamine-containing GABAergic amacrine cell type, some extending up to 5 mm from the cell body. The extensive spread of these processes means that, although there are less than 10 000 of these cells in the retina, they nevertheless cover its entire extent (Mariani et al 1984; Dacey 1990). Some have considered that this dopaminergic amacrine cell type may also represent one form of the interplexiform cell, a cell type that has been studied most extensively in non-mammalian species. These cells have cell bodies in the inner nuclear layer along with other amacrine cells and receive synaptic inputs in the inner plexiform layer but make synaptic output connections not only in that layer but also onto bipolar and horizontal cell processes in the outer plexiform layer (**Fig. 2.8**). This represents a potential path for retinal information feedback from the inner to the outer retina. The dopamine content of these cells in some primates (Dowling 1986) may serve not only to adjust the overall sensitivity of retinal mechanisms but also to regulate the gap junction coupling of horizontal cells (Hampson et al 1994) and thereby the spatial organization of receptive fields in the neurons of the outer retina.

Retinal outflow and the optic nerve, chiasm and tract

Retinal ganglion cell axons represent the output path from the retina and they form the nerve fibre layer, bounded at its innermost extent by the inner limiting membrane, a specialization of the end feet of the Müller glial cells.

The ganglion cell axons display a characteristic path across the inner retinal surface to their exit point posteriorly at the optic disc, the visuotopic position of the blind spot due to the absence of photoreceptors at this location. Axons from nasal locations in the retina take a path directly to the disc, as do axons from superior and inferior temporal quadrants in temporal retina. Those arising from ganglion cells nasal to the fovea also course directly to the optic disc, forming the papillomacular bundle. In contrast, those arising from points temporal to the fovea take an arcuate course above or below the fovea, depending on whether they originate from inferior or superior retinal locations respectively (Hogan et al 1971).

Optic nerve head

Approximately one million ganglion cell axons exit the retina to form the optic nerve (Potts et al 1972a; Balazsi et al 1984; Sanchez et al 1986; Mikelberg et al 1989; Jonas et al 1990, 1992). In doing so, their course takes them initially through the intraocular (or intrascleral) optic nerve, a 1 mm length also referred to as the optic nerve head, which represents a region of considerable specialization. The scleral organization is modified here to form a sieve-like meshwork, the cribriform plates, which support the axons in this part of their course, designated the lamina cribrosa (**Fig. 2.9A**). The cribriform plates are composed of various extracellular matrix components. The cores of these trabeculae comprise mainly elastin with collagen types I and III, while collagen type IV and laminin are found associated with their margins (Hernandez et al 1987; Rehnberg et al 1987; Morrison et al 1989; Hernandez 1992). Various proteoglycans have also been localized to the region of the lamina cribrosa (Caparas et al 1991).

Prior to their course through the lamina cribrosa, the unmyelinated axons are gathered into astrocyte-lined fascicles. These are continuous with the pores that penetrate the cribriform plates (**Fig. 2.9B**) (Anderson 1969; Hogan et al 1971; Ruskell 1988). These pores are variable in size, and the thickness of the connective tissue plates separating the axon bundles varies accordingly. The pore sizes are apparently generally larger in superior and inferior quadrants at the lamina cribrosa (Quigley et al 1990), suggesting that the physical support of axons is weaker in these locations, and hinting that there may be an increased likelihood

of axons in these locations being disrupted by elevated intraocular pressure.

In the postlaminar region of the optic nerve head, the ganglion cell axons are myelinated, accounting for the increase in the nerve diameter from 1.5 mm at the laminar level to approximately 3–3.5 mm. Given the central neural origin of the optic nerve, the myelin sheath of the axons derives from oligodendrocytes, while the general absence of myelination along the prior course of the axons has been ascribed to a possible barrier to the migration of oligodendrocyte precursor cells by the lamina cribrosa (Perry & Lund 1990).

It should be noted, prior to considering further proximal locations, that not all axons in the optic nerve originate from retinal ganglion cells. A few, maybe only a dozen, are centrifugal axons originating from cell bodies in the posterior hypothalamus and dorsal raphe nucleus. They arborize in the inner retinal layers and possibly function to regulate retinal interneuron activity and blood flow (Gastinger et al 2006; Repérant et al 2006).

Postlaminar optic nerve

The optic nerve at the postlaminar level is invested by a meningeal sheath; the dura mater, an outer, thick collagenous layer of connective tissue, envelops the arachnoid mater, a middle layer of trabeculae with collagen cores surrounded by meningothelial cells. The innermost layer, the pia mater, is a delicate connective tissue layer in which are embedded numerous blood vessels. Connective tissue septa of pial origin extend into the nerve to surround the axon fascicles at this postlaminar level of the nerve (**Fig. 2.9C**). The spaces between the meningeal layers, the subdural and subarachnoid spaces, are filled with cerebrospinal fluid. The latter is continuous with the intracranial subarachnoid space, meaning that increased intracranial pressure has the potential for direct compression on the optic nerve.

The optic nerve carries the myelinated retinal ganglion cell axons from the intraocular segment to the optic chiasm, a distance of 40–50 mm, which can be subdivided into three further segments. Firstly, the intraorbital part of the optic nerve is about 20–30 mm in length and extends to the optic foramen (canal). The path is not direct but arcs laterally near the orbital apex, resulting in about 6 mm of slack that enables compliant movement of the nerve during ocular rotation (Wolff 1948). Where the nerve enters the foramen the dural sheath fuses with the orbital periosteum, limiting potential movement along the subsequent intracanalicular part of the nerve. The path of the nerve through

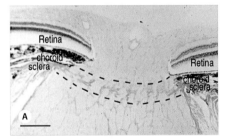

Figure 2.9A Section through the optic nerve head. The location of the lamina cribrosa is highlighted by the blue-stained plates extending through the nerve head at the level of the sclera (*indicated by broken lines*). Scale bar 0.5 mm.

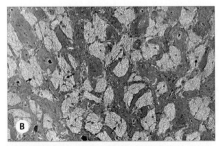

Fig. 2.9B Transverse section of the optic nerve at the peripheral margin of the lamina cribrosa. The lighter stained regions represent the pores occupied by ganglion cell axons, the darker regions being interfascicular tissue. The arrows indicate the cell bodies of astrocytes amongst the axon bundles.

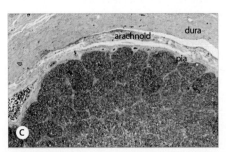

Figure 2.9C Transverse section of the postlaminar optic nerve showing the fascicular organization of the nerve and the location of the different meningeal layers.

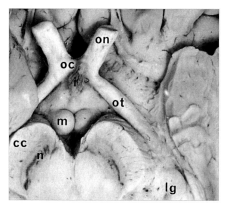

Figure 2.10 Gross dissection of the ventral aspect of the human brain showing the course of the intracranial optic nerve (on), the optic chiasm (oc), and the optic tract (ot) through to the major retinorecipient target, the lateral geniculate nucleus (lg). I, infundibular stalk; m, mammillary body; n, substantia nigra; cc, cerebral peduncle.

the optic canal carries it into the cranium, where, after an intracranial course that can vary in length considerably (average about 12 mm), the nerve joins with that from the opposite eye at the midline, the optic chiasm. Following their course through this region, ganglion cell axons pass into the optic tract on one or other of the brain's hemispheres (**Fig. 2.10**), and then onwards to their ultimate termination at one of the various central nervous targets of retinal ganglion cells, which will be discussed further below.

Optic chiasm and tract

The fascicular organization of the optic nerve axons changes along the pathway to the brain. The fascicle number is greatest distally in the nerve, this arrangement being lost at the optic chiasm and optic tract (Jeffery et al 1995). This may represent a further adaptation to ease compliant movement of the nerve during eye movements.

Retinal ganglion cell axons within the optic pathway do not have the same diameter. They can range from 0.1 μm to 8.3 μm in the nerve with a skewed unimodal distribution that peaks at approximately 0.5 μm (Potts et al 1972b; Jonas et al 1990). The different diameter ranges are represented across all parts of the optic nerve (**Fig. 2.11A**), although the inferotemporal region appears to contain a larger proportion of small-diameter axons than elsewhere across the nerve (Sanchez et al 1986; Reese & Ho 1988). This relatively even distribution of axons of different diameters across the optic nerve changes significantly at the level of the optic chiasm where the ganglion cell axons undergo a set of complex rearrangements that have been observed in all examined species including primates (Reese & Baker 1992).

By far the most widely recognized of these rearrangements is the segregation of crossing (decussating) and non-crossing optic axons. The decussating axons arise from ganglion cells in the nasal retina and take a path across the midline into the contralateral optic tract, while the axons originating from temporal retinal ganglion cells do not cross the midline, instead remaining uncrossed and coursing into the ipsilateral optic tract. The nasal:temporal split is normally about 53:47, possibly with some overlap (Kupfer et al 1967; Fukuda et al 1989) and this roughly hemi-decussation underlies the binocular representations of the visual field in the mammalian brain.

These proportions are considerably altered in hypopigmented individuals such as found in albinism. The proportion of non-crossing axons is greatly reduced as a consequence of many axons arising in the temporal retina taking an aberrant course into the contralateral hemisphere at the optic chiasm (Apkarian et al 1983; Guillery et al 1984; Morland et al 2002; Hoffmann et al 2005). This chiasmatic misrouting has significant consequences for the organization of further central projections in the visual pathways of albinos, and probably underlies some of the significant visual anomalies that they possess, although the effects of retinal abnormalities are also likely to be significant (Jeffery 1997).

A second reorganization of axons in the optic chiasm results in a distribution in the optic tract that partially

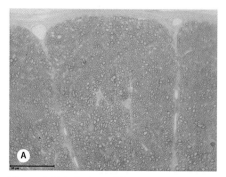

Figure 2.11A Section of the macaque optic nerve stained to show myelinated axons and indicating the presence of fibres of the entire range of diameters within a single fascicle, an arrangement that exists across the whole optic nerve.

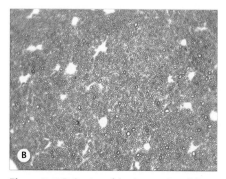

Figure 2.11B Section of the deep region of the macaque optic tract showing an absence of large-diameter axons from this part of the tract.

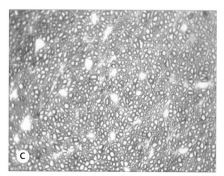

Figure 2.11C The superficial part of the tract is predominantly occupied by large-diameter axons with few of the smaller axons apparent in the deeper part of the tract.

segregates the large from the small-diameter axons. In the optic tract, the large-diameter axons accumulate towards the superficial border (**Figs 2.11B** and **2.11C**), unlike the nerve, where they are relatively evenly distributed (**Fig. 2.11A**) (Reese & Guillery 1987; Reese & Ho 1988; Reese 1993). Selective labelling of the distinct populations demonstrates that the superficially located axons arise mainly from the parasol ganglion cell type, while those axons deep in the optic tract arise from the midget type (Reese & Cowey 1990a) and which, as will be discussed further below, represent distinct functional pathways from the eye to the brain.

The segregation of the distinct axon populations in the optic tract, but the presence of their cell bodies overlapping across the entire retina (Perry et al 1984), indicates that there must be partially segregated representations of the retina in the optic tract (Reese & Cowey 1990b). Therefore, the tract cannot be considered as a single representation of the contralateral hemifield, which has been the classical explanation (e.g. Duke-Elder 1961; Polyak 1957), thereby providing an anatomical explanation for the incongruity in visual field defects of the two eyes following partial disruption of one optic tract (Bender & Bodis-Wollner 1978; Savino et al 1978). Further, the segregation of axons of different ganglion cell types indicates that the separate field representations can be expected to have distinct functional properties (Reese 1993), and therefore require particular perimetric approaches to fully define defects.

A third redistribution of axons concerns the segregation of axons arising from the dorsal versus the ventral retina. In the optic tract, this retinal axis is represented by the dorsal retinal axons in the caudomedial part of the tract while the ventral retinal axons travel in the rostrolateral region (Hoyt & Luis 1962; Naito 1994). The dorsal and ventral fibres are also generally segregated at the level of the optic nerve head, but between that distal location and the optic tract, the axons disperse such that the representation of that retinal axis becomes indistinct (Hoyt & Luis 1962, 1963; Naito 1989), reappearing during their passage through the optic chiasm (Naito 2000).

It is no understatement to describe the rearrangements of axons at the optic chiasm as complex, with axons from different retinal locations changing their relations between their exit from the retina at the optic nerve head and their passage along the optic tract. The changes that occur at the optic chiasm relate to a change from a roughly retinotopic order of axons to a chronotopic arrangement where the fibre order is a reflection of their sequence of addition during development (Reese & Baker 1992; Reese 1996). This distribution of axons along the pathway is significant for the retinotopic representation along the pathway, and important for our understanding of the development of the pathway and the effects of, for example, compressive lesions at different locations along its course.

The pathway is widely considered to be generally ordered in a retinotopic fashion at the optic nerve head, with the axon organization reflecting their characteristic course across the retina to the optic disc described above (Hogan et al 1971), although the degree of order has been questioned (Fitzgibbon & Taylor 1996). The large proportion of fibres arising from the central retina due to the greater density of ganglion cells in that region gives the macular region a proportionally greater fraction of the retinotopic representation in the pathway. The organization of the axons changes along the course of the optic nerve so that the papillomacular fibres come to occupy a location in the centre of the nerve (Brouwer & Zeeman 1926; Hoyt & Luis 1962; Hoyt & Tudor 1963, 1989).

This classical view also paints a picture of the temporal and nasal fibre distribution being largely segregated, but more recent evidence indicates that there is significant intermixing of the populations (Naito 1989). Nevertheless, these populations have divergent courses at the optic chiasm into the ipsilateral and contralateral optic tracts, respectively, and it appears that their segregation may be evident even prior to their chiasmatic course (Hoyt & Luis 1963; Unsold & Hoyt 1980; Naito 1989, 1994).

This has developmental and clinical implications. It suggests that, unlike non-primate mammals, interactions between the axons from each eye may not be necessary for pathway guidance at the optic chiasm during development (Neveu et al 2006). Also, the bitemporal hemianopia associated with tumours of the pituitary gland located inferior to the optic chiasm in the sella turcica is readily accounted for by compression of solely midline decussating fibres from the nasal retina. Further, it accounts anatomically for the nasal hemianopia resulting from lateral compression on the region as might accompany an aneurysm of the internal carotid artery (e.g. Day 1990).

Wilbrand's knee – a myth?

No description of the course of axons from the optic nerve and through the chiasm to the tract is complete without mention of Wilbrand's knee. This refers to a group of decussating fibres that take a looping path of 1–2 mm anteriorly into the contralateral optic nerve prior to coursing posteriorly into the optic tract. Disruption of this group of fibres was proposed to be associated with the superior temporal hemianopia exhibited as part of the anterior chiasmal syndrome, and that they course from the nasal part of the nerve. These fibres have been widely described but their presence, although previously queried (Strachan & Cleary 1972), has recently received a scholarly examination which failed to identify them in the chiasm of normal primates. Rather, the fibres that comprise Wilbrand's knee are present only following atrophy of one pathway following monocular enucleation, are of undefined retinal origin, and the degree of incursion of the fibres into the contralateral optic nerve increases with the period since enucleation (Horton 1997). It appears then that Wilbrand's knee is an artefact resulting from the degeneration of ganglion cell fibres from the contralateral eye. However, this proposal does not appear to have received universal acceptance (Karanjia & Jacobsen 1999).

Targets of retinal ganglion cell axons

The great majority of ganglion cell axons in primates are unbranched, and each projects to only one target in the brain (Rodieck 1998). There are a number of distinct targets and most of the ganglion cell axons (90%) course along the optic tract to one target in particular, the lateral geniculate nucleus.

Lateral geniculate nucleus

The lateral geniculate nucleus is the gateway to the primary visual cortex, and the retino-geniculo-cortical pathway is largely the substrate for our conscious awareness of the visual world. The nucleus is traditionally pictured as comprising six major cellular layers (**Fig. 2.12**) but this is variable, especially at rostral levels of the nucleus where layers merge (Hickey & Guillery 1979; Malpeli et al 1996). The cells of the nucleus are classified as either relay cells, each with an axon that projects to visual cortex, or interneurons, with an axon that is confined to the nucleus. Relay cells greatly outnumber interneurons.

The laminar organization is expressed in a number of ways. Firstly, the relay cells are layered according to their size, with the ventral two layers (layers 1 and 2) comprising mainly large cells while the remaining four major layers (layers 3–6) contain small cells. These layers are consequently the magnocellular and parvocellular layers, respectively. Each of these layers has an associated sublayer, a koniocellular layer, just below it containing sparsely distributed, very small cells (Hendry & Yoshioka 1994). In addition to soma size, the cells differ in their dendritic expanse and orientation in the layers as well as their calcium-binding protein content; the relay cells of the magno- and parvocellular layers contain parvalbumin while those of the koniocellular layers contain a calbindin (Casagrande 1994; Hendry & Reid 2000).

In addition to the segregation of the relay cells according to size, the different sublayers receive their retinal inputs from distinct ganglion cell types. The magnocellular layers receive from parasol ganglion cells while midget ganglion cells project onto the parvocellular layers, with the parvocellular layers 5 and 6 receiving from ON midget cells and the parvocellular layers 3 and 4 mainly from OFF midget cells (Schiller & Malpeli 1978). As for the koniocellular layers, the small, bistratified ganglion cell type projects to at least those sublayers associated with the parvocellular layers 3 and 4 (Hendry & Reid 2000).

The layers of the lateral geniculate nucleus also express ocular segregation. Each of the major layers, with its associated sublayer, receives its retinal inputs from the specific ganglion cell types in only one eye. Magnocellular layer 1 and parvocellular layers 4 and 6 receive from the contralateral retina, while magnocellular 2, and parvocellular layers 3 and 5 receive from the ipsilateral eye. The retinal input to each layer is retinotopically organized and therefore there are multiple retinal representations of the opposite hemifield with magnified representation of the central visual field. All of these retinotopic maps are in register so that a single point in the binocular field is represented at aligned points, producing a so-called line of projection that runs orthogonally through the layers (Malpeli & Baker 1975). In situations where the crossed–uncrossed divergence of ganglion cell axons at the optic chiasm is abnormal, as seen for example in albinism, the visual field representations are clearly abnormal and are associated with abnormal geniculate lamination (Guillery et al 1975; Guillery 1986).

Therefore, the lateral geniculate nucleus can be viewed as relaying various relatively independent, retinotopically organized, cell-type-specific and therefore potentially functionally different inputs to the visual cortex. However, it is simplistic to think of the nucleus as a mere relay. Although the great majority of retinal ganglion cell axons project to the relay neurons of the lateral geniculate nucleus, these retinal inputs are only a small minority of the afferents to the nucleus (approximately 10% in the cat: Van Horn et al 2000). They are far outnumbered by descending afferents from the primary visual cortex and inputs from brainstem regions such as the parabrachial nucleus. In addition, a significant proportion of the synaptic input comes from the thalamic reticular nucleus, a structure that surrounds the thalamus laterally and with which the relay cells are reciprocally connected. There is also a large synaptic contact from intrinsic interneurons of the nucleus (Sherman & Guillery 1996).

These anatomical relations alone hint at a more sophisticated role for the nucleus than a simple relay and new views of the neural circuitry point to its role as a gate or toggle, switching the relay between states that favour distinct modes of information transfer from the retina to the striate cortex (Sherman & Guillery 1998; Sherman 2001).

Superior colliculus

Of the 10% of retinal ganglion cells that do not terminate in the lateral geniculate nucleus, many continue their course along an extension of the optic tract, the brachium of the superior colliculus. The superior colliculus, where the axons terminate, is a laminated paired structure on the roof of the midbrain, but its individual layers are not as distinctive as those of the lateral geniculate nucleus (Hilbig et al 1999).

The axons from retinal ganglion cells terminate in the superficial layers of the superior colliculus, but unlike the lateral geniculate nucleus the inputs from the separate retinas are not segregated to separate layers. Instead, the ocular inputs interdigitate at largely overlapping depths (Pollack & Hickey 1979). These inputs, like the projection(s) to the lateral geniculate nucleus, are organized to produce a retinotopic representation that, contrary to early reports (e.g. Bunt et al 1975), includes the fovea (Cowey & Perry 1980). The retinal ganglion cells that send axons to the superior colliculus have comparatively extensive dendrites and have been considered to comprise three distinguishable groups on the basis of the organization of their dendritic arborizations (Rodieck & Watanabe 1993).

The deeper layers of the superior colliculus also receive auditory and somatosensory inputs, and by coordinating the sensory inputs with descending inputs from particular regions of the cortex, this structure serves to control visually guided eye movements.

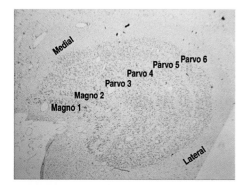

Figure 2.12 Frontal section through the human lateral geniculate nucleus. The distinct magnocellular and parvocellular layers are indicated and the koniocellular layers are the lightly stained regions between the major layers.

Pretectum

Several groups of cells in the midbrain, rostral to the superior colliculus, receive inputs from ganglion cell axons that leave the brachium. These mainly include the nucleus of the optic tract, involved in eye movement control, and the pretectal olivary nucleus, part of the circuitry underlying the pupillary light reflex. The pretectum receives axons from cells that have a dendritic extent among the largest of the retinal ganglion cells (Rodieck & Watanabe 1993). These cells were considered earlier in the context of their intrinsic photosensitive properties.

The pretectal olivary nucleus receives a bilateral retinal input and, in turn, its cells send axons predominantly to the contralateral Edinger–Westphal nucleus, the origin of the parasympathetic component of the oculomotor nerve (Gamlin & Clarke 1995; Kourouyan & Horton 1997). This circuit, via its subsequent synapse at the ciliary ganglion and projection onward to the iris sphincter muscle, regulates pupil size. The presence of direct and consensual pupillary light reflexes is likely due to the bilateral inputs to the pretectal olivary nuclei.

Accessory optic system

A small number of axons leave the optic tract via the transpeduncular tract to terminate in the dorsal, lateral or medial terminal nuclei. Unlike the retinorecipient structures described above, these nuclei predominantly receive input from the contralateral retina. Although the morphology of the ganglion cells from which the axons arise is unknown, the cells are sensitive to movement in a particular direction, and the inputs to each nucleus have a different preferred direction (Fredericks et al 1988; Cooper et al 1990; Baleydier et al 1990). These nuclei appear to coordinate eye and head movements.

Suprachiasmatic nucleus

Several hypothalamic nuclei, most notably the suprachiasmatic nucleus and the paraventricular nucleus, receive retinal input from axons that leave the main pathway dorsally at the optic chiasm to form the retinohypothalamic tract (Moore 1973; Sadun et al 1984; Schaecter & Sadun 1985). The paraventricular nucleus is concerned with neuro-endocrine function, while the suprachiasmatic nucleus is intimately involved in the light–dark entrainment of the circadian rhythm. The small subset of ganglion cells that give rise to the projection to the suprachiasmatic nucleus are probably photosensitive due to their melanopsin content (Hattar et al 2002; Berson et al 2002; Dacey et al 2005).

Connecting to striate cortex

The majority of the relay cells of the lateral geniculate nucleus send their axons to the striate cortex,[1] so named because of the presence of the stria of Gennari, a white layer visible in fresh sections of the region. The striate cortex is located mainly on the medial surface of the occipital lobe,

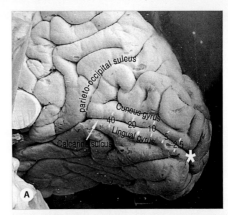

Figure 2.13A Photograph of the medial face of the occipital and parietal lobes separated by the parieto-occipital sulcus. The calcarine sulcus is indicated with approximate representation of the central 40 degrees of visual field mapped on to the anterior–posterior extent of the sulcus. The asterisk (*) indicates the location of the foveal representation at the posterior pole of the lobe.

where it folds to form the calcarine sulcus (**Fig. 2.13A**). Most of the striate cortex surface area is actually concealed on the walls of the sulcus, although it extends upwards and downwards onto the cuneus gyrus and the lingual gyrus, respectively (**Fig. 2.13B**). The surface area has been estimated at approximately 2500 mm^2 (Horton & Hoyt 1991), although a more recent report indicated up to a 2.5-fold difference across individuals (Dougherty et al 2003).

The axons of lateral geniculate cells that connect to the striate cortex form the optic radiation and their course passes initially from the thalamus, penetrating the thalamic reticular nucleus and continuing laterally into the internal capsule.

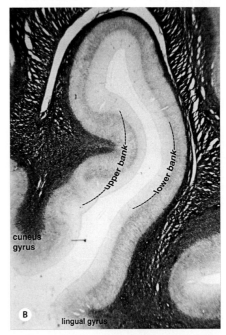

Figure 2.13B Micrograph of section through the region of the calcarine sulcus. The deep infolding of the sulcus between the cuneus and lingual gyri shows the extent of the striate cortex. The upper bank contains the representation of the lower visual field and the lower bank the upper visual field.

---

[1]Historically, a number of different labels have been assigned to the primary visual cortex. A histological classification of the region, 'area 17', followed Brodmann's categorization of distinct cerebral cortical zones. This term has often been used interchangeably with 'V1', a description having a more functional connotation but which may not precisely correspond to the histologically defined region. Here, therefore, the term 'striate cortex' will be applied.

The internal capsule, in the horizontal plane, comprises anterior and posterior limbs that meet at the genu. The posterior limb extends caudally beyond the adjacent lentiform nucleus, forming the retrolenticular portion of the posterior limb, and it is through this most posterior part of the internal capsule that the axons of the optic radiation course as a fairly compact bundle (Carpenter 1991). The limited spread of the axons at this point means that even relatively localized ischaemic tissue damage resulting from disorders of the middle cerebral artery branches that supply this part of the internal capsule can frequently result in complete contralateral hemianopia.

Fibre topography in the optic radiation

Beyond the internal capsule, the fibres of the optic radiation fan out along their course before terminating at the calcarine sulcus. Nevertheless, despite the relatively tortuous course taken by many, a crude retinotopic order remains within the arrangement of fibres along the pathway.

Axons from relay cells in the medial part of the lateral geniculate nucleus, which receive input from the superior retinal quadrants and therefore represent the lower visual field, form the superior portion of the optic radiation. The course of these axons takes them through the white matter underlying the parietal cortex and over the posterior horn of the lateral ventricle en route to the occipital lobe, where they terminate on the superior bank of the calcarine sulcus.

In contrast, the axons arising from cells in the lateral part of the nucleus, which receive inputs from inferior retinal quadrants and carry the superior visual field representation, distribute to the inferior bank of the sulcus. The axons of this inferior portion of the optic radiation take a very different path to that of the superior radiation. They initially pass anteriorly and ventrolaterally into the temporal lobe, where they fan out around the rostral tip of the inferior horn of the lateral ventricle. At this point along their course, known as Meyer's loop, the fibres turn posteriorly, taking a path adjacent to the outer wall of the lateral ventricle and subsequently into the occipital lobe.

The widespread distribution of the optic radiation fibres means that complete contralateral hemianopia is uncommon following lesions to this pathway. For example, temporal lobe lesions will produce defects solely in the upper visual field (e.g. Marino & Rasmussen 1968) and because limited disruption is usual, quadrantic field defects are more likely.

Retinotopic organization of striate cortex

Although the optic radiation pathway to the striate cortex, like the optic tract course to the lateral geniculate nucleus, contains a crude retinotopic map, the terminations produce a precise representation of the entire contralateral visual field. Both the monocular and binocular regions of the left visual field are represented in the right striate cortex, and vice versa.

In addition to the mapping of the inferior and superior retinal representations respectively to the inferior and superior walls of the calcarine sulcus that was discussed above, the central to peripheral retinal dimension is mapped in a caudal to rostral direction along the sulcus (**Fig. 2.13A**). The foveal representation is at the occipital pole extending slightly onto the lateral surface of the occipital lobe (Holmes & Lister 1916; Horton & Hoyt 1991; McFadzean et al 1994).

The striate representation of the retina is not a simple linear map of retinal or visual field spatial coordinates (Hubel & Wiesel 1974; Drasdo 1977). On average, in humans the representation of the central 20 degrees occupies approximately 75% of the striate cortex and the entire peripheral field beyond 40 degrees is represented within the most anterior 10% (Horton & Hoyt 1991). This 'over-representation' of the macular region is possibly a simple reflection of its greater retinal ganglion cell density (Wässle et al 1990) although alternative views have been proposed (e.g. Azzopardi & Cowey 1993).

The greatly magnified macular representation is also a potential explanation for the phenomenon of macular sparing, i.e. the retention of foveal vision in the presence of an otherwise extensive scotoma. Perhaps the mere extent of the foveal representation in the striate cortex means that there is often some intact part of the representation remaining. This explanation is in addition to those provided by the presence of foveal overlap of ipsilaterally and contralaterally projecting retinal ganglion cells indicated above (Fukuda et al 1989) or possible overlapping vascular supply from branches of both the posterior and middle cerebral arteries.

Cellular organization in the striate cortex

The striate cortex is histologically divisible into six primary layers and various sublayers on the basis of the distribution of cell bodies. These run from layer 1 closest to the pial surface through to the deepest layer 6 adjacent to the underlying white matter (**Fig. 2.14A**). In general, the upper layers are the sites of connections with other cortical regions, the middle layers receive the fibre inputs from the optic radiation, and the deep layers are the origins of outputs to the thalamus and brainstem.

In addition to this laminar division of striate cortex there is histochemical heterogeneity. Staining for the presence of metabolic enzymes, notably cytochrome oxidase (CO), shows a regular, patchy distribution of cytochrome-rich 'blobs' about 0.5 mm apart, most prominently in layers 2 and 3 but also faintly in layers 5 and 6 (Hendrickson et al 1981; Horton & Hubel 1981).

The optic radiation inputs are segregated into different sublayers and histochemical compartments in striate cortex, retaining the segregation of distinct retinal inputs produced at

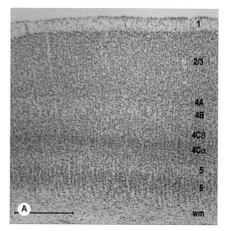

Figure 2.14A Micrograph of a section of striate cortex stained to indicate neuronal cell bodies. Layers 1–6 are indicated with layer 4 subdivided to show the locations of sublaminae 4A, 4B, 4Cα and 4Cβ. wm indicates the location of the underlying white matter. Scale bar 500 μm.

the lateral geniculate nucleus (see above). This organization has led to the suggestion of segregation of distinct visual functional characteristics from retina to striate cortex and beyond (e.g. Livingstone & Hubel 1988). The geniculate input to the striate cortex is mainly into layer 4, with the axons of magnocellular geniculate cells synapsing on cells in the upper division of layer 4C (4Cα) while those of parvocellular cells terminate on cells in the lower division (4Cβ). In addition, both of these cell types send sparser axon collaterals into layer 6 (Hubel & Wiesel 1972; Hendrickson et al 1978). The koniocellular cells of the lateral geniculate nucleus send their axons mainly to the CO blob regions in layer 3 (Hendry & Yoshioka 1994).

Anatomical segregation of the distinct konio-, magno- and parvocellular pathways seems to end there. There are cells in layer 4Cα that send axons to layer 4B and to the blob regions in layer 3. In addition, cells in layer 4Cβ project to the blob regions (Yabuta & Callaway 1998). The blob regions in layer 3 appear therefore to receive converging inputs from all three pathways, but this ignores their relative density or functional strength of input.

Columnar organization of striate cortex

Within the geniculorecipient layer 4C of striate cortex, the inputs to the two sublaminae are also segregated according to the represented eye (Hubel & Wiesel 1968; Horton & Hedley-Whyte 1984). Left eye and right eye representations are distinct, forming alternating 'ocular dominance columns' (**Fig. 2.14B**). Given the overall retinotopic precision of the inputs to the striate cortex this indicates that there are, in fact, two interleaved representations, one for each retina (Hubel & Wiesel 1972).

In addition to eye preference, all cells within a column aligned orthogonally to the surface of the striate cortex have receptive fields tuned to a particular stimulus orientation. Adjacent columns have slightly different preferences and there is an orderly progression through 180 degrees over a distance of approximately 1 mm (Hubel & Wiesel 1977; Hubel et al 1977).

The presence of these intersecting ocular dominance and orientation columns in striate cortex resulted in the concept of the hypercolumn (Hubel & Wiesel 1977), in which one of these cortical 'modules' represents all orientations at the same visual field position for each eye, and adjacent hypercolumns do the same for an adjacent point in the visual field.

The architecture of the hypercolumn has since required some remodelling, with the observation that blobs are found in the centre of ocular dominance columns (e.g. Humphrey & Hendrickson 1983). Nevertheless, the development of sensitive in vivo imaging techniques has uncovered the precise arrangement of orientation columns, and if such maps of iso-orientation contours are superimposed on the arrangement of ocular dominance bands, it is evident that adjacent ocular dominance columns share iso-orientation domains for a single point in the visual field (Obermayer & Blasdel 1993).

Other visual cortical inputs

The inputs to the striate cortex do not all arise from the lateral geniculate nucleus. Other cortical areas as well as other thalamic and brainstem nuclei provide input (Casagrande & Kaas 1994). In a mode comparable to the role of the extraretinal inputs to the lateral geniculate nucleus discussed above, in the striate cortex these may well act as the modulators of the primary driver inputs originating from the lateral geniculate nucleus (Sherman & Guillery 1998).

Further, although the large majority of the output from the lateral geniculate nucleus does terminate in the striate cortex, some cells send axons directly to other cortical visual areas (Yukie & Iwai 1981; Bullier & Kennedy 1983; Sincich et al 2004). The presence of these paths may be, at least partially, the substrate for residual visual function in individuals with damage to the striate cortex, such as is found in blindsight. Nevertheless, most of the retinal input is relayed via the lateral geniculate nucleus to the striate cortex, which represents the neural switching mechanism for routing different functional pathways towards distinct extrastriate cortical regions.

Acknowledgements

Professor Gordon Ruskell had an enormous influence on my thinking about the visual pathways and by way of acknowledging that influence I have incorporated some of his illustrations into this chapter. I would like to thank sincerely Gordon's wife, Valerie, for permitting their inclusion.

I would also like to thank my colleagues, Professors Ron Douglas and Glen Jeffery, for their substantial comments on an earlier draft.

References

Ahnelt P, Kolb H 1994a Horizontal cells and cone photoreceptors in primate retina: a Golgi-light microscopic study of spectral connectivity. Journal of Comparative Neurology 343:387–405

Ahnelt P, Kolb H 1994b Horizontal cells and cone photoreceptors in human retina: a Golgi-electron microscopic study of spectral connectivity. Journal of Comparative Neurology 343:406–427

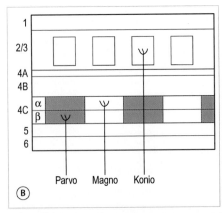

Figure 2.14B Schematic to show a summary of the locations of the major terminations for the three lateral geniculate cell types that send axons to the striate cortex. The alternating shaded and unshaded regions in layer 4C represent the arrangement of ocular dominance bands in the input layer from the lateral geniculate nucleus to the striate cortex. Boxed regions in layers 2/3 indicate the location of the CO-rich blob regions.

Anderson 1969 Ultrastructure of human and monkey lamina cribrosa and optic nerve head. Archives of Ophthalmology 82:800–814

Apkarian P, Reits D, Spekreijse H et al 1983 A decisive electrophysiological test for human albinism. Electroencephalography & Clinical Neurophysiology 55:513–531

Azzopardi P, Cowey A 1993 Preferential representation of the fovea in the primary visual cortex. Nature 361:719–721

Balazsi A G, Rootman J, Drance S M et al 1984 The effect of age on the nerve fiber population of the human optic nerve. American Journal of Ophthalmology 97:760–766

Baleydier C, Magnin M, Cooper H M 1990 Macaque accessory optic system: II. Connections with the pretectum. Journal of Comparative Neurology 302:405–416

Bender M B, Bodis-Wollner I 1978 Visual dysfunctions in optic tract lesions. Annals of Neurology 3:187–193

Berson D M, Dunn F A, Takao M 2002 Phototransduction by retinal ganglion cells that set the circadian clock. Science 295:1070–1073

Bok D 1985 Retinal photoreceptor-pigment epithelium interactions. Investigative Ophthalmology & Visual Science 26:1659–1694

Bok D 1990 Processing and transport of retinoids by the retinal pigment epithelium. Eye 4:326–332

Boycott B B, Kolb H 1973 The horizontal cells of the rhesus monkey retina. Journal of Comparative Neurology 148:115–139

Brouwer B, Zeeman W P C 1926 The projection of the retina in the primary optic neuron in monkeys. Brain 49:1–35

Bullier J, Kennedy H 1983 Projection of the lateral geniculate nucleus onto cortical area V2 in the macaque monkey. Experimental Brain Research 53:168–172

Bunt A H, Hendrickson, A E, Lund J S et al 1975 Monkey retinal ganglion cells: morphometric analysis and tracing of axonal projections, with a consideration of the peroxidase technique. Journal of Comparative Neurology 164:265–285

Calkins D J, Schein S J, Tsukamoto Y et al 1994 M and L cones in macaque fovea connect to midget ganglion cells by different numbers of excitatory synapses. Nature 37:70–72

Caparas V L, Cintron C, Hernandez-Neufeld M R 1991 Immunohistochemistry of proteoglycans in human lamina cribrosa. American Journal of Ophthalmology 112:489–495

Carpenter M B 1991 Core text of neuroanatomy. Lippincott Williams and Wilkins, Philadelphia

Casagrande V A 1994 A third parallel visual pathway to primate area V1. Trends in Neurosciences 17:305–310

Casagrande V A, Kaas J H 1994 The afferent, intrinsic, and efferent connections of primary visual cortex in primates. In: Peters A, Rockland K (eds) Primary visual cortex of primates, vol. 10, Cerebral Cortex. Plenum, New York, pp 201–259

Chu P G, Grunwald G B 1990 Identification of an adhesion-associated protein of the retinal pigment epithelium. Investigative Ophthalmology and Visual Science 31:856–862

Chun M H, Grünert U, Martin P R et al 1996 The synaptic complex of cones in the fovea and in the periphery of the macaque monkey retina. Vision Research 36:3383–3395

Cooper H M, Baleydier C, Magnin M 1990 Macaque accessory optic system: I. Definition of the medial terminal nucleus. Journal of Comparative Neurology 302:394–404

Cowey A, Perry V H 1980 The projection of the fovea to the superior colliculus in rhesus monkeys. Neuroscience 5:53–61

Crooks J, Kolb H 1992 Localization of GABA, glycine, glutamate and tyrosine hydroxylase in the human retina. Journal of Comparative Neurology 315:287–302

Curcio C A, Allen K A 1990 Topography of ganglion cells in human retina. Journal of Comparative Neurology 300:5–25

Curcio C A, Sloan K R, Kalina R E et al 1990 Human photoreceptor topography. Journal of Comparative Neurology 292:497–523

Curcio C A, Allen K A, Sloan K R et al 1991 Distribution and morphology of human cone photoreceptors stained with anti-blue opsin. Journal of Comparative Neurology 312:610–624

Dacey D M 1990 The dopaminergic amacrine cell. Journal of Comparative Neurology 301(3):461–489

Dacey D M 1993a The mosaic of midget ganglion cells in the human retina. Journal of Neuroscience 13:5334–5355

Dacey D M 1993b Morphology of a small-field bistratified ganglion cell type in the macaque and human retina. Visual Neuroscience 10:1081–1098

Dacey D M, Lee B B 1994 The 'blue-on' opponent pathway in primate retina originates from a distinct bistratified ganglion cell type. Nature 367:731–735

Dacey D M, Lee B B, Stafford D K et al 1996 Horizontal cells of the primate retina: cone specificity without spectral opponency. Science 271:656–659

Dacey D M, Liao H W, Peterson B B et al 2005 Melanopsin-expressing ganglion cells in primate retina signal colour and irradiance and project to the LGN. Nature 433:749–754

Day A L 1990 Aneurysms of the ophthalmic segment. A clinical and anatomical analysis. Journal of Neurosurgery 72:677–691

DeVries S H, Baylor D A 1995 An alternative pathway for signal flow from rod photoreceptors to ganglion cells in mammalian retina. Proceedings of the National Academy of Sciences USA 92: 10658–10662

Dougherty R F, Koch V M, Brewer A A et al 2003 Visual field representations and locations of visual areas V1/2/3 in human visual cortex. Journal of Vision 3:586–598

Dowling J E 1986 Dopamine: a retinal neuromodulator? Trends in Neuroscience 9:236–240

Drasdo N 1977 The neural representation of visual space. Nature 266:554–556

Duke-Elder S 1961 The anatomy of the visual system. In: Duke-Elder S, Wybar K C (eds) System of ophthalmology, vol 2. Henry Kimpton, London

Fitzgibbon T, Taylor S F 1996 Retinotopy of the human retinal nerve fibre layer and optic nerve head. Journal of Comparative Neurology 375:238–251

Fredericks C A, Giolli R A, Blanks R H et al 1988 The human accessory optic system. Brain Research 454:116–122

Fukuda Y, Sawai H, Watanabe M et al 1989 Nasotemporal overlap of crossed and uncrossed retinal ganglion cell projections in the Japanese monkey (*Macaca fuscata*). Journal of Neuroscience 9:2353–2373

Gamlin P D, Clarke R J 1995 The pupillary light reflex pathway of the primate. Journal of the American Optometric Association 66:415–418

Gamlin P D, McDougal D H, Pokorny J et al 2007 Human and macaque pupil responses driven by melanopsin-containing retinal ganglion cells. Vision Research 47:946–954

Gastinger M J, Tian N, Horvath T et al 2006 Retinopetal axons in mammals: emphasis on histamine and serotonin. Current Eye Research 31:655–667

Guillery R W 1986 Neural abnormalities of albinos. Trends in Neurosciences 9:364–367

Guillery R W, Okoro A N, Witkop C J 1975 Abnormal visual pathways in the brain of a human albino. Brain Research 96:373–377

Guillery R W, Hickey T L, Kaas J H et al 1984 Abnormal central visual pathways in the brain of an albino green monkey (*Cercopithecus aethiops*). Journal of Comparative Neurology 226:165–183

Hampson E C, Weiler R, Vaney D I 1994 pH-gated dopaminergic modulation of horizontal cell gap junctions in mammalian retina. Proceedings of the Royal Society London (Biological Sciences) 255:67–72

Hattar S, Liao H W, Takao, M et al 2002 Melanopsin-containing retinal ganglion cells: architecture, projections, and intrinsic photosensitivity. Science 295:1065–1070

Haverkamp S, Grünert, U, Wässle H 2000 The cone pedicle, a complex synapse in the retina. Neuron 27:85–95

Hendrickson A E, Wilson J R, Ogren M P 1978 The neuroanatomical organization of pathways between the dorsal lateral geniculate nucleus and visual cortex in Old World and New World primates. Journal of Comparative Neurology 182:123–136

Hendrickson A E, Hunt S P, Wu J Y 1981 Immunocytochemical localization of glutamic acid decarboxylase in monkey striate cortex. Nature 292(5824):605–607

Hendry S H, Reid R C 2000 The koniocellular pathway in primate vision. Annual Review of Neuroscience 23:127–153

Hendry S H, Yoshioka T 1994 A neurochemically distinct third channel in the macaque dorsal lateral geniculate nucleus. Science 264: 575–577

Hernandez M R 1992 Ultrastructural immunocytochemical analysis of elastin in the human lamina cribrosa. Changes in elastic fibers in primary open-angle glaucoma. Investigative Ophthalmology and Visual Science 33(10):2891–2903

Hernandez M R, Luo X X, Igoe F et al 1987 Extracellular matrix of the human lamina cribrosa. American Journal of Ophthalmology 104:567–576

Hickey T L, Guillery R W 1979 Variability of laminar patterns in the human lateral geniculate nucleus. Journal of Comparative Neurology 183:221–246

Hilbig H, Bidmon, H J, Zilles K et al 1999 Neuronal and glial structures of the superficial layers of the human superior colliculus. Anatomy and Embryology (Berlin) 200:103–115

Hoffmann M B, Lorenz B, Morland A B et al 2005 Misrouting of the optic nerves in albinism: estimation of the extent with visual evoked potentials. Investigative Ophthalmology and Visual Science 46:3892–3898

Hogan M J, Alvarado J A, Weddell J 1971 Histology of the human eye. Saunders, Philadelphia

Holmes G, Lister W T 1916 Disturbances of vision from cerebral lesions with special reference to the cortical representation of the macula. Brain 39:34–73

Hornstein E P, Verweij J, Schnapf J L 2004 Electrical coupling between red and green cones in primate retina. Nature Neuroscience 7:745–750

Horton J C 1997 Wilbrand's knee of the primate optic chiasm is an artefact of monocular enucleation. Transactions of the American Ophthalmological Society 95:579–609

Horton J C, Hedley-Whyte E T 1984 Mapping of cytochrome oxidase patches and ocular dominance columns in human visual cortex. Philosophical Transactions Royal Society London B Biological Sciences 304:255–272

Horton J C, Hoyt W F 1991 The representation of the visual field in human striate cortex. A revision of the classic Holmes map. Archives of Ophthalmology 109:816–824

Horton J C, Hubel D H 1981 Regular patchy distribution of cytochrome oxidase staining in primary visual cortex of macaque monkey. Nature 292(5825):762–764

Hoyt W F, Luis O 1962 Visual fiber anatomy in the infrageniculate pathway of the primate. Archives of Ophthalmology 68:94–106

Hoyt W F, Luis O 1963 The primate chiasm. Details of visual fiber organization studied by silver impregnation techniques. Archives of Ophthalmology 70:69–85

Hoyt W F, Tudor R C 1963 The course of parapapillary temporal retinal axons through the anterior optic nerve. A Nauta degeneration study in the primate. Archives of Ophthalmology 69:503–507

Hubel D H, Wiesel T N 1968 Receptive fields and functional architecture of monkey striate cortex. Journal of Physiology 195:215–243

Hubel D H, Wiesel T N 1972 Laminar and columnar distribution of geniculo-cortical fibers in the macaque monkey. Journal of Comparative Neurology 146:421–450

Hubel D H, Wiesel T N 1974 Uniformity of monkey striate cortex: a parallel relationship between field size, scatter, and magnification factor. Journal of Comparative Neurology 158:295–305

Hubel D H, Wiesel T N 1977 Ferrier lecture. Functional architecture of macaque monkey visual cortex. Proceedings of Royal Society London B Biological Sciences 198:1–59

Hubel D H, Wiesel T N, Stryker M P 1977 Orientation columns in macaque monkey visual cortex demonstrated by the 2-deoxyglucose autoradiographic technique. Nature 269:328–330

Humphrey A L, Hendrickson A E 1983 Background and stimulus-induced patterns of high metabolic activity in the visual cortex (area 17) of the squirrel and macaque monkey. Journal of Neuroscience 3:345–358

Jacoby R, Stafford D, Kouyama, N et al 1996 Synaptic inputs to ON parasol ganglion cells in the primate retina. Journal of Neuroscience 16:8041–8056

Jacoby R A, Wiechmann A F, Amara S G et al 2000 Diffuse bipolar cells provide input to OFF parasol ganglion cells in the macaque retina. Journal of Comparative Neurology 416:6–18

Jeffery G 1997 The albino retina: an abnormality that provides insight into normal retinal development. Trends in Neuroscience 20: 165–169

Jeffery G, Evans A, Albon J et al 1995 The human optic nerve: fascicular organisation and connective tissue types along the extra-fascicular matrix. Anatomy and Embryology (Berlin)191:491–502

Jonas J B, Müller-Bergh J A, Schlötzer-Schrehardt U M et al 1990 Histomorphometry of the human optic nerve. Investigative Ophthalmology and Visual Science 31:736–744

Jonas J B, Schmidt A M, Müller-Bergh J A et al 1992 Human optic nerve fiber count and optic disc size. Investigative Ophthalmology and Visual Science 33:2012–2018

Kalloniatis M, Marc R E, Murry R F 1996 Amino acid signatures in the primate retina. Journal of Neuroscience 16:6807–6829

Karanjia N, Jacobsen D M 1999 Compression of the prechiasmatic optic nerve produces a junctional scotoma. American Journal of Ophthalmology 128:256–258

Kolb H, Dekorver L 1991 Midget ganglion cells of the parafovea of the human retina: a study by electron microscopy and serial section reconstructions. Journal of Comparative Neurology 303:617–636

Kolb H, Marshak D 2003 The midget pathways of the primate retina. Documenta ophthalmologica (Advances in ophthalmology) 106:67–81

Kolb H, Linberg K A, Fisher S K 1992 Neurons of the human retina: a Golgi study. Journal of Comparative Neurology 318:147–187

Koontz M A, Hendrickson A E 1990 Distribution of GABA-immunoreactive amacrine cell synapses in the inner plexiform layer of macaque monkey retina. Visual Neuroscience 5:17–28

Koontz M A, Hendrickson L E, Brace S T et al 1993 Immunocyto-chemical localization of GABA and glycine in amacrine and dis-placed amacrine cells of macaque monkey retina. Vision Research 33:2617–2628

Kourouyan H D, Horton J C 1997 Transneuronal retinal input to the primate Edinger-Westphal nucleus. Journal of Comparative Neurology 381:68–80

Kouyama N, Marshak D W 1992 Bipolar cells specific for blue cones in the macaque retina. Journal of Neuroscience 12:1233–1252

Kupfer C, Chumbley L, Downer J C 1967 Quantitative histology of optic nerve, optic tract and lateral geniculate nucleus of man. Journal of Anatomy 101:393–401

Leventhal A G, Rodieck R W, Dreher B 1981 Retinal ganglion cell classes in the Old World monkey: morphology and central projections. Science 213:1139–1142

Livingstone M, Hubel D 1988 Segregation of form, color, movement, and depth: anatomy, physiology, and perception. Science 240 (4853):740–749

McFadzean R, Brosnahan D, Hadley D et al 1994 Representation of the visual field in the occipital striate cortex. British Journal of Ophthalmology 78:185–190

Malpeli J G, Baker F H 1975 The representation of the visual field in the lateral geniculate nucleus of *Macaca mulatta*. Journal of Comparative Neurology 161:569–594

Malpeli J G, Lee D, Baker F H 1996 Laminar and retinotopic organiza-tion of the macaque lateral geniculate nucleus: magnocellular and parvocellular magnification functions. Journal of Comparative Neurology 375:363–377

Mariani A P 1990 Amacrine cells of the rhesus monkey retina. Journal of Comparative Neurology 301:382–400

Mariani A P, Kolb H, Nelson R 1984 Dopamine-containing amacrine cells of rhesus monkey retina parallel rods in spatial distribution. Brain Research 322:1–7

Marino R, Rasmussen T 1968 Visual field changes after temporal lobectomy in man. Neurology 18:825–835

Martin P R, Grünert U 2003 Ganglion cells in mammalian retinae. In: Chalupa L M, Werner J S (eds) The visual neurosciences. MIT Press, Massachusetts, pp 410–421

Masland R H 2001 The fundamental plan of the retina. Nature Neuroscience 4(9):877–886

Mikelberg F S, Drance S M, Schulzer M et al 1989 The normal human optic nerve. Axon count and axon diameter distribution. Ophthalmology 96:1325–1328

Moore R Y 1973 Retinohypothalamic projection in mammals: a comparative study. Brain Research 49:403–409

Morland A B, Hoffmann M B, Neveu M et al 2002 Abnormal visual projection in a human albino studied with functional magnetic resonance imaging and visual evoked potentials. Journal of Neurology, Neurosurgery and Psychiatry 72:523–526

Morrison J C, Jerdan J A, Dorman M E et al 1989 Structural proteins of the neonatal and adult lamina cribrosa. Archives of Ophthalmology 107:1220–1224

Naito J 1989 Retinogeniculate projection fibers in the monkey optic nerve: a demonstration of the fiber pathways by retrograde axonal transport of WGA-HRP. Journal of Comparative Neurology 284:174–186

Naito J 1994 Retinogeniculate projection fibers in the monkey optic chiasm: a demonstration of the fiber arrangement by means of wheat germ agglutinin conjugated to horseradish peroxidase. Journal of Comparative Neurology 346:559–571

Naito J 2000 Changes in the retinotopical fiber order along the horizontal and dorsoventral axes of the nasal retina in the monkey optic chiasm. Cell and Tissue Research 302:387–390

Nelson R, Kolb H 2003 ON and OFF pathways in the vertebrate retina and visual system. In: Chalupa L M, Werner J S (eds) The visual neurosciences. MIT Press, Massachusetts, pp 260–278

Neveu M M, Holder G E, Ragge N K et al 2006 Early midline interactions are important in mouse optic chiasm formation but are not critical in man: a significant distinction between man and mouse. European Journal of Neuroscience 23:3034–3042

Obermayer K, Blasdel G G 1993 Geometry of orientation and ocular dominance columns in monkey striate cortex. Journal of Neuroscience 13:4114–4129

Østerberg G A 1935 Topography of the layer of rods and cones in the human retina. Acta Ophthalmologica 13 (Suppl 6):1–103

Oyster C W 1999 The human eye: structure and function, 1st edn. Sinaeur, Massachusetts

Perry V H, Lund R D 1990 Evidence that the lamina cribrosa prevents intraretinal myelination of retinal ganglion cell axons. Journal of Neurocytology 19:265–272

Perry V H, Oehler R, Cowey A 1984 Retinal ganglion cells that project to the dorsal lateral geniculate nucleus in the macaque monkey. Neuroscience 12:1101–1123

Peterson B B, Dacey D M 2000 Morphology of wide-field bistratified and diffuse human retinal ganglion cells. Visual Neuroscience 17:567–578

Pollack J G, Hickey T L 1979 The distribution of retino-collicular axon terminals in rhesus monkey. Journal of Comparative Neurology 185:587–602

Polyak S 1941 The retina. University of Chicago Press, Chicago

Polyak S 1957 The vertebrate visual system. University of Chicago Press, Chicago

Potts A M, Hodges D, Shelman C B et al 1972a Morphology of the primate optic nerve. I. Method and total fiber count. Investigative Ophthalmology and Visual Science 11:980–988

Potts A M, Hodges D, Shelman C B et al 1972b Morphology of the primate optic nerve. II. Total fiber size distribution and fiber density distribution. Investigative Ophthalmology and Visual Science 11:989–1003

Quigley H A, Brown A E, Morrison J D et al 1990 The size and shape of the optic disc in normal human eyes. Archives of Ophthalmology 108:51–57

Rao-Mirotznik R, Harkins A B, Buchsbaum G et al 1995 Mammalian rod terminal: architecture of a binary synapse. Neuron 14:561–569

Reese B E 1993 Clinical implications of the fibre order in the optic pathway of primates. Neurological Research 15:83–86

Reese B E 1996 The chronotopic reordering of optic axons. Perspectives on Developmental Neurobiology 3:233–242

Reese B E, Baker G E 1992 Changes in fiber organization within the chiasmatic region of mammals. Visual Neuroscience 9:527–533

Reese B E, Cowey A 1990a Fibre organization of the monkey's optic tract: I. Segregation of functionally distinct optic axons. Journal of Comparative Neurology 295:385–400

Reese B E, Cowey A 1990b Fibre organization of the monkey's optic tract: II. Noncongruent representation of the two half-retinae. Journal of Comparative Neurology 295:401–412

Reese B E, Guillery R W 1987 Distribution of axons according to diameter in the monkey's optic tract. Journal of Comparative Neurology 260:453–460

Reese B E, Ho K Y 1988 Axon diameter distributions across the monkey's optic nerve. Neuroscience 27:205–214

Rehnberg M, Ammitzboll T, Tengroth B 1987 Collagen distribution in the lamina cribrosa and the trabecular meshwork of the human eye. British Journal of Ophthalmology 71:886–892

Repérant J, Ward R, Miceli D et al 2006 The centrifugal visual system of vertebrates: a comparative analysis of its functional anatomical organization. Brain Research Reviews 52:1–57

Rodieck R W 1988 The primate retina. In: Steklis H D, Erwin J (eds) Comparative primate biology, vol 4. Alan R Liss, New York, pp 203–278

Rodieck R W 1989 Starburst amacrine cells of the primate retina. Journal of Comparative Neurology 285:18–37

Rodieck R W 1998 The first steps in seeing. Sinauer, Massachusetts

Rodieck R W, Marshak D W 1992 Spatial density and distribution of choline acetyltransferase immunoreactive cells in human, macaque, and baboon retinas. Journal of Comparative Neurology 321:46–64

Rodieck R W, Watanabe M 1993 Survey of the morphology of macaque retinal ganglion cells that project to the pretectum, superior colliculus, and parvicellular laminae of the lateral geniculate nucleus. Journal of Comparative Neurology 338:289–303

Ruskell G L 1988 Neurology of visual perception In: Edwards K, Llewellyn R (eds) Optometry. Butterworths London, pp 3–24

Sadun A A, Schaechter J D, Smith L E 1984 A retinohypothalamic pathway in man: light mediation of circadian rhythms. Brain Research 302:371–377

Sanchez R M, Dunkelberger G R, Quigley H A 1986 The number and diameter distribution of axons in the monkey optic nerve. Investigative Ophthalmology and Visual Science 27:1342–1350

Savino P J, Paris M, Schatz N J et al 1978 Optic tract syndrome. A review of 21 patients. Archives of Ophthalmology 96:656–663

Schaecter J D, Sadun A A 1985 A second hypothalamic nucleus receiving retinal input in man: the paraventricular nucleus. Brain Research 340:243–250

Schiller P H, Malpeli J G 1978 Functional specificity of lateral geniculate nucleus laminae of the rhesus monkey. Journal of Neurophysiology 41:788–797

Schneeweis D M, Schnapf J L 1995 Photovoltage of rods and cones in the macaque retina. Science 268:1053–1056

Sherman S M 2001 Tonic and burst firing: dual modes of thalamocortical relay. Trends in Neurosciences 24:122–126

Sherman S M, Guillery R W 1996 Functional organization of thalamocortical relays. Journal of Neurophysiology 76:1367–1395

Sherman S M, Guillery R W 1998 On the actions that one nerve cell can have on another: distinguishing 'drivers' from 'modulators'. Proceedings of the National Academy of Sciences USA 95:7121–7126

Sincich L C, Park K F, Wohlgemuth M J et al 2004 Bypassing V1: a direct geniculate input to area MT. Nature Neuroscience 7:1123–1128

Stafford D K, Dacey D M 1997 Physiology of the A1 amacrine: a spiking, axon-bearing interneuron of the macaque monkey retina. Visual Neuroscience 14(3):507–522

Steinberg R H, Fisher S K, Anderson D H 1980 Disc morphogenesis in vertebrate photoreceptors. Journal of Comparative Neurology 190:501–518

Sterling P, Demb J B 2004 Retina. In: Shepherd G M (ed.) The synaptic organization of the brain, 5th edn. Oxford University Press, New York, pp 217–269

Stockman A, Sharpe L T, Ruther K et al 1995 Two signals in the human rod visual system: a model based on electrophysiological data. Visual Neuroscience 12:951–970

Strachan I M, Cleary P E 1972 The study of the human optic nerve with elliptically polarised light. In: Cant, J S (ed.) The optic nerve. Henry Kimpton, London, pp 292–297

Telkes I, Distler C, Hoffmann K P 2000 Retinal ganglion cells projecting to the nucleus of the optic tract and the dorsal terminal nucleus of the accessory optic system in macaque monkeys. European Journal of Neuroscience 12:2367–2375

Unsold R, Hoyt W F 1980 Band atrophy of the optic nerve. The histology of temporal hemianopsia. Archives of Ophthalmology 98:1637–1638

Van Horn S C, Erisir A, Sherman S M 2000 Relative distribution of synapses in the A-laminae of the lateral geniculate nucleus of the cat. Journal of Comparative Neurology 416:509–520

Wässle H 2004 Parallel processing in the mammalian retina. Nature Reviews Neuroscience 5:1–11

Wässle H, Grünert U, Rohrenbeck J et al 1990 Retinal ganglion cell density and cortical magnification factor in the primate. Vision Research 30:1897–1911

Wässle H, Grünert U, Chun M H et al 1995 The rod pathway of the macaque monkey retina: identification of AII-amacrine cells with antibodies against calretinin. Journal of Comparative Neurology 361:537–551

Wässle H, Dacey D M, Haun T et al 2000 The mosaic of horizontal cells in the macaque monkey retina: with a comment on biplexiform ganglion cells. Visual Neuroscience 17:591–608

Watanabe M, Rodieck R W 1989 Parasol and midget ganglion cells of the primate retina. Journal of Comparative Neurology 289:434–454

Werblin F S, Dowling J E 1969 Organization of the retina of the mud-puppy, *Necturus maculosus*. II. Intracellular recording. Journal of Neurophysiology 32:339–355

Williams R W 1991 The human retina has a cone-enriched rim. Visual Neuroscience 6:403–406

Wolff E 1948 The anatomy of the eye and orbit. Lewis, London

Yabuta N H, Callaway E M 1998 Functional streams and local connections of layer 4C neurons in primary visual cortex of the macaque monkey. Journal of Neuroscience 18:9489–9499

Young R 1971 The renewal of rod and cone outer segments in the rhesus monkey. Journal of Cell Biology 49:303–318

Young R, Bok D 1969 Participation of the retinal pigment epithelium in the rod outer segment renewal process. Journal of Cell Biology 42:392–403

Yukie M, Iwai E 1981 Direct projection from the dorsal lateral geniculate nucleus to the prestriate cortex in macaque monkeys. Journal of Comparative Neurology 201:81–97

CHAPTER 3

Visual development

Carol Westall

Introduction

I write this chapter from my perspective as a vision scientist whose research encompasses investigations into visual development when the visual system has been compromised pre- or postnatally. Visual system development may be compromised by disease, drugs or other toxic insult. Thus, my choice of topics included in this chapter has been sculptured by my research interest.

During the first 6 months of life, in the absence of any insult to vision development, the way in which a child perceives a favourite toy changes from a poorly resolved and weakly coloured, low-contrast image (**Fig. 3.1**) into one that appears brightly coloured with high resolution (**Fig. 3.2**).

Although resolution is poor in the neonate, infants have been shown to orientate towards faces at birth. Typically, developing children will look longer at a face which engages them; that is, they prefer direct gaze versus averted gaze (Farroni et al 2002). The demonstration of a response to face stimuli at birth (Klaus et al 1970; Farroni et al 2002) is indicative of functional vision in the newborn. From birth onwards vision functions mature, as noted as long ago as 1877 by Darwin:

> . . . his eyes were fixed on a candle as early as the 9th day, and up to the 45th day nothing else seemed thus to fix them; but on the 49th day his attention was attracted by a bright-coloured tassel, as was shown by his eyes becoming fixed and the movements of his arms ceasing. It was surprising how slowly he acquired the power of following with his eyes an object if swinging at all rapidly; for he could not do this well when seven and a half months old.
>
> http://psychclassics.yorku.ca/Darwin/infant.htm

This description of the development of visual processing was published in *Mind* by Darwin (1877). Since then, observations of visual development have been superseded by descriptions of vision function using more quantitative methods, many of which can be found in documented accounts of the development of visual functions, such as those of Teller (1997) and Atkinson (2000).

This chapter will provide basic information on spatial and chromatic visual development and visual sensitivity. Techniques for measurement of vision function are described briefly and more details can be found in Leat et al (1999). The chapter will include examples of normal values according to age, and the neural substrates responsible for development. It will focus on selected forms of visual dysfunction in the early period of plasticity in human visual development. The examples of developmental dysfunction will be taken from the different stages of maturity.

Several methods have been used to assess visual function in infants. This chapter will focus on two techniques, namely behavioural and electrophysiological. Both of these techniques began over half a century ago. Behavioural methods are based on the observation that young infants will often stare fixedly at bold, high-contrast patterns, track the motion of such patterns, and exhibit compensatory eye and head movements to keep these patterns in their central vision. Techniques based on the observation of fixation patterns have been called *preferential looking* (PL) techniques and were developed from the original observations of Robert Fantz in the 1950s,

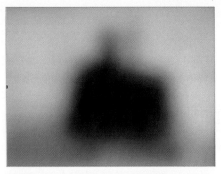

Figure 3.1 A coloured toy as seen by a neonate. (Infant vision simulation courtesy of TinyEyes.com)

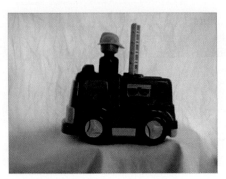

Figure 3.2 The same toy as in Figure 3.1 seen by a 5-year-old. (Infant vision simulation courtesy of TinyEyes.com)

who found that newborn infants consistently chose to look towards targets differing in spatial arrangement. He also demonstrated the ability of neonates to resolve structured targets (Fantz 1961).

Electrophysiological techniques such as visual evoked potentials (VEP) or electroretinograms (ERGs) come from the assessment of electrical responses to a specific stimulus recorded from electrodes placed over the visual cortex and cornea, respectively. Detection of the signals is achieved by isolating the visual signal from the background electrical noise. Around the same time that preferential looking techniques were being developed, electrophysiological procedures were emerging as an objective alternative to assess paediatric vision function. As shown later in the chapter, rates of development vary quite considerably between these two techniques.

Visual evoked potential (VEP) recordings were published first in 1934 (Adrian and Matthew, cited by Harding 1991). A VEP is an evoked potential produced by sensory stimulation within the visual field and is observed using electroencephalography (EEG). Commonly used visual stimuli are flashing lights or checkerboards on a video screen that flicker between black-on-white to white-on-black (inverted contrast).

VEPs are especially useful in determining visual function in those who cannot communicate, such as infants or patients with developmental disabilities. If repeated stimulation of the visual field produces no change in EEG potential, then this indicates that the subject's brain is probably not receiving any signal from the eyes.

Before entering into further discussion of testing vision functions and their development, a short discussion of retinal development is included, as the development of the cellular elements in the first stage of vision processing are essential for the interpretation of the developmental processes of vision functions.

Retinal development

Retinal cells are established before birth whereas the retinal layers are differentiated at birth (Abramov et al 1982; Hendrickson & Drucker 1992). Early in prenatal development a continuous layer of homogeneous neuroblasts increase in number by mitosis; these cells are multipotent with the capability of differentiating into any one of a specific retinal neurone type (Barnstable 2004; Candy 2006). The first differentiation into ganglion cells occurs around the third gestational month (Candy 2006). Subsequent to ganglion cell differentiation, cone differentiation occurs, followed by horizontal cells and amacrine cells. Around birth, the rod photoreceptors differentiate as do their connecting bipolar and Müller cells (Barnstable 2004).

At about 4.5 months gestational age the retinal layers form. At this time the ganglion cells in the central retina develop. This is followed, during the first 7 gestational months, by a 'wave' of development to the periphery. At this stage synchronized bursting activity of immature ganglion cells, coordinated between neighbouring cells, comprise the 'retinal waves' (Wong 1999). The bursting activity sweeps in waves across the retina (Meister et al 1991) in unpredictable and different directions (Meister et al 1991; Wong et al 1993; Feller et al 1996), avoiding areas that recently experienced depolarization and bursting activity (Feller et al 1996, 1997). The spontaneous, synchronized, bursting activity of immature ganglion cells is essential for retinal differentiation and subsequent visual system development (Catsicas & Mobbs 1995).

Neurotransmitters

Excitatory networks and synapses are established before inhibitory ones and the pre-natal brain is in a state of increased excitability. The excitatory neurotransmitter acetylcholine (ACh) and its receptors regulate early phases of neural migration and neurogenesis (Feller, Wellis et al. 1996). A temporary increased availability of ACh promotes more neurogenesis and transient circuit formation during late stages of prenatal development. During early postnatal development there is a switch in neurotransmitters driving retinal waves; if cholinergic activity is blocked the waves continue to spread and glutamate becomes the instigator of wave propagation. In the mature retina glutamate allows information to be transmitted vertical through the mature retina. This switch in the type of modulating transmitter occurs when the bipolar cells are making initial synaptic connections with ganglion cells and when the synapses between amacrine and ganglion cells become numerous and morphologically mature (http://webvision.med.utah.edu).

Postnatally, the inhibitory neurotransmitter gamma aminobutyric acid (GABA) takes over the modulation of retinal waves. The number of amacrine cells that are immunoreactive to GABA increases dramatically during the early postnatal period, showing higher levels than in the mature retina. This excess of GABA-reacting neurons suggests that GABA plays a transient role in circuit formation as ACh did in earlier development. GABA modulates the pattern of correlated spontaneous bursting activity between amacrine cells and ganglion cells (Karne et al 1997). Patterns of immunoreactivity of a GABAergic network in the inner plexiform layer of the neonatal retina coincide with the appearance of correlated bursting activity in the inner retina (Karne et al 1997).

GABA is the primary transmitter of most retinal amacrine cells. For infant eyes, unlike at maturity, GABA provides excitatory input for ganglion cells. Later in development, when the ganglion cells are differentiating into ON and OFF inputs to the lateral geniculate nucleus (see Ch. 2), GABA suppresses ganglion cell bursting activity. This role is maintained in the mature retina. In the neonate $GABA_A$ receptors play an important role in synaptogenesis between cones and horizontal cells (Sharma & Johnson 2000). Any blockade of spontaneous retinal activity and synaptogenesis disrupts the normal pattern of retinal ganglion cell axons to the lateral geniculate nucleus (Penn et al 1998).

Structural development

Once ocular development is complete, the foveal area is much thinner than the rest of the retina. The ganglion cells have migrated away from the centre so that the incident light does not have to pass through several layers of retinal cells to reach the cones. This area, the foveal pit, starts to appear at 24–26 weeks' gestational age. At birth, the foveal depression is still forming. The ganglion cell layer has started the process of thinning, but the fovea is still overlaid with one or two layers of ganglion cells. The very centre of the fovea is the rod-free foveola, which is larger at birth than in an adult and the cones are more widely spaced within it. The cone outer segments are much fatter and shorter than those of an adult, resulting in a smaller area of light-sensitive pigment available to capture light. Postnatally within the fovea, the cone outer segments thin and the cones move inwards, thereby increasing the density. This results in a decreased area of the foveola with thinner and more tightly packed cones. From birth to 45 months there is a 2.5 times increase in cone density followed by a further 35% increase to adulthood (Yuodelis & Hendrickson 1986). By 15 months the cone outer segments are seven times longer than at birth, but are still shorter than in the adult. By 45 months they are still 30–50% shorter than adult outer segments (Hendrickson 1993). During the early months of postnatal development the inner retinal layers move away from the fovea; by about postnatal month 4 the ganglion cells move away from the centre and the foveal pit is formed (Abramov et al 1982; Hendrickson & Drucker 1992). By 12 months postnatally the diameter of the foveola decreases to half its size with subsequent tighter cone packing (Floren & Hendrickson 1984). Between 15 and 45 months, the fovea has reached adult size.

Rod and cone receptors in the mid-periphery are more mature than foveal receptors (Hendrickson 1993). Further, by 13 months' postnatal age the rod outer segments are of a similar length to those found in adults (Hendrickson 1993).

The myelin sheath of the optic nerve and optic tract fibres mature rapidly during the first few postnatal months, reaching maturity over the first 2 years after birth (Friede & Hu 1967). The visual cortex continues to develop after birth. The number of synapses in the visual cortex remains constant for the first 2 months after birth, then increases rapidly to more than double by 8 months of age, reducing to adult levels over about the next 11 years, during which time the excessive number of connections is refined and pruned by eliminating those that are redundant.

The laterate geniculate nucleus (LGN) is the second major structure of the visual system that undergoes marked anatomical and physiological development during the prenatal and postnatal period. The LGN is characterized by its six layers: two contain relatively large neurons (magnocellular (M) layers) and four contain smaller neurons (parvocellular (P) layers) (see Ch. 2). Physiologically, neurons of the M-projecting pathway have high luminance contrast sensitivity and excellent temporal frequency resolution and are responsive to low luminance stimuli. In contrast, neurons of the P-projecting pathway show colour opponency, low sensitivity, and only moderate temporal resolution. The P and M layers of the LGN are separated further by layers of very small cells, the koniocellular (K) layers (Kaas et al 1978; Dacey & Lee 1994; Martin et al 1997). These layers receive inputs from a distinct ganglion cell type, the small bistratified ganglion cell, that carries excitatory input from S (blue) cones (Dacey & Lee 1994). This distinct ganglion cell type demonstrates an anatomically distinct pathway that conveys S-cone signals to the brain.

Inputs to each geniculate layer come from only one eye, and are arranged retinotopically. Development of the LGN during the first trimester involves cell migration and differentiation, and primary branching of axons and dendrites. By the second trimester, the LGN synapses with retinal axons, dendritic processes appear, and the cells of the P and M layers differentiate. At birth, the M and P layers are readily observed, but the cell bodies in each layer are smaller than in adults (Banks & Salapatek 1983). Therefore, if the processes involved in cell migration or differentiation are disrupted during prenatal life, functions specific to the LGN layers, such as contrast sensitivity or colour vision, may be compromised.

The primary visual cortex receives a wealth of incoming fibres from the LGN, which reflects its integral role in visual processing. The topographic lamination of the visual cortex, which begins to develop during the third trimester, is correlated with functional specializations that are beyond the scope of this chapter (see Ch. 2). It is sufficient to say that the cortical neurons respond selectively to different properties of visual stimuli, such as orientations, motion, spatial frequency or wavelengths.

Development of visual–ocular functions

Visual acuity

Visual acuity (VA) is a test of the spatial limit of visual discrimination at high contrast (Atkinson 2000). It is the predominant measure of visual function and is often used as an index of visual function integrity in clinical trials. VA is determined by finding the minimum angle of resolution, where resolution is the minimum distance between distinguishable objects in an image (see Ch. 12).

Units of visual acuity are typically cycles per degree (cpd) for a grating stimulus (in which 30 cycles per degree represent a resolution of 1 minute of arc). Visual acuity may also be quantified as the logarithm of the minimum angle of resolution (logMAR) in which 0 logMAR is equivalent to a minimum resolution of 1 minute of arc, or the traditional Snellen notation of 6/6 (20/20).

Behavioural assessment

The preferential looking technique was refined into a rigorous infant vision testing technique by Davida Teller (Teller 1979). The revised technique was called forced-choice preferential looking (FPL). The infant is held in front of a large, uniform visual display and then a visual stimulus is presented in one of two possible locations, to either the left or the right (see **Fig. 28.4A,B**). An observer, masked to the location of the visual stimulus, observes the infant's fixation and tracking behaviour. The observer then checks the left–right location of the stimulus. Testing requires 20 trials at each of a series of spatial frequencies. A psychometric function determines the highest spatial frequency cutoff to elicit 75% correct judgements from the observer. This limit is assumed to represent the resolution ability of the infant.

The acuity card procedure (McDonald et al 1986) is a commonly used and faster technique developed after the stringent FPL procedure. Acuity cards have been marketed and today are used around the world (see Ch. 28). Each card has a grating of a specific spatial frequency horizontally shifted from a central peephole. The observer presents a grating card, watches the infant's response through the peephole, flips the card such that the stripes are shifted horizontally and determines if the infant's response shifted. If the response shifted in response to the grating shift it is assumed that the infant could resolve the grating. A grating of a higher spatial frequency is then selected until consistent responses are no longer made.

Other cards have been developed for the child who has progressed from infancy to the toddler stage, which may stimulate children over 1 year old more than do stripes. Woodhouse et al developed the Cardiff Acuity Test (Adoh and Woodhouse 1994), which uses familiar pictures whose visibility depends on the spatial frequency of the border of the image (see **Fig. 28.6A**). A PL technique is used for visual acuity assessment. Once the spatial frequency of the border has surpassed the resolution limit, the picture vanishes.

One advantage of using acuity cards is that they are accessible to clinicians. Teller acuity cards (Stereo Optical Company, Chicago, IL) come with recommended testing strategies and normative data. Monocular values for this test can be found in Mayer et al (1995). Of note is the fact that data may vary if the card luminance exceeds the recommended values. When assessing visual acuity in infants one should be aware of the sharp improvement in grating acuity that occurs between 1 and 12 months of age (**Fig. 3.3**). Data recorded in the Westall lab show ongoing improvement in VA (using the Teller acuity cards and Cardiff Acuity Test) with ranges from approximately 0.4–0.8 logMAR at 12 to 18 months of age to 0.10–0.50 logMAR by 24 to 30 months. **Figure 3.3** shows a plot of Acuity Card resolution versus age (note these data are plotted as 1-logMAR to denote improvement in acuity as the child develops). The rate of VA

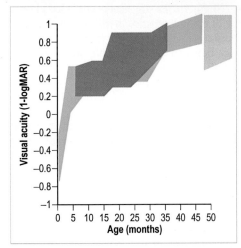

Figure 3.3 Ninety-five per cent confidence limits of visual acuity versus age. Plotted as 1-logMAR versus age in months. Green, Teller cards; purple, Cardiff Acuity Test; orange, logMAR Crowded Test. Note: if 1− logMAR is equal to 1 then logMAR = 0, which is equivalent to 1 minute of arc resolution.

development, as determined by acuity cards, plateaus by about 4–6 years and VA has generally reached adult levels by this age (Maurer & Lewis 2001).

VEP assessment

The sweep VEP (sVEP) is a frequently used method in studies of infant development (Regan 1977). This approach differs from conventional VEPs (Odom et al 2004) since the sweep VEP measures visual thresholds. VEPs are recorded from three active electrodes over the visual cortex. The signal is fed into an amplifier via three channels. The amplitude of the second harmonic (2F1) of the response is tracked over the sweep time (typically 10 seconds). The stimulus, typically a sine-wave grating, is increased or decreased in terms of contrast or spatial frequency. An assessment of visual acuity can be achieved by plotting the amplitude of the VEP signal against the stimulus parameter (e.g. the spatial frequency of the grating) and extrapolating the response to zero amplitude. The threshold of the visual parameter under investigation is taken as the intersection with the x-axis at 0 microvolts (**Fig. 3.4**).

Grating acuity as determined by the sweep VEP increases from 4.5 cpd at 1 month of age to between 20 and 30 cpd by 6–8 months of age (Norcia & Tyler 1985; Skoczenski & Norcia 2002) and reaches an asymptote at adult levels by 6 years of age (Skoczenski & Norcia 2002). Lauritzen et al (2004) showed a similar developmental trend (**Fig. 3.5**) in their description of visual acuity development in 92 infants, tested on two occasions, between the ages of 6 and 40 weeks. Although the average grating acuity is within adult levels by 6 years of age, there is considerable variability in the data across the different studies. **Figure 3.5** plots data from these studies with findings recorded from the Westall lab using the same technique. The variability remains with sweep VEP data recorded in adults. Ridder (2004) used sweep VEP assessment of grating acuity in 10 adult subjects. However, the data extracted had considerable variability, ranging from 16 to 45 cpd (95% confidence interval).

The Westall lab has data on sweep VEPs recorded from 147 typically developing children between 3 months and

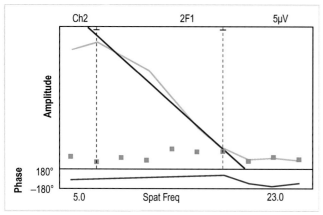

Figure 3.4 The VEP recorded for a range of decreasing evoked signal responses to increasing spatial frequencies (*yellow line*), forming a linear regression to zero amplitude. The line is extrapolated from the point at the peak of the signal. This is the point which separates deceasing amplitude values (from higher spatial frequencies) from the point at which the amplitude plateaus (ceiling effect reached). The peak is required to meet all scoring criteria. A linear regression line (*blue line*) is fit between this peak down to the point of zero amplitude (*abscissa*) to determine the spatial frequency threshold (grating acuity). The squares represent the noise response. The lower rectangular area of each function plots the phase (in radians) of the evoked response (*red line*). Phase consistency is a component of the scoring criteria. Ch 2, the recording channel; 2F1, the response recorded at the second harmonic of the stimulus frequency; 5 μV, the highest point on the y-axis. (Adapted from Chang et al 2007.)

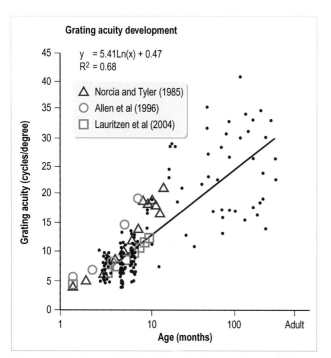

Figure 3.5 Grating acuity (c/deg) plotted against age in months. Blue dots are grating acuity data from the Westall lab graduate theses (Perron 2001; Mirabella 2003; Morong 2003; Bega 2005). Data are shown with data re-plotted from Norcia & Tyler 1985; Allen et al 1986; and Lauritzen et al 2004. Almost 68% of variability in the data is explained by the regression equation.

228 months of age. These results were included as part of a PhD thesis (Mirabella 2003) and three Masters theses (Perron 2001; Morong 2003; Bega 2005). Between 7 and 13 months of age, the mean grating acuity was about 50% of the mean

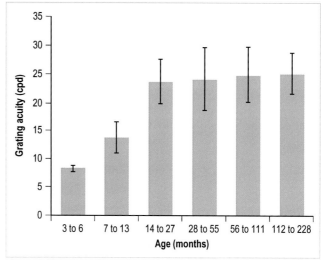

Figure 3.6 Grating acuity scores determined by sweep VEP, based on age (in months). The error bars are 95% confidence intervals. (Data from Perron 2001; Mirabella 2003; Morong 2003; Bega 2005.) In the 7 to 13 month age group 33% of infants have grating acuity within the 95% confidence intervals for the 11 plus year old age group. By 14 to 27 months 80% of data fall within the 11 plus year old data range.

finding (25 cpd) for the oldest group in our cohort (9 to 10 years of age); after 14 months, mean grating acuity was 92% of the mean value of the oldest group and 80% of the grating acuity values data fell within the normal adult limits. Data are re-plotted in the form of a histogram to depict the maturation of sweep VEP grating acuity (**Fig. 3.6**).

Contrast sensitivity

Contrast sensitivity, which refers to the capability to differentiate between an object and its background, measures the ability to discern between different luminosities in a static image (see Ch. 12). Contrast threshold is the lowest contrast discernable for a given spatial frequency. Contrast sensitivity is defined as the reciprocal of the percentage contrast required for detection and represents the minimum luminance difference (or contrast between light and dark areas) that the visual system can detect. The smaller the contrast necessary to detect the grating, the greater the sensitivity. Contrast sensitivity is usually assessed across different spatial frequencies to obtain a contrast sensitivity function (CSF), which provides an overall estimate of pattern detectability (see **Fig. 12.11**).

It is important to note that the spatial CSF varies with luminance level, retinal location, and temporal frequency. For high photopic luminances, the human CSF may peak at 5 to 6 cpd, and detection of spatial frequencies of 50 to 60 cpd is possible with high contrast and under optimal conditions (Cornsweet 1970). At low luminance levels, the peak sensitivity shifts to lower spatial frequencies. Regardless of luminance level, high-frequency attenuation is always seen, but the low-frequency attenuation is most obvious under photopic conditions. With respect to retinal locus, overall contrast sensitivity is reduced for a same size patch of grating which is shifted from the fovea onto the periphery. Finally, when temporal frequencies are increased, sensitivity to high spatial frequencies is decreased slightly, while sensitivity to low spatial frequencies shows a large increase

(Robson 1966). At high temporal frequencies (above 6 Hz), the spatial CSF becomes low-pass (not band-pass), as low-spatial frequency attenuation disappears.

Compared with adults, contrast sensitivity is reduced markedly in young infants, particularly at medium and high spatial frequencies (Atkinson et al 1979). In response to a sine-wave grating the resulting contrast sensitivity curve in 2-month-old infants is shifted to the left quite dramatically and the sensitivity at all spatial frequencies is reduced (Banks & Salapatek 1976). Contrast sensitivity varies between individuals, reaching its peak around 2–5 cpd at approximately 20 years of age.

Behavioural assessment

At Cardiff University, we (Westall et al 1992) used forced-choice preferential looking (FPL) to assess contrast sensitivity behaviourally in 30 infants and children ranging in age from 3 months to 5 years. Stimuli consisted of a sine-wave grating of fixed spatial frequency that was presented on one of two monitors and changed in contrast (using the staircase technique). At 3 months of age the peak contrast sensitivity was 5 at one cycle per degree. At 6–8 months the peak had shifted to 3 cycles per degree with contrast sensitivity close to 10, and in a cohort older than 30 months of age, the peak had reached the adult 5–6 cycles per degree with contrast sensitivity close to 100 (**Fig. 3.7**) (Westall et al 1992).

VEP assessment

Contrast sensitivity can also be estimated using the sweep VEP (Regan 1977) by increasing the contrast of the grating, plotting the amplitude of the VEP signal against contrast and extrapolating the response to zero amplitude (**Fig. 3.8**). The contrast threshold is taken as the intersection with the X-axis at 0 microvolts.

VEP contrast sensitivity to low spatial frequencies develops rapidly in the first few months of life. Between 4 and 9 weeks of age, contrast sensitivity at low spatial frequencies increases by a factor of 4 to 5, reaching a plateau at 10 weeks of age (Norcia et al 1990) and remains relatively constant from 10 to 40 weeks of age (**Fig. 3.9**). Norcia et al (1990) and Lauritzen et al (2004) both showed a similar developmental trajectory (see **Fig. 3.9**), though considerable variability in contrast sensitivity was observed between studies. Contrast sensitivity to high spatial frequencies, on the other hand, increases until at least 30 weeks of age (Norcia et al 1990). There is further gradual improvement in contrast sensitivity to both high and low spatial frequencies over the next few years (Norcia et al 1990).

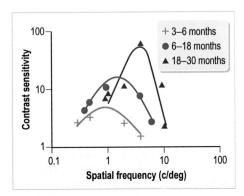

Figure 3.7 Mean contrast sensitivity recorded from three age groups: 3–6 months (*crosses*), 6–18 months (*circles*), and 18–30 months (*triangles*).

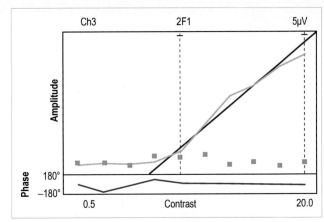

Figure 3.8 The VEP record for a range of increasing evoked signal responses to increasing contrast (*yellow line*) forming a linear regression to zero amplitude. The line is extrapolated from the peak to zero amplitude. The peak is the point which separates deceasing amplitude values (from higher contrast levels) from the point at which the amplitude plateaus (ceiling effect reached). The peak is required to meet all scoring criteria. A linear regression line (*blue line*) is fit between this peak down to the point of zero amplitude (*abscissa*) to determine the contrast threshold. The squares represent the noise response. The lower rectangular area of each function plots the phase (in radians) of the evoked response (*red line*). Phase consistency is a component of the scoring criteria. Ch 2, the recording channel; 2F1, the response recorded at the second harmonic of the stimulus frequency; 5 μV, the highest point on the y-axis. (Adapted from Chang et al 2007.)

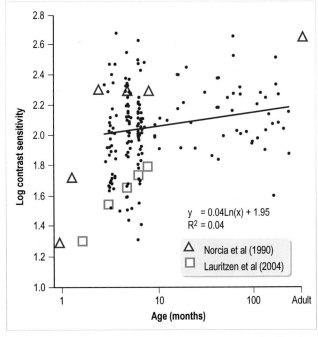

Figure 3.9 Contrast sensitivity plotted against age in months. Blue dots are contrast sensitivity data from graduate theses in the Westall lab (Perron 2001; Mirabella 2003; Morong 2003; Bega 2005). The youngest children are 3 months of age and it can be seen that there is little further development after this time. Data are shown with data re-plotted from Norcia et al 1990; and Lauritzen et al 2004.

Data from the Westall group, in which the sweep VEP was used to assess contrast sensitivity in 147 typically developing children from 3 months to 228 months of age, are shown in **Figure 3.9** and **Figure 3.10**. Even in the youngest

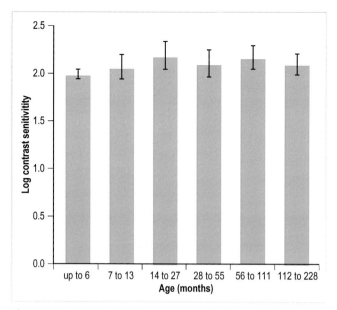

Figure 3.10 Contrast sensitivity scores determined by sweep VEP, based on age (in months). The error bars represent the 95% confidence interval. (Data from Perron 2001; Mirabella 2003; Morong 2003; Bega 2005.) The youngest age for these data was 3 months. In all age groups the data fall within the 95% confidence interval for 11 plus years age group.

age group tested (3–6 months) contrast sensitivity values are within the normal range of values for the oldest group.

Factors related to visual function development

The development of visual acuity and contrast sensitivity are expected with the maturation of the retina. Specifically, increased photoreceptor outer segment length would result in increased quantal catch and therefore greater sensitivity. Additionally, reduced cone spacing would result in the detection of finer detail, and the development of the fovea explains the increase in contrast sensitivity to high spatial frequencies. Several studies have used an 'ideal observer' model which estimates the ideal performance for detection using only the limitations of optics and photoreceptors, and which is insensitive to fluctuations of internal noise. An early human study by Banks and Bennett (1988) and a later macaque model by Kiorpes and Movshon (2004) compared the performances of ideal adult and neonatal observers with actual behavioural performance. They showed that a reasonable proportion of the differences between neonatal and adult contrast sensitivities and grating acuities is explained by age-related changes in optics and the foveal cone structure. The absolute sensitivity of the ideal observer exceeds that found by behavioural measurement. Candy et al reported that receptor and optical immaturities cannot explain fully the limitation of the neonate for either contrast sensitivity or visual acuity. They discounted the assumption that the neonate fovea might be functioning like that of an adult fixing from their parafovea (10° eccentricity) (Candy et al 1998). Post-receptor factors including increased myelination and cortical development must explain some of the developmental immaturities in vision.

From the retina, synapses at the ganglion cells send the visual signal to the LGN. Over the first year after birth in the macaque monkey, there is an overall improvement in responsiveness and spatial resolution in parvocellular and magnocellular cells (Blakemore & Vital-Durand 1986). Similar to human studies, earlier sensitivity and spatial resolution improves between birth and 6 months in the macaque, with the magnitude of the behavioural changes exceeding the electrophysiological LGN changes markedly (Movshon & Kiorpes 1997; Kiorpes & Movshon 2004). These researchers suggested that cellular development in the LGN (electrophysiological) parallels changes in vision function expected from an ideal macaque observer (Kiorpes & Movshon 2004). During early development in the macaque, the spacing between foveal cones decreases, both LGN and V1 (visual cortex) resolution increase and the receptive field size of V1 neurons in the macaque shrinks (Kiorpes & Movshon 2004). Kiorpes and Movshon surmise that cortical receptive field properties follow retinal development (Kiorpes & Movshon 2004).

Differences in human visual development as assessed by behavioural and VEP techniques

Both grating acuity and contrast sensitivity increase at a greater rate when VEP rather than behavioural techniques are used. There are several factors that might be responsible for this difference. Firstly, retinal illuminance is typically higher for VEP studies compared with behavioural testing. Candy and colleagues (Candy et al 1998) scaled the data to take account of these luminance differences between VEP and behavioural testing using published data from adults (Banks et al 1991) and 1-month-old infants (Banks & Salapatek 1978). Even when the factor of luminance differences between VEP and behavioural recordings is considered, a large difference remains and the improvement in grating acuity between the neonate and adult is 15 times for preferential looking and up to 9 times for VEPs. Contrast sensitivity improves by approximately 7.5 times for PL and 3 times for VEPs (numbers approximated from **Figure 3.6** (Candy et al 1998). Although both modes of testing are consistent with the earlier development of contrast sensitivity than visual acuity, there is still a lag in the development of preferential looking, compared with VEP thresholds for the vision function tested.

Animal models of electrophysiological versus behavioural differences might explain these observed variations. Changes in retinal receptor spacing and density contribute to the maturation of visual acuity, while shifts in the morphology of receptor outer segments contribute to the maturation of contrast sensitivity. Both of these changes match sweep VEP responses more closely than behavioural measurements. The difference between VEP and behavioural vision functions may be due to the VEP recording signals directly from the visual cortex compared with the greater number of cortical areas influencing the behavioural response; preferential looking responses are likely to depend on involvement of the extrastriate cortex and higher cognitive centres. Additionally, the presentation of stimuli differs for the two methods of testing. Patterns are generally static for preferential looking but temporally modulated for VEPs.

Development of scotopic sensitivity

Scotopic retinal function undergoes change from early infancy. A mini-review by Brown (1990) reported studies showing the rapid early development of scotopic (dark-adapted, rod-driven visual) sensitivity. The differences between electrophysiological and preferential looking measures of visual acuity and contrast sensitivity also apply to measurements of scotopic sensitivity. Data from Fulton and Hansen (1982) demonstrated that scotopic sensitivity measures, derived by ERG b-wave sensitivity, parallel those obtained using psychophysical techniques (Powers et al 1981; Hansen et al 1986). At about 1 month of age, rod sensitivity, as assessed by the b-wave of the ERG, is approximately 1.5 log units lower than adult levels, whereas FPL-obtained values range from 1.75 to 2.25 log units lower than adult findings (data from Brown 1990 Fig. 1). Using both ERG and FPL measurement techniques, scotopic sensitivity data approach adult values by 6 months of age (Brown 1990). Fulton and Hansen (2000) investigated the smaller change in dark-adapted, rod-mediated visual sensitivities compared with psychophysical sensitivity between infancy and adulthood. In the following statements, rod-mediated sensitivity represents sensitivity across the whole retina. Fulton and Hansen found that comparisons between rod sensitivity and peripheral (at 30° eccentricity) PL visual sensitivity are closer in values than rod sensitivity and parafoveal (10° eccentricity) PL sensitivities. Fulton and Hansen surmise that rod immaturities are responsible for the lower scotopic visual sensitivity in infants. They suggest that rod outer segment abnormalities, with a lowered probability of quanta capture, limit scotopic sensitivity in infants (Fulton & Hansen 2000).

Development of the electroretinograms

Electroretinograms (ERGs) show dramatic development within the first 6 months of life (Fulton & Hansen 1985) We recorded ERGs from infants using standards recommended by the International Society for Clinical Electrophysiology of Vision (ISCEV)(Marmor et al 2004). By 1 year of age, ERG amplitudes and implicit times begin to approach adult levels. **Figure 3.11** shows ERG responses from a 4-month-old infant and an adult. It is essential to have age-matched control data for correct interpretation of the ERG when recording from a paediatric population. ERGs which are diminished and delayed in typically developing infants compared with adult normal control data might be erroneously ascribed to retinal disease in the infant patients.

The rod response of the ERG is the slowest of the ISCEV-recommended ERG types to develop. At 1 month of age the rod response may not be measurable. With Anne Fulton (Boston's Children Hospital) we published normal data from 128 children. In the youngest group, aged 1–5 weeks, a quarter of the infants had no detectable ISCEV rod response (Fulton et al 2003). By 6 months of age, most data fall short of adult normal limits and it is not until 84 months of age that 95% of the data fall within adult limits (**Fig. 3.12**).

In addition to ISCEV standards, our lab recorded scotopic ERGs to increasing flash intensities. The resulting data are plotted as stimulus response functions; the maximum response is calculated as well as the retinal sensitivity derived from the semi-saturation constant of the function. The data showing maximum response and retinal sensitivity are shown in **Figure 3.13** and **Figure 3.14**, respectively.

The maximum b-wave response derived from the stimulus–response function is about 30% of the adult amplitude by 1 month of age and is approaching adult values by 6 months of age (**Fig. 3.13**). By 37 months 95% of data lie within adult limits.

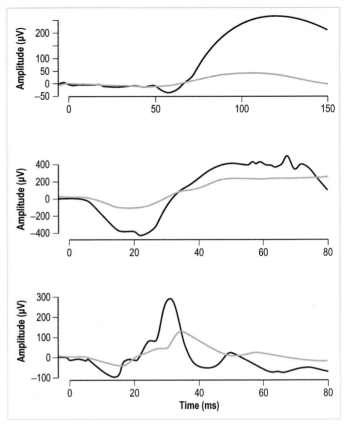

Figure 3.11 ERG rod response (*top*), mixed rod–cone response (*middle*) and cone response (*bottom*) recorded in a 4-month-old infant (*yellow line*) and adult (*purple line*). Positive deflection of the ERG is upward. The stimulus onset occurs at 0 ms.

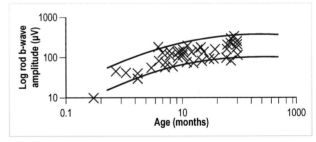

Figure 3.12 Rod response versus age in months. Solid lines represent the growth curve (Westall et al 1998) and contain 95% of normal data. Data points are raw data collected in Westall's lab, some of which were used in Westall et al 1998 and Fulton et al 2003.

Retinal sensitivity, as evaluated by the semi-saturation constant of the ERG dark-adapted b-wave stimulus response function collected from the Westall lab, shows the timescale for development (**Fig. 3.14**) (Westall et al 1998). After the first year most findings lie within normal adult limits. These data are clearly sparse for infants under 1 month of age; however, it is evident that by 6 months of age the data are approaching adult levels. As discussed earlier and by Brown (1990), the ERG sensitivity of the neonate is over one log unit lower than the adult. However, by 34 months of age 95% of data fall within adult limits.

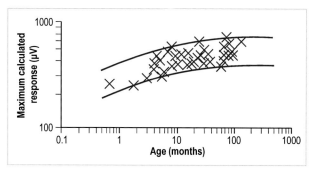

Figure 3.13 Maximum b-wave response versus age in months. Solid lines represent the growth curve (Westall et al 1998; Fulton et al 2003) and contain 95% of normal data. Data points are raw data collected in Westall's lab, some of which were used in Westall et al 1998 and Fulton et al 2003.

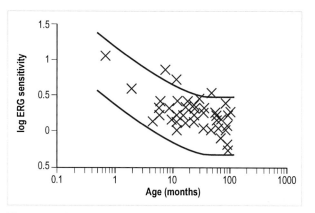

Figure 3.14 Log scotopic ERG sensitivity development. Normalized log sensitivity (relative to adult) versus age in months. Solid lines represent the growth curve and contain 95% of normal data (Westall et al 1998).

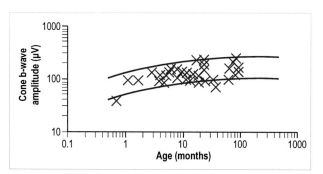

Figure 3.15 Cone b-wave response versus age in months. Solid lines represent the growth curve (Westall et al 1998) and contain 95% of normal data. Data points are raw data collected in Westall's lab, some of which were used in Westall et al 1998 and Fulton et al 2003.

After 10 minutes of light adaptation, photopic responses were measured in the paediatric cohort. The cone response b-wave develops in a similar time frame to scotopic responses with the most rapid development occurring within the first few months (**Fig. 3.15**). By 6 months the data are approaching adult values, with 95% of data within adult limits by 64 months of age (Westall et al 1998).

Colour vision

Using either behavioural or VEP testing, newborns demonstrate little or no colour vision. Peeles and Teller (1975), using a behavioural looking technique, found that 2-month-old infants were able to discriminate a red target from a white background in a condition likely to be void of luminance cues. Similar findings were revealed using VEPs, in response to low-frequency red–green (or long–medium (LM) wavelength) chromatic stimuli (Morrone et al 1990, 1993). Pathways mediating short-wavelength information may be functioning later than those responsible for LM wavelengths. It is estimated that red–green colour discriminations are present by about 2 months whilst blue–yellow (or short (S) wavelength) discrimination emerges somewhat later, at around 3–4 months (Teller 1997; Atkinson 2000; Suttle et al 2002). Techniques for measuring colour discrimination are more complex than achromatic mechanisms. Studies differ in the interpretation of the maturation of LM wavelength (red/green) mechanisms versus S mechanisms (blue/yellow). This may be due to a number of factors such as achromatic interference (i.e. luminance differences), use of broadband versus monochromatic stimuli and/or the effect of noisier visual systems or the response to contrast being poorer regardless of inferior colour discrimination. These factors are discussed in depth by Abramov and Gorden (2006).

Colour vision development

Of interest regarding the observation noted above that postnatally LM mechanisms develop before S-cone mechanisms is the finding that the prenatal retina has considerably more S cones than in the neonate, with peak numbers occurring between 14 and 17 weeks of gestation (Cornish et al 2004a, 2004b). Using an antibody against short-wavelength-sensitive opsin, Cornish (Cornish et al 2004a, 2004b) studied the changing distribution of short-wavelength-sensitive photoreceptors (S cones) between developing and adult human retinae. In the adult retina S cones are sparse (about 8% of the cone population) and are most dense in the foveal rim. During gestation there are major changes in cone patterning. Specifically, in early development (before 20 weeks), S cones have a random distribution and are distributed more peripherally, whereas in later development, the S cones shift to a more central placement. There is also a large population of cones in the fetal retina expressing both S and LM opsins (Cornish et al 2004a, 2004b). These S and LM cones are detected mainly at peripheral sites in early gestation, then near the fovea by week 17. By the end of gestation, S and LM cones have diminished greatly in number (Cornish et al 2004a).

Chromatic VEPs (cVEP)

At The Hospital for Sick Children in Ontario, Canada, we used VEPs to assess colour vision and its development in 46 infants (less than 1 year old) and 26 children. These data are contained in three theses (Elia et al 2005; Till et al 2005; Lafoyiannis 2006). Stimuli were sinusoidal equiluminant chromatic gratings presented in an onset–offset pattern mode (onset at 100 ms followed by offset at 400 ms) at a repeat rate of 2 Hz. Data from typically developing controls from our extensive data base were composed of chromatic VEPs from children aged 3 months to 12 years of age (Elia 2004; Till 2004; Lafoyiannis 2006). In adults, chromatic VEPs typically consist of a negative–positive complex

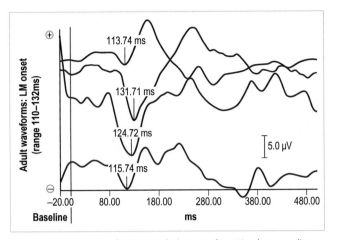

Figure 3.16 Examples of VEPs recorded to stimuli exciting long–medium wavelength chromatic mechanisms. The timing of the responses is shown for four adult subjects. The vertical scale depicts 5 microvolts and the horizontal scale is time in milliseconds (ms). Positive deflection of the VEP is upward. The stimulus onset occurs at 0 ms. (Data collected as part of PhD thesis, Till 2004.)

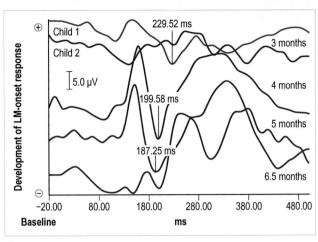

Figure 3.18 Examples of VEPs recorded to stimuli exciting medium–long wavelength chromatic mechanisms in two children: child 1 at 3 months of age and in child 2 tested longitudinally from 3 months up to 6.5 months. The vertical scale depicts 5 microvolts and the horizontal scale is time in milliseconds (ms). Positive deflection of the VEP is upward. The stimulus onset occurs at 0 ms. (Data collected as part of PhD thesis, Till 2004.)

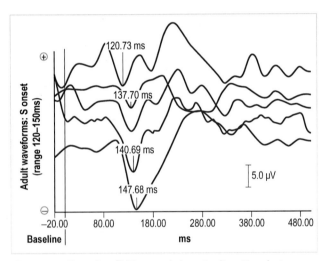

Figure 3.17 Examples of VEPs recorded to stimuli exciting short wavelength chromatic mechanisms. The timing of the responses is shown for four adult subjects. The vertical scale depicts 5 microvolts and the horizontal scale is time in milliseconds (ms). Positive deflection of the VEP is upward. The stimulus onset occurs at 0 ms. (Data collected as part of PhD thesis, Till 2004.)

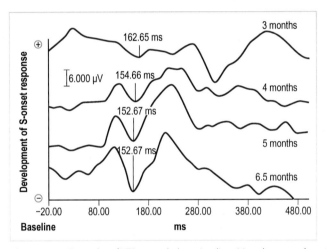

Figure 3.19 Examples of VEPs recorded to stimuli exciting short wavelength chromatic mechanisms in a child tested longitudinally between the ages of 3 and 6.5 months. The vertical scale depicts 6 microvolts and the horizontal scale is time in milliseconds (ms). Positive deflection of the VEP is upward. The stimulus onset occurs at 0 ms. (Data collected as part of PhD thesis, Till 2004.)

(**Figs 3.16** and **3.17**) (Rabin et al 1994; Crognale et al 1998; Suttle & Harding 1999) whereas infants show a positive–negative complex (**Figs 3.18** and **3.19**) (Crognale & Jacobs 1988; Suttle et al 1997).

In older children and adults, the latency for the S-axis (blue–yellow) response lags behind that of the LM-axis (red–green) (Crognale et al 2001; Crognale 2002; Till 2004). In a group of 22 typically developing children from 7 to 12 years of age the mean LM and S response latencies were 123.15 ms (SD = 8 ms) and 137 ms (SD = 7.49 ms), respectively (Elia 2004).

Limited data suggest that in young infants, the timing of LM- and S-cone mechanisms is reversed. During the preparation for PhD data collection by Christine Till (Till 2004), data were collected from two children at monthly intervals (**Figs 3.18** and **3.19**). At 3 months of age, it was difficult to define the waveforms from child 2; however, by 4 months of age the response was clear. Child 1, when tested at 3 months, showed a much clearer response (**Fig. 3.18**).

Over the first few months of life a clear VEP is evident, becoming more complex at the 6.5 month testing time.

Figure 3.19 illustrates the development of the short wavelength mechanism when tested longitudinally (child 2). The latencies of the responses are faster than those found for the long–medium wavelength mechanisms in this child. In another thesis, chromatic VEPs were recorded in 6-month-old infants. Constantina Lafoyiannis collected data from 27 typically developing children as the control cohort for her thesis (Lafoyiannis 2006). The data showed that at 6 months of age the mean for the short wavelength mechanism (153.3 ms, SD = 7.5) was comparable to that of the LM wavelength mechanism (152.33 ms, SD = 29). Note, however, that the standard deviation is much higher for the LM wavelength mechanism. It is conceivable that in early development the short wavelength mechanism has a faster latency than that for long–medium wavelengths. However, around 6 months of age, the LM mechanism becomes faster.

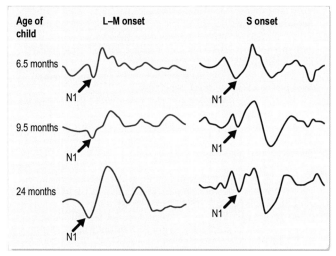

Figure 3.20 Visual evoked responses to LM-onset and S-onset stimuli recorded from typically developing children of different ages. Typical chromatic peaks are shown. (Adapted from Till 2004.)

Figure 3.20 shows VEP responses from three typically developing children to chromatic pattern-onset stimuli (Till 2004). The upper two traces show the responses from a 6.5- and a 9.5-month-old infant. The infant response to the LM wavelength stimulus is characterized by one prominent negative component occurring around 125 ms whereas the response to the short wavelength stimulus is delayed in latency compared with the LM stimulus response. The bottom trace shows the isoluminant chromatic response from a 24-month-old child. Consistent with previous reports using low spatial frequency stimuli with young children (Crognale 2002), the waveform becomes more complex with maturation. Our data are consistent with previous reports and demonstrate a change in morphology as the chromatic waveforms become more complex with development. The latencies of the chromatic negative component responses decrease with age.

This chapter has described spatial and chromatic vision development from birth through childhood. Tools for measurement have been outlined. The chapter will conclude with examples of developmental dysfunction taken from different stages of maturity.

Selected forms of visual dysfunction in the early period of plasticity

Electrophysiological vision measures have also been used to identify deficits in populations where knowledge of visual problems was previously unknown. Over the years our lab has collected data when the human visual system is compromised, pre- or postnatally, by disease, drugs or toxic insult.

In adults, vision functions such as visual acuity, contrast sensitivity and colour vision have proved useful in the assessment of toxic-related injury to the central nervous system (Mergler 1995). Animal studies have shown that a variety of solvents readily cross the placenta and have the potential to disrupt neurodevelopment in the neonatal rodent (Stoltenburg-Didinger et al 1990). The human fetus

lacks mature detoxification mechanisms and may be more susceptible than children or adults to visual toxic damage since its visual system is undergoing critical development at the time of exposure. Using the sweep VEP technique, Till and colleagues found significant compromise to the visual systems of children exposed prenatally to organic solvents (Till et al 2003, 2005; Till 2004). Prenatal exposure may occur as a result of maternal exposure to solvents in the workplace during pregnancy. Examples of such workplaces include dry cleaning and paint industries. The findings also included a significant reduction in contrast sensitivity compared with controls. Using a chromatic VEP it was found that 26.3% of infants in the exposed group versus 0% of the controls produced abnormal VEP responses to a red–green onset stimulus (Thompson et al 1996; Till et al 2005). The results confirm that neonates are at risk for prenatal exposure to organic solvents and it is likely that the developing ganglion cells are compromised.

Another example of pre- and postnatal insult to the visual system is early thyroid dysfunction. Infants may be born with insufficient thyroid hormone or to mothers with thyroid insufficiencies. Animal models demonstrate that thyroid hormone is critical for the normal development of the visual pathway. This is particularly true in the retina, where thyroid hormone is required for the differentiation of cones and rods (Kelley et al 1995; Gamborino et al 2001) and specific cone subtypes (Ng et al 2001). In humans, thyroid hormone deficiency during critical periods of fetal and neonatal development may be due either to an insufficient maternal supply during gestation or to a congenital thyroid hormone disorder where the infant is unable to produce its own hormone. When these groups are examined, VEP measures have identified both contrast sensitivity (Mirabella 2003) and red–green colour vision deficits (Rovet et al 2006).

Other insults to the developing visual system studied by our group are the effects of seizures and antiseizure medication on the developing visual system. The anticonvulsive medication vigabatrin results in visual toxicity in some patients. This toxicity is identified by restriction of visual field and/or abnormalities of the ERG. We compared the frequency of ERG defects before treatment with that during and after treatment (Westall et al 2002, 2003; Morong 2003). The ERG surrogate of toxicity was found in 30% of infants taking vigabatrin, with no improvement after cessation of the drug.

An unexpected result was found during the investigation of vision deficit in patients taking vigabatrin. Using sweep VEPs we observed that children with infantile spasms had reduced contrast sensitivity compared with children with other seizure types (Hammoudi et al 2005; Mirabella et al 2007). However, the drug itself had little impact on contrast sensitivity.

Studies after the period of rapid visual development demonstrate the utility of the parameters described in this chapter in the detection of vision dysfunction not found during the standard clinical examination. For example, contrast sensitivity recorded with VEP shows deficits in children with optic nerve glioma (Chang et al 2007). Additionally, some children with early diabetes have abnormal timing of the short-wavelength VEP, suggesting that the chromatic VEP is a very useful marker in detecting early dysfunction related to diabetes (Elia et al 2005).

This chapter has demonstrated the feasibility of assessing a range of vision and retinal functions from visual acuity to contrast sensitivity and colour vision at every stage of the developing infant's life. The results provide valuable information on growth and provide sensitive markers to early, often preclinical, visual system insult.

References

Abramov I, Gordon J 2006 Development of color vision in infants. In: Duckman R (ed.) Visual development, diagnosis, and treatment of the pediatric patient. Lippincott, Williams & Wilkins, Philadelphia, pp 143–170

Abramov I, Gordon J, Hendrickson A et al 1982 The retina of the newborn human infant. Science 217(4556):265–267

Adoh T O, Woodhouse J M 1994 The Cardiff acuity test used for measuring visual acuity development in toddlers. Vision Research 34(4):555–560

Allen D, Norcia A M, Tyler C W 1986 Comparative study of electrophysiological and psychophysical measurement of the contrast sensitivity function in humans. American Journal of Optometry and Physiological Optics 63(6):442–449

Atkinson J 2000 The developing visual brain. Oxford University Press, Oxford

Atkinson J, Braddick O, French J 1979 Contrast sensitivity of the human neonate measured by the visual evoked potential. Investigative Ophthalmology and Visual Science 18(2):210–213

Banks M S, Bennett P J 1988 Optical and photoreceptor immaturities limit the spatial and chromatic vision of human neonates. Journal of the Optical Society of America A 5(12):2059–2079

Banks M S, Salapatek P 1976 Contrast sensitivity function of the infant visual system. Vision Research 16(8):867–869

Banks M S, Salapatek P 1978 Acuity and contrast sensitivity in 1-, 2-, and 3-month-old human infants. Investigative Ophthalmology and Visual Science 17(4):361–365

Banks M S, Salapatek P 1983 Infant visual perception. Wiley & Sons, Toronto

Banks M S, Sekuler A B, Anderson S J 1991 Peripheral spatial vision: limits imposed by optics, photoreceptors, and receptor pooling. Journal of the Optical Society of America A 8(11):1775–1787

Barnstable C J 2004 Molecular regulation of vertebrate retinal development. In: Chalupa L M, Werner J S (eds) The visual neurosciences. The MIT Press, Cambridge, Massachusetts, pp 33–45

Bega S 2005 Is seizure onset related to visual deficits in pediatric epilepsy patients exposed to vigabatrin and can a visual evoked potential be used to follow vigabatrin therapy in this group? MSc thesis, University of Toronto, Toronto, p 124

Blakemore C, Vital-Durand F 1986 Organization and post-natal development of the monkey's lateral geniculate nucleus. Journal of Physiology 380:453–491

Brown A M 1990 Development of visual sensitivity to light and color vision in human infants: a critical review. Vision Research 30(8):1159–1188

Candy T R 2006 Development of the visual system. In: Duckman R (ed.) Visual development, diagnosis, and treatment of the pediatric patient. Lippincott, Williams & Wilkins, Philadelphia, pp 7–33

Candy T R, Crowell J A, Banks M S 1998 Optical, receptoral, and retinal constraints on foveal and peripheral vision in the human neonate. Vision Research 38(24):3857–3870

Catsicas M, Mobbs P 1995 Retinal development. Waves are swell. Current Biology 5(9):977–979

Chang B C, Mirabella G, Yagev R et al 2007 Screening and diagnosis of optic pathway gliomas in children with neurofibromatosis type 1 by using sweep visual evoked potentials. Investigative Ophthalmology and Visual Scieice 48(6):2895–2902

Cornish E E, Hendrickson A E, Provis J M 2004a Distribution of short-wavelength-sensitive cones in human fetal and postnatal retina: early development of spatial order and density profiles. Vision Research 44(17):2019–2026

Cornish E E, Xiao M, Yang Z et al 2004b The role of opsin expression and apoptosis in determination of cone types in human retina. Experimental Eye Research 78(6):1143–1154

Cornsweet T N 1970 Contrast sensitivity and visual acuity. Visual perception. Academic Press, New York

Crognale M A 2002 Development, maturation, and aging of chromatic visual pathways: VEP results. Journal of Vision 2(6):438–450

Crognale M, Jacobs G H 1988 Temporal properties of the short-wavelength cone mechanism: comparison of receptor and postreceptor signals in the ground squirrel. Vision Research 28(10):1077–1082

Crognale M A, Teller D Y, Motulsky A G et al 1998 Severity of color vision defects: electroretinographic (ERG), molecular and behavioral studies. Vision Research 38(21):3377–3385

Crognale M A, Page J W, Fuhrel A 2001 Aging of the chromatic onset visual evoked potential. Optometry and Vision Science 78(6):442–446

Dacey D M, Lee B B 1994 The 'blue-on' opponent pathway in primate retina originates from a distinct bistratified ganglion cell type. Nature 367(6465):731–735

Darwin C R 1877 A biographical sketch of an infant. Mind 2:285–294

Elia Y 2004 Visual evoked potentials to investigate the effects of long-term glucose control on the chromatic mechanisms of pre-teen children with type 1 diabetes. Institute of Medical Sciences. University of Toronto, Toronto, p 146

Elia Y T, Daneman D, Rovet J et al 2005 Color visual evoked potentials in children with type 1 diabetes: relationship to metabolic control. Investigative Ophthalmology and Visual Science 46(11):4107–4113

Fantz R L 1961 The origin of form perception. Scientific American 204:66–72

Farroni T, Csibra G, Simion F et al 2002 Eye contact detection in humans from birth. Proceedings of the National Academy of Science USA 99:9602–9605

Feller M B, Wellis D P, Stellwagen D F et al 1996 Requirement for cholinergic synaptic transmission in the propagation of spontaneous retinal waves. Science 272(5265):1182–1187

Feller M B, Butts D A, Aaron H L et al 1997 Dynamic processes shape spatiotemporal properties of retinal waves. Neuron 19(2):293–306

Floren I, Hendrickson A 1984 Indoleamine-accumulating horizontal cells in the squirrel monkey retina. Investigative Ophthalmology and Visual Science 25(9):997–1006

Friede R L, Hu K H 1967 Proximo-distal differences in myelin development in human optic fibers. Z Zellforsch Mikrosk Anat 79(2):259–264

Fulton A B, Hansen R M 1982 Scotopic adaptation in human infants. Documenta Ophthalmologica Proceedings Series 31(3):191–197

Fulton A B, Hansen R M 1985 Electroretinography: application to clinical studies of infants. Journal of Pediatric Ophthalmology and Strabismus 22(6):251–255

Fulton A B, Hansen R M 2000 The development of scotopic sensitivity. Investigative Ophthalmology and Visual Science 41(6):1588–1596

Fulton A B, Hansen R M, Westall C A 2003 Development of ERG responses: the ISCEV rod, maximal and cone responses in normal subjects. Documenta Ophthalmologica 107(3):235–241

Gamborino M J, Sevilla-Romero E, Munoz A et al 2001 Role of thyroid hormone in craniofacial and eye development using a rat model. Ophthalmic Research 33(5):283–291

Hammoudi D S, Lee S S, Madison A et al 2005 Reduced visual function associated with infantile spasms in children on vigabatrin therapy. Investigative Ophthalmology and Visual Science 46(2):514–520

Hansen R M, Fulton A B, Harris S J 1986 Background adaptation in human infants. Vision Research 26(5):771–779

Harding G F A 1991 History of visual evoked cortical testing. In: Heckenlively J R and Arden G B (eds) Principals and practice of clinical electrophysiology of vision. Mosby Year Book, St Louis, pp 17–22

Hendrickson A 1993 Morphological development of the primate retina. In: Simmons K (ed.) Early visual development, normal and abnormal. Oxford University Press, Oxford, pp 287–295

Hendrickson A, Drucker D 1992 The development of parafoveal and mid-peripheral human retina. Behavioral Brain Research 49(1):21–31

Kaas J H, Huerta M F, Weber J T et al 1978 Patterns of retinal terminations and laminar organization of the lateral geniculate nucleus of primates. Journal of Comparative Neurology 182(3):517–553

Karne A, Oakley D M, Wong G K et al 1997 Immunocytochemical localization of GABA, GABAA receptors, and synapse-associated proteins in the developing and adult ferret retina. Visual Neuroscience 14(6):1097–1108

Kelley M W, Turner J K, Reh T A 1995 Ligands of steroid/thyroid receptors induce cone photoreceptors in vertebrate retina. Development 121(11):3777–3785.

Kiorpes L, Movshon J A 2004 Neural limitations on visual development in primates. In: Chalupa L M, Werner J S (eds) The visual neurosciences. The MIT Press, Cambridge Massachusetts, pp 159–173

Klaus M H, Kennell J H, Plumb N 1970 Human maternal behavior at the first contact with her young. Pediatrics 46:187–192

Lafoyiannis C 2006 Chromatic VEPs on offspring of women with thyroid disease in pregnancy. Institute of Medical Sciences, University of Toronto, Toronto, p 160

Lauritzen L, Jorgensen M H, Michaelsen K F 2004 Test-retest reliability of swept visual evoked potential measurements of infant visual acuity and contrast sensitivity. Pediatric Research 55(4):701–708

Leat S, Shute R, Westall C 1999 Assessing children's vision – a handbook. Butterworth-Heinemann, Oxford

McDonald M, Ankrum C, Preston K et al 1986 Monocular and binocular acuity estimation in 18- to 36-month-olds: acuity card results. American Journal of Optometry and Physiological Optics 63(3):181–186

Marmor M F, Holder G E, Seeliger M W et al 2004 Standard for clinical electroretinography (2004 update). Documenta Ophthalmologica 108(2):107–114

Martin P R, White A J, Goodchild A K et al 1997 Evidence that blue-on cells are part of the third geniculocortical pathway in primates. European Journal of Neuroscience 9(7):1536–1541

Maurer D, Lewis T L 2001 Visual acuity: the role of visual input in inducing postnatal change. Clinical Neuroscience Research 1:239–247

Mayer D L, Beiser A S, Warner A F et al 1995 Monocular acuity norms for the Teller Acuity Cards between ages one month and four years. Investigative Ophthalmology and Visual Science 36(3):671–685

Meister M, Wong R O, Baylor D A et al 1991 Synchronous bursts of action potentials in ganglion cells of the developing mammalian retina. Science 252(5008):939–943

Mergler D 1995 Color vision: replication, rather than nonreplication of findings. Journal of Occupational and Environmental Medicine 37(7):789–790

Mirabella G 2003 Development of contrast sensitivity in infants with prenatal and neonatal thyroid hormone insufficiencies. PhD thesis, University of Toronto, Toronto, p 140

Mirabella G, Morong S, Buncic J R et al 2007 Contrast sensitivity is reduced in children with infantile spasms. Investigative Ophthalmology and Visual Science 48(8):3610–3615

Morong S E 2003 Sweep visual evoked potentials in children with West syndrome before and during vigabatrin treatment. MSc thesis, University of Toronto, Toronto, p 169

Morrone M C, Burr D C, Fiorentini A 1990 Development of contrast sensitivity and acuity of the infant colour system. Proceedings of the Royal Society B. Biological Sciences 242(1304):134–139

Morrone M C, Burr D C, Fiorentini A 1993 Development of infant contrast sensitivity to chromatic stimuli. Vision Research 33(17):2535–2552

Movshon J A, Kiorpes L 1997 Sensitivity of LGN neurons in infant macaque monkeys. Perception 26:S:2

Ng L, Hurley J B, Dierks B et al 2001 A thyroid hormone receptor that is required for the development of green cone photoreceptors. Nature Genetics 27(1):94–98

Norcia A M, Tyler C W 1985 Spatial frequency sweep VEP: visual acuity during the first year of life. Vision Research 25(10):1399–1408

Norcia A M, Tyler C W, Hamer R D 1990 Development of contrast sensitivity in the human infant. Vision Research 30(10):1475–1486

Odom J V, Bach M, Barber C et al 2004 Visual evoked potentials standard. Documenta Ophthalmologica 108(2):115–123

Peeles D R, Teller D Y 1975 Color vision and brightness discrimination in two-month-old human infants. Science 189(4208):1102–1103

Penn A A, Riquelme P A, Feller M B et al 1998 Competition in retinogeniculate patterning driven by spontaneous activity. Science 279(5359):2108–2112

Perron A M 2001 The effect of vigabatrin treatment on contrast sensitivity in a pediatric population. MSc thesis, University of Toronto, Toronto, p 178

Powers M K, Schneck M, Teller D Y 1981 Spectral sensitivity of human infants at absolute visual threshold. Vision Research 21(7):1005–1016

Rabin J, Switkes E, Crognale M et al 1994 Visual evoked potentials in three-dimensional color space: correlates of spatio-chromatic processing. Vision Research 34(20):2657–2671

Regan D 1977 Rapid methods for refracting the eye and assessing the visual acuity in amblyopia using steady-state visual evoked potentials. In: Desmedt J E (ed.) Visual evoked potentials in man: new developments. Clarendon Press, Oxford, pp 418–426

Ridder W H 3rd 2004 Methods of visual acuity determination with the spatial frequency sweep visual evoked potential. Documenta Ophthalmologica 109(3):239–247

Robson J G 1966 Spatial and temporal contrast-sensitivity functions of visual system. Journal of the Optical Society of America 56(1):1141–1142

Rovet J, Lafoyiannis D, Simic N et al 2006 Color vision in infants lacking TH gestationally. Endocrine Society Abstracts, 492

Sharma R K, Johnson D A 2000 Molecular signals for development of neuronal circuitry in the retina. Neurochem Research 25(9–10):1257–1263

Skoczenski A M, Norcia A M 2002 Late maturation of visual hyperacuity. Psychological Science 13(6): 537–541

Stoltenburg-Didinger G, Altenkirch H, Wagner M 1990 Neurotoxicity of organic solvent mixtures: embryotoxicity and fetotoxicity. Neurotoxicol Teratology 12(6):585–589

Suttle C M, Harding G F 1999 Morphology of transient VEPs to luminance and chromatic pattern onset and offset. Vision Research 39(8):1577–1584

Suttle C M, Anderson S J, Harding G F 1997 A longitudinal study of visual evoked responses to tritan stimuli in human infants. Optometry and Vision Science 74(9):717–725

Suttle C M, Banks M S, Graf E W 2002 FPL and sweep VEP to tritan stimuli in young human infants. Vision Research 42(26):2879–2891

Teller D Y 1979 The forced-choice preferential looking procedure: a psychophysical technique for use with human infants. Infant Behavior and Development 2:135–153

Teller D Y 1997 First glances: the vision of infants. the Friedenwald lecture. Investigative Ophthalmology and Visual Science 38(11):2183–2203

Thompson D A, Moller H, Russell-Eggitt I et al 1996 Visual acuity in unilateral cataract. British Journal of Ophthalmology 80(9):794–798

Till C 2004 Visual functioning following prenatal exposure to organic solvents. PhD thesis, University of Toronto, Toronto, p 257

Till C, Rovet J F, Koren G et al 2003 Assessment of visual functions following prenatal exposure to organic solvents. Neurotoxicology 24(4–5):725–731

Till C, Westall C A, Koren G et al 2005 Vision abnormalities in young children exposed prenatally to organic solvents. Neurotoxicology 26(4):599–613

Westall C A, Woodhouse J M, Saunders K et al 1992 Problems measuring contrast sensitivity in children. Ophthalmic and Physiological Optics 12(2):244–248

Westall C A, Panton C M, Levin A V 1998 Time courses for maturation of electroretinogram responses from infancy to adulthood. Documenta Ophthalmologica 96(4):355–379

Westall C A, Logan W J, Smith K et al 2002 The Hospital for Sick Children, Toronto, longitudinal ERG study of children on vigabatrin. Documenta Ophthalmologica 104(2):133–149

Westall C, Nobile R, Morong S et al 2003 Changes in the electroretinogram resulting from discontinuation of vigabatrin in children. Documenta Ophthalmologica 107(3):299–309

Wong R O 1999 Retinal waves and visual system development. Annual Review of Neuroscience 22:29–47

Wong R O, Meister M, Shatz C J 1993 Transient period of correlated bursting activity during development of the mammalian retina. Neuron 11(5):923–938

Yuodelis C, Hendrickson A 1986 A qualitative and quantitative analysis of the human fovea during development. Vision Research 26(6):847–855

CHAPTER 4

The psychology of vision

James M Gilchrist

Introduction

The *psychology of vision* is about trying to understand how vision works and how it relates to knowledge (*cognition*) and *behaviour*. The topic was introduced previously (Gilchrist 1988) as a bridge spanning three disciplines: *physics*, providing methods for the specification and measurement of visual stimuli; *physiology*, providing methods for objective measurement of neural responses; and *psychophysics*, providing methods for measuring subjective perceptual responses. Each of these may be studied in isolation but questions on visual perception can generally be answered more effectively by considering how they act together. A similar approach presented recently by Goldstein (2005) emphasizes further the importance of relationships between the disciplines, in particular between physiology and psychophysics (**Fig. 4.1**).

Goldstein (2005) gives examples of how psychophysical results have guided physiological research by providing researchers with specific goals. One is the conclusion based on psychophysical measurement by Hecht, Shlaer and Pirenne (1942) that a single visual pigment molecule is enough to excite a response from a retinal receptor. It was many years before this was confirmed physiologically and the biochemical mechanism involved was fully described (Stryer 1986). The converse, that the search for psychophysical results may be inspired by physiology, is also true. Hubel and Wiesel, (1959,1962) showed that many cells in the cat visual cortex would respond only when the visual stimulus contained lines of a certain orientation. Later, Campbell and Kulikowski (1966) demonstrated similar pattern-orientation selectivity in humans using psychophysical methods. There followed a great many psychophysical studies of spatial patterns which characterized perceptual responses in humans similar to many of the physiological responses obtained from animals. Thus, 'from the seed planted by electrophysiological research ... grew a vast literature of interlocking physiological and psychophysical research (Goldstein 2005, p 11).

In recent years this multidisciplinary approach to the study of perception has developed into *cognitive neuroscience* (Ward 2006), which includes visual neurosciences (Chalupa & Werner 2004). Section headings from this work are listed in **Figure 4.1**. This recognizes that vision may be studied in many ways, through biochemistry and physiology to psychophysics and computational modelling, but all place a principal emphasis on attempting to understand the neural activity that underlies visual perception, that is, on the relationship between physiological and perceptual responses. Considerable progress has been achieved in recent years, much of it due to the emergence of technologies that enable noninvasive study of physiological activity in humans, notably: event-related potentials – ERP (Luck & Girelli 1998), positron emission tomography – PET (Corbetta 1998) and, most significantly, functional magnetic resonance imaging – fMRI (Courtney & Ungerleider 1997; Haxby et al 1998; Raichle 1998; Heeger & Ress 2002).

The view taken previously (Gilchrist 1988) was that an overview of the psychology of vision should present some aspects of low-level or *basic visual processing*, represented by topics enclosed in red in **Figure 4.1**, because: (1) these provide foundations for understanding higher-level processing, (2) some aspects

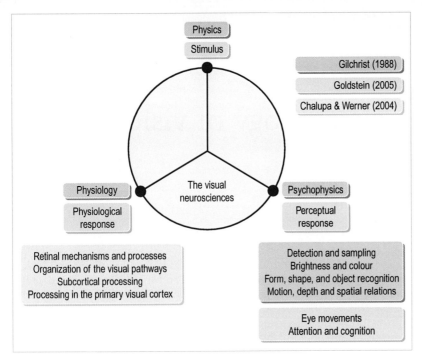

Figure 4.1 The psychology of vision is a very broad area of study, which may be thought of as a bridge spanning the disciplines of *physics*, *physiology* and *psychophysics* (Gilchrist 1988). These disciplines, in turn, are concerned with the specification of the *visual stimulus*, and the study of *physiological* and *perceptual responses* to the stimulus (Goldstein 2005). Relationships between physiological and perceptual responses are of particular importance in the psychology of vision and have been studied from many different perspectives, under the general heading of *visual neurosciences* (Chalupa & Werner 2004).

of basic vision, such as spatial and temporal contrast sensitivity, are important in clinical assessment of visual function, and (3) it then seemed timely to attempt a summary of the wealth of physiological and psychophysical vision research that occurred during the 1960s and 1970s (Frisby 1979), and the important 'paradigm shift' during the 1980s towards research guided by computational theory (Marr 1982). Now, 20 years later, further advances in understanding basic vision have been realized, often in terms of the 'linking relationships' between psychophysics and physiology described above, and many topics discussed previously are now well represented in introductory texts (Palmer 1999; Levine & Shefner 2000; Norton et al 2002; Wolfe et al 2005; Blake & Sekuler 2006; Mather 2006; Snowden et al 2006) as well as in more advanced volumes (Chalupa & Werner 2004). The present chapter therefore introduces the psychology of vision from a perspective that acknowledges a recent resurgence of interest in the psychological side of cognitive neuroscience, that is, *cognitive psychology*.

Cognitive psychology is concerned not only with how we perceive the world, but also with how we learn through perception, retain perception and learning in memory, and make active use of perception, learning and memory. There is broad agreement that the modern form of the discipline emerged during the 1950s and 1960s alongside the early development of computer technology, artificial intelligence and the exciting idea of perception as information processing (Kazdin 2000), and the book by Neisser (1967) is widely regarded as the seminal work of that period. The cognitive psychology of vision encompasses all of the topics listed under perceptual responses in **Figure 4.1** (as well as others not listed, notably memory and language: Braisby & Gellatly 2005; Eysenck & Keane 2005) but the role of *attention* is of particular importance. Attention and *eye movements* are also prominent components in an approach to the study of vision that is emerging currently. This has been called

active vision, a term borrowed from research on computer vision (Aloimonos et al 1988), and it contrasts the relatively passive process of *seeing* (Frisby 1979) with the more active process of *looking* (Findlay & Gilchrist 2003).

The idea of active vision appears in work by Goodale & Humphrey (2005), who identify two broad purposes in vision: recognition of objects and their relationships in space and time (e.g. some cups and a teapot on a kitchen table), and the control of actions directed at those objects (making a cup of tea). These two purposes may be described as *vision for perception* and *vision for action*. Although there have long been advocates of the need to study vision in the context of action (Gibson 1979), much research has concentrated on object perception, which has been studied with particular emphasis on the ideas that the visual system operates by analysing scenes into primitive elements such as edges and surfaces, and constructing from these elements internal (mental) representations of scenes and the objects within them (Marr 1982; DeValois & DeValois 1988; Graham 1989; Watt 1991; Wandell 1995; Ullman 1996; Regan 2000). Although this side of visual perception involves a great deal of neural activity, it has been described as passive vision (Findlay & Gilchrist 2003) because it takes no account of eye movements or other forms of motor activity that are an essential part of interaction with the visual world.

This chapter introduces some aspects of our current understanding of cognitive/active vision, including feature detection and organization (basic visual processes), memory and attention. Eye movements are discussed in terms of how they integrate with perceptual processes; space limitations prevent any more detailed coverage. References to findings from neurophysiological studies are included where these seem particularly relevant. An extremely useful online laboratory resource for studying many of the phenomena of visual cognition is *CogLab* (http://coglab.wadsworth.com; also Sternberg 2003; Reed 2004).

Understanding cognitive/active vision

Concepts, metaphors and models

Our ability to understand vision relies heavily upon the development of an appropriate conceptual approach. If we can describe what vision does using familiar *concepts*, then the complex workings of the visual system become more approachable. Most of us are at ease with concepts such as attention and memory; we understand in a common-sense way what it means to 'pay attention' and the difference between short-term and long-term memory, even if we have no idea how these processes actually work. In studying the psychology of vision we must be willing to use familiar concepts and, if necessary, to extend them in unfamiliar ways. For example, if we understand the concept of paying attention to a visual stimulus, then we might extend the idea to consider whether vision is possible without attention (*inattentive*), or whether some useful visual processing might occur before attention comes into play (*preattentive*). By this extended reasoning we introduce new concepts that may be useful in thinking about how vision works.

Concepts help us to build descriptions. To enrich these descriptions, and to develop them into explanations, it is useful to adopt concepts that have some explanatory power. Often, this involves finding analogies or *metaphors*; for example, 'spotlight of attention', which likens visual attention to a spotlight that selectively illuminates a particular area of the scene. Of course, this is not a literal explanation of how attention works, but it provides an idea that we can use to prompt further questions which might be tested by experiment; for example, if attention acts like a spotlight then it should have only one beam, not many beams, prompting the question of whether we can attend to just one location at a time, or to many different locations.

Since different aspects of vision must be described using different concepts, a very important part of psychology is concerned with how concepts are related. Some concepts such as memory and attention represent *processes*; that is, mechanisms/procedures for handling information. Others, such as locations and objects, represent *entities* that provide the information to be processed. Ideas about how entities and processes may be organized into systems capable of describing and explaining perception are called *models*. These may be simple, involving just a few concepts and a description of how they are related, or they may be very complex, involving many concepts with mathematical rules governing the organization of visual information and its transformation by perceptual processes. Mathematical models are generally the most powerful because they give quantitative predictions of the end results of processing which can be tested in the laboratory, but they are also the most difficult for non-specialists to understand. However, most if not all models of vision can be presented using schematic, block diagrams which help to make the ideas more accessible.

The remainder of this chapter will introduce some important concepts in cognitive/active vision, in a couple of different model arrangements. The first is a simple processing sequence that is particularly common in everyday vision.

Simple active vision model: selection–fixation–recognition

If the study of passive vision is concerned mainly with what we see, then active vision is concerned with where we look as well as what we look at. The basic processing structure in active vision might be stated as the sequence: *Selection–Fixation–Recognition* (SFR). An example from clinical optometry shows the application of this principle, and provides some insight into the distinction between passive seeing and active looking.

Suppose you are presented with a series of single-letter targets, one after another, as part of a procedure for measuring visual acuity (**Fig. 4.2A**). When the first letter appears it must be actively located, selected and fixed. Subsequent letters are selected and fixed with little active effort, because each is presented at the same location, without a need for any active effort to isolate the target letter from other surrounding letters. There is also no need for any action following recognition of the target, such as moving fixation to the next letter or line of letters. In this example letter recognition occurs in a relatively passive manner.

Alternatively, suppose you are presented with a conventional visual acuity letter chart (**Fig. 4.2B**). First, a starting letter must be selected and fixation moved to that letter. This involves an effort of active concentration (attention) in order to isolate the target letter from those around it. After fixation has moved to the target and a recognition decision made, a new target must be selected and the whole process repeated. These extra 'overheads' of target selection and

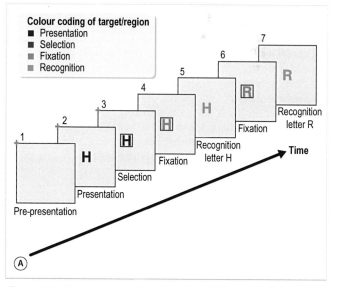

Figure 4.2A The *Selection–Fixation–Recognition* (*SFR*) principle for sequential presentation of single letters at a constant location is represented by a series of image frames in which visual processing over time proceeds from left to right. Colour-coding differentiates between initial target presentation prior to processing (*dark-blue*), selection (*orange*), fixation (*green*) and identification (*light-blue*). Sequence: (1) blank field pre-presentation with fixation set at upper left corner as indicated by the green cross, (2) target presentation brings no change in fixation initially, (3) while fixation is maintained (upper left corner) target is selected by covert attention, (4) fixation moves to target location, which is now selected by overt attention, (5) recognition is completed, (6) a new target presented at same location is automatically selected and fixed, and (7) recognition follows.

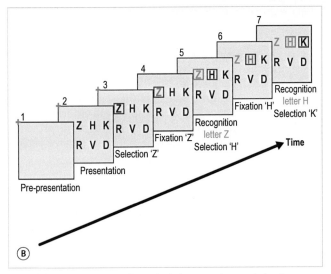

Figure 4.2B SFR sequence for multiple letters, colour-coded as in Figure 4.2a. Sequence: (1) blank field pre-presentation, (2) target presentation brings no change in fixation initially, (3) while fixation is maintained, first (*upper left*) letter Z selected by covert attention, (4) fixation moves to letter Z, now selected by overt attention, (5) fixation maintained on letter Z and recognition is completed, while next letter H is selected by covert attention, (6) fixation moves to letter H, (7) fixation maintained on letter H and recognition is completed, while next letter K is selected by covert attention, and so on.

fixation suggest that the letter chart presents a greater visual processing challenge than the single-letter test.

It is evident that these two methods of visual acuity assessment involve different perceptual abilities. The first, to a large extent, isolates the process of letter recognition, while the second combines letter recognition with the additional processes of selection and fixation. The selection–fixation–recognition sequence is represented schematically in **Figure 4.2C**.

This scheme is based upon common observations: (1) when we want to decide whether a stimulus can be recognized we shift our gaze to inspect it using foveal fixation, (2) when there are multiple stimuli or many regions of potential interest within one stimulus, we shift gaze repeatedly to enable foveal inspection of each region in turn, with each being selected by peripheral attention while another is under fixation. There is evidence that this is a

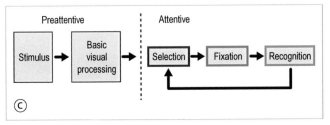

Figure 4.2C Five concepts combined to form a simple model of active vision: *stimulus*, the familiar entity that provides the information for perception; *basic visual processing*, which extracts some useful information from the image and is thought of as a preattentive stage of processing; *selection* of a particular region of the stimulus; and subsequent *fixation* on that region to enable full *recognition*. The selection–fixation–recognition stage involves attentive processing.

reasonable description of natural visual behaviour. Land et al (1999) used a head-mounted video camera designed to give simultaneous images of eye position and the scene to which gaze was directed, and found that fixation behaviour during ordinary tasks, such as making a cup of tea, consisted almost entirely of a sequential stream of actions. Furthermore, the eye movement record showed that gaze was generally directed to locations where activity was taking place and anticipated locations where activity was about to begin, indicating a repeating cycle of selection–fixation. The repositioning of gaze occurred with great frequency, often several times each second, and the authors described this eye movement record as having 'the frenetic appearance of a movie that has been greatly speeded up'.

Selection–fixation–recognition in action

In spite of its simplicity the SFR model of visual processing is useful and can be applied to many complex tasks. These include:

Reading

Reading involves repetition of the SFR sequence to enable words in lines of text to be recognized in a standard left-to-right, top-to-bottom order. In addition, reading requires visual memory to hold letter and word groups pending their interpretation, and also involves cognitive processes associated with word recognition and semantic interpretation of phrases and sentences. There is a large literature on the psychology of reading (Rayner & Pollatsek 1989), which has increasingly emphasized the importance of attention and eye movements (Inhoff et al 1989, 2000; O'Regan 1990; Rayner 1998; McConkie & Yang 2003).

One recent influential model of the reading process (Reichle et al 2003) closely resembles our simple SFR sequence model in its assumptions that: (1) word recognition involves a preattentive processing stage followed by an attentive stage, (2) attention is allocated serially, one word at a time, (3) some process of selection is involved in programming eye movements for word fixation, and (4) recognition of one word is the signal for repeating the sequence and moving fixation to the next word. Reichle et al (2003) review other reading models which also incorporate SFR principles to varying degrees.

Visual search

Visual search tasks involve inspecting images or scenes in order to locate and identify targets of specific interest. There are many different types of search task, including: simple search of an image for an object or shape, search of a text passage for specific keywords, and inspection of manufactured goods for faults and imperfections. There are also search tasks that have the characteristic of 'foraging', such as selecting books from library shelves or beachcombing. Like reading, visual search involves repetition of the SFR sequence but the regularity of this varies with task type. Keyword search or fault inspection, for example, might employ SFR in a fairly regular, systematic manner, whereas foraging-type tasks may be more likely to mix some systematic SFR repetition such as looking at the titles of a series of books on one shelf, with some random (or quasi-random) repetition such as quickly scanning library shelves to find the location of a subject of interest. Visual search has been studied extensively within cognitive psychology, with particular emphasis on the roles of attention (Wolfe 1998) and eye movements (Findlay & Gilchrist 1998, 2005).

Scene evaluation

Scene evaluation resembles the foraging form of visual search in which there are potential targets rather than specific predefined targets. Scene evaluation serves a wide range of purposes from generally 'weighing-up' or 'getting the gist' of the scene (Underwood 2005a) without any particular preconceptions as to its content, to question-specific evaluations such as judging the layout of the environment or scanning the faces of people in a room to identify who is present, known or of interest. Relevant reviews of this topic are provided by Henderson & Hollingworth (1999) and Henderson (2003).

Driving

Driving a vehicle involves a particularly complex and important form of scene evaluation. Drivers rely very heavily on visual information (Sivak 1996) and the driving task presents both specific and potential targets, with the added complications that the content of the scene changes from moment to moment and the costs of performance errors may be fatally high. This means that the driving task places a significant demand on attention for effective target selection, and also on the memory processes required to support effective action. Understanding the looking behaviour of drivers and the factors that affect it is an important issue for road safety (Green 2002).

Limitations of the SFR model

In spite of its general applicability, the SFR model suffers from a number of limitations.

Stimulus-driven versus knowledge-driven processing

All information in the SFR model comes from the stimulus. In other words, SFR processing is entirely *stimulus-driven*. There is no provision for the introduction of knowledge or purpose as occurs with many natural visual tasks. For example, in visual search and scene evaluation we may use knowledge of what we are interested in to influence selection of regions for fixation. Yarbus (1967), for example, made a now-famous study of the eye movement patterns of observers who had been given different instructions for looking at a picture of a visitor arriving into a family dining room. Observers were asked to estimate the ages of people in the picture, remember the clothes worn, remember the locations of people and objects in the room, and so on. The result was that eye movement patterns differed markedly depending upon the question asked, indicating that the selection–fixation sequence was being determined not only by information in the stimulus but also, predominantly, by the particular goals set for the task and the knowledge of the observer. Models of active vision must therefore incorporate both *stimulus-driven* and *knowledge-driven* processing (Hayhoe & Ballard 2005).

The need for memory

As soon as we recognize that selection, fixation and recognition must be driven by knowledge as well as stimulus information, it becomes obvious that vision must have access to the memory structures in which such knowledge is stored. Indeed, it quickly becomes difficult to think of real-world tasks that do not make use of memory-based knowledge. Reading, for example, might use a simple word-by-word sequence of SFR. However, word recognition is impossible without long-term memory of words learned previously (*mental lexicon*), but word recognition alone will be meaningless unless the process is closely linked to long-term knowledge of sentence structure and meaning. Memory must also be able to handle short-term needs such as holding a word sequence for just as long as is required to interpret it.

Serial versus parallel processing

The SFR sequence operates in a *serial* manner, with the implication that one stage must be completed before another begins. There is no suggestion of any *parallel* activity, in which a number of processes occur at the same time. This may conflict with reality in various ways. First, although it is clear that successive gaze shifts from one fixation point to another must occur serially, it is also apparent that we do not have to fix many points in a scene in order to gather at least an impression of its whole content. Even the briefest glimpse of a scene will provide information from many different locations at the same time, so parallel processing must be available at some stage. A second serious limitation of the serial SFR structure is that *recognition* can only be achieved by going through all the other processes first. There is no option for stimuli to be recognized without selection and fixation whereas, in reality, we know that we can often recognize something or someone that we glimpse out of the 'corner of the eye' and to which we may not be attending. Indeed, if this were not possible then undertaking complex tasks such as driving would be extremely difficult. Everyone who drives a vehicle is familiar with the experience of arriving at a destination without being aware of all the visual information (road junctions, traffic lights, etc.) that must have been recognized correctly en route. Recognition is certainly possible without fixation, and possibly without attentive selection, so processing models must accommodate these possibilities.

Where and what: spatial and object perception

The SFR sequence implies that, since each fixation gaze shift must be directed to a specific location in the stimulus/scene, the purpose of attention is to select the next location for fixation and that recognition will naturally relate to a region centred on that location. This view, that processing is geared to the locations of stimulus features, places main emphasis on the spatial (*where*) aspects of visual processing. On the other hand, there are situations in which the emphasis is on attending not to different spatial locations but to different ways of looking at the content (*what*) of the scene. Some of these will be discussed later.

There is therefore a distinction to be made between spatial perception and object perception, and there is good evidence that these are handled by separate physiological pathways or processing streams. The *dorsal stream*, projecting from the primary visual cortex to the posterior parietal cortex, is concerned with localization of objects in space (*where*), while the *ventral stream*, projecting from the primary visual cortex to the inferotemporal cortex, is important in object identification (*what*) (Ungerleider & Mishkin 1982; Ungerleider & Haxby 1994).

Extended active vision model

In an effort to overcome the limitations discussed above, **Figure 4.2D** introduces an extended version of the SFR model. This is still merely a schematic attempt to show the principal concepts in active visual processing and to represent relationships between them in a way that accords reasonably with our everyday experience of vision in action, as well as with the findings of experimental studies over the past 20–30 years.

This extended model incorporates:

Recognition System: Instead of treating basic visual processing and attention as precursors of recognition in a purely serial system (see **Fig. 4.2C**), we now consider that these processes actually work as components *within* a recognition system so that, in principle, recognition may occur at any stage. In some situations recognition might be achieved using only preattentive processing, while others will require attention before a decision can be reached. Each component of the recognition system shows a clear division of aspects relating to spatial (*where*) processing and object (*what*) processing.

Basic Visual Processing: This is the early, low-level stage of visual processing in which basic stimulus information is encoded. Traditionally, this processing stage has been assumed to precede attention, so it is generally referred to as *preattentive* vision.

Visual Working Memory: This is included because: (1) recognition always involves relating what we see to what we already know, that is, information held in long-term memory, and (2) when we attend to various characteristics of an image to gather information for recognition, that information must be held in short-term working memory so that we may act on the results of a series of fixations. For this reason, the output of the

recognition system is shown emerging from visual working memory. This is not to imply that the final stage of visual recognition necessarily happens within the memory system, but that wherever it happens the decision must be closely involved with memory processing. Here, visual working memory is positioned on the boundary between preattentive and attentive processes. This idea will be discussed later.

The model incorporates two forms of control. *Stimulus-driven* processing, as the name suggests, means that the observer responds purely to information contained in the stimulus, while *knowledge-driven* processing means that the observer uses information from memory to direct actions using knowledge of specific processing goals along with interpretation of stimulus information.

Attention System: This combines selection (covert attention) and fixation (overt attention) on the principles that: (1) the anatomy of the visual system ensures that covert attention of non-foveal areas is always available alongside foveal fixation – indicated by the circular graphic (orange), representing the idea that covert attention is effective within an area of the visual field outside of the central fovea (green), where overt attention is effective, (2) it is possible to switch between covert and overt attention – indicated by the double-headed arrows linking the selection and fixation processes, (3) the covert nature of selection means that it is assumed to occur while fixation is engaged elsewhere and, as explained in **Figure 4.2B**, it will often be followed by *fixation* of the selected item (*overt attention*) by execution of a gaze-shifting saccadic eye movement (Findlay & Gilchrist 2003) – indicated by the curved arrow linking covert selection to overt fixation. Attention is crucial for locating potential targets and mentally

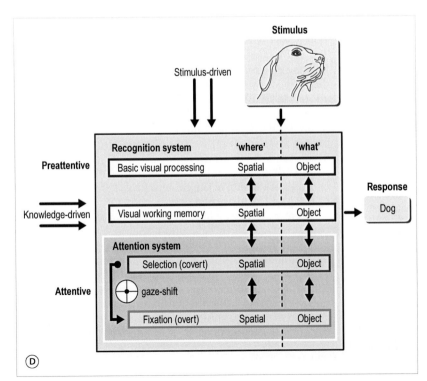

Figure 4.2D An extended conceptual model of active vision, which addresses some limitations of the approach represented by Figure 4.2C. Here, both *basic (preattentive) visual processing* and *attentive processing* are represented as part of a *recognition system*, which also incorporates a component of *visual working memory*. The combination of these processing components enables the visual system to respond to both *stimulus-driven* and *knowledge-driven* influences, while maintaining a distinction between *spatial* (where) and *object* (what) characteristics of the stimulus.

isolating them from their surroundings (*selection*), and for orienting saccadic eye movements for *fixation* of targets. In a sense, therefore, attention is the key to active vision. [Note on terminology: a distinction is made here between selection and fixation in terms of covert and overt forms of attention. Some authors, however, use the general term *selection* to cover both processes, or may distinguish between them by referring to *visual selection* (covert) and *oculomotor selection* (overt)].

Basic visual processing

The term *basic visual processing* refers to the low-level stage of perception where information in the retinal image is encoded for transmitting to higher levels (Frishman 2005). This includes much of the processing referred to previously (see **Fig. 4.1** and Gilchrist 1988); sampling of the image by retinal photoreceptors (Williams & Hofer 2004), adaptation to changes of luminance level (Reeves 2004), processing of brightness and lightness (Fiorentini 2004), colour perception (Gordon & Abramov 2005) and spatial pattern perception (Wandell 1995; Palmer 1999).

The extended model represents *basic visual processing* as the first stage in the recognition system. It is shown as having connections to working memory and hence to the attention system, but it must be capable of functioning in some useful way without necessarily invoking either of these additional components. If we assume that basic visual processing occurs before information reaches the attention system, then we can think of it as *preattentive*. This concept appears to have been introduced by Neisser (1967), who suggested that 'since the processes of attention cannot operate on the whole field simultaneously, they can come into play only after preliminary operations have already segregated the figural units involved. I will call … (these preliminary operations) … preattentive processes.' This view makes it clear that preattentive processing is assumed to operate in parallel, and that its function is to segregate the scene into 'figural units' that can be attended.

Preattentive parallel processing

A striking characteristic of preattentive vision is that it seems to be automatic and effortless. This impression comes from the observation that certain features, such as a sudden stimulus change, can capture our attention such that we immediately look to where the change has occurred. This happens involuntarily and, indeed, the reflex urge to attend to an abrupt change may be difficult to ignore (Remington et al 1992). Inasmuch as this capture of attention seems to occur automatically and without effort, so any processing of the stimulus that occurs prior to attention would also seem to have the same characteristic.

Figure 4.3A illustrates effortless preattentive processing. Patterns 1 and 2 contain one element that differs from the others by the value of a single *feature*. Pattern 1 shows a red line within a group of blue lines of the same orientation, and Pattern 2 shows a horizontal line within a group of vertical lines of the same colour. In both cases the *singleton* (red or horizontal line) can be located without the need for attentive consideration; that is, it 'pops out' automatically and without effort. Pattern 3 has one vertical red line among vertical blue lines and horizontal red lines. Here, the

distinctive element differs not on a single feature value but on the *conjunction* of two features – it is vertical AND red. In this case it does not pop out automatically, but requires attention and a longer processing time to identify the distinctive feature conjunction.

The fact that simple feature differences can be seen automatically and effortlessly, and that such stimuli have the effect of capturing attention, has been interpreted as evidence that the processing involved in pop-out occurs preattentively (Treisman & Gelade 1980). The same authors also provide evidence that single-feature processing occurs over the entire visual field simultaneously (in parallel) because the time taken to find a pop-out element in a visual search task is the same whatever the *set size*, that is, the number of other *distractor* elements. However, if the search target is defined by a conjunction of features, and does not pop out automatically, then the time taken to find it increases with the total set size (**Fig. 4.3B**). Treisman & Gelade (1980) suggested that this result indicated that processing of feature conjunctions must be carried out serially by attending to each item in turn. Thus, we can identify some conditions under which recognition might be achieved preattentively, and others in which attention must be engaged in order to achieve recognition.

Wolfe (1998, 2000) provides a list of *basic features* that can be processed preattentively and in parallel, including: colour, orientation, curvature, vernier offset, size/scale/spatial frequency, motion, pictorial (monocular) depth cues and stereoscopic depth. So, for example, a curved line can be seen effortlessly if it is surrounded by straight lines. Note that all the features listed are stimulus primitives, and preattentive pop-out of certain feature differences is very much a stimulus-driven phenomenon. Generally, a stimulus element will attract attention if it is markedly different to its surroundings. This quality that makes certain stimuli immediately visible is called *salience*.

Preattentive salience map

The three patterns of **Figure 4.3A** may be placed in different positions on a hypothetical salience scale according to how readily the distinctive element appears to *pop out*. The concept of salience therefore represents the degree to which information contained within the stimulus itself can drive the processes of attention 'from the bottom up', that is, without the need for any conscious decision to inspect the pattern. It is easy to see how this aspect of basic processing works within our extended processing model (see **Fig. 4.2D**); salient features attract attention automatically and are selected covertly as a precursor to overt fixation, which follows naturally. This happens frequently in everyday life in a compelling reflex manner. If some feature in a scene is distinctly different from everything else, then we are naturally inclined to look at it. This is why techniques for salience enhancement of visual stimuli are so effective, for example, use of colour or font highlighting to distinguish and draw attention to key words or passages within text, use of specific colours as warning lights or safety indicators, use of flashing lights as hazard indicators, and so on. Abrupt luminance changes, such as flashing or sudden onset of a stimulus are especially salient and may capture attention even when they provide little information about where the stimulus is located or, remarkably, even when observers

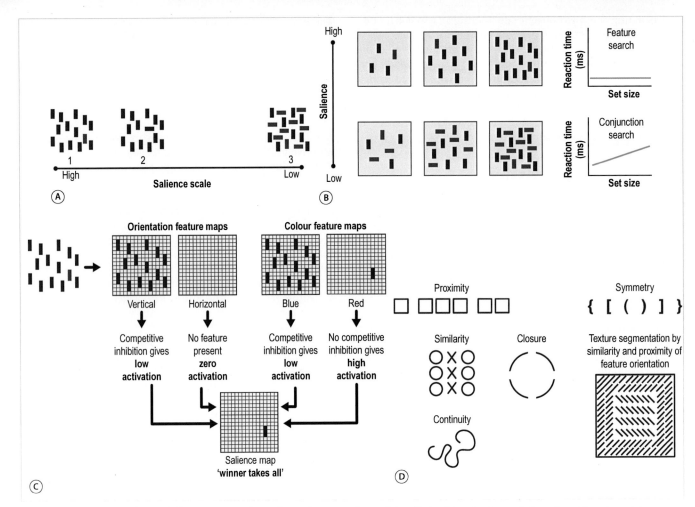

Figure 4.3 (A) Visual search stimuli illustrate preattentive and attentive processing and the effects of target salience. Patterns 1 and 2 each contain one element (target) that differs from the others (distractors) by the value of a single *feature*: a red target with blue distractors (pattern 1), and a horizontal target with vertical distractors (pattern 2). In both cases the target element seems to 'pop-out' automatically and without effort. Thus, when salience is high, target recognition appears to occur preattentively. Pattern 3 involves search for a target that is a *conjunction* of two features: vertical and red. Here the target salience is low and recognition therefore requires attentive processing. (B) Recognition of high-salience targets in *feature search* occurs automatically, and increasing the number of distractors does not increase the time required for recognition. This has been interpreted as evidence that recognition of high-salience targets occurs preattentively. Recognition time for low-salience targets in *conjunction search* increases in proportion as the number of distractors is increased. This 'set-size effect' has been interpreted as evidence that recognition of low-salience targets requires attentive processing. (C) Illustration of the principle by which spatial *maps* of different stimulus features may be formed independently and then combined to create a general *salience map* for visual target recognition. In the visual system, salience will be represented by the level of neural *activation*, and the feature (or conjunction of features) giving the highest activation will appear most salient. (D) Illustration of the notion that target recognition may sometimes depend upon perceptual *grouping* of features or structures instead of (or in addition to) their salience. A number of different grouping principles are shown here.

are instructed to ignore them (Jonides & Yantis 1988; Remington et al 1992; Theeuwes et al 1998).

Salience of stimulus features plays such a fundamental role in controlling visual attention that many current theories and models of attention employ the idea that the visual system encodes salience (or saliency) in a map-like representation of visual space (Koch & Ullman 1985; Treisman, 1988; Wolfe 1998; Parkhurst et al 2002). The concept of the *salience map* allows the most distinct object to be identified, whatever its features (Itti & Koch 2000, 2001). **Figure 4.3C** shows the basic principle: the stimulus pattern is analysed by different pools of neurons that respond to specific features, in this example orientation and colour.

Each neuron pool contains feature-detection mechanisms; that is, the receptive fields of the neurons are tuned to respond to particular features (see Frisby 1979; Gilchrist

1988 and recent texts such as Snowden et al 2006 and Wolfe et al 2005 for introductory explanations of how receptive fields detect features). The feature detectors produce distinct topographic maps of visual space in which all occurrences of their particular features are encoded. Within each *feature map* there will be competitive inhibition between multiple stimuli: when two stimuli are presented at the same time the neural response to one tends to suppress that to the other. This means that the neural response or *activation* produced by each specific feature will be low when there are many and high when there are few. By selecting the feature that produces the highest activation ('winner takes all') the system is able to determine the most salient location in the scene, whatever features may be present at that location.

This approach to understanding how the visual system determines salience is based on sound principles of neural computation (Itti & Koch 2001) but the same result may be achieved in other ways. Li (2000, 2002) and Zhaoping (2005), for example, have proposed that the primary visual cortex could provide a saliency map signalled in the responses of feature-selective cells without the need for separate feature maps or any subsequent combination of them, and Li and Snowden (2006) report results of psychophysical experiments supporting this proposal. There may also be alternative sites in the visual system where feature salience is encoded. Fecteau and Munoz (2006) review the neurophysiological evidence for the salience map and suggest that a good candidate, theoretically and in terms of neural activity patterns, is the oculomotor network, which is spread across several regions of the brain, including the frontal eye fields, superior colliculus and brainstem reticular formation. This suggestion is especially interesting since there is evidence that the role of feature salience in automatically capturing attention is important for programming of fixation eye movements (Findlay & Walker 1999; Findlay & Gilchrist 2001; Tehovnik et al 2003).

Feature grouping and binding

Neisser's conception (1967) was that preattentive processing is responsible for segregation (now often called *segmentation*) of the visual stimulus into 'figural units'. In other words, the visual system needs to work out which elements of a stimulus belong together so that objects may be differentiated from each other and from their backgrounds. It is now accepted that preattentive processing does not produce a complete 'picture in the brain', but constructs a patchy, dispersed series of sketches with different stimulus features represented in different cortical maps. To achieve figural unity we require *feature integration* (Treisman & Gelade 1980) or *binding* (von der Malsburg 1995; Ashby et al 1996; Treisman 1996, 1998; Humphreys 2001), because 'to identify an object, we must specify not only its parts and properties, but also how those parts and properties are combined' (Treisman 1996). There are various types of binding, notably: form-binding, which involves grouping stimulus elements to define object shapes, and surface-binding, which involves associating shapes with their surface properties such as colour, shading and texture (Grossberg & Pessoa 1998).

The concept of form-binding or *grouping* concerns the relationships between stimulus elements that have different locations in space. It has long been of interest in cognitive psychology, and is particularly associated with the Gestalt tradition of the 1930s (Koffka 1935; Köhler 1940), which proposed a general principle that vision tends to group stimulus elements so as to produce the simplest and most stable form. This is supported by a number of specific principles that characterize much of our current understanding of grouping (Palmer 1999, 2000). Stimulus elements tend to be grouped together by: proximity, similarity, continuity (to create continuous forms rather than broken or disrupted forms), closure (to create complete rather than incomplete forms) and symmetry (to create forms that are symmetrical about some axis). Segmentation through spatial grouping of form features is an essential step in determining what objects are present in the stimulus (Marr 1982; Regan 2000).

The effortless, preattentive nature of grouping is evident in **Figure 4.3D**, which illustrates various principles described above. In each case figural unity emerges automatically without any apparent need for attentional effort, and there is evidence that this form-binding can be achieved preattentively (Moore & Egeth 1997; Humphreys et al 2000). However, it is thought that preattentive processing is not able to deliver complete object shapes (Wolfe & Bennett 1997) but constructs *proto-objects* which provide short-lived local descriptions of scene structure (Rensink 2000) and these must receive attention to turn them into coherent, longer-lasting representations.

Note that the automatic texture segmentation of the stimulus in **Figure 4.3D** is not due to any particular feature having greater salience, as was the case in **Figure 4.3A**. Rather, the patterns are segregated into groups which may be seen as separate 'perceptual surfaces' (Watt & Phillips 2000). Thus, we may distinguish two apparently distinct forms of preattentive segmentation: one based on *salience*, which depends on feature contrast, the other based on *grouping*, which depends on finding regions that are homogeneous in certain features.

Perceptual grouping (form-binding) is a basic step in solving the related second-stage problem of *surface-binding*, in which object shapes are integrated with surface details. **Figure 4.3A** shows why this is a significant issue. Here, Pattern 3 has one element that differs from all the others by its unique *conjunction* of feature values; the only line that is both red and vertical. As discussed previously, this element does not pop out but requires an effort of attention, suggesting that preattentive vision is not able to process the binding together of two (or more) features automatically (Treisman & Gelade 1980), so *surface-binding* is assumed to require attention (Humphreys et al 2000; Humphreys 2001).

Basic visual data – object files

Although preattentive processing is very fast in providing a panoramic whole-field view, what it delivers is somewhat sketchy and fragmented. A study of the type of data resulting from basic visual processing concludes that overall object shapes are not available preattentively (Wolfe & Bennett 1997), and suggests that preattentive vision delivers 'shapeless bundles of basic features'. These authors also propose that, although this information is not enough to represent complete objects, it can be thought of as a set of object files.

The concept of *object files* has become increasingly popular since Kahneman et al (1992) showed that people can associate a set of features with a particular object and maintain this association as the object moves or disappears temporarily. They suggested that the visual system forms object files, which are abstract structures in which the features of an object are stored together as a single representation. The appeal of this concept is that it allows a visual object to be represented even if some of its feature information is missing: the object does not have to be 'all or nothing'. These object files are created by the *binding* processes described previously. The object file concept has recently been extended to encompass the *active vision* principle, suggesting that just as stimulus perception requires integration of visual features, so there is also evidence of some sort of feature integration process in planning an action (Hommel 2004). Thus, it is possible to think more generally in terms of *event files*, in which object features and action-planning features may be bound together.

An important aspect of these ideas is that preattentive *object files* are assumed to be constructed in *episodic memory*, a temporary storage memory that is capable of integrating information from a variety of sources, and which may possibly be enriched by object-related knowledge from long-term memory (Hommel 2004). This is our first indication of a direct link between basic visual processing and visual memory, and of a possible mechanism for introducing knowledge-driven influences into what we have so far assumed to be stimulus-driven processing (see **Fig. 4.3** and Soto et al 2006).

Visual attention

The importance of attention in human perception and behaviour has long been appreciated (Hatfield 1996). Scientific interest in attention grew with the early development of psychology in the late nineteenth and early twentieth centuries (James 1890; Pillsbury 1908; Titchener 1908), but the increase in research since the 1980s has been remarkable. There are now hundreds of published articles on many aspects of attention, including a number of books and reviews covering perceptual/cognitive aspects (Posner & Petersen 1990; Desimone & Duncan 1995; LaBerge 1995; Egeth & Yantis 1997; Pashler 1998; Behrmann & Haimson 1999; Wolfe 2000; Findlay & Gilchrist 2001; Chun & Wolfe 2005) and physiological aspects (Luck 1998; Motter 1998; Kanwisher & Wojciulik 2000; Kastner & Ungerleider 2000).

What drives attention?

Our extended model (see **Fig. 4.2D**) identifies two modes in which attention may be driven, which James (1890) called *involuntary* and *voluntary*, and which have also been called *exogenous* and *endogenous* (Posner 1980). Now these are usually called *stimulus-driven* (or *bottom-up*) and *knowledge-driven* (*top-down* or *goal-directed*).

Stimulus-driven (bottom-up) attention

This is simply the idea that, when we look at any scene, there may some object or feature that immediately 'catches the eye'. The important thing is that the stimulus itself captures attention, without any prior decision or reason to attend to it. In Basic Visual Processing above, we established that feature *salience* and *grouping* may capture attention automatically.

Figure 4.3A includes the concept of a hypothetical salience scale to represent the fact that salience is not a discrete quality but lies on a continuum, so that the higher the salience of a feature the more likely it is to capture attention and influence behaviour. Note that the salience of a feature depends not simply on its presence within a stimulus but on the extent to which it differs from (*contrasts* with) other features. A solitary red line within a group of blue lines has high salience; one red line within a group of blue and red lines has low salience. A red traffic light may not succeed in attracting attention if the scene also contains many red vehicle lights, unless either some (bottom-up) action is taken to increase the salience of the stimulus itself such as switching from another colour, flashing the light and/or positioning it so that it occupies a separate area of visual space, and/or some knowledge-driven (top-down) action is taken such as scanning the scene looking for red traffic lights.

Similarly, with feature grouping (**Fig. 4.3D**) there must be sufficient contrast between figural units that one is perceived as being distinct from another. Therefore, grouping might be considered not as being fundamentally different to salience but rather as a mechanism for extracting a higher level of salience. Without grouping we must rely upon salient features to capture attention, but with grouping we may also find salient units or objects.

Note that a salient feature or object is not necessarily relevant or meaningful. Salience is a stimulus (bottom-up) characteristic, whereas *relevance* is a knowledge- or goal-related (top-down) characteristic.

Knowledge-driven (top-down) attention

It is obvious that one cannot rely upon salience to guide selection and fixation in everyday life. The natural world presents some situations in which relevant features/objects are also salient, but many in which they are not. For example, animals often use camouflage to hide from predators. The predators therefore must search for relevant targets of low salience. This necessitates attentive search that is directed by the goal of obtaining the next meal and the knowledge gained from previous searches. Likewise, those being preyed upon cannot rely on the salience of the predator to alert them but, rather, must maintain a state of vigilance (Parasuraman 1986) directed by the goal of staying alive and the knowledge of how to survive. The ability to control attention using *knowledge-driven* processing is fundamental for survival and appears to dominate over stimulus-driven control in the real world (Einhauser & König 2003; Turano et al 2003; Chen & Zelinsky 2006).

Knowledge-related (cognitive) factors are therefore extremely important in the control of active vision and many examples of this are discussed in two volumes edited by Underwood (1998, 2005b). An obvious difficulty in understanding the principles that may be used by the visual system for top-down control of attention is that, whereas the number of possibilities in a stimulus-driven salience map might be constrained by a limited combination of common stimulus features, the number of possibilities for a knowledge-driven relevance map appears exceedingly large. Different individuals in any situation may consider different aspects of the scene to be relevant for selection and fixation, so there is a need to ask whether there are certain organizing principles that may help to limit the number of possibilities. How do we determine relevant objects and events in complex scenes?

One aspect of all visual scenes that is most likely to constrain top-down selection and fixation is *context*. Objects and events rarely occur in isolation, but appear with other objects and events in some well-defined context: words organized into passages of meaningful text, pieces positioned on a chess board, the layout of a road junction, and so on. This is helpful because: (1) context imposes some constraints on what is valid and what might be expected in a given situation, (2) new contexts can be learned and knowledge of existing contexts can be adapted so that observers can benefit from re-using familiar contextual information, (3) familiar context imposes structure and stability for the processes of active vision. A context-based approach to understanding goal-directed control of active vision is not yet well developed, but holds promise for future research (Chun 2000).

What do we attend to?

The stimulus-driven capture of attention by features and fig-ural units highlights a distinction between attending to spe-cific feature locations (see **Fig. 4.3A**) and attending to regions corresponding to figural units (see **Fig. 4.3D**). The former is called space-based or *spatial attention*, the latter is *object-based attention*.

Spatial attention

Two experimental paradigms have contributed most of our knowledge of spatial attention. These are *visual search* (Treisman & Gelade 1980; Findlay & Gilchrist 1998, 2005; Wolfe,1998, 2003; Palmer et al 2000) referred to in Basic Visual Processing (above) (**Figs 4.3A and B**), and *spatial cueing* (Posner 1980).

The principle of cueing is to use some signal or *cue* to direct the observer's attention towards the location where a target stimulus may appear a short time later. The observer's task is to respond as quickly as possible to the appearance of the target, and the measure of performance is reaction time. Cues may take different forms; brightening of an outline object, onset of some simple stimulus, or a symbol such as an arrow to indicate where attention should be deployed (Chun & Wolfe 2005). Cues may also act to control atten-tion in different ways; a cue that appears suddenly at the potential target location draws attention to that location automatically (exogenously), whereas an arrow that points in the direction of where a target may appear directs the observer (endogenously) to 'look there'.

Posner (1980; see also Posner et al 1980) ran detection trials using three different configurations of cue and target: *valid cue* trials, in which an arrow cue pointed towards the correct target location; *neutral cue* trials, in which no indica-tion was given of the likely target location; and *invalid cue* trials, in which the cue pointed towards an incorrect location. Results showed that valid cues gave the fastest reac-tion times and invalid cues the slowest, while times for neu-tral cues fell between these two. This provided compelling evidence that attending to the likely location of a target enhanced processing of the target, and it led Posner (1980) to suggest that attention operates like a *spotlight* that is localized in space and can move to facilitate processing in different parts of the scene.

The idea that attention can be moved around a scene, clarifying objects or regions at will, is simple and intuitively appealing, not least because movement of fixation (overt attention) around a scene literally does clarify the objects of fixation. The spotlight is perhaps the most popular meta-phor for attention but not necessarily the most useful. Some difficulties of the concept are discussed by Chun and Wolfe (2005; see also Cave & Bichot 1999).

Object-based attention

It is also possible to direct attention in a non-spatial manner (Findlay & Gilchrist 2003). There are different ways of thinking about this. One is to assume that attention is more likely to be captured by salient characteristics of objects, or driven by knowledge-directed selection of objects, than by characteristics of arbitrary locations in space. To put it another way, 'it is hard to imagine that it would be useful to have an attentional system that deployed attention to

the location of a toddler at one moment but then left atten-tion at that location while the toddler toddled off' (Wolfe 2000). In the real world, it seems more natural to attend to objects than locations (Cave & Bichot 1999). In one sense, there seems to be no major difference between spa-tial- and object-based attention, since objects occupy loca-tions in space and moving attention from one object to another will often be equivalent to moving from one loca-tion to another. However, the significance of the distinction becomes more apparent in the situation where two objects overlap or occupy the same spatial location.

Neisser and Becklen (1975) tested this by showing two overlapping film presentations in which people were carry-ing out different activities. The two action streams were coincident in space, yet observers could shift attention from one to the other at will, so this use of attention was not based on spatial location but on objects and events within one film or the other. A similar result using static overlap-ping stimuli was demonstrated by Duncan (1984, see also Bayliss & Driver 1993; Vecera & Farah 1994). In the case of overlapping stimuli it seems natural that attention must be directed by grouping features together to form objects, and a number of studies have confirmed the general princi-ple that object-based attention is indeed strongly influenced by perceptual grouping (Kramer & Jacobson 1991; Gross-berg et al 1994; Moore et al 1998).

Perceptual grouping introduces a scaling effect in the sense that small elements will always be grouped within larger elements. Thus object-based attention must be able to change its operating scale in the manner of a zoom lens (Eriksen & St James 1986). Natural examples of stimuli in which the scaling of attention is a significant issue are reading text, in which researchers have debated whether readers attend to individual letters, whole words or even groups of words according to their meaning, and face recog-nition, which raises similar questions of whether attention is to whole faces or parts of faces (Martelli et al 2005).

Object-based attention is apparent in **Figure 4.4A**, which shows stimuli (Items 1 & 2) in which attention to the larger-scale structure leads to one recognition outcome (H or △), while attention to the smaller leads to another (E or ▮). Since elements at both scales have familiar identities, there is some perceptual interference between the two (Navon 1977), and an important function of attention in this case is to overcome this interference. Similarly, Item 3 shows a larger-scale structure made up of orientated line segments. Here, as in Item 4 (the familiar Necker cube), the figure is perceived as a three-dimensional structure that presents two forms, either rising or dropping towards the front edge. When one form is perceived, an effort of attention is required to switch to the other.

Another classic example of interference between stimulus interpretations is the Stroop effect, **Figure 4.4B** (Stroop 1935; MacLeod 1991; MacLeod & MacDonald 2000). The task is to identify the items in each column as quickly as possible. The requirements are to say the words in columns 1 and 2, and to name the colours of the stimuli in columns 3 and 4. Generally, reading the words is easier than naming the colours, and there is not much difference for columns 1 and 2 even though there is some interference between word names and colour names. In column 3, colours can be named with relatively little interference from the letters, but colour naming in column 4 is much slower due to

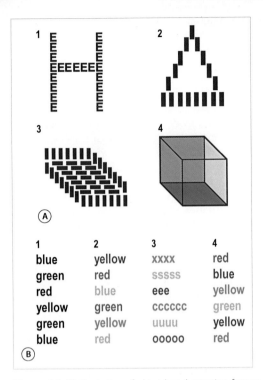

Figure 4.4 (A) Illustration of *object-based attention*: feature grouping results in the formation of perceptual *objects*, and therefore visual attention may be directed to whole objects or objects within objects, rather than to specific locations in visual space. (B) The Stroop effect is a classic example of how attention is required to overcome *perceptual interference* between competing stimulus interpretations. The task is to name the words in columns 1 & 2, and to name the colours of the stimuli in columns 3 & 4. The task is most difficult, and requires greatest attention, in column 4 because the word name tends to dominate the interpretation.

strong interference from words, which tend to be recognized more automatically. The task provides a measure of the ability of observers to attend selectively to either colour names or word names.

What does attention do?

We introduced attention (**Figs 4.2C and 4.2D**) as a system encompassing the actions of covert selection and overt fixation. In Basic Visual Processing we established that preattentive processing cannot always provide representations that are adequate for recognition and/or action, and attention must be called upon to bind features into more complete representations. This is a very powerful strategy; preattentive vision uses just enough processing power for us to get the gist of what we are looking at, then attention is brought in so that more processing can be directed to where it is needed. In addition to its role in facilitating feature binding, attention offers a number of other benefits.

Attention enhances visual processing

Attention not only increases the speed of visual processing (Posner 1980; Carrasco & McElree 2001) but also increases sensitivity (Bashinski & Bacharach 1980; Carrasco et al 2000; Pestilli & Carrasco 2005), enhances resolution (Yeshurun & Carrasco 1999; Carrasco et al 2002), improves accuracy in identifying characteristics of visual stimuli (Shulman & Wilson 1987; Downing 1988) and even alters the appearance of stimuli by changing their perceived contrast (Carrasco et al 2004). Generally, visual enhancement may be thought of as the result of amplifying a visual signal and/or reducing the

effects of background noise that may interfere with that signal, and it has been shown that attention can influence visual processing in both respects (Di Russo et al 2001; Lu et al 2002).

Attention resolves competition between multiple stimuli

'*[Attention] is the taking possession of the mind, in clear and vivid form, of one out of what seem several simultaneously possible objects or trains of thoughts. . . . It implies withdrawal from some things in order to deal effectively with others.*'

(James 1890)

In everyday life the visual system is presented with an enormous amount of information and, since its processing capacity is limited (Broadbent 1958; Tsotsos 1990), we need mechanisms for limiting access to some pieces of information and giving priority to others. Researchers generally agree that this is the main role of attention (Chun & Wolfe 2005). The problem can be thought of as one of competition between multiple stimuli (Kastner & Ungerleider 2000). When two stimuli are presented at the same time, competition for processing resources means that the neural response to one tends to suppress that to the other. The effect of selectively attending to one stimulus is to bias the response in favour of the attended stimulus.

The idea of *biased competition* between stimuli is the basis of an influential model of attention (Desimone & Duncan 1995). One way to understand this is to imagine a horizontal flat sheet that represents the baseline response or *activation* level of the visual system looking at a blank field. Next, a single stimulus is introduced and this produces a response, which can be visualized as the sheet being pushed up by some object underneath it; the width or spread of the activation peak will depend upon the size of the object, and the height upon how strongly it pushes. A second stimulus is then introduced which produces its own response and this corresponds to another activation peak somewhere on the sheet. Now, to make sense of the competition idea, suppose the sheet is tied down along its edges, limiting how far it can be pushed up (analogous to limited processing resources). This means that if adding the second stimulus threatens to push the sheet beyond its limit, then the peak for the first stimulus will need to be reduced. When the sheet is at its limit, additional peaks can only be accommodated by reducing one or more of those already present. Under this analogy it is easy to appreciate how attention might work in a variety of ways to give priority to a selected stimulus. One way is to enhance the neural response to the attended stimulus, like pushing the sheet up further in one area, forcing it to push down in others. A second way is by filtering out unattended stimuli, like forcing the sheet down so that unattended stimuli produce lower peaks and that of the selected stimulus appears higher. A third way is to increase the baseline activation for the attended stimulus, like allowing more 'slack' in the sheet so that it can be pushed up further in the area of attention. Physiological studies have shown that all of these effects may occur (Kanwisher & Wojciulik 2000; Kastner & Ungerleider 2000).

Covert attention prepares the way for overt fixation

One of the findings of Kastner and Ungerleider (2000) was that the stimulus that wins the competition for access to the visual cortex will not only benefit from enhanced processing but also gain access to other brain areas, including motor systems involved with guiding action and behaviour. This ties in with other studies which suggest that the neural mechanisms of covert attention (selection) are largely overlapping with those that control the programming of saccadic eye movements for fixation (Rizzolatti et al 1987; Kowler et al 1995; Kustov & Robinson,1996). Schall (2004), for example, states that 'Saccade target selection cannot be discussed without consideration of the allocation of visual attention. In fact, it can be argued that visual target selection and the allocation of visual attention amount to the same thing', and he continues to outline a number of lines of evidence that selection and fixation depend on a common mechanism. Hoffman and Subramaniam (1995) instructed subjects to fix on (make saccades to) specific locations while they also attended to (detected targets at) the same or different locations. They found that subjects were unable to attend to one location while preparing to shift their gaze to another, suggesting that attention was always directed to the intended fixation point. Deubel and Schneider (1996) presented similar evidence and concluded that a single mechanism drives both selection of objects and the information needed to drive the appropriate fixation responses. Results such as this support the idea that covert selection may generally be regarded not just as an end in itself but as preparation for an expected fixation shift to the same location (Findlay & Gilchrist 2001, 2003), and there now seems to be a broad consensus among neurophysiologists that the systems for visual selection (attention) and oculomotor selection (fixation) are largely, though not inextricably, associated (Corbetta et al 1998; Awh et al 2006). Such observations help to validate our descriptive framework (**Fig. 4.2**), in which selective attention is assumed to be a natural precursor of fixation.

Visual working memory

Memory is extremely important at most if not all stages of processing in active vision. Most texts on visual perception, however, have little if anything to say about the role of memory. Our processing model (**Fig. 4.2D**) includes a *visual working memory* component situated at the interface between preattentive and attentive processing. It is not yet clear exactly where memory fits in such a scheme, or how it integrates with other processing components. However, evidence is emerging in support of the idea that basic visual processing, visual working memory and attention are closely linked.

Structure of working memory

Working memory is a theoretical construct, introduced by Baddeley and Hitch (Baddley & Hitch 1974; Baddeley 1986, 2005) as a model for thinking about how the brain deals with temporary information storage in performance of complex tasks. The concept developed from earlier models of short-term memory (Broadbent 1958; Atkinson and Shiffrin 1968) but differed in two ways. First, instead of assuming a single memory store it suggested a multi-component system. Second, it emphasized the importance of memory in cognition. The working memory model comprises: (1) *visuospatial sketchpad* (visual working memory), which holds information about spatial and object characteristics of visual data,

(2) *phonological loop*, which holds verbal and acoustic information such as word sounds, and (3) *central executive*, which is assumed to be an attention control system.

Consider the use of working memory in searching an image for a specific target. Information about the target must be held in memory for comparison to items in the image. In addition, details of locations searched and data found must be kept in memory in order to improve search efficiency by avoid unnecessary repetition. Here the value of the sketchpad analogy can be appreciated; it is as though the brain makes a sketch of the search pattern that it can refer back to at any stage and, when search is finished, the sketch can be thrown away. Similarly, many other forms of visuospatial task will benefit from availability of a 'memory sketch', such as visualizing a landscape, a route, a road layout, or a three-dimensional object.

Baddeley and Hitch (1974) initially treated *working (short-term) memory* as something quite separate from *long-term memory*, largely because there are many clinical examples of patients with short-term memory loss whose long-term memories are intact. However, more recent studies have suggested that some long-term learning, such as language, may depend upon effective short-term memory and there may be an analogue of this for visuospatial learning and memory. For this reason, Baddeley (2000) has extended the working memory concept to include a long-term component linked via an episodic buffer. The concept of episodic memory as a store for preattentive object files was outlined earlier. A more detailed discussion of the non-visual and extended components of working memory is beyond the scope of this chapter, but **Figure 4.5** illustrates its structure.

Working memory, preattentive and attentive vision

Evidence of a close association between basic visual processing and working memory is found in a number of recent studies summarized by Pasternak & Greenlee (2005) which show that fundamental stimulus features such as contrast, orientation, spatial frequency and vernier offset can be retained in memory for many seconds with little or no loss of information. Furthermore, it seems that these distinct elements of the stimulus are stored by separate, feature-selective mechanisms located early in the visual processing stream (Magnussen 2000). Indeed, the association between encoding and storage of stimulus features appears to be so close that memory and perception should not be regarded as entirely separate processes.

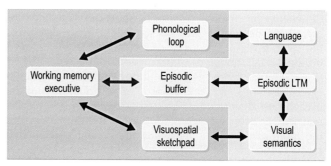

Figure 4.5 Illustration of the conceptual structure of *working memory*, as represented in the influential model developed by Alan Baddeley and colleagues.

Similarly, a recent review by Awh & Jonides (2001) points out that spatial working memory and spatial selective attention are also often treated as separate processes and studied in isolation, in spite of the fact that they must cooperate in some manner for active vision. In fact, some results in studies of visual working memory bear a clear resemblance to those from studies of visual attention. For example, memory representations can be biased by top-down control. In a classic study, Sperling (1960) presented observers with rows of letters and numbers followed by a cue to indicate which row should be reported, and found that observers could selectively transfer data representation from the cued row into short-term memory. Also, Rensink et al (1997) studied the ability of observers to see changes in scenes. Their finding that changes are most likely to be perceived in the regions considered most relevant indicates a top-down influence of long-term memory on the control of working memory. Conversely, evidence of bottom-up influence on the storage of information in visual working memory comes from Schmidt et al (2002), who tested observers ability to remember visual objects, some of which were preceded (cued) by a highly salient, peripheral flash of light. They found that the cued objects were more likely to be remembered than those that were not cued, even though the cues presented no information relevant to the task. These results show that the processes of attention and working memory are both susceptible to top-down and bottom-up influences and may even share the same control mechanisms. Other studies suggest an even closer association; just as it has been shown that visual processing is enhanced at attended locations, so it is also the case that processing is enhanced at memorized locations. This suggests that memorized and attended locations may be the same. Furthermore, if observers are forced to direct their attention away from locations they have remembered, then their memory for those locations is impaired (Smyth & Scholey 1994). This suggests that attention is actually an essential part of the spatial memory process, and Smyth and Scholey (1994) even propose that covert shifts of attention to different locations are necessary for maintaining information about them in working memory. There is therefore a clear functional overlap of the mechanisms of working memory with those of selective attention and early encoding of visual features (Awh & Jonides 2001), and working memory may be thought of as a short-term memory system with the addition of a central executive component to manage the memory data through the control of attention (Cowan 1995).

Capacity of working memory

Generally, information persists in short-term memory for periods of between 1 and 60 seconds. During that time, the memory trace gradually decays unless it is preserved through rehearsal of the information to be remembered (for example, repeating a telephone number to oneself before dialling), but the amount of information lost by decay is less than that lost by interference from other information. The more interfering (*distractor*) items there are, and the more similar these are to the item being remembered (*target*), the greater the loss of information (Waugh & Norman 1965).

The capacity of short-term memory is limited. A notable article by Miller (1956) suggested that it could hold approximately seven items, though recent research suggests that the general capacity limit may be closer to four items (Cowan 2001). Evidence of a capacity limit of four or five has also been reported for visual working memory and, significantly, this limit appears to be set in terms of the number of visual objects, not features (Luck & Vogel 1997; Vogel et al 2001; Alvarez & Cavanagh 2004). It has also been shown that the number of items held in visual working memory is related to how efficiently it can be used, since people who can remember more objects are also better at excluding irrelevant objects, and that this ability depends on filtering by visual attention (Cowan & Morey 2006).

The capacity limit in visual memory may be related to our ability to divide attention to track multiple objects simultaneously, which has practical relevance for activities such as playing team sports and video games, and driving. Here it has also been found that it is generally possible to track no more than about four objects simultaneously (Pylyshyn & Storm 1988; Cavanagh & Alvarez 2005).

Conclusion

This chapter has introduced a number of important topics that are currently prominent in research on cognitive/active vision. We have really just 'scratched the surface' and there are many interesting and important aspects that it has not been possible to discuss, particularly in relation to memory and attention. We end with a brief mention of two of these.

The first concerns various phenomena that demonstrate limitations in normal memory and attentional processing, with implications for the relationship between attention, awareness and consciousness: (1) *inattentional blindness* is the failure to notice a salient object or event when attention is focused on some other object or event (Mack & Rock 1998; Simons 2000) and is relevant to the study of attentional load and the effect of distractors (Lavie 2005), (2) the *attentional blink* refers to impaired performance in detecting an item shortly after a different item has been detected (Shapiro et al 1997), (3) *repetition blindness* is impaired performance in detecting a second presentation of the same item, even when a different item is presented between the repetitions (Kanwisher 1987) and (4) *change blindness* is the surprising failure to notice substantial change in a visual scene (Beck et al 2001; Simons & Rensink 2005).

The second, of particular interest to clinicians, is the variety of ways in which the ability to attend to objects and/or locations may be impaired by trauma or pathology (Robertson & Rafal 2000): (1) *unilateral (or hemispatial) neglect and extinction*, in which objects are missing from one half of the visual scene, usually the left as a result of damage to the right parietal cortex (Esterman et al 2000; Rizzolatti et al 2000), (2) *Balint's syndrome*, characterized by the inability to see more than one object at a time and to reach for a perceived object in the correct direction (Rizzo & Vecera 2002), (3) *integrative agnosia*, in which objects can be seen but their relationships in space are disturbed. This often reflects a problem with attending correctly to local and global structure (see **Fig. 4.4A** and Ivry & Robertson 1998). A comprehensive account of these and other clinical disorders is given by Robertson (2004, see also Humphreys & Riddoch 2005).

If the psychology of vision sometimes seems remote from the study and practice of optometry, then perhaps the clinical accounts given in this last reference will help to discourage insularity; observing how vision sometimes goes wrong is an important part of understanding how it works normally, and studying how it works normally helps us to make sense of what is happening when it goes wrong.

References

Aloimonos J, Bandopadhay A, Weiss I 1988 Active vision. International Journal of Computer Vision 1:333–356

Alvarez G A, Cavanagh P 2004 The capacity of visual short-term memory is set both by visual information load and by number of objects. Psychological Science 15:106–111

Ashby F G, Prinzmetal W, Ivry R B et al 1996 A formal theory of feature binding in object perception. Psychological Review 103:165–192

Atkinson R C, Schiffrin R M 1968 Human memory: a proposed system and its control processes. In: Spence K W (ed.) The psychology of learning and motivation: advances in research and theory. Academic Press, Philadelphia, pp 89–195

Awh E, Jonides J 2001 Overlapping mechanisms of attention and spatial working memory. Trends in Cognitive Sciences 5(3):119–126

Awh E, Armstrong K M, Moore T 2006 Visual and oculomotor selection: links, causes and implication for spatial attention. Trends in Cognitive Sciences 10(3):124–130

Baddeley A D 1986 Working memory. Clarendon Press, Oxford

Baddeley A D 2000 The episodic buffer: a new component of working memory? Trends in Cognitive Sciences 4(11):417–423

Baddeley A D 2005 Human memory: theory and practice, revised edn. Psychology Press, Hove, UK

Baddeley A D, Hitch G J 1974 Working memory. In: Bower G H (ed.) The psychology of learning and motivation, vol 13. Academic Press, New York, pp 47–89

Bashinski H S, Bacharach V R 1980 Enhancement of perceptual sensitivity as the result of selectively attending to spatial locations. Perception and Psychophysics 28:241–248

Baylis G C, Driver J 1993 Visual attention and objects: evidence for hierarchical coding of location. Journal of Experimental Psychology: Human Perception and Performance 19:451–470

Beck D M, Rees G, Frich C D et al 2001 Neural correlates of change detection and change blindness. Nature Neuroscience 4:645–650

Behrmann M, Haimson C 1999 The cognitive neuroscience of visual attention. Current Opinion in Neurobiology 9:158–163

Blake R, Sekuler R 2006 Perception. McGraw-Hill, Boston

Braisby N, Gellatly A (eds) 2005 Cognitive psychology. Oxford University Press, Oxford

Broadbent D E 1958 Perception and communication. Pergamon, London

Campbell F W, Kulikowski J J 1966 Orientational selectivity of the human visual system. Journal of Physiology 187:437–445

Carrasco M, McElree B 2001 Covert attention accelerates the rate of visual information processing. Proceedings of the National Academy of Sciences USA 98:5363–5367

Carrasco M, Penpeci-Talgar C, Eckstein M 2000 Spatial covert attention increases contrast sensitivity across the CSF: support for signal enhancement. Vision Research 40:1203–1215

Carrasco M, Williams P E, Yeshurun Y 2002 Covert attention increases spatial resolution with or without masks: support for signal enhancement. Journal of Vision 2:467–479

Carrasco M, Ling S, Read S 2004 Attention alters appearance. Nature Neuroscience 7:308–313

Cavanagh P, Alvarez G A 2005 Tracking multiple targets with multifocal attention. Trends in Cognitive Sciences 9(7):349–354

Cave K R, Bichot N P 1999 Visuospatial attention: beyond a spotlight model. Psychonomic Bulletin and Review 6:204–223

Chalupa L M, Werner J S 2004 The visual neurosciences. MIT Press, Cambridge, MA

Chen X, Zelinsky G J 2006 Real-world visual search is dominated by top-down guidance. Vision Research 46:4118–4133

Chun M 2000 Contextual cueing of visual attention. Trends in Cognitive Sciences 4(5):170–178

Chun M, Wolfe J M 2005 Visual attention. In: Goldstein E B (ed.) Blackwell handbook of sensation and perception. Blackwell Publishing, Malden, MA, pp 272–310

Corbetta M 1998 Functional anatomy of visual attention in the human brain: studies with positron emission tomography. In: Parasuraman R (ed.) The attentive brain. MIT Press, Cambridge, MA, pp 95–122

Corbetta M, Akbudak E, Conturo T E et al 1998 A common network of functional areas for attention and eye movements. Neuron 21:761–773

Courtney S M, Ungerleider L G 1997 What fMRI has taught us about human vision. Current Opinion in Neurobiology 7:554–561

Cowan N 1995 Attention and memory: an integrated framework. Oxford University Press, Oxford

Cowan N 2001 The magical number 4 in short-term memory: a reconsideration of mental storage capacity. Behavioral and Brain Sciences 24:87–185

Cowan N, Morey C C 2006 Visual working memory depends on attentional filtering. Trends in Cognitive Sciences 10(4):139–141

Desimone R, Duncan J 1995 Neural mechanisms of selective visual attention. Annual Review of Neuroscience 18:193–222

Deubel H, Schneider W X 1996 Saccade target selection and object recognition: evidence for a common attentional mechanism. Vision Research 36:1827–1837

DeValois R L, DeValois K K 1988 Spatial vision. Oxford University Press, Oxford

Di Russo F, Spinelli D, Morrone M C 2001 Automatic gain control contrast mechanisms are modulated by attention in humans: evidence from visual evoked potentials. Vision Research 41:2435–2447

Downing C J 1988 Expectancy and visual spatial attention: effects on perceptual quality. Journal of Experimental Psychology: Human Perception and Performance 14:188–202

Duncan J 1984 Selective attention and the organization of visual information. Journal of Experimental Psychology: General 113(4):501–517

Egeth H E, Yantis S 1997 Visual attention: control, representation, and time course. Annual Review of Psychology 48:269–297

Einhauser W, König P 2003 Does luminance-contrast contribute to a saliency map for overt visual attention? European Journal of Neuroscience 17:1089–1097

Eriksen C W, St James J D 1986 Visual attention within and around the field of focal attention – a zoom lens model. Perception and Psychophysics 40:225–240

Esterman M, McGlinchey-Berroth R, Milberg W P 2000 Parallel and serial search in hemispatial neglect: evidence for preserved preattentive but impaired attentive processing. Neuropsychology 14:599–611

Eysenck M W, Keane M T 2005 Cognitive psychology: a student's handbook. Psychology Press, Hove, UK

Fecteau J H, Munoz D P 2006 Salience, relevance, and firing: a priority map for target selection. Trends in Cognitive Sciences 10(8):382–390

Findlay J M, Gilchrist I D 1998 Eye guidance and visual search. In: Underwood G (ed.) Eye guidance in reading and scene perception. Elsevier, Amsterdam, pp 295–312

Findlay J M, Gilchrist I D 2001 Visual attention: the active vision perspective. In: Jenkin M, Harris L R (eds) Vision and attention. Springer-Verlag, New York, pp 83–103

Findlay J M, Gilchrist I D 2003 Active vision: the psychology of looking and seeing. Oxford University Press, Oxford

Findlay J M, Gilchrist I D 2005 Eye guidance and visual search. In: Underwood G (ed.) Cognitive processes in eye guidance. Oxford University Press, Oxford, pp 259–281

Findlay J M, Walker R 1999 A model of saccade generation based on parallel processing and competitive inhibition. Behavioral and Brain Sciences 22:661–674

Fiorentini A 2004 Brightness and lightness. In: Chalupa L M, Werner J S (eds) The visual neurosciences, vol 2. MIT Press, Cambridge, MA, pp 881–891

Frisby J P 1979 Seeing: illusion, brain and mind. Oxford University Press, Oxford

Frishman L J 2005 Basic visual processes. In: Goldstein E B (ed.) Blackwell handbook of sensation and perception. Blackwell, Malden, MA, pp 53–91

Gibson J J 1979 The ecological approach to visual perception. Houghton Mifflin, Boston

Gilchrist J 1988 The psychology of vision. In: Edwards K, Llewellyn R (eds) Optometry. Butterworth, London, pp 25–43

Goldstein E B 2005 Crosstalk between psychophysics and physiology in the study of perception. In: Goldstein E B (ed.) Blackwell handbook of sensation and perception. Blackwell, Malden, MA, pp 1–23

Goodale M A, Humphrey G K 2005 Separate visual systems for action and perception. In: Goldstein E B (ed.) Blackwell handbook of sensation and perception. Blackwell, Malden, MA, pp 311–343

Gordon J, Abramov I 2005 Color vision. In: Goldstein E B (ed.) Blackwell handbook of sensation and perception. Blackwell, Malden, MA, pp 92–127

Graham N 1989 Visual pattern analyzers. Oxford University Press, New York

Green P 2002 Where do drivers look while driving (and for how long)? In: Dewar R E, Olson P L (eds) Human factors in traffic safety. Lawyers and Judges Publishing, Tucson, AZ, pp 77–110

Grossberg S, Pessoa L 1998 Texture segregation, surface representation and figure–ground separation. Vision Research 38:2657–2684

Grossberg S, Mingolla E, Ross W D 1994 A neural theory of attentive visual search: interactions of boundary, surface, spatial and object representations. Psychological Review 101(3):470–489

Hatfield G 1996 Attention in early scientific psychology. In: Wright R D (ed.) Visual attention. Oxford University Press, New York

Haxby J V, Courtney S M, Clark V P 1998 Functional magnetic resonance imaging and the study of attention. In: Parasuraman R (ed.) The attentive brain. MIT Press, Cambridge, MA, pp 123–142

Hayhoe M, Ballard D 2005 Eye movements in natural behavior. Trends in Cognitive Sciences 9(4):188–194

Hecht S, Shlaer S, Pienne M H 1942 Energy, quanta and vision. Journal of General Physiology 25:819–840

Heeger D J, Ress D 2002 What does fMRI tell us about neuronal activity? Nature Reviews Neuroscience 3:142–151

Henderson J M 2003 Human gaze control in real-world scene perception. Trends in Cognitive Sciences 7:498–504

Henderson J M, Hollingworth A 1999 High-level scene perception. Annual Review of Psychology 50:243–271

Hoffman J E, Subramaniam B 1995 The role of visual attention in saccadic eye movements. Perception and Psychophysics 57:787–795

Hommel B 2004 Event files: feature binding in and across perception and action. Trends in Cognitive Sciences 8(11):494–500

Hubel D H, Wiesel T N 1959 Receptive fields of single neurons in the cat's striate cortex. Journal of Physiology 148:574–591

Hubel D H, Wiesel T N 1962 Receptive fields, binocular interaction and functional architecture in the cat's visual cortex. Journal of Physiology 160:106–154

Humphreys G W 2001 A multi-stage account of binding in vision: neuropsychological evidence. Visual Cognition 8:381–410

Humphreys G W, Riddoch M J 2005 The neuropsychology of visual object and space perception. In: Goldstein E B (ed.) Blackwell handbook of sensation and perception. Blackwell, Malden, MA, pp 204–236

Humphreys G W, Cinel C, Wolfe J M et al 2000 Fractionating the binding process: neuropsychological evidence distinguishing binding of form from binding of surface features. Vision Research 40:1569–1596

Inhoff A W, Pollatsek A, Posner M I et al 1989 Covert attention and eye movements during reading. Quarterly Journal of Experimental Psychology 41A:63–89

Inhoff A W, Radach R, Starr M et al 2000 Allocation of visuo-spatial attention and saccade programming during reading. In: Kennedy A, Radach R, Heller D et al (eds) Reading as a perceptual process. North Holland, Amsterdam, pp 221–246

Itti L, Koch C 2000 A saliency-based search mechanism for overt and covert shifts of visual attention. Vision Research 40:1489–1506

Itti L, Koch C 2001 Computational modelling of visual attention. Nature Reviews Neuroscience 2(3):194–203

Ivry R B, Robertson L C 1998 The two sides of perception. MIT Press, Cambridge, MA

James W 1890 The principles of psychology. Dover Publications, Mineola, NY

Jonides J, Yantis S 1988 Uniqueness of abrupt visual onset in capturing attention. Perception and Psychophysics 43:346–354

Kahneman D, Treisman A, Gibbs B J 1992 The reviewing of object files: object-specific integration of information. Cognitive Psychology 24(2):175–219

Kanwisher N 1987 Repetition blindness: type recognition without token individuation. Cognition 27:117–143

Kanwisher N, Wojciulik E 2000 Visual attention: insights from brain imaging. Nature Reviews Neuroscience 1:91–100

Kastner S, Ungerleider L G 2000 Mechanisms of visual attention in the human cortex. Annual Review of Neuroscience 23:315–341

Kazdin A E (ed.) 2000 Encyclopedia of psychology. American Psychological Association, Washington, DC

Koch C, Ullman S 1985 Shifts in selective visual attention: towards the underlying neural circuitry. Human Neurobiology 4(4): 219–227

Koffka K 1935 Principles of gestalt psychology. Harcourt Brace, New York

Köhler W 1940 Dynamics in psychology. Liveright, New York

Kowler E, Anderson E, Dosher B et al 1995 The role of attention in the programming of saccades. Vision Research 35:1897–1916

Kramer A F, Jacobson A 1991 Perceptual organisation and focused attention: the role of objects and proximity in visual processing. Perception and Psychophysics 50:267–284

Kustov A A, Robinson D L 1996 Shared neural control of attentional shifts and eye movements. Nature 384:74–77

LaBerge D 1995 Attentional processing: the brain's art of mindfulness. Harvard University Press, Cambridge, MA

Land M F, Mennie N, Rusted J 1999 The roles of vision and eye movements in the control of activities of everyday living. Perception 28:1311–1328

Lavie N 2005 Distracted and confused? Selective attention under load. Trends in Cognitive Sciences 9(2):75–82

Levine M W, Shefner J M 2000 Fundamentals of sensation and perception. Oxford University Press, Oxford

Li Z 2000 Pre-attentive segmentation in the primary visual cortex. Spatial Vision 13(1):25–50

Li Z 2002 A saliency map in primary visual cortex. Trends in Cognitive Sciences 6(1):9–16

Li Z, Snowden R J 2006 A theory of a saliency map in primary visual cortex (V1) tested by psychophysics of color-orientation interference in texture segmentation. Visual Cognition 14:911–933

Lu Z-L, Lesmes L A, Dosher B A 2002 Spatial attention excludes external noise at the target location. Journal of Vision 2:312–323

Luck S J 1998 Neurophysiology of selective attention. In: Pashler H (ed.) Attention. Psychology Press, Hove, UK, pp 257–295

Luck S J, Girelli M 1998 Electrophysiological approaches to the study of selective attention in the human brain. In: Parasuraman R (ed.) The attentive brain. MIT Press, Cambridge, MA, pp 71–94

Luck S J, Vogel E K 1997 The capacity of visual working memory for features and conjunctions. Nature 390:279–281

McConkie G W, Yang S-N 2003 How cognition affects eye movements during reading. In: Hyona J, Radach R, Deubel H (eds) The mind's eye: cognitive and applied aspects of eye movement research. Elsevier, Oxford, pp 413–427

Mack A, Rock I 1998 Inattentional blindness: perception without attention. MIT Press, Cambridge, MA

MacLeod C M 1991 Half a century of research on the Stroop effect: an integrative review. Psychological Bulletin 109(2):163–203

MacLeod C M, MacDonald P A 2000 Interdimensional interference in the Stroop effect: uncovering the cognitive and neural anatomy of attention. Trends in Cognitive Sciences 4(10):383–391

Magnussen S 2000 Low-level memory processes in vision. Trends in Neuroscience 23:247–251

Marr D 1982 Vision. W H Freeman, San Francisco

Martelli M, Majaj N J, Pelli D G 2005 Are faces processed like words? A diagnostic test for recognition by parts. Journal of Vision 5:58–70

Mather G 2006 Foundations of perception. Psychology Press, Hove, UK

Miller G A 1956 The magical number seven, plus or minus two: some limits on our capacity for processing information. Psychological Review 63:81–97

Moore C M, Egeth H E 1997 Perception without attention: evidence of grouping under conditions of inattention. Journal of Experimental Psychology: Human Perception and Performance 23:339–352

Moore C M, Yantis S, Vaughan B 1998 Object-based visual selection: evidence from perceptual completion. Psychological Science 9: 104–110

Motter B C 1998 Neurophysiology of visual attention. In: Parasuraman R (ed.) The attentive brain. MIT Press, Cambridge, MA, pp 51–69

Navon D 1977 Forest before the trees: the precedence of global features in visual perception. Cognitive Psychology 9:353–383

Neisser U 1967 Cognitive psychology. Appleton-Century-Crofts, New York

Neisser U, Becklen R 1975 Selective looking: attending to visually specified events. Cognitive Psychology 7:480–494

Norton T, Corliss D, Bailey J 2002 Psychophysical measurement of visual function. Butterworth-Heinemann, New York

O'Regan J K 1990 Eye movements and reading. In: Kowler E (ed.) Eye movements and their role in visual and cognitive processes. Elsevier, Amsterdam, pp 395–453

Palmer S E 1999 Vision science: photons to phenomenology. MIT Press, Cambridge, MA

Palmer S E 2000 Perceptual organization. In: Kazdin A E (ed.) Encyclopedia of psychology, vol 6. American Psychological Association, Washington DC, pp 93–97

Palmer J, Verghese P, Pavel M 2000 The psychophysics of visual search. Vision Research 40:1227–1268

Parasuraman R 1986 Vigilance, monitoring, and search. In: Boff K R, Kaufmann L, Thomas J P (eds) Handbook of human perception and performance, vol 2. John Wiley, New York, pp 43.1–43.39

Parkhurst D, Law K, Niebur E 2002 Modeling the role of salience in the allocation of overt visual attention. Vision Research 42(1):107–123

Pashler H 1998 The psychology of attention. MIT Press, Cambridge, MA

Pasternak T, Greenlee M W 2005 Working memory in primate sensory systems. Nature Reviews Neuroscience 6:97–107

Pestilli F, Carrasco M 2005 Attention enhances contrast sensitivity at cued and impairs it at uncued locations. Vision Research 45: 1867–1875

Pillsbury W B 1908 Attention. Arno Press, New York

Posner M I 1980 Orienting of attention. Quarterly Journal of Experimental Psychology 32:3–25

Posner M I, Petersen S 1990 The attention system of the human brain. Annual Review of Neuroscience 13:25–42

Posner M I, Snyder C R R, Davidson B J 1980 Attention and the detection of stimuli. Journal of Experimental Psychology: General 109:160–174

Pylyshyn Z W, Storm R W 1988 Tracking multiple independent targets: evidence for a parallel tracking mechanism. Spatial Vision 3: 179–197

Raichle M E 1998 Behind the scenes of functional brain imaging: a historical and physiological perspective. Proceedings of the National Academy of Sciences USA 95:765–772

Rayner K 1998 Eye movements in reading and information processing: 20 years of research. Psychological Bulletin 124:372–422

Rayner K, Pollatsek A 1989 The psychology of reading. Prentice Hall, Englewood Cliffs, NJ

Reed S K 2004 Cognition: theory and applications. Wadsworth, Belmont, CA

Reeves A 2004 Visual adaptation. In: Chalupa L M, Werner J S (eds) The visual neurosciences, vol 1. MIT Press, Cambridge, MA, pp 851–862

Regan D 2000 Human perception of objects: early visual processing of spatial form defined by luminance, color, texture, motion and binocular disparity. Sinauer Associates, Sunderland, MA

Reichle E D, Rayner K, Pollatsek A 2003 The E-Z reader model of eye movement control in reading: comparison to other models. Behavioral and Brain Sciences 26:445–476

Remington R W, Johnston J C, Yantis S 1992 Involuntary attentional capture by abrupt onsets. Perception and Psychophysics 51:279–290

Rensink R A 2000 Seeing, sensing, and scrutinizing. Vision Research 40:1469–1487

Rensink R A, O'Regan J K, Clark J J 1997 To see or not to see: the need for attention to perceive changes in scenes. Psychological Science 8:368–373

Rizzo M, Vecera S P 2002 Psychoanatomical substrates of Balint's syndrome. Journal of Neurology, Neurosurgery and Psychiatry 72:162–178

Rizzolatti G, Riggio L, Dascola I et al 1987 Reorientating attention across the horizontal and vertical meridians: evidence in favor of a premotor theory of attention. Neuropsychologia 25:31–40

Rizzolatti G, Berti A, Gallese V 2000 Spatial neglect: neurophysiological bases, cortical circuits and theory. In: Boller F, Grafman J, Rizzolatti G (eds) Handbook of neuropsychology, vol 1. Elsevier, Amsterdam, pp 503–537

Robertson L C 2004 Space, objects, minds, and brains. Psychology Press, Hove, UK

Robertson L C, Rafal R 2000 Disorders of visual attention. In: Gazzaniga M (ed.) The new cognitive neuroscience. MIT Press, Cambridge, MA, pp 633–649

Schall J D 2004 Selection of targets for saccadic eye movements. In: Chalupa L M, Werner J S (eds) The visual neurosciences, vol 2. MIT Press, Cambridge, MA, pp 1369–1390

Schmidt B K, Vogel E K, Woodman G F et al 2002 Voluntary and automatic attentional control of visual working memory. Perception and Psychophysics 64:754–763

Shapiro K L, Arnell K M, Raymond J E 1997 The attentional blink. Trends in Cognitive Sciences 1(8):291–296

Shulman G L, Wilson J 1987 Spatial frequency and selective attention to local and global information. Perception 16:89–101

Simons D J 2000 Attentional capture and inattentional blindness. Trends in Cognitive Sciences 4(4):147–155

Simons D J, Rensink R A 2005 Change blindness: past, present, and future. Trends in Cognitive Sciences 9(1):16–20

Sivak M 1996 The information that drivers use: is it indeed 90% visual? Perception 25:1081–1089

Smyth M M, Scholey K A 1994 Interference in immediate spatial memory. Memory and Cognition 22:1–13

Snowden R J, Thompson P, Troscianko T 2006 Basic vision: an introduction to visual perception. Oxford University Press, Oxford

Soto D, Humphreys G W, Heinke D 2006 Working memory can guide pop-out search. Vision Research 46:1010–1018

Sperling G 1960 The information available in brief visual presentations. Psychological Monographs 74:1–29

Sternberg R J 2003 Cognitive psychology. Wadsworth, Belmont, CA

Stroop J R 1935 Studies of interference in serial verbal reactions. Journal of Experimental Psychology 18(6):643–662

Stryer L 1986 Cyclic GMP cascade of vision. Annual Review of Neuroscience 9:87–119

Tehovnik E J, Slocum W M, Schiller P H 2003 Saccadic eye movements evoked by microstimulation of striate cortex. European Journal of Neuroscience 17(4):870–878

Theeuwes J, Kramer A F, Hahn S et al 1998 Our eyes do not always go where we want them to go: capture of the eyes by new objects. Psychological Science 9(5):379–385

Titchener E B 1908 Lectures on the elementary psychology of feeling and attention. Macmillan, New York

Treisman A 1988 Features and objects, the Fourteenth Bartlett Memorial Lecture. Quarterly Journal of Experimental Psychology 40:201–237

Treisman A 1996 The binding problem. Current Opinion in Neurobiology 6:171–178

Treisman A 1998 Feature binding, attention and object perception. Philosophical Transaction of the Royal Society, Series B 353:1295–1306

Treisman A M, Gelade G 1980 A feature-integration theory of visual attention. Cognitive Psychology 12(1):97–136

Tsotsos J K 1990 Analyzing vision at the complexity level. Behavioral and Brain Sciences 13:423–469

Turano K A, Geruschat D R, Baker F H 2003 Oculomotor strategies for the direction of gaze tested with a real-world activity. Vision Research 43:333–346

Ullman S 1996 High-level vision. MIT Press, Cambridge, MA

Underwood G (ed.) 1998 Eye guidance in reading and scene perception. Elsevier, Amsterdam

Underwood G 2005a Eye fixations on pictures of natural scenes: getting the gist and identifying the components. In: Underwood G (ed.) Cognitive processes in eye guidance. Oxford University Press, Oxford, pp 163–187

Underwood G (ed.) 2005b Cognitive processes in eye guidance. Oxford University Press, Oxford

Ungerleider L G, Haxby J V 1994 'What' and 'where' in the human brain. Current Opinion in Neurobiology 4(2):157–165

Ungerleider L G, Mishkin M 1982 Two cortical visual systems. In: Ingle D J, Goodale M A, Mansfield R J W (eds) Analysis of visual behavior. MIT Press, Cambridge, MA, pp 549–586

Vecera S P, Farah M J 1994 Does visual attention select objects or locations? Journal of Experimental Psychology: General 123:146–160

Vogel E K, Woodman G F, Luck S J 2001 Storage of features, conjunctions, and objects in visual working memory. Journal of Experimental Psychology: Human Perception and Performance 27(1):92–114

von der Malsburg C 1995 Binding in models of perception and brain function. Current Opinion in Neurobiology 5:520–526

Wandell B A 1995 Foundations of vision. Sinauer Associates, Sunderland, MA

Ward J 2006 The student's guide to cognitive neuroscience. Psychology Press, Hove, UK

Watt R J 1991 Understanding vision. Academic Press, London

Watt R J, Phillips W A 2000 The function of dynamic grouping in vision. Trends in Cognitive Sciences 4(12):447–454

Waugh N C, Norman D A 1965 Primary memory. Psychological Review 72:89–104

Williams D R, Hofer H 2004 Formation and acquisition of the retinal image. In: Chalupa L M, Werner J S (eds) The visual neurosciences, vol 1. MIT Press, Cambridge, MA, pp 795–810

Wolfe J M 1998 Visual search. In: Pashler H (ed.) Attention. University College London Press, London, pp 13–74

Wolfe J M 2000 Visual attention. In: DeValois K K (ed.) Seeing. Academic Press, San Diego, pp 335–386

Wolfe J M 2003 Moving towards solutions to some enduring controversies in visual search. Trends in Cognitive Sciences 7(2):70–76

Wolfe J M, Bennett S C 1997 Preattentive object files: shapeless bundles of basic features. Vision Research 37(1):25–43

Wolfe J M, Levi D, Kluender K et al 2005 Sensation and perception. Sinauer Associates, Sunderland, MA

Yarbus A L 1967 Eye movements and vision. Riggs L A, transl. Plenum Press, New York

Yeshurun Y, Carrasco M 1999 Spatial attention improves performance in spatial resolution tasks. Vision Research 39:293–306

Zhaoping L 2005 The primary visual cortex creates a bottom-up saliency map. In: Itti L, Rees G, Tsotsos J K (eds) Neurobiology of attention. Elsevier, London, pp 570–575

CHAPTER 5

Visual performance

W Neil Charman

Introduction

Previous chapters have outlined the characteristics of the optical and neural parts of the visual system. It is clear that the system has remarkable flexibility, particularly in its neural arrangements for acquiring and analysing the optical image over a wide range of lighting conditions. In this chapter we shall be concerned with the resultant capability of the normal human visual system to carry out a range of tasks, concentrating on those aspects that are clinically most relevant. Since, however, this visual capability is always a function of the light level available to perform the task, we need first to define a measurement system for specifying light levels.

Illumination and the eye

Basic concepts: radiometry

Light is, of course, only one of the many forms of electromagnetic radiation, exceptional only in that its wavelengths lie within the range capable of stimulating the visual system. Radiometry is concerned with the quantification of any electromagnetic radiation in purely physical, energy-related terms, while in photometry, quantification takes into account the ability of the radiation to stimulate the human visual system. Radiometry is obviously of ocular importance when we are discussing ultraviolet or infrared wavelengths, which may damage or otherwise affect the eye even though they are invisible. Four important descriptors of the characteristics of radiation can conveniently be defined:

1. *Radiant flux,* **F**: This describes the rate of energy flow. It would normally be measured in watts (joules/sec). However, we can also measure it in photons/sec, since each photon carries an energy of hc/λ joules, where h is Planck's constant ($6.63 \cdot 10^{-34}$ Joule sec), c is the velocity of light ($3 \cdot 10^8$ m/sec) and λ is the wavelength of the light. At visible wavelengths, each photon carries only a very small amount of energy. To give an example of this, consider the beam from a 0.5 milliwatt red laser pointer. Assuming that the wavelength is 600 nm, the equivalent photon flux is about $1.5 \cdot 10^{15}$ photons/sec. At shorter, ultraviolet wavelengths, individual photons may carry enough energy to cause damage to the molecules of the cornea, a fact that is made use of in procedures such as excimer laser refractive surgery (see Ch. 23).

2. *Radiant intensity,* **I**: If, in a specified direction, a source sends out a radiant flux dF uniformly into a solid angle $d\omega$, the radiant intensity, I, is given by:

$$I = dF/d\omega$$

i.e. the intensity is a measure of the radiant energy flux per unit solid angle in a given direction.

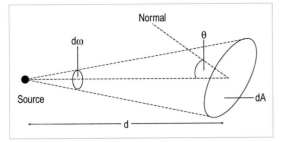

Figure 5.1 Relationships between radiant flux, radiant intensity and irradiance. In photometry, the same relationships apply between luminous flux, luminous intensity and illuminance.

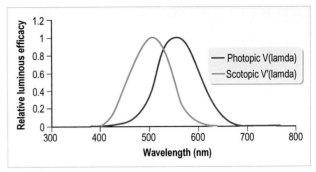

Figure 5.2 Relative luminous efficacy curves adopted by the Commission Internationale de l'Eclairage (CIE) for photopic and scotopic conditions. In the mesopic range the peak of the luminous efficiency function shifts gradually between these extremes. At the peak of the V_λ curve (555 nm, $V_\lambda = 1$) a radiant energy flux of 1 watt ($2.8.10^{18}$ photons/sec) gives a luminous flux of 683 photopic lumens. For the peak of the scotopic curve (509 nm, $V'_\lambda = 1$), 1 watt of radiant energy corresponds to 1700 scotopic lumens.

3. **Irradiance, E**: Suppose that a radiant flux dF is emitted by a small source within a solid angle dω and falls on a small area dA, where the area is inclined at an angle θ to the direction of the incident flux. The irradiance E is then given by:

$$E = dF/dA$$

Note that it follows from the geometry of **Figure 5.1** that:

$$E = dF/dA = (dF.\cos\theta.d^2)/(dA.\cos\theta.d^2)$$

$$\text{Since } d\omega = (dA.\cos\theta)/d^2$$

$$E = (dF.\cos\theta)/d\omega.d^2 = I\cos\theta/d^2$$

This is the well-known inverse square law. The important feature of irradiance is that it describes the radiation falling onto a surface.

4. **Radiance, L**: We have so far assumed that our radiation source is a point. In practice this will rarely be the case: our source will have an extended area. If I is the radiant intensity of the source in a given direction and A_s is the projected area of the source perpendicular to that direction, the radiance is given by:

$$L = I/A_s$$

i.e. it expresses the intensity per unit area of the source.

Visible radiation: photometry

The above terms can be applied to electromagnetic radiation of any wavelength. In the case of 'visible light', however, we are concerned only with the interaction of wavelengths of about 380 to 760 nm with the visual system. Radiation at other wavelengths may be present but the eye cannot detect it. Thus, to determine the visual effect we need to consider not only the radiant energy emitted by any source at a given wavelength but also the way in which that wavelength stimulates the eye.

The sensitivity of the eye to different wavelengths is usually expressed by the relative luminous efficacy function (**Fig. 5.2**): this expresses, in relative terms, the sensitivity to a constant amount of light energy as a function of wavelength, the curve being normalized to unity at its peak. However, the situation is complicated by the fact that the retina contains two different types of photoreceptor. As a result, under photopic ('bright') conditions, when the retinal cones are the dominant receptors, the efficacy curve (V_λ) peaks at 555 nm, while under scotopic ('dim') conditions, when rods are the most effective receptors, the curve (V'_λ) peaks at 509 nm. As the light level is reduced under intermediate mesopic (twilight) conditions, when both cones and rods contribute to vision, the efficacy curve shifts gradually between the two extreme V_λ and V'_λ cases: this effect is known as the 'Purkinje shift', after its discoverer, the Czech Johannes Purkinje (1787–1869).

Under photopic conditions, if one has an energy flux ε_λ of wavelength λ entering the eye the corresponding photopic luminous flux will be proportional to the product ε_λ. V_λ. In fact, at the peak of the V_λ curve, where the wavelength is 555 nm, 683 lumens are produced by each watt of radiation. Hence, if ε_λ is measured in watts per unit wavelength interval, for a broadband source of radiation the luminous flux F in photopic lumens will be given by:

$$F = 683 \int_0^\infty \varepsilon_\lambda.V_\lambda.d\lambda$$

In practice, the relative luminous efficacy curve changes not only with the absolute level of the flux (photopic, mesopic, scotopic) but also with the measurement method used and such factors as the angular size and location of the image of the stimulus on the retina, since the relative spatial densities of retinal rods and cones are affected by these parameters. It also shows some variation with the individual observer, particularly with colour vision. In quantitative photometry it is usual to assume that standardized photopic and scotopic conditions prevail, and that the V_λ and V'_λ curves take standard values. For example, the photopic curve (see **Fig. 5.2**) adopted by the Commission Internationale de l'Eclairage (CIE) is based on average data obtained with foveal fields 2 degrees in diameter, and the scotopic curve only applies to observers whose age is less than 30 when observing at angles of not less than 5 degrees from the fovea.

If, then, we weight the wavelength distribution of our radiant flux with the appropriate luminous efficacy curve to obtain the luminous flux, we can move from our basic radiometric parameters to the corresponding photometric quantities, as shown in **Table 5.1**.

There is one other unit which is occasionally used in relation to the eye. When viewing a surface of constant luminance, the resultant illuminance on the retina depends on the area of the pupil of the eye: the larger the pupil area the higher the retinal illuminance. Since the response of the retinal receptors is likely to depend upon the illuminance falling on them, we therefore

Table 5.1 Corresponding radiometric and photometric quantities

Radiometric quantity	Corresponding photometric quantity
Radiant flux (watts)	Luminous flux (lumens)
Radiant intensity (watts.sr^{-1})	Luminous intensity (lumens.sr^{-1} or candelas)
Irradiance (watts.m^{-2})	Illuminance (lumens.m^{-2} or lux)
Radiance (watts.sr^{-1}.m^{-2})	Luminance (candelas.m^{-2})

need a unit which takes into account the pupil area. This unit is the troland, where 1 troland is the retinal illuminance produced by viewing a surface of 1 cd.m^{-2} through a pupil of area 1 mm^2, i.e. the retinal illuminance in trolands is the product of the scene luminance and the pupil area.

The real-world luminous environment

Before discussing some aspects of visual performance it is helpful to be able to relate them to the lighting levels that might be encountered in everyday life. Obviously, these vary considerably with the individual's exact environment, but **Table 5.2** gives some representative values of illuminance and luminance under various circumstances, together with the recommended lighting levels for optometric test charts. Note that if a diffusely reflecting surface has a reflectance R (where R is the fraction of luminous flux that is reflected) and the illuminance is E, the corresponding luminance of the surface as seen by reflection is RE.

The striking aspect of **Table 5.2** is how much higher lighting levels are under outdoor daylight conditions, even on dull winter's days. The approximate luminance range for scotopic vision is 10^{-6} to 10^{-3} cd.m^{-2}, that for mesopic vision 10^{-3} to 3 cd.m^{-2} and finally for photopic vision ≥ 3 cd.m^{-2}.

Factors affecting visual performance

As described in Chapter 1, in the absence of refractive or accommodative errors of focus, the optics of the eye can deliver an in-focus retinal image that, on axis under daylight photopic conditions, has a quality which approaches that of a system limited only by diffraction. Off axis, and under scotopic conditions, increasing levels of optical aberration result in a decline in image quality but, even so, the image quality remains reasonable. The characteristics of the optical image must, however, be explored by a neural retina and subsequent higher levels of the visual system whose characteristics are strongly dependent on not only the retinal location but also the retinal illuminance produced by the visual stimulus (see Ch. 2). Broadly speaking, neural performance at higher light levels will be dominated by the spatial distribution and other properties of retinal cones and their processing arrangements, and that at scotopic levels by those of rods. We shall now consider how optics and neural aspects of the visual system combine to control performance in a variety of visual tasks.

Dark and light adaptation

As discussed in Chapter 2, in both rods and cones light must be absorbed by a visual pigment in order to initiate the chain of photochemical and neural activity which leads to the sensation of vision. Suppose an individual is exposed to a large, achromatic (white), photopic luminance field for long enough for complete adaptation to occur. Under these conditions substantial 'bleaching' of the visual pigments results, that is, a significant proportion of the photopigment molecules in each receptor has undergone light-induced change so that the receptor no longer responds at maximal efficiency to weak stimuli. If now the adaptation field is switched off and replaced by a smaller test field, the rest of the visual environment being dark, what luminance is required for the test field to be just detectable? Although the exact results vary with the conditions of the experiment

Table 5.2 Typical values of illuminance and some corresponding values of surface luminance, together with recommended lighting levels for externally and internally illuminated optometric test charts

Situation	Illuminance on horizontal surface (lux)	Corresponding luminance of typical surface (cd.m^{-2})
Clear sky in summer at noon (UK)	150 000	Grass 2900
Overcast sky in summer at noon (UK)	16 000	Grass 300
Light overcast sky in winter (UK)	5000	Brick 200
Textile inspection	1500	Light grey cloth 140
Office work	500	White paper 120
Heavy engineering	300	Steel 20
Good street lighting	10	Concrete road surface 1.0
Moonlight	0.1	Asphalt road surface 10^{-2}
Overcast night sky	10^{-4}	Grass 2.10^{-6}
Optometric test chart	600	150

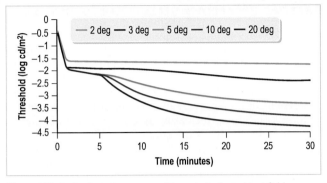

Figure 5.3 Dark adaptation curves with centrally fixated test fields subtending the angles indicated at the eye. With the inclusion of more peripheral areas of retina, rods make a progressively larger contribution to the sensitivity, giving the marked break in the adaptation curves. (After Hecht et al 1937.)

(e.g. the luminance, wavelength, size and retinal location of the adaptation and test stimuli and the psychophysical methods used to establish the thresholds), it is found that the threshold luminance gradually decreases as time goes on. Some typical results for centrally fixated test fields of different angular diameters are shown in **Figure 5.3**. It can be seen that, for a small 2 degree field, there is a rapid decrease in threshold over the first few minutes (i.e. an increase in sensitivity), after which the threshold does not fall much farther. For larger test fields, however, curves with two distinct branches develop: an initial rapid fall in threshold followed by near constancy is then succeeded by a second stage in which threshold falls at a somewhat lower rate to reach a low, constant level after some 30 minutes in the dark.

Although dilation of the pupil in the dark must contribute in part to the improvement in sensitivity, the maximal possible change in pupil area is only about $16\times$, which is obviously inadequate to explain the threshold changes in **Figure 5.3**; moreover, pupil dilation is largely complete after about a minute (Wyszecki & Stiles 1982). The general form of these data can be better explained in terms of the spatial distribution of rods and cones across the retina and their different characteristics (see Ch. 2). With the small, 2 degree, central test field, the light falls mainly on cone receptors, there being few rods in the central fovea. These central cones attain their maximal sensitivity through regeneration of photopigment at a relatively rapid rate, after which there is little further improvement. In contrast, with the larger test fields, substantial numbers of rods as well as cones are included in the retinal areas affected by the test stimulus. In these areas, the initial period of cone adaptation (the first branch of the curve) is followed by one of rod adaptation, which evidently takes considerably longer to complete. Under dark-adapted conditions, faint objects are more likely to be detected by using the rod-rich peripheral retina rather than cone-rich foveal vision. Thus, the process of dark adaptation provides good evidence for what is often called the duplex (i.e. rod and cone) theory of vision.

It follows from the above that individuals born with only rods in their retina (rod monochromats) will show only the rod branch of the dark adaptation curve, while patients with certain diseases, such as retinitis pigmentosa, in which the retinal rods are destroyed, will progressively lose the rod

branch of the dark adaptation curve and find it difficult to cope under low levels of lighting.

If we reverse this process and suddenly expose the dark-adapted retina to photopic levels of light, the process of light adaptation takes place much more rapidly than dark adaptation, since the rods become saturated and only the more rapidly adapting cones remain sensitive.

The absolute threshold

Suppose we allow a subject to fully dark adapt. What is the faintest level of light that can be detected? We can see from the field dependence of the data in **Figure 5.3** that the answer is likely to depend upon the characteristics of the test stimulus used: it will also depend upon the psychophysical methods used to establish the threshold. However, a fascinating insight into the ability of the visual system to detect low levels of light was given by the classic study of Hecht et al (1942): their results have subsequently been supported by various other authors. Briefly, Hecht and his colleagues used a small (10 minute of arc diameter) circular test stimulus located at a peripheral angle of 20 degrees so that it fell on a rod-rich area of retina. The test field was of wavelength 510 nm to match the peak of the scotopic V'_λ curve (see **Fig. 5.2**) and was flashed on for 1 ms. An artificial pupil 2 mm in diameter was used to avoid the influence of natural fluctuations in pupil diameter on retinal illuminance. The result was that their fully dark-adapted subjects could detect the test stimulus when the light energy measured at the cornea before the light entered the eye was roughly 4.10^{-17} Joules. As will be discussed in more detail below, this is a very small amount of energy. Pirenne (1967) sets it in context in his charming comment:

The mechanical energy of a pea falling from a height of one inch would, if transformed into luminous energy, be sufficient to give a faint impression of light to every man that ever lived.

We can, in fact, explore further the factors underlying the absolute threshold if we convert the energy of the threshold stimulus to the corresponding number of photons. Photons of wavelength 510 nm each have an energy of about $3.9.10^{-19}$ Joules, so our energy threshold corresponds to about 100 photons being incident at the relevant area of the cornea. Not all of these will, of course, reach the retina: around 50% will be reflected, absorbed or scattered by the anterior structures (see **Fig. 1.11**), leaving about 50 photons. Again, not all of these will be absorbed by the rhodopsin in the retinal rods: the best estimate is that only about 20% are absorbed, i.e. around 10 photons (Pirenne 1967). These photons are, of course, spread out randomly across the retinal area corresponding to the image of the 10 minutes of arc test patch, which it is estimated contains about 500 rods when the effects of optical diffraction and aberration are allowed for. Statistically, there is a low probability that 2 or more of our 10 photons have been absorbed by any one of the 500 possible rods. Thus, it follows that our threshold must result from the near-simultaneous absorption of single photons by several different rods, each absorption being in a single rhodopsin molecule. A retinal rod is therefore capable of reaching the absolute limit of sensitivity set by the quantum nature of light. Presumably, summation of the outputs of a group of rods occurs later in the neural circuitry and the 'firing' of around 10 of the rods is required in order for the signal to break the synaptic barrier and be transmitted to the higher levels of the system. In practice, the statistical fluctuations associated with the quantum nature of light result in a 'frequency of seeing' curve rather than an abrupt threshold (e.g. Pirenne 1967; Davson 1990) but the basic concept of pooled responses from rods which are individually excited by single photons remains valid. For small areas and short times, spatial and temporal integration occur, for example:

$$\text{Threshold luminance} \times \text{stimulus area}$$
$$= \text{constant (Ricco's law)}$$

$$\text{Threshold luminance} \times \text{stimulus presentation time}$$
$$= \text{constant (Bloch's law)}$$

These 'laws' only apply over limited ranges of the parameters, which vary with such factors as retinal location (e.g. Hood & Finkelstein 1986).

The perception of contrast

If for simplicity we ignore the effects of colour, our ability to see objects in the surrounding environment generally depends upon the difference between their luminance and that of their surroundings. If we carry out a simple experiment in which a small circular field of luminance $L + \Delta L$ is to be detected against a uniform background of luminance L, we can find the threshold value of ΔL (the liminal differential threshold) for different values of L. A plot of $\Delta L/L$ against L then typically takes the form shown in **Figure 5.4**. It can be seen that as the background luminance is increased the relative threshold falls, to reach an approximately constant value at low and moderate photopic levels. At high values of background luminance, as would be encountered under good daylight conditions, the relative threshold starts to rise slightly. Over quite a wide range the fraction $\Delta L/L$ is almost independent of L, the value typically being about 0.02 to 0.03. This constancy of the ratio between the differential threshold and the background luminance is often known as the Weber–Fechner law and is an example of Weber's law, which applies in a number of sensory modalities. The fraction $\Delta L/L$ is known as the Weber–Fechner

fraction. Thus, what matters is not the absolute value of ΔL but its relation to L, i.e. our ability to see objects depends upon the contrast between them and their surroundings rather than on the absolute differences in luminance (although note that different definitions of contrast may be used in other circumstances).

Since for objects seen by reflected light the luminance difference will depend upon differences in reflectance, changes in the level of illumination will not affect the contrast between objects and their surroundings. This can easily be understood. Suppose the reflectances of the object and its surround are R_o and R_s respectively and the illuminance is E. The apparent luminances will be proportional to ER_o and ER_s, so that $\Delta L/L$ becomes:

$$(ER_o - ER_s)/ER_s = (R_o - R_s)/R_s = \Delta R/R_s$$

Clearly, then, the contrast is independent of the illuminance, so that within the range of illuminances within which the Weber–Fechner law is valid, the visibility of objects is likely to remain unchanged.

As might be expected, values of $\Delta L/L$ vary not only with luminance level but also with the size of the test field (bigger stimuli are generally easier to see), the location on the retina (since the rod and cone densities affect the luminance dependence), whether vision is binocular or monocular (binocular Weber–Fechner fractions are lower) and other factors.

Form vision and the acuities

Visual acuity (minimum resolvable acuity)

Central to many visual tasks is the ability to recognize the shape of objects. A familiar clinical example is the test of visual acuity in which progressively smaller letters or other optotypes must be correctly identified (see Ch. 12) until a angular subtense limit is reached, beyond which no further recognition is possible (even though the presence of the symbols may still be detected). Remembering the more general characteristics of the visual system, it is not surprising to find that performance in acuity tasks depends upon such factors as the light level, the colour, contrast and form of the task, its location with respect to the fovea, the duration of its presentation, movement, and the adaptation of the individual. Since visual acuity depends upon both optical and neural performance it is, in general, degraded by any defocus due to refractive error.

Figure 5.5 summarizes typical results showing the general effect of some of these factors. Visual acuity here is expressed in decimal terms, where the decimal rating corresponds to the reciprocal of the angular subtense in minutes of arc (1 degree contains 60 minutes) of the significant detail (e.g. the width of each limb of a Snellen letter). Thus, a decimal acuity of 0.5 means that the subject can just recognize symbols with a detail size of 2 minutes arc. The angular subtense at which the test object can just be recognized is often called the minimum angle of resolution or MAR (i.e. decimal acuity = 1/MAR).

While the absolute levels of peak acuity vary somewhat between the different studies, due to the differing test objects and other conditions involved, it is evident that acuity declines with contrast, luminance and target movement: there are also falls with age (see Ch. 12).

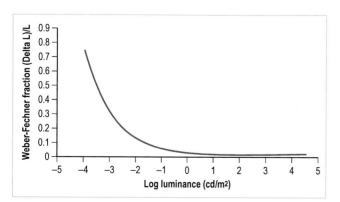

Figure 5.4 Typical plot of the value of $\Delta L/L$ as a function of the background luminance L. (After Weston 1962.)

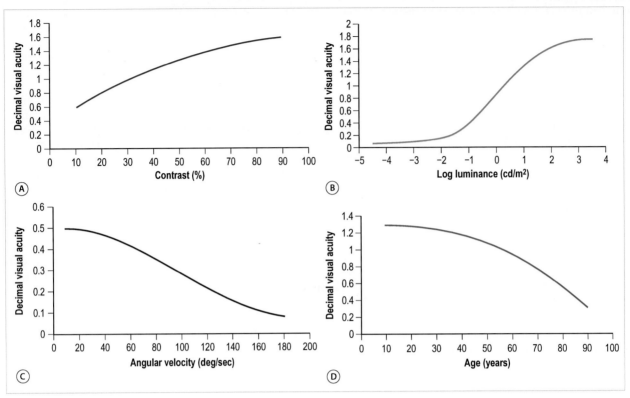

Figure 5.5 Examples of the effects on visual acuity of changes in **(A)** test contrast (after Regan & Neima 1983), **(B)** luminance (Koenig, after Hecht 1928), **(C)** target motion (dynamic acuity, after Ludvigh and Miller 1958), and **(D)** age (based on Owsley et al 1983). Any refractive error in the subjects has been corrected.

The contrast sensitivity function

While visual acuity tests are widely used in clinical practice, they have been criticized because they concentrate on spatial vision for objects near the threshold of resolution and fail to yield information on the ability to see larger, low-contrast objects. The contrast sensitivity function (CSF) overcomes this criticism by specifying performance over a range of object sizes (see Ch. 12).

To measure the CSF, grating test objects, in which the luminance varies sinusoidally in the direction perpendicular to the grating bars, are used. Each grating is specified in terms of its spatial frequency (i.e. the reciprocal of the angular separation in degrees of neighbouring peaks of the grating) and its modulation or contrast, defined as $(L_{max} - L_{min})/(L_{max} + L_{min})$, where L_{max} and L_{min} are, respectively, the luminances at the peaks and troughs of the grating. The measurement procedure consists of determining the threshold modulation of the just-perceptible sinusoidal grating as a function of its spatial frequency, at a constant space-averaged luminance. The sensitivity at each frequency is the reciprocal of the contrast threshold and the plot of sensitivity against spatial frequency is the CSF. The frequency at which the contrast sensitivity falls to zero is related to (but not identical to) the visual acuity as determined with high-contrast targets, since it is an indication of the highest spatial

frequency detail that the visual system can detect. The CSF again depends upon the measurement conditions. **Figure 5.6** shows typical data for the effect of luminance on the foveal CSF and the effect of field angle on the photopic CSF. Not surprisingly, like visual acuity, CSF falls as the light level is reduced and is lower in the peripheral field.

The vernier acuities

Vernier acuity concerns the ability to detect small lateral offsets in the alignment of two parallel lines or other figures. The two lines are initially collinear, with the ends together. One of them is then moved in a direction perpendicular to its length until the subject reports a break in contour. The smallest detectable angular offset is taken as the threshold, which typically has a value of about 5 seconds of arc (60 arc seconds = 1 arc minute). This is considerably less than the angular diameter of a foveal cone (around 20 arc seconds). Vernier acuity is one of a wider group of so-called hyperacuities which also includes tasks such as the detection of changes in the orientation or movement of a line. The hyperacuities are relatively robust against blur caused by defocus or cataract and have therefore been recommended for the clinical assessment of neural function in the presence of these conditions (Enoch et al 1985; McKee et al 1990).

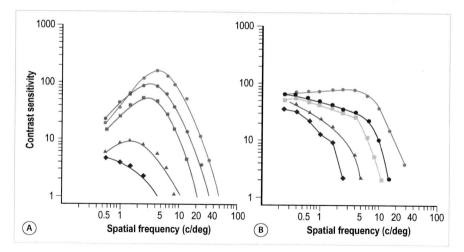

Fig. 5.6 Examples of CSF data for young adult observers. **(A)** Effect of luminance on foveal CSF. Curves (from the top) are for space-averaged luminances of 17, 1.7, 0.17, 0.017 and 0.0017 cd/m². (After deValois et al 1974.) **(B)** Effect of field angle on photopic CSF. Contrast sensitivity tends to decrease with eccentricity (starting from the top the angles are 0, 5, 10, 20 and 40 degrees). (After Banks et al 1991.)

Temporal effects

Vision is almost always a dynamic activity, involving frequent changes in fixation to bring different objects onto the fovea for detailed examination. It is not surprising, then, to find that the temporal characteristics of stimuli may have a strong effect on such tasks as their detection and recognition.

As discussed above, at very low light levels the ability to detect a stimulus is governed by the number of photons detected. Temporal summation then leads to Bloch's law. However, as we move away from absolute thresholds, more complex behaviour is observed.

The critical fusion (or flicker) frequency (CFF)

Suppose we have a test field which alternates regularly between dark and light (a temporal square-wave stimulus). What rate of alternation is required before the flicker can no longer be detected and the stimulus is perceived as being continuous? A typical result for rod-free foveal vision is shown by the black line in **Figure 5.7**. The critical flicker fusion frequency is, over a wide range (about 0.5 to 10 000 trolands), proportional to the logarithm of the retinal illuminance and stimulus luminance (the Ferry–Porter law). Note that the CFF is only a few Hz (cycles/sec) at scotopic luminances and rises to a maximum of 50–60 Hz at high photopic levels. If the stimulus is displaced from the fovea so that rods are included in the stimulated region of the retina, the Ferry–Porter law breaks down, as shown by the yellow and blue curves of **Figure 5.7**, where the stimulus is centred at peripheral angles of 5 and 15 degrees. The non-linearity is particularly noticeable at lower scotopic luminances where the rods maintain the CFF at higher values than would be found with cones alone: the highest values of scotopic CFF are therefore found when the stimulus falls away from the fovea. In addition, the CFF is found to depend on other factors such as stimulus area, colour and duty cycle.

The temporal contrast sensitivity function

If, rather than alternating between dark and light, we modulate the luminance of a test field sinusoidally with

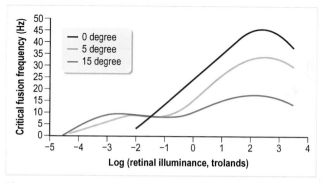

Figure 5.7 Critical fusion frequency (alternatively called critical flicker frequency) as a function of retinal illuminance for a small (2 degree) stimulus, centred at 0°, 5° and 15° in the visual field. (After Hecht & Verrip 1933.)

time, we can establish a temporal contrast sensitivity function which is analogous to the spatial contrast sensitivity function discussed earlier. Some typical data are shown in **Figure 5.8A**. Note that, at high values of retinal illuminance, the sensitivity peaks at about 20 Hz, although the absolute cutoff (corresponding approximately to the CFF) is at about 70 Hz. These values decrease as the illuminance is lowered, and the lower-frequency peak disappears at scotopic levels.

It is clear that in the real world stimuli vary in both space and time. This has led to interest in the determination of complete spatiotemporal contrast sensitivity functions (**Fig. 5.8B**) in which both the spatial and the temporal frequencies of a stimulus are varied. These show that, at photopic levels, the visual system shows maximal sensitivity at intermediate spatial and temporal frequencies.

Colour vision and stereoscopic vision

These topics will be discussed in Chapters 19 and 16, respectively.

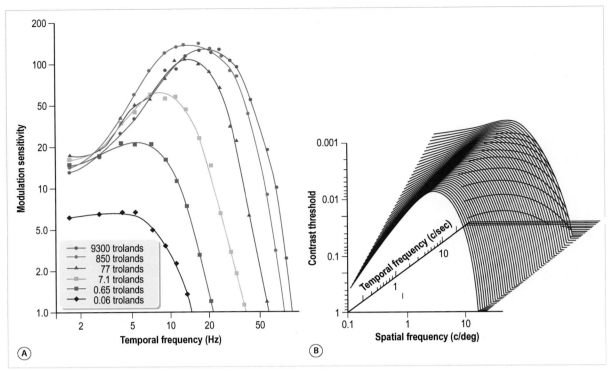

Figure 5.8 (A) Temporal contrast sensitivity functions at various levels of retinal illuminance. (After Kelly 1961.) **(B)** Combined photopic spatiotemporal CSF, representing luminance contrast sensitivity for different combinations of spatial and temporal modulation. (After Kelly 1979.)

References

Banks M S, Sekuler A B, Anderson S J 1991 Peripheral vision: limits imposed by optics, photoreceptors, and receptor pooling. Journal of the Optical Society of America A 8:1775–1787

Davson H 1990 Physiology of the eye, 5th edn. Macmillan, London, pp 264–278

deValois R L, Morgan H, Snodderly D M 1974 Psychophysical studies of monkey vision III. Spatial luminance contrast sensitivity tests of macaque and human observers. Vision Research 14:75–81

Enoch J M, Essock E A, Fendick M 1985 Hyperacuity: a promising means of evaluating vision through cataract. In: Osborne N N, Chader G J (eds) Progress in retinal research, vol 4. Pregamon, Oxford, pp 67–89

Hecht S 1928 The relation between visual acuity and illumination. Journal of General Physiology 11:255–281

Hecht S, Verrip C D 1933 Intermittent stimulation by light, III. The relationship between intensity and critical fusion frequency for different1 retinal locations. Journal of General Physiology 17:251

Hecht S, Haig C, Chase A M 1937 The influence of light adaptation on subsequent dark adaptation of the eye. Journal of General Physiology 20:831–850

Hecht S, Shlaer S, Pirenne M H 1942 Energy, quanta and vision. Journal of General Physiology 25:819–840

Hood D C, Finkelstein M A 1986 Sensitivity to light. In: Boff K R, Kaufman L, Thomas J P (eds) Handbook of perception and human performance, vol 1. Wiley, New York, pp 5.1–5.66

Kelly D H 1961 Visual responses to time-dependent stimuli. I Amplitude sensitivity measurements. Journal of the Optical Society of America 51:422–429

Kelly D H 1979 Motion and Vision. II Stabilised spatio-temporal threshold surface. Journal of the Optical Society of America 69:1340–1349

Ludvigh E, Miller J W 1958 Study of visual acuity during the ocular pursuit of moving test objects. I Introduction. Journal of the Optical Society of America 48:799–802

McKee S P, Welch L, Taylor D G et al 1990 Finding the common bond: stereoacuity and the other hyperacuities. Vision Research 30: 879–891

Owsley C, Sekuler R, Siemsen D 1983 Contrast sensitivity throughout adulthood. Vision Research 23:689–699

Pirenne M H 1967 Vision and the eye, 2nd edn. Chapman & Hall, London, pp 76–109

Regan D, Neima D 1983 Low-contrast letter charts as a test of visual function. Ophthalmology 90:1192–1200

Weston H C 1962 Sight, light and work, 2nd edn. Lewis, London, p 13

Wyszecki G, Stiles W S 1982 Color science. Wiley, New York, Table 1, p 2.4.5

CHAPTER 6

Basic pharmacology relevant to the action of drugs on the eye

Michael J Doughty

Nomenclature for drugs, pharmaceutical agents and medicines

A drug can be considered as a chemical substance that has been shown to have a specific action on various functions in the human body, e.g. on the iris muscles. Within the context of this chapter, such a drug has been approved for human use and, in the form presented to the human body (e.g. as eyedrops) has been shown to have a predictable action. Furthermore, its use in the form presented is relatively free of substantial unwanted effects, also known as side effects or adverse reactions.

Drugs for ophthalmic use are known by a common name, also known as the International Nonproprietary Name (INN) or simply as the Non-Proprietary Name (NPN). An example of a common name for a drug with an action on the iris tissue would be tropicamide. This drug is presented to the eye in the form of eyedrops and tropicamide is the active ingredient of these drops. A commonly used product, as identified by its BRAND name, would be MINIMS® TROPICA-MIDE with the ® indicating that that BRAND name was registered with a particular company (which was (and still is) Chauvin Pharmaceuticals in Europe, but the drug is now registered with Bausch & Lomb Surgical in the UK).

An unusual situation existed in the UK until law changes were implemented in 2005 for the naming of drugs, in that there were a number of British Approved Names (or BANs) as opposed to INNs. Examples included the topical ocular anaesthetics such as benoxinate (now renamed oxybuprocaine, a name which is now consistent with many European countries), amethocaine (now renamed tetracaine) and lignocaine (now renamed lidocaine).

Characteristics of sites of drug action on tissues and cells

Drugs usually work in the human body by interaction with specific 'receptors'. This attribute can often be an advantage in that a drug will selectively affect one receptor and not another so as to produce readily identified and specific effects. This interaction can be characterized in three inter-related ways (**Fig. 6.1**). These can be by in vitro laboratory studies (in which the amount of drug binding to tissues or parts of cells can actually be measured in relation to the amount of drug), by ex vivo studies (in which the effect of a drug on the physiological response of a tissue can be measured in relation to the drug concentration) and lastly by in vivo studies (in which the magnitude of a clinical effect can be measured, again in relation to the amount or dose of a particular drug). A good example to illustrate these slightly different measures will be to consider the action of the drug phenylephrine.

For an in vitro method, the steps would be as follows (Nathanson 1981; Mittag & Tormay 1985). Parts of the iris (or other) tissue could be removed from eyes

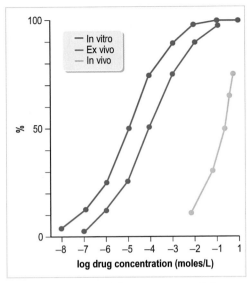

Figure 6.1 Principals of drug interaction with 'receptors' as assessed by drug binding to iris muscle membranes in test tube experiments (in vitro), drug-induced contraction of iris muscle tissue in laboratory experiments (ex vivo) and drug-induced dilation of the pupil after presentation of a drug to the eye as eyedrops (in vivo). In the in vitro experiments, the y-axis is the proportion (%) of receptors occupied by bound drug. In the ex vivo experiments, the y-axis is the relative tension (%) of the contracted muscle, while in in vivo (living eye) studies the y-axis is the relative diameter of the pupil. Note that the x-axis is the concentration of the drug in moles/L on a logarithmic scale.

and the cells separated out and broken up into extremely small pieces. Following very-high-speed centrifugation, fragments of cell membranes (including those from iris muscle and neural tissue) can be obtained. These could be dispersed in an aqueous solution and incubated for a few hours, essentially in a test tube, with different amounts of phenylephrine. The fragments are again obtained by very-high-speed centrifugation so that a pellet and a supernatant are obtained. The pellet will contain membrane fragments to which some of the phenylephrine will have bound, while the supernatant contains the amount of the drug that did not bind to the membrane fragments. By comparing the amount of drug in the pellet versus the supernatant, one can produce a drug binding profile in relation to the concentration of phenylephrine in the original aqueous solution. This is shown as a graph in **Figure 6.1** (in vitro), and it should be noted that the x-axis has a logarithmic scale while the y-axis is the amount of bound drug (in this case presented as a percentage value). The plot is S-shaped and has an inflexion point at threshold (10%) and at saturation (90%) while the midpoint along the 'S' represents 50% binding. Each of these corresponds to a certain concentration of phenylephrine, and this type of plot tells us that the amount of drug that binds to a specific receptor (in this case on membranes of the iris dilation muscle tissue) is strictly proportional to the concentration of the drug. Furthermore, there is only a narrow range of concentrations over which this binding profile can be observed. In this example, the concentration at 50% binding is 10^{-5} M (or 0.01 mM), which is also equivalent to a solution concentration of 0.00025 g/100 mL or 0.00025% w/v of the drug. A little of the phenylephrine has bound at 10^{-7} M and almost all of the

binding sites are occupied at 10^{-3} M. If, for example, the membrane fragment had been only incubated with phenylephrine concentrations of between 10^{-10} and 10^{-6} M, then only partial binding would have been observed at the highest concentration. If the drug concentrations had been between 10^{-4} and 10^{-1} M, then it might even appear that the drug binding was independent of concentration since most or all the sites would be occupied at all concentrations tested. In neither case would the S-shaped curve be obtained. The most important concentration, for the in vitro binding, is that at which 50% of the receptor sites are occupied with the drug. It is also often known as the dissociation constant (or K_D) value.

For an ex vivo method, the whole iris tissue could be carefully dissected out from an eye (Van Alphen 1976; Matheny et al 1977). Narrow strips of tissue containing the dilator muscle could be mounted into an experimental chamber which supports both ends of the muscle strip and a small amount of tension applied. If the muscle strip was immersed for approximately 1 hour in an experimental solution that resembled the aqueous humour of the eye, then the iris muscle tissue would adopt a particular length and have a certain natural tension that could be measured with a strain or tension gauge. If phenylephrine were now added to the experimental solution, then it should cause the iris dilator muscle to contract and the tension to increase. This is the expected result of phenylephrine binding to those same receptors that were measured in the in vitro binding assay. The muscle strip could also be made to contract if a part of the long ciliary nerve were still attached, and a small electrical signal sent into the tissue. For phenylephrine, which is a specific alpha$_1$-adrenergic drug that binds to sympathetic nerve endings on the ciliary nerves (see later for explanation), the drug-induced contraction and increase in tension can be shown to be proportional to the concentration of the drug (phenylephrine). So, a similar response curve to the drug binding assay can be developed (**Fig. 6.1**, ex vivo) in which the y-axis could now be muscle tension. The x-axis is again logarithmic and the drug concentration that produces a just-measurable increase in muscle tension noted, as well as that which produced maximal or near maximal contraction (tension increase) and the concentration required to produce a 50% effect. These three concentrations are likely to be slightly higher than those measured in the in vitro assay simply because cell and tissue components other than the iris dilator muscle strip will non-specifically absorb some of the drug. These other tissue components include the melanin pigment characteristic of the posterior aspect of the iris tissue. Notwithstanding these non-specific effects, it should again be possible to demonstrate a distinct S-shaped dose–response plot for phenylephrine-induced contraction of the iris dilator muscle. If it were possible to dissect out small strips of iris tissue that only contained dilator muscle without any functional portions of iris sphincter muscle, then incubation of the iris muscle strip with tropicamide should produce no change in muscle tension. In reality, there might be a very slight relaxation (reduction in tension). This would be because tropicamide, as a specific blocker of muscarinic receptors on the iris sphincter muscle normally innervated by parasympathetic branches of the ciliary nerves, might relax any small parts of functional sphincter muscle in the isolated strip of tissue.

For an in vivo approach on a living eye, the same principles of specific drug interaction with receptors can be applied (Matsumoto et al 1982; Buckley et al 1987) (**Fig. 6.1**, in vivo). In this case, the iris tissue is inside the eye and surrounded by aqueous humour. If an eyedrop containing phenylephrine at a certain concentration were applied to the corneal surface, then some of the phenylephrine will permeate into the aqueous humour and reach the iris tissue. When the drug binds with the receptor sites, it would be expected to produce contraction of the iris dilator muscle, but not affect the iris sphincter because of its selective action. When the iris dilator muscle is stimulated, it contracts, pupil diameter increases and mydriasis occurs. Just as with the in vitro and ex vivo approaches, it can be shown that the increase in pupil diameter is proportional to the concentration of phenylephrine. When eyedrops are used, it is usual for the concentration to be expressed in w/v terms rather than molar terms. For example, if the eyedrop contained 0.125% w/v phenylephrine (i.e. 0.125 g/ 100 mL), little or no effect ($\leq$10% effect) on the pupil diameter can be observed. If the eyedrop contained 10% phenylephrine, the net increase in pupil diameter would be close to the maximal amount, while at 2.5% concentration approximately a 50% effect would be likely. In molar concentration terms, these amounts are higher than those shown to be effective in the in vitro or ex vivo assays. For example, phenylephrine 2.5% is equivalent to a 0.12 M (1.2×10^{-1} M) solution. The reason for the difference in effective concentrations is because only a very small amount of a drug in eyedrops actually gets into the aqueous humour. Even less reaches the iris muscles because of non-specific interaction with melanin and other tissue components (see later). Notwithstanding, the dose–response plot for phenylephrine-induced mydriasis is very similar in shape to the other two plots because of the specific binding to receptor sites.

Many of the drugs currently used as diagnostic pharmaceutical agents by optometrists have actions on the ocular end plates of the autonomic nervous system. As such, their actions can be described as outlined above. Notable exceptions are the actions of topical ocular anaesthetics (e.g. oxybuprocaine) (Doughty 2005). While these drugs have fairly selective effects on nerve activity in the cornea and conjunctiva, current evidence indicates that they achieve this by changing the characteristics of the nerve membranes themselves. A specific anaesthetic-binding receptor molecule has yet to be clearly identified. Similarly, certain antiinfective drugs (e.g. polymyxin B) also alter the permeability characteristics of cell membranes rather than act through a receptor protein, with the target in this case being bacterial cell membranes (Doughty 2008).

Not all drugs work by interacting with membrane-associated receptors or even cell membranes. Some drugs (e.g. the antibacterial agent chloramphenicol) bind to protein molecules inside the bacterial cells, namely the ribosome protein complexes (Doughty 2008). Some other antibacterial drugs (e.g. sulphacetamide) bind to the site of enzymes inside the bacterial cells. As with many drugs in systemic medications, these enzyme sites may be either inside or on the surface of cells. While the principles of drug interaction with enzymes are very similar to those described for membrane-associated receptor molecules, there are some differences. Notwithstanding, a drug interaction with an enzyme generally results in a clearly defined dose–response effect which can also be characterised by an S-shaped plot.

Pharmacological actions versus toxic effects

In modern-day medicine, the use of a well-described and defined drug in a pharmaceutical product generally carries little risk of toxic effects. However, since many of the drugs used in optometry work on the autonomic nervous system, overstimulation or extended suppression can result in a general imbalance in the control between the sympathetic and parasympathetic systems. These control mechanisms may be influenced secondarily by individual genetic make-up (Doughty & Lyle 1992a) but can produce a general malaise. Since such adverse reactions generally occur when the doses given are much higher than recommended, they are sometimes referred to as toxic effects, intoxication or even as a type of poisoning (Gray 1979). In most instances, spontaneous recovery of the autonomic balance will occur provided there is no repeated administration of the drug (Norden 1978; Yolton et al 1980; Applebaum & Jaanus 1983; Wildsoet 1985). It was once common for a small child to experience mild poisoning from having been given excess atropine eyedrops prior to a refraction (Gray 1979).

Additionally, there are other reasons for toxic effects. As outlined in the previous section, a remarkable property of many drugs is that they show a predicable interaction with a receptor molecule (or enzyme) over a fairly narrow range of concentrations. If the concentration of a drug within the vicinity of a target site is substantially higher than that needed to occupy all the binding sites then there is a risk of toxic effects. Similarly, for drugs that generally interact with cell membranes, there is always an inherent risk of toxic effects. In either case, these occur because the drug exerts non-specific effects on cells. For example, if all the receptors on a cell are saturated with a particular drug and this state is sustained, then the mechanisms of homeostasis (i.e. a balance between all the activities in a cell) can become upset and the cell is unable to adjust. If cell membranes are substantially affected by a drug (due to its chemical characteristics), general control of ionic permeability is lost, the cell is unable to adjust and will die. In some clinical situations, cell-based toxic effects can be evident if the ingredients of a pharmaceutical product alter cell homeostasis. An example is the presence of a cleaning agent or surfactant in a contact lens solution that dissolves part of the cell membranes of the corneal or conjunctival epithelia, resulting in punctate staining visible with fluorescein dye (see later). A more pronounced toxic effect on the ocular surface would occur if a chemical designed to kill bacteria (by rapidly oxidizing their cell membranes and so destroying permeability control mechanisms) was inadvertently placed on the eye. A 3% hydrogen peroxide solution, intended for contact lens disinfection, could be brought into contact with the eye if the peroxide was not neutralized and/or washed off the contact lens before insertion. In such a case, the extent of the damage to the cells is likely to be substantial, with large areas of epithelium removed. However, in many such toxic events, recovery of the ocular surface will occur as the dead cells are replaced by freshly dividing cells in the absence of the toxic agent.

Ingredients of ophthalmic pharmaceutical products

Drugs for diagnostic or therapeutic use can be presented to the eye in various forms. These contain a range of ingredients and are usually made available as a single- or multi-dose unit contained in a bottle or tube. The nature of the mixture of ingredients is termed the formulation, while the form of the container is known as the presentation of the product. Most ophthalmic products are liquids, dispensed in the form of eyedrops, but viscous drops, gels and ointments are also available.

For eyedrops, the liquid is an aqueous (water) solution containing saline and sometimes additional salts to produce an osmolality similar to the natural tear film (Mullen et al 1973; Sasaki et al 1996). The product contains the drug (the active ingredient) and a chemical agent both to produce a given pH level and to maintain that value. This pH can range from as low as 5.0 (e.g. for some topical ocular anaesthetics) to 8.0 (e.g. for some contact lens re-wetting solutions) but most products are formulated to have a pH between 6.5 and 7.5. The pH buffers are typically chemical compounds such as a mixture of sodium phosphate salts (referred to as a phosphate buffer), borate salts with boric acid (referred to a borate buffer), acetate or citrate salts. They are generally stable so that the product can be prepared and then kept for many months before being used. The product labelling may also indicate that small quantities of acid (e.g. hydrochloric acid) or alkali (e.g. sodium hydroxide) have been added to adjust the pH of the buffer mixture.

Many ophthalmic solutions also contain small quantities of 'polymers' or 'viscolizers' that increase the viscosity of the eyedrops to exceed that of natural tears. The actual increase in viscosity is dependent on the polymer used and the amount included (Sasaki et al 1996). Typical polymers include cellulose derivatives (e.g. hydroxypropylmethylcellulose, also known as hypromellose or HPMC), polyvinyl alcohol (also known as PVA), polyvinylpyrrollidone (also known as polyvidone or povidone) and sodium hyaluronate (also known as hyaluronan). Ophthalmic gels can be considered as very viscous solutions which also have an aqueous base with saline, but with a special type of polymer such as polyacrylic acid (generally referred to as a Carbomer base) (Doughty 2008).

Ophthalmic ointments are non-aqueous. The active ingredient is dispersed into a mixture of oily chemicals such as petrolatum, paraffin oils and wool fat (also known as a form of lanolin) and is generally immiscible with water or saline. This formulation will cause them to have a greasy texture.

The length of time for which a product can be kept is commonly referred to as the shelf life, and is the period between the date of manufacture (sometimes marked as D.O.M. on a bottle or package) and a use-by date (usually referred to as the expiration date, or as EXP on the product). This will usually be around 2 years. A few specialized products contain bicarbonate or carbonate salts as buffers but these are less stable and may require special packaging around the plastic container to ensure a good shelf life. Once opened, single-dose units (SDUs) should be used immediately and then discarded straight away. Other products (e.g. 5–15 mL bottles of eyedrops or 4 or 5 g plastic tubes) are for multiple or repeated use and it is a common recommendation for any such product to be discarded after 3 or 4 weeks of use. This multiple usage may be on different patients (e.g. diagnostic drugs) or on the same patient (e.g. a therapeutic drug product).

SDUs are for single use only because they contain no ingredients to stop microbial growth, and are often referred to as preservative-free (or PF) products. Solutions for multiuse will usually contain a preservative, as do many ophthalmic gels and ointments. A preservative is a chemical with antimicrobial actions (i.e. it will rapidly limit the growth of or even kill many common microorganisms), and is included in multi-dose products to reduce the chance of microorganisms multiplying in the product. Since ophthalmic products, by law, have to be prepared under sterile conditions, the source of the microorganisms is usually from external contamination. This is commonly the result of accidental contact of the opened end of the bottle or tube with the eyelashes, eyelid margin skin or the periocular skin. Even in a healthy eye, these sites are commonly colonized by bacteria, while in an infected eye there are much higher levels of the microorganism causing the infection. The commonest preservative in eyedrops is benzalkonium chloride (sometimes referred to as BAC). This is a quaternary ammonium compound. Alternatives to BAC include polidronium, cetrimide, the biguanide compounds (such as polyhexylmethylbiguanide, also known as PHMB), chlorhexidine or similar chemicals such as polyhexanide. Mercurial compounds such as thimerosal (also known as thiomersal) were once commonly used. While less prevalent nowadays, it should be noted that some very widely used ophthalmic products (e.g. chloramphenicol eyedrops) are preserved with a mercurial compound, in this case phenylmercuric acetate. While a necessity for any multiuse product, the presence of a preservative carries the risk of adverse reactions (since these chemicals are toxic to cells, especially at higher concentrations) and/or allergic reactions. The preservatives used in ophthalmic products are also widely used in other non-therapeutic products so a patient may develop an allergy to a skin cream which becomes manifest when an eyedrop containing the same preservative is instilled.

Drug delivery to the ocular tissues from ophthalmic pharmaceuticals

The active pharmaceutical agents in ophthalmic products are generally presented to the surface of the eye by instillation of eyedrops or application of gels or ointments. Both are best presented by first pulling down the lower eyelid. The drop, gel or ointment should be delivered into the lower cul-de-sac and then the eyelids closed for a short while (e.g. 30 seconds). A notable exception is the use of an ophthalmic strip (also known as a wafer) which has been pre-soaked in a solution, allowed to dry and then placed in sterile packaging. Just before use, the package is opened, the end of the strip re-wetted (preferably with a drop of sterile saline) and the flat surface of the strip briefly touched onto the surface of the bulbar conjunctiva. Care should be taken to avoid scraping the strip or its edge across the corneal surface. This method can be used to deliver a dye such as fluorescein to the surface of the eye, although eyedrops of fluorescein are also available.

Ocular pharmaceutical agents are generally designed so that the active ingredient either briefly covers the surface of the eye after mixing with the tear film (e.g. a dye such as fluorescein) or essentially coats the surface of the eye for a few minutes so that the drug can be absorbed into the corneal and conjunctival tissue and then permeates through the cornea into the anterior chamber. Once inside the eye, the drugs can produce their effects on the pupil or ciliary body. The drug will subsequently be washed out of the eye by the normal flow of aqueous humour through the trabecular meshwork and outflow facility to reach the peripheral ocular circulation and systemic circulation. Any of the pharmaceutical agents that fail to penetrate into the eye will normally pass down the nasolacrimal duct, where they can be absorbed into the systemic vasculature (Urtti & Salminen 1993; Sasaki et al 1996).

After presentation onto the surface of a generally healthy eye, only a small proportion of the active drug is actually absorbed into the cornea and conjunctiva (around 5%) and even smaller amounts get into the aqueous humour (around 1%). Therefore, most of the ingredients (>90%) of an ophthalmic product are available for systemic absorption via the nasolacrimal duct. The application of slight pressure over the puncta and/or the region over the nasolacrimal ducts for a short period of time after the pharmaceutical was used (e.g. for 30–60 s) will slow down the rate of systemic absorption (and even cause some of the product to spill onto the periocular skin) but cannot prevent the ultimate systemic absorption of the ingredients. Since the practice of 'punctal occlusion', or even just closing the eyelids for 30 s, is so often not performed, each time the patient blinks it will be promoting nasolacrimal drainage (White et al 1991).

If the intended action of the active ingredient is actually on the surface of the eye, then the effects will be immediate and often last for just a few minutes (Sasaki et al 1996; Doughty 2008). The rate of wash-out of simple aqueous solutions, even those containing a small amount of polymer, is usually between 15 and 40% per minute. If higher concentrations of a polymer are used, this may be reduced to just 5% per minute, providing the product itself does not elicit reflex lacrimation, which will increase the wash-out rate. With the use of an ophthalmic ointment, the time required for half of the ingredients to be washed from the ocular surface should be at least 15 minutes (i.e. the wash-out rate is now down to around 5% per minute or less) even if there is some reflex tearing, and can be as long as an hour. Accordingly, ophthalmic ointments provide a very effective means of prolonging contact of the active ingredient of the pharmaceutical with the surface of the eye (Doughty 2008).

Mechanisms of action of selected drugs for ophthalmic use

Drugs, as included in pharmaceutical products, can produce effects on the eye (or exogenous microorganisms on the eye) by a wide range of mechanisms (**Table 6.1**).

Table 6.1 Pharmacological mechanisms and clinical categories of drugs for ophthalmic use

Name of drug (chemical)	Pharmacological mechanism	Clinical use (category)
Fluorescein	Non-specific	Non-toxic dye
Rose bengal	Non-specific	Vital stain
Lissamine green	Non-specific	Vital stain (?)
Oxybuprocaine (benoxinate)	Blocks nerve Na^+ channels	Topical ocular anaesthetic
Proxymetacaine (proparacaine)	Blocks nerve Na^+ channels	Topical ocular anaesthetic
Tetracaine (amethocaine)	Blocks nerve Na^+ channels	Topical ocular anaesthetic
Lidocaine (lignocaine)	Blocks nerve Na^+ channels	Topical ocular anaesthetic
Tropicamide	Cholinergic blocking drug	Mydriatic (cycloplegic)
Phenylephrine	Adrenergic drug	Mydriatic
Cyclopentolate	Cholinergic blocking drug	Cycloplegic (mydriatic)
Atropine	Cholinergic blocking drug	Cycloplegic (mydriatic)
Pilocarpine	Cholinergic drug	Miotic
Dapiprazole	Adrenergic blocking drug	Miotic
Moxisylyte (thymoxamine)	Adrenergic blocking drug	Miotic
Propramidine	Antiinfective drug	Blocks bacterial ribose uptake
Sulphacetamide	Antiinfective drug	Inhibitor of bacterial metabolism
Polymyxin B	Antibiotic	Permeabilizes bacterial membranes
Bacitracin zinc	Antibiotic	Inhibits bacterial cell wall synthesis
Chloramphenicol	Antibiotic	Inhibits bacterial protein synthesis
Fusidic acid	Antibiotic	Inhibits bacterial protein synthesis

Eyewashes and ophthalmic irrigation solutions

If there is a need to remove a drug (pharmaceutical) from the ocular surface, tap water is definitely not the recommended option. Rather, it is best to use a small 20 or 25 mL ampoule of sterile, isotonic, non-preserved saline, i.e. 0.9% NaCl solution. The solution is osmotically balanced to the tear film (unlike tap water), and any unused amount is simply discarded. A contact lens 'saline' solution could be used as an alternative but this contains preservatives, and the use of the nozzle (or tube) on a saline aerosol canister is generally not a good way of trying to wash the surface of the eye.

Ophthalmic dyes and stains (fluorescein, rose bengal, lissamine green)

Ophthalmic dyes and stains are discussed in Chapters 7 and 17.

Topical ocular anaesthetics (oxybuprocaine, proxymetacaine, tetracaine, lidocaine)

A topical ocular anaesthetic can be used to block the sensory nerves on the surface of the eye and thereby facilitate examination. There are several slightly different drugs that can be used, classified according to their chemical structure (**Table 6.2**) (Doughty 2008). These drugs work by selectively blocking the ionic conductivity of the nerve membranes, notably to that of Na^+ ions. The mechanism of the ion channel blockade appears to be based on anaesthetic-induced changes in the phospholipid bilayer of cell membranes, and the net result is a slowing or complete block of the nerve signals (Doughty 2005). The clinical use of these topical ocular anaesthetics produces two remarkable changes, namely to reduce the eye blink reflex that will normally accompany a touch to the ocular surface, and can almost completely remove (albeit temporarily) the touch sensation from the ocular surface.

The anaesthetics, presented to the ocular surface in the form of eyedrops, will very quickly permeate through the most superficial cell layers of the corneal and conjunctival epithelia to reach the nerve endings. This takes only a couple of minutes in most individuals and the changes are temporary and reversible, as the anaesthetic will slowly be washed out of the tissues as well as being metabolized (broken down to inactive molecules). The clinical effects are dose-dependent (Polse et al 1978), but one usually uses only a single concentration of the drug with the option of using more than one drop if needed.

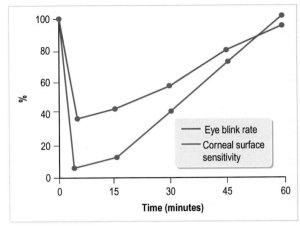

Figure 6.2 Expected effects of instillation of a topical ocular anaesthetic (e.g. oxybuprocaine 0.4%) on the spontaneous eye blink rate and on ocular surface sensitivity. The y-axis for eye blink activity is the relative (%) eye blink rate (SEBR, in eye blinks/min), while for the ocular surface sensitivity it is the relative value (%) for the sensitivity to a mechanical (touch) stimulus made to the corneal surface.

The first action of the topical ocular anaesthetic is to reduce the blink reflex (**Fig. 6.2**, eye blink rate). Normal healthy subjects usually blink 10 to 15 times per minute, and will attempt to close their eyes whenever the ocular surface is touched. However, within 5 minutes after instillation of a topical ocular anaesthetic, it can be expected that the spontaneous eye blink rate will be reduced along with the reflex blink. While some recovery occurs fairly quickly, it will generally take 10 to 15 minutes before a full reflex blink can be induced. The complete restoration of normal blink rate may take over an hour (Naase et al 2005).

With a single drop, it can be shown that there is a time-dependent reduction in the touch sensitivity of the ocular surface (**Fig. 6.2**, corneal surface sensitivity). This is not usually assessed per se, although some practitioners might advocate touching the edge of the cornea or the eyelid margin with a cotton bud applicator (or a wisp of cotton wool) to check that touch sensitivity has been reduced before making further contact with the cornea with instruments. However, from an experimental perspective it is possible to ascertain how much mechanical sensitivity is still present using a Cochet–Bonnet aesthesiometer (see Ch. 17). This instrument has a very fine nylon filament that can be adjusted in length. If fully extended to 60 mm in length, the filament is very pliable and a normal individual can just detect when this touches the central region of the cornea, i.e.

Table 6.2 Chemical classes of anaesthetic drugs and their uses

Chemical class (group) for anaesthetic drug	Examples (common names)	Uses
p-aminobenzoic acid esters	Tetracaine, oxybuprocaine, benzocaine, procaine	Topical and local
Benzoic acid amides	Lidocaine, mepivacaine, etidocaine, bupivacaine, prilocaine	Topical and local
m-aminobenzoic acid esters	Proxymetacaine	Topical
Benzoic acid esters	Cocaine	Topical
Phenoxymorpholines	Pramocaine	Topical
Quinoline carboxyamides	Cinchocaine	Topical

the sensitivity threshold is the 60 mm filament. As the anaesthetic takes effect, the fully extended filament cannot be felt but a much shorter and more rigid length of the filament can be felt. When using the Cochet–Bonet aesthesiometer, a good indication that the filament has been felt is when slight eyelid closure is attempted, i.e. the reflex blink occurs in response to a certain magnitude of stimulus. Within 5 minutes after instillation of an anaesthetic, the threshold sensitivity to the aesthesiometer is reduced to about 5 mm, and with this reduction in contact sensitivity other instruments (e.g. an applanation tonometer) can be placed on the surface of the eye. Once this peak effect is reached, some sensitivity starts to return almost immediately but it is usually 10 or 15 minutes before a patient can feel gentle contact with an applanation probe (when the sensitivity might be around 25 mm with the aesthesiometer filament). It usually takes about 30 minutes for full (normal) sensitivity to return.

As commercially available, usually in the form of eyedrops in single-dose units (Minims®), there is no substantial difference in efficacy between the different anaesthetics (Draeger et al 1984; Lawrenson et al 1998). However, there are two major reasons for multiple products being available, namely to avoid adverse reactions (due to allergy) and for patient and practitioner comfort and/or preference. The issue of possible allergy is very important and should always be checked for. The same or similar drugs are also widely used for other purposes (e.g. topical skin anaesthetics as well as in many dental procedures as injectable anaesthetics) (see **Table 6.1**) (Doughty 2008). This widespread use means that many patients will have already been exposed to these drugs and so could have become sensitized to the drug or other ingredients of the pharmaceutical agents. As outlined in **Table 6.1**, these drugs fall into different chemical classes. If a patient reports allergy to lidocaine (e.g. from a dental procedure), then an anaesthetic from a different chemical class should be used in the optometric assessment (e.g. proxymetacaine). If a patient reports an allergy to tetracaine, then lidocaine will likely be a good alternative. The issue of comfort should also be considered as these eyedrops produce a brief but sometimes quite substantial stinging sensation. This probably results from the eyedrops being acidic (pH around 5.0). However, the stinging will usually wear off in 5 minutes or less, especially if the eyes are closed for 30 s after the eyedrops are instilled. In terms of practitioner preferences beyond simply choosing to use the eyedrop that seems to sting less, some topical ocular anaesthetics are marketed as drops that also contain fluorescein. These options are useful if applanation tonometry is being performed (e.g. use proxymetacaine with fluorescein) or if slit-lamp assessment is being carried out on eyes where injury has occurred or is suspected (e.g. use lidocaine with fluorescein).

Topical ocular anaesthetics are often referred to as local anaesthetics. While the effect produced is local (to the ocular surface), the use of such a term carries the considerable risk of associating the use of a topical anaesthetic with that administered by injection, e.g. lidocaine for dental work. The injection of local anaesthetics (e.g. in dental procedures) is usually uneventful but in rare cases can result in very serious adverse reactions (e.g. on cardiac function) and even death (Wildsoet 1985). A case cannot be made that the same degree of risk, no matter how rare, can be logically applied to the topical use of such anaesthetics. If there were such risks to the use of topical ocular (or skin or mouthwash) anaesthetic products, then surely fewer would be available as over-the-counter non-prescription products (Doughty 2008).

Mydriatics (tropicamide, phenylephrine)

Two drugs are used routinely as mydriatics in optometric practice to dilate the pupil. One (tropicamide) is generally used alone and is often adequate. The other drug (phenylephrine) is better used in combination with tropicamide when adequate pupil dilation may be difficult to achieve (Doughty 2008).

Tropicamide binds specifically with receptors on the iris sphincter muscle which are located on the postsynaptic membranes of the parasympathetic nerves that drive the pupillary light reflex (i.e. pupil constriction when a bright light is shone into the eye). The drug acts to block these postsynaptic receptors so that the neurotransmitter being released from the parasympathetic nerves cannot activate these receptors to produce contraction of the sphincter muscle. As this blocks parasympathetic receptors, it is termed a parasympatholytic drug and, since it falls into the same chemical class as muscarine, it is also often referred to as an antimuscarinic drug. The preferred terminology is to describe it as a cholinergic blocker, as the parasympathetic nerves use the neurotransmitter acetylcholine. The net effect of tropicamide is to dilate the pupil due to relaxation of the iris sphincter muscle.

Just like topical ocular anaesthetics, tropicamide has to permeate through the cornea, but it also has to diffuse to the iris tissue. This permeation and diffusion takes time, and so the mydriatic response is slower than that of topical anaesthesia. Generally, it will take around 15 to 20 minutes for adequate dilation to be achieved (**Fig. 6.3**). This dilation is rarely complete (i.e. the pupil has not opened to its fullest extent) and this can be partly attributed to the fact that insufficient drug has reached the receptors to saturate all of them fully. The mydriatic effect of tropicamide is dose dependent (Yoshida & Mishima 1975), with 1.0% concentration generally producing slightly greater dilation than 0.5% w/v (**Fig. 6.3**). For most patients, at least 3 or 4 mm net dilation should be possible from the pre-mydriatic pupil diameter (under bright light) of approximately 3 mm. That

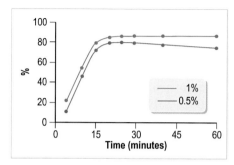

Figure 6.3 Expected time-dependent effects of the instillation of different doses of a mydriatic drug (e.g. tropicamide) on the pupil diameter of adults where 0.5% indicates use of an eyedrop with a concentration of 0.5% and 1% indicates the use of an eyedrop containing 1% tropicamide. The y-axis is the relative diameter of the pupil where 100% indicates the maximal dilation possible.

full dilation is not achieved is not usually a problem since a 6 mm pupil generally allows an acceptable view inside the eye (see Ch. 18). It should also be remembered that the drug has blocked the pupil light reflex so the pupil does not constrict when light from an ophthalmoscope or slit lamp are shone in the eye. While the mydriasis is incomplete, the maximum dilation should be maintained for at least 30 minutes before recovery begins. This is because suitable concentrations of drug persist in the vicinity of the iris tissue before it is slowly washed out of the eye by the normal flow of aqueous humour. In many patients, a notable recovery of pupil diameter has occurred within a couple of hours, and it is common for the pupil to return to its pre-mydriatic size between 6 and 12 hours post-instillation, and sometimes in significantly shorter time periods (Doughty & Lyle 1992b). The net effect of tropicamide eyedrops also varies with iris pigmentation, with patients having dark-brown irides exhibiting less dilation with the standard dose of tropicamide.

Phenylephrine binds to postsynaptic alpha$_1$-adrenergic receptors that are present on the sympathetic nerves that supply the dilator muscle. It activates these receptors and therefore augments the normal sympathetic response that dilates the pupil (e.g. when a subject is frightened or emotionally aroused by anger or pleasure). Phenylephrine is a sympathomimetic drug, and the preferred terminology is that it is an adrenergic agonist. The net effect of phenylephrine is to dilate the pupil due to contraction of the dilator muscle (Doughty 2008).

Again, phenylephrine must permeate through the cornea and diffuse to the iris before pupillary dilation can occur. Indeed, after presentation of phenylephrine 2.5% w/v eyedrops to the ocular surface, there is often a delay of 20 to 30 minutes before any dilation is noted. It is not unusual for the dilation to take 60 minutes to reach its maximum. As with tropicamide, when used at the normally available concentrations, phenylephrine produces only partial dilation, with a net change of only 2 to 3 mm (rather than the 3 to 4 mm normally seen with tropicamide) (Doughty et al 1988). Furthermore, since phenylephrine has no effect on the light reflex of the pupil, some pupil closure will occur when a bright light is shone into the eye. Therefore, when using phenylephrine 2.5% alone there is less chance of obtaining a 6 mm pupil. A partial dilation will generally be maintained for at least an hour, followed by a slow recovery, so the pupil (at least under dim light) may still be slightly dilated 12 or even 24 hours later. It should be noted that if phenylephrine 10% eyedrops are used, the net pupil dilation can be expected to be much greater (see **Fig. 6.1**, in vivo). However, in routine optometric practice, the use of this high concentration of phenylephrine is not recommended as it carries a risk of unwanted systemic sympathetic reactions (e.g. increased pulse, flushing, raised blood pressure, etc.) and such effects could be serious for those with pre-existing cardiovascular problems.

With tropicamide and phenylephrine acting on different iris muscles, their combined use will be expected to produce more substantial mydriasis (Doughty & Lyle 1992b). For example, instillation of one drop of phenylephrine 2.5% followed 5 minutes later by a drop of tropicamide 0.5% or 1% is likely give a 1 mm greater net dilation than either drug used on its own (Kergoat et al 1989), so that a net dilation of 4 or 5 mm can be achieved. This can be advantageous in patients whose pupils are difficult to dilate, such as elderly diabetics (providing they do not have substantial cardiovascular disease that would contraindicate the use of the phenylephrine).

The use of tropicamide and/or phenylephrine eyedrops for mydriasis is usually uneventful. Both may produce a transient stinging sensation but this is usually less than for a topical ocular anaesthetic. Some phenylephrine products may be stabilized with bisulphites and these can be a cause of notable allergic reactions including bronchoconstriction.

Cycloplegics (cyclopentolate, tropicamide, homatropine, atropine)

For routine optometric practice, there is really only one drug that is used as a cycloplegic, namely cyclopentolate. It is used in children of all ages (Stolovitch et al 1992). Tropicamide has some cycloplegic action and can be used as an alternative to cyclopentolate in teenagers and adults should a cycloplegic refraction be needed (albeit rather unusually). Tropicamide might also be used in childhood screening clinics where an autorefractor is being used, but merely as an aid to reducing the child's accommodative function rather than obtaining a true measure of their refractive error. Homatropine was widely used before cyclopentolate and tropicamide became available in the late 1950s. While atropine eyedrops have been used for cycloplegic refractions for over 100 years, there are few instances nowadays where a practitioner can justify subjecting a young child to the potentially unpleasant experience of being 'atropinized' (Gray 1979; Doughty 2008).

Cyclopentolate, like tropicamide, is a cholinergic blocking drug and therefore may also be referred to as an antimuscarinic agent. In addition to blocking receptors on the iris sphincter muscle, it has a substantial affinity for the parasympathetic nerve endings in the ciliary body muscles. The net result of the block is a relaxation of the ciliary body, and a relative state of cycloplegia is produced. The same mechanism applies to tropicamide except it has relatively poor efficacy as a cycloplegic, whereas both homatropine and especially atropine produce greater (and longer lasting) cycloplegia than cyclopentolate.

The cycloplegic drug is used to stop a child accommodating during retinoscopy. Assessment of accommodative ability can be made by measuring the amplitude of accommodation to a near visual stimulus, e.g. by using an RAF rule or similar near-point target (see Ch. 15) (Gimpel et al 1994). The penetration of cyclopentolate into the eye is generally slightly slower than for tropicamide and it usually takes 20 to 30 minutes for maximum cycloplegia to be achieved. The response to cyclopentolate is usually dose dependent (**Fig. 6.4**). With the use of cyclopentolate 0.5% w/v or 1.0% w/v eyedrops, the relaxation of accommodation is not complete, i.e. some accommodation is still possible. This is again partly due to the incomplete occupation of all receptors on the ciliary muscles. After 30 minutes, the residual amplitude of accommodation is generally around 10% of the original value or below 2 D. At this level of accommodation, any involuntary but slight accommodation during retinoscopy is unlikely to have a measurable clinical effect during the measurement of refractive error. The state

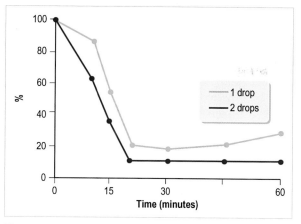

Figure 6.4 Expected time-dependent effects of the instillation of different doses of a potent cycloplegic (e.g. cyclopentolate) on the amplitude of accommodation of children where an eyedrop with a concentration of 0.5% was used with the total dose being either 1 drop or 2 drops, as indicated. The y-axis is the relative magnitude of the near-point amplitude of accommodation, where 100% indicates the maximal value possible in the absence of the cycloplegic drug. Note that the lesser dose may leave a significant residual accommodation.

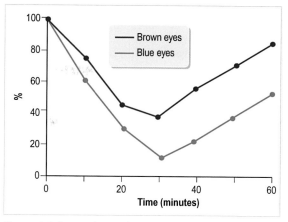

Figure 6.5 Expected time-dependent effects of the instillation of a less potent cycloplegic (e.g. tropicamide 1%) on the amplitude of accommodation of adults with lightly pigmented (blue eyes) or darkly pigmented (brown eyes) irides. The y-axis is the relative magnitude of the near-point amplitude of accommodation, where 100% indicates the maximal value possible in the absence of the cycloplegic drug. Note the rapid recovery of near-point accommodation (reading ability) especially in those with dark irides (brown eyes).

of cycloplegia should persist for at least 1 hour, or even 2 hours if the 1% concentration was used, after which time the drug dissociates and is slowly washed out of the eye, so that recovery of accommodative ability occurs over the next 6 to 12 hours. The efficacy of cyclopentolate as a cycloplegic is usually reduced in patients with highly pigmented eyes, but it is acceptable to use two drops of either concentration. As cyclopentolate has a stronger effect on the iris sphincter muscle, it is not unusual for the pupil to be visibly dilated on the morning after instillation. The use of cyclopentolate eyedrops, especially in young children, may be regarded with some apprehension as they will sting upon instillation. If the resultant episode of crying is to be avoided, then parental cooperation and practitioner expertise are needed, otherwise the drug will simply be washed from the ocular surface and inadequate cycloplegia will be obtained (see Ch. 28). Some practitioners advocate the use of a topical anaesthetic, to be administered a few minutes before the cyclopentolate.

The use of cyclopentolate eyedrops as an aid to refraction is generally without consequence. While the drug is a strong cholinergic blocker, it is uncommon for systemic parasympatholytic adverse effects to occur in children (but see later section on atropine). However, in infants even a small amount of systemic absorption of cyclopentolate may cause slight gastrointestinal disturbance which can manifest as feeding intolerance. In young children, the same absorption may cause small changes in the regularity of toilet routine, e.g. slight constipation or difficulty in urinating, but this is usually for less than a day.

Cyclopentolate 0.5% may be used in teenagers requiring a cycloplegic refraction, but in these and older individuals the weaker cycloplegic tropicamide may also be used. This is justified since the amplitude of accommodation decreases substantially with age (see Ch. 15), and tropicamide is adequate to give residual accommodation of 2 D. However, the cycloplegic effect is not usually sustained and some recovery can start almost immediately after the lowest amplitude has

been reached (Mordi et al 1986) (**Fig. 6.5**). For this reason, the timing of the refraction is more critical to ensure that the ciliary muscle is maximally relaxed when tropicamide is used as a cycloplegic.

As noted earlier, homatropine and atropine were routinely used cycloplegics before cyclopentolate became available. As a result of its poor penetration into the eye (as eyedrops or ointment), effective cycloplegia with atropine requires several doses over a 2- or 3-day period, e.g. one drop morning and night for 2 days and then again on the morning of the scheduled refraction. It might be argued that the cycloplegic effect produced is remarkable (i.e. no residual accommodation at all) and that this is the only way to determine the true refractive error in a hyperopic child. However, such repeated dosing with an antimuscarinic drug carries the almost unavoidable risk of systemic side effects and these can be substantial. The risk of adverse reactions is far greater than for cyclopentolate (even those associated with the use of a stronger concentration of cyclopentolate eyedrops, such as the 2% concentration which is marketed in some countries). Beyond any gastrointestinal disturbances of the type noted for cyclopentolate, the parasympatholytic side effects of atropine may extend to palpitations, racing pulse and skin flushing, leading to the one time-honoured caution of the practitioner needing to be on the lookout for 'Hot as a hare, Red as a beet, Dry as a bone, Blind as a bat, Mad as a wet hen' (Gray 1979). These effects, to varying degrees, are both predictable and almost unavoidable since some of each dose of atropine administered to the eye will be absorbed systemically (both via the nasolacrimal duct and through the conjunctival circulation). When dosing is extended over 2 or 3 days, it is not surprising that some children present with so-called atropine 'poisoning' after such therapy. Even more importantly from the perspective of patient management, the effects of atropine on the eye are not only substantial but sustained. Reading ability may be lost for 2 or 3 days after the administration, while the pupil may take a week or more to return to normal.

Two closing notes on the use of cyclopentolate and possible adverse reactions are appropriate, within the context of what has been presented for atropine. In rare cases, the use of any antimuscarinic eyedrops has been associated with what might be referred to as central nervous system (CNS) disturbances. Under such circumstances, a patient may report disorientation, confusion or even experience hallucinations. The net result, especially for a child, could be unexpected and potentially alarming behaviour. Powerful antimuscarinic drugs such as benztropine are used systemically for patients with CNS-based disturbances in (motor) coordination. Therefore, the pharmacology of the CNS adverse reaction should ease the mind of the practitioner unfortunate enough to experience such an episode of uncontrolled behaviour following administration of antimuscarinic eyedrops. It is unknown why it should occur more frequently with cyclopentolate but perhaps it is because the drug is rapidly and effectively absorbed into the body after the eyedrops are administered (Urtti & Salminen 1993). This presents a further issue to all practitioners for there is an increasing recent trend to 'place pressure over lacrimal sac' after instillation of eyedrops. If cyclopentolate is being absorbed by the conjunctiva, then no amount of punctal occlusion will stop such a reaction.

Miotics (pilocarpine, dapiprazole, moxisylyte)

As part of a diagnostic evaluation of the eye, there is rarely any need for a miotic. However, it was once common practice to at least offer the patient a miotic after a mydriatic had been used (to prompt recovery), while a practitioner in a rural area may want the support of having access to a miotic in the unlikely event of an angle closure following pupillary mydriasis. It is beyond the scope of this chapter to address either of these in detail (see Ch. 7).

The time-honoured miotic, in use for well over a hundred years, is pilocarpine. It is a parasympathetic agonist, better known as a cholinergic drug. It specifically binds to the postsynaptic membranes of the parasympathetic nerves supplying both the iris and ciliary muscles. It also has a substantial relaxing effect on the smooth muscles surrounding the vasculature of the conjunctiva. In response to pilocarpine binding, the postsynaptic receptors are activated and so the parasympathetic response is augmented, the sphincter muscle contracts and the pupil constricts. In addition, as a result of an indirect action on the ciliary body (which will contract, at least in younger patients), aqueous outflow facility is increased so the net rate of aqueous humour drainage should increase. The net result should be a lowering of the intraocular pressure. The effects of pilocarpine on the pupil are very much dose dependent, with threshold effects being easily observable at concentrations as low as 0.5%, with maximal and sustained miosis being achievable with the use of eyedrops containing 10% or even 12% pilocarpine w/v (Yoshida & Mishima 1975; Rengstorff & Royston 1976; Doughty & Lyle 1991). At lower concentrations, the effects should start to wear off in a few hours, while a much longer time will be required for the pupil to return to normal if high concentrations or repeated doses are used. Since pilocarpine will often be used after a mydriatic, it should be noted that this could produce miosis in two different ways. If the pupil had been dilated with tropicamide (or another antimuscarinic agent), then pilocarpine has to displace tropicamide from the postsynaptic receptors so that it can then enhance the effects of acetylcholine. However, if the pupil had been dilated with an adrenergic drug such as phenylephrine, then the postsynaptic receptors on the sphincter muscle are still accessible to the pilocarpine without the need to displace the phenylephrine. As a result, pilocarpine will be expected to display slightly superior efficacy in constricting a phenylephrine-dilated pupil than one dilated with tropicamide (since there is no direct competition for the receptors) (Doughty & Lyle 1991).

Two other miotics deserve brief note, namely dapiprazole and moxisylyte (also known by its BAN as thymoxamine). Dapiprazole eyedrops are marketed in some countries, while moxisylyte was once marketed in the UK. Both have been advocated for the purpose of constricting a pupil after the use of a mydriatic and work differently from pilocarpine (Doughty & Lyle 1992b). Both of these drugs are alpha-adrenergic antagonists, i.e. sympatholytic drugs. They bind to the postsynaptic receptors on the dilator muscle and so will block the action of the sympathetic transmitter. Therefore, the dilator muscle cannot contract and, even under even modest illumination, the pupil should close as the light reflex mechanism is still intact via the iris sphincter muscle. If used after an adrenergic mydriatic, these adrenergic blockers will need to displace the mydriatic from the dilator, and the action of the adrenergic blocker drugs on the dilator will be working against the drugs on the sphincter. In either case, when used after a mydriatic, these adrenergic blocking drugs have been shown to have some efficacy in enhancing the rate of return of the pupil to normal size but the miotic effect is not as substantial as that observed with pilocarpine.

Topical ocular antiinfectives (propamidine, sulphacetamide, polymyxin B, bacitracin, chloramphenicol, fusidic acid)

Based on the law in different countries, some optometrists or the general public may have access to or be allowed to use certain drugs categorized as topical ocular antiinfectives. This term means that drugs which work against bacteria causing an infection of the external eye or adnexa are presented to the external surface of the eye (as eyedrops) or to the eyelid margins (usually as an ointment). The term anti-infective is the most appropriate term, rather than antibiotics. This is because an antibiotic is a drug that has been identified in and then extracted from a microorganism (e.g. a fungus or mould) and shown to have an adverse effect on another microorganism (e.g. a bacterium). The best-known example of this is penicillin, which was first isolated and used for treatment of bacterial infections of the eye in the 1950s. However, before that time, there were other chemicals, which were synthesized in a laboratory, and these are therefore not antibiotics although they were known to have antibacterial effects. Examples of these antiinfective drugs are propamidine and sulphacetamide.

Antibacterial drugs work by a range of mechanisms which allow one to combat a bacterial infection of the eye (Hugo & Russell 1998; Doughty 2008). If one drug product fails to work, there is a good chance that another will be successful because it is rare for a bacterium to develop multiple mechanisms of resistance to a range of antibiotics currently used for eye infections.

Propamidine and its derivative dibromopropamidine are synthetic drugs with an antiinfective action. These drugs exert general membrane effects that reduce the ability of bacteria to absorb essential nutrients (such as ribose sugars) from their environment (e.g. on the moist skin around the eye or on the mucous membranes of the eye). If the bacteria are deprived of ribose sugars, for example, then their ability to produce energy and synthesize DNA is impaired. As a result, the bacteria fail to thrive and so these drugs are bacteriostatic as the rate of replication of the bacteria is slowed down (Doughty 2008). These drugs have been used for many years to treat minor infections of the external eye. They can be available as non-prescription, over-the-counter products for treatment of both eye and skin infections.

Sulphacetamide and related 'sulpha' drugs became widely available in the 1940s and were once used very extensively before resistance to them developed. These drugs inhibit an enzyme activity called dihydrofolate reductase, which is present inside bacteria and required for what is called the intermediate metabolism of these cells. By this folic acid-related activity, the bacteria synthesize many molecules, some of which are required for making DNA (Hugo & Russell 1998; Doughty 2008). As with propamidine, if bacteria are exposed to high enough levels of sulpha drugs, they fail to thrive.

Polymyxin B is a true antibiotic that has an adverse effect on the membranes of susceptible bacteria, including many that occur on the skin and mucous membranes. The drug inserts itself into the lipid membrane bilayer and, as a result, makes these membranes 'leaky' to ions and essential metabolites (Doughty 2008). If the bacteria cannot control their internal ion concentrations then, just like mammalian cells, they will die fairly quickly. Polymyxin B, if used at high concentrations, is therefore bactericidal. Bacitracin is another antibiotic which works on the cell walls of bacteria rather than on their cell membranes (Doughty 2008). Bacteria that have a substantial cell wall are known as Gram-positive organisms because, when a sample containing these bacteria is stained with a Gram stain and then viewed under a microscope, the cell wall can be seen to be visibly coloured by this stain. The cell wall serves to protect these bacteria against a harsh or changing environment. Bacitracin, as a zinc complex, interferes with the internal synthetic process by which bacteria make their cell walls. In this sense, bacitracin is similar in action to penicillin except that it affects a different part of the synthetic process. Notwithstanding, if a bacterium is unable to synthesize and assemble an effective cell wall, it will be stressed and even killed the next time it encounters a change in its environment. Bacitracin, as usually used, is certainly bacteriostatic but can be indirectly bactericidal if used often enough. Both drugs can be used alone, but it is more common for them to be used together. In some countries there are non-prescription, over-the-counter products containing both polymyxin B and bacitracin for treating minor eye and skin infections.

Chloramphenicol is another true antibiotic, first isolated in the 1950s and has been in widespread clinical use for eye infections since that time. Unlike the other antiinfectives and antibiotics so far mentioned, chloramphenicol is a good broad-spectrum antibiotic. This means that it can be expected to be active against many types of bacteria. A case can be made that, since its use has been largely restricted to ocular infections (although it can still be used systemically for very severe life-threatening bacterial infections unresponsive to other antibiotics), the development of resistance has been small. It achieves its broad-spectrum action by inhibiting certain stages in the sequence of protein synthesis in bacteria. Since such synthesis is essential for the bacteria to replicate, exposure of bacteria to chloramphenicol results in a prompt slowing of the rate of division and so the spread of the infection; thus chloramphenicol is bacteriostatic. Beyond having been available in the form of eyedrops and ointments as prescription-only medicines for 50 years, recent changes in UK law (for example) mean that it is also available to the public from a pharmacy (without a prescription) for the treatment of bacterial conjunctivitis. All optometrists in the UK are allowed to use this antibiotic.

The last antibiotic is chosen as another example of a protein synthesis inhibitor (i.e. it achieves the same net effect as chloramphenicol although it works at a slightly different site in the protein synthesis mechanism; Doughty & Dutton 2006), but one with a narrow spectrum of action. This means that it can only be expected to work on certain types of bacteria, but these include those commonly causing infections of the conjunctiva and eyelid margins, provided there are no concurrent infections of the nose, throat or lungs. The bacteria that often cause the latter conditions are generally more resistant or completely resistant to fusidic acid. Fusidic acid is also widely used for bacterial infections of the skin, and so there is also a higher chance of general resistance to this antibiotic. Notwithstanding, it is worthy of mention as the only antibiotic preparation available as a viscous eyedrop, i.e. it is presented to the eye neither as a conventional eyedrop (that is readily washed away) nor an ointment (which is eminently suitable for providing antibiotic cover for the overnight period following a single application at bedtime). The viscous eyedrop can be expected to stay on the surface of the eye to provide antibacterial action for a time period somewhere between conventional eyedrops and an ophthalmic ointment. Recent changes in law (2005) mean that all optometrists in the UK are also allowed to use this antibiotic as soon as they have completed their training.

Products used in first aid and emergency procedures

In routine optometric practice, there are really only two special products that might be considered for first aid or emergency procedures. It is unlikely that either will be found in a normal optometric practice (unless specific legislation requires this).

The first is that of an emergency eye wash. Large bottles (e.g. 500 mL or even 1 L) of buffered saline should be used to irrigate the surface of the eye following accidental exposure or contact with any toxic chemical. The same would likely be used at an accident and emergency (A&E) department of a hospital but they, just as any factory using toxic chemicals, may also have an emergency eyewash station. This is a sink fitted with special taps that will direct jets of water into the eyes, which will be used for copious irrigation of the external eye. If emergency eyewash is used in an optometric practice, it should only be as a first measure before getting the patient to an A&E department at a hospital as soon as possible.

A second pharmaceutical appropriate for emergency treatment is injectable adrenaline for management of severe anaphylactic shock. Very rarely, a patient develops an acute and severe systemic bronchopulmonary reaction following instillation of an eyedrop. The systemic reaction follows from systemic absorption through the nasolacrimal duct, and the reaction can be so severe as to be life threatening. A single systemic administration, by subcutaneous injection of adrenaline from an EpiPen (or similar) will counter the anaphylactic reaction at least to the extent that the patient can breathe. As with emergency eyewash, the optometric administration of adrenaline is a remedial measure prior to getting paramedical support or getting the patient to hospital in an ambulance.

References

Applebaum M, Jaanus S D 1983 Use of diagnostic pharmaceutical agents and incidence of adverse effects. American Journal of Optometry & Physiological Optics 60:384–388

Buckley C, Curin D M, Docherty J et al 1987 Ageing and apha₁ adrenoceptors in the iris. Eye 1:211–216

Doughty M J 2005 Diagnostic and therapeutic pharmaceutical agents relevant to contact lens practice. In: Bennett E, Weissman B A (eds) Clinical contact lens practice. Lippincott-Williams & Wilkins, Philadelphia, pp 773–825

Doughty M J 2008 Drugs, medications and the eye. Smawcastellane Information Services, Helensburgh, Dunbartonshire G84 7HL, Scotland. 17th edition

Doughty M J, Dutton G N 2006 Fusidic acid viscous eyedrops – an evaluation of pharmacodynamics, pharmacokinetics and clinical use for UK optometrists. Ophthalmic and Physiological Optics 26:343–361

Doughty M J, Lyle W M 1991 Dapiprazole, an alpha adrenergic blocking drug, as alternative miotic to pilocarpine or moxisylyte (thymoxamine) for reversing tropicamide mydriasis. Canadian Journal of Optometry 53:111–117

Doughty M J, Lyle W M 1992a Ocular pharmacogenetics. In: Fatt H V, Griffin J R, Lyle W M (eds) Genetics for primary eye care practioners. Butterworth-Heinemann, Toronto, pp 179–193

Doughty M J, Lyle W M 1992b A review of the clinical pharmacokinetics of pilocarpine, moxisylyte (thymoxamine) and dapiprazole in the reversal of diagnostic pupillary dilation. Optometry and Vision Science 69:358–368

Doughty M J, Lyle W M, Trevino R et al 1988 A study of mydriasis produced by topical phenylephrine 2.5% in young adults. Canadian Journal of Optometry 50:40–60

Draeger J, Langenbucher H, Banert C 1984 Efficacy of topical anaesthetics. Ophthalmic Research 16:135–138

Gimpel G, Doughty M J, Lyle W M 1994 Large sample study of the effects of phenylephrine 2.5% eyedrops on the amplitude of accommodation in man. Ophthalmic and Physiological Optics 14:123–128

Gray L G 1979 Avoiding adverse effects of cycloplegics in infants and children. Journal of the American Optometric Association 50: 465–470

Hugo W B, Russell A D 1998 Pharmaceutical microbiology, 6th edition. Blackwell Science, Oxford

Kergoat H, Lovasik J V, Doughty M J 1989 A pupillographic evaluation of a phenylephrine 5% – tropicamide 0.8% combination mydriatic. Journal of Ocular Pharmacology 5:199–216

Lawrenson J G, Edgar D F, Tanna G K et al 1998 Comparison of the tolerability and efficacy of unit-dose, preservative-free topical ocular anaesthetics. Ophthalmic and Physiological Optics 18:393–400

Matheny J L, Carrier G O, Ahlquist R P 1977 Role of neuronal and extraneuronal uptake in responses of rabbit iris dilator muscle to levoarterenol and phenylephrine. Journal of Pharmaceutical Sciences 66:93–95

Matsumoto S, Tsuru T, Araie M et al 1982 Pharmacokinetics of phenylephrine hydrochloride in the normal human eye. Japanese Journal of Ophthalmology 26:338–344

Mittag T W, Tormay A 1985 Adrenergic receptor subtypes in rabbit iris–ciliary body membranes. Classification by radioligand studies. Experimental Eye Research 40:239–249

Mordi J A, Lyle W M, Mousa G Y 1986 Does prior instillation of a topical anesthetic enhance the effect of tropicamide? American Journal of Optometry and Physiological Optics 63:290–293

Mullen W, Shepherd W, Labovitz J 1973 Ophthalmic preservatives and vehicles. Survey of Ophthalmology 17:469–483

Naase T, Doughty M J, Button N F 2005 An assessment of the pattern of spontaneous eyeblink activity under the influence of topical ocular anaesthesia. Graefe's Archives Clinical and Experimental Ophthalmology 243:306–312

Nathanson J A 1981 Human ciliary process adrenergic receptors: pharmacological characterization. Investigative Ophthalmology and Visual Science 21:798–804

Norden L C 1978 Adverse reactions to topical autonomic agents. Journal of the American Optometric Association 49:75–79

Polse K A, Kener R J, Jauregui M J 1978 Dose–response effects of corneal anesthetics. American Journal of Optometry and Physiological Optics 55:8–14

Rengstorff R, Royston M 1976 Miotic drugs. A review of ocular, visual and systemic complications. American Journal of Optometry and Physiological Optics 53:70–80

Sasaki H, Yamamura K, Nishida K 1996 Delivery of drugs to the eye by topical application. Progress in Retinal and Eye Research 15:583–620

Stolovitch C, Lowenstein A, Nemet P et al 1992 The use of cyclopentolate versus atropine cycloplegia in Caucasian children. Binocular Vision Quarterly 7:93–96

Urtti A, Salminen L 1993 Minimizing systemic absorption of topically administered drugs. Survey of Ophthalmology 37:435–456

Van Aphen G W H M 1976 The adrenergic receptors of the intraocular muscles of the human eye. Investigative Ophthalmology 15:502–505

White W L, Glover A T, Buckner A 1991 Effect of blinking on tear elimination as evaluated by dacryscintigraphy. Ophthalmology 91:367–369

Wildsoet C 1985 Diagnostic drugs – what are the risks? Australian Journal of Optometry 68:85–95

Yolton D P, Smith Kandell J, Yolton R L 1980 Diagnostic pharmaceutical agents: side effects encountered in a study of 15 000 applications. Journal of the American Optometric Association 51:113–118

Yoshida S, Mishima S 1975 Pharmacokinetic analysis of the pupil response to topical pilocarpine and tropicamide. Japanese Journal of Ophthalmology 19:121–138

CHAPTER 7

Diagnostic drugs

Carly S Y Lam

Introduction

Ophthalmic drugs are administered to the eye for three main purposes: diagnostic, therapeutic or prophylactic. Optometrists use drugs to investigate, diagnose and differentiate clinical conditions. Optometrists in countries such as the United States and Australia and more recently in the United Kingdom also use drugs for therapeutic purposes to treat conditions primarily in the anterior segment of the eye. In addition, in many states in the US, optometrists are also permitted to treat glaucoma. Several recent overviews have summarized both the dynamic changes and the current scene in optometric practice for the use of both diagnostic and therapeutic drugs (Edgar 1998; Mason & Mason 2002; Soroka et al 2006).

With the extended scope of optometry practice and the increasingly recognized importance of the primary eye care provider, optometrists are relying more on the use of ophthalmic drugs to assist them in making an accurate judgement of clinical conditions. Drugs that dilate the pupil aid in examination of the fundus (see Ch. 18), while agents that temporarily anaesthetize the cornea facilitate contact tonometry (Ch. 24), gonioscopy (Ch. 17) and ultrasound biometry measurement (Ch. 19). This chapter covers the diagnostic drugs used by optometrists, namely cycloplegics, mydriatics, local anaesthetics and diagnostic staining agents. The characteristics of the pharmaceuticals, adverse reactions, uses and administration outlined here are based on a number of well-documented references (Bartlett 2006; Rhee & Deramo 2001; Sweetman 2007), and the pharmacology is further discussed in Chapter 6.

The use of drugs by optometrists is governed by law, and the choice and availability of drugs will change from time to time. In addition, legislation varies from country to country. Indeed, within the United States, the use of drugs by optometrists varies between states. In the UK, the use of drugs by optometrists is determined by the Opticians Act (1989) and the Medicines Act (1968). The College of Optometrists (UK) have published the *Optometrists' Formulary*, which provides the most updated list of drugs along with guidelines for application (2007).

Cycloplegic drugs

The primary action of cycloplegics is paralysis of the ciliary muscle, resulting in a reduction or loss of accommodation. In addition to the cycloplegia, mydriasis or dilation of the pupil occurs. When a patient is suspected of having latent hyperopia, accommodative spasm or esotropia, a cycloplegic refraction is highly recommended.

Mechanism of action

Cycloplegic drugs are anticholinergic in action (Manny & Jaanus 2001). They act by preventing the neurotransmitter acetylcholine (ACh) from reaching the final receptor site. During normal innervation of the cholinergic synapse in the parasympathetic system, ACh is released from the vesicles into the synapse, where it binds to the muscarinic receptors of the innervated structure. ACh is then metabolized to acetic acid and choline by the enzyme acetylcholinesterase (AChE). Cycloplegic drugs compete with acetylcholine for the postsynaptic receptor site on the smooth muscle fibre of the ciliary body. They do not offset nerve impulses nor prevent the release of acetylcholine. They are also named antimuscarinic agents.

Cycloplegia always occurs concurrently with mydriasis and loss of the pupil reflex, as the muscarinic antagonists will also prevent access of acetylcholine to its receptors in the sphincter muscle of the iris.

Drugs available for cycloplegia

The ideal cycloplegic drug should include the following characteristics: rapid onset of action, quick recovery of normal accommodation, sufficient cycloplegia and no local or systemic side effects (Hopkins & Pearson 2007).

An eye with a residual accommodation of less than 2 dioptres (D) is regarded as having an adequate level of cycloplegia. The major cycloplegic agents used in optometric practice, in order of decreasing strength, are atropine, homatropine, cyclopentolate and tropicamide. In the UK, the drug of choice for cycloplegia is cyclopentolate, with tropicamide primarily used in older children. The situation in the US is similar, with cyclopentolate being the first choice for cycloplegia. In the UK, as a result of recent legislative changes, atropine and homatropine are no longer available to all optometrists, but only to those with additional training and accreditation.

Atropine

Atropine is a powerful cycloplegic and mydriatic agent. It is the most potent cycloplegic available for optometrists and a number of adverse systemic effects have been documented including effects on the central nervous system (CNS), gastrointestinal tract, heart and the eye (Sweetman 2007).

Atropine is found naturally in plant species such as *Atropa belladonna*. In the form of atropine sulphate, it is available in 0.5%, 1%, 2% and 3% solutions as well as 0.5% and 1% ointments.

Atropine used to be used commonly in the refraction of young children because of its ability to produce complete paralysis of accommodation. It has also been used in amblyopia therapy to blur the vision in the good eye as a form of penalization. Although the outcome was found to be as good as conventional occlusion (Kaye et al 2002), it should be used with caution due to its potency.

The ointment form of atropine is favoured for young children as a systemic toxic reaction is less likely to occur with this method of administration compared with a solution. The usual dosage for cycloplegic refraction in children is 1% ointment to be administered twice each day for up to 3 days before the examination. If parents are asked to administer the drug, 0.5% atropine ointment is usually prescribed. Maximum mydriasis is reached typically in 30 to 40 minutes while recovery may take a week or more. Cycloplegia commences after 30 minutes, with marked cycloplegia being reached in 1 to 3 hours. The effect may last up to 6–12 days before normal accommodation is restored (Sweetman 2007). The different time courses of mydriasis and cycloplegia make pupil dilation a poor indicator of cycloplegic effect (Amos 1978). Auffarth and Hunold (1992) suggested that two drops of 0.5% or 1% atropine

solution is just as effective as 3 days of atropine ointment in inducing cycloplegia. The decline in amplitude of accommodation is only 0.5 D less with this regimen when compared with 3 days of ointment; however, the recovery time is much shorter.

Homatropine

Homatropine in the form of homatropine hydrobromide, a colourless crystal, can be used for cycloplegia. It is available in concentrations of 1%, 2% and 5% for cycloplegia. For use as a mydriatic, 0.25% and 0.5% are usually used. While the cycloplegic effect is weaker than atropine, the recovery time is much shorter. Homatropine of 1–2% acts maximally in 30–60 minutes with recovery occurring within 1 to 3 days (Sweetman 2007). To determine refractive error, one or two drops may be instilled initially; repeated instillation may be necessary 5 or 10 minutes later. Currently, homatropine is more commonly used for alleviation of ciliary spasm rather than for cycloplegic refraction.

Cyclopentolate

Cyclopentolate is the preferred choice for cycloplegia over atropine and homatropine. Ophthalmic solution is in the form of cyclopentolate hydrochloride, a white crystalline powder. Cyclopentolate works faster and the duration of action is shorter than the two drugs described above.

It is available as 0.5% and 1% solutions in both single-dose and multi-dose form, as well as a spray application for use under a closed eye condition. Spray application of cycloplegic drugs can be a satisfactory route of topical administration for children (Ismail et al 1994; Goodman et al 1999). Ismail et al (1994) found no significant difference in cycloplegic refraction using conventional eyedrops and the spray in a group of hyperopic children aged between 18 months and 6 years, while the spray was assessed to be more comfortable for most patients.

The recommended dosage for cycloplegic refraction is two drops given 5 minutes apart, 30 to 45 minutes before the examination. The recommended concentrations are 0.5% for adults, 1% for young children and no more than 0.5% for infants during the first 3 months of life (Sweetman 2007).

Fifteen minutes after instillation, the mydriatic and cycloplegic effects are obvious, reaching a maximum cycloplegic effect around 20 to 40 minutes. The recovery time from cyclopentolate is shortest amongst the three agents, with accommodation returning to normal within 6 to 12 hours, though in some cases it may take up to 24 hours before accommodation returns to normal. Some studies suggest a more accurate measure of the time course may be found by monitoring the residual distance accommodative ability and reported a shorter time course (Rosenfield & Linfield 1986; Manny et al 1993). For example, Rosenfield and Linfield (1986) reported that just 8.67 minutes were required to reach maximum cycloplegia in young adults as defined by a near point of accommodation of less than 2.00 D. Manny et al (1993) measured the time course of cycloplegia with 1% cyclopentolate hydrochloride using an objective measurement of residual accommodation and found that it varied with different iris pigmentation. Their results on both adults and children confirmed that individuals with light irides may attain maximal cycloplegia 10 minutes after the instillation of 1% cyclopentolate, whereas those with dark irides require 30 to 40 minutes before maximal cycloplegia is achieved. They further suggested that it is unnecessary to wait 30 to 60 minutes after drug instillation before the refraction is carried out.

Tropicamide

Tropicamide is a synthetic derivative of tropic acid. Its lipid solubility allows a greater penetration through the cornea and therefore a more rapid effect and shorter duration of action than cyclopentolate. It is available in 0.5% and 1% concentrations. Cycloplegia occurs in 10–15 minutes and lasts up to 6 hours. However, its efficacy is lower than cyclopentolate. For example, Pollack et al (1981) demonstrated the dose–response effects of tropicamide within the range of concentrations from 0.25% to 1.0%; the mean residual accommodation was 2.50 D for one drop of 0.25% tropicamide and 1.5 D for one drop of both 0.75% and 1% tropicamide. However, the time taken to reach maximum cycloplegia was similar for all concentrations.

Choice of concentration/dosage

Longer-acting agents are thought to provide more effective cycloplegia. Cyclopentolate provides cycloplegia for 6 to 12 hours (and up to 24 hours in some cases), while tropicamide is expected to provide 4 to 10 hours of cycloplegia. Hofmeister et al (2005) found cyclopentolate 1% was more effective than tropicamide in reducing accommodative amplitude in adult myopes although patients strongly preferred tropicamide 1% for comfort; there was, in fact, no statistically significant difference in mean cycloplegic refraction between the two agents.

Some studies have suggested that cyclopentolate and tropicamide might be equally efficacious for cycloplegic refractions in children (Egashira et al 1993; Mutti et al 1994; Lin et al 1998; Owens et al 1998; Manny et al 2001). Fan et al (2004) compared the safety and efficacy of cycloplegia in three combination solutions of (1) tropicamide 0.5% and phenylephrine 0.5%, (2) tropicamide 1.0% and cyclopentolate 1.0% and (3) atropine 1.0% in young, dark-pigmented irides. They concluded that in children older than 5 years, the lower concentration of combination solution of (1) was as effective as (2) and can be used to avoid cyclopentolate toxicity. They recommended that atropine 1% is still the most effective cycloplegic agent in children younger than 5 years who may have strabismus in combination with dark-pigmented irides. However, the toxicity of this drug should be carefully considered and atropine should be regarded as the last choice for use.

It has been claimed that a combination of several drugs has improved efficacy. Hamasaki et al (2007) reported that the cycloplegic effect of a mixed eyedrop containing 0.5% tropicamide and 0.5% phenylephrine is an effective cycloplegic agent in Japanese myopic children. The mean residual accommodation was 0.21 D, which is insignificant and acceptable. Ebri et al (2007) suggested a combination of cyclopentolate and tropicamide should be the recommended agent for routine cycloplegic refraction in African children. This combined regimen was more effective than cyclopentolate alone, was less expensive, and was also preferable to atropine.

Twelker and Mutti (2001) compared retinoscopy results in a group of infants from 4 to 7 months with both tropicamide 1% and cyclopentolate 1%. They found no statistically significant difference between the two drug conditions, and suggested that tropicamide is as effective as cyclopentolate for the measurement of refractive error in healthy, non-strabismic infants.

Adverse reactions

Adverse reactions are related to the pharmacological action at muscarinic receptor sites. These effects are dose related and reversible. The use of stronger cycloplegics, particularly atropine and homatropine, can lead to systemic toxicity, which is manifested with skin redness, dry mouth, irregular and rapid pulse, hallucination, speech difficulty and loss of coordination. Tear secretion is also reduced substantially by atropine (Crandall & Leopold 1979). Practitioners should be aware of these symptoms and alert parents when cycloplegics are given to children. The risk of toxic effects increases with conditions such as Down's syndrome (Davies et al 2007). Other risks include angle-closure glaucoma; cycloplegic drugs have been reported to cause a significant rise in intraocular pressure (IOP) in patients with narrow anterior chamber angle (Harris et al 1971), and primary open-angle glaucoma (Shaw & Lewis 1986; Marchini et al 2003). Allergic reactions to cyclopentolate hydrochloride, manifested as a facial rash and redness around the eyelid region in young children, have been reported, although these usually subside in a few hours (Jones & Hodes 1991).

Loewen and Barry (2000) reported their results of a questionnaire on cycloplegia protocol. Among 57 centres with 1112 cumulated years of experience in using cycloplegia, with an average of 34 patients cyclopleged per week in each centre, there may be, in total, 2 to 10 severe or very severe complications overall. Accordingly, the risk of severe complications is very small. They commented further that patients should be informed about frequent occurrence of harmless side effects in order to achieve a good compliance of cycloplegia, and not necessarily mention the life-threatening complications which were previously associated with use of a higher dose.

In choosing the most suitable cycloplegic, optometrists should consider the age and ocular condition of the patient, whether patients are likely to have an allergic response towards the intended drug, weigh up the benefits and risks associated with the choice of pharmaceutical agent, and select the least toxic drug available when used with the minimal effective dosage.

Clinical indications and procedures

Cycloplegia is necessary when refracting young children, especially in cases of high hyperopia and patients with strabismus and accommodative spasm (see Ch. 28) (Bujara et al 1981). When maximum cycloplegia is required, for example, in the case of accommodative esotropia, a stronger drug or a greater dosage is indicated. Rosenbaum et al (1981) recommended that atropine refraction should be conducted for all esotropic children who show two or more dioptres of hyperopia. Atropine cycloplegia is said to uncover about 0.4 D more hyperopia than cyclopentolate (Fulton et al 1980). Nevertheless, cyclopentolate is more extensively used today, and has generally replaced atropine to avoid the long duration and inconvenience of prolonged blurred vision at near found with atropine, as well as its greater risk of toxicity.

Reaction after drug instillation

Mild transient stinging is normal following drug instillation due to its acidic pH. When patients are cyclopleged, they may experience blurred vision, glare and photosensitivity due to the dilated pupil. Judging depth may be less accurate. Patients will not be able to focus at near; the duration of this inability to read at close distances will depend upon the drug and dosage used.

Precautions prior to instillation

During history taking, information should be obtained related to any previous adverse reactions to cycloplegic or mydriatic drugs, other ocular or systemic medications, and family history of glaucoma, as well as ocular and general health.

All patients who are to undergo cycloplegia should first have their anterior chamber angle depth evaluated to ascertain the risk of angle closure. IOP should also be measured for baseline. While these measurements may be difficult to perform on very young children, they should certainly be carried out on older children, teenagers and all adult patients. As with all the topical ocular medication, punctal occlusion should be used to avoid systemic absorption (see Ch. 6), especially with children, the elderly and in the presence of certain medical conditions. Caution must be taken when performing other activities such as driving or operating moving machinery while eyes remain dilated and cyclopleged (Woodard & Woodard 1991).

Shah et al (1997) proposed the use of local anaesthetics prior to instillation of cycloplegia to minimize the discomfort and distress in young children. They reported that 70% of the 88 children who received cyclopentolate alone cried and were unhappy whereas 91% of the children who received cyclopentolate after proxymetacaine showed no traumatic reaction to the cycloplegia and remained happy.

Postcycloplegic examination

Drug effects are usually allowed to wear off naturally. The patient should be provided with sunglasses while the pupil is still dilated. They should be advised not to drive or operate moving machinery until the effects of the drug have worn off, as well as cautioned as to difficulties in performing near work. It is important that the patient be advised of the expected time course for cycloplegia and mydriasis to wear off.

Hancox et al (2002) studied the changes in intraocular pressure following mydriasis with cyclopentolate 1% in patients with cataract, retinal changes and glaucoma. They recommended that due to individual variability in the effects on aqueous dynamics, intraocular pressure should be rechecked after dilation in glaucoma patients with significantly damaged optic nerves. In a review of published research, between 1933 and 1999, the risk of glaucoma being induced following mydriasis with tropicamide alone is close to zero, with no cases being identified. The presence of chronic glaucoma does not constitute an additional risk (Pandit & Taylor 2000). Patients should also be assessed for signs and symptoms of systemic toxicity to the cycloplegic agent.

Mydriatics

Mydriatics are used to dilate the pupil to allow an easier and more comprehensive examination of structures in the posterior segment of the eye (see Ch. 18). The ideal mydriatic is an agent that does not affect accommodation, and thus will not disturb the patient's near vision.

Mechanism of action

The ideal mydriatic drugs exert their effect only on the iris musculature to dilate the pupil. There should be little or no effect on the ciliary musculature so that accommodative function would not be affected. Drugs that match this requirement of mydriasis without cycloplegia are in two main groups: either weak muscarinic antagonists or sympathetic agonists. Muscarinic antagonists act by blocking receptors on smooth muscle. They paralyse the pupil sphincter and ciliary muscle, resulting in pupil dilation and varying degrees of reduced accommodation. The split between mydriasis and cycloplegia is relative; the weaker antimuscarincs such as tropicamide can also be used as mydriatics. The relative effects in the muscarinic antagonists can be explained by the fact that the pathway to the ciliary muscle is longer than that to the pupil sphincter. When a weak antagonist is used, the majority of the drug interacts with the closer receptors in the iris, leaving insufficient amount of drug to act on the ciliary muscle receptors, resulting in less effect on accommodation (Vale & Cox 1985).

The sympathetic agonist agent has a different mechanism, with mydriasis and cycloplegia being totally separated (Portello & Jaanus 2001). The effects of a sympathetic agonist are contraction of the pupil dilator muscle, resulting in mydriasis, constriction of the conjunctival blood vessels and elevation of the upper eyelid. Accommodation is not affected.

Drugs available for mydriasis

The two most commonly used mydriatics are tropicamide hydrochloride, a muscarinic antagonist, available as 0.5% and 1% drops (including single-dose units), and phenylephrine hydrochloride, a sympathetic agonist available as 2.5% and 10% drops (and single-dose units).

Tropicamide

The lower concentration of 0.5% is used for mydriasis only. Pupil dilation commences within a few minutes and reaches a maximum within about 30 minutes. Pupil response to light is minimal. Full return of the pupil response to normal occurs in around 6 hours (Sweetman 2007). The effect on accommodation varies between patients, and residual accommodation averages around 2 D.

The dose effect of tropicamide for mydriasis is not apparent as in cycloplegia when comparing concentrations between 0.25% and 1.0% under normal and bright illuminance. Thus, 0.25% tropicamide is effective in providing mydriasis (Pollack et al 1981). Siderov and Nurse (2005) compared instillation of one and two drops of tropicamide in young healthy subjects and suggested that a single drop of 0.5% tropicamide is adequate to produce a pupillary diameter of at least 6 mm, which should be sufficient for a dilated fundus examination.

Phenylephrine

Phenylephrine is a direct-acting sympathomimetic agent. As a mydriatic, it is available in concentrations up to 10%, although for mydriatic purposes, 2.5% solution is recommended. Onset of pupil dilation commences 10–20 minutes following the instillation of one drop of 2.5% solution and can take up to 60 minutes to reach its maximum effect. Full recovery from mydriasis occurs in approximately 6 hours (Bartlett 2006).

The 10% concentration has been associated with serious cardiovascular reactions, including an increase in systolic and diastolic blood pressure (Hakim et al 1990; Baldwin & Morley 2002; Fraunfelder et al 2002). Accordingly, practitioners should be cautious when using this drug in hypertensive patients. Phenylephrine should be avoided in patients with hyperthyroidism as they show excessive reactions to sympathetic drugs. As phenylephrine stimulates only the dilator muscle of the iris, mydriasis may be less effective in patients with dark-pigmented irides. Additionally, patients may complain of blurring even though accommodation is minimally affected. This is probably due to increased spherical aberration with the larger pupil size. In addition to pupil dilation, phenylephrine may cause widening of the palpebral aperture and blanching of the conjunctiva due to alpha$_1$-receptor agonist action on alpha receptors present in Muller's smooth muscle in the upper and lower eyelids and conjunctival vessels.

Choice of concentration/dosage

In comparing these two drugs, tropicamide would seem to give more reliable mydriasis in a shorter time with the complete demolition of the light reflex. In healthy adults, the first choice for mydriasis would be 0.5% tropicamide or 2.5% phenylephrine. Additionally, a combination of the two agents can be used to produce adequate mydriasis. Combinations of tropicamide and phenylephrine, cyclopentolate and phenylephrine are commercially available in North America but not currently in the UK.

Effects of the combination of two or more mydriatics have been studied widely in various populations (Kergoat et al 1989; Wesson et al 1993; Benavides et al 1997; Eyeson-Annan et al 1998). Krumholz et al (2006) reported that combination preparations of reduced concentrations of tropicamide and phenylephrine can also produce clinically adequate mydriasis. Their results indicated that a combination solution containing 0.5% tropicamide and 1.25% phenylephrine is sufficient to dilate pupils adequately for internal ocular examination. This has the advantage of reducing both the number of drop administrations and the total amount of drug delivered to the patient.

Prior administration of a topical anaesthetic was shown to improve patient comfort, but did not produce any significant change in the level of mydriasis produced by 0.5% tropicamide (Haddad et al 2007). However, low concentrations of phenylephrine, when used in conjunction with a topical anaesthetic, produce the same degree of mydriasis as higher concentrations of the drug alone (Keller & Chang 1976). Chung and Feder (2005) reported that pupil dilation after instillation of 1% tropicamide was significantly faster after LASIK surgery and further suggested that the resulting corneal thinning enhanced the penetration of tropicamide.

Some conditions render the pupil less responsive to mydriatics. For example, elderly patients are more difficult to dilate due to senile miosis. The denervated pupil in a diabetic patient may respond poorly to tropicamide, especially in those patients who have had laser treatment for proliferative retinopathy (Huber et al 1985); a combination of tropicamide 0.5% and phenylephrine 10% is recommended rather than tropicamide alone for these patients. However, in a double-blind study comparing 0.5% and 1% tropicamide for annual retinal screening in diabetic adolescents without diabetic miosis, all pupils in this young cohort dilated to 6 mm with either drug concentration (Hassler-Hurst et al 2004).

As with cycloplegia, a heavily pigmented iris may require a higher concentration of mydriatic, although a lower concentration is recommended for young children and infants (Khoo et al 2000; Chew et al 2005). Khoo et al found the single-combination eyedrops of cyclopentolate 0.2% and phenylephrine 1% is as effective and safe a mydriatic for infants with dark irides as both tropicamide 0.5% and phenylephrine 2.5%. Mydriatic sprays on closed eyelids can be as efficacious as the use of mydriatic drops for children (Benavides et al 1997) while causing less ocular discomfort.

Adverse reaction

Possible adverse reactions from tropicamide have been discussed under the cycloplegia section, and, being a less potent drug, these are rare. Since phenylephrine is absorbed through the mucosa, the 10% concentration may produce systemic effects following absorption through the conjunctiva and nasolacrimal duct. It may cause a prolonged rise in blood pressure due to an excessive vasopressor response. Additionally, tachycardia or reflex bradycardia may be induced and therefore this drug should be avoided in patients with severe hyperthyroidism and ischaemic heart disease (Sweetman 2007). Steps should always be taken to reduce absorption via the canaliculi and the use of the lower concentration (2.5%) considered in patients with known cardiovascular problems. As with tropicamide, the possibility of a rise in intra-ocular pressure should not become a problem if patients are carefully selected. Pukrushpan et al (2006) suggested that post-dilation IOP in open-angle, non-glaucoma patients undergoing routine diagnostic mydriasis with tropicamide is equivalent to pre-dilation IOP, although there is significant anterior chamber angle narrowing. Therefore, these authors suggested that it is not necessary to recheck IOP following dilation in every patient as routine practice but recommended performing gonioscopy to assess the angle width before dilation and rechecking IOP only in selected cases.

Mydriasis can be reversed using a miotic although this is generally not recommended. Physostigmine (an anticholinesterase) or pilocarpine (a parasympathomimetic) can be used following administration of an antimuscarinic drug. Phenylephrine can be reliably reversed with dapiprazole, which is used infrequently by US optometrists but is not available in the UK.

Clinical indications for mydriasis

When a comprehensive examination of structures in the posterior segment of the eye is indicated, dilation of the pupil will provide better observation (see Ch. 18). Patients with small pupils or ocular media opacities should be examined under mydriasis. Occasionally, mydriatics are used as provocative tests for glaucoma and in the assessment of anisocoria.

Precautions, pre-mydriatic and post-mydriatic examination

The pre-mydriatic examination aims to identify those patients who might potentially suffer serious side effects from the mydriatic eyedrops. The procedures to be carried out are the same as the pre- and post-cycloplegic tests. The anterior chamber angle should be checked for any possibility of an acute increase in IOP. This can be done with the flashlight or oblique illumination test (Pophal & Ripkin 1995), the Van Herick test (Van Herick et al 1969) or gonioscopy.

Local anaesthetics

Clinical indications

Local anaesthetics are used in optometric practice for a number of purposes. The surface of the cornea is highly sensitive due to the numerous nerve endings and any assessment or treatment procedures requiring contact with the cornea can be made more comfortable if a local anaesthetic is instilled. This reduces the sensitivity and provides a transient numbness of the localized region where it is applied. Procedures requiring temporary corneal desensitization include applanation tonometry, certain types of contact lens fitting, ocular media examination using a contact format such as gonioscopy, ultrasound pachymetry, ultrasound biometry, specular microscopy, confocal microscopy, insertion of punctual plugs and superficial foreign body removal.

Occasionally, contact lens fitting requires the use of local anaesthetic, especially for the very apprehensive patients or the rare occasion of taking an impression of the eye for construction of a scleral lens. Some optometrists also use a local anaesthetic before fitting rigid gas-permeable (RGP) lenses. A number of practitioners use a local anaesthetic to reduce the reflex tearing before a Schirmer test and prior to the insertion of a punctual plug. Other diagnostic procedures are enhanced by prior instillation of local anaesthetics. Depending on the duration of the procedure, the choice of local anaesthetics varies; for example, longer anaesthesia is required when performing gonioscopy compared with pachymetry.

The use of local anaesthetics makes confocal microscopy more comfortable and does not alter the morphology of the cornea when viewed with the confocal microscope (Perez-Gomez et al 2004). By removing the discomfort, there is less chance of capturing a poor-quality image. Procedures such as the removal of a foreign body would be nearly impossible for the patient to endure if the cornea was not anaesthetised first; the associated blepharospasm would make foreign body removal very difficult.

Some practitioners instil one drop of local anaesthetic prior to pupillary dilation or cycloplegia to reduce the stinging sensation of the drops and produce an enhanced and quicker effect. Siu et al (1999) reported that prior application of local anaesthetics could shorten the time to full cycloplegia for Chinese patients with dark irides. A local anaesthetic is sometimes used prior to the instillation of rose bengal stain for the assessment of corneal integrity to reduce stinging.

Mechanism of action

Jackson and McLure (2006) and McLure and Rubin (2005) have recently reviewed the pharmacology of local anaesthetics. The physiology of nerve conduction, mechanism of action, chemistry and toxicity of most available local anaesthetics were included in these reviews, as well as in Chapter 6.

Drugs available for anaesthesia

There are two main groups of local anaesthetics; ester and amide groups. The ester group includes cocaine, proparacaine, procaine, chloroprocaine, tetracaine and oxybuprocaine while the amide group includes lidocaine, mepivacaine and bupivacaine. They are usually formulated in the form of their hydrochloride salt, which is water soluble. Amide anaesthetics can penetrate both fat-soluble tissues and water-soluble tissues due to their chemical structure, making them ideal for application to the surface of the eye. The ester anaesthetic is commonly associated with increased allergies (Blaschke & Fuchs 2003).

A wide range of local anaesthetics is available to optometrists for clinical use. These include tetracaine (amethocaine), proxymetacaine (proparacaine), oxybuprocaine (benoxinate) and lidocaine (lignocaine). Most of them are in commercial preparations and a few are available in single-dose units.

Proxymetacaine/proparacaine hydrochloride

Proxymetacaine HCl is available in ophthalmic solutions at a 0.5% concentration in both multi-dose and preservative-free unit-dose form, either alone or in combination with 0.25% fluorescein (Minims, Chauvin Pharmaceuticals). It is should be stored at a refrigerated temperature of 4–8°C and kept away from light. Stiles et al (2001) reported that short-term storage of proxymetacaine at room temperature did not affect efficacy, but storage at room temperature for more than 2 weeks decreased the effectivity of the drug.

Instillation of one drop of 0.5% proxymetacaine produces anaesthesia in 10 to 20 seconds, which lasts about 15 minutes. A comparative study of oxybuprocaine 0.4%, amethocaine 0.5% and proxymetacaine 0.5% using a slit-lamp-mounted Cochet–Bonnet aesthesiometer showed all three agents produce anaesthesia of rapid onset within 1 minute of instillation and complete recovery for all subjects after 45 minutes (Lawrenson et al 1998). Both Polse et al (1978) and Jauregui et al (1980) demonstrated that the anaesthetic effect varies with drug concentration. Lower concentrations of proparacaine (0.25%) and oxybuprocaine (0.2%) were as effective as the commercially available concentrations (0.5% and 0.4% respectively) in providing sufficient duration to carry out standard optometric procedures. Complete recovery of corneal sensation from the lowest dose of 0.125% proparacaine occurs after 20 minutes and from the two higher doses of 0.25% and 0.5% after about 30 minutes (Polse et al 1978).

Proxymetacaine appears to produce the least discomfort or stinging upon instillation (Bartfield et al 1994; Lawrenson et al 1998; Shafi & Koay 1998). Bartfield et al (1994) compared proxymetacaine directly with tetracaine, noting that 86% of the patients reported that proxymetacaine caused less pain on administration and lasted slightly longer. These properties make proxymetacaine preferable to tetracaine. Further, Shafi and Koay (1998) compared proxymetacaine and amethocaine and concluded that proxymetacaine is more comfortable. They suggested the pH of the anaesthetic agents affects the degree of comfort following instillation. Amethocaine has a pH of 4.54 and proxymetacaine a pH of 4.64. Lawrenson et al (1998) compared oxybuprocaine, amethocaine and proxymetacaine in preservative-free unit-dose solutions and also concluded that proxymetacaine was significantly better tolerated than the other two anaesthetics.

In a prospective, masked, double-blind study, proxymetacaine–fluorescein and lignocaine–fluorescein were compared during applanation tonometry. Several aspects of the tonometry process were evaluated including the duration of the stinging, the degree of discomfort, the extent of reflex lacrimation and the time required to complete the measurement. Proxymetacaine–fluorescein was preferred over lignocaine–fluorescein by 98% of the study patients (Birchall & Kumar 2001). Proxymetacaine–fluorescein caused significantly less discomfort and reflex tearing, and a shorter time to complete the tonometry.

Using pachymetry, an increase in the central corneal thickness due to the development of corneal oedema was observed after the use of two drops of 0.5% proxymetacaine (Herse & Siu 1992). However, one drop of 0.5% proxymetacaine did not produce any significant change in central corneal thickness (Lam & Chen 2007). Nam et al (2006) reported that oxybuprocaine and proxymetacaine also produced temporary increases in corneal thickness, which returned to baseline within 80 seconds, but proxymetacaine produced values that were more variable for 5 minutes after application. They recommended corneal thickness should be measured 80 seconds after instillation to ensure greater accuracy prior to refractive surgery or in glaucoma patients.

Proxymetacaine has few side effects; the most common are mild corneal oedema and epithelial staining. These usually subside quickly. Anaesthetics also stimulate some reflex tearing and moderate conjunctival hyperaemia. Such hyperaemia usually subsides within a few minutes and the bulbar conjunctiva returns to its normal colour (Norden 1976; Jose et al 1984).

Wilson and Fullard observed the effects of 0.5% proxymetacaine on the rate of corneal epithelial desquamation and found that the drug initially reduces the rate of normal cell sloughing (Fullard & Wilson 1986; Wilson & Fullard 1988). Increased epithelial cell desquamation was apparent for at least 6 hours. They proposed that proxymetacaine might cause desquamation by interfering with normal epithelial cell membrane activity. Similar effects were also observed with tetracaine (Boljka et al 1994).

Oxybuprocaine (benoxinate) hydrochloride

Oxybuprocaine HCl is available in ophthalmic solutions at a 0.4% concentration in combination with 0.25% fluorescein. It belongs to the same ester group of para-aminobenzoic acid (PABA) and so has an onset, intensity, and duration of anaesthesia similar to proxymetacaine 0.5% and tetracaine 0.5%. It produces rapid onset (15–20 seconds) of anaesthesia, which lasts for 15 to 20 minutes.

The combination solution has been shown to have substantial antibacterial properties (Yolton & German 1980), which makes it a preferred choice of local anaesthetic for applanation tonometry. Comparison of an oxybuprocaine/fluorescein combination with a proparacaine/fluorescein combination showed that the oxybuprocaine combination caused marginally more stinging but less corneal desquamation than the proparacaine combination after Goldmann applanation tonometry (Yeung et al 2000). Both caused corneal desquamation at 20 minutes after instillation. Therefore, Yeung et al (2000) suggested that corneal integrity should be evaluated even 20 minutes after applanation tonometry procedures.

Fluctuations in corneal thickness before and after instillation of oxybuprocaine 0.4% have been reported (Asensio et al 2003; Nam et al 2006). The effect of anaesthetic eyedrops should be considered if the corneal thickness measurement is for used for LASIK surgery.

Tetracaine hydrochloride (amethocaine hydrochloride)

Tetracaine hydrochloride is available in 0.25–1% solutions. Upon instillation, there is an initial burning sensation, which disappears within minutes. Anaesthesia persists for 10–20 min depending on the concentration used. Tetracaine is relatively stable in solution but may be hydrolysed by light. Therefore, it should be stored in a dark bottle or cupboard.

There is a cumulative effect following repeated instillations; superficial corneal epithelial lesions can be commonly seen with the slit-lamp microscope after use of this pharmaceutical agent. Epithelial regeneration, both mitosis and cellular migration, have been shown to be affected.

Lignocaine hydrochloride

Lignocaine is a white crystalline powder; a concentration of 2–4% is adequate to anaesthetize the cornea. Onset of anaesthesia occurs after about 1 minute with a duration of 30 minutes. It is also marketed as a mixture with fluorescein. It is an alternative agent in individuals sensitive to ester-type local anaesthetics (Ritchie & Cohen 1975).

Choice of local anaesthetics

In the UK, proxymetacaine, either alone or in combination with fluorescein in single-dose units, is the most popular local anaesthetic as it causes less stinging for the patient. Oxybuprocaine is another frequently used anaesthetic, particularly when performing applanation tonometry.

Adverse reactions

All anaesthetics have a potential to become toxic in higher doses. There is a possibility of both local and systemic adverse effects. The typical overdose symptoms are lightheadedness, ringing in the ears, or blurred vision.

Allergic responses to local anaesthetics are more likely to occur with the older ester-linked compounds, i.e. proxymetacaine, oxybuprocaine and tetracaine, than with lignocaine, which is an amide (Rosenwasser et al 1990). Systemic effects occur less frequently. Hypersensitivity can range from mild, transient blepharoconjunctivitus to a diffuse necrotizing epithelial keratitis, which may be sufficient to reduce visual acuity significantly (Lyle & Page 1975).

Repeated instillation of a local anaesthetic can cause a number of ocular reactions, for example, keratopathy in dry eye patients (Jallet et al 1980; Penna & Tabbara 1986; Chen et al 2004), cytotoxic effects on the cornea (Sturrock & Nunn 1979; Boljka et al 1994) and a lower finding on a Schirmer's test (see Ch. 17) (Shiono 1989). Local anaesthetic drops are never prescribed for a patient to use at home. Frequent use interferes with the healing process and can cause corneal melting.

Precaution prior to instillation

A history should be taken to assess any contraindications to local anaesthetics. Consider apprehension, as a nervous patient may benefit from use of a local anaesthetic to ease reaction or anxiety during certain optometric procedures. Patients should be warned not to rub their eyes after instillation of local anaesthetics. As the cornea now lacks sensation, the patient could conceivably rub hard enough to cause a corneal abrasion.

Post-examination

The cornea should be examined for punctate staining. Patients should be advised to avoid touching the eye until anaesthesia has worn off. In the case of any allergic or toxic response, medical attention is generally required to prevent the condition from becoming more serious.

Staining agents

Staining agents are used in assessing ocular conditions such as the integrity of the ocular surface, presence of hypersensitivity of the ocular surface or any lacrimal drainage problems. They are also used in certain diagnostic procedures such as contact lens fitting, Goldmann tonometry, blockage of the lacrimal system and observation of wound healing. Commonly used staining agents include fluorescein, rose bengal and lissamine green. The three dyes stain different structures; fluorescein stains epithelial lesions, rose bengal stains degenerate cells and lissamine green stains mucus.

Fluorescein sodium

Fluorescein is a chemical dye that has the property to emit fluorescent light when exposed to light. It is orange-red in colour. The absorbed light energy in a dilute concentration of fluorescein excites the molecules to emit fluorescent light. The light appears green, having its highest intensity at a wavelength between 525 and 530 mm (Schnider 2001; Hopkins & Pearson 2007). The intensity of fluorescence is affected by factors such as the pH, concentration and other solutes in the solution. For best observation of the fluorescence, a cobalt blue filter is used. A yellow Wratten number 15 filter has also been suggested to enhance the detection of fluorescein staining of the cornea.

When used as a topical ophthalmic dye, fluorescein is in the form of a 2% solution or as 1 mg fluorescein-impregnated filter paper strips and is available in single-dose sterile pipettes to prevent bacterial contamination.

Clinical use

Fluorescein is used to assess the integrity of the ocular surface. It will stain any cell it enters and temporarily marks any damaged areas. The stain differs according to which part of the eye is affected. For example, damage to the lining of the conjunctiva will stain yellow or orange whereas damage to the cornea appears green. This bright yellow-green fluorescence allows the detection of abrasions, ulcers and oedema in the cornea and conjunctiva resulting from trauma or infection. Lesions in the corneal epithelium will allow the dye to penetrate into the stroma. If the dye penetrates to the anterior chamber, it appears as a green flare in the anterior chamber. Fluorescein can also be used to identify foreign bodies in the eye as they will be surrounded by a green boundary.

When examining the integrity of the ocular surface, one or two drops of the solution is instilled into the lower conjunctival fornix or the paper strip is moistened with sterile water or saline and the lower conjunctiva is gently touched with the strip.

If the corneal epithelium is intact it will be impermeable so the fluorescein diffuses into the tear layer, which is visible as a green layer. Staining of the tear film allows assessment of tear break-up time, tear flow and nasolacrimal duct patency (see Ch. 17) and measurement of intraocular pressure with applanation tonometry (see Ch. 24), as well as the evaluation of fitting of rigid gas-permeable contact lenses. For the evaluation of soft lens fitting, a large molecule of fluorescein known as Fluorexon can be used to stop fluorescein being absorbed by the soft contact lens.

Measurement of IOP with the Goldmann tonometer requires the applanation probe to contact the corneal surface (see **Fig. 24.1**). The concentration of fluorescein recommended for tonometry is 0.25% with a local anaesthetic such as oxybuprocaine 0.4%. A mixture of 4% lignocaine with 0.25% fluorescein and 0.5% proxymetacaine with 0.25% fluorescein are available in single-use units (Hopkins & Pearson 2007).

Tear break-up time and tear flow can be measured by making the tears visible with fluorescein. Lacrimal patency can be assessed with the Jones test (Zappia & Milder 1972a,b; Hagele et al 1994). After instillation of one or two drops of 2% fluorescein into the conjunctival fornix, the patient is then asked to blow the nose with a tissue and observe whether there are any yellow stains on the tissue. Lack of staining on the tissue indicates a blockage in the lacrimal drainage system.

Fluorescein is also used for performing Seidel's test to observe corneal wound healing after cataract or glaucoma surgery (Romanchuk 1979; Cain & Sinskey 1981).

Precautions

Fluorescein in solution is highly susceptible to bacterial contamination, especially by *Pseudomonas aeruginosa*. Preservatives used to prevent growth of microorganisms in fluorescein solutions include chlorobutanol and thimerosal. Sterile single-does vials of fluorescein solution or filter paper strips are recommended for topical use if a preservative is clinically contraindicated. For combination of fluorescein–anaesthetic solutions, for example oxybuprocaine with fluorescein, such solutions are resistant to bacterial contamination. Since fluorescein will discolour soft contact lenses, it is important to rinse or irrigate the eye thoroughly before inserting any soft lenses.

Rose bengal

Rose bengal stains devitalized epithelial cells of the cornea and conjunctiva (Norn 1970). It also stains mucous strands of the precorneal tear film. This diagnostic agent is commonly used for ocular surface disease such as in the diagnosis of keratitis, keratoconjunctivitis sicca, abrasions and for the detection of foreign bodies (see Ch. 17).

Rose bengal is a derivative of fluorescein and is photo-reactive. It stains tissues with a vivid pink or magenta colour when viewed with white light (see **Fig. 17.14**). There is an initial irritation to the surface of the eye, especially in patients with dry eye. Rose bengal has been formulated as a 1% solution and in the form of 1.3 mg sterile impregnated paper strips that require moistening with sterile saline or ocular irrigating solution (Bartlett 2006).

Clinical use

Rose bengal is used in the differential diagnosis of dry eye syndromes (Sjogren & Bloch 1971). In addition, it has also been recommended for the evaluation of corneal and conjunctival lesions, abrasions, ulcerations, detection of foreign bodies and dendritic ulcers (Schnider 2001). A mixture of stains containing 1% fluorescein sodium and 1% rose bengal was investigated by Norn (1970), who concluded that it was superior to the individual stains alone.

Feenstra and Tseng (1992) suggested that rose bengal is not truly a vital stain as it actually contributes to the death of those cells unprotected by a coating of mucin and albumin. They observed a toxic response to rose bengal in normal rabbit corneas. Cells exposed to the dye demonstrated instantaneous morphologic changes, loss of cellular motility, cell detachment and cell death. In fact, rose bengal staining could occur due to the loss of the protective preocular tear film. The ability of rose bengal to stain cells is also dose related.

Adverse reactions

Adverse reactions include mild stinging, irritation and discomfort, particularly in higher concentrations. This discomfort may be relieved with a topical anaesthetic. Rose bengal can also stain eyelids, cheeks, fingers and clothing. Accordingly, the eye should be irrigated and rinsed thoroughly to avoid subsequent staining of skin or clothing.

Lissamine green

Lissamine green is a vital stain that stains degenerate or dead cells and mucus in much the same way as rose bengal, and 1% of lissamine green is similar to 1% rose bengal. It is commonly used by practitioners in the convenient form of impregnated sterile paper strips. Lissamine green stains membrane-damaged epithelial cells and corneal stroma in a similar manner to fluorescein. Like rose bengal, it binds to the nuclei of severely damaged cells (Chodosh et al 1994). However, the staining effect lasts longer than rose bengal. Lissamine green stains mucus strands in a bluish-green colour, and is particularly useful for assessing dry eye conditions. Lissamine green is better tolerated by

patients than rose bengal and is equally effective in evaluating the ocular surface in keratoconjunctivitis sicca (Manning et al 1995).

Unlike rose bengal, lissamine green does not possess significant antiviral activity (Stroop et al 2000) and is therefore recommended for detecting recurrent corneal erosions and herpetic ulcers. It has also been recommended for evaluating ocular surface disorders (Kim & Foulks 1999) as rose bengal affects corneal epithelial cell viability adversely and can stain normal proliferating cells. No adverse effects or irritation following instillation of lissamine green have been reported (Bartlett 2006).

References

Amos D M 1978 Cycloplegics for refraction. American Journal of Optometry and Physiological Optics 55(4):223–226

Asensio I, Rahhal S M, Alonso L et al 2003 Corneal thickness values before and after oxybuprocaine 0.4% eye drops. Cornea 22(6): 527–532

Auffarth G, Hunold W 1992 Cycloplegic refraction in children: single-dose-atropinization versus three-day-atropinization. Documenta Ophthalmologica 80(4):353–362

Baldwin F J, Morley A P 2002 Intraoperative pulmonary oedema in a child following systemic absorption of phenylephrine eyedrops. British Journal of Anaesthesia 88(3):440–442

Bartfield J M, Holmes T J, Raccio-Robak N 1994 A comparison of proparacaine and tetracaine eye anesthetics. Academic Emergency Medicine 1(4):364–367

Bartlett J D 2006 Ophthalmic drug facts. Wolters Kluwer Health, St Louis

Benavides J O, Satchell E R, Frantz K A 1997 Efficacy of a mydriatic spray in the pediatric population. Optometry and Vision Science 74(3):160–163

Birchall W, Kumar V 2001 A comparative study of proxymetacaine-fluorescein and lignocaine-fluorescein use during applanation tonometry. The British Journal of Ophthalmology 85(4):477–479

Blaschke V, Fuchs T 2003 [Relevant allergens by periorbital allergic contact dermatitis. Oxybuprocain, an underestimated allergen]. 100(8):628–632

Boljka M, Kolar G, Vidensek J 1994 Toxic side effects of local anaesthetics on the human cornea. The British Journal of Ophthalmology 78(5):386–389

Bujara K, Schulz E, Haase W 1981 [Retinoscopy under cycloplegic and non-cycloplegic conditions in children. Comparison of measurements of three examiners (author's transl)]. Albrecht von Graefes Archiv fur klinische und experimentelle Ophthalmologie 216 (4):339–343

Cain W Jr, Sinskey R M 1981 Detection of anterior chamber leakage with Seidel's test. Archives of Ophthalmology 99(11):2013

Chen H T, Chen K H, Hsu W M 2004 Toxic keratopathy associated with abuse of low-dose anesthetic: a case report. Cornea 23(5): 527–529

Chew C, Rahman R A, Shafie S M et al 2005 Comparison of mydriatic regimens used in screening for retinopathy of prematurity in preterm infants with dark irides. Journal of Pediatric Ophthalmology and Strabismus 42(3):166–173

Chodosh J, Dix R D, Howell R C et al 1994 Staining characteristics and antiviral activity of sulforhodamine b and lissamine green b. Investigative Ophthalmology and Visual Science 35(3):1046–1058

Chung H S, Feder R S 2005 Pupil response to tropicamide following laser in situ keratomileusis. Journal of Cataract and Refractive Surgery 31(3):553–556

Crandall D C, Leopold I H 1979 The influence of systemic drugs on tear constituents. Ophthalmology 86(1):115–125

Davies P H O C, Hopkins G A, Pearson R M 2007 Ophthalmic drugs: Diagnostic and therapeutic uses, 5th edn. Butterworth Heinemann/Elsevier, Edinburgh

Ebri A, Kuper H, Wedner S 2007 Cost-effectiveness of cycloplegic agents: results of a randomized controlled trial in Nigerian children. Investigative Ophthalmology and Visual Science 48(3):1025–1031

Edgar D F 1998 An overview of the current drugs scene. Ophthalmic and Physiological Optics 18(2):97–102

Egashira S M, Kish L L, Twelker J D et al 1993 Comparison of cyclopentolate versus tropicamide cycloplegia in children. Optometry and Vision Science: Official Publication of the American Academy of Optometry 70(12):1019–1026

Eyeson-Annan M L, Hirst L W, Battistutta D et al 1998 Comparative pupil dilation using phenylephrine alone or in combination with tropicamide. Ophthalmology 105(4):726–732

Fan D S, Rao S K, Ng J S et al 2004 Comparative study on the safety and efficacy of different cycloplegic agents in children with darkly pigmented irides. Clinical and Experimental Ophthalmology 32(5):462–467

Feenstra R, Tseng S 1992 What is actually stained by rose Bengal. Archives of Ophthalmology 110(7):984–993

Fraunfelder F W, Fraunfelder F T, Jensvold B 2002 Adverse systemic effects from pledgets of topical ocular phenylephrine 10%. American Journal of Ophthalmology 134(4):624–625

Fullard R J, Wilson G S 1986 Investigation of sloughed corneal epithelial cells collected by non-invasive irrigation of the corneal surface. Current Eye Research 5(11):847–856

Fulton A B, Dobson V, Salem D et al 1980 Cycloplegic refractions in infants and young children. American Journal of Ophthalmology 90(2):239–247

Goodman C R, Hunter D G, Repka M X 1999 A randomized comparison study of drop versus spray topical cycloplegic application. Binocular Vision and Strabismus Quarterly 14(2):107–110

Haddad D E, Rosenfield M, Portello J K et al 2007 Does prior instillation of a topical anaesthetic alter the pupillary mydriasis produced by tropicamide (0.5%)? Ophthalmic and Physiological Optics 27(3):311–314

Hagele J E, Guzek J P, Shavlik G W 1994 Lacrimal testing. Age as a factor in Jones testing. Ophthalmology 101(3):612–617

Hakim O J, Orton R B, Cadera W 1990 Topical 2.5% and 5% phenylephrine: comparison of effects on heart rate and blood pressure. Canadian Journal of Ophthalmology 25(7):336–339

Hamasaki I, Hasebe S, Kimura S et al 2007 Cycloplegic effect of 0.5% tropicamide and 0.5% phenylephrine mixed eye drops: objective assessment in Japanese schoolchildren with myopia. Japanese Journal of Ophthalmology 51(2):111–115

Hancox J, Murdoch I, Parmar D 2002 Changes in intraocular pressure following diagnostic mydriasis with cyclopentolate 1%. Eye 16(5):562–566

Harris L S, Galin M A, Mittag T W 1971 Cycloplegic provocative testing after topical administration of steroids. Archives of Ophthalmology 86(1):12–14

Hassler-Hurst J, Wadham C, Rayman G 2004 A double-blind study comparing 0.5% and 1% tropicamide for annual retinal screening in diabetic adolescents. Diabetic Medicine 21(5):434–439

Herse P, Siu A 1992 Short-term effects of proparacaine on human corneal thickness. Acta Ophthalmologica 70(6):740–744

Hofmeister E M, Kaupp S E, Schallhorn S C 2005 Comparison of tropicamide and cyclopentolate for cycloplegic refractions in myopic adult refractive surgery patients. Journal of Cataract and Refractive Surgery 31(4):694–700

Hopkins G, Pearson R 2007 Ophthalmic drugs: diagostic and therapeutic uses, 5th edn. Butterworth Heinemann/Elsevier, Edinburgh, pp 85–106

Huber M J, Smith S A, Smith S E 1985 Mydriatic drugs for diabetic patients. The British Journal of Ophthalmology 69(6):425–427

Ismail E E, Rouse M W, De Land P N 1994 A comparison of drop instillation and spray application of 1% cyclopentolate hydrochloride. Optometry and Vision Science: Official Publication of the American Academy of Optometry 71(4):235–241

Jackson T, McLure H A 2006 Pharmacology of local anesthetics. Ophthalmology Clinics of North America 19(2):155–161

Jallet G, Cleirens S, Girard E et al 1980 [Particularly rapid appearance of a severe toxic keratopathy caused by oxybuprocaine]. Bulletin des societes d'ophtalmologie de France 80(4–5):385–387

Jauregui M J, Sanders T J, Polse K A 1980 Anesthetic effects from low concentrations of proparacaine and benoxinate. Journal of the American Optometric Association 51(1):37–41

Jones L W, Hodes D T 1991 Possible allergic reactions to cyclopentolate hydrochloride: case reports with literature review of uses and adverse reactions. Ophthalmic and Physiological Optics 11(1):16–21

Jose J G, Polse K A, Holden E K 1984 Optometric pharmacology. Grune & Stratton, Orlando, FLA

Kaye S B, Chen S I, Price G et al 2002 Combined optical and atropine penalization for the treatment of strabismic and anisometropic amblyopia. J AAPOS 6(5):289–293

Keller J T, Chang F W 1976 An evaluation of the use of topical anesthetics and low concentrations of phenylephrine HCl for mydriasis. Journal of the American Optometric Association 47(6):752–754

Kergoat H, Lovasik J V, Doughty M J 1989 A pupillographic evaluation of a phenylephrine HCl 5%–tropicamide 0.8% combination mydriatic. Journal of Ocular Pharmacology 5(3):199–216

Khoo B K, Koh A, Cheong P et al 2000 Combination cyclopentolate and phenylephrine for mydriasis in premature infants with heavily pigmented irides. Journal of Pediatric Ophthalmology and Strabismus 37(1):15–20

Kim J, Foulks G N 1999 Evaluation of the efffect of lissamine green and rose bengal on human corneal epithelial cells. Cornea 18(3):328–332

Krumholz D M, Portello J K, Rosenfield M et al 2006 A combination solution for routine pupillary dilation. Optometry 77(7):350–353

Lam A K, Chen D 2007 Effect of proparacaine on central corneal thickness values: an evaluation using noncontact specular microscopy and pentacam. Cornea 26(1):55–58

Lawrenson J G, Edgar D F, Tanna G K et al 1998 Comparison of the tolerability and efficacy of unit-dose, preservative-free topical ocular anaesthetics. Ophthalmic and Physiological Optics 18(5):393–400

Lin L L, Shih Y F, Hsiao C H et al 1998 The cycloplegic effects of cyclopentolate and tropicamide on myopic children. Journal of Ocular Pharmacology and Therapeutics: the official journal of the Association for Ocular Pharmacology and Therapeutics 14(4): 331–335

Loewen N, Barry J C 2000 The use of cycloplegic agents. Results of a 1999 survey of German-speaking centers for pediatric ophthalmology and strabology. Strabismus 8(2):91–99

Lyle W M, Page C 1975 Possible adverse effects from local anesthetics and the treatment of these reactions. American Journal of Optometry and Physiological Optics 52(11):736–744

McLure H A, Rubin A P 2005 Review of local anaesthetic agents. Minerva Anestesiologica 71(3):59–74

Manning F J, Wehrly S R, Foulks G N 1995 Patient tolerance and ocular surface staining characteristics of lissamine green versus rose Bengal. Ophthalmology 102(12):1953–1957

Manny R E, Jaanus S D 2001 Cycloplegics. In: Bartlett J D et al (eds) Clinical ocular pharmacology, 4th edn. Butterworth-Heinemann, Boston, pp 149–166

Manny R E, Fern K D, Zervas H J et al 1993 1% cyclopentolate hydrochloride: another look at the time course of cycloplegia using an objective measure of the accommodative response. Optometry and Vision Science 70(8):651–665

Manny R E, Hussein M, Scheiman M et al 2001 Tropicamide (1%): an effective cycloplegic agent for myopic children. Investigative Ophthalmology and Visual Science 42(8):1728–1735

Marchini G, Babighian S, Tosi R et al 2003 Comparative study of the effects of 2% ibopamine, 10% phenylephrine, and 1% tropicamide on the anterior segment. Investigative Ophthalmology and Visual Science 44(1):281–289

Mason A, Mason J 2002 Optometrist prescribing of therapeutic agents: findings of the AESOP survey. Health Policy (Amsterdam, Netherlands) 60(2):185–197

Mutti D O, Zadnik K, Egashira S et al 1994 The effect of cycloplegia on measurement of the ocular components. Investigative Ophthalmology and Visual Science 35(2):515–527

Nam S M, Lee H K, Kim E K et al 2006 Comparison of corneal thickness after the instillation of topical anesthetics: proparacaine versus oxybuprocaine. Cornea 25(1):51–54

Norden L C 1976 Adverse reactions to topical ocular anesthetics. Journal of the American Optometric Association 47(6):730–733

Norn M S 1970 Rose Bengal vital staining. Staining of cornea and conjunctiva by 10 percent rose Bengal, compared with 1 percent. Acta Ophthalmologica 48(3):546–559

Optometrists' formulary 2007 College of Optometrists

Owens H, Garner L F, Yap M K et al 1998 Age dependence of ocular biometric measurements under cycloplegia with tropicamide and cyclopentolate. Clinical and Experimental Optometry: Journal of the Australian Optometrical Association 81(4):159–162

Pandit R J, Taylor R 2000 Mydriasis and glaucoma: exploding the myth. A systematic review. Diabetic Medicine 17(10):693–699

Penna E P, Tabbara K F 1986 Oxybuprocaine keratopathy: a preventable disease. The British Journal of Ophthalmology 70(3):202–204

Perez-Gomez I, Hollingsworth J, Efron N 2004 Effects of benoxinate hydrochloride 0.4% on the morphological appearance of the cornea using confocal microscopy. Contact Lens and Anterior Eye 27(1):45–48

Pollack S L, Hunt J S, Polse K A 1981 Dose-response effects of tropicamide HCl. American Journal of Optometry and Physiological Optics 58(5):361–366

Polse K A, Keener R J, Jauregui M J 1978 Dose–response effects of corneal anesthetics. American Journal of Optometry and Physiological Optics 55(1):8–14

Pophal M, Ripkin D 1995 Assessment of anterior chamber depth. Oblique illuminatin test. Annals of Ophthalmology 27:171–174

Portello J K, Jaanus S D 2001 Mydriatics and mydriolytics. In: Bartlett J D et al (eds) Clinical ocular pharmacology, 4th edn. Butterworth-Heinemann, Boston, pp 135–148

Pukrushpan P, Tulvatana W, Kulvichit K 2006 Intraocular pressure change following application of 1% tropicamide for diagnostic mydriasis. Acta Ophthalmologica Scandinavia 84(2):268–270

Rhee D J, Deramo V A 2001 The Wills eye drug guide: diagnostic and therapeutic medications, 2nd edn. Lippincott Williams & Wilkins, Philadelphia

Ritchie J M, Cohen P J 1975 Local anesthetics. In: Goodman L S, Gilman A (eds) The pharmacological basis of therapeutics, 5th edn. Macmillan, New York, pp 379–403

Romanchuk K G 1979 Seidel's test using 10% fluorescein. Canadian Journal of Ophthalmology 14(4):253–256

Rosenbaum A L, Bateman J B, Bremer D L et al 1981 Cycloplegic refraction in esotropic children. Cyclopentolate versus atropine. Ophthalmology 88(10):1031–1034

Rosenfield M, Linfield P B 1986 A comparison of the effects of cycloplegics on accommodation ability for distance vision and on the apparent near point. Ophthalmic and Physiological Optics 6 (3):317–320

Rosenwasser G O, Holland S, Pflugfelder S C et al 1990 Topical anesthetic abuse. Ophthalmology 97(8):967–972

Schnider C 2001 Dyes. In: Bartlett J and Jaanus S (eds) Clinical ocular pharmacology, 4th edn. Butterworth-Heinemann, Boston, pp 349–366

Shafi T, Koay P 1998 Randomised prospective masked study comparing patient comfort following the instillation of topical proxymetacaine and amethocaine. The British Journal of Ophthalmology 82 (11):1285–1287

Shah P, Jacks A S, Adams G G 1997 Paediatric cycloplegia: a new approach. Eye (London, England) 11(6):845–846

Shaw B R, Lewis R A 1986 Intraocular pressure elevation after pupillary dilation in open angle glaucoma. Archives of Ophthalmology 104 (8):1185–1188

Shiono T 1989 Effect of topical anesthesia on secretion of lysozyme and lysosomal enzymes in human tears. Japanese Journal of Ophthalmology 33(3):375–379

Siderov J, Nurse S 2005 The mydriatic effect of multiple doses of tropicamide. Optometry and Vision Science 82(11):955–958

Siu A W, Sum A C, Lee D T et al 1999 Prior topical anesthesia reduces time to full cycloplegia in Chinese. Japanese Journal of Ophthalmology 43(6):466–471

Sjogren H, Bloch K 1971 Keratoconjunctivitis sicca and the Sjogren syndrome. Survey of Ophthalmology 16:145–159

Soroka M, Krumholz D, Bennett A 2006 The practice of optometry: national board of examiners in optometry survey of optometric patients. Optometry and Vision Science 83(9):625–636

Stiles J, Krohne S, Rankin A et al 2001 The efficacy of 0.5% proparacaine stored at room temperature. Veterinary Ophthalmology 4(3):205–207

Stroop W G, Chen T M, Chodosh J et al 2000 PCR assessment of HSV-1 corneal infection in animals treated with rose Bengal and lissamine green b. Investigative Ophthalmology and Visual Science 41 (8):2096–2102

Sturrock J E, Nunn J F 1979 Cytotoxic effects of procaine, lignocaine and bupivacaine. British Journal of Anaesthesia 51(4):273–281

Sweetman S E 2007 Martindale: the complete drug reference 35. Pharmaceutical Press, London

The Medicine Act 1968 Chapter 67

The Opticians Act 1989 Chapter 44, and as now modified by statutory instrument 1999 no. 3267

Twelker J D, Mutti D O 2001 Retinoscopy in infants using a near noncycloplegic technique, cycloplegia with tropicamide 1%, and cycloplegia with cyclopentolate 1%. Optometry and Vision Science 78(4):215–222

Vale J, Cox B 1985 Drugs and the eye, 2nd edn. Butterworths, London

Van Herick W, Shaffer R N, Schwartz A 1969 Estimation of width of angle of anterior chamber. Incidence and significance of the narrow angle. American Journal of Ophthalmology 68(4):626–629

Wesson M D, Bartlett J D, Swiatocha J et al 1993 Mydriatic efficacy of a cycloplegic spray in the pediatric population. Journal of the American Optometric Association 64(9):637–640

Wilson G, Fullard R J 1988 Cell sloughing with proparacaine. Journal of the American Optometric Association 59(9):701–702

Woodard D R, Woodard R B 1991 Handbook of drugs in primary eyecare. Appleton & Lange, Norwalk, CONN.

Yeung K K, Kageyama J Y, Carnevali T 2000 A comparison of fluoracaine and fluorox on corneal epithelial cell desquamation after Goldmann applanation tonometry. Optometry 71(1):49–54

Yolton D P, German C J 1980 Fluress, fluorescein and benoxinate: recovery from bacterial contamination. Journal of the American Optometric Association 51(5):471–474

Zappia R J, Milder B 1972a Lacrimal drainage function. 1. The Jones fluorescein test. American Journal of Ophthalmology 74(1): 154–159

Zappia R J, Milder B 1972b Lacrimal drainage function. 2. The fluorescein dye disappearance test. American Journal of Ophthalmology 74(1):160–162

CHAPTER 8

Therapeutic drugs

Graham Hopkins

Introduction

Topical application remains the preferred administration route for drugs to treat conditions concerning the anterior segment of the eye. Other routes are used for deeper problems such as macular degeneration secondary to subfoveal neovascularization, but this chapter will concentrate purely on agents administered as drops, gels or ointments to the conjunctival sac.

Therapeutic drugs are administered to produce one or more of the following effects:

- resolving infections caused by a variety of microorganisms
- reducing inflammation, whether exogenous or endogenous in origin
- reducing the effects of an allergic reaction
- reducing IOP
- ameliorating the problems caused by tear deficiency.

Antiinfectives

Ocular infections can result from the invasion of a variety of organisms, such as protozoa, fungi, bacteria, rickettsiae and viruses, and their treatment is partly determined by the causative organism and partly by the locus of infection. A deep infection with *Pseudomonas* will require a radically different approach to a mild conjunctivitis.

However, the basic goal of all treatments is the same, i.e. to maintain the minimum concentration necessary to kill (or inhibit the growth of) the infecting organism for sufficient time for the infection to be eradicated. Antiinfectives produce their effect by the competitive inhibition of some biochemical process in the microorganism, and thus concentration of the agent is all important.

The emergence of so-called 'superbugs' which have the ability to resist a wide variety of antiinfectives has been a great stimulus to the discovery and development of new agents and therefore the examples listed below may become obsolete in the future.

Antibacterials

The use of any antibacterial is aimed at the swift eradication of the invading organism, with a minimum of side effects to the host. Three factors are important in achieving this goal:

1. Drug: This should be based on knowing which organism is causing the infection. Unfortunately, this would normally involve taking a swab and identifying the organism. This involves costs and time and could delay treatment. To avoid these problems antibacterials with broad spectra are generally used.

2. Dose: This should be high enough to allow the maintenance of the minimum inhibitory concentration for the probable invading organism. This varies according to the antibacterial used, but is normally achievable with the

concentrations found in ophthalmic drops, providing the dosing is frequent enough. The half-life of a drop in the conjunctival sac is very short and after 60 minutes little of the active ingredient is present. To obtain sufficiently high levels, hourly dosing is often required.

3. Duration: Often, the clinical signs of infection will disappear before the organism is completely eradicated. If treatment is discontinued at this stage, the infection can reappear, but this time with a strain of the organism resistant to the antibacterial. It is important that treatment is continued for a period after the apparent resolution of the problem. It is difficult to be precise about exactly how long to continue treatment but a general rule of thumb would appear to be 3 days after the eye is symptomless.

With the use of antibacterial agents, there is always a danger of the emergence of resistant strains resulting from the previous use of the agent to treat an infection somewhere else in the body. With the two principal agents used generally to treat surface infections of the eye, this is not such a problem. Chloramphenicol has very little systemic use because of its toxicity, causing fatal blood dyscrasias. It is only used for treating life-threatening infections. Fusidic acid, although it is available in an oral form and is widely used in the topical treatment of skin infections, is another agent which has found favour in ophthalmic treatments.

Chloramphenicol

Chloramphenicol has a wide spectrum, being effective not only against ophthalmic pathogenic bacteria such as *Corynebacterium* and *Haemophilus* species but also some rickettsiae and spirochaetes. It produces its antibacterial effect by inhibiting protein synthesis by bacterial ribosomes. Resistance to it can occur by the production of an inactivating enzyme, chloramphenicol acetyltransferase, but for the reasons stated above resistance is relatively uncommon (Seal et al 1982).

Chloramphenicol is ideally suited to ophthalmic use being lipid soluble and thus penetrating the cornea well, leading to high levels in the cornea (Ismail & Morton 1987) and aqueous humour. It is available as drops (0.5%) or ointment (1%). In order to maintain sufficiently high levels, the drops should be administered at a maximum of 2-hourly intervals, especially in the initial stage of treatment. Ointment, which has a significantly longer half-life, can be administered four times a day.

Even after many decades, in the UK chloramphenicol has remained in the front line in the treatment of bacterial conjunctivitis and fears of the development of the toxic effects associated with systemic infections have proved unfounded (Titcomb 1997). In fact, in the UK it is now available to the public without prescription.

Fusidic acid

Like the previous agent, fusidic acid produces its effect by inhibiting protein synthesis, but not by binding to ribosomes. It is effective against a range of Gram-positive bacteria, including some strains of methicillin resistant *Staphylcoccus aureus* (MRSA). Most Gram-negative bacteria are resistant, although activity has been demonstrated against some *Neisseria* species. Resistant strains can develop quickly.

It is used as a 1% viscous eyedrop, requiring only twice-a-day application and now equals chloramphenicol as the front-line choice in the treatment of bacterial conjunctivitis. It has demonstrated better compliance than chloramphenicol (James et al 1991).

Polymixin

This is an older antibacterial, which is normally found in combination with other agents such as bacitracin or trimethoprim. It is similar to gentamicin (see Aminoglycosides, below) in its antibacterial properties, being effective against many strains of *Pseudomonas aeruginosa* and many other Gram-negative rods.

Quinolones: ciprofloxacin and ofloxacin

These are relatively recent introductions into the field of broad-spectrum antibiotics and are extensively used in the treatment of many systemic infections, such as those affecting the respiratory and urinary tract. They interfere with the production of DNA. The emergence of resistance is low and there is no cross-resistance with other groups of antibacterials. Ciprofloxacin and ofloxacin are produced as 0.3% eyedrops. Both agents are well absorbed and effective levels are achieved in the aqueous humour. They have both been shown to be effective in the treatment of bacterial conjunctivitis.

Aminoglycosides: neomycin and gentamicin

These are a group of effective, but toxic, antibiotics which produce their effects by inhibiting protein synthesis involving a combination with mRNA and by disrupting cell membranes. They have had systemic use in the past but the main use today is topical. They have a wide antibacterial spectrum affecting Gram-positive and Gram-negative bacteria, including *Pseudomonas*. Resistance occurs as a result of the development of mutations in the ribosome binding sites, decreased uptake by the cell or by the development of enzymes which inactivate the antibiotic.

Neomycin is often found in combination eyedrops with steroids such as prednisolone and betamethasone. It is rarely used on its own today. An isomer of neomycin (neomycin B) is also known as framycetin and has a wide antibacterial spectrum against Gram-positive and Gram-negative bacteria.

Gentamicin is probably the most effective of the aminoglycosides, being effective against many strains of *Pseudomonas aeruginosa* and is often the treatment of choice for infections caused by this organism. Resistant strains, however, have been found. For this reason it should not be used for trivial infections.

Tobramycin is one of the newer aminoglycoside antibiotics and has a better antibacterial spectrum than gentamicin. It is effective against most strains of *Pseudomonas aeruginosa* and many of the staphylococci found on the surface of the eye. It is available in combination with dexamethasone in eyedrop form.

Propamidine and dibromopropamidine

These are antimicrobial compounds which as well as antifungal properties possess activity against some Gram-positive and a few Gram-negative bacteria. Their action is not inhibited by pus or serum. These compounds form the active ingredients of over-the-counter preparations for the treatment of bacterial conjunctivitis. Dibromopropamidine has been used in conjunction with neomycin in the treatment of *Acanthamoeba* infections. It is effective against the active trophozite but is ineffective against the dormant cyst form.

Antivirals

The eye is susceptible to infection from a variety of viruses, but the ones that respond to treatment are from the herpes group, in particular herpes simplex, which causes dendritic ulcer, and herpes zoster, which is responsible for ophthalmic shingles. Many of the older compounds, e.g. idoxuridine and trifluorothymidine, have fallen into disuse, and today only two are in regular use.

Acyclovir

Acyclovir (acycloguanosine) owes its ability to attack only virus-infected cells due to the difference in the structure and functioning of thymidine kinase (an enzyme necessary to activate the drug) found in viruses to that found in uninfected host cells. The form of thymidine kinase found in virus-infected cells can metabolize acyclovir while the form found in uninfected host cells cannot. Acycloguanosine is phosphorylated to acycloguanosine triphosphate, which competes with guanosine triphosphate for incorporation into the DNA chain. When the phosphorylated drug is taken up, it prevents further growth of the DNA chain.

This selectivity of action is important because it is necessary not only to eradicate the virus but also to allow growth and repair of the damaged cornea. Acyclovir does not interfere with corneal regrowth and re-epithelization (Lass et al 1979). It is available as a 3% ointment.

Ganciclovir

Concern about the growth of HIV infection has led to the search for new antivirals. Additionally, the discovery of the problems caused by cytomegalovirus (CMV) in the retina has stimulated further research. As a result, a new antiviral ganciclovir has been marketed, which is a close relative of acyclovir, being a derivative of guanine. Like acyclovir, it must be phosphorylated to produce the inhibition of viruses. CMV does not produce thymidine kinase, but cells infected with this virus phosphorylate the antiviral at a much greater rate than uninfected cells. Once activated, ganciclovir inactivates all herpes virus DNA polymerases, thus preventing replication. Although developed to treat CMV infections, ganciclovir is effective in the treatment of herpes simplex and herpes zoster infections.

Antifungals

Although many parts of the body are susceptible to fungal infections, e.g. oral and vaginal thrush, athlete's foot and fungal infections of the nails, the eye appears to be relatively resistant to this type of infection. When ophthalmic fungal infections do occur they are potentially serious, sight-threatening events and will require specialist attention. Some of the antibacterial agents have antifungal actions, but there are no specific antifungals generally available.

Antiinflammatory agents

The effects of inflammation of the ocular structures can be serious and sight threatening. Thus, several potent antiinflammatory agents have been developed to reduce these effects. However, inflammation can be the body's response to infections and it is important in these cases that the infection is treated at the same time by the use of a concurrent antiinfective or the use of a combination product.

Steroids

The term 'steroid' refers to the chemical structure shared by a group of biologically important compounds which includes cholesterol, vitamin D, the male and female sex hormones, and the adrenocorticoid hormones. The latter has several important actions. Firstly, they can affect electrolyte balance – mineralocorticoid action. They can also affect blood glucose levels and have an antiinflammatory effect – glucocorticoid. Some compounds, e.g. aldosterone and fludrocortisone, are predominantly mineralocorticoids, while others such as hydrocortisone have both effects.

Chemical research has led to the development of more potent and effective compounds with greater antiinflammatory effects and less mineralocorticoid effects. Corticosteroids reduce inflammation, whatever the cause – infection, radiation, immunological, chemical or trauma. They act on many of the effects of inflammation. They reduce the vasodilation that normally accompanies inflammation and which is responsible for the characteristic redness. They act as mast cell stabilizers and reduce the production of histamine. Part of their action is due to the inhibition of the conversion of arachidonic acid to prostaglandin by the enzyme cyclooxygenase.

Of course, these potent therapeutic effects come at a price. Steroids are well known for their side effects when taken systemically, not least of which is the development of a posterior subcapsular cataract. They can also produce effects when applied topically, including cataract. They can inhibit wound healing, changing the relationship between cells and collagen, which reduces the tensile strength of wounds. Steroids can also produce a rise in intraocular pressure (IOP) in a small number of individuals, so-called 'steroid responders'. The ocular hypertension is caused by a reduction in outflow facility resulting from morphological and biochemical changes (Clark 1995). There are similarities between steroid glaucoma and primary open-angle glaucoma and it has been postulated that there is a causal relationship. All topical steroids have this ability. Some are claimed to produce a lesser effect but this is probably due to differences in absorption. The effect is dose related and normally occurs after high doses for prolonged periods. It is reversible in the early stages, but if treatment continues, the condition becomes permanent.

Hydrocortisone

Hydrocortisone is a naturally occurring corticosteroid with marked glucocorticoid and mineralocorticoid actions. Its principal use today is as a treatment for skin inflammations such as those occurring from allergic reactions or insect bites. It has been formulated with neomycin as an eye ointment but its ophthalmic use has to a large extent been superseded by more modern compounds.

Prednisolone

Prednisolone has five times the antiinflammatory potency of hydrocortisone and reduced mineralocorticoid actions. It has a longer half-life than the naturally occurring compound, but a shorter one than other synthetic drugs such as betamethasone and dexamethasone. It is extensively used orally in the treatment of asthma and other atopic conditions. It has also been formulated as a 0.5% and 1.0% eyedrop. The weaker strength is available on its own or in combination with an antibiotic.

Betamethasone

Betamethasone has marked antiinflammatory actions with minimal mineralocorticoid effects. It is effective in low concentrations and, like prednisolone, is formulated on its own or with an antibiotic.

Dexamethasone

Dexamethasone is a potent antiinflammatory steroid with minimal mineralocorticoid effects. It has the greatest effect on IOP.

Fluorometholone

The principal advantage of this agent is a reduced effect on IOP.

Rimexolone

Used short term for acute inflammations, it has similar effects to fluorometholone.

Nonsteroidal antiinflammatory drugs

Nonsteroidal antiinflammatory drugs (NSAIDs) are potent inhibitors of cyclooxygenase, i.e. the enzyme responsible for producing prostaglandins, which are implicated in the process of inflammation. Prostaglandins increase the permeability of the ciliary epithelium, thereby allowing large amounts of protein to pass into the aqueous humour. This will produce aqueous flare. Prostaglandins are also thought to be involved in corneal neovascularization. They have three principal effects:

- antiinflammatory
- analgesic
- antipyretic.

NSAIDs do not produce the same side effects as steroids. They do not cause a rise in IOP or posterior subcapsular cataracts. However, the reduction in prostaglandin levels does produce problems in the gastrointestinal tract, initially dyspepsia and later gastritis and gastric ulcer. This is not a direct irritant effect, and can be produced irrespective of the route of administration. A new generation of NSAIDs has been developed, those acting principally on cyclooxygenase-2 (COX-2 inhibitors), to avoid this problem, but these agents are not without problems.

The principal systemic use of these agents has been in the treatment of autoimmune conditions such as rheumatoid arthritis and, because of the prevalence of these conditions, many agents have been introduced for systemic use. A few of these have been formulated for ophthalmic use.

Diclofenac

This is one of the most commonly used NSAIDs for systemic use, marketed under the trade name of Voltarol. It is a potent inhibitor of cyclooxygenase. In the eye it has been used for the prevention of intraoperative miosis (Bonomi et al 1987), a prostaglandin-mediated effect, and the reduction of postoperative inflammation, either alone or with steroids such as prednisolone (Struck et al 1994). It can be as effective as dexamethasone for this purpose. Its effectiveness in more everyday inflammations such as vernal conjunctivitis, giant papillary conjunctivitis and seasonal allergic conjunctivitis has not been proven.

Ketorolac

Ketorolac has indications similar to those of diclofenac. It penetrates the eye well and is an effective antiinflammatory agent.

Flurbiprofen

Flurbiprofen has similar properties and indications to ketorolac.

Cycloplegics

Part of the treatment of inflamed muscles is rest. If inflamed muscles (whether skeletal or smooth) continue to be used, discomfort will result and healing will be delayed. If the inflamed muscle is attached to a limb, it is a relatively straightforward matter to immobilize it. Intraocular muscles can be immobilized by paralysing them, using a long-acting antimuscarinic agent such as atropine or cyclopentolate. In addition to the relief of discomfort, antimuscarinics reduce the formation of posterior synechiae (adhesions between the posterior surface of the iris and the anterior surface of the lens).

Antimuscarinics are rarely used alone and are normally accompanied by steroid drops. Occasionally, with very darkly pigmented eyes, a synergistic sympathomimetic mydriatic may be necessary to dilate the pupil (see Chs 6 and 7).

Atropine

Theoretically, this should be the drug of choice, being the longest-acting antimuscarinic agent in use. However, its toxicity and central nervous system (CNS) effects have led to the use of more modern drugs.

Cyclopentolate

The modern drug of choice, it is relatively long acting. It also has CNS effects (see Chs 6 and 7), but these are not normally seen when excessive doses are avoided.

Antiallergic agents

Antiinflammatory agents are used to reduce the effects of inflammation resulting from trauma, infection or autoimmune conditions. Antiallergic agents are used to combat the effects of allergy resulting from the interaction between an external allergen and the body's antibodies to that allergen. The effects of this reaction involve histamine and other related compounds.

Histamine produces the well-defined triple response when it is injected into the skin. Firstly, a local vasodilation at the injection site, which manifests itself as a red spot. This is followed by an increase in capillary permeability to plasma proteins, which results in oedema which is seen as localized swelling. Lastly, diffuse redness appears as a result of reflex vasodilation. This triple response is accompanied by stimulation of pain and itch fibres.

There is more than one type of histamine receptor; H_2 receptors are involved in gastric acid secretion. Accordingly, H_2-blocking drugs such as cimetidine and ranitidine are used in the treatment of dyspepsia. However, the triple response is mediated by H_1 receptors.

The allergic symptoms caused by histamine can be alleviated by one of three methods:

- using an H_1 antagonist – antihistamine
- preventing the release of histamine – mast cell stabilizer
- using an agonist on a receptor with an opposite effect to histamine – usually a sympathomimetic.

Antihistamines

Antihistamines are best known for their systemic use in the treatment of hay fever. They are divided into the older, sedating and the more modern non-sedating products. The former are still used because they are very effective. Many antihistamines have antimuscarinic actions and this is responsible for some of the side effects.

Some of the drugs are topically active and this has led to their incorporation into eyedrops. This has the advantage of being faster in action because the drug is delivered directly to the affected structure, the conjunctiva, and there is less chance of systemic effects.

Antazoline

Antazoline has been available for many years in combination with a sympathomimetic (xylometazoline). The combination is a synergistic mixture of a pharmacological and physiological antagonist. The antihistamine relieves the itching while the sympathomimetic is a powerful vasoconstrictor and reduces the redness.

Azelastine

Some antihistamines possess mast cell stabilizing actions, in that they prevent the release of histamine as well as antagonizing its effects. Azelastine also prevents the release of other agents involved in the allergic response, such as leucotrienes and serotonin.

Emedastine

Emedastine drops are licensed for the treatment of seasonal allergic conjunctivitis.

Epinastine

Epinastine is a very selective H_1 blocker, having little antimuscarinic action.

Ketotifen

Ketotifen is similar to azelastine, having mast cell stabilizing properties. It is quick in onset and is very effective in reducing the signs and symptoms of allergic conjunctivitis.

Levocabastine

This one of the newer antihistamines which has been used for the treatment of allergic conjunctivitis (Zuber & Pecaud 1988).

Olopatadine

Olopatadine has no antimuscarinic actions, but it does stabilize mast cells, preventing the release of histamine. It compares favourably with sodium cromoglicate and nedocromil.

Mast cell stabilizers

The reaction of an antigen with an antibody sets in motion a chain of reactions which ultimately leads to the release of histamine and other chemical mediators from mast cells. This process can be inhibited by mast cell stabilizers which prevent the influx of calcium necessary for histamine release. They are best used prophylactically and patients should ideally instil the drops before symptoms are experienced and continue until after there is no danger of exposure to the allergen. If symptoms have appeared before the commencement of treatment, then an antihistamine can be used in conjunction with the mast cell stabilizer unless the mast cell stabilizer has inherent antihistamine activity.

Nedocromil sodium

Nedocromil sodium is effective against many of the cells involved in the inflammatory process such as macrophages and eosinophils as well as mast cells. It is fast in onset and has the advantage over the older drug, cromoglicate, in that it only requires a twice-a-day dosage as compared with four times a day, when used in the treatment of seasonal allergic conjunctivitis (Blumenthal et al 1992). It is effective also in the treatment of perennial allergic conjunctivitis, but this may require a more frequent dosage. It has few side effects.

Sodium cromoglicate

This drug was originally developed for the treatment of asthma, when the cause was allergenic and steroids could not be used. Its use for this purpose has to a large extent been superseded by newer agents. Its major use today is as a treatment for seasonal allergic conjunctivitis and it is available in a variety of over-the-counter preparations. It has no intrinsic vasoconstrictor or antiinflammatory action and does not act as an antihistamine.

Lodoxamide

Lodoxamide is another mast cell stabilizer with no intrinsic antihistamine effect which is indicated for the treatment of giant papillary conjunctivitis, vernal conjunctivitis and other forms of noninfective conjunctivitis. It is applied four times a day and has a faster onset than cromoglicate (Fahy et al 1988).

Topical vasoconstrictors

Topical vasoconstrictors are solutions of sympathomimetics designed to reduce the vasodilation of conjunctival blood vessels resulting from a variety of stimuli such as allergenic, chemical, and traumatic. They act directly on the smooth muscle of the blood vessels. The concentrations applied for this purpose are much lower than those used for producing mydriasis and thus the contraindication for patients with closed-angle glaucoma is more theoretical than actual.

Xylometazoline

It is used in combination with antazoline (see above) at a concentration of 0.05% as treatment for allergic conjunctivitis.

Combination products

There are several combination products containing a steroid and an antiinfective. Although their use should be restricted to the treatment of infections where the cause of the infection is known, they are often employed as 'antibiotic cover'. If the cause of the inflammation is not certain, then the treatment with a steroid alone could be disastrous. The incorporation of the two agents into one product could be justified in that it aids patient concordance, as they only have to apply one drop instead of two. Patients often find it difficult applying drops and giving them more than one to put in may reduce compliance. However, the British National Formulary (www. bnf.org) states that their use 'is rarely justified'.

Ocular hypotensive agents

Glaucoma continues to be a very serious problem and is a major cause of preventable blindness. The last two decades have seen a great increase in the number and types of topical glaucoma treatments. In addition, increased life expectancy has led to the prospect of these products being used for much longer periods and the possibility of the development of chronic local and systemic effects. In selecting an anti-glaucoma preparation, certain criteria should be considered:

1. Reduction of intraocular pressure
   Reduction of IOP is the aim of all glaucoma treatments, but the questions are by how much and what level of IOP constitutes 'control'? A figure of 20 mmHg is often taken as the figure below which it should be reduced, but for a patient with low-tension glaucoma the disease would continue to progress at this level (see Ch. 10). It is probably more important that the pressure remains steady and there is little variation throughout the day.

2. Duration of effect
   Drugs with a long duration of action have a double benefit. Not only is administration easier for the patient as they require fewer instillations per day but compliance is improved if the drug only needs to be administered twice a day rather than four times a day.

3. Preservation of visual field
   This is obviously the most important aim of treatment. Modern diagnostic methods (see Ch. 20) often detect the problem before extensive damage to the visual field has occurred.

4. Maintenance of effect
   On occasion, a treatment which is initially successful may lose its effect with continued use, necessitating either a replacement or additional therapy. Both will have implications for patient concordance.

5. Compatibility
   For the reason stated above, as it is often necessary to administer more than one product, it is vital that they are compatible, both chemically and pharmacologically.

6. Lack of topical adverse effects
   Often, with early diagnosis, the condition may be symptomless and unpleasant side effects from the medication may affect patient compliance adversely. It is difficult to persuade patients to use eyedrops which are causing discomfort for a condition that is currently asymptomatic.

7. Lack of systemic effects
   Although the treatments are applied topically, they have the ability to produce systemic effects. Many therapies produce their effects by modifying the actions of the autonomic nervous system, and thus can affect other autonomically innervated structures in the body.

8. Patient compliance
   Many factors affect patient compliance. Apart from the nature of the active ingredient and the adjuvants contained in the formulation, the design of the container can also make a difference.

Glaucoma treatments have evolved over several decades. The impetus has been towards the reduction of side effects as much as the enhancement of therapeutic action. Some of the early treatments were effective but the side effects made them difficult to use. The groups are arranged below in roughly chronological order, illustrating the evolution of treatment.

Parasympathomimetics

Previously referred to as miotics, parasympathomimetics are the same agents that are used to reverse the effects of mydriatic drops (see Ch. 7). They produce their hypotensive effect by contracting the longitudinal ciliary muscle, which puts tension on the trabecular meshwork. The accompanying miosis is an annoying side effect, unless, of course, it is angle-closure glaucoma that is being treated.

At the height of their use, many different miotics were tried, not only other parasympathomimetics but also anticholinesterases as well. Some of the latter, the irreversible anticholinesterases, were very potent and had long durations of action. The contraction of the ciliary muscle was sufficiently strong as to increase the possibility of retinal detachment in susceptible patients.

Due to the improved diagnostic techniques that have allowed the differential diagnosis of open- and closed-angle glaucoma and the advent of newer treatments, miotics have fallen into disuse and the only one used today is pilocarpine.

Pilocarpine

Pilocarpine was first used in ophthalmology in the nineteenth century and is a natural alkaloid found in species of *Pilocarpus* (including *P. microphyllus*, the jaborandi bush). It is available in a range of concentrations from 0.5% to 4%. Its effects last for about 6 hours and thus require a four-times-a-day regimen, if used alone. When used as adjunct therapy, it is often used just twice a day. It increases outflow and has little effect on aqueous production.

Developments in the formulation of pilocarpine have been aimed at prolonging its action, thus requiring less frequent administration and less IOP variation over the course of the day. Methods employed include using viscolized solutions, gels, oily solutions and controlled delivery devices. This latter method consisted of a viscous solution surrounded by a membrane that allowed a slow but constant delivery of pilocarpine. To date, it has failed to find widespread use.

Sympathomimetics

Sympathomimetics reduce IOP by reducing aqueous production and increasing outflow. However, their introduction into the treatment of glaucoma was dependent on the discovery of techniques for assessing the depth of the anterior chamber angle, such as the gonioscope. Sympathomimetics have the ability to dilate the pupil and therefore are obviously contraindicated in narrow-angle glaucoma.

The first sympathomimetic used was adrenaline (epinephrine) and its introduction produced two immediate advantages. Firstly, no miosis is produced and secondly it can be administered only twice a day. Its action on IOP is complex, involving an initial fall, followed by a rise, followed by more persistent fall. The action is mediated by both alpha and beta receptors.

The use of adrenaline is not without its problems. Its vasoconstrictor action eventually leads to reactive hyperaemia and a red eye. Adrenaline is inherently unstable and is liable to oxidation to a black breakdown product, adrenochrome, which can be deposited in the cornea (Madge et al 1971). Maculopathy can occur in aphakic patients (Kolker & Becker 1968). Adrenaline is no longer used in the treatment of glaucoma.

The problems of adrenaline have led to the introduction of newer sympathomimetics: apraclonidine, brimonidine and dipivefrin.

Apraclonidine

Apraclonidine is a derivative of clonidine, a centrally acting systemic antihypertensive agent. It is a selective alpha$_2$ agonist which produces a marked fall in IOP by reducing secretion. It is well tolerated but unfortunately it is subject to rapid tachyphylaxis and can only be used short term. It is used in a 1% unit-dose preparation for the treatment or prevention of increased IOP following surgery or as a 0.5% multi-dose for adjunct therapy.

Brimonidine

Brimonidine has no vasoconstrictor or mydriatic actions, being a highly selective alpha$_2$ agonist. It acts both on secretion and outflow and can be used on its own or as an adjunct therapy. It is used as a 0.2% multi-dose preparation.

Dipivefrin

Dipivefrin is a prodrug in that it is inactive in vitro and only becomes active when it is acted upon by enzymes which split it into adrenaline and pivalic acid. The advantage of the prodrug is that it has good lipid solubility and passes through the cornea easily. Theoretically, it should have less vasoconstrictor effect on the conjunctival blood vessels but reactive hyperaemia (Azuma & Hirumo 1981) and follicular conjunctivitis (Coleiro et al 1988) have been noted.

Beta blockers

Beta blockers are widely used in the treatment of cardiovascular problems such as hypertension. The discovery that some of them lowered IOP led to their use for the treatment of glaucoma. At the time of their introduction they represented an advance in therapy, being an effective, well-tolerated, twice-daily treatment. The hypotensive effect is due a reduction in secretion rather than an increase in outflow.

However, they are not without problems. Beta-stimulant drugs are used in the treatment of asthma and chronic obstructive pulmonary disease and their effects can be inhibited by the use of beta blockers, thus leading to airway constriction in affected patients. Cardio-selective beta$_1$ blockers were thought to avoid this problem but they still have the ability to cause difficulties.

The use of these medications for the treatment of cardiovascular problems means they have the ability to cause cardiovascular side effects when applied topically. Some beta blockers have been claimed to have intrinsic sympathomimetic activity. In other words, they are acting as partial agonists and should cause less bradycardia and bronchoconstriction.

Some of the early beta blockers were found to have membrane stabilizing actions on nerve fibres and acted as local anaesthetics. If this property were present in topically applied drugs, it would have the potential to cause corneal damage. Although most beta blockers do indeed act in this fashion, it is not usually clinically significant.

Betaxolol

Betaxolol is a cardio-selective (beta$_1$) blocker, which is available as both a 0.5% solution and a 0.25% suspension. It has demonstrated a reduction in visual field loss, although its hypotensive effect is modest.

Carteolol

Carteolol is available in a 1% and a 2% solution and has a lower potency than other available drugs.

Levobunolol

Levobunolol is very similar to timolol (see below) (Savelsbergh-Fillette & Demailly 1988), which, being the first beta blocker to be introduced, is the standard against which all others are compared.

Metipranolol

Metipranolol is available only as single-use units. Unfortunately, it has a higher incidence of stinging on instillation than other agents (Krieglstein et al 1987).

Timolol

Timolol, the first beta blocker to be introduced for the treatment of glaucoma, is well tolerated when applied topically. It is interesting that upon instillation it produces an effect in the contralateral eye as well as the treated eye. This observation calls into question the practice of using the contralateral eye as a control when monitoring the effects of the drug.

Applied twice a day, the effect is rapid in onset and the maximum effect is seen within 2 hours, with some hypotensive effect being detected after 24 hours. Unfortunately, over the long term the effects appear to decline (Steinert et al 1981) and adjunct therapy is sometimes required. It is available in both multi-dose and single-dose solutions of 0.25% and 0.50% as well as eye gels at the same concentrations.

Carbonic anhydrase inhibitors

Carbonic anhydrase is an enzyme located in the ciliary epithelium which is responsible for the active secretion of bicarbonate ions into the aqueous humour. It is also found in many other locations in the body, including the kidney. Drugs which interfere with the action of this enzyme, the carbonic anhydrase inhibitors, were originally developed as diuretics for the systemic treatment of oedema. They have now been replaced by more modern agents. They were also used for the systemic treatment of glaucoma, obviating the need for patients to instil eyedrops.

Acetazolamide

Not active topically, this drug was originally used in the form of tablets. Unfortunately, this led to serious side effects such as lack of appetite, fatigue and gastrointestinal disturbances. It is now used mainly for the prophylaxis of altitude sickness.

Brinzolamide

The lack of topical efficacy of acetazolamide led to the search for topically active carbonic anhydrase inhibitors with improved lipid solubility which could penetrate the cornea more easily. The modern agents are effective and are used either alone or as adjunct agents, but unfortunately they have similar side effects to the systemically administered drugs. They should be used with caution in patients with a compromised corneal endothelium and patients with keratoplasty. Brinzolamide is available as a 1% solution.

Dorzolamide

This was the first topically active carbonic anhydrase inhibitor to be introduced. It can be used on its own or as an adjunct therapy. It is available on its own as a 2.0% solution or in combination with timolol.

Prostaglandin analogues

Prostaglandins are best known as mediators of inflammation but in the eye they can produce reductions in IOP of around 25% by increasing uveoscleral outflow. Their action is prolonged, allowing for once-a-day treatment. All prostaglandins currently used have the peculiar side effect of increasing pigmentation in the eyelashes and iris, which is a problem if the patient is being treated monocularly.

Bimatoprost

Bimatoprost is slightly different from the other two drugs listed below in that it is a prostamide, which mimics the effects of prostaglandins without acting on any known prostaglandin receptor. Its effect is maximal within 8 to 12 hours and lasts for at least 24 hours.

Latanoprost

Latanoprost is a prodrug which releases a prostaglandin analogue on administration. This acts on a specific prostaglandin receptor to produce a fall in IOP, mainly by increasing uveoscleral outflow, although it has some effect on the trabecular meshwork. Its time course is similar to that of bimatoprost. Its effects are additive to those of miotics, sympathomimetics, beta blockers and carbonic anhydrase inhibitors.

Travoprost

Travoprost is similar to latanoprost but has the advantage of being stable at room temperature.

Combination products

It is often necessary to prescribe more than one antiglaucoma medication. In the early stages, this is achieved by the co-prescription of two separate drops, but as the practice continues there is an impetus to provide combined drops. There are advantages to the patient in the use of combined drops. Primarily, it is easier administering one drop instead of two, especially if they have to be administered at the same time. Given the size of the conjunctival sac, it is pointless to instil a second drop until the first has drained away. This involves a delay of at least 10 minutes.

There are, of course, disadvantages to combined drops. Some drugs are best used at night while others are given twice daily. It is also impossible to vary independently the concentrations of the drugs used.

To be beneficial, the two agents must have different pharmacological modes of action. In the past, a combination of two miotics was used containing physostigmine and pilocarpine. Since pilocarpine is not broken down by cholinesterase, the combination was pointless and merely served to increase the incidence of side effects.

Today, the principal combining agent is timolol, which, as well as being available on its own in various formulations, is available combined with the following drugs:

* sympathomimetic
  (i) brimonidine – Combigan
* prostaglandin analogues
  (i) latanoprost – Xalacom
  (ii) bimatoprost – Ganforth
  (iii) travoprost – Duo-Trav
* carbonic anhydrase inhibitors
  (i) dorzolamide – Cosopt.

Tear replacement therapy

The tear film is a complex tri-laminar structure which results from the secretions of several glands. It has several important functions:

* It prevents desiccation of the corneal epithelium.
* It provides an optically smooth surface.
* It lubricates the passage of the lids across the cornea.
* It helps remove debris and foreign bodies.
* It contains antibacterial systems to inhibit bacterial invasion.
* It helps to provide oxygen and nutrients to the avascular cornea.

We become aware of the importance of tears when their flow is deficient through ageing, the effects of drugs, excessive evaporation or other pathological causes. The extent of the lack of tears can range from minor irritation to a serious, potentially sight-threatening condition. A variety of treatments is available to ameliorate the condition. None of them comes close to emulating natural tears, but help in reducing the worst effects of dry eye. A good artificial tear replacement therapy should:

- have a good lubricating action
- be retained in the eye for a long time
- produce a smooth surface to the tear film
- be pleasant and easy to use
- be inexpensive (as dry eyes require frequent applications).

The problems caused by preservatives are particularly important when they are incorporated into artificial tears. Not only is there the possibility of allergy, which is more likely to occur with frequent applications, but also agents such as benzalkonium chloride can affect the stability of the tear film and lead to a shortening of the tear break-up time. Thus, it is often necessary to use single-dose, unpreserved drops.

Simple viscolized solutions

These are formulations of a viscolizer incorporated in a vehicle with the normal adjuvants. Some of the commonly used viscolizers are derivatives of methyl cellulose while others are based on water-soluble polymers.

Hypromellose

This is probably the most commonly used viscolizer and is available in a variety of formulations which vary in pH and the concentration of hypromellose. It is more viscous than polyvinyl alcohol and has good surface-wetting properties. The choice of an artificial tear drop is often based on empirical choice and hypromellose 0.3% is usually the starting point.

Carmellose

Carmellose is another derivative of methyl cellulose which produces a satisfactory viscous drop. It is available for single-dose use.

Hydroxyethylcellulose

Used in 0.44% solution in a single-dose unit, it increases tear break-up time and acts as a lubricant.

Povidone

Povidone is best known as a carrier for iodine (povidone-iodine, a well-known antiseptic which has been used in contact lens solutions). Povidone at a concentration of 5% increases viscosity of solutions and is available as a single-use unit.

Polyvinyl alcohol

Polyvinyl alcohol has wetting properties which led to its inclusion in contact lens wetting solutions and it is incorporated in a number of therapeutic drops as well as artificial tears as a viscolizer.

Carbomers

Carbomers have superior properties to ordinary viscolizers as they produce thixotropic solutions. These have variable viscosities, being less viscous when shearing forces are applied. Therefore, they produce less drag during blinking.

They are longer lasting and reduced dosing is required. In addition, they can work overnight, obviating the need for the nocturnal use of ointments. They are available as eye gels in both multi- and single-use units.

Ointments

Ointments produce a blurry film on the eye and are thus not used regularly during the day, except for serious cases. They are often used at bedtime to give protection during sleep when tear production is reduced. They are mixtures of wool fat, liquid paraffin and yellow soft paraffin in the correct proportions to produce an ointment which is retained well in the conjunctival sac but melts at body temperature.

Mucolytics

N-acetylcysteine is able to break down the molecule of mucin in order to reduce its viscosity. In keratoconjunctivitis sicca, it used to remove filaments of mucus strands attached to the cornea and mucus plaques which contain mucus, epithelial cells and other debris.

References

Azuma I, Hirumo T 1981 Long term topical use of DPE solution in open angle glaucoma. Acta Society Ophthalmology Japan 85:1157–1164

Blumenthal M et al 1992 Efficacy and safety of nedocromil sodium ophthalmic solution in the treatment of seasonal allergic conjunctivitis. American Journal of Ophthalmology 113:56–63

Bonomi L et al 1987 Prevention of trauma-induced miosis during cataract extraction by diclofenac eye drops. New Trends in Ophthalmology II:513–519

Clark A F 1995 Steroids ocular hypertension and glaucoma. Journal of Glaucoma 4:354–369

Coleiro J A, Sigurdsson H, Lockyer J A 1988 Follicular conjunctivitis on dipivefrin therapy for glaucoma. Eye 2:440–442

Fahy G et al 1988 Double masked efficacy and safety evaluation of lodoxamide 0.1% ophthalmic solution versus opticrom 2% – a multicentre study. Ophthalmology Today 341–342

Ismail B, Morton D J 1987 Ophthalmic uptake of chloramphenicol from proprietary preparations using an in vitro method of evaluation. International Journal of Pharmacology 37:1113

James M R, Brogan R, Carew-McColl M 1991 A study to compare the use of fusidic acid viscous eye drops and chloramphenicol eye ointment in an accident and emergency department. Archives of Emergency Medicine 8:125–129

Kolker A E, Becker B 1968 Epinephrine maculopathy. Archives of Ophthalmology 79:552–562

Krieglstein G K et al 1987 Levobunolol and metipranolol. Comparative ocular hypotensive effects. British Journal of Ophthalmology 71:250–253

Lass J H, Pavan-Langston D, Park N H 1979 Acyclovir and corneal wound healing. American Journal of Ophthalmology 88:102–108

Madge G E, Geeraets W J, Guerry D 1971 Black cornea secondary to topical epinephrine. American Journal of Ophthalmology 71:402–405

Savelsbergh-Fillette M P, Demailly P 1988 Levobunolol compared with timolol for control of elevated IOP. Journal of French Ophthalmology 11:587–590

Seal D V, Barrett S P, McGill J T 1982 Aetiology and treatment of acute bacterial infection of the external eye. British Journal of Ophthalmology 66:357–360

Steinert R F, Thomas J V, Boger W P 1981 Long term drift and continued efficacy after multi-year timolol therapy. Archives of Ophthalmology 99:100–103

Struck H G et al 1994 Influence of diclofenac and flurbiprofen eye drops on the inflammation after cataract extraction. Ophthalmology 31:482–485

Titcomb L 1997 Ophthalmic chloramphenicol and blood – a review. Pharmacology Journal 258:28–35

Zuber P, Pecaud A 1988 Effect of levocabastine, a new H_1 antagonist, in a conjunctival provocation test with allergens. Journal of Allergy and Clinical Immunology 82:590–594

CHAPTER 9

The optometric management of ocular adverse reactions to systemic medication

Bernard Gilmartin

Introduction

The physician, botanist and mineralogist William Withering (1741–1799) published in 1785 what is considered to be the most elegant and definitive description of an adverse drug reaction:

> *The foxglove, when given in very large and quickly repeated doses, occasions sickness, vomiting, purging, giddiness, confused vision, objects appearing green or yellow, increased secretion of urine with frequent motions to part with it, and sometimes inability to retain it; slow pulse, even as low as 35 in a minute, cold sweats, convulsions, syncope and death*
> (Davidson & Hickey-Dwyer 1991).

Over two centuries later the well-known plant species foxglove (*Digitalis purpurea*) is still farmed to produce the cardiac glycoside digoxin used for the treatment of supraventricular tachycardia. Withering would no doubt be pleased to see that the systemic and visual side effects listed in the British National Formulary (BNF 2006) for digoxin bear a remarkable resemblance to those he observed and intrigued by the number of pharmaceutical agents currently prescribed. In 2001, nearly 600 million prescriptions for medicines were dispensed in the UK and some 700 million packages of non-prescription medicines were supplied (National Audit Office 2003). Each agent has at least the propensity to produce adverse effects and the purpose of this chapter is to facilitate the management of ocular adverse reactions (OARs) by the optometrist by first, reviewing the contribution that can be made in terms of monitoring, detecting and reporting OARs; second, outlining methods to increase the probability of identifying a genuine OAR; and finally providing a compendium of selected OARs that demonstrates the nature and range of OARs encountered in general practice.

National Health Service (NHS) prescribing in both primary care and hospitals in England cost about £10.7 billion in 2005 (around £210.92 per person) and hence it is clear that a large proportion of the UK population will be taking prescribed medication at any given time (Hospital Prescribing 2006). All concerned with the formulation, administration and efficacy of drugs have therefore become increasingly aware that drugs can produce adverse effects. An adverse drug reaction is any unwanted or unintended effect of a drug that occurs during its normal therapeutic use, and collectively adverse drug reactions are considered to be a major cause of morbidity in the community, accounting possibly for up to 5% of all medical admissions to hospital (Aronson & White 1996). Adverse drug reactions can occur generally in two forms: type A, the more common at around 75% of reactions, and type B, which can be present in very low concentrations. Type A reactions are dose related and represent an accentuation of a drug's normal effect. Type B reactions are unpredictable, idiosyncratic reactions that are often of sudden onset and may involve anaphylaxis (Routledge 2004).

This chapter will be concerned principally with OARs to systemic drugs prescribed by a patient's general medical practitioner that are most likely to come to the attention of the optometrist in general practice (Gilmartin 1987, 1999; Edgar & Gilmartin 1997; Lawrenson 2001; Santodomingo-Rubido et al 2003; Cox & Gilmartin 2006). Although more rare and of less general significance, adverse reactions may also arise from diagnostic and therapeutic drugs used topically by the optometrist. Examples include the hypersensitive responses to corneal anaesthetics or the interaction between topically instilled drugs and concurrent medication (e.g. the potential for interaction between topical sympathomimetic phenylephrine and systemic monamine oxidase inhibitors used for depressive states). Topical drugs may also have systemic adverse effects of which the optometrist should be aware (Polak 2000). For example, the respiratory problems associated with the use of the beta adrenoceptor antagonist timolol for primary open-angle glaucoma (an example of a type A reaction) and the risk, albeit very small, of aplastic anaemia with the antibiotic chloramphenicol (an example of a type B reaction). Recent and prospective legislative changes in the UK pertaining to additional supply, supplementary and independent prescribing of topical therapeutic agents will extend substantially the role of the optometrist in this area. OARs can also be associated with over-the-counter (OTC) pharmacy medicines such as artificial tear substitutes, contact lens preparations, ocular nutritional supplements (Bartlett & Eperjesi 2005) and herbal remedies. Regarding the latter, of special note is the crystalline retinopathy associated with canthaxanthine, a carotenoid used in cosmetics, as a food colouring and to produce an artificial suntan when administered orally (Fraunfelder 2004). Commonly ingested substances such nicotine, alcohol, caffeine, and the use of other recreational drugs can each produce OARs, particularly in excess, that are exacerbated by concurrent systemic medication together with respective treatments for addiction.

The central role of the pharmacist as a portal for detecting and managing both ocular and systemic adverse reactions to all forms of medication is widely recognized by the general public and acknowledged by all healthcare professionals. The optometrist also has a responsibility to be particularly aware of the various factors that predispose patients to an OAR. The eye is unique in that it is a relatively small structure made up of a variety of very specialized tissues which have specific metabolic requirements, affinities and storage characteristics. Systemic drugs enter the eye principally via its rich vascular network and with certain drugs via the tear secretion system. Indirect effects on visual performance, particularly at near, can occur if the drug affects the central nervous system (CNS) oculomotor control centres. The cornea, the retina and the uvea are particularly important target tissues principally because the cornea is in such close apposition with the tear layer, and the retina and the uvea have high levels of melanin relative to other tissues in the body.

The role of the optometrist

Fortunately, the majority of ocular changes induced by systemic drugs are reversible if detected in the early stages of toxicity and consequently the detection and reporting of OARs to systemic medication is an important and continuing aspect of primary eye care (College of Optometrists 2002). The inherent nature of adverse reactions is that their detection is often based on circumstantial evidence and it is rare that an OAR can be unequivocally linked to a particular drug. An informed suspicion that an OAR has occurred is probably the most that can be achieved. Nevertheless, the optometrist is in a special position to monitor, detect and report OARs.

Monitoring OARs

As the numbers of patients used in pre-marketing drug trials may only average several thousands (Rawlins & Jeffreys 1991) the final test on the safety of a drug is in fact the period following its release for general use, and so the large patient sample seen by optometrists, approximately 16 million eye examinations in 2004, is of great value in terms of the pharmacosurveillance of OARs. Although many drugs have been implicated in causing adverse effects in the eye, it should be emphasized that the majority of patients will experience no problems whatsoever. Nevertheless, the number of OARs reported to the Medicines and Healthcare Products Regulatory Agency's (MHRA) Yellow Card scheme in the UK (see below) were relatively high between 1964 and 2004 and totalled 4.3% of all reports (Cox 2006). A reasonable estimate of the likely occurrence of OARs in a full-time general optometric practice would be around one per month. The wide age distribution of patients seen in optometry, typically 5 years to 85 years, also means that a broad range of drugs and systemic conditions is encountered. An additional and important aspect is that patient databases allow the optometrist to examine patients on a regular basis over a long period of time; continuity of data collection and comparison facilitates greatly the monitoring of OARs.

Detecting OARs

Optometrists are in a position to compile and record basic reference data on, for example, fundus appearance, visual acuity, oculomotor status and accommodative/pupil responses, all of which can be affected by systemic drugs. Importantly, the optometrist is in a position to be specific in the description of OARs: a major problem for drug reporting schemes is that general qualitative terms are often used such as 'poor' vision or 'dim' vision rather than quantitative indexes of ocular effects. Letter charts incorporating logarithmic scaling and variations in letter contrast (see Ch. 14) are particularly well suited to assessing subtle changes in visual acuity. In addition, most optometrists now have access to further investigative techniques, such as binocular indirect ophthalmoscopy, slit-lamp microscopy, central (including Amsler charts) and peripheral visual fields, tonometry, colour vision tests, assessment of tear function and fundus photography, all of which provide comprehensive information on ocular structure and function. The additional imaging and archiving facilities provided by digital technology are also important features of modern methods of ophthalmic examination.

Reporting OARs

Should the optometrist detect any changes in ocular tissues or visual performance that resemble an OAR it is essential that the appropriate reporting procedures are adopted. In the first instance the details of the suspected OAR should be fully recorded in the patient's record together with any advice given and recommendations made. The incident can be reported independently, in which case it is essential that the patient's physician is informed fully of the course of action taken, or the optometrist may choose first to consult with the patient's physician to agree an appropriate course of action. There should be no implied criticism of a patient's medical management when informing either the patient or the medical prescriber of the possibility of a reaction: the prescriber may be well aware of the possibility of a reaction but has the responsibility for taking into account the risk: benefit ratio of a given medication. The course of action will depend on the disease being treated, the net benefit to the patient of the drug and the nature of the OAR, and is a matter for the prescriber to decide.

Of particular importance is that the optometrist should ensure that the reporting procedure does not cause undue alarm to the patient with the attendant risk that essential medication might be stopped abruptly or the dose altered. Further, it should be pointed out that a drug reaction or side effect does not of necessity imply toxicity, detriment to the patient, permanent damage or that the drug itself does not conform to manufacturing specifications.

Reporting procedures for OARs

Medicines and Healthcare Products Regulatory Agency

In the UK the Medicines and Healthcare Products Regulatory Agency (MHRA) is the principal route for the reporting of adverse drug reactions but this does not supersede the need to complete a full clinical record and inform or consult appropriately the patient's medical prescriber. The MHRA and the Commission on Human Medicines (CHM) operate the Yellow Card scheme of reporting adverse drug reactions, including OARs, and collect information on reactions to prescription medicines, herbal remedies and OTC medicines. The equivalent reporting scheme in the United States is administered by the Department of Health and Human Service's Food and Drug Administration (FDA) via the FDA Medical Products Reporting Program, MedWatch (http://fda.gov/medwatch).

The MHRA and its predecessor organizations have collected reports of suspected adverse drug reactions through the Yellow Card reporting scheme for over 40 years, during which time over 500 000 reports have been received. Reports can be submitted by health professionals or patients (or patients' parents or carers as part of an ongoing pilot scheme) using one of the Yellow Cards at the rear of the British National Formulary (BNF, see below), by downloading a pdf of a Yellow Card from the MHRA website, or by using the MHRA website to submit reports online. Optometrists can log in as a Healthcare Professional (http://www.mhra.gov.uk). An acknowledgement will be sent to the practitioner when the MHRA receives a report, together with a unique identification number assigned to the report; a copy of the report will also be provided, for inclusion in the patient's notes. The scheme is confidential and reports are not available to others without the reporter's consent, other than as anonymous aggregated data.

Physicians, pharmacists and scientists working in the Pharmacovigilance Group of the MHRA Post Licensing Division use data from Yellow Card reports to assess the causal relationship between the drugs and reported reactions and to identify possible risk factors contributing to the occurrence of reactions, for example, age or underlying disease. When new medicines come onto the market, there is relatively limited information about their safety from clinical trials. New medicines are therefore intensively monitored in order to confirm the risk:benefit profile. The CHM and the MHRA encourage the reporting of all suspected reactions to these newer drugs and vaccines and these products are identified by the inverted black triangle symbol in the BNF. Although there is no standard time for a product to retain black triangle status an assessment is usually made following 2 years of post-marketing experience and the black triangle symbol is not removed until the safety of the drug is well established.

A Yellow Card should be completed, either independently or, if preferred, in consultation with the patient's medical prescriber, when it is suspected that an OAR may be related to a drug, or a combination of drugs. Although attention is directed here to ocular adverse reactions a report may also be prompted by the possibility of a systemic adverse reaction. Importantly, practitioners should not be deterred from submitting a report if the reaction seems to be an isolated case, there is uncertainty as to causality of the adverse reaction or some details requested by the Yellow Card are not known.

For all 'black triangle' drugs all suspected reactions are reported, including those considered to be trivial in nature.

For established drugs and herbal remedies taken by adults, only serious reactions adverse reactions are reported.

For established drugs and herbal remedies taken by children (defined as less than 18 years of age), all serious and minor reactions are reported.

Sources of information

Patient history

A comprehensive patient history is the most important information source (see Ch. 26). Although most patients are aware that adverse reactions to drugs can occur, many are often unaware that the eye can be affected by systemic medication: the functioning of the eye may appear to be quite remote from, for example, their tablets for arthritis or angina. Patients frequently attribute their visual problems to the need for stronger spectacles or just simply to normal ageing processes. During history-taking the optometrist should establish whether or not drugs are being taken regularly and, if so, determine their identity. Some patients, however, may not be able to remember drug names correctly or have them in their possession. In such cases they are usually able to inform the optometrist of the reason for taking the drug(s) and it is essential therefore to possess reliable and comprehensive sources of information (see below) which indicate the drugs or groups of drugs used in different conditions. When questioning patients about medicines use, it should be remembered that some drugs capable of inducing side effects are available from a pharmacy without a prescription and patients may be using these on a regular basis without thinking of them as medicines and thus neglect to mention them.

Armed with the above information and knowledge of local prescribing habits, optometrists may immediately refer to a standard reference source to find out whether OARs have been previously reported; others may proceed as normal, referring back to the possibility of a drug reaction when an ocular problem cannot be fully accounted for in other ways.

Profile of local medical prescribing

Lawrenson (1999) has indicated that a typical medical practice would have the major therapeutic drug groups ranked in weighted descending order (highest = 1) of number of annual prescriptions issued as follows: Cadiovascular (1.00); Central Nervous System (0.81); Respiratory (0.46); Gastrointestinal (0.45); Infection (0.40); Endocrine (0.35). Whilst not affecting the inherent incidence of OARs for a particular therapeutic group these weightings will affect the probability of the optometrist encountering an OAR linked to a specific therapeutic group. Cardiovascular and CNS drugs constituted therefore the majority of OAR reports submitted to the College of Optometrist's 'green card' reporting scheme in the UK between 1990 and 1997 (the precursor to entry into the Yellow Card scheme). OARs for the major therapeutic drug groups ranked in weighted descending order (highest = 1) were as follows: Cadiovascular (1.00); Central Nervous System (0.68); Endocrine (0.29); Respiratory (0.19); Musculoskeletal (0.19); Gastrointestinal (0.08); Malignant disease (0.08); Infection (0.08); Obstetrics (0.06); Nutrition/blood (0.02) (Edgar & Gilmartin 1997; Lawrenson 1999). One in three of the cardiovascular OAR reports to the College were related to the use of the antiarrhythmic drug amiodarone.

Despite the high prevalence of cardiovascular and CNS drug prescribing in most areas, the overall prescribing profile will depend on whether the geographical location of the optometrist's practice is rural, suburban or urban. Thus, a simple and effective strategy for detection of OARs is for the optometrist to collate an in-practice log book of the range of medications commonly reported by patients that comprise the practice list. Information on previously reported OARs specific to a particular drug or therapeutic drug group can then be compiled from the variety of information sources detailed below.

British National Formulary

The British National Formulary (BNF) is published by the British Medical Association and the Royal Pharmaceutical Society of Great Britain and is aimed at the health professions involved with prescribing, monitoring, supplying and administering medicines. It is an essential reference source for optometrists to obtain information on drug management of common conditions together with details of the medicines currently used. The BNF is based on the latest information from clinical literature, regulatory authorities and professional bodies and is issued every 6 months (currently September and March) in print form or is accessible via the internet following a simple registration process (http://bnf.org). *BNF for children* contains detailed information on the use of medicines in children as well as copies of Yellow Cards.

The BNF includes clinically relevant systemic and ocular side effects for all drugs other than those used by specialists (e.g. cytotoxics and drugs used in anaesthesia). As all medicines are prone to hypersensitivity reactions these are not listed in the BNF unless a special predisposition has been reported. It should be noted that information on possible OARs to a particular agent may not be restricted to the 'Side effects' section of the respective BNF entry: relevant information can also be included in the juxtaposed sections on 'Cautions' and 'Contraindications'. The internet site provides a useful and simple search facility for OARs.

Monthly Index for Medical Specialties

The Monthly Index for Medical Specialties (MIMS), published monthly by Haymarket Publishing, is the most up-to-date and widely used prescribing guide used on subscription by doctors, pharmacists and nurses in the UK. All major medicines available on prescription are listed by therapeutic area, and key information is provided about each product's active ingredients, uses, dosages, warnings, important licensing changes and reviews of new products.

Medicines and Healthcare Products Regulatory Agency

Practitioners can access via the MHRA internet site Drug Analysis Prints (DAPs), which are collections of information from Yellow Card reports submitted on a particular medicine. DAPs are, however, of limited value to the practitioner as, although very detailed and up to date, they do not provide a complete overview of the risks associated with specific medicines.

It should be noted that the reports record the suspicions of reporters without formal proof of causality. Also, the high level of under-reporting means not all reactions are listed. DAPs do not help one estimate the incidence of adverse reactions for a particular drug since information is not provided on how many prescriptions were issued.

Electronic Medicines Compendium

The Electronic Medicines Compendium (eMC) was launched in 1999 and provides free and continuously updated information on UK medicines, both prescription medicines and those that can be bought over the counter in a pharmacy. The eMC internet site (http://emc.medicines.org.uk) provides electronic Data Sheets, Summaries of Product Characteristics (SPCs) and Patient Information Leaflets (PILs), all of which are submitted directly from the pharmaceutical company that manufactures the medicine. PILs are intended for the patient and are included in the medicine packaging. All PILs include a section on reported side effects, which may alert the patient to the possibility of an ocular adverse reaction and be presented to the optometrist during the consultation.

Dedicated information sources

Whereas the BNF and eMC will provide information on OARs that are of special significance, more dedicated sources will need to be consulted for a comprehensive listing of reported OARs. Textbooks providing detailed information on general adverse reactions (incorporating OARs) would include those of Davies et al (1998), Aronson (2006) and Martindale (2007). Specific chapters on OARs can be found in optometric drug textbooks such as Bartlett & Jaanus (2001) and Hopkins & Pearson (2007). Textbooks specific to OARs are Grant and Schuman (1993) and Fraunfelder and Fraunfelder (2001). The latter is distinctive as its format is particularly suitable for use by the practising optometrist and is due to be superseded by a text on clinical ocular toxicology (Fraunfelder et al 2008). Fraunfelder and his son founded The National Registry of Drug Induced Ocular Side-Effects (www.eyedrugregistry.com) in 1976 based in Oregon, USA. In addition to collecting spontaneous reports from clinicians, the Registry accumulates data from the World Health Organization's Uppsala Monitoring Center, the Food and Drug Administration, pharmaceutical companies, and periodic screening of the world's literature (Fraunfelder et al 2004).

Of special note and utility is the UK-based powerful and rapid search facility for OARs designed specifically for the practising optometrist (Thomson Software Solutions 2006). The system can be installed at modest cost on standard computers and allows OARs to be located with reference to OAR suspected, drug name (full or part), drug category or the condition that the drug is being used to treat. Registered users of the database can download updates over the internet for a period of 1 year post-registration and thereafter for a small annual fee. Professional magazines also play an important role in their ability to publish breaking news on OARs and continuing professional development articles that accrue points for continuing optometric registration.

Assessing the probability of ocular adverse reactions

In the product literature the frequency of side effects is generally described as follows: Very Common – greater than 1 in 10; Common – 1 in 100 to 1 in 10; Uncommon – 1 in 1000 to 1 in 100; Rare – 1 in 10 000 to 1 in 1000; Very rare – less than 1 in 10 000. An approach taken by the World Health Organization's Causality Assessment of Suspected Adverse Reactions Guide (Edwards & Biriell 1995) is to categorize medicines into side-effect profiles defined as Certain; Probable/Likely; Possible; Unlikely; Conditional and/or Unclassified; Inaccessible/Unclassifiable. Of most practical use is the system used by the BNF: side effects are generally listed in order of frequency and arranged broadly by body systems. Following the initial listing, designations range from 'less common', 'very rarely' to 'other reported side effects', although occasionally a rare and serious side effect may be listed first (British National Formulary 2006). Nevertheless, it should be noted that a single case presenting to the optometrist may be the first indication of a new adverse effect to a medication (Aronson 2003).

Deciding whether an OAR is likely to be genuine or feasible requires clinical initiative, awareness and judgement, and has to take full account of major case features concerning the condition being treated, the patient's clinical profile, the nature of the drug prescribed and, importantly, the complex interactions that can occur between these features.

The condition

Chronic conditions, for example rheumatic and cardiovascular problems, often require medication over a long period, which may increase the probability that the optometrist will encounter an OAR to respective therapeutic groups. Fortunately, much care is taken to ensure that medications are judiciously prescribed (and dispensed) for use over short periods with optimum doses for the clinical effect required and hence minimal chance for cumulative effects to occur.

Ocular pathology associated with a given condition can sometimes confound the situation, in that the pathology may be associated with the condition being treated concurrently by the drug rather than being directly induced by the drug itself. Metabolism and excretion of a drug can also be affected by certain conditions (particularly those affecting the kidney and liver) and thus the potential for drug toxicity may be increased.

Furthermore, the nature of the condition being treated may determine the route of administration of a drug and hence indirectly affect its potential to induce adverse effects. Acute ocular reactions are more likely to follow parenteral, that is, intramuscular or intravenous, administration whereas chronic ocular reactions tend to be more often associated with oral medication. Topical preparations for ocular, nasal and skin conditions can also result in sufficient systemic absorption to lead to OARs.

The patient

The age of the patient receiving therapy is a very significant factor in the incidence of adverse reactions, particularly for very young and very elderly patients. It appears that the rate of systemic adverse reactions (and probably OARs) peaks at around 70 to 75 years of age and is possibly linked to impaired liver or kidney function or multiple drug therapy. The glomerular filtration rate (GFR) is a useful marker for renal dysfunction and declines progressively with age to reach on average 30% of normal at 80 years of age. Other factors include slower metabolic processes and reduction in brain mass, neuron density and cerebral blood flow (Routledge 2004). Young adult patients are more likely to be candidates for contact lens fitting or refractive surgery and account may need to be taken of OARs with certain therapeutic groups.

Contact lens wear

Both topical and systemic drugs can produce adverse effects in patients who wear contact lenses, in particular those that affect the quantity and quality of tears. There is the potential for antimicrobial preservatives in topical multi-dose preparations to accumulate in the hydrogel material of soft contact lenses and induce toxic reactions. Therefore, unless especially indicated, the lenses should be removed before instillation and not worn during the treatment period. Alternatively, single-dose, unpreserved eyedrops can be used.

A number of drugs used systemically can also have adverse effects on contact lens wear, for example: oral contraceptives (particularly those with higher oestrogen content), drugs which can reduce blink rate (e.g. anxiolytics, hypnotics, antihistamines and muscle relaxants); drugs which can reduce lacrimation (e.g. antihistamines, antimuscarinics, phenothiazines, some beta blockers, diuretics and tricyclic antidepressants); and drugs that can increase lacrimation (e.g. ephedrine and hydrazaline). Other drugs that may affect contact lens wear are isotretinoin, which can cause conjunctival inflammation; aspirin, where the salicylic acid can be present in tears and absorbed by the contact lens with subsequent irritation; rifampicin and sulfasalazine, which can discolour soft contact lenses (British National Formulary 2006).

Refractive surgery

The agents listed above that affect contact lens wear may also need to be considered in those patients opting for laser eye surgery (Hanratty 2005). In addition, certain $5HT_1$ agonists may cause an increased risk of vascular occlusion when the intraocular pressure is raised during treatment. The patient can be reconsidered for surgery if, with the medical practitioner's consent, a change to an alternative drug can be made at least 1 month before treatment. The retinoid isotretinoin, used for severe acne, can cause marked dry eye but the patient can be considered for surgery if the drug is stopped or substituted with the practitioner's consent for 6 months before treatment (Hanratty 2005).

Of special note, of course, is an indication that a systemic adverse reaction to a prescribed drug has occurred as this can be accompanied by an ocular adverse reaction. For example, a dry mouth with certain neuroleptic drugs will invariably be accompanied by reports of dry eye. A history of previous reactions to drugs is important and may well indicate a predisposition to drug allergy (often known as hypersensitivity reactions). The basis of the common type I hypersensitivity response is the combination of a drug with an endogenous protein to form an antigenic complex. Subsequent exposure to the drug or similar agent results in an antigen–antibody interaction which triggers the release of a variety of endogenous substances, for example histamine, leucotrienes and prostaglandins that produce the signs and symptoms of an allergic reaction.

The extent to which an individual metabolizes a drug is linked chiefly to genetic factors (Weinshilboum 2003). In particular, there is normally a genetic basis to idiosyncratic, unpredictable type B adverse responses (that is, they cannot be deduced from the pharmacological action of the drug), for example, the rapid rise in intraocular pressure that can occur with topical steroids. Genetically determined rates of drug metabolism can also influence the incidence of adverse effects, an example being the peripheral neuropathy and optic neuritis that can occur with isoniazid. Around 60% of the European population have a slow rate of metabolism of isoniazid and are hence more likely to experience problems. Although not confirmed for OARs, it has been reported that women have a greater risk than men of general adverse drug reactions (Kando et al 1995) related to differences in pharmacokinetic profile, body size and associated fat:water ratio, hormonal changes and increased longevity. It has been reported that patients from different ethnic groups have different risks in relation to important adverse drug reactions to cardiovascular drugs either because it acts as a surrogate measure of genetic make-up or because cultural factors alter the risk (McDowell et al 2006). There appear, however, to be no reports to date of a well-defined link between ethnicity and susceptibility to OARs.

The drug

The nature of the drug itself can determine the probability of an OAR. The inherent pharmacological properties of a drug determine its pharmacokinetic fate in terms of its absorption, metabolism and excretion. Similarly, the probability of a particular drug affecting ocular tissue and function will depend on its ability to penetrate the blood–brain, blood–aqueous or blood–retina barrier. Melanin is present in the uveal tract and retinal pigment epithelium and, being a free radical, can bind with certain drugs to produce ocular toxicity, for example, the psychotopic drugs such as chlorpromazine and haloperidol. Some drugs have the potential to affect ocular structures more than others, for example, the cardiac glycoside digoxin and corticosteroids. The chemical structure of the drug can also be important in this respect; for example, the ring structure of phenothiazine may determine the nature of the OAR produced. Pharmacogenetics is a developing discipline which aims to increase the effectiveness of drugs and minimize the risk of side effects by matching drugs to people according to their genetic make-up (McLeod & Evans 2001; Routlege 2004).

Drug dosage is very important with regard to the incidence of adverse reactions: although reactions do occur when the drug-serum concentration is within the therapeutic range, many reactions reported only occur when the dose is outside this range. A useful indicator is whether the onset of the reaction coincides with commencement of the medication, but the reaction can also occur when a course of medication is terminated. For example, adverse effects associated with certain medications, e.g. chloroquine, can persist for up to 7 years after cessation. Drugs with a low therapeutic ratio (i.e. the difference between the therapeutic dose and toxic dose is low) are associated with increased risk of adverse reactions or interactions; examples include oral hypoglycaemic agents, corticosteroids and digoxin.

Interactions between several drugs being taken concurrently also confound the situation and can both affect the efficacy of a given drug and increase the risk of adverse reactions. It has been estimated that drug interactions account for between 6% and 30% of all adverse reactions (Orme 1991). The basis for interaction may be altered pharmacodynamic or pharmacokinetic properties; the former is more common and concerns the interaction between drugs that have similar or antagonistic pharmacological effects or side effects; the latter concerns interaction that alters the absorption, distribution, metabolism or excretion of another drug. The BNF can be consulted for details concerning the current range of known significant interactions. Although more than 1000 drug interactions have been described, the number that are clinically important is much smaller and involves a relatively small number of pharmacological drug groups (Seymour & Routledge 1998). Significant interactions can also occur with commonly ingested drugs such as alcohol and nicotine and possibly with pollutants and radiation in the environment.

Taxonomy of ocular adverse reactions

There exists a multitude of reports linking OARs to certain drugs. All therapeutic groups have been implicated and the effects range from minor disturbances in pupil size and accommodation, which are fully reversible on withdrawal of the drug, through to permanent damage to ocular tissues with accompanying deterioration in visual function. The approach taken to the taxonomy of reported OARs varies between information sources and can range from classification by specific drug name, therapeutic group, condition being treated or ocular structure affected. An exhaustive list of all the drugs which have been implicated in causing OARs is outside the scope of this chapter and is, in any event, available from the information sources cited earlier. Considered to be of overriding importance are the principles presented above, which govern the likelihood of identifying a genuine OAR in terms of the condition, patient and drug.

The approach taken here is pragmatic and acknowledges that, in general optometric practice, the possibility of an OAR may only be seriously considered in the absence of a more explicable cause of a particular ocular sign or symptom. Often patients will not know the specific name of the drug that has been prescribed and, in any event, signs and symptoms that constitute an OAR can be associated with a number of drugs. Patients are mostly aware of the condition for which the drug has been prescribed, which, with the aid of the BNF or one of the information sources listed above, will assist in identifying at least the subclass of therapeutic agent prescribed.

Stevens–Johnson syndrome

Stevens–Johnson syndrome is one of the most commonly cited side effects in the BNF that has ocular effects. It is an acute, generally self-limiting, severe, mucocutaneous, vesiculobulbous disease, which primarily occurs in young healthy individuals. The condition occurs more often in males than females, with the most common precipitating factor being a hypersensitivity reaction to a drug (**Fig. 9.1**). The basic lesion is an acute vasculitis, which affects the skin in all patients and the conjunctiva in 90% of patients, with 35% experiencing permanent visual damage (Harrison 1996). The inflammation is generally self-limiting but subsequent conjunctival scarring and damage to lacrimal ductules and goblet cells can lead to an intractable eye syndrome (Kanski 2003; Cox 2006). Over 200 drugs are associated with Stevens–Johnson syndrome. Betalactam antibiotics, tetracyclines, sulphonamides and nonsteroidal antiinflammatory drugs (NSAIDs) are among the most common causes, but other drugs include macrolides, carbamazepine, lamotrigine and phenothiazines (Lee & Thomson 2006).

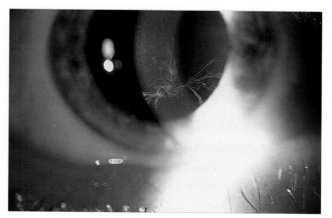

Figure 9.2 Amiodarone keratopathy. (From Kanski 2003 Clinical ophthalmology: a systematic approach, 5th edn, p 137, Fig. 5.135.)

Corneal verticillata

Also of special note is that a number of drugs can cause a characteristic whorl-like vortex pattern of deposition within the corneal epithelium, often referred to as corneal verticillata: e.g. amiodarone, chloroquine, chlorpromazine, indometacin and tamoxifen (**Fig. 9.2**). The deposits may be indicative of a generalized toxic response and possibly an associated maculopathy; they are best seen with a dilated pupil and slit-lamp retroillumination.

Compendium of ocular adverse reactions

Given that fortunately most OARs are transient and clinically insignificant, the compendium below lists only those previously reported OARs that are significant in terms of tangible effects on structure or function relevant to the general optometric practitioner. The principal BNF therapeutic classes of drugs are listed together with details of OARs reported for selected subgroups of each class. Although a particular OAR may have been associated with one or more members of a subgroup, all members have been listed to facilitate monitoring of the drug group. A selection of principal systemic side effects (SSEs) based on current BNF entries are given as, if reported by the patient, they may be indicative of a concurrent OAR. Most entries are accompanied by a clinical commentary where an OAR is especially significant, has specific advice listed in the BNF or demonstrates a special general or specific feature of interest.

Gastrointestinal system

As many gastrointestinal drugs are formulated to remain in the gut, systemic absorption is minimal and hence prevalence of OARs is low.

Antispasmodics

Direct relaxants of intestinal smooth muscle.

Antispasmodics (antimuscarinics)

Formerly termed anticholinergics, antimuscarinics reduce intestinal motility. They are used occasionally for the management of irritable bowel syndrome and diverticular disease.

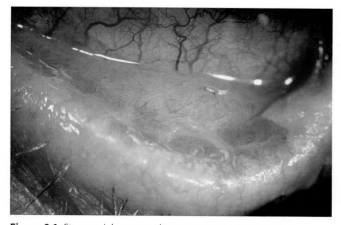

Figure 9.1 Stevens–Johnson syndrome. (From Kanski 2003 Clinical ophthalmology: a systematic approach, 5th edn, p 79, Fig. 4.58.)

Examples: Tertiary amines: atropine sulphate, dicycloverine hydrochloride. Quaternary ammonium compounds: propantheline bromide, hyoscine butylbromide.
SSEs: Constipation, transient bradycardia (followed by tachycardia, palpitation and arrhythmias), reduced bronchial secretions.
OARs: Mild and transitory mydriasis and cycloplegia, induced closed-angle glaucoma (very rare).

Ulcer-healing drugs

H₂-receptor antagonists

Heal gastric and duodenal ulcers by reducing gastric acid output and are also used to relieve symptoms of gastro-oesophogeal reflux.
Examples: Cimetidine, famotidine, nizatidine, ranitidine.
SSEs: Gastrointestinal disturbance, altered liver function, headache and dizziness.
OARs: Visual disturbances (ranitidine).
Clinical commentary: Despite the relatively high level of prescribing of this class of agents few OARs of significance have been reported. Nevertheless, transient myopia, a yellow or pink tinge to objects and sicca-like symptoms have been recorded (Fraunfelder & Fraunfelder 2001).

Proton pump inhibitors

Inhibit the secretion of gastric acid by blocking the hydrogen–potassium adenosine triphosphatase enzyme system (the 'proton pump') of the gastric parietal cell. Proton pump inhibitors are effective short-term treatments for gastric and duodenal ulcers; they are also used in combination with antibacterials for the eradication of *Helicobacter pylori*.
Examples: Esomeprazole, lansoprazole, omeprazole, pantoprazole, rabeprazole sodium.
SSEs: Gastrointestinal disturbance, headache, dizziness.
OARs: Blurred vision (infrequent), photosensitivity, Stevens–Johnson syndrome (rare).

Chronic bowel disorders

These include ulcerative colitis and Crohn's disease and treatment involves a combination of drug therapy, nutritional advice and, when severe, surgery.

Aminosalicylates

Examples: Balsalazide sodium, mesalazine, olsalazine sodium, sulfasalazine.
SSEs: Nausea, abdominal pain, headache.
OARs: Sulfasalazine: transient myopia, photosensitization, ocular complications (including periorbital oedema), staining of soft contact lenses, Stevens–Johnson syndrome.
Clinical commentary: Although a number of OARs have been associated with this group most are rare and reversible. Bilateral transient myopia, possibly induced by ciliary body oedema, can occur and may exceed several dioptres (Santodomingo-Rubido et al 2003).

Corticosteroids

Used as adjunct treatment in refractive or moderate bowel disease.
Examples: Budesonide, hydrocortisone, prednisolone.
SSEs: See entry under Endocrine System.
OARs: See entry under Endocrine System.

Cardiovascular system

Positive inotropic drugs

Increase the force of contraction of the myocardium.

Cardiac glycosides

Used in the treatment of supraventricular tachycardia, especially for controlling ventricular response in persistent atrial fibrillation. Digoxin is now rarely used for the rapid control of heart rate.
Examples: Digoxin, digitoxin.
SSEs: Anorexia, nausea, vomiting.
OARs: Usually associated with excessive dose. Retinal effects produce altered colour perception (sometimes a yellow-blue tinge to objects) and glare phenomena, visual field defects, corneal oedema.
Clinical commentary: It has been estimated that OARs occur in 11–25% of patients taking cardiac glycosides although nearly all are reversible (Fraunfelder & Fraunfelder 2001). Normal therapeutic doses can cause OARs (Hobley & Lawrenson 1991) with acquired colour vision defects found along the blue–yellow axis being the most commonly recorded with a 100-hue test, although patients do not normally complain of impaired colour perception. The colour vision defects can occur in 80% of patients on long-term therapy. Reducing the dose or stopping therapy produces a marked reduction in the error score on the 100-hue test. A later study (Lawrenson et al 2002) used a battery of colour vision tests to show slight to moderate red–green impairment in around 20–30% of elderly patients taking a maintenance therapy of digoxin, with approximately 20% showing a severe tritan deficiency. There was no correlation between colour vision impairment and serum digoxin level. Visual field defects are invariably central or paracentral.

Diuretics

Thiazides and related diuretics

Used to relieve oedema due to chronic heart failure and, in lower doses, to reduce blood pressure.
Examples: Bendroflumethiazide, chlortalidone, cyclopenthiazide, indapamide, metolazone, xipamide.
SSEs: Gastrointestinal problems, headache, fatigue.
OARs: Bendroflumethiazide: photosensitivity; indapamide: photosensitivity, reversible acute myopia.
Clinical commentary: OARs due to the thiazides are infrequent and transitory. The myopia that has been reported may be linked to changes in lens volume or choroidal effusions (Soylev et al 1995).

Antiarrhythmic drugs

Arrhythmic conditions include ectopic beats, atrial fibrillation, atrial flutter, paradoxysmal supraventricular tachycardia, arrhythmias after myocardial infarction, ventricular tachycardia.

Supraventricular arrhythmia and ventricular arrhythmias

Examples: Amiodarone, disopyramide, flecainide acetate, procainamide hydrochloride, propafenone hydrochloride, quinidine.
SSEs: Nausea, vomiting, taste disturbances.

OARs: Corneal microdeposits (amiodarone), optic neuropathy, blurred vision, visual disturbances, lens changes, photosensitivity, antimuscarinic effects, angle-closure glaucoma.

Clinical commentary: amiodarone is used in the treatment of arrhythmias, particularly when other drugs are ineffective or contraindicated, and optometrists need to be especially aware of its potential for OARs (Mantyjarvi et al 1998). It may also be used for tachyarrhythmias associated with Wolff–Parkinson–White syndrome. The BNF states that amiodarone treatment should be initiated only under hospital or specialist supervision.

Most patients taking amiodarone develop corneal microdeposits which are reversible on withdrawal of treatment; these rarely interfere with vision, but drivers may be dazzled by headlights at night. However, if vision is impaired or if optic neuritis or optic neuropathy is apparent, the patient must be referred immediately. Because of the possibility of phototoxic reactions, patients should be advised to shield the skin from light during treatment and for several months after discontinuing amiodarone; a wide-spectrum sunscreen to protect against both long-wave ultraviolet and visible light should be used. The deposits are characteristic whorl-like vortex patterns of deposition within the corneal epithelium, sometimes described as corneal verticillata. The drug is thought to form complexes with cellular phospholipids which cannot be metabolized in the normal way by lysosomal phospholipidases; hence, they are deposited in the superficial layers of the cornea. The vortex pattern formed by the deposits is thought to be due to abnormal basal epithelia cells migrating towards the central cornea, and although the deposits are not considered to be sight-threatening and normally reverse on withdrawal of the drug, they should be reported as they may underlie a more general toxic response (see **Fig. 9.2**).

The pattern of deposition is seen in between 70% and 100% of patients treated with amiodarone, to such an extent that they could be used as an indication that the drug is being taken correctly. The deposits can occur as early as 2 weeks after starting the course of treatment and it seems that most patients will probably have some form of deposit after 3 months of taking the drug. In the initial stages, greyish or light-brown deposits appear in the mid-peripheral inferior epithelium just anterior to Bowman's membrane. The deposits do not stain with fluorescein. Progression to the second stage takes around 6 months, such that the deposits coalesce to form a horizontal line set usually at the junction of the middle and lower third of the cornea, although several lines can branch out towards the periphery without actually reaching the limbus. In the tertiary stage the lines increase in density to form the characteristic whorl-like vortex pattern. The changes are usually bilateral and clear within 3 to 7 months once medication is finished. Vision is not usually affected, apart from complaints of haloes around bright lights.

Amiodarone has also been associated with the formation of small, anterior, subcapsular, yellow-white, punctuate opacities within the pupillary zone. The opacities can be detected in 50–60% of patients between 5 and 22 months after starting treatment and, although they persist after treatment has been discontinued, vision is not usually affected (Flach & Dolan 1990).

Patients on amiodarone treatment often carry risks for developing non-arteritic ischaemic optic neuropathy, which has signs and symptoms very similar to that of amiodarone neuropathy (Macaluso et al 1999). A patient presenting to the optometrist with any sign of optic neuropathy should be referred immediately.

Beta-adrenoceptor blocking drugs

Used in hypertension, angina pectoris, myocardial infarction, arrhythmias, heart failure and thyrotoxicosis, anxiety and migraine.

Examples: Propranolol hydrochloride, acebutolol, atenolol, bisoprolol fumarate, carvedilol, celiprolol hydrochloride, esmolol hydrochloride, labetalol hydrochloride, metoprolol tartrate, nadaolol, nebivolol, oxprenolol hydrochloride, pindolol, sotalol hydrochloride, timolol maleate.

SSEs: Asthma, coldness of extremities, sleep disturbances.

OARs: Dry eyes (rare and reversible on withdrawal), transient diplopia, difficulty with contact lenses.

Clinical commentary: Current beta-blocking drugs have relatively innocuous OARs. Nevertheless, they need to be monitored owing to the reports from 30 years ago that linked the beta blocker practolol with a severe oculocutaneous syndrome characterized by corneal and conjunctival scarring, keratinization and a loss of the conjunctival fornices (Wright 1975).

Hypertension and heart failure

Angiotensin-converting enzyme inhibitors

The angiotensin-converting enzyme (ACE) inhibitors inhibit the conversion of angiotensin I to angiotensin II and are indicated in heart failure, hypertension, diabetic nephropathy, prophylaxis of cardiovascular events.

Examples: Captopril, cilazapril, enalapril maleate, fosinopril sodium, imidapril hydrochloride, lisinoprilmoexipril hydrochloride, perindopril erbumine, quinapril, ramipril, trandolapril.

SSEs: Dizziness, vertigo, headache.

OARs: Blurred vision, Stevens–Johnson syndrome (occasionally).

Clinical commentary: Oedema of ocular vasculature has been reported along with conjunctivitis and (rarely) photosensitivity (Goodfield & Millard 1985).

Calcium channel blockers

Influence myocardial cells and cells of vascular smooth muscle by interfering with the inward displacement of calcium ions through the slow channels of active cell membranes. Used in the treatment of vasospastic angina and chronic stable angina.

Examples: Amlodipine, diltiazem hydrochloride, felodipine, isradipine, lacidipine, lercanidipine, nicardipine hydrochloride, nifedipine, nimodipine, nisoldipine, verapamil hydrochloride.

SSEs: Abdominal pain, nausea, palpitation.

OARs: Blurred vision (amlodipine), photosensitivity (diltiazem), visual disturbance and eye pain (nifedipine, nisoldipine), Stevens–Johnson syndrome (verapamil).

Antifibrinolytic and haemostatics

Slow the dissolution of fibrin and help blood loss in conditions such as menorrhagia and epistaxis.

Examples: Aprotinin, etamsylate, tranexamic acid.
SSEs: Nausea, vomiting, diarrhoea.
OARs: Tranexamic acid: disturbances in colour vision.
Clinical commentary: Treatment should be discontinued if colour vision problems are reported.

Lipid-regulating drugs

Nicotinic acid group

Used to lower cholesterol as well as for the treatment of peripheral vascular disease.
Examples: Acipimox, nicotinic acid.
SSEs: Flushing, rash, headache.
OARs: Nicotinic acid: blurred vision, sicca syndromes, eyelid oedema, cystoid macular oedema.
Clinical commentary: The maculopathy is more common in males between 30 and 60 years of age who were taking more than 3 g of the drug daily (Fraunfelder & Fraunfelder 2001).

Respiratory system

Bronchodilators

Antimuscarinic bronchodilators

Used for the short-term relief of chronic asthma (ipratropium) and management of chronic obstructive pulmonary disease (tiotropium).
Examples: Ipratropium bromide, tiotropium.
SSEs: Dry mouth, nausea, constipation.
OARs: Acute angle-closure glaucoma (with nebulized ipratropium).
Clinical commentary: The risk of acute angle-closure glaucoma with nebulized ipratropium is increased when given with nebulized salbutamol and possibly other beta$_2$ agonists. Care is therefore needed to protect a patient's eyes from nebulized drug or drug powder.

Corticosteroids

For the management of reversible and irreversible airways disease. Effective in asthma as they reduce airway inflammation and its associated oedema and secretion. Also used in chronic obstructive pulmonary disease.
Examples: Beclometasone dipropionate, budesonide, ciclesonide, fluticasone propionate, mometasone furoate.
SSEs: See entry under Endocrine System.
OARs: Inhaled corticosteroids have significantly fewer systemic effects than oral corticosteroids although there is a small but increased risk of glaucoma and cataract with prolonged high doses (see entry under Endocrine System).
Clinical commentary: See entry under Endocrine System.

Antihistamines

H$_1$ receptor antagonists are used topically in the treatment of nasal allergies, seasonal allergic rhinitis (hay fever), and systemically for urticaria, pruritus, insect bites and stings and drug allergy.
Examples: Acrivastine, cetirizine, desloratadine, fexofenadine hydrochloride, levocetirizine hydrochloride, loratadine, mizolastine, alimemazine tartrate, chlorphenamine maleate, clemastine, cyproheptadine hydrochloride, hydroxyzine hydrochloride, ketotifen, promethazine hydrochloride.
SSEs: Drowsiness, headache, dry mouth.
OARs: Antimuscarinic effects leading to blurred vision.
Clinical commentary: OARs are uncommon and invariably disappear when treatment is finished. The antimuscarinic effects can, however, accumulate over time to produce a dry eye sufficient to interfere with contact lens wear and produce clinically significant effects on accommodation function and pupil.

Central nervous system

Hypnotics and anxiolytics

Axiolytics ('sedatives') and hypnotics will both induce sleep, the latter when given at night and the former when given during the day. Both agents are reserved for short courses of treatment to alleviate acute conditions after causal factors for the anxiety have been established.

Anxyolytics (benzodiazepines)

Are sometimes referred to incorrectly as 'minor tranquillizers'. Can be used as both hypnotics (e.g. nitrazepam and flurazepam) or for short-term relief of severe anxiety. They act at benzodiazepine receptors which are associated with gamma-aminobutyric acid (GABA) receptors.
Examples: Diazepam, alprazolam, chlordiazepoxide hydrochloride, lorazepam, oxazepam.
SSEs: Drowsiness, confusion, ataxia.
OARs: Visual disturbances (occasional), diplopia, allergic conjunctivitis.
Clinical commentary: Generalized but low-level antimuscarinic effects may be evident (see further comment below under Antidepressants).

Drugs used in psychoses and related disorders

Antipsychotic drugs

Also known as neuroleptics and may be referred to incorrectly as 'major tranquillizers'. They are principally phenothiazine derivatives and their short-term use is to quieten disturbed patients with psychopathology associated with schizophrenia, brain damage, mania, toxic delirium, agitated depression.
Examples: Benperidol, chlorpromazine hydrochloride, flupentixol, fluphenazine hydrochloride, haloperidol, levomepromazine, pericyazine, perphenazine, pimozide, prochlorperazine, promazine hydrochloride, sulpiride, trifluoperazine, zuclopenthixol acetate, zuclopenthixol dichloride.
SSEs: Tremor, abnormal face and body movements, restlessness.
OARs: Antimuscarinic symptoms (e.g. dry eye), blurred vision. Rare: corneal and lens opacities, purple pigmentation of cornea, conjunctiva and retina.
Clinical commentary: Whereas the overall rate of OARs for this group has been estimated at 3%, OARs will be present in 30% of patients that have been treated for a number of years and in 100% of patients that have been treated for

more than 10 years (Fraunfelder & Fraunfelder 2001). Generalized but medium-level antimuscarinic effects are common (see further comment below under Antidepressants). The most prevalent OARs associated with chlorpromazine therapy are anterior capsular and subcapsular lens pigmentation and corneal endothelial pigmentary changes. The lens opacities can progress from being dot-like to a white, yellow or tan stellate pattern, at which point the corneal changes become evident (Rasmussen et al 1976).

Antidepressant drugs

Effective in the treatment of major depression of moderate and severe degree and dythymia (i.e. lower-grade chronic depression).

Tricyclic and related antidepressant drugs

Examples: Amitriptyline hydrochloride, clomipramine hydrochloride, dosulepin hydrochloride, imipramine hydrochloride, lofepramine, nortriptyline, trimipramine, mianserin hydrochloride, trazodone hydrochloride.
SSEs: Arrhythmias, convulsions, dry mouth.
OARs: Antimuscarinic effects: (less with mianserin and trazodone) dry eye, blurred vision, disturbance of accommodation. Very rare: angle-closure glaucoma.
Clinical commentary: Muscarinic antagonists (that is, atropine-like) have the potential when used systemically to cause relaxation of the ciliary and sphincter muscles and cause dry eye. The patient may thus experience difficulties with accommodation and be disturbed by bright lights because of the pupil dilation and diminished light reflex; contact lens wear may also become difficult. These generalized anticholinergic effects may result in the need for a modified reading addition or a tinted lens and, owing to an increase in pupil size, may render ocular structures more susceptible to damage by ultraviolet radiation. If the reduction in accommodation is substantial then, in young patients, there may be a concomitant alteration in the AC/A ratio or a decompensation of an existing hyperphoria; very occasionally oculomotor status may be sufficiently challenged to cause diplopia.

Selective serotonin re-uptake inhibitors (SSRIs)

Examples: Citalopram, escitalopram, fluoxetine, fluvoxamine, paroxetine, sertraline.
SSEs: Gastrointestinal effects (dose-related and fairly common), anorexia with weight loss and hypersensitivity reactions including rash.
OARs: Weak antimuscarinic effects: dry eye, blurred vision, disturbance of accommodation.
Clinical commentary: Although SSRIs have weak anticholinergic activity compared with tricyclic antidepressants, there are reports of angle closure (Eke et al 1997; Tripathi et al 2003).

Antiepileptic drugs

Control of epilepsy

Examples: Carbamazepine, lamotrigine, oxcarbazepine, sodium valporate and topiramate are the drugs of choice for partial (focal) seizures. Ethosuximide, gabapentin, pregabalin, levetiracetam, phenobarbital, primidone, phenytoin, tiagabine, vigabatrin, zonisamide, clobazam, clonazepam.
SSEs: Nausea, vomiting, dizziness, drowziness.

OARs: Visual disturbances: carbamazepine (especially diplopia and often associated with peak plasma concentrations, Stevens–Johnson syndrome), primidone, clonazepam. Visual field defects: vigabatrin carries CHM advice (see below). Acute angle-closure glaucoma: topiramate.
Clinical commentary: Vigabatrin is used for partial epilepsy with or without secondary generalization in combination with other antiepileptic treatment. Its use is restricted to patients in whom all other combinations are inadequate or not tolerated. About one-third of patients treated with vigabatrin have visual field defects, with onset varying from 1 month to several years after starting treatment. The defect is bilateral, usually asymptomatic and characteristically presents as concentric peripheral field loss with temporal and macular sparing. Invariably, the defect persists after discontinuation. Visual acuity and colour vision can be affected (Miller et al 1999). The product literature advises visual field testing before treatment and at 6-month intervals. Patients should be referred immediately if any new visual symptoms are reported.

Topiramate has been associated with acute myopia with secondary angle-closure glaucoma, typically occurring within 1 month of starting treatment. Choroidal effusions resulting in anterior displacement of the lens and iris have also been reported. The CHM advises that if raised intraocular pressure occurs seek specialist ophthalmological advice; use appropriate measures to reduce intraocular pressure; stop topiramate as rapidly as feasible (Committee on Safety of Medicines 2002). Acute angle-closure glaucoma with topiramate is usually bilateral and occurs from 3 to 14 days after the start of oral therapy (Fraunfelder et al 2004).

Dopaminergic drugs used in parkinsonism

Dopaminergic drugs

Examples: Levodopa, co-beneldopa, co-careldopa, amantadine hydrochloride, apomorphine hydrochloride, bromocriptine, carbergoline, entacapone, lisuride maleate, pergolide, pramipexole, rasagiline, ropinirole, rotigotine, selegiline hydrochloride, tolcapone.
SSEs: Nausea, anorexia, drowsiness.
OARs: Visual disorders (pramipexole), blurred vision (amantadine), conjunctivitis (rasagiline).
Clinical commentary: Pramipexole: ophthalmological testing recommended by the BNF owing to the risk of visual disorders.

Antimuscarinic drugs

Examples: Benzatropine mesilate, orphenadrine hydrochloride, procyclidine hydrochloride, trihexyphenidyl hydrochloride.
SSEs: Constipation, dry mouth, nausea.
OARs: Blurred vision, angle-closure glaucoma (rare).

Infections

Viruses, bacteria and other unicellular and multicellular organisms that exist in the environment can also live in the human body to produce beneficial as well as unwanted biological responses within the host. Antiinfective agents account for around 12% of prescriptions a year issued by a typical medical practice, of which the majority are antibiotic preparations which have a high therapeutic index. Fortunately, relatively few commonly used antiinfective preparations, apart from ethambutol, chloroquine and didandosine have OARs of special clinical significance (Gilmartin 1999).

Antibacterial drugs

Antituberculous drugs

Examples: Capreomycin, cycloserine, ethambutol hydrochloride, isoniazid, pyrazinamide, rifabutin, rifampicin, streptomycin.
SSEs: Urticaria, rashes, pruritus.
OARs: Optic neuritis, red–green colour defects, visual field defects (ethambutol); optic neuritis (isoniazid).
Clinical commentary: Ethambutol is a tuberculostatic agent effective against *Mycobacterium tuberculosis* whose toxic effects are more common where excessive dosage is used or if the patient's renal function is impaired. A daily dose of up to 15 mg/kg appears to be relatively safe. Symptoms of optic neuritis become evident 3 to 6 months after the commencement of therapy. Axial and periaxial neuritis can occur, the former being associated with macular degeneration, the latter with visual field defects such as paracentral scotomas (i.e. central acuity remains normal) and red–green colour vision defects. The BNF states that the earliest features of toxicity are subjective and patients should be advised to discontinue therapy and seek advice immediately at the first sign of visual deterioration. Early discontinuation invariable results in recovery from the visual disturbances. Contrast sensitivity changes can be a very early indication of toxicity and occur prior to colour vision defects identified by 100-hue or D15 tests (Russo & Chaglasian 1994).

Quinolones

Are effective in uncomplicated urinary tract infections.
Examples: Ciprofloxacin, levofloxacin, moxifloxacin, nalidixic acid, norfloxacin, ofloxacin.
SSEs: Nausea, vomiting, dyspepsia.
OAR: Dyschromatopsia (nalidixic acid).
Clinical commentary: Disturbances of colour vision with nalidixic acid involve a green, yellow, blue or violet tone to objects; there may also be flashing lights or a glare phenomenon.

Other antibacterials

Used for pneumonia, complicated skin and soft-tissue infections caused by Gram-positive bacteria (initiated under expert supervision).
Examples: Chloramphenicol, fusidic acid, vancomycin, teicoplanin, daptomycin, linezolid, quinupristin, dalfopristin, polymyxins.
SSEs: Diarrhoea, nausea, vomiting.
OAR: Optic neuropathy (linezolid).
Clinical commentary: Linezolid: severe optic neuropathy may occur rarely, particularly if is used for longer than 28 days. The CHM recommends that: patients should be warned to report symptoms of visual impairment (including blurred vision, visual field defect, changes in visual acuity and colour vision) immediately; patients experiencing new visual symptoms (regardless of treatment duration) should be evaluated promptly, and referred to an ophthalmologist if necessary; visual function should be monitored regularly if treatment is required for longer than 28 days (Commission on Human Medicines/MHRA 2006).

Antiviral drugs

Viruses cannot replicate independently and must occupy cells to gain energy from DNA, RNA and protein-synthesizing mechanisms. For antiviral drugs to be effective, therefore, they need to engage cells which in certain circumstances may not be affected by the virus, a feature which forms the basis of toxic reactions.

HIV infection (nucleoside reverse transcriptase inhibitors)

Examples: Abacavir, didanosine, emtricitabine, lamivudine, stavudine, tenofovir disoproxil, zidovudine.
SSEs: Hypersensitivity reactions.
OARs: Didanosine: dry eye, retinal and optic nerve changes (especially in children).
Clinical commentary: Didanosine: a mydriatic eye examination is recommended (especially in children) every 6 months or if visual changes occur (Whitcup et al 1994).

Antiprotozoal drugs

Antimalarials

Chloroquine is generally used in low dose over a short term for the prophylaxis of malaria in areas of the world where the risk of chloroquine-resistant *Falciparum* malaria is still low.
Examples: Chloroquine.
SSEs: See entry under Musculoskeletal and Joint Diseases.
OARs: See entry under Musculoskeletal and Joint Diseases.
Clinical commentary: See entry under Musculoskeletal and Joint Diseases.

Endocrine system

Corticosteroids

Physiologically, steroids are involved in all aspects of metabolism (fat, protein, carbohydrate and electrolyte) and therefore the propensity for ocular and general adverse effects is closely monitored.

Glucocorticoid therapy

Examples: Prednisolone, cortisone acetate, deflazacort, dexamethasone, hydrocortisone, methylprednisolone, triamcinolone.
SSEs: Dyspepsia, osteoporosis, adrenal suppression, depression.
OARs: Glaucoma, papilloedema, posterior subcapsular cataracts, corneal or scleral thinning, exacerbation of ophthalmic fungal or viral disease, blurred vision, difficulty with contact lens wear.
Clinical commentary: Steroids have the potential to induce changes in almost all ocular structures. A well-documented affect on the crystalline lens is the tendency for corticosteroids used over prolonged periods, particularly in rheumatoid conditions, to cause the formation of posterior subcapsular cataracts. The opacities are typically bilateral, and irreversible (Urban & Cotlier 1986). Although it is rare for the opacities to cause significant reduction in acuity, patients may report photophobia, reading problems or difficulty with glare. Corneal oedema may also occur and affect the wearing of contact lenses.

Systemic steroids have the potential, in susceptible individuals, to raise intraocular pressure to a level sufficient to cause glaucomatous changes at the optic disc and concomitant visual field changes (McDonnell & Muir 1985).

Sex hormones

Female sex hormones (oestrogens and HRT)

Used to alleviate female menopausal symptoms.
Examples: Range of conjugated oestrogens with and without progestogen.
SSEs: Dyspepsia, osteoporosis, adrenal suppression, depression.
OARs: Contact lenses may irritate, dry eye.

Drugs affecting bone metabolism

Bisphosphonates

Inhibit bone reabsorption in the management of hypercalcaemia of malignancy. Also used in the treatment of Paget's disease.
Examples: Alendronic acid, disodium etidronate, disodium pamidronate, ibandronic acid, risedronate sodium, sodium clodronate, tiludronic acid, zoledronic acid.
SSEs: Oesophageal disorders, abdominal pain, dyspepsia.
OARs: Photosensitivity, uveitis, scleritis, episcleritis, dry eye, corneal lesions.
Clinical commentary: Pamidronate has been associated with both unilateral and bilateral scleritis usually within 6 to 48 hours of administration. If there is persistent visual disturbance or ocular pain the patient should be referred to an ophthalmologist (Fraunfelder & Fraunfelder 2003).

Obstetrics, gynaecology and urinary tract disorders

Contraceptives

Combined hormonal contraceptives

Examples: A range of products containing an oestrogen and a progestogen.
SSEs: Nausea, vomiting, headache.
OARs: Contact lenses may irritate, dry eye.
Clinical commentary: The evidence for a definite link between dry eye and contraceptive use is equivocal and few significant OARs have been associated with this group (Vessey et al 1998).

Drugs for genitourinary disorders

Drugs for urinary retention (alpha blockers)

Relax smooth muscle in benign prostatic hyperplasia, thus producing an increase in urinary flow rate.
Examples: Alfuzosin hydrochloride, doxazosin, indoramin, prazosin hydrochloride, tamsulosin hydrochloride, terazosin.
SSEs: Drowsiness, hypotension, syncope.
OARs: Pupil disorders, amblyopia, blurred vision.

Malignant disease and immunosuppression

Sex hormones and hormone antagonists

Hormone antagonists (breast cancer)

Examples: Anastrozole, exmestane, fulvestrant, letrozole, tamoxifen, toremifene.
SSEs: Hot flushes, gastrointestinal disturbances, abdominal pain.
OARs: Corneal opacities, cataract (letrozole), retinopathy, blurred vision.
Clinical commentary: The antioestrogen agent tamoxifen competes with the hormone oestrogen at receptor sites within tumour cells. As a large proportion of human breast cancers are oestrogen-dependent for growth, tamoxifen is prescribed following surgery for breast cancer, as a prophylactic therapy against recurrence of the tumour and as a preventative therapy for patients who do not have breast cancer but have a strong family history of the condition. Tamoxifen is associated with a bilateral superficial maculopathy which presents as fine yellow-white crystal-like refractile opacities surrounding the macula (Bentley et al 1992; Dulley 1999) (**Fig. 9.3**). Visual acuity is usually reduced and there may be an associated cystoid macular oedema. The OAR may be reversible if detected in the early stages but reversal of the retinopathy becomes increasingly unlikely in the later stages of toxicity and appears to be dependent on the cumulative dose (Ah-Song & Sasco 1997). Mild to moderate tritanomalous colour defects have been recorded and central scotomas that fall within the Amsler chart area. A keratopathy similar to that found with amiodarone has also been reported. Posterior subcapsular cataracts have also been linked to tamoxifen (Gorin et al 1998). Incidence levels for OARs with tamoxifen appear to be around 1–2% of patients. Dulley (2001) emphasizes that patients with retinopathy and keratopathy may be asymptomatic and recommends a baseline check prior to therapy that incorporates the Amsler grid, D15 or City University colour vision assessment, slit-lamp examination and binocular indirect fundus examination.

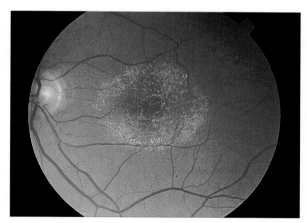

Figure 9.3 Tamoxifen retinopathy. (From Kanski 2003 Clinical ophthalmology: a systematic approach, 5th edn, p 433, Fig. 13.106.)

Nutrition and blood

Anaemias

Drugs used in hypoplastic, haemolytic, and renal anaemias (iron overload)

Examples: Deferiprone, desferrioxamine mesilate.
SSEs: Hypotension, disturbances of hearing, gastrointestinal problems.
OARs: Desferrioxamine: visual disturbances, blurred vision, poor night vision, lens opacities, retinopathy.
Clinical commentary: Patients who require regular blood transfusions can suffer from iron overload, and desferrioxamine acts as a chelating agent to break the iron down to ferrioxamine. The BNF recommends eye and ear examinations before treatment and at 3-month intervals during treatment (Rubinstein et al 1985).

Musculoskeletal and joint diseases

Drugs used in rheumatic diseases and gout

Nonsteroidal antiinflammatory drugs

Nonsteroidal antiinflammatory drugs (NSAIDs) are methylated indole derivatives used as antipyretic, analgesic or antiinflammatory agents in the treatment of rheumatoid arthritis, rheumatoid spondylitis and degenerative joint disease.
Examples: Aceclofenac, celecoxib, dexibuprofen, dexketoprofen, diclofenac sodium, diflunisal, etodolac, etoricoxib, fenbufen, fenoprofen, flurbiprofen, ibuprofen, indometacin, ketoprofen, lumiracoxib, mefenamic acid, meloxicam, nabumetome, naproxen, piroxicam, sulindac, tenoxicam, tiaprofenic acid.
SSEs: Gastrointestinal problems, bronchospasm, headache.
OARs: Blurred vision, conjunctivitis, corneal deposits.
Clinical commentary: Indometacin: ophthalmic examination is advised during prolonged therapy. The prevalence and nature of OARs associated with this group are, however, not well established (Fraunfelder & Fraunfelder 2001). Nevertheless, of note is the reported occurrence of corneal opacities, similar to those seen in chloroquine keratopathy, which diminish or disappear within 6 months of discontinuing therapy (Burns 1968). Cases of loss of vision or disturbances of vision associated with cyclooxygenase-2 (COX-2) inhibitors, such as celecoxib, have been reported (Fraunfelder et al 2006). The possible mechanism is reduction in retinal blood flow; the effect appears to be reversible (Coulter et al 2003).

Corticosteroids

Treatment with corticosteroids in rheumatic diseases is reserved for specific indications, e.g. when other antiinflammatory drugs are unsuccessful.
Examples: Prednisolone, hydrocortisone, dexamethasone.
SSEs: See entry under Endocrine System.
OARs: See entry under Endocrine System.
Clinical commentary: See entry under Endocrine System.

Drugs which suppress the rheumatic disease process (antimalarials)

Hydroxychloroquine is used to treat rheumatoid arthritis of moderate inflammatory activity and mild systemic lupus erythematosus, particularly when involving cutaneous and joint manifestations. Chloroquine is only considered for treating chronic inflammatory conditions where other drugs have failed. Mepacrine hydrochloride (an antigiardial drug) is also used for antimalarial therapy but has negligible OARs.
Examples: Chloroquine, hydroxychloroquine.
SSEs: Gastrointestinal disturbances, headache, skin reactions (rashes, pruritus).
OARs: Corneal deposits, pigment deposits at macula.
Clinical commentary: Chloroquine can induce in 1–2% of patients retinal and macular changes, narrowing of retinal vessels and deterioration in vision. In these patients, a high proportion of chloroquine is retained in the melanin of the retinal pigment epithelium and produces a perimacular 'bull's-eye' ring of pigment. The depth of the associated annular scotoma can be monitored with red targets on most visual field screening devices. Importantly, central visual acuity can be retained until the late stages of toxicity. Patients at greatest risk are those on hydroxychloroquine therapy for longer than 5 years or those with liver or renal disease. In the elderly it may be difficult to distinguish drug-induced changes from ageing changes although there is no evidence to show that hydroxychloroquine therapy will worsen pre-existing macular degeneration.

Corneal deposits similar to those reported for amiodarone, chlorpromazine and tamoxifen have also been reported for chloroquine. The deposits may be seen as early as 3 weeks after the start of medication and, importantly, may be an indicator of maculopathy. The corneal changes may first appear as a Hudson–Stähli line or as an increase in a pre-existing Hudson–Stähli line (Easterbrook 1988).

Guidelines for screening to prevent ocular toxicity on long-term treatment with hydroxychloroquine were published by the UK Royal College of Ophthalmologists in 2004 (Royal College of Ophthalmologists 2004).

In the context of optometric screening, the guidelines recommend assessment by an optometrist before treatment followed by referral to an ophthalmologist if an ocular problem is present. During treatment, the monitoring of near visual acuity using a standard reading chart is recommended. If a reduction in acuity occurs or visual symptoms are reported, the patient should be advised to stop the treatment and seek the prescribing doctor's advice.

Skin

Acne and rosacea

Oral preparations for acne (oral retinoid)

Retinoids are used to treat cystic acne, psoriasis and various skin disorders.
Example: Isotretinoin.
SSEs: Dry skin and lips.
OARs: Dry eye syndrome, blepharitis, conjunctivitis, keratitis, visual disturbances, transitory myopia, papilloedema, corneal

opacities, anterior subcapsular cataracts, decreased dark adaptation, photophobia, colour vision defects, optic neuritis.

Clinical commentary: Isotretinoin is secreted in the tears via the lacrimal gland to produce the reported blepharoconjunctivitis and corneal irritation and may also have a direct effect on meibomian gland function to increase tear evaporation and osmolarity. These adverse responses will determine the success or otherwise of contact lens wear. The effects are thought to underlie the fine, rounded subepithelial opacities found in the central and peripheral areas of the cornea although these do not normally interfere with vision (Fraunfelder et al 2001).

Conclusion

Future therapeutic agents will be linked to advances in genomics and proteomics and are likely to produce some remarkable new agents for the treatment of viral, psychiatric, malignant and autoimmune disease. All will have at least the potential to generate adverse effects, and therefore the management of OARs will be a continuing and developing aspect of primary care for the optometrist.

Acknowledgements

Anthony R Cox MRPharmS of the West Midlands Centre for Adverse Drug Reactions, City Hospital, Birmingham, UK for critical review of the draft manuscript.

References

Ah-Song R, Sasco A J 1997 Tamoxifen and ocular toxicity. Review. Cancer Detection and Prevention 21:522–531

Aronson J K 2003 Anecdotes as evidence. British Medical Journal 326:1346

Aronson J K 2006 Meyler's side effects of drugs: the international encyclopedia of adverse drug reactions and interactions, 15th edn. Elsevier, London

Aronson J K, White N J 1996 Principles of clinical pharmacology and drug therapy. In: Weatherall D, Ledingham J G, Warrel J (eds) 3rd edn. Oxford Textbook of Medicine, Oxford University Press, Oxford, pp 1235–1263

Bartlett H, Eperjesi F 2005 Possible contraindications and adverse reactions associated with the use of ocular nutritional supplements. Ophthalmic Physiological Optics 25:179–194

Bartlett J D, Jaanus S D 2001 Ocular effects of systemic drugs. In: Bartlett J D, Jaanus S D (eds) Clinical Ocular Pharmacology, 4th edn. Butterworth-Heinemann, Boston, pp 903–948

Bentley C R, Davies G, Aclimandos W A 1992 Tamoxifen retinopathy: a rare but serious complication. British Medical Journal 304:495–496

British National Formulary 2006 B M J Publishing Goup Ltd and R P S Publishing

Burns C A 1968 Indomethacin, reduced retinal sensitivity and corneal deposits. American Journal of Ophthalmology 66:825–835

College of Optometrists UK 2002 Optometrist's Formulary 6–8. Online. Available:http://www.college-optometrists.org/coo/download.cfm?uuid=ACA41B0C–9ED5–12E2–8F1CAC2347AC79DA&type=members_handbook

Commission on Human Medicines/MHRA 2006 Linezolid (Zyvox) severe optic neuropathy. Current Problems in Pharmacovigilance 31:2–3

Committee on Safety of Medicines 2002 Topiramate (Topamax): acute myopia and raised intraocular pressure. Current Problems in Pharmacovigilance 28:4

Coulter D M, Clark D W J, Savage R L 2003 Celecoxib, rofecoxib, and acute temporary visual disturbance. British Medical Journal 327:124–125

Cox A 2006 Prevention and management of drug-induced ocular disorders. The Prescriber June:39–42

Cox A, Gilmartin B 2006 Drug-induced ophthalmic adverse reactions. Adverse Drugs Reactions Bulletin 241:923–926

Davidson S T, Hickey-Dwyer M 1991 Eye disorders. In: Davies D M (ed.) Textbook of adverse drug reactions, 4th edn. Oxford University Press, Oxford, pp 567–576

Davies D M (ed.) 1991 Textbook of adverse drug reactions, 4th edn. Oxford University Press, Oxford

Davies D M, Ferner R E, de Glanville H 1998 Davies's textbook of adverse drug reactions, 5th edn. Chapman and Hall Medical, London

Dulley P 1999 Ocular adverse reactions to tamoxifen – a review. Ophthalmic Physiological Optics (Suppl:Clinical Optometry Update) 19: S2–S9

Dulley P 2001 The ocular effects of tamoxifen – a review and update. The Optician 221(No. 5792):32–35

Easterbrook M 1988 Ocular effects and safety of antimalarial agents. American Journal of Medicine 85(Supp 4A):23–29

Edgar D, Gilmartin B 1997 Ocular adverse effects of systemic medication. Ophthalmic Physiological Optics (Suppl:Clinical Optometry Update)17:S2–S8

Edwards I R, Biriell C 1995 Harmonisation in pharmacovigilance. Drug Safety 10:93–102

Eke T, Bates A K, Carr S 1997 Acute angle closure glaucoma associated with paroxetine. British Medical Journal 314:1387

Flach A J, Dolan B J 1990 Amiodarone-induced opacities: an 8-year follow-up study. Archives of Ophthalmology 108: 1668–1669

Fraunfelder F W 2004 Ocular side effects from herbal medicines and nutritional supplements. American Journal of Ophthalmology 138:640–648

Fraunfelder F T, Fraunfelder F W 2001 Drug-induced ocular side effects, 5th edn. Butterworth Heinemann, Boston

Fraunfelder F W, Fraunfelder F T 2003 Bisphosphonates and possible ocular adverse drug reactions. New England Journal of Medicine 348:1187–1188

Fraunfelder F W, Fraunfelder F T 2004 Adverse ocular drug reactions recently identified by the national registry of drug-induced ocular side effects. Ophthalmology 111:1275–1279

Fraunfelder F T, Fraunfelder F W, Edwards R 2001 Ocular side-effects possibly associated with isotretinoin usage. American Journal of Ophthalmology 132:299–305

Fraunfelder F W, Keates E U, Fraunfelder F T 2004 Topiramate associated acute, bilateral, secondary angle-closure glaucoma. Ophthalmology 111:109–111

Fraunfelder F W, Solomon J, Mehelas T J 2006 Ocular adverse effects associated with cyclooxygenase-2 inhibitors. Archives of Ophthalmology 124:277–279

Fraunfelder F T, Fraunfelder F W, Chambers W 2008 Clinical ocular toxicology. Saunders, Philadelphia

Gilmartin B 1987 The Marton Lecture: Ocular manifestations of systemic medication. Ophthalmic Physiological Optics 7: 449–459

Gilmartin B 1999 The ocular side-effects of anti-infective agents. The Optician 218(No. 5715):20–25

Goodfield M J, Millard L G 1985 Severe cutaneous reactions to captopril. British Medical Journal 290:1111

Gorin M B, Day R, Constantino J P et al 1998 Long-term tamoxifen citrate use and potential ocular toxicity. American Journal of Ophthalmology 125:493–501

Grant W M, Schuman J S 1993 Toxicology of the eye, 4th edn. Charles C Thomas Publisher Ltd, Springfield, IL

Hanratty M 2005 LASIK – a handbook for optometrists. Butterworth-Heinemann, Oxford, pp 14–17

Harrison R J 1996 Ocular adverse reactions to systemic drug therapy. Adverse Drug Reaction Bulletin 180:683–686

Hobley A, Lawrenson J 1991 Ocular adverse effects to the therapeutic administration of digoxin. Ophthalmic Physiological Optics 11:391–393

Hopkins G, Pearson R 2007 Adverse ocular reactions to systemic drug treatment. In: Ophthalmic drugs, 5th edn. Butterworth-Heinemann, Oxford, pp 288–313

Hospital Prescribing 2006: England. Online. Available:http://www.ic. nhs.uk/webfiles/publications/hospres06/Hospital%20Prescribing%202006%20England%20Bulletin%202006.pdf 4 December. 2007

Kando J C, Yonkers K A, Cole J O 1995 Gender as a risk factor for adverse events to medications. Drugs 50:1–6

Kanski J J 2003 Clinical ophthalmology, 5th edn. Butterworth-Heinemann, Oxford

Lawrenson J 1999 The ocular effects of cardiovascular drugs. The Optician 217(No. 5697):30–33

Lawrenson J 2001 Identifying and reporting of ocular adverse reactions. The Optician 222(No. 5829):18–21

Lawrenson J G, Kelly C, Lawrenson A L et al 2002 Acquired colour vision deficiency in patients receiving maintenance therapy. British Journal of Ophthalmology 86:1259–1261

Lee A, Thomson J 2006 Drug-induced skin reactions. In: Lee (ed.) Adverse drug reactions, 2nd edn. Pharmaceutical Press, London, pp 125–156

Macaluso D C, Shults W T, Fraunfelder F T 1999 Features of amiodarone-induced optic neuropathy. American Journal of Ophthalmology 127:610–612

McDonnell P J, Muir M G K 1985 Glaucoma associated with systemic corticosteroid therapy. Lancet 2(8451):386–387

McDowell S E, Coleman J J, Ferner R E 2006 Systematic review and meta-analysis of ethnic differences in risks of adverse reactions to drugs used in cardiovascular medicine. British Medical Journal 332:1177–1181

McLeod H L, Evans W E 2001 Pharmacogenomics: unlocking the human genome for better drug therapy. Annual Review of Pharmacology and Toxicology 41:101–121

Mantyjarvi M, Tuppurainen K, Ikaheimo K 1998 Ocular side effects of amiodarone. Survey of Ophthalmology 42:360–366

Martindale 2007 Sweetman S C (ed.) The complete drug reference, vol 1, 35th edn. Pharmaceutical Press, London

Miller N R, Johnson M A, Paul S R et al 1999 Visual dysfunction in patients receiving vigabatrin: clinical and electrophysiological findings. Neurology 53:2082–2087

National Audit Office 2003 Safety, quality, efficacy: regulating medicines in the UK. Report by the Comptroller and Auditor General HC 255 Session. 2002–2003: 16 January. 2003. The Stationary Office, London

Orme M L'E 1991 Drug interactions of clinical importance. In: Davies D M (ed.) Textbook of adverse drug reactions, 4th edn. Oxford University Press, Oxford, pp 788–810

Polak B C D 2000 Drugs used in ocular treatment. In: Meyler's side effects of drugs, 14th edn. Elsevier Amsterdam, Oxford, pp 1636–1648

Rasmussen K, Kirk L, Faurbye A 1976 Deposits in the lens and cornea of the eye during long-term chlorpromazine medication. Acta Psychiatrica Scandinavica 53:1–6

Rawlins M D, Jeffreys D B (1991) Study of UK product licence applications containing new active substances, 1987–9. British Medical Journal 302:223–225

Routledge P A 2004 Adverse drug reactions and interactions: mechanisms, risk factors, detection, management and prevention. In: Talbot J, Waller P (eds) Stephen's detection of new adverse drug reactions, 5th edn. Wiley, Chichester, pp 91–125

Royal College of Ophthalmologists 2004 Ocular toxicity and hydroxychloroquine: guidelines for screening. 2004. Online. Available: http://www.rcophth.ac.uk/docs/ publications/Oculartoxicity2004.pdf 8 May 2007

Rubinstein M, Dupont P, Doppee J P 1985 Ocular toxicity of desferrioxamine. Lancet 1(8432):817–818

Russo P A, Chaglasian M A 1994 Toxic optic neuropathy associated with ethambutol: implications for current therapy. Journal of the American Optometric Association 65:332–338

Santodomingo-Rubido J, Gilmartin B, Wolffsohn J S 2003 Drug-induced bilateral transient myopia with the sulphonamide sulfasalazine. Ophthalmic Physiological Optics 23:567–570

Seymour R M, Routledge P A 1998 Important drug–drug interactions in the elderly. Drugs Aging 12:484–494

Soylev M F, Green R L, Feldon S E 1995 Choroidal effusion as a mechanism for transient myopia induced by hydrochlorthiazide and triamterene. American Journal of Ophthalmology 120:395–397

Thomson Software Solutions 2006 Ocular adverse reactions of drugs database. Online. Available: www.thomson-software-solutions.com

Tripathi R C, Tripathi B J, Haggerty C 2003 Drug-induced glaucomas: mechanism and management. Drug Safety 26:749–767

Urban R C, Cotlier E 1986 Corticosteroid-induced cataracts. Survey of Ophthalmology 31:102–110

Vessey M P, Hannaford P, Mant J et al 1998 Oral contraception and eye disease: findings in two large cohort studies. British Journal of Ophthalmology 82:538–542

Weinshilboum R 2003 Inheritance and drug response. New England Journal of Medicine 348:529–537

Whitcup S M, Dastgheib K, Nussenblatt R B et al 1994 A clinicopathologic report of the retinal lesions associated with didanosine. Archives of Ophthalmology 112:1594–1598

Wright P 1975 Untoward effects associated with practolol administration: oculo-mucocutaneous syndrome. British Medical Journal 1:595–598

CHAPTER 10

Ocular disease

Christopher Bentley • Ranjit Sandhu

Introduction

This chapter on ocular disease is intended to act as an introduction to the subject. Space constraints simply do not allow for a comprehensive treatment of the whole of ocular disease; as far back as the 1960s Sir Stewart Duke-Elder needed 15 volumes (Duke-Elder System of Ophthalmology 1961–69). Similarly we cannot hope to provide great depth for each topic covered, although we have attempted to provide more depth when a disorder is more likely to be encountered in primary care or illustrates a wider point. Where possible, the reader is encouraged to dig deeper and use the references available as a starting point to lifelong learning.

External disease

Blepharitis

Probably the most common condition of the eyelids seen in normal optometric practice is blepharitis. This results in chronic ocular irritation. There is thickening of the lids, abnormal vessel formation along the margins (*telangiectasis*) and meibomian gland dysfunction. Commonly, lash crusting is seen. The most likely causative organism will be *Staphylococcus* species.

Blepharitis accounts for 4.5% of all ophthalmological problems presenting in primary care. About 2–5% of general practitioner consultations are related to eye problems and new episodes of blepharitis are reported as 1.8 per 1000 population per year (Manners 1997).

Good lid hygiene with mechanical scrubbing of the lid margins, warm compresses, and antibiotic ointment at bedtime using bacitracin or erythromycin is the standard treatment for blepharitis. Patients whose blepharitis responds poorly to these simple measures, those who have rosacea, or those who have corneal complications such as marginal infiltrates may benefit from the use of systemic tetracycline (250 mg, orally four times each day for 1 week, then twice daily) or doxycycline (100 mg, orally twice daily for 1 week, then once daily). Systemic erythromycin is an alternative to systemic doxycycline, especially in children, where tetracyclines should be avoided because of the risk of developing permanent staining of the teeth. The mechanism of action of systemic tetracycline may in part be due to the inhibition of bacterial lipases and subsequent reduction in free fatty acid production. Inhibition of keratinization and antimicrobial activity may also be important.

Blepharitis is often associated with a poor-quality tear film and dry eye syndrome; artificial tears can often provide symptomatic relief (Frith et al 2001).

Conjunctivitis

The conjunctiva is a thin protective membrane that covers the ocular surface and reflects around the inside surface of the eyelids. There are a variety of conditions that affect the conjunctiva.

Allergic conjunctivitis is an inflammation of the conjunctiva that occurs due to hypersensitivity reactions following sensitization and re-exposure to an allergen.

In general:

- *Type I hypersensitivity* reactions occur immediately following contact with an allergen, causing mast cells to degranulate, leading to conjunctivitis.
- *Type IV hypersensitivity* reactions develop 24–48 hours after contact with an allergen and lead to inflammation without degranulation of mast cells.

When mast cells degranulate, they release histamine and other inflammatory mediators. These mediators cause:

- conjunctival blood vessels to dilate and the eye to appear red
- increased permeability of blood vessels, resulting in oedema
- itching and pain

Pure type I hypersensitivity reactions are frequently associated with allergic rhinitis and hay fever; they are caused by airborne allergens and rarely involve the cornea.

Seasonal allergic conjunctivitis is caused mostly by pollens, which occur seasonally.

Perennial allergic conjunctivitis is caused by allergens that are present in the environment year-round, primarily house dust mites (Friessler et al 1997).

These conditions are common; about 15% of all general practice eye consultations are allergic conjunctivitis related, of which about half will be seasonal allergic conjunctivitis. Optometrists in practice will see these conditions along with contact dermatitis. Most likely, though, they will see *giant papillary conjunctivitis* (GPC) related to contact lens wear (see **Fig. 21.7**).

This group of conditions is characterized by itching, burning and occasionally mild photophobia. Signs include conjunctival injection (due to engorged blood vessels) and chemosis. There may be some watery discharge and papillae (cobblestone-like swellings), and lid swelling does occur. In contact lens wearers, symptoms of GPC tend to manifest as contact lens intolerance in addition to the symptoms above, with the appearance of giant papillae.

Management

Always exclude potentially serious causes of a red eye. There should not be significant pain; if there is moderate to severe pain or moderate to severe photophobia, a secondary cause for the conjunctivitis must be excluded. Be alert for deep ciliary injection, particularly circumlimbal, which may indicate an underlying uveitis. Visual loss is also *not* a feature of conjunctivitis, although transient blur, clearing with a blink, is acceptable.

Topical antihistamines and mast cell stabilizers are the mainstay of treatment if conservative measures are not effective. Topical antihistamines directly block the action of histamine in the conjunctiva, and have a rapid onset of action. Topical mast cell stabilizers prevent the release of histamine and other inflammatory mediators from mast cells but, due to their mode of action, take several weeks to be effective when used as a single agent (Owen et al 2004). Combination agents are available. Oral antihistamines are commonly used in the treatment of allergic conjunctivitis. They have a role in suppressing type I (IgE)-mediated associated hypersensitivity, and are often helpful in the presence of allergic rhinitis.

Infective conjunctivitis

Viral

Acute follicular conjunctivitis is often caused by adenovirus. It is often associated with an upper respiratory tract infection and preauricular lymphadenopathy. Usually both eyes are involved, but the picture may be quite asymmetric. Less common causes of acute follicular conjunctivitis include herpes simplex infection and acute haemorrhagic conjunctivitis. Patients will present with sudden onset of diffuse lid swelling and conjunctival injection. They will complain of ocular discomfort, with watery discharge. Often, the foreign body sensation is intense. Follicles are present along with subconjunctival haemorrhage, while in severe cases there may be pseudomembrane formation.

The pattern of corneal involvement typically starts with intraepithelial microcysts appearing during the first few days, followed by fluorescein-staining epithelial hyperplasia. Clinical diagnosis is confirmed by the appearance of subepithelial infiltrates during the second week as the eye becomes less red. The subepithelial infiltrates usually fade and get smaller, resolving in most cases over several weeks to months.

Viral conjunctivitis is extremely contagious, and occasionally outbreaks occur in eye departments. Strict hand washing and surface disinfection are required. Patients should use separate towels at home.

Treatment for viral conjunctivitis is supportive, such as cool compresses and artificial tears. In severe cases associated with acute incapacitating discomfort, pseudomembranes, corneal erosions, or significantly reduced vision as a result of subepithelial infiltrates, topical corticosteroids may be used under ophthalmic supervision.

Bacterial conjunctivitis

This is characterized by conjunctival injection, papillary reaction, and purulent or mucopurulent discharge. It is caused by a wide variety of microorganisms. The patient notices a red eye with discharge which is usually worse in the morning and the lids may be stuck together. Epiphora and irritation are present, but significant pain is not typical. The condition is usually unilateral but may be bilateral. There is widespread injection of the conjunctiva, and a papillary reaction is seen in the inferior palpebral conjunctiva. There may be anything from scant mucopurulent excretion to frank pus frequently crusting the lashes. The most common bacteria associated with acute conjunctivitis are *Staphylococcus*, *Streptococcus*, and *Haemophilus influenzae*.

Bacterial conjunctivitis is best treated topically with a broad-spectrum antibiotic such as chloramphenicol or fucithalmic. The fluoroquinolones, such as ofloaxacin, and aminoglycosides, such as gentamicin, are probably best left for more serious situations such as an infected corneal ulcer.

Microbiology is not usually indicated in this self-limiting condition but in persistent disease, or if there is corneal involvement, culture and sensitivity studies are indicated (Sheikh & Hurwitz 2006). Underlying dacryocystitis can cause refractory mucopurulent conjunctivitis requiring systemic antibiotics.

In chronic conjunctivitis a high level of suspicion for *Chlamydia* infection should be entertained. Trachoma is also a possibility for patients from countries where the disease is endemic. In the neonate, *Chlamydia* infection is potentially serious and a multidisciplinary approach is recommended as there is a risk of pneumonitis.

Contact lenses should not be worn if conjunctivitis is present or during a course of topical therapy. Soft lenses should not be worn within 5–10 minutes of instilling eye drops containing the preservative benzalkonium chloride.

Acute dendritic herpes simplex keratitis

Acute dendritic herpes simplex keratitis (HSK) presents with the sudden onset of superficial corneal ulceration in the form of a dendritic ulcer after infection with the herpes simplex virus (HSV). A dendrite is a branching epithelial ulceration with swollen, raised edges and terminal bulbs caused by active infection of the corneal epithelium with HSV type 1 (**Fig. 10.1**). Primary infections with HSV often pass unnoticed and the virus becomes latent in the trigeminal ganglion. Factors precipitating virus 'reactivation' include fever, ultraviolet exposure, trauma, and stress. The use of topical or systemic corticosteroids is associated with the aggravation of dendritic keratitis and their use without close ophthalmic supervision should be discouraged.

Patients will have epiphora, pain and/or foreign body sensation, redness and photophobia. Fluorescein staining demonstrates the typical tree-branching appearance. Occasionally, multiple, small dendrites may be present.

Acute HSV dendritic keratitis is treated with topical antiviral medication such as acyclovir ointment five times each day for 10 to 14 days. Topical steroids are contraindicated except under strict ophthalmic supervision (Wilhelmus 2007).

Further manifestations of ocular HSV infections include lid blisters, follicular conjunctivitis, conjunctival dendrites, and geographic ulcers. Primary infection (usually in childhood) can present in dramatic fashion as an unwell child with an extensive vesicular lid eruption. Lid margin involvement can affect the adjacent tissues (cornea and conjunctiva), often resulting in a follicular conjunctivitis (also seen in recurrent infection). In this case, the involved eye should also be treated with topical antiviral medications.

Geographic ulcers are large dendrites with similar epithelial borders but larger central epithelial defects. Geographic ulcers are treated with topical antivirals, but care must be taken to avoid the toxic effects of prolonged use, usually seen as a superficial punctate keratitis. Systemic acyclovir

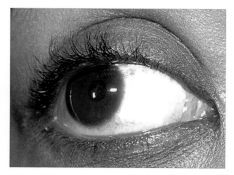

Figure 10.1 Typical dendritic ulcer (HSV-1) showing swollen, raised edges stained with fluorescein.

alone is effective in the treatment of dendritic keratitis but is not indicated unless standard topical antiviral therapy is unsuccessful.

Trophic herpetic disease

Patients with a history of recurrent HSV keratitis are prone to trophic epithelial defects which are non-infectious. These defects are epithelial erosions with smooth, rolled edges. They are thought to occur as a result of decreased corneal sensitivity in recurrent HSV disease. Unfortunately, they may be complicated by corneal melting and perforation and with secondary bacterial infection.

Trophic ulcers usually respond to lubrication and topical antibiotics when required.

Occasionally, a more invasive approach is required such as tarsorrhaphy (lid suturing) to promote epithelial healing when lubrication is insufficient. Corneal melting and small perforations are best managed with tissue adhesives and a bandage contact lens, but a patch graft or a penetrating keratoplasty or other corneal procedure may be required (Green & Pavan-Langston 2006).

Stromal keratitis

HSV stromal keratitis is divided into non-necrotizing and necrotizing diseases. Non-necrotizing HSV stromal keratitis appears as localized corneal oedema. Disciform keratitis is a common form of non-necrotizing HSV stromal keratitis associated with a round area of full-thickness corneal oedema that is often accompanied by localized granulomatous keratic precipitates.

The Herpetic Eye Disease Study (HEDS) (Barron et al 1994) study showed that topical corticosteroids (Wilhelmus et al 1994) accompanied by antiviral prophylaxis are safe and effective treatment for non-necrotizing HSV stromal keratitis, shortening the time until resolution. It is usually necessary to taper topical steroids quite slowly, often using decreasing concentrations of topical steroid. The HEDS treatment studies showed that systemic acyclovir is not effective in the treatment of stromal HSV keratitis. However, the HEDS prevention studies demonstrated a beneficial effect for systemic acyclovir in reducing recurrences with resultant scarring and visual loss.

Necrotizing stromal keratitis

Necrotizing HSV stromal keratitis has areas of white stromal infiltrates in addition to corneal oedema. Neovascularization of the cornea is frequently present.

When patients with recurrent HSV keratitis develop staining infiltrates, it is important to rule out microbial superinfection with bacteria or unusual organisms by performing scrapes and cultures. Treatment is with topical steroid and antivirals unless there is associated microbial superinfection, which would be treated with appropriate antibiotics, depending on the results of the laboratory investigations.

Ultimately, HSV keratitis can lead to sight-threatening corneal opacification which may require surgical intervention, such as penetrating keratoplasty, the details of which are outside the scope of this chapter.

Herpes zoster ophthalmicus

Typically, herpes zoster ophthalmicus (HZO) presents as a vesicular skin eruption with scarring. HZO follows the distribution of the trigeminal nerve, with the first or ophthalmic division most commonly involved. Occasionally, the rash is very mild or absent, which may present diagnostic difficulties.

Herpes zoster is caused by the organism responsible for chickenpox, namely the herpes varicella virus. Once infected (usually in childhood) the virus lies 'dormant' in the trigeminal ganglion or sensory ganglion of the spinal cord. Herpes zoster infection may develop many years later, when there is virus reactivation. The key risk factor for the development of herpes zoster is waning of the cell-mediated immune system associated with ageing. The lifetime risk of herpes zoster is estimated to be 10–20%; there is a much increased risk in immunocompromised individuals.

The individual will notice increasing discomfort or pain on the affected side in the scalp, forehead, temple area, and behind the eye. The pain is often seen several days prior to the rash, which is vesicular and results in scarring (Fig. 10.2).

A consistent feature of herpes zoster is that skin involvement strictly obeys the midline. The anatomy helps the clinician in that the globe shares innervation with the tip of the nose via the nasociliary branch of the ophthalmic division of the trigeminal nerve. Involvement of the tip of the nose increases the likelihood of ocular involvement to 75% (Hutchinson's sign). Conjunctival injection and discharge is common even without intraocular involvement. If the rash involves the eyelid, cicatricial contraction may result in corneal exposure and/or trichiasis.

Patients with acute herpes zoster ophthalmicus are treated with acyclovir (800 mg, five times daily) for 7 to 10 days. Alternative treatment includes famciclovir (500 mg three times daily) or valacyclovir (1000 mg three times daily), but the latter is not used in immunocompromised hosts. Topical antibiotics and cold compresses are helpful

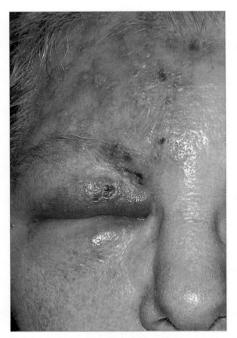

Figure 10.2 Herpes zoster showing a typical rash that obeys the midline but in this case does not involve the tip of the nose (nasociliary branch).

for conjunctivitis. A dermatologist may be consulted for additional topical treatment of the vesicular lesions (Severson et al 2003).

Ocular involvement

The acute presentation of a patient with herpes zoster ophthalmicus with eye involvement is usually one of a marked conjunctivitis and punctate keratitis. Sometimes the punctate keratitis may appear dendritiform in nature, so-called pseudodendrites, which mimic HSV dendritic keratitis. The typical skin rash of herpes zoster usually serves to differentiate the two, but it may be delayed or atypical, such as when there is hard palate involvement.

Zoster epithelial keratitis

Classic zoster pseudodendrites tend to be seen later during the disease, often after the skin rash has settled. Zoster pseudodendrites are mucous plaques that are elevated, stain with fluorescein, and have tapered ends. This is in contrast to the dendrites of herpes simplex, which are epithelial ulcerations with a depressed centre and terminal bulbs. Zoster dendrites are treated with lubrication, using frequent preservative-free drops and ointment. Topical antivirals are not helpful. Topical steroids can be used as required to treat zoster keratouveitis, which is also frequently seen.

Zoster stromal keratitis

Herpes zoster is associated with various forms of stromal keratitis occurring several weeks or more after the acute infection.

A disciform keratitis that is similar in appearance to herpes simplex disciform keratitis is seen with zoster. In fact, it may follow both chickenpox or zoster. Lesions that are similar but more variable in size than the subepithelial infiltrates seen in adenoviral keratoconjunctivitis may appear.

Interstitial keratitis with localized corneal oedema and deep corneal neovascularization and lipid infiltrates may be seen.

Topical corticosteroids are used to treat stromal keratitis, often of seemingly very low dose. In general, great care is required and they must be tapered over many months or years. It is not uncommon to see patients on maintenance doses of 0.125% prednisolone on alternate days or even one drop per week to prevent reactivation.

Neurotrophic keratitis

Neurotrophic keratitis that may be associated with corneal melting is a late manifestation of herpes zoster. The cornea has permanently decreased sensation.

Trophic epithelial defects are erosions that form with smooth borders inferocentrally. Persistent epithelial defects can be complicated by a corneal melt, resulting in impending or frank perforation plus the danger of bacterial superinfection.

Once such at-risk individuals are identified, a regimen of lubrication, often in the form of bland ointments, is required with or without antibiotics. If there is recurrent surface breakdown, tarsorrhaphy (suturing of lids together) or botulinum toxin may be used to promote healing.

Corneal melts are managed in a similar fashion to trophic defects in order to ensure healing of the epithelium. A combination of tissue adhesives, bandage contact lenses and patch grafts are used. Topical steroids may exacerbate the problem and must be used with care.

Zoster uveitis

Uveitis may be seen with keratitis or occur de novo. Granulomatous keratic precipitates are usual and frequently there is a hypertensive uveitis with raised intraocular pressure (IOP). Zoster uveitis can cause sector iris atrophy and an irregular pupil. Hyphaema is occasionally seen in severe cases.

Zoster uveitis responds to cycloplegia and topical steroids on a gradually tapering regimen without topical antivirals. Raised IOP is treated as required.

Zoster episcleritis and scleritis

Episcleritis and scleritis are both associated with zoster. They share the features of pain, localized redness, tenderness and swelling of the conjunctiva, episclera, and sclera seen in non-zoster patients. The normally fairly benign course of nodular episcleritis can evolve into nodular scleritis in zoster. Scleritis may be accompanied by localized stromal keratitis.

Zoster-related episcleritis responds to topical steroids, but zoster scleritis requires systemic nonsteroidal antiinflammatory agents or systemic steroids. Sclerokeratitis usually requires topical steroids for the cornea and systemic medication for the scleritis.

Apart from the ocular involvement of HZO, the most frequent and debilitating complication of herpes zoster, regardless of dermatomal distribution, is postherpetic neuralgia (PHN), a neuropathic pain syndrome that persists or develops after the zoster rash has resolved. The main risk factor for PHN is advancing age; other risk factors include severe acute zoster pain and rash, a painful prodrome, and ocular involvement (Liesegang 2008).

Epithelial corneal dystrophies

Cogan's microcytic dystrophy is an anterior corneal dystrophy affecting the epithelium and its basement membrane. It is one of the epithelial basement membrane corneal dystrophies. It may be inherited but can occur de novo.

The features are of intraepithelial cysts ranging in size from very small spots to larger, oval and irregularly shaped cysts, all within the corneal epithelium in all layers. The cysts are generally found centrally, unilaterally or bilaterally. The cornea remains clear around the lesions with no vascularization. If the cysts are numerous, large and on the visual axis, they may cause blurred vision from irregular astigmatism. These patients are subject to corneal erosions. The cysts are accompanied by map-like or fingerprint lines that are fine, linear changes surrounding the cysts.

If patients are symptomatic, treatment is by lubrication, surgical debridement (including anterior stromal puncture) and occasionally excimer laser.

Map-dot fingerprint dystrophy is an anterior, epithelial basement membrane dystrophy that includes Cogan's microcysts, map-like changes produced by areas of basement membrane present within the epithelium, and fingerprints, which are parallel rows of basement membrane within the epithelium. It tends to be symptomatic between the third and sixth decades.

Patients again have recurrent erosions which generally respond to lubricants but may require excimer phototherapeutic keratectomy or anterior stromal puncture.

Meesmann's dystrophy affects the corneal epithelium and is inherited in an autosomal dominant pattern. Multiple, fine, small cysts are seen in the corneal epithelium. Histology reveals a fibrogranular substance that stains for mucopolysaccharide within the epithelial cells. The cysts are numerous, involving almost all the epithelium from limbus to limbus but do not encroach into the stroma. They appear early in life and are usually stationary. Acuity is near normal.

Corneal dystrophies of Bowman's layer

Reis-Buckler corneal dystrophy is dominantly inherited and usually appears in the first decade of life. The main symptoms are painful corneal erosions and moderately to significantly reduced vision due to opacities in the region of Bowman's layer and superficial stroma. In time, there is scarring with corneal anaesthesia. Reis-Buckler corneal dystrophy is now considered by many authors to be the same as a superficial variant of granular dystrophy. It is still confused with the honeycomb dystrophy of Thiel and Benhke. This has led to a slight dichotomy of opinion in naming the Bowman's layer dystrophies and some divide them into two groups: corneal dystrophy of Bowman's layer type I (CDB-I, 'true' Reis-Buckler dystrophy) and corneal dystrophy of Bowman's layer type II (CDB-II), or the honeycomb dystrophy, also of dominant inheritance.

In the early stages of both CDB-I and CDB-II, treatment consists of lubricating drops, occasional bandage soft contact lenses, and antibiotics. With time, as vision decreases with increased scarring, surgical intervention may be required, usually in the form of superficial keratectomy, often with the excimer laser. Unfortunately, it tends to recur after laser but vision is improved for several years prior to keratoplasty.

Stromal dystrophies

Granular dystrophy is a quite a common, dominantly inherited condition. Symptoms tend to occur later as the dystrophy progresses. Pathology is central rather than peripheral and there is no inflammation or vascularization of the cornea.

A key feature of this dystrophy is the clear areas between the stromal hyaline deposits, with good vision late in the disease (although this is not universal for all pedigrees). As with most of these conditions, recurrent corneal erosions can occur later in the course of the disease. Excimer laser phototherapeutic keratectomy and lamellar keratoplasty are not generally indicated in granular dystrophy as the lesions are deep in the stroma. Keratoplasty may be indicated and the grafts tend to do quite well, although recurrence is fairly common.

The genetics of granular, lattice, and macular dystrophy have revealed that they all involve a mutation at the BIGH-3 gene (Bron & Rabinowitz 1996; Afshari et al 2001).

Lattice corneal dystrophy is another dominantly inherited stromal dystrophy which features amyloid deposition in the cornea. Recurrent erosions may appear in the fourth decade and beyond, which lead to decreased corneal sensation, scarring and decreased vision.

Lattice corneal dystrophy is a bilateral corneal dystrophy with linear deposits of hyaline in the stroma, which are sometimes confused with prominent corneal nerves and blood vessels in the cornea. More superficial structures are spared until the fourth decade. At this stage, painful erosions arise along with marked irregular astigmatism and confluent scar formation, which result in decreased acuity. Once symptomatic, the irregular astigmatism that occurs can be managed with a soft or rigid gas-permeable contact lens. Later, the superficial cornea may be removed by superficial keratectomy or phototherapeutic keratectomy with excimer laser. Eventually, penetrating or deep lamellar keratoplasty is required.

Macular corneal dystrophy is the only major autosomal recessive stromal dystrophy. It presents early (first or second decade) with visual loss. It results from abnormal synthesis of keratin sulfate proteoglycan; two types are described, i.e. with and without systemic involvement. Clinically, there is widespread haze due to accumulation of glycosaminoglycans within stromal keratocytes, the endothelium, and the stroma. Paradoxically, there is corneal thinning. Central, discrete, white deposits are seen in the stroma against a background of variable haze. Erosions are not a feature and while the corneal surface remains smooth, vision is normal. In time the glycosaminoglycan deposits build up and corneal opacification increases. Corneal transplantation is indicated at this stage. Recurrence does happen but, unlike the other dystrophies, it seems to be less aggressive and occurs later.

Schnyder's crystalline dystrophy is an autosomal dominant dystrophy that is less common than granular, lattice and macular stromal dystrophies. It is characterized by crystals (cholesterol) appearing in irregular, central, ring-like deposits early in life. With time, more cholesterol crystals are deposited in the stroma, along with triglycerides and cholesterol esters. There is more diffuse corneal opacification, and the entire stroma, from limbus to limbus, is involved. Keratoplasty is usually indicated in the fifth decade due to visual loss. Repeat keratoplasty may be required with graft haze in time (often >20 years).

Endothelial dystrophies

Corneal guttata (endothelial dystrophy) are mushroom-shaped excrescences on Descemet's membrane which occur with decreased cell numbers and flattening of the endothelia layer. Thickening of Descemet's membrane may be seen, which progresses with ageing, to further endothelial cell 'drop out' and increasing numbers of guttata. Most patients with cornea guttata do not progress to full-blown Fuchs' dystrophy. This condition is important in terms of co-morbidity, as many patients who undergo cataract surgery have endothelial dystrophy and are prone to develop postoperative corneal oedema which may be persistent even in uncomplicated surgery.

Fuchs' endothelial dystrophy consists of stromal corneal swelling with evidence of epithelial oedema in the presence of endothelial guttata. It is thought to be an autosomal dominant trait in some families (around 10%). Fuchs' dystrophy is more common in women.

The earliest diagnosis of Fuchs' dystrophy can be made in patients with corneal guttata who have stromal swelling seen at the slit lamp (or by pachymetry). Early epithelial oedema may be present only on wakening because of overnight corneal decompensation.

Later in the disease, as endothelial cell function diminishes, epithelial and stromal oedema are constant, with poor vision. Macroedema is then observed and eventually may lead to bullous keratopathy. Initially the oedema often responds to hypertonic saline and lowering of IOP. In the latter stages, a bandage contact lens is useful and occasionally the warm air from a hairdryer can improve vision in the morning. Persistent oedema will require keratoplasty, which has a good prognosis.

Posterior polymorphous dystrophy is an autosomal dominant dystrophy not usually found until later in life, when unusual single or groups of vesicles are seen on routine examination.

Most patients have good vision until later. This condition is best demonstrated via retroillumination against the red reflex in a dilated pupil. In most cases, stromal and epithelial oedema do not occur, but when the endothelium is compromised sufficiently, corneal stromal and epithelial oedema are features. About a quarter of patients may develop peripheral anterior synechiae (viewed gonioscopically). There is an increased risk of glaucoma in these individuals that is often refractory to treatment.

One should be aware of potential confusion with iridocorneal endothelial (ICE) syndrome. Posterior polymorphous dystrophy is bilateral and dominantly inherited, but ICE syndrome is not inherited and is unilateral. All patients with ICE syndrome develop glaucoma, although this is not the case with posterior polymorphous dystrophy. In general, it is acceptable simply to observe posterior polymorphous dystrophy. If significant corneal stromal and epithelial oedema occurs, it should be managed as for Fuchs' dystrophy. Keratoplasty is sometimes required and has a high degree of success in the absence of glaucoma.

Congenital hereditary endothelial dystrophy may demonstrate either autosomal dominant or recessive inheritance. Significant corneal oedema and visual loss is a feature during the first few years of life.

This disease, which can be seen at birth, is part of the differential diagnosis for a 'cloudy cornea'. Congenital glaucoma must be excluded and is usually done so on the basis of a normal intraocular pressure in congenital hereditary endothelial dystrophy with a normal-sized but thickened cornea. Treatment with keratoplasty can be difficult.

Degenerations

Keratoconus is a relatively common (4–100 per 10 000) corneal ectasia. There is no gender preponderance and it has a wide variation in symptoms and morbidity. Keratoconus can be associated with Down's syndrome, atopy and vernal disease. It also occurs with retinitis pigmentosa, aniridia and Marfan's syndrome.

Optometrists are in the front line for early recognition of this disorder, as the earliest manifestation is a frequently changing prescription. Inferior corneal steepening is a feature, best demonstrated with corneal topography (Kaya et al 2007). With progression, various clinical signs appear, such as apical protrusion and thinning. There are various eponymous signs such as Vogt's striae, which are folds in Descemet's membrane that disappear in response to pressure. A Fleischer's ring may be visible around the cone or at the base; this is an iron line that is deposited because of corneal surface irregularity. With more protrusion, apical scarring occurs, which can make contact lens use increasingly difficult. Eventually, with continuing protrusion, Descemet's membrane stretches and ruptures. This leads to egress of aqueous into the stroma, leading to corneal hydrops (with marked swelling and visual loss).

The mainstay of management is conservative, in the form of spectacles and contact lenses (particularly rigid gas-permeable; see Ch. 21). Various alternatives to corneal transplantation for the management of keratoconus aim to enhance corneal rigidity by means of nonsurgical collagen cross-linking, or with the use of intrastromal corneal ring segments (see Ch. 23), and these treatments may reduce astigmatism or ectatic progression to varying degrees.

Recent developments in anterior lamellar keratoplasty enable targeted replacement or augmentation of corneal stroma without replacement of endothelium (heavily implicated in rejection), and include procedures such as deep anterior lamellar keratoplasty, microkeratome or laser-assisted anterior lamellar surgery, and peripheral tectonic lamellar keratoplasty procedures which demonstrate successful reinforcement of peripheral stroma to reduce astigmatism (Tan & Por 2007).

Pellucid marginal degeneration is similar to keratoconus in that there is marked corneal steepening and anterior protrusion of the inferior cornea near the 6 o'clock limbus. It is rarer than keratoconus and is more peripheral, with the central cornea remaining clear until late in the disease. Management is generally with contact lenses.

A *pterygium* is a 'wing-like', fibrovascular, degenerative tissue that extends from the conjunctiva onto the cornea. They are usually found on the nasal side but can arise in other areas. Risk factors are said to be ultraviolet (UV) light and dusty, dry environments, especially those near the equator.

Capillaries in the head of the pterygium may grow further onto the cornea and lead to more opacification. Pterygia are slightly unpredictable in that they may advance onto the cornea and then become dormant, never affecting acuity, or they may advance across the visual axis, causing significant visual loss (**Fig. 10.3**).

Simple lubricants are sufficient in many cases, with occasional short courses of topical steroid (under supervision). If the visual axis is threatened, then removal is required. The preferred technique is surgical removal with a conjunctival autograft, which reduces the risk of recurrence although adjunctive agents such as mitomycin C are also used (Ang et al 2007).

Pinguecula formation is common with increasing age. It is considered a degenerative process and is common in some racial groups (Lee et al 2005). Typically, a yellowish deposit occurs in the nasal conjunctiva adjacent to the limbus. These deposits are elastotic degeneration of the substantia propria

and may represent abnormal elastic fibres. As with pterygia, exposure to UV light, drying and dust can cause pinguecula formation. Pingueculae may become inflamed and vascularized, causing pingueculitis, which again usually responds to a short course of topical steroids. Surgical excision is an option and recurrence is relatively rare.

Ocular adnexa

Besides being important to facial expression, the eyelids play an integral part in corneal protection. The muscles for opening the eyelid are the levator palpebrae superiori and Müller's muscle in the upper eyelid, and the lower eyelid retractors in the lower eyelid. The ideal upper eyelid height should be 2–3 mm above the visual axis but covering the superior corneal limbus. The ideal lower eyelid position should be within 1–2 mm above or below the lower corneal limbus. The orbicularis muscle closes the eyelid and forms an integral part of the lacrimal pump that enables efficient tear drainage from the ocular surface.

Eyelid disease can be broadly divided into five areas:

1. Eyelid height: eyelid ptosis or retraction.
2. Eyelid malposition: the eyelid is divided into the anterior and posterior lamella, the anterior lamella consisting of the skin and orbicularis muscle and the posterior consisting of the tarsal plate and conjunctiva.

   The eyelashes grow from the anterior lamella lid margin. If there is an imbalance between the two lamellae, e.g. in entropion (**Fig. 10.4**) the eyelashes are rolled inwards, abrading the cornea, and in ectropion (**Fig. 10.5**) the posterior lamella is rolled out and exposed, causing discomfort and epiphora (watering). This is because the lacrimal puncta are located in the medial aspect of the posterior lamella and require contact with the tear lake to allow normal drainage of tears.

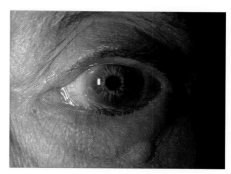

Figure 10.4 Senile entropion. There is pooling and staining of fluorescein inferiorly.

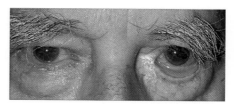

Figure 10.5 Left ectropion. There has been previous medial canthal surgery.

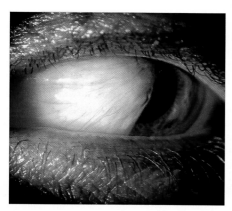

Figure 10.3 Advanced pterygium that involves the visual axis.

3. Poor eyelid closure.

Both eyelid malposition and retraction can impair eyelid closure and impair corneal protection.

A weakened orbicularis due to facial nerve palsy or other myopathic conditions can also contribute to poor eyelid closure and corneal exposure.

Orbital proptosis, e.g. from thyroid eye disease (TED), may similarly result in poor eyelid closure.

4. Eyelid tumours.

As the eyelids contain a mucocutaneous junction, all types of benign and malignant neoplasia that affect skin and mucosal surfaces can give rise to eyelid tumours.

5. Dystonias.

Conditions such as blepharospasm, hemifacial spasm and aberrant regeneration of the facial nerve can cause periocular spasm and may lead to involuntary eyelid closure.

Treatment of eyelid disorders depends on aetiology, the severity of the symptoms and whether or not vision is affected.

Ptosis

A drooping eyelid (**Fig. 10.6**) may have neurogenic, myogenic, aponeurotic or mechanical causes and may be associated with several syndromes.

Clinical features

Not all drooping of the upper lid is a true ptosis. It may be secondary to blepharospasm, apraxia of lid opening, pseudoptosis from ocular misalignment and high anisometropia. Other conditions involving the eyelid, such as chalazia, tumours, and preseptal cellulitis, may result in a ptotic lid.

Evaluation of the patient with ptosis should first determine if the condition is *congenital* or *acquired*. Old photographs are helpful in this regard. If acquired, a neuro-ophthalmologic problem must be sought before the diagnosis of levator dehiscence secondary to old age is made. The most important neuro-ophthalmic entities are Horner's syndrome, cranial nerve III palsy, and myasthenia gravis.

Less frequently encountered causes of ptosis are Fisher's variant of the Guillain–Barré syndrome, botulism, and chronic progressive external ophthalmoplegia.

Eyelid tumours

Approximately 5% to 10% of all skin cancers occur in the eyelid (Bernardini 2006).

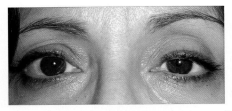

Figure 10.6 Left ptosis in a contact lens wearer. The skin crease is high, suggesting a levator aponeurotic defect.

Basal cell carcinoma

Basal cell carcinomas (BCCs) typically occur in middle-aged or older patients, especially in fair-skinned individuals. In young patients they tend to behave more aggressively. Although BCCs usually do not metastasize, such behaviour has been reported in 0.02% to 1% of cases. Distant spread may occur through both haematogenous and lymphatic pathways.

Periocular basal cell carcinomas occur most frequently on the lower eyelid, followed in order of frequency by the medial canthus, upper eyelid, and lateral canthus. Clinically, periocular BCCs can present as:

- localized (nodular, ulcerative, cystic), which accounts for 75% of all BCC
- diffuse (morpheaform, sclerosing), which accounts for approximately 15% of all BCC and has a tendency to invade deep into the dermis
- superficial, multifocal BCCs, which exhibit diffuse multicentric involvement of the epidermis and superficial dermis. It may be difficult to confirm histological clearance of diffuse and superficial types of BCC.

Squamous cell carcinoma

Periocular squamous cell carcinoma (SCC) is a potentially lethal tumour. Precursor clinical presentations include actinic keratosis, Bowen's disease, and radiation dermatoses. Like BCCs, they occur most frequently on the lower eyelid.

SCCs have a variable clinical presentation and may mimic many other types of benign and malignant skin lesions, and a biopsy is critical to establish the diagnosis. SCCs have a tendency to metastasize to regional lymph nodes and distant sites through haematogenous and lymphatic pathways. Perineural infiltration by SCC of the eyelids facilitates spread into the orbit, intracranial cavity, and periorbital structures.

Squamous cell carcinoma typically occurs in fair-skinned, elderly individuals who have a history of chronic sun exposure and skin damage.

Sebaceous gland carcinomas

Sebaceous gland carcinomas (SGCs), which account for less than 1% of all eyelid tumours, may have varied clinical presentations, depending whether they arise from the meibomian glands in the tarsus, the Zeis glands in the eyelashes or the caruncle. The tumour typically occurs in the elderly but may occur in younger patients, especially those with a history of radiation exposure. This tumour has the potential to metastasize via lymphatic and vascular channels as well as aggressive local spread. Any atypical presentations of unilateral blepharoconjunctivitis or chronic chalazion, especially with madarosis, merit a biopsy to exclude this tumour.

The more common form of SGC is the nodular type which is minimally infiltrative and located on the tarsus or eyelid margin. It easily can be mistaken for a BCC, SCC, chronic chalazion or even as blepharitis; hence it is known as the 'the great masquerader'. SGC can also present as a non-nodular tumour that is typically moderately to highly infiltrative.

SGCs can spread into the epithelium of the conjunctiva, cornea and eyelid skin in two ways. Pagetoid spread involves neoplastic cells invading the epithelium as single cells or as small clusters of cells that are devoid of intercellular bridges. Intraepithelial conjunctival extension has been reported in 44% to 80% of patients with SGC. Secondly, SGC cells replace the full thickness of the surface epithelium, which may mimic squamous cell carcinoma in situ and can display multifocal involvement with skip areas.

Malignant melanoma

Periocular malignant melanoma is extremely rare. Three of the four forms of cutaneous melanoma (nodular, superficial spreading melanoma and lentigo maligna melanoma) can present in the eyelids. A biopsy should be performed if there is enlargement, increased pigmentation, bleeding or ulceration of an eyelid lesion.

Treatment of eyelid tumours

Basal cell carcinoma and squamous cell carcinoma

An evidence rating of I (strong supporting evidence) was applied to only two treatments: Mohs' micrographic surgery and excision with frozen-section or permanent-section control. These two treatment recommendations yielded the highest cure rate, lowest frequency of recurrence and had the greatest record of use.

Sebaceous gland carcinoma

An evidence rating of I was applied to the recommendation of either Mohs' micrographic surgery or excision with frozen-section control combined with conjunctival map biopsies.

Malignant melanoma

Recommendations for treatment of malignant melanoma are legion and often conflicting (Cook and Bartley 2001).

Thyroid eye disease

The most common cause for proptosis (both bilateral and unilateral) is thyroid eye disease (TED). This is an autoimmune process that results in orbital inflammation and scarring. It is much more common in women than men and is most often seen in middle age.

This may generate anything from mild swelling to severe proptosis, lid retraction, corneal exposure and motility disturbance. In severe cases there may be visual loss as a result of optic nerve compression.

Most patients have or have previously had a systemic thyroid abnormality; however, at presentation of eye signs the thyroid status may be hyperthyroid, hypothyroid or occasionally euthyroid.

Clinical features

Thyroid-related ophthalmopathy features chronic orbital inflammation and scarring. As might be expected, it is generally bilateral but may be highly asymmetric and this is a pitfall for the unwary. The extraocular muscles and orbital fat are infiltrated by inflammatory cells in the short term and in the longer term by mucopolysaccharide and collagen. The disease process is marked by early inflammation and long-term fibrosis and scarring. Other diagnostic difficulties are that the early manifestations of TED are often subtle, with non-specific redness, irritation, chemosis and eyelid swelling.

The early signs of lid retraction, lid lag or systemic thyroid symptoms (which are outside the scope of this chapter) help confirm the diagnosis. With progression, lid signs, such as retraction and lag, become more obvious. If marked, corneal exposure can become an urgent management issue. Proptosis and restriction of motility are also later signs. The most commonly involved muscle is the inferior rectus muscle, followed by the medial rectus, making restriction of upgaze and lateral gaze the most common motility disturbances.

While various grading systems are in use for TED, an indication of activity is provided by the Mourits score (Mourits et al 1997). This gives a value to each of the following signs and symptoms: orbital pain or pain during ocular movement, redness (eyelid or conjunctiva), swelling (proptosis, lid oedema, chemosis or caruncle oedema), limitation of ocular movements, and visual dysfunction (acuity, field and colour). Of a total of 10 scores, patients with a score of 3 and higher and/or an increasing score on follow-up are judged to be active. Rundle staging may be applied to record the severity of the ocular involvement (Rundle 1964), ranging from Grade 1 (mild) ophthalmopathy with ocular discomfort, transient oedema and mild proptosis to Grade 4 (severe) ophthalmopathy presenting with optic nerve dysfunction with reduction of colour vision and visual acuity loss. Imaging (CT or MRI with fat suppression) shows muscle belly involvement and sparing of the tendons (Mayer et al 2001). After 12 to 24 months, patients may be left with optic nerve damage, double vision, lid retraction and proptosis. TED should not be underestimated; it is a serious eye condition with a considerable threat to vision.

Management of TED is complex and may benefit from a multidisciplinary approach. Patient education as to the potential dangers is important (Kendall-Taylor 1998; Weetman & Wiersinga 1998). Mild disease usually responds to simple lubricants but those with more severe disease and particularly sight-threatening compression will require much more. This often involves orbital irradiation, which appears to stop progression of thyroid-related ophthalmopathy in a significant percentage of patients. It has a delayed onset of action, so acute disease will, in addition, require other treatment such as high-dose steroids and/or orbital decompression surgery. Once stabilized, selective or cosmetic orbital decompression (24 mm proptosis or more), extraocular muscle surgery and finally eyelid surgery (levator recession, blepharoplasty) may be considered (Steel & Potts 1999).

Orbital cellulitis

Bacterial infection of the orbit, most often associated with sinus disease, may result in orbital cellulitis. Patients present with a short history (1–2 days) of progressive redness and swelling involving the ocular adnexae.

Clinical features

Preseptal (less severe) and orbital cellulitis present with swollen, red, and warm lids, sometimes with fever and a raised white cell count.

Orbital cellulitis may be differentiated from preseptal cellulitis by orbital signs such as chemosis, limited motility, proptosis, orbital resistance to retropulsion, an afferent pupillary defect, and decreased acuity. This is an emergency referral.

Onset of infection is likely to have been preceded by an upper respiratory infection, especially in children. Fever and leukocytosis are more common in children but not universal. Associated sinus disease is thought to cause 85% of cases. Other causes include external wounds or bites, recent dental work, and dacryocystitis. Imaging (usually CT scan) is essential for these patients to exclude orbital/subperiosteal abscess or mass and to assess the paranasal sinuses. Treatment involves high-dose antibiotics (usually intravenous in hospital) and surgical drainage of abscesses. Recently, concerns have been raised regarding the emergence of community-acquired methicillin-resistant *Staphylococcus aureus* (MRSA) in orbital infection (Bilyk 2007).

Internal disease

Cataract

Cataract surgery is not only one of the most common operations performed worldwide but also one of the most successful. For this reason, and the fact that increasingly optometrists are involved in the shared care of cataract, it is worth considering cataract assessment along with some of the pitfalls. Also discussed are the potential complications of its treatment in some detail and to a lesser extent the mechanics of its treatment.

The classification of cataract is varied and at times confusing. Older texts tended to be rather descriptive whereby opacities were described by their appearance; more recently, cataracts tend to be classified by anatomic location (**Fig. 10.7**). It is common to see more than one type of cataract in the crystalline lens.

It is not possible to give an exhaustive account of cataract in this chapter but it is useful to remember that cataract is associated with certain specific diseases such as diabetes and drugs such as corticosteroids. The overwhelming risk factor for the development of cataract is, however, increasing age (**Table 10.1**). It will not have escaped the reader that as we move forward in the twenty-first century the population is ageing (see Ch. 31) and cataract incidence is inevitably increasing.

Assessment of the patient with cataract

During the history and examination of a patient with cataract it is important to ask about a family history of cataract.

Table 10.1 Risk factors for cataract

Medical	Diabetes
	Drugs
	Family history
Environmental	Nutrition
	Radiation
	Smoking
Others	Myopia
	Systemic hypertension
	Severe diarrhoea
	Renal failure
	Various biochemical markers

The Framingham Eye Study (FES) showed that of 2500 participants with visual acuity of 6/9 (20/30) or worse due to cataract 18% were aged 65–74 years and 46% were 75–85 years. Although visually significant cataracts are rare before the fifth decade of life, FES data suggested that half of the population had visually significant opacities by the eighth decade. The risk of cataract at age 70 years is about 13-fold that at age 50 (Leibowitz et al 1980).

Other factors to consider are symptoms such as glare and duration, previous ophthalmic history and surgery and other medical conditions such as glaucoma. Ocular medications are important but some systemic medications, e.g. tamsulosin (Schwinn & Afshari 2006), can have adverse effects on pupillary dilatation.

Refractive error is important, particularly in patients with unilateral cataract and those who wish to consider a 'monovision' correction postoperatively.

Most authorities would agree that, whilst important, simple acuity-based assessments are not sufficient to make an informed decision on cataract surgery. The patient should be asked about the effect on lifestyle in terms of employment, leisure pursuits including driving, and about the effects of glare, which may be either:

- Discomfort glare: photophobic sensation without measurable effects on visual function
- Disability glare: causes reduction in visual function due to presence of a bright light source. This is a specific type of glare caused by light scattered by the ocular media and is commonly tested by devices developed to document glare.

Slit-lamp examination

Slit-lamp examination should include inspection of lids and lashes for blepharitis, lash and lid malposition (especially trichiasis and ectropion (see **Fig. 10.5**), and other lid abnormalities as these may increase the risk of infection after cataract surgery.

Pupils

Evaluation of the pupils should not only determine the presence or absence of an afferent pupillary defect, but also pupil shape, size (before and after dilation) and reactivity. Photopic and scotopic pupil size are important when

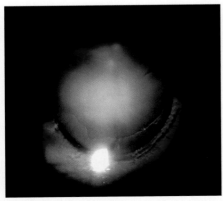

Figure 10.7 Nuclear sclerotic cataract. Inferiorly there is a frill of pseudoexfoliative material on the anterior lens capsule and on the pupil margin, which may mean cataract surgery is hazardous.

determining intraocular lens (IOL) size and it may help the surgeon select the implant style as well, especially when considering a multifocal IOL. A relative afferent pupillary defect indicates either optic neuropathy or diffuse retinal disease. The origin should be sought before considering cataract surgery, because it will likely have an impact on subsequent vision.

Fundus examination

With mild to moderate cataract, the fundus examination generally presents little problem in a dilated patient when using indirect ophthalmoscopy at the slit lamp with hand-held lenses (see Ch. 18). Any fundus abnormality should be excluded, with particular attention to the optic disc and the macula. Recognition of co-morbidity such as glaucoma or age-related macular degeneration is important at this point, as this may well have a bearing on prognosis.

In a mature cataract, the crystalline lens is white as there is complete opacification of the cortex. Sometimes, a sclerotic nucleus can be seen through the cortex on slit-lamp examination. The fundus cannot be adequately visualized ophthalmoscopically. Before cataract surgery, some assessment of retinal function is prudent. One should be particularly careful to look for an afferent pupil defect. Two-point light discrimination and light projection in each quadrant should be tested. Other tests of macular function might include blue-field entoptic phenomena and the use of a potential acuity meter and laser interferometry. Unfortunately, these tests are not reliable in cases of very dense cataracts and are rarely performed outside of the laboratory. B-scan ultrasonography should be done to rule out other posterior segment pathology, especially if there is any suggestion of trauma.

Treatment of cataract

A full treatment of modern, small-incision cataract surgery is beyond the scope of this chapter. However, there are two main types of cataract surgery, i.e. intra- and extracapsular. Extracapsular cataract extraction involves the removal of almost the entire natural lens while the elastic lens capsule (posterior capsule) is left intact to allow implantation of an intraocular lens.

Extracapsular cataract extraction (ECCE) involved manual expression of the nucleus through a large (usually 10–12 mm) incision made in the cornea or sclera. ECCE is rarely performed in the UK at the time of writing although it is still used in some 'third-world' environments as it is generally less equipment dependent and is therefore both easier to perform in such environments and less expensive.

Phacoemulsification ('Phaco') is now the preferred method in most cases in modern health economies. It involves the use of a specialized piece of equipment (partly a disadvantage) with an ultrasonic handpiece with a titanium or steel tip. The tip vibrates at ultrasonic frequency (40 000 Hz) and the lens material is simply emulsified and aspirated. A second fine instrument (sometimes called a manipulator, chopper or simply second instrument) may be used via a side incision to facilitate cracking or chopping of the nucleus into smaller pieces. Breaking the hard central nucleus into smaller pieces makes emulsification easier, thus decreasing the energy required to remove the cataract, leading to earlier postoperative rehabilitation (Devgan 2007).

After phacoemulsification of the lens nucleus a dual irrigation–aspiration (I–A) probe or a bimanual I–A system is used to aspirate the remaining peripheral cortical material also known as 'soft lens matter'.

Intracapsular extraction is an out-dated method of cataract surgery, rarely performed today. Latterly, it would be recommended for use in the presence of an unstable capsular bag, often post trauma. However, in recent years surgeons have developed capsular stabilizing techniques that allow phacoemulsification in cases that previously would not have been considered suitable.

Intraocular lens implantation: After cataract removal, an IOL is generally implanted into the eye, normally through a small incision (1.8–2.8 mm) using a foldable IOL, or through an enlarged incision, using a polymethyl methacrylate (PMMA) lens. Foldable IOLs are made of silicone or acrylic material that may be hydrophobic or hydrophillic. The IOLs come in a wide range of powers and it is not uncommon to see implants > +30D in high hyperopes or even negatively powered implants used in high myopia. There are a variety of instruments available to place the IOL, from simple folding forceps to 'pre-loaded' cartridges with dedicated introducers.

The IOL is inserted through the incision into the capsular bag within the posterior chamber, so-called 'in-the-bag implantation'. In complicated cataract surgery, especially if there has been posterior capsular tear with vitreous loss, a sulcus-fixated lens may be placed in front of the capsular bag but behind the iris. In cases of zonulodialysis where there is interruption of the supporting capsular ligaments (zonules), an implant may prove to be unstable but may be assisted by the placement of a capsular tension ring to stabilize the capsular bag (Hasanee and Ahmed 2006).

Implantation of posterior-chamber IOLs in infants is possible but remains controversial due to rapid ocular growth at this age. Young children also tend towards florid postoperative inflammation, which may be very difficult to control. Treatment of congenital cataract remains a highly specialized branch of cataract surgery where amblyopia is a constant threat.

In the last few years a plethora of new designs for IOLs has appeared. Such designs include specially tinted IOLs, multifocal and even accommodating IOLs. These implants allow simultaneous focusing of rays from distant as well as near objects. Of course, preoperative patient selection is extremely important to avoid unrealistic expectations and postoperative patient dissatisfaction. Acceptability for these lenses has become better and studies have shown good results in selected patients where astigmatism is controlled (Leyland et al 2002).

Complications of cataract surgery

Whilst the outcomes of modern, small-incision cataract surgery have improved dramatically in recent years, it should not be forgotten that any surgical procedure carries inherent risks. It is incumbent on the surgeon to minimize these risks. Thus, attention to detail is a key part of this branch of microsurgery. This starts with the initial assessment, as described above, but continues with a careful discussion with the patient as to visual requirements and, not least, expectations. Improved biometry to calculate the implant power (based on measurements of axial length and corneal curvature) has enabled surgeons to make accurate predications of postoperative refraction and may include planned procedures to reduce astigmatism (especially important if multifocal implants are used). Inaccurate biometry or placement of an inappropriate implant (type or power) is a risk and can be considered a complication of cataract surgery.

Implant and wound problems

Pupillary capture occurs when a portion of the implant is 'caught' by the iris, giving a distorted or 'peaked pupil'. It is often associated with other complications such as posterior capsular rupture (see below) or postoperative trauma. Wound leaks often gave rise to this but, as incisions have decreased in size, this has become less common. Occasionally, in a very dense cataract where ultrasound times are prolonged, a corneal burn is sustained, which can lead to a wound leak.

Implants may become decentred with time (**Fig. 10.8**), giving rise to so-called 'sunrise' or 'sunset' syndromes. This most often occurs when a lens is placed in the bag and a zonular dehiscence is present, or the lens haptic goes through a capsular tear. As the capsule contracts, the lens is drawn 'off centre'. Capsular contraction de novo may also cause implant problems as well as reduced vision and glare in the 'capsular phimosis syndrome' (Gimbel et al 2005).

Residual cortical and nuclear fragments

Occasionally, remnants of cortical lens material (soft lens matter) or fragments of the harder nucleus remain following cataract surgery.

Soft lens matter (SLM) may be hidden by the iris perioperatively but later swells into larger, fluffy, white opacities. It often migrates into the anterior chamber, where it usually follows a benign course, melting away over several weeks. SLM that is located between the intraocular lens and the posterior capsule or between the peripheral anterior and posterior capsule takes longer to be reabsorbed and may result in early opacification of the capsule. SLM in the vitreous also takes longer to resolve. Increased inflammatory reactions sometimes develop in these eyes.

Nuclear fragments in the anterior chamber or vitreous will remain for an extended period and cause marked inflammation. One of the most serious perioperative complications is a posterior capsular tear, with loss of a large nuclear fragment or even the entire nucleus into the vitreous. If vitreous gel presents through the posterior capsular tear, this may prevent normal implant placement, and anterior vitrectomy is required (usually performed at the time by

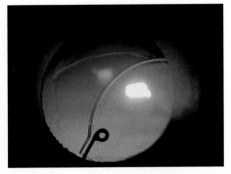

Figure 10.8 An implant is seen displaced inferiorly with the edge of the optic, close to the visual axis ('sunsetting').

the anterior segment surgeon). As well as technical difficulties with cataract surgery, it may increase the likelihood of other complications such as cystoid macular oedema, infection and retinal detachment.

Management: In general, cortex in the anterior chamber reabsorbs. The inflammatory reaction and any elevation of intraocular pressure respond to topical and/or systemic medication. Nuclear fragments may be troublesome depending on size, position and associated inflammatory reaction. Fragments in the anterior chamber may cause depression of the endothelial cell count. Small nuclear fragments in the vitreous can be observed, but larger ones should be removed by vitrectomy (removal of the vitreous gel with specialized vitreous cutting equipment in the hands of a vitreoretinal surgeon (Kim and Miller 2002).

Cystoid macular oedema describes the accumulation of fluid within the sensory retina around the macular. It may occur after intraocular surgery, such as cataract (especially if complicated), glaucoma procedures and after retinal detachment surgery. Several other conditions, particularly diabetic retinopathy, posterior uveitis and retinitis pigmentosa, are associated with cystoid macular oedema.

Clinical features: The patient will complain of visual loss, often after a period of good vision initially. Refraction may show a positive shift (hyperopic) and observation of the macular may show a loss of fine detail. However, the classic characteristic of cystoid macular oedema is a petaloid appearance during fundus fluorescein angiography (FFA) caused by leakage of the fluorescein dye in the outer plexiform layer. More recently optical coherence tomography (OCT) (see Chs 18 and 19) has given the clinician a noninvasive method of visualizing macular oedema. The cause is obscure, but there is evidence suggesting that inflammatory mediators play a role (Ray & D'Amico 2002).

Endophthalmitis

This is a potentially devastating complication of cataract surgery.

Clinical features: Patients with endophthalmitis occurring within the first week after intraocular surgery usually present with pain, redness and visual loss. In the early phase there will be cellular activity in the anterior chamber and minimal hypopyon.

The fundus may still be easily visualized and it is often quite difficult to differentiate between a purely inflammatory process and an infectious one. The level of discomfort, degree of ciliary injection and chemosis, as well as the presence or absence of vitreous cells, are all factors that are considered. If there is any doubt in the mind of the practitioner, immediate referral should be made. In mild cases, a trial of hourly topical steroids may be tried with close observation to determine if the condition improves. In more severe cases, a view of the retina may be difficult because of vitreous involvement.

The results of the Endophthalmitis Vitrectomy Study Group (EVSG) were published in 1995. The study showed that for patients with hand motion or better vision, there was no difference in outcomes between immediate three ports pars plana vitrectomy versus anterior chamber and vitreous taps followed by injection of intravitreal antibiotics. However, when visual acuity at presentation was light perception only, better visual results were obtained when an immediate vitrectomy was done (a threefold increase in the frequency of achieving 6/12 (20/40) or better acuity, i.e. 33% vs 11%). The EVSG treatment outcomes demonstrated no difference in final visual acuity or media clarity outcomes whether or not systemic antibiotics were used.

Posterior capsular opacification

This is normally associated with uncomplicated modern cataract surgery where an implant (IOL) is placed in the capsular bag. In order to do this the anterior capsule must be partially removed but in most cases the posterior capsule remains (in fact, as stated above, posterior capsular rupture is associated with increased complications in cataract surgery). The proliferation of lens epithelial cells across the posterior capsule causes clouding. If allowed to progress, vision may be worse than it was prior to cataract surgery in some cases, and will require treatment. Historically this was difficult but fortunately, with the advent of the YAG (Yttrium Aluminium Garnet) laser, treatment of posterior capsule opacity is relatively safe and highly effective. This is done as an outpatient procedure under local anaesthetic. A high-powered contact lens is used to help focus the beam and prevent corneal damage.

The procedure is not entirely risk free. Problems described include IOL damage (usually pitting), which does not normally have any effect on vision. Rarely, if the capsulotomy is made too large, posterior displacement of the implant is seen; this was more common with some older-style IOLs that have been superseded. There is also a risk of retinal detachment following YAG laser capsulotomy (Charles 2001) and occasionally macular oedema. Patients should be warned to report symptoms of floaters, flashes, and a curtain-like vision loss to their ophthalmologist immediately (Sheard et al 2003).

Retinal detachment

Retinal detachment is fortunately a rare occurrence but one that may have serious sight-threatening consequences. It may be defined as a separation of the sensory retina from the retinal pigment epithelium by subretinal fluid (SRF). Depending on the mechanism of subretinal fluid accumulation, retinal detachments traditionally have been classified into rhegmatogenous, tractional, and exudative.

Rhegmatogenous retinal detachment

Rhegmatogenous retinal detachment is one in which SRF derived from liquefied vitreous gains access to the subretinal space through a retinal break. It is associated with certain ocular features such as high myopia, posterior vitreous detachment and trauma (Lewis 2003). Incidence varies between 7 and 10 cases per 100 000, depending on the population studied (Wong et al 1999).

Posterior vitreous detachment

This represents a separation of the vitreous gel from points of attachment on the posterior retina. The patient usually complains of photopsia (flashes of light) with 'floaters' which generally represent condensations of the collagen fibres or haemorrhage. In some cases a well-demarcated ring of tissue is seen anterior to the optic disc (Weiss ring). The clinical significance of posterior vitreous detachment (PVD) is the small but significant incidence of retinal tear, which is approximately 15%, but much higher in the presence of vitreous haemorrhage.

The firm adhesions between retina and vitreous can cause vitreoretinal traction. This is particularly seen at such points as vitreoretinal tufts, meridional folds, or areas of lattice degeneration. The retina can be torn and become free floating, giving rise to an operculated tear. If the torn retina stays attached, the tear is designated a horseshoe tear. Horseshoe tears are more likely to progress to retinal detachment than are operculated tears, because vitreous traction remains and helps to separate the retina from the underlying pigment epithelium.

Management

Careful fundus examination is essential to exclude associated retinal tears (see Ch. 18). These are then usually treated with laser photocoagulation. Breaks are most common in the superior temporal quadrant.

In acute rhegmatogenous retinal detachment, liquefied vitreous gains access to the subretinal space through a retinal break (Greek: rhegma). This then leads to separation of the sensory retina from the retinal pigment epithelium (RPE). More than 95% of patients with rhegmatogenous retinal detachment have a clinically demonstrable retinal break. Vitreous haemorrhage is common in cases caused by a flap tear. In cases of recent onset, the detached retina is opaque and corrugated. If the macula is detached, it frequently develops cystoid macular oedema that may be confused with a full-thickness macular hole. Intraocular pressure should be checked as it is often decreased. Nonrhegmatogenous retinal detachment, retinoschisis, and choroidal detachment must be ruled out.

For uncomplicated, primary rhegmatogenous retinal detachments, treatment approaches include scleral buckling, pneumatic retinopexy and, increasingly, pars plana vitrectomy with an internal approach (Azad et al 2007).

If there is significant vitreous haemorrhage, a giant tear or significant proliferative vitreoretinopathy, an internal approach with vitrectomy will be performed. These techniques are outside the scope of this chapter.

Tractional retinal detachment

If no retinal break is present, retinal detachment is still possible in the form of tractional retinal detachment (TRD). TRD may occur in a number of ocular pathologic conditions, such as proliferative diabetic retinopathy (PDR), sickle haemoglobinopathies, retinal vein occlusion, and retinopathy of prematurity (ROP). Retinal ischaemia leads to release of growth factors such as vascular endothelial growth factor (VEGF), which cause neovascularization, which in turn may lead to strong vitreoretinal adhesions. In time, these may physically pull the neurosensory retina away from the underlying RPE.

Exudative retinal detachment

Normally, water flows from the vitreous to the choroid. The direction of flow is influenced by the relative hyperosmolarity of the choroid with respect to the vitreous, and the RPE actively pumps ions and water from the vitreous into the choroid. When there is an imbalance between inflow and outflow of fluid the normal compensatory mechanisms cannot cope and fluid accumulates in the sub-retinal space, leading to an exudative retinal detachment. Conditions that predispose to exudative retinal detachment include age-related macular degeneration, idiopathic central serous chorioretinopathy and choroidal melanoma plus rare conditions such Vogt–Koyanagi–Harada syndrome and Coats' disease.

It should not be forgotten that there is a small but significant incidence of retinal detachment following laser refractive surgery (Ruiz-Moreno et al 1999).

Glaucoma

This is a relatively common condition affecting millions across the world (Thylefores & Negrel 1994). What is glaucoma? It is a disease entity that represents the process whereby damage results to ocular structures as a result, at least in part, from an increase in intraocular pressure (IOP).

Those individuals who have the classic characteristics of this condition, namely visual field defects and/or an optic neuropathy, are said to have glaucoma whereas those that merely have some risk factor, be that a positive family history or some other aspect such as pigment dispersion syndrome, are currently described as glaucoma suspects.

Ocular hypertension (OHT) is a term used for individuals in whose eyes IOP lies above the normal population range but whose optic nerve and visual field show no signs of glaucomatous damage. There are various estimates as to the conversion rate from OHT to primary open-angle glaucoma (POAG). It is likely that approximately 10% of individuals with persistent OHT will convert to POAG over a 10-year period. Risk factors for the conversion of OHT to POAG can be divided into ocular and systemic, as follows:

Ocular risk factors:

- IOP: the greater the IOP the greater the risk
- large vertical cup:disc ratio (**Fig. 10.9**) (indicating reduced neuroretinal rim area:volume)
- cup:disc (C:D) ratio inter-eye asymmetry >0.2
- previous history of disc haemorrhage
- retinal nerve fibre layer defect in the absence of morphometric optic nerve head changes

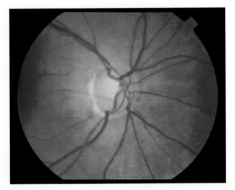

Figure 10.9 This right optic disc shows advanced glaucomatous cupping, with marked thinning of the neuroretinal rim.

- thinner than average central corneal thickness (note: excimer laser procedures on the cornea can result in artefactually lowered IOPs on measurement).

Systemic risk factors:

- increasing age
- individuals of black African or Caribbean origin (Tielsch et al 1991)

Also, the following additional risk factors have been cited as playing a role in the development of POAG:

- positive family history in a first-degree relative
- high myopia
- diabetes (although the evidence is equivocal (Rudnicka & Owen 2007))

Classification of glaucoma has important implications for treatment and prognosis. Primary glaucoma is unrelated to other ocular disease; secondary glaucoma occurs as a consequence of other ocular pathology.

Glaucoma may also be identified by anterior chamber tissue alterations (e.g. congenital, neovascular glaucoma), by accumulation of abnormal substances (including macrophages, degraded lens protein, tumour cells, altered blood cells, and melanin pigment) in the anterior chamber angle, and by the anatomical configuration of the anterior chamber angle (open- or closed-angle glaucoma).

The understanding of the relationship between IOP and glaucoma has changed considerably and is still evolving. Convincing evidence has finally arrived to implicate IOP in the pathogenesis of the disease, yet clinical impressions indicate that IOP is not the only factor. Genetic defects, blood flow defects, optic nerve structural defects or problems related to ocular neurotoxins and neurotrophic growth factors may yet prove to be implicated in the pathogenesis of glaucoma (Quigley et al 1994).

Evaluation of the glaucoma patient

This is an exciting area, with much progress in recent years. Previously, clinicians relied on clinical impressions of optic nerve appearance and noncomputerized visual fields. Recently, computer-aided optic nerve head (ONH) evaluation has become integral to the diagnosis and management of glaucoma for several reasons. Glaucoma causes characteristic, although not pathognomonic, defects in the ONH, which aids in diagnosis. Disease progression also results in progressive changes in the ONH that occur slowly, typically over months to years.

Thus, careful observation and, more importantly, perhaps the recording of disc appearance is a good indicator for recognition of progression (and disease management). As such documentation of the ONH is objective, it may prove to be more reliable than visual field analysis.

Therefore, increasing emphasis has been placed upon the morphological changes occurring at the optic nerve head and retinal nerve fibre layer. Traditionally, the disc appearance would be documented by the clinician in terms of:

- cup:disc ratio with consideration as to the size of the disc
- disc pallor
- presence or absence of disc haemorrhage (may be a marker of progressive disease)

- nasalization, bayoneting and baring of the circumlinear vessel
- peripapillary atrophy and notching of the neural rim

These are best evaluated using high-powered convex lenses such as 90D, 78D, Superfield® and 66D with the slit-lamp biomicroscope.

However, ascertaining progression of the ONH by clinical examination and photography involves subjective interpretation by the clinician, which is susceptible to intra- and interobserver variability. Newer imaging techniques attempt to limit this variability to increase the sensitivity of detecting subtle change. The optic disc and the retinal nerve fibre layer (RNFL) are the principal sites of apparent damage from glaucoma. Defects in the RNFL occur in patients with glaucoma. Recent evidence suggests that RNFL defects may pre-date visual field or ONH changes. Changes as small as 10–20 µm may indicate disease progression before visual field changes are noted. RNFL imaging technology's potential for earlier diagnosis and finer sensitivity to disease progression is actively being evaluated. Its exact clinical role has not yet been established.

The principal modalities involved are confocal scanning laser ophthalmoscopy, scanning laser polarimetry and optical coherence tomography (see Chs 18 and 19).

Confocal scanning laser ophthalmoscopy provides rapid and reproducible measurements of optic disc topography and various optic disc parameters, including disc and cup area, maximum cup depth and volume, neuroretinal rim volume and area. The Heidelberg Retina Tomograph (HRT; Heidelberg Engineering GmbH) has been extensively evaluated to assess its ability to produce reproducible data on these parameters and to demonstrate glaucomatous progression (see **Figs 18.28 and 18.29**).

Scanning laser polarimetry is based on assessing the phase shift (retardation) caused by the birefringent properties of the RNFL. It has been shown that retardation is linearly related to RNFL thickness (see Ch. 18). The GDx VCC instrument (Laser Diagnostic Technologies Inc.) incorporates variable corneal compensation for corneal birefringence and has a rapid acquisition time and produces a map of RNFL thickness. Inbuilt software then calculates the probability of abnormality and, as is the norm in these instruments, produces a colour-coded printout (see **Figs 18.26 and 18.27**).

Optical coherence tomography (OCT) uses light in a manner akin to medical ultrasound to produce cross-sectional images of the ocular microstructure. The OCT (Zeiss Humphrey Systems) performs a linear scan of the retina with a near infrared light beam and resolution of <10 µm. Like the GDx, acquisition time is approx 1 s and it gives volumetric analysis of the optic nerve head. RNFL measurements may also be selected, again with colour coding for assessment of progression (Reus & Lemij 2005) (see **Figs 18.17, 18.20 and 18.21**).

Visual fields in glaucoma

There is, of course, still a vital role for standard 'white on white' perimetry in the management of glaucoma. The principal change in visual function in glaucoma is a loss of sensitivity of the visual field. This can be demonstrated by measuring sensitivity to light at repeatable points in the visual field. Due to the specific arrangement of the retinal nerve fibres (see Ch. 20) characteristic loss of the visual field

may be observed in glaucoma. Thus, glaucomatous field defects (which may be relative or absolute) initially comprise isolated paracentral scotomata. Paracentral scotomata may then increase in size to form arcuate defects which, if large enough, may include the blind spot. Due to the discrete nature of the horizontal raphe, which obeys the horizontal midline in the temporal periphery, a so-called nasal step may form, giving dramatic asymmetry in retinal sensitivity above and below the horizontal midline, which is almost pathognomonic for POAG. In advanced disease, all these scotomata may coalesce and 'break through' to the periphery, leaving a very small island of central vision, which occasionally is extinguished altogether.

Visual fields are likely to remain important in glaucoma management as they are a measure of function rather than damage that has occurred, or is likely to occur, to the optic nerve. Further studies will determine appropriate combinations of tests, both functional and anatomical. At the moment, it is obvious that no one modality provides a complete solution (Shah et al 2006).

Treatment: The only proven strategy to slow down the progression of glaucoma has been reduction of IOP (Nouri-Mahdavi et al 2004). Traditionally, this has been performed with medication. More recently laser and incisional surgery have also been shown to be effective methods of IOP reduction. Generally, medical treatments are still the 'first line' in glaucoma therapy but there are some obvious exceptions; the management of closed- or narrow-angle glaucoma is usually treated (at least initially) with laser iridotomy, whereas infantile glaucoma is mainly treated surgically (Migdal 1995).

Glaucoma therapy aims to maintain visual function during the patient's lifetime. To achieve this, it is assumed that patients will agree to monitoring (possibly optometrist led) and intervention when appropriate.

Target IOP

In recent years, the concept of setting a 'target' IOP for an individual patient has become popular, whilst acknowledging that this may need to be adjusted in the clinical course. For a review of IOP measurement, see Chapter 24.

The 'target' IOP is usually thought of as the 'optimum' IOP for a particular eye; it would be set at a level designed to minimize the risk of disease progression. It is, of course, difficult in an individual patient at the outset to know the IOP level that might be required to do this. As a guide, however, the lower the presenting IOP and the more severe the damage at presentation, the lower the 'target' IOP is likely to be. Conversely, if the IOP is higher at presentation (e.g. over 40 mmHg) together with evidence of early damage, then an initial target IOP of 20 mmHg or less may suffice. The status of the fellow eye and the patient's life expectancy are useful pointers.

The results from the Advanced Glaucoma Intervention Study (AGIS 2000) suggest that for 'high-pressure glaucoma' the visual field is better preserved when all IOP readings are below 18 mmHg, with the majority below 15 mmHg. It has also been demonstrated that the IOP can rise during sleep, so attention needs to be given to those glaucoma treatments that are effective over 24 hours. There is also recent independent evidence that shows better field preservation with smaller diurnal fluctuations in IOP (Nouri-Mahdavi et al 2004) although some later studies appear to refute this (Bengtsson et al 2007).

There is evidence that IOP is part of the pathogenic process in normal-tension glaucoma. Therapy that is effective in lowering IOP and free of adverse effects would be expected to be beneficial in patients who are at risk of disease progression (Collaborative Normal-Tension Glaucoma Study Group 1998).

Medical treatment

For most patients, the first line of treatment of glaucoma is medical. A detailed discussion of these agents is outside the scope of this chapter, although it is reviewed in Chapter 8. However, it is worth considering the broad picture.

Topical treatment with prostaglandin analogues or a beta blocker is usually the first choice today, with carbonic anhydrase inhibitors and alpha agonists being utilized as second-choice agents.

Combination therapy drops are increasingly used, and it is argued with some justification that compliance is improved. Systemic treatment with carbonic anhydrase inhibitors such as acetazolamide is highly effective. Unfortunately, the side effect profile precludes maintenance therapy with these drugs, except as a temporizing measure perhaps prior to a more definitive intervention.

Side effects are not confined to systemic agents, and topical antiglaucoma drugs can have significant side effects, which may be life threatening, especially in the elderly. A full medical and drug history may identify possible risks. Allergic individuals or those with dry eyes are more prone to problems with long-term use of topical antiglaucoma therapy. Patients should be informed of important potential side effects when starting treatment. Practitioners must stay vigilant, as some side effects may only appear after prolonged treatment.

Laser surgery in treatment of glaucoma

Argon laser trabeculoplasty

Introduced in 1979, the published results of argon laser trabeculoplasty (ALT) have shown IOP to be reduced in most eyes with POAG, by an average IOP of 30%.

Unfortunately, this is not generally replicated in clinical practice. Also, with time, the effect of ALT tends to decrease in some patients, and IOP control can escape quite quickly. This has implications for management as these patients need more frequent follow-up. Furthermore, if surgery is required, previous ALT may limit surgical outcomes. Increasingly, ALT would appear to be used (if at all) as a temporizing measure prior to more definitive surgery or in the very infirm.

YAG laser iridotomy

Laser iridotomy is increasingly popular and may have a role in the absence of symptoms of intermittent angle closure. However, it is only likely to lower the IOP in those eyes with an open but narrow drainage angle where there is some iris–trabecular contact (Stein & Challa 2007).

Cyclodiode laser

This may be very effective in selected patients, often in those where other treatments have failed. It is a partially ablative therapy and may be applied externally transsclerally or more recently via an endoscopic approach (Vernon et al 2006).

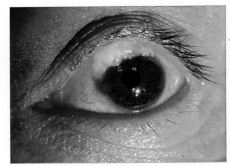

Figure 10.10 This patient has undergone previous trabeculectomy (glaucoma filtration surgery). Superiorly, there is a raised drainage 'bleb', which can give rise to foreign body sensation.

Surgery

For more than 40 years, the operation of choice in POAG has been trabeculectomy. Modifications to the size and shape of the scleral flap and internal osteum have not been associated with reduced success rates. Various additional techniques have been introduced such as laser suture lysis, releasable or adjustable sutures. These techniques are aimed mainly at preventing complications such as overdrainage and 'flat anterior chamber'. Drainage bleb (**Fig. 10.10**) failure may be treated with postoperative bleb manipulation (also called 'needling'). This is an outpatient procedure.

Patients who have risk factors for 'bleb failure' due to fibrosis and scarring of the drainage bleb should be considered for antimetabolite supplementation. Risk factors for late failure include previous ocular surgery, a long history of using certain topical medications, black African or Caribbean origin, pre-existing uveitis and diabetes mellitus (especially with retinopathy).

The optimum antimetabolite regimen will vary from patient to patient, and caution should be exercised as the topical antimetabolites currently in use, 5-flurouracil and mitomycin C (MMC), have potentially catastrophic side effects (especially MMC). These high-risk patients will benefit from supervision from a glaucoma specialist (Jones et al 2005).

The 2003 European Glaucoma Society treatment algorithm is presented in **Figure 10.11**.

Neuro-ophthalmology

The neurosensory layer of the retina is the beginning of the visual pathway and it extends to the visual cortex. Familiarity with the neuroanatomy of the visual pathway helps to understand the localizing value of the visual field test.

For generations of practitioners, the central visual field was measured with the tangent screen, and the full peripheral visual field with the Goldmann perimeter. Nowadays, visual field analysis is more often done by an automated method that measures a variable amount of the central field (see Ch. 20). Whilst this is more reproducible, the peripheral field is less well documented.

Normal visual field

The 'normal' monocular visual field is generally considered to be 60 degrees nasally, 100 degrees temporally, 60 degrees superiorly, and 70 degrees inferiorly (dependent upon the

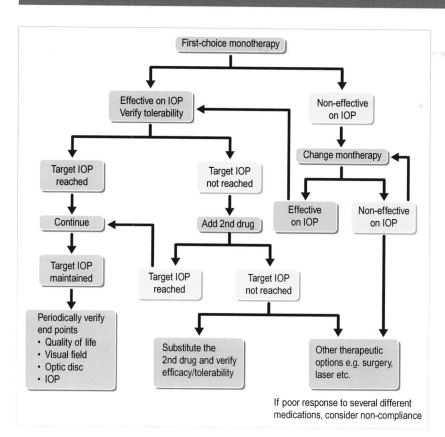

Figure 10.11 The 2003 European Glaucoma Society treatment algorithm. (Reproduced from European Glaucoma Society, 2nd edn, Chart VIII.)

size and colour of the test target). The physiological blind spot, corresponding to the optic disc, is quite consistent in its dimensions and projects into the temporal visual field. It is usually at 15.5 degrees temporal to fixation and 1.5 degrees below the horizontal and is 5.5 degrees wide and 7.5 degrees high. The blind spot is an absolute scotoma, remaining undetected with both eyes open due to the overlapping of the binocular field.

The diagnosis of lesions involving the visual pathways was traditionally made by associated neuro-ophthalmic signs. For instance, the patterns of visual field loss can be highly localizing, guiding the clinician to specific anatomic areas (see **Fig. 20.4**).

The advent of modern neuroimaging techniques such as computed tomography (CT) and magnetic resonance imaging (MRI) have perhaps reduced the importance of determining the visual field. However, it remains a valuable, inexpensive diagnostic procedure and is useful for monitoring disease progression and function.

Optic neuritis

Clinical features: Patients affected are usually younger than 45 years of age. Women are affected more often than men. It is second only to glaucoma as the most common acquired optic nerve disorder in persons younger than 50 years of age. The visual changes are characterized by a sudden decrease in visual acuity, usually in one eye, preceded or accompanied by pain on movement of the eye. Pain on eye movements is an extremely important sign that occurs in more than 90% of patients with optic neuritis (Beck et al 1995).

The visual acuity may be anything from normal to the level of no light perception in optic neuritis. Visual field abnormalities in the form of a centrocecal scotoma or an altitudinal defect are common, as are acquired dyschromatopsia and a relative afferent pupillary defect (RAPD). The optic disc may appear normal in the retrobulbar variety of optic neuritis or may be swollen with a few cells overlying the swollen disc in cases of papillitis. Over time, optic atrophy may be seen, especially after recurrent attacks.

Optic neuritis is a common cause of visual loss in young patients, typically presenting with painful monocular visual loss and decreased colour vision. Visual function generally improves spontaneously over weeks, and 95% of patients return to visual acuity of at least 6/12 (20/40) within 12 months. The initial MRI helps stratify the risk of multiple sclerosis (MS) in patients with acute isolated optic neuritis. In the Optic Neuritis Treatment Trial (ONTT), the 10-year risk of MS in the group of patients with at least one MRI T2 lesion was 56%, whereas the 10-year risk with a normal baseline MRI was 22% (Beck et al 1994).

A normal MRI in concert with painless optic neuritis, severe optic nerve head oedema, peripapillary haemorrhages or a macular star defines a very low MS risk subgroup. The probability of a recurrence of optic neuritis in either eye within 5 years is 28%. Visual recovery after a second episode in the same eye is generally very good (Beck et al 1994).

High-dose steroids hasten the rate, but not the final extent, of visual recovery in optic neuritis, and the decision to use this therapy is individualized (Atkins et al 2006). In the ONTT, standard-dose oral prednisone alone did not improve the visual outcome and was associated with an increased rate of new attacks of optic neuritis. Treatment with an intravenous followed by oral corticosteroid regimen provided a short-term reduction in the rate of development of multiple sclerosis, particularly in patients with brain MRI changes consistent with demyelination. However, after 3 years of follow-up, this treatment effect had subsided. The treatments were generally well tolerated, and side effects during the treatment period were mild. Interferon beta-1a therapy should be considered in selected high-risk patients. Routine blood tests, chest X-ray, brain MRI and lumbar puncture are of limited value for diagnosing optic neuritis in a patient with typical features of optic neuritis.

Myasthenia gravis

This is an autoimmune disorder whereby antibodies to acetylcholine receptors are raised, resulting in a decreased number of these receptors available at the neuromuscular junction.

Clinical features: A drooping eyelid or double vision may be the initial ocular symptom of myasthenia gravis. Unilateral or bilateral ptosis, with or without other ocular signs, occurs as the initial manifestation of myasthenia in as many as 75% of patients. Myasthenic ptosis is absent or minimal on awakening but may become more pronounced as the day goes on. It is often possible to demonstrate progressive fatigability on prolonged upgaze and waiting for an increase in ptosis. The variable nature of signs in myasthenia can delay diagnosis, so variable ptosis, fatigability, and periods of exacerbation and remission are common. The lid signs of myasthenia are often accompanied by ocular misalignment which may mimic other recognized patterns of incomitant strabismus.

The diagnosis of myasthenia gravis (MG) is often difficult as the condition can be generalized or confined to the extraocular muscles. There are a variety of tests available (Rivero et al 1995). The demonstration of elevated serum acetylcholine receptor antibodies is highly specific for myasthenia and has a sensitivity >90% in patients with systemic disease (Vincent & Newsom-Davis 1985). However, the sensitivity drops to 45% to 65% in patients with ocular myasthenia.

The tensilon test consists of injecting up to 10 mg edrophonium chloride intravenously in divided doses and detecting an improvement of ptosis. An unequivocal resolution of the ptosis is compelling evidence for myasthenia, although false-negative results occur. False-positive test results are encountered more rarely. The tensilon test sensitivity is 95% for systemic MG, falling to 86% in ocular MG. There are risks of serious cardiorespiratory complications so the test should be carried out in a controlled environment with resuscitation facilities available.

A relatively novel test for MG is 'the ice test', which involves placing ice on a ptotic lid for 2 minutes. A 2 mm or greater improvement in ptosis has a high (90%) sensitivity and is close to 100% specific for MG. Single-fibre electromyography is positive in 88% to 92% of patients with ocular myasthenia but electromyography is invasive with the attendant risks involved.

Management: All newly diagnosed myasthenics must have chest imaging to search for thymic hyperplasia or a thymoma and it is sensible to check thyroid status. The management of the disease is best left to neurologists or neuro-ophthalmologists. MG is controllable with cholinesterase-inhibiting medications. Edrophonium is used primarily as a diagnostic tool because its half-life is so brief.

Pyridostigmine may be used for long-term maintenance. High doses of corticosteroids are commonly employed. Patients with MG also may be taking other immunosuppressive drugs (e.g. azathioprine, ciclosporin). Bronchodilating drugs may be useful in overcoming the bronchospasm associated with a cholinergic crisis (Richman & Agius 2003).

Incomitant squint as a result of MG that demonstrates long-term stability may respond quite well to strabismus surgery and/or botulinum toxin treatment (Bentley et al 2001).

The pupil

Innervation to the pupils is via the autonomic nervous system. The parasympathetic system produces pupillary constriction, and the sympathetic system pupillary dilation. It follows that a decrease in parasympathetic input produces pupillary mydriasis (dilatation), and sympathetic lesions result in miosis (constriction). Often, these abnormalities are unilateral, so the examiner will note anisocoria (difference in pupil size). Pupillary asymmetry is not always a sign of underlying pathology as approximately one-fifth of the normal population demonstrate clinically observable anisocoria (physiological).

Examination pearls

The relative difference of pupillary size remains constant in varying illumination in physiological anisocoria. The amount of anisocoria due to sympathetic paresis is greater in dim illumination, whereas parasympathetic lesions tend towards anisocoria that is greater in bright light. Remember that some pupil abnormalities do not cause anisocoria but produce changes to pupillary reactivity, shape, or position.

Damage to significant numbers of afferent visual fibres will reduce pupillary light reactions; this may result from a disease process in the retina, optic nerve, optic chiasm, or optic tract.

Note: Lesions that destroy retinal function or involve the optic disc are normally visible on standard ophthalmoscopic examination. However, with retrobulbar lesions the fundus is usually normal.

An abnormal pupil reaction to the 'swinging flashlight test' is a *relative afferent pupillary defect* (RAPD). When present, this sign indicates impaired function of the retina or optic nerve of one eye relative to the other eye. It provides objective evidence of anterior visual pathway dysfunction. Only one working iris sphincter is required to perform the test, which can be carried out in the presence of unilateral posterior synechiae, third nerve palsy, corneal opacities, or hyphaema. Interestingly, opacities of the ocular media, such as cataracts and corneal opacities do not produce a RAPD even though they filter a significant proportion of incoming light.

The swinging flashlight test is ideally carried out in a dimly lit room, using a bright light source. The patient should fixate in the distance to avoid the miosis associated with accommodation.

Shine the test light along the visual axis to illuminate first one pupil and then the other.

The illumination should pause 3 to 5 seconds for each eye, and this manoeuvre should be repeated several times.

In general, the pupils are round and practically equal in diameter and are briskly and symmetrically reactive to light stimuli. After an initial, prompt pupil constriction, a slight 'escape' dilation usually occurs.

Thus, in the presence of a right afferent defect, the pupillary diameters are equal and slightly larger bilaterally when the right eye is stimulated and bilaterally smaller when the normal left eye is illuminated. If only the illuminated pupil is observed, the other pupil being hidden in darkness, the following is seen: the normal left pupil constricts promptly on illumination; as the light is moved rapidly to the right, the right pupil actually is seen to dilate or 'escape'; as the light moves again to the left, the left pupil again constricts briskly.

An abnormal dilated pupil

Tonic or Adie's pupil

The patient is usually asymptomatic or has vague complaints of blurred reading vision and asthenopia. The pupil is dilated, constricts minimally or not at all in response to direct light, but does constrict slowly to sustained near effort. The re-dilation phase is equally slow and tonic. Slit-lamp examination of the iris sphincter demonstrates areas of sector paresis, giving so-called vermiform movements of the pupil in response to bright light.

Adie's pupil may appear in isolation or be associated with decreased deep tendon reflexes in the lower extremities (Adie's syndrome). Adie's pupil is thought to result from a lesion in the ciliary ganglion. Denervation hypersensitivity is demonstrated by pupillary constriction to weak (0.1%) pilocarpine solution. Before denervation hypersensitivity occurs, the pupil may not constrict even in response to 1% pilocarpine, causing a diagnostic conundrum with pharmacologic blockade.

In time, the Adie's pupil tends to become bilateral (50% at 10 years), and affected pupils become smaller.

Dorsal midbrain lesions producing light–near dissociation

Dorsal midbrain lesions often produce pupillary light–near dissociation, a poor direct light reflex with relative preservation of the near response. The most frequent cause is a tumour of the pineal gland. The pupils are usually quite dilated, and are often oval. Light–near dissociation is only one component of the dorsal midbrain syndrome (Parinaud's syndrome). Other features include a supranuclear upgaze palsy, impaired convergence and convergence–retraction nystagmus on attempted upgaze.

A rare form of light–near dissociation is the so-called Argyll Robertson pupil. Argyll Robertson pupils are small, often irregular in shape and dilate poorly to all mydriatics. The condition is due to neurosyphilis.

Small pupil

Sympathetic paresis or Horner's syndrome

The syndrome of ptosis, miosis, and facial anhidrosis was first attributed to a lesion of the sympathetic pathway by Friedrich Horner in 1858. Because the lower eyelid has an equivalent to

Müller's muscle (i.e. retractors of lower lid), the lower eyelid is higher on the side of the sympathetic paresis. Lesions distal to the superior cervical ganglion usually spare the sweating and vasoconstrictor fibres, leaving only ptosis and miosis. Other inconsistent or transitory findings include increased accommodation, and ocular hypotony. Iris heterochromia generally implies congenital Horner's syndrome.

Anisocoria that does not increase in darkness is unlikely to be due to Horner's syndrome. In addition to increased anisocoria in darkness, the Horner pupil dilates more slowly than normal, often requiring 10 to 15 seconds to dilate completely.

Lesions of the sympathetic pathway to the eye can be classified anatomically as central, preganglionic, or postganglionic, and localization is useful in making an underlying diagnosis. Horner's syndrome may occur with a lesion at any point along the three-neuron sympathetic chain. An isolated, third-order, Horner's syndrome is most likely to be caused by a benign condition. However, the presence of trigeminal hypaesthesia and the more or less continuous characteristic of the pain may be associated with paratrigeminal masses. Lesions of the first neuron usually produce other neurologic signs or symptoms, and second-order Horner's syndrome caused by superior pulmonary sulcus malignancies (i.e. Pancoast's syndrome) are accompanied by arm or scapular region pain.

The distinction between a preganglionic (i.e. first- and second-order Horner's syndrome) and a postganglionic (i.e. third-order Horner's syndrome) lesion can be made pharmacologically. Cocaine drops dilate normal pupils but not pupils with sympathetic paresis independent of the level of the lesion. Hydroxyamphetamine does not dilate the miotic pupil in Horner's disease if it results from a third-order neuron lesion but does dilate normal and first- and second-order Horner's pupils. Unfortunately, both these medications may be difficult (or even illegal) to obtain. Increasingly, with improved access to MRI, Horner's patients undergo MRI of the head and chest and magnetic resonance angiography (MRA) of the neck.

An acquired Horner's syndrome in the first few years of life is an ominous occurrence and may be caused by a neuroblastoma involving the sympathetic chain in the chest or neck. These tumours may be difficult to detect, and the assistance of a paediatric oncologist should be sought in children with acquired Horner's syndrome (Woodruff et al 1988). Horner's syndrome that is present at birth, on the other hand, is almost always benign and a cause is rarely found.

Anterior ischaemic optic neuropathy

Anterior ischaemic optic neuropathy (AION) is the result of an infarction of the optic nerve head caused by compromise of the posterior circulation of the globe. This principally involves vessels supplying the optic nerve at its exit from the eye, mainly the short posterior ciliary arteries as the connective tissue support is poor in this region (Collignon-Robe et al 2004).

Two forms of AION are described: a nonarteritic or idiopathic form, and an arteritic form, secondary to giant cell arteritis.

Clinical features

Anterior ischaemic optic neuropathy occurs in the vasculopathic age group, and may result in decreased acuity, visual field defects, and a swollen, variably pale optic disc.

Nonarteritic AION (NAION) occurs typically in patients older than 45 years of age. It is sudden in onset, and painless. Visual loss varies from mild to severe. Typically, disc swelling is seen in the superior or inferior portion of the nerve, which is pale, and classically there is an altitudinal visual field defect.

Visual acuity is usually better preserved than in the arteritic variety, and the visual field defects tend to be stable. The fellow eye usually shows an optic disc with no cup (the 'crowded disc'); patients with small discs having smaller or nonexistent cups have an anatomical predisposition for NAION.

The incidence of subsequent infarction in the second eye ranges from 14% to 35%. The risk of a recurrent event in the same eye is 4% (Hattenhauer et al 1997).

Arteritic AION results from giant cell (temporal) arteritis. The optic disc is usually paler (classically described as 'chalky white') than in the nonarteritic variety, and some areas of retinal ischaemia may be seen. The visual loss is often profound and usually worse than in the nonarteritic variety. The patients are generally older than 65 years of age.

The symptoms associated with giant cell arteritis (GCA) include those of polymyalgia rheumatica (e.g. stiffness and pain of the neck and shoulder muscles, weight loss and fever). Other common symptoms include pain in the jaw muscles on chewing, chronic headache, and tenderness in the forehead and temporal scalp areas. Sometimes a tender, rope-like, nonpulsatile temporal artery can be felt. Occasionally, tongue and scalp ulceration may be seen. The erythrocyte sedimentation rate (ESR) is usually elevated along with the C-reactive protein (an inflammatory marker).

Cupping of the optic disc is the most common end-stage disc appearance of arteritic AION, but is not commonly seen in nonarteritic AION.

Management

Visual loss from giant cell arteritis is an ophthalmic emergency and requires immediate referral to hospital. Oral steroids are of little or no use in NAION and are usually of little benefit in established arteritic AION.

However, in GCA it is vital that high-dose systemic steroids are initiated early, particularly if involvement is unilateral. Unfortunately, even with optimal, timely treatment, vision may be lost in the fellow eye. Optic nerve fenestration was advocated for AION until the completion of the Ischemic Optic Neuropathy Decompression Trial (IONDT 1995). This study conclusively showed no effect of the surgery.

Paralytic strabismus

It is worth noting that the optometrist may be the first person to examine the patient with a recent-onset incomitant deviation, and in view of the possible life-threatening aetiologies, it is essential that these patients be referred urgently.

Paralysis of the sixth cranial nerve is a common entity in the very young and old. In children, causes commonly include trauma, post-viral syndrome (which usually resolves, but frequently recurs) and neoplasia. In fact, a third of brainstem gliomas present as isolated, unilateral sixth nerve palsy (Freeman & Farmer 1998).

Clinical features

Patients usually present with horizontal diplopia. The decreased abduction gives rise to increased separation of the uncrossed diplopic images, especially when looking to the affected side.

The commonest cause in older adults is microvascular disease, leading to the so-called microvascular mononeuropathy, where generally the patient is >50 years of age; there is improvement after 1 month and recovery of function after 2–3 months. Neuroimaging is normal when performed and there is usually a history of hypertension, diabetes mellitus, hypercholesterolaemia and smoking.

Investigations

The erythrocyte sedimentation rate should be checked to exclude GCA and diabetes, while hypertension should also be screened for. Follow up with serial orthoptic examinations and Hess chart plots. Neuroimaging is required if there is no sign of recovery after 3 months, or there is progression of palsy, especially with development of additional neurological signs.

Care needs to be taken in the 'atypical age group' as a retrospective study in 2001 demonstrated that the most common cause of non-traumatic sixth nerve palsies in patients between 20 and 50 years of age was a central nervous system mass lesion (Peters et al 2002; Table 10.2).

Management of sixth nerve palsy

Previously, in children under 16 years of age, it was usual to observe those who had no associated neurological signs, especially following a 'flu-like' illness or vaccination. However, increasingly, children with a documented sixth nerve palsy will undergo MRI scanning as will the adult between 20 and 50 years (see above).

If the scan is negative, a thorough medical and neurologic examination and other laboratory studies to exclude hypertension, collagen vascular disease, MS, Lyme disease and syphilis should be undertaken. Only in the so-called 'microvascular group' is it reasonable to observe and treat symptomatically.

Table 10.2 Causes of non-traumatic sixth nerve palsies in patients 20–50 years of age

Cause (20–50yrs)	n (%)
Central nervous system mass lesion	15 (33%)
Multiple sclerosis	11 (24%)
Idiopathic	6 (13%)
Viral infection	4 (9%)
Idiopathic intracranial hypertension	3 (7%)
Meningitis	3 (7%)
Microvascular	2 (4%)
Progressive spinocerebellar degeneration	1 (2%)

Peters et al 2002

Treatment may be conservative in the form of occlusion or prisms (usually temporary 'Fresnel' prisms). Botulinum toxin chemodenervation is often used, particularly to aid in differentiation of a partial versus a complete unrecovered palsy. This is important, as a partial sixth nerve palsy will respond to a horizontal recess/resect procedure whereas a complete palsy will require full vertical muscle transposition (Dawson et al 2001). Surgery should generally not be considered until measurements are stable for 6 months and the underlying cause is stable. Young children are at risk of developing amblyopia and may require alternate occlusion. Surgery cannot restore lost function and is mainly aimed at correction of diplopia, elimination of a face turn and enhancement of the usable field of binocular single vision (Riordan-Eva and Lee 1992).

Trochlear (fourth) nerve palsy

The fourth nerve is the only cranial nerve to cross to the opposite side and exit the brainstem dorsally. It has a long intracranial course and its relation to the anterior medullary velum and the tip of the temporal lobe makes it vulnerable to a variety of insults, especially trauma.

Clinical features

Paresis or paralysis of the trochlear nerve produces a hypertropia that is worse when looking down and to the opposite side with the head tilted up and to the same side. The patient will also have an esodeviation. Trauma is the most frequent cause of a fourth nerve paresis. A unilateral fourth nerve palsy has a torsional component but it is usually <5 degrees of excyclotorsion.

A blow to the top of the head can produce bilateral fourth nerve lesions which may be characterized by alternating hypertropias on gaze to the left and right. There is a large torsional component that may be as large as 15–20 degrees of excyclotorsion.

Congenital fourth nerve palsy is quite commonly seen in otherwise healthy individuals who may present with a compensatory head tilt and or facial asymmetry (Tollefson et al 2006). Older patients tend to present with neck pain. They usually have good binocular vision, and amblyopia is uncommon; bilaterality is rare. Most patients describe rather vague asthenopic symptoms. Usually, patients have only intermittent diplopia and have developed the ability to fuse abnormally large amounts of vertical ocular misalignment. A vertical fusional amplitude >5 degrees usually indicates a congenital fourth nerve palsy. In fact, a patient with a large vertical fusional amplitude needs no further evaluation as they have a decompensating congenital fourth nerve palsy.

In the absence of trauma, fourth nerve palsies that are isolated are generally vasculopathic in origin in patients >45–50 years of age. In these cases it may be reasonable to defer imaging as long as the patient follows the 'typical course' of a microvascular mononeuropathy (see above). For patients in the nonvasculopathic age group, if they do not have increased vertical fusional amplitudes, or any patient with a motility disorder that is not quite 'classic', imaging should be performed. It is also worth remembering that myasthenia gravis can mimic any extraocular motility disorder and should be excluded.

Management

Nonsurgical therapy: No optical measures such as lenses or prisms can improve torsion; cylindrical lenses with offset axis have been tried. Occlusive lenses may be used to improve symptoms of diplopia.

Surgical considerations are dependent on the relative contributions of vertical or horizontal deviations. Surgery on oblique muscles causes a greater torsional effect than surgery on rectus muscles. Inferior oblique surgery will usually result in significant vertical effects as well as its effects on torsion. The options for superior oblique weakness with torsion further include the Harada Ito procedure ± Fells modification, and a superior oblique tuck, contralateral inferior rectus recession can be used when torsion is not a problem (Simons et al 1998).

Oculomotor (third) nerve palsy

This is the largest of all the extraocular nerves and supplies all the extraocular muscles except the lateral rectus and the superior oblique. It has paired and unpaired nuclei:

- unpaired levator subnucleus with bilateral innervation
- paired superior rectus subnuclei with contralateral innervation (i.e. crossed)
- paired medial and inferior recti and inferior oblique subnuclei with ipsilateral innervation.

In the anterior cavernous sinus, the third nerve divides into a superior division (levator and superior rectus) and an inferior division (medial and inferior rectus, inferior oblique muscles and the parasympathetic pupillary fibres). Remember that partial, even divisional, involvement may occur anywhere along its course.

Clinical features are ptosis, decreased adduction, elevation and depression and adduction plus or minus internal ophthalmoplegia. Involvement of the third cranial nerve can represent a life-threatening situation. **Figure 10.12** shows the typical appearance of a third nerve palsy with pupil involvement.

Common lesions include trauma, rupture/expansion of a posterior communicating or internal carotid aneurysm and small vessel disease. Other causes include pituitary apoplexy

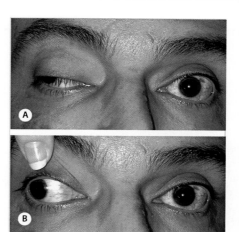

Figure 10.12 Typical appearance of a third nerve palsy. The eye is exotropic and hypertropic with ptosis **(A).** On lifting the lid, the pupil is seen to be involved (dilated) **(B).**

and intracavernous lesions such as a meningioma, a caroticocavernous fistula and granulomatous infection. The presentation may vary depending on the site affected such as in the orbital apex syndrome (proptosis/visual loss/multiple oculomotor nerve palsies).

Practically, when faced with a third nerve palsy in practice, one should evaluate for pupil sparing and, as a general rule, pupil sparing equates with microvascular aetiology. However, 10–20% of diabetic third nerve palsies affect the pupil (Jacobson 1998) and unfortunately pupil sparing has been described in midbrain lesions and aneurysms (Nadeau and Trobe 1983).

Accordingly, great care is required in evaluating these patients and not only should they be quickly assessed in the hospital setting but appropriate and timely imaging is essential.

In terms of surgical management of the ocular misalignment, this can be very challenging (Lee et al 2001) and is outside the scope of this chapter. In partial third nerve palsy, a (relatively) simple horizontal recess/resect procedure may suffice but in complete palsy the challenge is to obtain parallelism in the primary position.

Age-related macular degeneration

Age-related macular degeneration (AMD) is the leading cause of blindness in individuals over 50 years of age in the Western world. It accounts for nearly 50% of blind registrations in the UK. AMD is a bilateral but often asymmetrical disease of the macular area of the retina. It may be defined as:

1. Non-exudative (dry, atrophic) with the presence of drusen (**Fig. 10.13**) and progressive atrophy of the overlying retinal pigment epithelium. This is the commonest form of the disease, accounting for 90% of cases.
2. Exudative (wet, neovascular), which is characterized by choroidal neovascularization (CNV). The vessels may bleed, resulting in a retinal haemorrhage which later progresses to form a fibrous disciform scar (**Fig. 10.14**). CNV may be further classified as classic or occult according to their well-demarcated or ill-defined appearance during a fundus fluorescein angiogram (FFA).

AMD may also be defined as:

1. Early age-related maculopathy (ARM) with the presence of drusen associated with degeneration of the retinal pigment epithelium or increased pigment in the macular area.

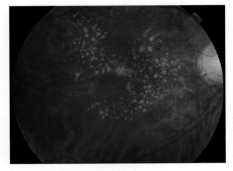

Figure 10.13 Widespread drusen.

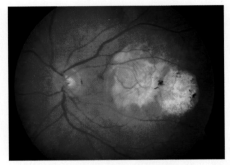

Figure 10.14 A large 'disciform' scar, which is most likely the result of exudative age-related macular degeneration.

2. Late ARM or AMD with the presence of geographic atrophy or exudative disease or both.

Risk factors for age-related macular degeneration

Age

Various epidemiological studies including the Beaver Dam eye study (Klein et al 1992), Rotterdam study (Vingerling et al 1995) and the Blue Mountains eye study (Mitchell et al 1995) have found end-stage (blinding) AMD prevalent in about 1.7% of all people aged over 50 years, the incidence rising with age (0.7–1.4% in people aged over 65 and 11.0–18.5% in people aged over 85).

Smoking

Recent evidence from the Age-Related Eye Disease Study Research Group (AREDS 2000) suggests that smoking is a recognized risk factor for both dry and wet AMD.

Family history

The lifetime risk of developing late-stage macular degeneration is 50% for people who have a relative with macular degeneration compared with only 12% for people who do not have relatives with macular degeneration, i.e. a fourfold higher risk.

Genetic

Various genes have now been identified which are closely linked to the development of AMD. One of these, identified as complement system protein factor H (CFH), has been associated with a sevenfold increase in risk for the disease. This gene inhibits the inflammatory response via the complement pathway (Klein et al 2005).

Cardiovascular risk factors

There is increasing evidence that atherosclerosis, high blood pressure, obesity and raised cholesterol are all associated with an increased risk for development of AMD.

Race

The prevalence of AMD has been found to be higher in whites than in blacks.

Other factors

Other risk factors such as alcohol consumption, oestrogen replacement and lifetime light exposure require further study.

Symptoms

The atrophic type has a progressive, gradual loss of central vision, producing a central scotoma, leading to difficulty in reading, seeing distant objects, distortion of straight lines, micropsia or macropsia (object size perceived as being smaller or larger than the original).

For the exudative type, the symptoms may be similar to those for atrophic AMD but may rapidly deteriorate to profound central visual loss.

Signs

Fundoscopy may show dry AMD in the form of either atrophic, pale areas or drusen which appear as discrete yellow deposits in the macular area. These may become paler, larger and confluent in patients at a higher risk for developing wet AMD. Wet AMD is characterized by growth of choroidal new vessels into the retina, resulting in a neovascular membrane (**Fig. 10.15**), with accumulation of serous fluid causing a localized retinal detachment. These may bleed and appear as a dark-red, well-defined haemorrhagic patch in the macular area. In the late stages of the disease, the choroidal neovascular membrane becomes fibrosed to form a disciform scar (known as the end stage) (see **Fig. 10.14**).

Management

Drug therapy

Dry AMD Unfortunately, no medical or surgical treatment is currently available for dry AMD. However, patients may benefit from low-vision aid assessment. Counselling may play an important role in understanding that the disease primarily affects the central vision with relative preservation of the peripheral field. Patients should be advised to stop smoking. High-dose vitamin supplements such as vitamin A (beta-carotene), C, E, zinc and copper have been shown to slow the progression of dry AMD to more advanced stages and should be recommended to patients (AREDS 2001).

Wet AMD

Laser photocoagulation Earlier trials by the Macular Photocoagulation Study Group showed laser photocoagulation to be effective for extrafoveal lesions, destroying the CNV before ingrowth to the fovea had occurred (MPS 1986). The limitations of laser treatment are the central scotoma produced as a consequence of treatment and the high recurrence rate, which limits its use to only small, classic extrafoveal lesions.

Photodynamic therapy with verteporfin Two-year results of two randomized clinical trials (TAP 2001) showed photodynamic therapy (PDT) with verteporfin to be effective in destroying CNV without damaging the neurosensory retina, thereby proving to be of benefit in treating subfoveal lesions. Verteporfin acts by occluding newly formed vessels and has been shown to be effective in patients with classic and predominantly

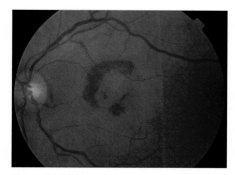

Figure 10.15 Deep haemorrhage associated with a choroidal neovascular membrane.

classic subfoveal lesions. These two patient groups are those recommended for verteporfin treatment following current UK guidelines (National Institute for Clinical Excellence). The TAP study showed 53% of verteporfin-treated patients lost fewer than 15 letters of vision compared with 38% of placebo-treated patients. However, significant visual loss may still result in some patients after PDT for subfoveal CNV as PDT may be ineffective for some lesion types including minimally classic CNV.

Antivascular endothelial growth factor As vascular endothelial growth factor (VEGF) plays a significant role in the development and maintenance of CNV, substances which block VEGF have been developed as a treatment for wet AMD. Anti-VEGF therapies are a major advancement in the treatment of wet AMD and are effective in all types and sizes of CNV lesions: classic, predominantly classic, minimally classic and occult lesions including serous retinal pigment epithelial detachments (PED). Two specific agents have been developed for use as intravitreal injections. These are Pegaptanib (Macugen, Pfizer/OSI Eyetech) and Ranibizumab (Lucentis, Genentech/Novartis Pharma). These have been licensed for use in the UK recently (Macugen, May 2006; Lucentis, February 2007). The VISION Clinical Trial Group has shown Pegaptanib to be effective for neovascular age-related macular degeneration (D'Amico et al 2006). The MARINA Study Group found a significant benefit in patients treated with Ranibizumab for neovascular age-related macular degeneration, with 94.5% of the patients losing less than 15 letters of vision when compared with 62.2% receiving sham injections. This acuity difference was maintained after 2 years. Visual acuity improved by 15 or more letters in 24.8–33.8% of the treated patients as compared with 5.0% of the sham-injection group (Rosenfeld et al 2006). Similar results were shown by the ANCHOR Study Group (Brown et al 2006).

A third agent, Bevacizumab (Avastin, Genentech/Roche), is licensed for the treatment of colorectal or breast cancer. However, it has effects similar to Ranibizumab (results from pilot studies) when given intravitreally, which has led to the widespread 'off-label' use of the drug in the UK. It has been found to be effective but no randomized, controlled trials exist to date. Comparison of AMD Treatments Trial (CATT) started in February 2008 and is currently recruiting participants verified by the National Eye Institute. This will compare Avastin to Lucentis. This study aims to recruit 1200 patients.

Visual rehabilitation and support

Refraction, low-vision aid (magnifiers for near vision, telescopes for distance vision) assessments, large-print books, talking tapes and advice on good lighting are vital in maximizing an individual's visual potential in the performance of daily tasks. Low-vision therapies are discussed in Chapter 30.

Optometrists plays an important role as they may be the first to see patients with sudden visual loss which may result in an emergency referral to the hospital eye clinic. UK practitioners may use this occasion to provide a low-vision leaflet (LVL) enabling them to self-refer to social services and contact the sources of advice and support included in the leaflet (see **Fig. 10.16**).

In the UK Hospital Eye Service, a Certificate of Vision Impairment (CVI August 2007) may be used for registration of patients with sight impairment or severe sight impairment (previously termed as partial sightedness or blindness, respectively). A Referral of Vision Impairment (RVI) form may be used, with the consent of the patient, to request an assessment for social needs where CVI registration is inappropriate or the patient has declined registration.

Figure 10.16 illustrates the referral pathway for vision-impaired people.

Hypertensive retinopathy

Hypertension is a worldwide problem affecting approximately one billion people worldwide. It affects the microcirculation, acting as a silent killer for many years before overt end-organ damage is clinically apparent.

There have been numerous attempts to reclassify hypertensive retinopathy but the most widely accepted classification is shown in **Table 10.3** (Grosso et al 2005). A mild grade of retinopathy with generalized arteriolar narrowing, focal arteriolar narrowing, arteriovenous nicking, copper wiring of arteriolar wall (exaggerated arteriolar light reflex due to arteriosclerosis), or a combination of these have been associated with a mild increase of incident clinical stroke, coronary heart disease and death. Moderate grade of retinopathy with haemorrhages (blot, dot, or flame shaped), microaneurysms, cottonwool spots, hard exudates or a combination of these signs are more strongly associated with risk of incident stroke and mortality from cardiovascular causes (Wong et al 2003). WHO International Society of

Table 10.3 The Keith, Wagener, and Barker hypertensive retinopathy classification (grade I–IV), based on the level of severity of the retinal findings

Grade	Classification	Symptoms
Grade I (mild hypertension)	Mild, generalized retinal arteriolar narrowing or sclerosis.	No symptoms
Grade II (more marked hypertensive retinopathy)	Definite focal narrowing and arteriovenous crossings. Moderate to marked sclerosis of the retinal arterioles. Exaggerated arterial light reflex.	Asymptomatic
Grade III (mild angiospastic retinopathy)	Retinal haemorrhages, exudates and cotton wool spots. Sclerosis and spastic lesions of retinal arterioles.	Symptomatic
Grade IV	Severe grade III and papilloedema	Reduced survival

Keith et al 1939

Hypertension (WHO-ISH) 2003 statement 14 and the British Hypertension Society 2004 Guidelines (BHS IV)15 consider retinopathy as target organ damage, although only for grades III and IV.

Management

For grades I and II hypertensive retinopathy, a routine referral to a general medical practitioner for assessment and management of cardiovascular risk including lifestyle measures and periodic monitoring of blood pressure may be adequate. For grades III and IV, in addition to a referral for a more aggressive approach to the cardiovascular risk reduction, a referral should be made to the ophthalmologist for the evaluation and treatment of moderate to severe hypertensive retinopathy and any associated retinal vascular complications (venous and arterial occlusion, non-arteritic AION) (**Figure 10.17**).

Diabetic retinopathy

Diabetes mellitus is classified according to two distinct groups of patients: type 1 diabetes (previously known as 'insulin dependent' or 'juvenile onset') and type 2 diabetes (non-insulin dependent, adult onset). The new WHO classification also recognizes other types of secondary diabetes, e.g. after pancreatic disease and gestational diabetes. Complications of diabetes can be largely divided into macrovascular and microvascular. The macrovascular complications include cerebrovascular disease, coronary heart disease and peripheral vascular disease. The microvascular complications include diabetic retinopathy, neuropathy and nephropathy. The risk of developing cataract is greater in diabetics.

Diabetic retinopathy is the leading cause of severe visual loss in the working-age group in the Western world. Recent major population studies such as the Diabetes Control and Complications Trial (DCCT 1993) and a UK-based study (UKPDS 1998) have highlighted the significance of optimal

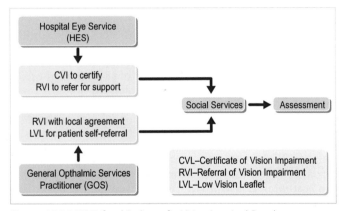

Figure 10.16 UK Referral Pathway for Vision Impaired People.

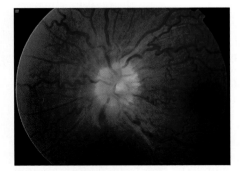

Figure 10.17 Bilateral disc swelling associated with raised intracranial pressure (papilloedema).

control of diabetes and blood pressure on the development and progression of long-term complications of diabetes.

Risk factors for retinopathy

Duration of diabetes is a recognized risk factor and a clear relationship between the duration and the development of retinopathy has been demonstrated in the results of the DCCT and the UKPDS trial. Improved glycaemic control, as measured by glycosylated haemoglobin (HbA1c), and tightly controlled blood pressure in the studies also showed a reduction in the development and progression of retinopathy. Other significant risk factors are increasing age, pregnancy, renal disease, smoking and hyperlipidaemia.

Classification and clinical features

The original classification is based on the Airlie House/EDTRS classification with grading according to the severity of ophthalmoscopic signs (ETDRS 1991). The more recent classification has been devised by National Screening Committee (NSC) of England and Wales for use in population screening aimed at detection of grades of retinopathy sufficiently severe to merit referral for an ophthalmological opinion and possible treatment (Harding et al 2003) (Tables 10.4 and 10.5).

Clinical features of diabetic retinopathy Classifications are difficult to use in clinical practice. Therefore, for the purposes of defining those patients at risk of developing new vessels, it is useful to categorize nonproliferative retinopathy (NPDR) as 'low risk' or 'high risk'.

Clinical features of 'low-risk' (mild/moderate) NPDR (**Fig. 10.18**) or background retinopathy are:

- mildly dilated veins
- microaneurysms

Table 10.4 International Classification by the American Academy of Ophthalmology. International Clinical Diabetic Retinopathy (DR) Disease Severity Scale

Proposed disease severity level	Findings observable with dilated ophthalmoscopy
No apparent DR	No abnormalities
Nonproliferative DR: mild	Microaneurysms only
Nonproliferative DR: moderate	More than 'mild' but less than 'severe'
Nonproliferative DR: severe	Any of the following:
	• 20 or more intraretinal haemorrhages in 4 quadrants
	• Definite venous beading in 2 or more quadrants
	• Prominent IRMA in 1 or more quadrants and no neovascularization
Proliferative DR	One or more of the following:
	• Definite neovascularization
	• Preretinal or vitreous haemorrhage

IRMA, intraretinal microvascular abnormalities.

Table 10.5 Current Proposed Grading in use by the National Screening Committee (NSC) UK. Disease grading protocol in National Guidelines on Screening for Diabetic Retinopathy

Retinopathy (R)	
Level 0	None
Level 1	Background microaneurysm(s) Retinal haemorrhage(s) ± any exudate
Level 2	Preproliferative venous beading Venous loop or reduplication Intraretinal microvascular abnormality (IRMA) Multiple deep, round or blot haemorrhages
Level 3	Proliferative new vessels on disc (NVD) New vessels elsewhere (NVE) Preretinal or vitreous haemorrhage Preretinal fibrosis ± tractional retinal detachment

Maculopathy (M)

Exudate within 1 disc diameter (DD) of the centre of the fovea

Circinate or group of exudates within the macula

Retinal thickening within 1 DD of the centre of the fovea or any microaneurysm or haemorrhage within 1 DD of the centre of the fovea only if associated with a best VA of 6/12

Photocoagulation (P)

Focal grid to macula

Peripheral scatter

Unclassifiable (U)

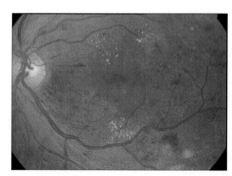

Figure 10.18 Nonproliferative diabetic retinopathy.

- dot haemorrhages
- exudates
- occasional cotton wool spots.

Clinical features of 'high-risk' (severe) NPDR (**Figs 10.19 and 10.20**) or pre-proliferative retinopathy are:

- IRMAs
- venous beading and loops
- clusters of large 'dot' or 'blot' haemorrhages
- multiple cotton wool spots.

Maculopathy may be defined as focal, diffuse, ischaemic or mixed. The characteristic features of focal maculopathy are well-circumscribed, leaking areas associated with rings of hard exudates. Diffuse maculopathy comprises

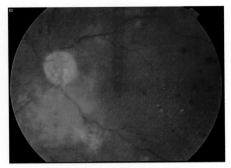

Figure 10.19 Severe proliferative diabetic retinopathy.

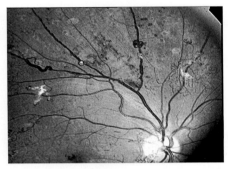

Figure 10.20 A 'red free' image of severe proliferative diabetic retinopathy which highlights the vascular changes seen in this condition.

generalized oedema of the central macula caused by widespread leakage with exudation of lipid in the macular area.

Management

1. Treatment of systemic risk factors

   The progression of nonproliferative diabetic retinopathy including maculopathy is significantly delayed by attention to general measures such as diabetes and blood pressure control. Control of diet (especially lipid intake) and regular exercise, along with regular clinical observation, may slow the progression of complications.

2. Treatment of proliferative retinopathy

   Laser treatment in the form of scattered, peripheral, panretinal photocoagulation (PRP) has been shown to be effective in significant reduction of severe visual loss which may occur due to complications of proliferative retinopathy (DRS 1981).

3. Treatment of diabetic maculopathy

   Diabetic maculopathy is the major cause of gradual progressive and largely irreversible loss of central vision. Treatment of diabetic maculopathy is indicated when there is clinically significant macular oedema involving the centre of the macula, and is performed in the form of focal or grid laser for focal and diffuse maculopathy, respectively (ETDRS Group 1985).

4. Treatment of complications

   Vitreous haemorrhage is the result of bleeding into the vitreous cavity from ruptured normal or new retinal vessels, usually caused by forward detachment of the vitreous gel leading to loss of vision. The fibrovascular membranes may progressively contract, leading to

tractional retinal detachments. Vitrectomy is performed to relieve retinal traction and to clear prolonged vitreous haemorrhage whilst allowing panretinal laser photocoagulation at the same time.

5. New treatments

   There is increasing evidence that the use of intravitreal steroids such as triamcinolone may be effective in the treatment of refractory macular oedema which has not responded to laser therapy.

Screening for diabetic retinopathy

The development of screening in Europe was first encouraged by the St Vincent Declaration, which set a target in 1992 for reduction of new blindness by one-third in the following 5 years. In late 2002, the National Service Framework for Diabetes was published, which includes the specific requirement for the introduction of a national programme for screening for diabetic retinopathy in England and Wales (NICE 2002) (**Table 10.6**). At the time of publication, an implementation process was underway in all four UK nations with the aim of 80% coverage by 2006 and 100% coverage by the end of 2007. The NSC recommendations are for the use of digital fundus photography with dilated pupils.

Two options exist for the delivery of NSC standard screening:

1. ambulant primary-care-based screening by teams of retinal-screening technicians
2. optometry based with digital photography in optometry practices.

Table 10.6 Grading and referral. Disease grading protocol in National Guidelines on Screening for Diabetic Retinopathy

Retinopathy (R)	R0 None	Annual screening
	R1 Background	Annual screening
	R2 Pre-proliferative	Refer to HES
	R3 Proliferative	Fast-track referral to HES
Maculopathy (M)	M0 None	
	M1 Present	Refer to HES
Photocoagulation (P)	P0 None	
	P1 Present	New: refer to HES Quiescent, post treatment: annual screening
Unclassifiable (U)		Poor view but gradable: refer to HES

HES, hospital eye service.

Uveitis

Uveitis is characterized by intraocular inflammation primarily involving the uveal tract (i.e. the iris, ciliary body and choroid) although inflammation of adjacent tissues such as the retina, optic nerve and vitreous humour can cause significant sight-threatening complications. Uveitis occurs mainly in the 20–50-year age group, and can affect one or both eyes. The incidence of uveitis varies from 14 to 52.4/100 000 with the overall prevalence around the world approximately 0.73%.

Pathogenesis of uveitis remains unclear but many cases are labelled as idiopathic. Infectious agents, the HLA-B27 positive group of diseases and being a part of a systemic disease process have been considered as well-recognized associations. The complement system has been implicated in the pathogenesis of autoimmune uveitis.

The International Uveitis Study Group (Bloch-Michel & Nussenblatt 1987) and the Standardization of Uveitis Nomenclature (SUN) Working Group (Jabs et al 2005) have classified uveitis based on the anatomical structures involved and the clinical features.

Anatomic classification of uveitis

Anterior uveitis: Primary site of inflammation: anterior chamber

Intermediate uveitis: Primary site of inflammation: vitreous

Posterior uveitis: Primary site of inflammation: retina or choroid

Panuveitis: Primary site of inflammation: anterior chamber, vitreous, retina or choroid.

Clinical classification of uveitis

Infectious: Bacterial, viral, fungal, parasitic

Non-infectious: Known systemic association, no known systemic association

Masquerade: Neoplastic, non-neoplastic.

Clinical features

Acute anterior uveitis is characterized by the symptoms of photophobia, pain, redness, lacrimation and decreased vision, whereas the eye may be white with minimal symptoms in chronic anterior uveitis. The signs of anterior uveitis are circumcorneal ciliary injection, corneal endothelial cellular deposits called keratic precipitates (KPs), iris nodules, inflammatory cells in the aqueous humour and anterior vitreous, aqueous flare and posterior synechiae, which are adhesions between the anterior lens surface and the iris. Large KPs and iris nodules indicate granulomatous inflammation. Flare results from leakage of protein into the aqueous from damaged iris blood vessels and may occur in the absence of active inflammation. Intermediate uveitis presents with floaters due to cellular infiltration of the vitreous (vitritis). Posterior uveitis presents with floaters due to vitritis and indicates severe inflammation with the involvement of choroid (choroiditis), retina (retinitis) and blood vessels (vasculitis). Significantly reduced vision in intermediate and posterior uveitis is usually caused by cystoid macular oedema.

Acute anterior uveitis

The most common form of uveitis with inflammation of the iris and ciliary body and is often episodic and recurrent. HLA-B27 antigen is associated in 50% of cases while the rest are considered idiopathic.

Ankylosing spondylitis Prevalence is 0.1–2% of the general population with peak onset at 15–25 years of age, with a male:female ratio of 5:1. HLA-B27 is associated in 92% of patients compared with 6% of the general population. Approximately 1–2% of all people who are positive for HLA-B27 develop ankylosing spondylitis (Brown et al 1997).

This usually presents before the age of 30 years with symptoms of inflammatory back pain. Ankylosing spondylitis is characterized by inflammation primarily involving the axial skeleton (e.g. sacroiliitis and spondylitis). Acute anterior uveitis occurs in 20–30% of patients. Of all patients with acute anterior uveitis, 30–50% either have or will develop ankylosing spondylitis.

Psoriatic arthropathy This affects 7% of patients with psoriasis, with involvement of the distal joints being most common. It affects males and females equally and is associated with an increased prevalence of HLA-B27. Conjunctivitis occurs in 20%, while 10% of patients with psoriatic arthropathy develop acute anterior uveitis.

Reactive arthritis Previously known as Reiter's syndrome, this is more common in males and 70–90% of cases are HLA-B27 antigen positive. Acute anterior uveitis develops in 25% of patients with reactive arthritis. There is frequent mucocutaneous involvement with conjunctivitis, oral ulcers and circinate balanitis.

Chronic anterior uveitis

Juvenile idiopathic arthritis (JIA)/juvenile chronic arthritis (JCA)/juvenile rheumatoid arthritis (JRA) Juvenile chronic arthritis is a group of systemic inflammatory disorders of unknown aetiology causing chronic joint inflammation in children under the age of 16 years. Its prevalence is 1 per 1000 children (Edelsten et al 2002). It is classified according to its mode of onset as:

- *Oligoarticular/pauciarticular onset*: with four or fewer joints involved.
  It is the commonest type (40–60%), being more common in girls (5:1). Peak age of onset is at age 2 years. Often asymmetric, it commonly involves the knees and less frequently the ankles and wrists. Approximately 75% of these patients test positive for antinuclear antibody (ANA). This mode of onset is rarely associated with systemic signs. A high risk for uveitis exists.

- *Polyarticular onset*: with more than four joints involved (20–40%)
  It is more common in girls (3:1). Peak age of onset is at 3 years of age. It commonly involves the small joints of the hand and less frequently the larger joints of the knee, ankle or wrist. Often asymmetric, arthritis may be destructive in 15% of patients. Immunoglobulin M (IgM) rheumatoid factor (RF) is present in 10% of children. Approximately 40% of these patients test positive for ANA. Systemic symptoms, including anorexia, anaemia, and growth retardation, are moderate. An intermediate risk for uveitis exists.

- *Systemic onset*: (10–20%)
  It occurs with equal frequency in boys and girls, and can present at any age. Symmetric polyarthritis is present and may be destructive in 25% of patients. It may involve hands, wrists, feet, ankles, elbows, knees, hips, shoulders, and cervical spine, and even the jaw may be involved. ANA is positive in only 10% of the patients. Systemic onset is associated with fever, rash and arthritis. A low risk for uveitis exists.

Management includes physiotherapy and occupational therapy to maintain function and prevent deformities.

Drugs

Topical steroids are indicated in uveitis. Nonsteroidal antiinflammatory drugs (ibuprofen) and analgesics can be used for control of pain and fever. Disease-modifying drugs (DMARDs) are now used early in the disease process. All have significant potential toxicity and require careful monitoring. Methotrexate is now considered by many experts to be the most effective agent. Other agents used include hydroxychloroquine, gold, penicillamine, sulfasalazine and immunosuppressants such as ciclosporin A, azathioprine, cyclophosphamide and chlorambucil.

Systemic corticosteroids are indicated in children with life-threatening complications. The tumour necrosis factor inhibitor, etanercept, has been shown to be effective and well tolerated (Lovell et al 2000). The prognosis is usually good depending on the specific subtype, with resolution occurring in up to 80% of affected children, who regain normal function.

Fuch's heterochromic cyclitis

It is usually unilateral and characterized by a classic triad of heterochromia, cataract and keratitic precipitates (KPs). It is equally common in males and females, and the mean age of presentation is 40 years. Patients are usually asymptomatic with minimal signs of inflammation. The eye is typically white with stellate KPs and absent posterior synechiae.

Patients may have symptoms of floaters due to vitritis. Inflammation is unilateral in 90% of patients and bilateral in 10%. Low-grade inflammation usually persists over many years and generally does not require treatment. In a few patients, inflammation flares up to a moderate level, requiring a short course of topical corticosteroid therapy but high-dose or chronic topical corticosteroids have not been found to be of any benefit.

Common complications of Fuch's heterochromic cyclitis include posterior subcapsular cataracts and secondary glaucoma.

Viral uveitis

Viruses such as herpes simplex (HSV), herpes zoster (HZV) and varicella zoster (VZV) can all cause non-granulomatous uveitis. HZV commonly causes iris atrophy and secondary glaucoma may occur, which may be difficult to treat. HSV can cause a necrotizing retinitis in the immunocompromised.

Posterior uveitis

Toxoplasmosis

Toxplasmosis is caused by *Toxoplasma gondii*, an obligate intracellular parasite. Cats are the main source of infection. Infectious oocysts are excreted by the cat for up to 2 weeks after the initial infection, and can survive in warm, moist soil for more than 1 year. The active proliferating forms of the organism are called tachyzoites. They can be found in any organ but occur most commonly in the brain, skeletal muscle, and heart muscle. Humans acquire infection from domestic cats or from eating raw or undercooked meat from another intermediate host. Human-to-human transfer only occurs via the maternal–fetal route but is being seen with increasing frequency in immunocompromised patients.

Toxoplasma infections may present in four main ways:

1. Acquired infection in non-compromised patients
   Commonly present as asymptomatic lymphadenopathy. The condition is usually mild, resolving within 1 to 3 months but can last up to a year.
2. Congenital infection in non-compromised patients
   Transmission to a fetus from the mother results in more severe infection if it occurs in the first trimester. Severe congenital toxoplasmosis is marked by the classic triad of chorioretinitis, intracranial calcifications, and *hydrocephalus*.
3. Acquired infection in immunocompromised patients
   Severe disseminated toxoplasmosis can occur in immunocompromised patients and may lead to multi-organ failure.
4. Ocular manifestations
   Symptoms include a painful red eye, blurred vision, floaters, photophobia, and metamorphopsia (image distortion). Cysts are deposited in the retina, causing focal necrotizing retinitis due to a hypersensitivity reaction causing a retinal *vasculitis* and granulomatous or non-granulomatous anterior uveitis. The most common finding in congenital toxoplasmosis is retinochoroiditis with a predilection for the posterior pole. It is seen in 75–80% of cases and is bilateral in 85% of cases. Severe bilateral impairment has been found in 9% of children with congenital toxoplasmic retinochoroiditis. Ocular toxoplasmosis-acquired infection is rare.

Management The immunoglobulin M (IgM) immunofluorescent antibody test (IgM-IFA) is used as a standard for the diagnosis of acute toxoplasmosis, with a titre of 1:160 or greater considered diagnostic of recently acquired *T. gondii* infection. In cases of diagnostic difficulty, IgG (Suzuki et al 2001) and polymerase chain reaction (PCR) have been used. Toxoplasmosis is a self-limiting condition. Therefore, treatment of systemic acquired toxoplasmosis is not usually recommended. In the case of ocular toxoplasmosis, several therapeutic regimens have been recommended. Triple and quadruple drug therapy involves the use of three or more of the following drugs: pyrimethamine, sulfadiazine, and prednisone and clindamycin.

Sarcoidosis

This is a multisystem chronic inflammatory condition characterized by the formation of non-caseating epithelioid granulomata. It affects young adults with up to 50% being asymptomatic. Symptoms include fever, night sweats, lymphadenopathy including hilar lymph node (lung) involvement in 90% of cases. Skin rashes are common and seen as erythema nodosum on the lower limbs. Ocular involvement occurs in 20% of the patients, presenting as a granulomatous anterior and posterior uveitis. Central nervous system involvement (neurosarcoid) and cranial nerve palsies may also occur. Diagnosis is aided by a frequently raised ESR (65% cases), elevated serum angiotensin-converting enzyme (ACE) levels (60%) and plain chest X-ray showing bilateral hilar lymphadenopathy.

Behçet's disease

This is an idiopathic, multisystem disorder commonly affecting men between 30 and 40 years of age and characterized by oral and genital ulceration with ocular abnormalities occurring in 70–85% of patients (International Study Group for Behçet's

Disease 1990). These include acute recurrent iritis, vitritis, retinitis and vasculitis. Systemic vascular complications occur in 25–48% of cases and are the main cause of mortality.

Infective causes

Human immunodeficiency virus, tuberculosis and syphilis are some of the systemic diseases which can cause chronic inflammation involving any part of the uveal tract.

Complications of uveitis

These include cataract, glaucoma and cystoid macular oedema.

Principles of management of uveitis

Medical management

Topical steroids are used for anterior uveitis, with the frequency depending on the severity of the inflammation being treated. Periocular steroids (sub-Tenon or orbital floor) are considered when a more posterior delivery for a long-lasting effect is required (e.g. triamcinolone acetonide). Systemic steroids are indicated in the presence of systemic disease or for vision-threatening uveitis. Both the short- and long-term adverse effects of corticosteroid use should be discussed with the patient, and may require the help of a general physician. Prednisone is the most commonly used oral corticosteroid.

Immunosuppressive agents include three main categories of therapy: antimetabolites, T-cell suppressors and cytotoxic agents. Antimetabolites include azathioprine, methotrexate and mycophenolate mofetil. T-cell inhibitors include ciclosporin and tacrolimus. Cytotoxic agents are alkylating agents and include cyclophosphamide and chlorambucil. Most agents take several weeks to achieve efficacy; therefore, they initially are used in conjunction with oral corticosteroids. Once the disease is under control, corticosteroids can be tapered. These agents require regular monitoring of adverse events in conjunction with a specialist with expertise in this area (Jabs et al 2000).

The new treatment modalities are medications that target specific mediators of the immune response. In particular, molecules that block the tumour necrosis factor-α (TNF-α), e.g. etanercept, infliximab and the interleukin-2 receptor (e.g. daclizumab) have been found to modulate the immune response effectively in patients with uveitis.

Intravitreal therapies include injection of steroids (e.g. triamcinolone, usually 4 mg in 0.1 mL (Baath et al 2007), anti-VEGF agents (e.g. bevacizumab (Wu et al 2008)) and surgically placed implants (e.g. fluocinilone or retisert (Jaffe et al 2006)). The treatment may be beneficial for the management of refractory cystoid macular oedema. However, cataract formation and elevated IOP are common, and the risk of endophthalmitis (usually sterile) is approximately 0.1%.

Surgical management

Posterior and intermediate uveitis may be associated with significant vitreous opacification that is unresponsive to medical therapy. Other complications of vasculitis such as vitreous haemorrhage may necessitate therapeutic vitrectomy.

Intraocular malignancy

It is not possible in this chapter to give a detailed account of the diagnosis and management of intraocular tumours. New techniques have emerged in recent years that require an understanding of pathology, especially in the field of tumour markers and genetics, that is outside the scope of this text. The reader is referred to the outstanding work of Drs Jerry and Carol Shields (Shields & Shields 2007).

The most common form of intraocular malignancy is a metastasis to the uvea. As many cases are visually asymptomatic in the context of primary or advanced systemic disease, these often remain undiagnosed. Therefore, in a clinical practice, uveal metastasis is probably not as common as primary uveal melanoma. This may appear anywhere along the uveal tract and may involve primarily the ciliary body or the choroid and may be pigmented or amelanotic (without the typical pigmentary appearance). Early tumours may be difficult to differentiate from a benign naevus; features that may help are whether the tumour is obviously raised and the presence of orange pigment on the surface (lipofucin). Serial photography may be acceptable in small lesions but there is no substitute for an experienced observer, and early referral is recommended if there is any doubt.

References

Afshari N A, Mullally J E, Afshari M A et al 2001 Survey of patients with granular, lattice, avellino, and Reis-Bücklers corneal dystrophies for mutations in the BIGH3 and gelsolin genes. Archives of Ophthalmology Jan 119(1):16–22

The AGIS Investigators 2000 The Advanced Glaucoma Intervention Study (AGIS), 7. The relationship between control of intraocular pressure and visual field deterioration. American Journal of Ophthalmology 130:429–440

Ang L P, Chua J L, Tan D T 2007 Current concepts and techniques in pterygium treatment. Current Opinions in Ophthalmology Jul 18(4):308–313

Age-Related Eye Disease Study Research Group (AREDS) 2000 Risk factors associated with age-related macular degeneration. A case-control study in the age-related eye disease study: Age-related Eye Disease Study Report Number 3. Ophthalmology 107: 2224–2232

Age-Related Eye Disease Study Research Group (AREDS) 2001 A randomised, placebo-controlled, clinical trial of high dose supplementation with vitamins C and E, bete-carotene, and zinc for age-related macular degeneration and vision loss: AREDS report no. 8. Archives of Ophthalmology 119:1417–1469.

Atkins E J, Biousse V, Newman N J 2006 The natural history of optic neuritis. Review of Neurological Disease Spring 3(2):45–56

Azad R V, Chanana B, Sharma Y R 2007 Primary vitrectomy versus conventional retinal detachment surgery in phakic rhegmatogenous retinal detachment. Acta Ophthalmologica Scandinavica Aug 85(5): 540–545

Baath J, Ells A L, Crichton A et al 2007 Safety profile of intravitreal triamcinolone acetonide. Ocular Pharmacological Therapy Jun 23(3): 304–310

Barron B A, Gee L, Hauck W W, Herpetic Eye Disease Study 1994 A controlled trial of oral acyclovir for herpes simplex stromal keratitis. Ophthalmology 101:1871–1882

Beck R W, Cleary P A, Backlund J C, Optic Neuritis Study Group 1994 The course of visual recovery after optic neuritis. Experience of the Optic Neuritis Treatment Trial. Ophthalmology 101:1771–1778

Beck R W, Trobe J D, Optic Neuritis Study Group 1995 The Optic Neuritis Treatment Trial: putting the results in perspective. Journal of Neuro-ophthalmology 15:131–135

Bengtsson B, Leske M C, Hyman L et al 2007 Fluctuation of intraocular pressure and glaucoma progression in the early manifest glaucoma trial. Early Manifest Glaucoma Trial Group. Ophthalmology Feb 114(2):205–209. Epub 2006 Nov 13

Bentley C R, Dawson E, Lee J P 2001 Active management in patients with ocular manifestations of myasthenia gravis. Eye 15(1):18–22

Bernardini F P 2006 Management of malignant and benign eyelid lesions. Current Opinions in Ophthalmology Oct 17(5):480–484

Bilyk J R 2007 Periocular infection. Current Opinions in Ophthalmology Sep 18(5):414–423

Bloch-Michel E, Nussenblatt R B 1987 International Uveitis Study Group recommendations for the evaluation of intraocular inflammatory disease. American Journal of Ophthalmology 103:234–235

Bron A J, Rabinowitz Y S 1996 Corneal dystrophies and keratoconus. Current Opinions in Ophthalmology Aug 7(4):71–82

Brown D M, Kaiser P K, Michels M et al 2006 ANCHOR Study Group. Ranibizumab versus verteporfin for neovascular age-related macular degeneration. New England Journal of Medicine 355(14):1432–1444

Brown M A, Kennedy L G, MacGregor A J et al 1997 Susceptibility to ankylosing spondylitis in twins: the role of genes, HLA, and the environment. Arthritis and Rheumatism Oct 40(10):1823–1828

Charles S 2001 Vitreoretinal complications of YAG laser capsulotomy. Ophthalmology Clinics of North America 14:705–709

Collaborative Normal-Tension Glaucoma Study Group 1998 Comparison of glaucomatous progression between untreated patients with normal-tension glaucoma and patients with therapeutically reduced intraocular pressures. American Journal of Ophthalmology 126:487–497

Collignon-Robe N J, Feke G T, Rizzo J F 3rd 2004 Optic nerve head circulation in nonarteritic anterior ischemic optic neuropathy and optic neuritis. Ophthalmology Sep 111(9):1663–1672

Cook B E, Bartley G B 2001 Treatment options and future prospects for the management of eyelid malignancies: an evidence-based update. Ophthalmology 108:2088–2098

D'Amico D J et al, VISION Clinical Trial Group 2006 Pegaptanib sodium for neovascular age-related macular degeneration: two year safety results of the two year prospective, multicentre, controlled clinical trials. Ophthalmology 113:992–1001

Dawson E, Bentley C, Lee J 2001 Squint surgery in the over sixties. Strabismus 9:217–220

Devgan U 2007 Surgical techniques in phacoemulsification. Current Opinions in Ophthalmology Feb 18(1):19–22

Diabetes Control and Complications Trial Research Group 1993 The effect of intensive treatment of diabetes on the development and progression of long-term complications in insulin-dependent diabetes mellitus. New England Journal of Medicine 329:977

Diabetic Retinopathy Study Research Group 1981 Photocoagulation treatment of proliferative diabetic retinopathy. Clinical application of Diabetic Retinopathy Study (DRS) findings, DRS Report Number 8. Ophthalmology 88:583

Early Treatment Diabetic Retinopathy Study Research Group 1985 Photocoagulation for diabetic macular oedema. Archives of Ophthalmology 103:1796

Early Treatment Diabetic Retinopathy Study Research Group 1991 Grading diabetic retinopathy from stereoscopic color fundus photographs – an extension of the modified Airlie House classification. ETDRS report number 10. Ophthalmology 98:786

Edelsten C, Lee V, Bentley C R et al 2002 An evaluation of baseline risk factors predicting severity in juvenile idiopathic arthritis (JIA) associated uveitis and other chronic anterior uveitis in early childhood. British Journal of Ophthalmology 86:51–56

Endophthalmitis Vitrectomy Study Group 1995 Results of the Endophthalmitis Vitrectomy Study. A randomized trial of immediate vitrectomy and of intravenous antibiotics for the treatment of postoperative bacterial endophthalmitis. Archives of Ophthalmology 113:1479–1496

Freeman C R, Farmer J-P 1998 Pediatric brain stem gliomas: a review. International Journal of Radiation Oncology Biology Physics January 40(2):265–271

Freissler K, Lang G E, Lang G K 1997 Allergic diseases of the lids, conjunctiva and cornea. Current Opinion in Ophthalmology 8 (4):25–30

Frith P, Gray R, MacLennan A H et al (eds) 2001 The eye in clinical practice, 2nd edn. Blackwell Science, London

Gimbel H V, Condon G P, Kohnen T et al 2005 Late in-the-bag intraocular lens dislocation: incidence, prevention, and management. Journal of Cataract Refractory Surgery Nov 31(11):2193–2204

Green L K, Pavan-Langston D 2006 Herpes simplex ocular inflammatory disease. International Ophthalmology Clinics Spring 46(2):27–37

Grosso A, Veglio F, Porta M et al 2005 Hypertensive retinopathy revisited: some answers, more questions. British Journal of Ophthalmology 89:1646–1654

Harding S, Greenwood R, Aldington S et al 2003 Grading and disease management in national screening for diabetic retinopathy in England and Wales. Diabetic Medicine 20:965

Hasanee K, Ahmed I I 2006 Capsular tension rings: update on endocapsular support devices. Ophthalmology Clinics of North America Dec 19(4):507–519

Hattenhauer M G, Leavitt J A, Hodge D O et al 1997 Incidence of nonarteritic anterior ischemic optic neuropathy. American Journal of Ophthalmology Jan 123(1):103–107

International Study Group for Behçet's Disease. 1990 Criteria for diagnosis of Behçet's diasease. Lancet 335:1078–1080

Ischemic Optic Neuropathy Decompression Trial Research Group 1995 Optic nerve decompression surgery for nonarteritic anterior ischemic optic neuropathy (NAION) is not effective and may be harmful. The Ischemic Optic Neuropathy Decompression Trial Research Group. Journal of the American Medical Association 273(8):625–632

Jabs D A, Rosenbaum J T, Foster C S et al 2000 Guidelines for the use of immunosuppressive drugs in patients with ocular inflammatory disorders: recommendations of an expert panel. American Journal of Ophthalmology Oct 130(4):492–513

Jabs D A, Nussenblatt R B, Rosenbaum J T, Standardization of Uveitis Nomenclature (SUN) Working Group 2005 Standardization of Uveitis Nomenclature for reporting clinical data. Results of the First International Workshop. American Journal of Ophthalmology 140:509–516

Jacobson D M 1998 Pupil involvement in patients with diabetes-associated oculomotor nerve palsy. Archives of Ophthalmology 116:723–727

Jaffe G J, Martin D, Callanan D et al, Fluocinolone Acetonide Uveitis Study Group 2006 Fluocinolone acetonide implant (Retisert) for noninfectious posterior uveitis: thirty-four-week results of a multicenter randomized clinical study. Ophthalmology Jun 113(6): 1020–1027. Epub 2006 May 9

Jones E, Clarke J, Khaw P T 2005 Recent advances in trabeculectomy technique. Current Opinions in Ophthalmology Apr 16(2):107–113

Kaya V, Karakaya M, Utine C A et al 2007 Evaluation of the corneal topographic characteristics of keratoconus with orbscan II in patients with and without atopy. Cornea Sep 26(8):945–948

Keith N M, Wagener H P, Barker N W 1939 Some different types of essential hypertension: their course and their prognosis. American Journal of Medical Science 197:332–343

Kendall-Taylor P 1998 Current management of thyroid-associated ophthalmopathy. Clinical Endocrinology 49:11–12

Kim I K, Miller J W 2002 Management of dislocated lens material. Seminars in Ophthalmology Sep–Dec 17(3–4):162–166

Klein R, Klein B E K, Linton K L P 1992 Prevalence of age-related maculopathy: the Beaver Dam Eye Study. Ophthalmology 99:933–943

Klein R J, Zeiss C, Chew E Y et al 2005 Complement factor H polymorphism in age-related macular degeneration. Science 308:385–389

Lee E T, Russell D, Morris T et al 2005 Visual impairment and eye abnormalities in Oklahoma Indians. Archives of Ophthalmology Dec 123(12):1699–1704

Lee V, Bentley C R, Lee J P 2001 Strabismus surgery in congenital third nerve palsy. Strabismus 9(2):91–99

Leibowitz H M, Krueger D E, Maunder L R et al 1980 The Framingham Eye Study monograph: an ophthalmological and epidemiological study of cataract, glaucoma, diabetic retinopathy, macular degeneration, and visual acuity in a general population of 2631 adults, 1973–1975. Survey of Ophthalmology May–Jun 24(Suppl):335–610

Lewis H 2003 Peripheral retinal degenerations and the risk of retinal detachment. American Journal of Ophthalmology 136:155–160

Leyland M D, Langan L, Goolfee F et al 2002 Prospective randomised double-masked trial of bilateral multifocal, bifocal or monofocal intraocular lenses. Eye Jul 16(4):481–490

Liesegang T J 2008 Herpes zoster ophthalmicus natural history, risk factors, clinical presentation, and morbidity. Ophthalmology Feb 115(2 Suppl):S3–S12

Lovell D J, Giannini E H, Reiff A et al 2000 Etanercept in children with polyarticular juvenile rheumatoid arthritis. Pediatric Rheumatology Collaborative Study Group. New England Journal of Medicine Mar 342(11):763–769

Macular Photocoagulation Study Group 1986 Argon laser photocoagulation for neovascular maculopathy. Three year results from randomised clinical trials. Archives of Ophthalmology 104:694–701

Manners T 1997 Managing eye conditions in general practice. British Medical Journal 315(7111):816–817

Mayer E, Herdman G, Burnett C et al 2001 Serial STIR magnetic resonance imaging correlates with clinical activity score in thyroid eye disease. Eye 15:313–318

Migdal C 1995 What is the appropriate treatment for patients with primary open-angle glaucoma: medicine, laser or primary surgery? Ophthalmic Surgery 26(2):108–110

Mitchell P, Smith W, Attebo K et al 1995 Prevalence of age-related maculopathy in Australia. The Blue Mountains Eye Study. Ophthalmology 102:1450–1460

Mourits M P, Prummel M F, Wiersinga W M et al 1997 Clinical Activity Score as a guide in the management of patients with Graves' ophthalmopathy. Clinical Endocrinology (Oxford) 47(1):9–14

Nadeau S E, Trobe J D 1983 Pupil sparing in oculomotor palsy: a brief review. Annals of Neurology 13(2):143–148

NICE. 2002 Management of type 2 diabetes retinopathy – screening and early management (NICE guideline). Inherited clinical guideline E. National Institute for Health and Clinical Excellence, London, www.nice.org.uk

Nouri-Mahdavi K, Hoffman D, Coleman A L et al 2004 Predictive factors for glaucomatous visual field progression in the Advanced Glaucoma Intervention Study. Ophthalmology 111(9):1627–1635

Owen C G, Shah A, Henshaw K et al 2004 Topical treatments for seasonal allergic conjunctivitis: systematic review and meta-analysis of efficacy and effectiveness. British Journal of General Practice 54(503):451–456

Peters G B III, Bakri S J, Krohel B G 2002 Cause and prognosis of nontraumatic sixth nerve palsies in young adults. Ophthalmology October 109(10):1925–1928

Quigley H A, Enger C, Katz J et al 1994 Risk factors in the development of glaucomatous field loss in ocular hypertension. Archives of Ophthalmology 112:644–649

Ray S, D'Amico D J 2002 Pseudophakic cystoid macular edema. Seminars in Ophthalmology Sep–Dec 17(3–4):167–180

Reus N J, Lemij H G 2005 Relationships between standard automated perimetry, HRT confocal scanning laser ophthalmoscopy, and GDx VCC scanning laser polarimetry. Investigative Ophthalmology and Visual Science Nov 46(11):4182–4188

Richman D P, Agius M A 2003 Treatment of autoimmune myasthenia gravis. Neurology Dec 61(12):1652–1661

Riordan-Eva P, Lee J P 1992 Management of VIth nerve palsy – avoiding unnecessary surgery. Eye 6:386–390

Rivero A, Crovetto L, Lopez L et al 1995 Single fiber electromyography of extraocular muscles: a sensitive method for the diagnosis of ocular myasthenia gravis. Muscle Nerve 18:943

Rosenfeld P J, Brown D M, Heier J S et al, MARINA Study Group 2006 Ranibizumab for neovascular age-related macular degeneration. New England Journal of Medicine Oct 355(14):1419–1431

Rudnicka A, Owen C G 2007 Epidemiology of primary open angle glaucoma. In: Edgar D, Rudnicka A (eds) Glaucoma identification and co-management. Butterworth Heineman, London, pp 1–16

Ruiz-Moreno J M, Pérez-Santonja J J, Alió J L 1999 Retinal detachment in myopic eyes after laser in situ keratomileusis. American Journal of Ophthalmology 128:588–594

Rundle F F 1964 Eye signs of Graves' disease. In: Pitt-Rivers R, Trotter WR et al (eds) The thyroid gland, vol 2. Butterworths, London, pp 171

Schwinn D A, Afshari N A 2006 Alpha(1)-adrenergic receptor antagonists and the iris: new mechanistic insights into floppy iris syndrome. Surveys in Ophthalmology Sep–Oct 51(5):501–512

Severson E A, Baratz K H, Hodge D O et al 2003 Herpes zoster ophthalmicus in Olmsted county, Minnesota: have systemic antivirals made a difference? Archives of Ophthalmology Mar 121(3):386–390

Shah N N, Bowd C, Medeiros F A et al 2006 Combining structural and functional testing for detection of glaucoma. Ophthalmology Sep 113(9):1593–1602

Sheard R M, Goodburn S F, Comer M B et al 2003 Posterior vitreous detachment after neodymium: YAG laser posterior capsulotomy. Journal of Cataract and Refractory Surgery 29:930–934

Sheikh A, Hurwitz B 2006 Antibiotics versus placebo for acute bacterial conjunctivitis. Cochrane Database of Systematic Reviews Issue 2. Art. No.: CD001211. DOI: 10.1002/14651858.CD001211.pub2

Shields J A, Shields C L 2007 Intraocular tumors: an atlas and textbook, 2nd edn. Lippincott Williams & Wilkins, Philadelphia

Simons B D, Saunders T G, Siatkowski R M et al 1998 Outcome of surgical management of superior oblique palsy: a study of 123 cases. Binocular Vision and Strabismus Quarterly 13(4):273–282

Steel D H, Potts M J 1999 Thyroid eye disease. In: Easty D (ed.) Text book of ophthalmology. Oxford University Press, Oxford, pp 722–730

Stein J D, Challa P 2007 Mechanisms of action and efficacy of argon laser trabeculoplasty and selective laser trabeculoplasty. Current Opinions in Ophthalmology Mar 18(2):140–145

Suzuki L A, Rocha R J, Rossi C L 2001 Evaluation of serological markers for the immunodiagnosis of acute acquired toxoplasmosis. Journal of Medical Microbiology Jan 50(1):62–70

Tan D T, Por Y M 2007 Current treatment options for corneal ectasia. Current Opinions in Ophthalmology Jul 18(4):284–289

Thylefores B, Negrel A D 1994 The global impact of glaucoma. Bulletin of the World Health Organization 3:323–326

Tielsch J M, Sommer A, Katz J et al 1991 Racial variations in the prevalence of primary open angle glaucoma. The Baltimore Eye Study. Journal of the American Medical Association 266:369–374

Tollefson M M, Mohney B G, Diehl N N et al 2006 Incidence and types of childhood hypertropia: a population-based study. Ophthalmology Jul 113(7):1142–1145. Epub 2006 Apr 27

Treatment of Age-Related Macular Degeneration with Photodynamic Therapy (TAP) Study Group 2001 Photodynamic therapy of subfoveal choroidal neovascularisation in age related macular degeneration with verteporfin: two-year results of 2 randomised clinical trials – TAP report 2. Archives of Ophthalmology 119:198–207

UK Prospective Diabetes Study Group 1998 Tight blood pressure control and risk of macrovascular and microvascular complications in type 2 diabetes: UKPDS 38. British Medical Journal 317:703

Vernon S A, Koppens J M, Menon G J et al 2006 Diode laser cycloablation in adult glaucoma: long-term results of a standard protocol and review of current literature. Clinical and Experimental Ophthalmology Jul 34(5):411–420

Vincent A, Newsom-Davis J 1985 Acetylcholine receptor antibody as a diagnostic test for myasthenia gravis: results in 153 validated cases and 2067 diagnostic assays. Journal of Neurology Neurosurgery and Psychiatry 48:1246

Vingerling J R, Dielemans I, Hofman A et al 1995 The prevalence of age-related maculopathy in the Rotterdam study. Ophthalmology 102:205–210

Weetman A, Wiersinga W M M 1998 Current management of thyroid-associated ophthalmopathy in Europe. Results of an international survey. Clinical Endocrinology 49:21–28

Wilhelmus K R 2007 Therapeutic interventions for herpes simplex virus epithelial keratitis. Cochrane Database of Systematic Reviews Issue 1. Art. No.: CD002898. DOI: 10.1002/14651858.CD002898.pub2

Wilhelmus K R, Gee L, Hauck W W 1994 Herpetic Eye Disease Study: a controlled trial of topical corticosteroids for herpes simplex stromal keratitis. Ophthalmology 101:1883–1896

Wong T Y, Tielsch J M, Schein O D 1999 Racial difference in the incidence of retinal detachment in Singapore. Archives of Ophthalmology Mar 117(3):379–383

Wong T Y, Klein R, Nieto F J et al 2003 Retinal microvascular abnormalities and ten-year cardiovascular mortality. A population-based case-control study. Ophthalmology 110:933–940

Woodruff G, Buncic J R, Morin J D 1988 Horner syndrome in children. Journal of Pediatric Ophthalmology and Strabismus 25:41–44

Wu L, Martínez-Castellanos M A, Quiroz-Mercado H et al 2008 Twelve-month safety of intravitreal injections of bevacizumab (Avastin(R)): results of the Pan-American Collaborative Retina Study Group (PACORES). Graefe's Archives of Clinical and Experimental Ophthalmology Jan 246(1):81–87. Epub 2007 Aug 3

CHAPTER 11

The development of refractive error

Nicola Logan

Introduction

Before optometrists can manage refractive error they must first understand the optical and structural development of the eye in order to identify the nature of normal refractive development and its aetiology. This chapter describes the ocular components in terms of their growth during infancy through to adulthood and how changes in the ocular components relate to refractive error development. Myopia is the most common refractive error encountered in optometric practice and therefore further attention is given to the development of myopia, discussion of its aetiology and possible associations.

Emmetropia in the human eye is dependent upon the optimum correlation between the radii of curvature of the cornea and the crystalline lens surfaces, the refractive indices of the ocular media, the anterior and vitreous chamber depths and the crystalline lens thickness. As the eye grows it must, in order to remain emmetropic, maintain a coordinated relationship between these components, so that the focal length of the optics is conjugate with the axial length of the eye. Any discrepancy between coordination of the ocular components results in a refractive error (Sorsby et al 1957; Sorsby & Leary 1970; Edwards 1998).

The refractive error of the eye is an anomaly of the refractive state in which, in the absence of accommodation, the image of objects at infinity is not formed on the retina. Myopia exists if the image falls in front of the retina and hyperopia occurs when the image falls behind the retina. The eye is deemed emmetropic when the image of an object at infinity falls on the retina. **Figure 11.1** shows the classical depiction of an emmetropic and a myopic eye.

The majority of infants are born with significant refractive errors. However, these refractive errors generally disappear with development. This process of reduction of refractive error is termed emmetropization, and while at least part of the refractive changes can be explained as an optical consequence of normal development as the eye enlarges, there is now convincing evidence from animal studies that eye growth is actively regulated and vision dependent (Wildsoet,1998). Specifically, emmetropization is dependent on normal visual experience, and if this is impeded, refractive error will result.

Refractive error

It has long been recognized that infants, on average, are hyperopic, and that the hyperopia decreases gradually during infancy and early childhood. These changes in normal refractive error, or emmetropization, are presumed to reflect finely regulated eye growth, controlled at least in part by the retina. Studies of early refractive development have shown the average newborn infant to be hyperopic with a mean refractive error of around $+2$ D (SD±2 D). A rapid decline in hyperopia occurs between 6 months and 2 years of age in normally developing eyes. A further, more gradual, decrease towards emmetropia is then seen up until the age of 6 years (**Fig.11.2**). This process of emmetropization has been described as

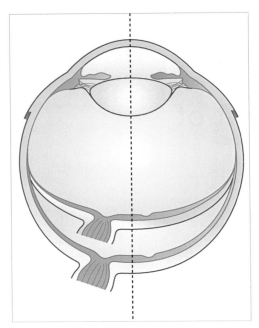

Figure 11.1 Classical depiction of an emmetropic eye and the larger, myopic eye. (From Heine 1899 Beitrage zur Anatrine des myopischen Auges. Archives Augenheilkd 38: 277.)

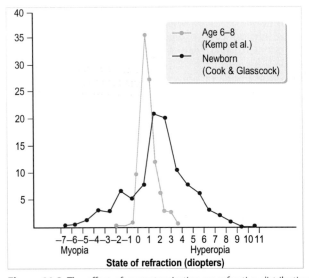

Figure 11.2 The effect of emmetropization on refractive distribution from birth to the age of 6 to 8 years. (Redrawn from Hirsch and Weymouth 1991.)

operating to produce a greater frequency of emmetropic eyes than would otherwise occur on the basis of chance. This mechanism coordinates the development of the optical system's various components to prevent ametropia.

Growth of the ocular components

The cornea

Research has indicated that the majority of corneal growth occurs prenatally (Scammon & Wilmer 1950) and nearly all postnatal growth has been found to occur within the first few years of life (Sorsby et al 1961). The cornea of the neonate is generally assumed to be 3 to 5 D steeper than that of a child. The mean corneal radius of curvature for 19 infants aged 3 to 18 months has been reported to be 7.76 mm (43.5 D), with a range from 7.35 to 8.46 mm (Wood et al 1996). This finding is in conflict with another report which recorded steeper corneal powers in 22 infants with a gestational age of 37–43 weeks in whom the mean corneal power was 7.05 mm (range 6.63–7.74 mm) (Inagaki et al 1985).

Cross-sectional results from a longitudinal study of myopia were reported by Zadnik et al (2003). In a large cohort of 2583 children, the researchers found that the corneal power did not change with age; mean corneal power was 43.767 D at 6 years of age and 43.37 D at 14 years of age.

A longitudinal study (which has the advantage of assessing intra-individual variations over time) of ophthalmic changes in 67 full-term subjects from 10 to 18 years of age found no significant change in corneal radius over this period (Fledelius 1982). The average value of corneal radius for the 36 male subjects was 7.93±0.27 mm for the 10-year-olds and 7.95±0.27 mm for the 18-year-olds. At both ages the range of corneal radius was 7.5 to 8.5 mm.

The investigations suggest that adult values of corneal radius are reached by the age of 3 years and remain relatively stable throughout life. Consequently, the crystalline lens was thought to succeed the cornea as the compensatory mechanism to maintain emmetropia in a growing eye. However, recent evidence has suggested that although the cornea does flatten during infancy (for infants between 3 and 9 months of age), it does so at a lower rate than the lens (Mutti et al 2005). Other studies have shown a longitudinal flattening of the cornea until late teenage years (Friedman et al 1996), although at a much slower rate than during the first 2 years of life.

Whether the cornea differs in power with refractive error is equivocal. Some studies have found that in myopes the cornea was more powerful and steeper compared with that in emmetropes (Goss et al 1997; Jones et al 2005), whereas other studies have observed the cornea in myopes to be both flatter and thinner than in emmetropes (Chang et al 2001). Although the data remain equivocal it is generally accepted that the cornea plays a relatively minor role in offsetting axial elongation compared to the crystalline lens.

The crystalline lens

The decrease in ocular power that occurs during the first year of life cannot be accounted for by the changes in axial length and corneal curvature. The crystalline lens must therefore contribute to the decrease in overall power of the eye.

Although the crystalline lens continues to grow throughout life, studies in children have shown a sagittal thinning of the lens during emmetropization (Brown et al 1999), explained by the observation that as the eyeball expands, it stretches the lens in an equatorial plane, making it thinner and thereby reducing its dioptric power (Mutti et al 1998;

Brown et al 1999). Values for a calculated equivalent refractive index within the lens have also been shown to decrease with age (Mutti et al 1998), leading to a loss of lens power. It is thought that the lens is the primary compensative component to axial elongation and becomes less powerful (Gernet 1981) and thinner with age to maintain a sharp image on the retina via either a passive (Mutti et al 2005) or an active feedback system (Garner et al 1992). In children, lens thinning has been shown to offset normal ocular elongation up to the age of 9–10 years (Zadnik et al 2004; Jones et al 2005) and has been found to follow temporally the growth in axial length (Mutti et al 2005) as a compensatory adjustment to maintain emmetropia. Myopia occurs once the compensatory lens flattening can no longer offset the growth in axial length and the eye becomes too long for light to focus on the retina (Garner et al 1992; Mutti et al 2005). Any supposed flattening of the lens may be an incomplete attempt to compensate for an increased axial length as the eye progresses to myopia (Wildsoet 1998).

In adults, the crystalline lens increases in thickness and the surfaces become steeper (Brown 1974; Koretz et al 1989). Theoretically, these changes would incur a myopic shift in the older eye. The fact that the majority of these ageing eyes do not become more myopic suggests a compensatory mechanism is involved. Those adults who do develop myopia typically have a corresponding increase in axial length of the eye (Hemenger et al 1995; McBrien & Adams 1997). Age-related changes in the refractive index distribution of the human ocular lens have been calculated using a gradient index parameter for two age groups using biometric data and a gradient index model of the lens (Hemenger et al 1995). For the older cohort (49 to 61 years) the gradient index was found to be flatter near the lens centre and steeper towards the lens surface than that for the younger age group (19 to 31 years). The researchers concluded that in the crystalline lens, the variations in gradient index compensated for the changes in surface curvatures and thickness that occur with age.

The anterior chamber depth

Cross-sectional studies have shown that the anterior chamber depth (ACD) increases from birth to adolescence while the eye is growing. Larsen (1971) measured ACD using ultrasound on 80 neonates and 846 children aged 6 months to 13 years. He reported that the ACD increased 0.9–1.0 mm from birth to 1.5 years, 0.3–0.4 mm from the age of 1 to 7 years and almost 0.1 mm from 8 to 13 years. Several studies have shown that the anterior chamber has normally reached its maximum depth by approximately 15 years of age (Sorsby et al 1961; Sorsby & Leary 1970; Larsen 1971). Few changes have been recorded in the ACD from adolescence to about 30 years of age. From 30 years of age onwards, a monotonic decrease in ACD has been found to occur as crystalline lens fibres are continually added (Weale 1982). Typical values for anterior chamber depth are 3 to 4 mm.

The effects of changes in ACD on refractive error have been investigated by calculating these effects using a schematic eye (Goss & Erickson 1990). Typical changes in ACD in the human eye were found to be approximately 0.1 mm in magnitude. Changing the ACD by this amount in the schematic eye produced small changes in refractive error

(<0.2 D). The findings suggest that the ACD does not appear to be a major contributing factor in the development of refractive error.

The axial length

The eye grows rapidly in early childhood with an increase in axial length from approximately 18 mm at birth to 23 mm by the age of 3 years (Sorsby et al 1961). Based on visual optics principles, a 1 mm increase in axial length is known to correlate with a myopic shift of approximately 2 to 3 D (Erickson 1991). According to Sorsby and colleagues, growth of the eye during infancy incurs a change in axial length of 5 mm; theoretically, this increase in axial length would induce 10 to 15 D of myopia (Sorsby et al 1961). This degree of myopic shift is not observed in normal development, suggesting that a compensatory mechanism by the other ocular components exists, such as thinning of the crystalline lens and corneal flattening.

The average axial length of the adult eye is approximately 24 mm. This suggests that the eye grows only 1 mm from the age of 3 to around 13 years of age. It is interesting that this relatively slow phase of ocular growth coincides with the period of maximum body growth. Irrespective of the initial refractive error, the effect of this ocular growth along the axial dimension on refractive error is normally countered by a compensatory change in corneal and/or lenticular power, such that the ocular refraction progresses towards emmetropia. However, it is the growth of the axial length, specifically the vitreous chamber depth, that is thought to be the primary structural correlate driving myopia (Gernet 1981; McBrien & Adams 1997). Work by Jones and colleagues showing the longitudinal growth of ocular components between the ages of 6 and 14 years demonstrated an increase in axial growth, specifically in the vitreous chamber depth, in myopes whilst the growth rates in other refractive groups slowed, most noticeably after the age of 10 years (Jones et al 2005). In addition, it has recently been reported that the eye experiences an accelerated ocular growth in the year preceding myopia onset (Mutti et al 2007), which immediately decelerates once myopia is manifest. It is evident that ocular growth is not monotonic but rather a multistage process.

Prevalence of refractive errors in children

Estimates of prevalence depend on the definition of the disease or disorder, on the study population, especially with regard to ethnicity, and on the measurement methods. Consequently, study of the prevalence of refractive error reveals a wide variation in figures reported in the published literature. In refractive error research in particular the lack of standard definitions makes comparisons between different studies difficult. For example, hyperopia may be defined as greater than or equal to +2.00 D in one study whereas in another a definition of greater than or equal to +0.50 D may be used (Ojaimi et al 2005b). The refractive error data has been summarized in **Table 11.1**. In addressing the lack of representative and comparative data, a series of population-based surveys of refractive error and visual impairment in school-aged children was initiated, beginning in 1998 and adhering to the same protocol. These Refractive Error

Table 11.1 Selection of recent studies on the prevalence of myopia and hyperopia in children and young adolescents

Country	n	Age (years)	Prevalence of myopia		Prevalence of hyperopia	
			Criteria	%	Criteria	%
UK[1]	7600	7	<-1.00 D	1.1	$>+2.00$ D	5.9
			≤-0.50 D	13.6		
Sweden[2]	1045	12–13	≤-0.50 D	45	$\geq+1.00$ D	8.4
USA[3]	2583	6–14	≤-0.75 D	10.1	$\geq+1.25$ D	8.6
USA[4]	2523	5–17	≤-0.75 D	9.2	$\geq+1.25$ D	12.8
African-American	534			6.6		6.4
Asian	491			18.5		6.3
Hispanic	463			13.2		12.7
White	1035			4.4		19.3
Australia[5]	1765	6	<-0.50 D	1.43	$\geq+0.50$ D	91.0
Australia[6]	2353	12	<-0.50 D	11.9	$>+2.00$ D	3.5
Hong Kong[7]	7560	5–16	≤-0.50 D	36.7	$\geq+2.00$ D	4.0
Singapore[8]	1453	7	≤-0.50 D	29.0	Data not reported	
		8	≤-0.50 D	34.7		
		9	≤-0.50 D	53.1		
Hong Kong[9]					Data not reported	
Local school	335	13–15	≤-0.50 D	85–88		
International school	789	13–15	≤-0.50 D	43	in non-Chinese	
				65	in mixed Chinese	
				80	in Chinese	

[1]Barnes et al 2001; [2]Villarreal et al 2003; [3]Zadnik et al 2003; [4]Kleinstein et al 2003; [5]Ip et al 2007; [6]Ojaimi et al 2005a; [7]Fan et al 2004; [8]Saw et al 2002a; [9]Lam et al 2002
After Gilmartin 2004 with the permission of Blackwell Publishing.

Study in Children (RESC) surveys were conducted in populations with different ethnic origins and environments. Data from these studies are summarized in **Table 11.2**.

Refractive error changes throughout the lifetime of an individual and these changes depend in part on age. In newborn infants refractive error has a wide distribution with myopia being present in approximately 19% of Caucasian infants and hyperopia in 74% (Cook & Glassock 1951; Banks 1980; Hirsch & Weymouth 1991). The high prevalence of hyperopia in infants is also accompanied by a high prevalence of astigmatism (Atkinson et al 1980; Fulton et al 1980; Gwiazda et al 1984). However, the distribution of the

Table 11.2 Studies on the prevalence of myopia in children (<-0.50 D spherical equivalent cycloplegic autorefraction in either eye) using the Refractive Error Study in Children sampling and measurement protocols (Negrel et al 2000)

Country	Region	Sample size	Myopia prevalence (%; [95% CI])	
			5 years	15 years
China[1]	Shunyi District (rural)	5884	M + F: 0.0	M: 36.7 [29.9–43.4] F: 55.0 [49.4–60.6]
Nepal[2]	Mechi Zone (rural)	5067	M + F: ≈ 0.5	M: ≈ 2.9; F: ≈ 1.0*
Chile[3]	La Florida (suburban)	5303	M + F: 3.4 [1.72–5.05]	M: 19.4 [13.6–25.2] F: 14.7 [10.1–19.2]
India[4]	Andra Pradesh (rural)	4074	M + F: 2.80 [1.28–4.33]	M + F: 6.72 [4.31–9.12]
India[5]	New Delhi (urban)	6447	M + F: 4.86 [2.54–6.83]	M + F: 10.80 [6.71–14.80]
South Africa[6]	Durban (metropolitan)	4890	M + F: 3.2 [0.6–5.7]	M + F: 9.60 [6.4–12.7]
China[7]	Guangzhou (urban)	4363	M + F: 3.3 [0.4–6.3]	M + F: 73.1 [68.0–78.2]
Malaysia[8]	Gombok district (urban)	4634	M + F: 10.0 [6.8–13.1]**	M + F: 32.5 [25.5–39.6]

[1]Zhao et al 2000; [2]Pokharel et al 2000; [3]Maul et al 2000; [4]Dandona et al 2002; [5]Murthy et al 2002; [6]Naidoo et al 2003; [7]He et al 2004; [8]Goh et al 2005
M, male; F, female; *Extrapolated data; **no data for 5 years of age, data at 7 years of age.
After Gilmartin 2004 with the permission of Blackwell Publishing.

refractive status of the infant does not appear to differ significantly between races or geographical locations (Fulton et al 1980; Edwards 1991). As refractive error development depends, in part, on visual feedback (Smith & Hung 1999), it is not surprising that there is little variation in infant refraction across races, as generally there is little variation in the near world of an infant. The refractive error in premature infants differs from that of full-term infants, with a higher frequency and magnitude of myopia demonstrated in premature infants; 39% of pre-term infants are myopic at birth compared with 17.5% of full-term infants (Dobson et al 1981; Saunders et al 2002). The mean spherical equivalent of pre-term infants has been found to be more myopic than full-term infants (Dobson et al 1981).

Emmetropization

The hyperopia seen in infants gradually decreases during infancy and early childhood (Mayer et al 2001). As previously mentioned, this relative myopic shift is presumed to reflect finely regulated eye growth and the processes involved are termed emmetropization. In preschool children, emmetropization is thought to reduce the level of refractive error, with the prevalence of myopia reducing from approximately 19% to 2–3% (for Caucasian children), but by the age of 6 years the prevalence of myopia rises to approximately 6% with the majority of the children being hyperopic (Robinson 1999; Junghans et al 2002; Zadnik et al 2002). However, a very low prevalence of myopia (approximately 1.5%) has been reported recently in 6-year-old Australian children (Ojaimi et al 2005a). The high prevalence of astigmatism that is seen in infants is greatly reduced or eliminated by 4 years of age (Gwiazda et al 1984). Myopia is the only type of refractive error that commonly develops during school age (Goss & Winkler 1983). Therefore, by the time these Caucasian children become young adults approximately 25% will have developed myopia (Sperduto et al 1983). High levels of myopia (greater than 5 D) in young children (less than 10 years of age) may indicate an associated systemic or ocular disorder, with myopia often being the first presenting symptom (Marr et al 2001; Logan et al 2004).

One possibility when examining a young hyperopic patient is that emmetropization may still be active. The optometrist may consider monitoring whether the child will grow out of the hyperopia before deciding on whether or not to prescribe (see Ch. 28). However, data from several studies suggest that this may not be an effective strategy as the time course of emmetropization is rapid (Mayer et al 2001; Pennie et al 2001; Mutti et al 2005).

The majority of refractive error change appears to take place in the first year of life, with substantial refraction change after this period much less likely. This pattern of refractive change can be seen in Berkeley Infant Biometry Study (BIBS) longitudinal data (Mutti et al 2005) and in cross-sectional data (Mayer et al 2001). There is a significant loss of hyperopia and decrease in the variability of refractive error between 3 and 9–12 months of age, with subsequent minor change up to at least 3 years of age (Mutti et al 2005). Emmetropization shows the expected bidirectional behaviour, i.e. a loss of hyperopia for most infants, with a few recovering from low myopic refractive errors (Ehrlich et al 1994; Saunders et al 1995). Most infants' refractive error is in the range of plano to +3.00 D by the age of 18 months. One of the reasons for rapid emmetropization is the concurrent rapid growth of the eye during that period. Between 3 and 9 months of age, the average infant eye increases in axial length by 1.20±0.51 mm and decreases in lens power by 3.62±2.13 D to reach values that are 90% of the average axial length and 155% of the average lens power of a child at 6 years of age (Mutti et al 2005).

Development of ametropia

Ametropia is generally believed to develop when there is a failure in the emmetropization process. An anomaly in the correlation of the ocular components will result in refractive error. Sorsby et al (1957) found that the majority of refractions within the range of +6 to −4 D showed values for individual components that were within the range seen in emmetropia. They described these refractive errors as correlation ametropias as they believed that it was a failure in the correlation between the components that produced the ametropia. In high refractive errors, the value of one component was found to fall outside the emmetropic range. This anomalous component was usually axial length and the degree of ametropia was found to correspond with the anomaly in axial length. This group of refractive errors was termed component ametropias.

Development of myopia

Myopia develops when either an increase in axial length is not compensated by a decrease in corneal power or the crystalline lens power is too great for the cornea and axial length correlation. The dioptric error in myopia has been found to be consistently related to an increase in axial length or, more specifically, the vitreous chamber depth (Erickson 1991). In contrast to the large decrease in ocular power that occurs during the first year of life, myopia usually develops during a period of relatively slower ocular growth, the prevalence of myopia increasing substantially from when children enter school to around 15 years of age (see **Table 11.2**).

Population studies of prevalence of refractive error

In the United Kingdom it is over 40 years since comprehensive data on refractive error in children has been collected (Sorsby et al 1961) and the data for the prevalence of refractive error in the UK is extrapolated principally from the findings in the USA, Scandinavia and Australia. However, as part of an ongoing study in the UK, the refractive error of 7600 children aged 7 years was obtained (Barnes et al 2001). The Avon Longitudinal Study of Parents and Children, based at Bristol University, enrolled 14 541 mothers during pregnancy in 1991–2 and has monitored the medical history of the children and parents ever since. In this birth cohort of children aged 7 years a prevalence of 1.1% for myopia less than −1.00 D was found, while hyperopia greater than +2.00 D was observed in 5.9% of the children. However, as the refraction data was obtained without cycloplegia and measured using an autorefractor, this is likely to overestimate the prevalence of myopia and underestimate the prevalence of hyperopia. Of note was the finding that 13.4% of the myopic children and 28.9% of the hyperopes did not have spectacles. In a survey of a birth cohort in one health district of the UK, 5.1% of the children were diagnosed, between the ages of 2 and 5 years, as having an ocular and/or vision defect (Stayte et al 1993). The vision defect in 2.1% of these children was attributable to refractive error which required correction with spectacles. In a retrospective study to examine the number of children referred with ocular defects to a hospital orthoptic service, an ocular or visual defect was found in 8.9% of 6-year-old children (Kendall et al 1989). The prevalence of refractive error was 6.5% with the majority being hyperopic (5.7%) and only a few were myopic (0.8%). However, the criteria used to define myopia and hyperopia were not reported. An ongoing study at Aston University is investigating the prevalence of refractive errors in a large, multi-ethnic population in Birmingham, specifically to look at differences in refraction with age and ethnicity. Interim data show that approximately 1 in 10 of 12-year-old children and 1 in 20 of 6-year-old children require but currently do not have the provision of spectacles (Logan et al 2007).

A study in Australia has investigated the prevalence of myopia in a large, representative sample of Sydney schoolchildren aged 6 and 12 years of age (Ojaimi et al 2005a; Ip et al 2007). The prevalence of myopia in 6-year-old Australian children was found to be very low by international standards for all the major ethnic groups (European, Caucasian, East Asian and South Asian), but that children from those communities that place heavy emphasis on education, such as East Asian and South Asian, develop more myopia. Myopia (spherical equivalent (SE) −0.50 D or less) was found in 11.9% and moderate hyperopia (SE +2.00 D) in 3.5% of the 12-year-old cohort. For the younger cohort, myopia (SE −0.50 D or less) was found in 1.43% and hyperopia (SE +0.50 D) in 91%. The results suggest that the Australian environment and lifestyle may to some extent protect from myopia, but that environmental risk factors such as frequent near work and education may still be effective.

In Sweden, a comprehensive nationwide screening programme for both ocular disease and visual dysfunction has been in operation for over 20 years and has provided detailed information on the prevalence of refractive error and other visual dysfunctions in children. In 12–13-year-old Swedish children, a prevalence of 45% for myopia (−0.50 D or more) was recorded, with hyperopia (+1 D or more) occurring in 8.4% of the 1045 children (Villarreal et al 2003). However, the high level of myopia found in this study may not indicate the true prevalence, as the participation rate was only 67%.

Photorefraction data from 14 000 US primary school children (age 3 to 8 years) indicated that 4.6% displayed significant anomalies, consisting of hyperopia ≥2.5 D, myopia ≥1.0 D, anisometropia ≥1.0 D, media opacities and ocular misalignment ≥10Δ (Morgan & Kennemer 1997). Another 6.7% had findings that were possibly significant; that is, the anomaly was present but the magnitude narrowly missed the level deemed significant. The most common refractive error was myopia, seen in 4.5% of the children, with 2.9% hyperopic. The proportion of children with hyperopia varies by sample, ethnicity, and by level of hyperopia. In a slightly older cohort of schoolchildren, aged 5 to 17 years, from four ethnic groups, 9.2% were found to be myopic (0.75 D or more) and 12.8% were hyperopic (+1.25 D) (Kleinstein et al 2003). Significant differences in the prevalence of refractive errors were found between the ethnic groups.

Variation of refractive errors with ethnicity

Ethnicity is a factor likely to affect the ocular characteristics within various populations. The prevalence of refractive error varies considerably with ethnicity; this is most evident in the data for the prevalence of myopia, with much higher values reported for Chinese (Lam et al 2002), Japanese (Matsumura & Hirai 1999) and Singaporean (Saw et al 2002a) populations. For example, the prevalence of myopia in Hong Kong for 6-year-old children is 30% (Lam & Goh 1991) compared with a prevalence of myopia of 4% for a similar age group in San Francisco (Zadnik et al 1993). In Asian populations the prevalence of myopia increases rapidly with age; 30% of 6–7-year-old Chinese children and up to 70% of 16–17-year-old Chinese males are myopic (Lam & Goh 1991). Similarly, 15–20% of Japanese 7-year-olds are myopic and a prevalence of 66% has been observed in Japanese 17-year-olds (Matsumura & Hirai 1999). Other Chinese population studies have also recorded a high prevalence of myopia; values of 11.8% for 6-year-old Taiwanese children have been noted (Lin et al 1996b), and this prevalence was found to increase to 55.5% by the age of 12 and to 75.9% at 15 years of age. In Taiwanese medical students aged 18–21 years, 92.8% were myopic (>0.25 D).

The prevalence of refractive error using non-cycloplegic refraction was investigated in 946 Singapore adolescents aged 15 to 19 years (Quek et al 2004). Whereas the prevalence of myopia (spherical equivalent of −0.50 D or more) reported was high at 73.9%, the prevalence of hyperopia (spherical equivalent of +0.50 D) was found to be only 1.5%; that of anisometropia was 11.2% for a spherical error difference of at least 1 D and 2.7% for a spherical error difference of at least 2 D. In contrast, anisometropia ≥2 D in Caucasian populations has a prevalence of around 1.5%. (Logan et al 2004). Of interest is that the ethnicity-specific prevalence of myopia in Malays, Chinese and Indians living in Singapore is higher than that in Malaysian Malays, Chinese and Indians (Saw et al 2006). As Malays, Chinese and Indians in Malaysia have genetic make-up similar to that of Malays, Chinese and Indians in Singapore, the researchers suggested that differences in environmental factors may contribute to the higher myopia rates.

However, not all Asian populations have a high prevalence of myopia. In Tibet and Melanesia the prevalence of myopia in children has been found to be much lower than that in Hong Kong, Japan and Taiwan. In Tibetan children aged 6 to 16 years, a prevalence of myopia of 3.9% has been reported (Garner et al 1995), with a similar finding in Melanesian children (Garner et al 1985). Epidemiological studies on remote populations in Arctic regions have revealed an inordinately high increase in myopia prevalence in the present generation compared to previous generations (Johnson 1988). Both a change to a more Westernized diet and the introduction of more formal schooling have been implicated as causations in the increased prevalence of myopia (Cordain et al 2002).

Ocular biometry: age, gender and ethnicity

Refractive error and ocular components in a large group of US children aged 6 to 14 years has been described as a function of age and gender (Zadnik et al 1993). Of these 2583 children, 10.1% were myopic (−0.75 D or more in both meridians) and 8.6% were hyperopic (+1.25 D or more in both meridians). No significant difference in mean refractive error between boys and girls was found. As expected, the authors found a significant effect of age on refractive error, with the younger children more hyperopic than the older children; similar findings were reported in the Australian study on epidemiology of myopia (Ip et al 2007). The most rapid changes in the ocular components were found to take place between 6 and 9 years of age. Additionally, this study on US schoolchildren investigated racial variations in refractive error (Kleinstein et al 2003). The investigation was a multicentre, longitudinal, observational study of refractive error and ocular development in children from four ethnic groups. The study population included 2523 children, of which 534 were African-American, 491 Asian, 463 Hispanic and 1035 white, all were aged 5–17 years. Myopia was defined as −0.75 D or more and hyperopia as +1.25 D or more in each principal meridian and the refractive error was assessed by cycloplegic refraction. As expected, Asians had the highest prevalence of myopia (18.5%) followed by Hispanics (13.2%). Whites had the lowest prevalence of myopia (4.4%), which was not significantly different from African-Americans (6.6%). Whites had the highest prevalence of hyperopia (19.3%), followed by Hispanics (12.7%). Asians had the lowest prevalence of hyperopia (6.3%), which was not significantly different from African-Americans (6.4%).

Myopia progression

Progression of myopia is influenced by a variety of factors such as age of onset, ethnicity, sex and visual environment (Zadnik et al 2004). One important question is whether myopia prevalence in Europe, Australia and the USA will increase to levels similar to those currently seen in East Asia (Rose et al 2003). Identification of factors that affect the rate of progression of myopia would further increase our understanding of myopia development and may facilitate advancement in the amelioration of myopia.

Myopia progression in children

Progression of myopia has been found to vary with age, with myopia progressing more rapidly in younger children (Parssinen & Lyyra 1993; Fulk et al 2000). Myopia progression has been found to be approximately 0.50 D per annum in myopic Caucasian children aged 8 to 13 years (Parssinen & Lyyra 1993), whereas Chinese children, aged 5 to 16 years, living in Hong Kong have been reported to have a mean myopic progression of 0.63 D per annum (Fan et al 2004). These studies were carried out on the general population and consequently myopic progression in children as seen by the optometrist may have a different trend from that of a general population. Due to self-selection, the characteristics of an optometric population will differ from those of a more general population even when considered within the same geographical region (Pointer 2000). One longitudinal study has analysed the refractive error change in UK Caucasian children aged between 7 and 13 years seen in routine optometric practice over a period of 6 years (Pointer 2001). All children were visually normal and were examined annually. The majority (73.2%) of the 41 children who attended all 7 annual refractions showed an increase in myopic refraction (spherical equivalent refraction, SER) between visits 1 and 7: mean change −0.80±0.80 D, equivalent to a myopic shift per annum of −0.13 D. If all children were included in the analysis, a mean change in SER was found to equate to −0.54±0.82 D (per annum −0.09 D). If only myopic children were considered, then a greater myopic shift in SER is observed: mean change −1.32±0.99 D (per annum −0.22 D). It is interesting that the values for annual rate of progression of myopia are much lower for UK Caucasian children than for Chinese children (Fan et al 2004).

Myopia progression in young adults

Although it is generally accepted that coordinated biological growth of the eye ceases around 15 years of age (Sorsby & Leary 1970), there is a proportion of myopes, estimated between 8% and 15%, who have an onset of myopia typically between 15 and 18 years of age (Gilmartin 2004). This late-onset myopia has a slow progression (≈0.16 D) and rarely exceeds a level of 2 D (Kinge et al 1999).

Myopia progression in adults

In children and young adults, axial elongation and in particular an increase in vitreous chamber depth accounts for the majority of myopia development and progression (Grosvenor & Scott 1993; Lin et al 1996a). In older adults, nuclear sclerosis of the lens may cause a myopic shift due to changes in lenticular power; however, an increase in axial length with progression of myopia has also been found in this age group (McBrien & Adams 1997). A longitudinal study on the development of myopia in a specific occupational group (clinical microscopists) recorded that 45% of the people (age range 21 to 63 years) in the study became myopic (> 0.37 D) during the 2-year period (McBrien and Adams 1997).

A retrospective study on myopia progression in adult contact lens wearers, age 20 to 40 years, determined that approximately 20% had a progression of at least −1.00 D over a period of 5 years, with progression being more common in subjects in their twenties (Bullimore et al 2002). Unfortunately, no data on axial length were given for this subject cohort.

It is well known that there is significant individual variation in the progression of myopia; however, it is interesting that for individuals developing myopia a Gompertz double exponential growth function closely fits the change in refractive error over time (Thorn et al 2002). The onset of myopia in most people has been shown to be abrupt but not instantaneous. Myopia progression also slows more rapidly than predicted by a simple ballistic asymptote, suggesting that there is a dampening factor causing the rapid cessation of myopia progression (Thorn et al 2002).

Risk factors for the development of myopia

It has long been debated whether myopia is under genetic or environmental control (Mutti et al 1996; Goldschmidt 2003). The consensus appears to be that some form of interaction exists between the two components (Wu & Edwards 1999). One proposal is that myopia has a biphasic aetiology, i.e. high myopia with a very young age of onset is inherited whereas a lower level of school myopia is determined by environmental risk factors (Guggenheim et al 2000; Morgan & Rose 2005).

A second mode of interaction is thought to be due to a genetic susceptibility of individuals to environmental risk factors (Saw et al 1996; Mutti et al 2002a).

A third, more established theory for low myopia is that a person's genes are responsible for growth of ocular components although the correlation between these may be influenced by the environment (Goldschmidt 1981).

Genetic factors

Evidence exists to suggest that genetics is a fundamental determinant of the refractive state. The distribution of myopia among races and ethnic groups, its prevalence in families and comparative studies in twins all support the idea that hereditary factors influence the development of ocular refraction (Curtin 1985). Detection of the genetic factors involved in complex traits is complicated. However, several research groups have identified genetic regions of interest with respect to myopia. Much of the current information on the molecular genetics of nonsyndromic human myopia can be drawn from studies of relatively few families affected by high and/or pathological myopia. To date, molecular genetic studies of predominantly families with two or more individuals with 6.00 D or more of myopia have found significant linkage with 13 different regions on a number of different chromosomes (Young et al 2007); however, one of these loci relates to low to moderate levels of myopia. Loci identified to date for isolated nonsyndromic high myopia are predominantly AD and highly penetrant. The 'family study of myopia' is a current investigation at Cardiff University, where the aim is to identify genes responsible for high myopia in the UK population. Preliminary results suggest that a gene on chromosome 12q is responsible for high myopia in at least 25% in the UK (Farbrother et al 2003). Different linked loci may play a role in the more common forms of low to moderate levels of myopia. Genetic analysis of DNA from children and their families participating in a longitudinal US study on myopia, the Orinda study, revealed that the genetic loci for high myopia were not associated with the lower levels of myopia that are more commonly seen in children (Mutti et al 2002b). However, a recent study on a cohort of white Australians has provided evidence that some high myopia loci may contribute to all levels of myopia (Chen et al 2007).

An important population study by Young and colleagues (Young et al 1969) reported a dramatic increase in the prevalence of myopia in the generation of Alaskan Eskimos first exposed to compulsory education and a 'Westernized' environment during their childhood. In the Eskimo families, the parents were illiterate whereas the children attended schools which followed a similar curriculum to the rest of the USA. Only 2 of the 130 parents were myopic whereas 60% of the children were myopic. The cause of the increase in myopia cannot solely be attributed to the introduction of formal schooling, as both diet and lifestyle changes occurred. Similar studies examining other isolated communities that had been exposed to changes in their environment corroborated the findings of greater myopia amongst the younger generation (Alsbirk 1979; Johnson 1988).

Human clinical data also support a genetic basis for myopia. Myopic parents tend to have myopic children in higher proportions than non-myopic parents (Mutti & Zadnik 1995; Pacella et al 1999; Mutti et al 2002a; Saw et al 2002b). The prevalence of myopia in children with two myopic parents is 30% to 40%, decreasing to 20% to 25% in children with only one myopic parent and to less than 10% in children with no myopic parents. An increasing number of myopic parents increases the odds of being myopic, with odds ratios of between 5 and 7.3 (Pacella et al 1999; Mutti et al 2002b) reported for having two myopic parents versus no parents with myopia.

The relative effect of heredity and environment on refractive error can best be investigated using co-twin controls. Identical twins are single-ovum (monozygotic) individuals, the product of a single conception, which splits in two at an early stage within the womb, thus leading to two individuals with identical genetic make-up. Binovular twins develop from two separately fertilized ova (dizygotic). Their genetic similarity is generally equivalent to that of ordinary siblings. The consensus is that if a significant amount of similarity, or concordance, exists between a pair of twins then this would indicate that genetic background is a major factor in determining ametropia (Chen et al 1985). Monozygotic twins tend to resemble each other in both ocular component values and refractive error more than dizygotic twins. Twin studies have provided high values for refractive error heritability (0.82 or greater), i.e. the proportion of phenotypic variance that may be accounted for by genetic factors, and this implies that the environmental impact on refraction is not significant (Hammond et al 2001; Lyhne et al 2001). However, the epidemiological association between near work and myopia, the increase in myopia prevalence within a few generations, and the theory of gene–environment interaction suggest that some individuals may be genetically susceptible to myopia if exposed to certain environmental factors.

Environmental factors

In the development of myopia, evidence exists from 'form-deprivation' myopia to suggest that environmental factors can override genetic inputs. Form-deprivation myopia occurs when clear vision is severely compromised during a critical period of postnatal development. This has been shown with both animals (Wildsoet 1997) and human infants (Mohney 2002). Furthermore, experimental findings from animal studies show that the refractive state of the eyes of young chicks or rhesus monkeys will adapt to compensate for refractive errors induced by spectacle lenses (Wildsoet 1997). Human clinical data also contain evidence for the influence of the environment. The prevalence of myopia in Hong Kong Chinese has increased from approximately 30% to 70% in just one generation, providing strong suggestion for an environmental causal factor (Lam & Goh 1991; Goh & Lam 1994; Lam et al 1994). Cross-sectional studies conducted in Sydney, Boston, California and Singapore suggest that myopic children spend less time in outdoor activities compared with nonmyopic children. The mechanism for the apparent protective effect of time spent outdoors against myopic development is unknown (McBrien et al 2009).

One assumed link between animal and human studies is that the human accommodative response is inaccurate, thereby creating hyperopic defocus during near work that simulates the effect of blur induced by spectacle lenses in animal experiments (Goss 1991; Gwiazda et al 1993; O'Leary & Allen 2001). This hyperopic blur is a hypothetical stimulant to eye growth, increasing the rate of axial elongation and myopia progression. The major correlate of myopia in children is an increase in axial length of the eye (Sorsby et al 1961).

However, the significance of hyperopic blur as a risk factor may need to be re-examined. Recent clinical trials in children and young adults aimed at reducing the exposure to hyperopic defocus through the use of bifocal spectacles or progressive addition lenses produced only a modest reduction in the progression of myopia, which was not of clinical significance (Fulk et al 2000; Edwards et al 2002; Gwiazda et al 2004).

Association with near work

Excessive and sustained near work has been cited for many years as a factor that predisposes a child to myopia, especially if combined with high levels of cognitive demand. The association between myopia and near work has been comprehensively reviewed in the book *Myopia and Nearwork* (Rosenfield & Gilmartin 1998). The book concludes that although near work does not appear to cause myopia, an association between them does exist.

Level of education is often used as a surrogate measure for near work, with a higher prevalence of myopia found among the more educated (Angle & Wissmann 1978; Sperduto et al 1983; Rosner & Belkin 1987). Researchers in East Asia have suggested that it is their rigorous schooling system and the long hours that the children spend studying that are responsible for the high rates of myopia in East Asia (Au Eong et al 1993; Zhao et al 2000). However, recent work from the Genes in Myopia Twin Study has shown that educational attainment is strongly influence by genes (Dirani et al 2008). The researchers concluded that educational attainment should not be solely considered as an environmental risk factor associated with myopia.

The complexity of examining and quantifying near work is further confounded by the association between myopia and intellectual ability. Children with myopia have been found to have higher intelligence test scores and higher achievement test scores, with better grades in school than do non-myopes (Hirsch 1959; Grosvenor 1970; Young et al 1970; Teasdale et al 1988). Unravelling the relative importance of near work, intelligence and heredity is impossible without examining all three factors in the same

subjects. In the Orinda longitudinal study on myopia, the association between children's myopia and parental myopia, as well as the children's visual activities and performance on a standardized achievement test, has been evaluated (Mutti et al 2002a). Both heredity and near work were found to be significantly associated with myopia, with heredity being the more important factor.

Visual display units

There has been a dramatic increase in use of computers in recent years and with this there is often an assumption that visual display units (VDUs) use may be associated with the development of myopia. However, a review of the literature (Mutti & Zadnik 1996) revealed that there was a high prevalence of asthenopia amongst computer users but no clear evidence of any association with myopia progression.

Night lighting

One study that received much publicity relates to the use of night-lights to the development of myopia (Quinn et al 1999). We know from research in animals that postnatal eye growth and refractive development are governed by a vision-dependent retinal mechanism (Wallman et al 1987; Wildsoet & Schmid 2001). The basis for the night-light study in humans was research on chick eyes that showed eye growth was modified by the duration of the light cycle (Stone et al 1995), with myopia progressing with light exposure and less ocular growth in the dark. The human study found that exposure to ambient lighting at night before 2 years of age indicated a tendency for myopia development (Quinn et al 1999). The researchers found that 55% of the children who slept with some light before the age of 2 were myopic. Other researchers have been unable to confirm this link between myopia development and ambient lighting at night (Gwiazda et al 2000; Zadnik et al 2000; Saw et al 2002b). However, these subsequent studies have found that myopic parents are more likely to use night-time lighting aids for their children, possibly to aid their own poor acuity in the dark. The well-documented association between parental myopia and their child's refractive error was not taken into consideration in the Quinn et al study.

Under-correction of myopia

It is feasible to assume that under-correction of myopia may be a possible method of slowing myopia progression. Chung et al (2002) assessed the progression of myopia over a 2-year period in 94 Malaysian and Chinese myopic children between 9 and 14 years of age. The children were randomly assigned to a group in which the myopia was fully corrected or to a group where the myopia was under-corrected. The children's myopia was under-corrected by approximately +0.75 D, thereby blurring their visual acuity to 6/12. After 2 years, the myopia progression in the fully corrected group was −0.77 D whereas in the under-corrected group the myopia had progressed by −1.00 D. Similar findings have been reported by Adler and Millodot (2006). Controversially, Chung et al stated that under-correction of myopia was a common procedure in clinical practice. Discussions with many optometry colleagues and academic optometrists responsible for teaching the modules of refraction and prescribing to students have not revealed any evidence of under-correction of myopes in current UK optometry practice.

These research findings are contrary to the findings in animal studies, where under-correction of the myopia slows myopia development (Hung et al 1995). Previous investigations in children did not find any effect on myopia progression if spectacles were removed for close work (Parssinen et al 1989; Ong et al 1999).

High myopia

The importance of myopia greater than 6 D as a category is evident from Curtin (1985) and from the work of Marr and coworkers (Marr et al 2001), who found high myopia to be strongly associated with ocular and systemic disease in young children attending a hospital eye department. Ocular problems associated with high myopia include retinal dystrophies (e.g. achromatopsia, congenital stationary night blindness), lenticular or zonular abnormalities (e.g. microspherophakia, ectopia lentis, lenticonus) and amblyopia (Curtin, 1985; Marr et al 2001). In addition, there are important systemic ramifications. Marfan's syndrome is probably the disorder most frequently thought of in association with high myopia; however, other disorders include homocystinuria, Stickler's syndrome and Down's syndrome (Curtin 1985; Ainsworth & Marr 2000; Marr et al 2001). High myopia in early childhood is not specifically identified in current UK ophthalmology, optometry or orthoptic protocols for screening, referral or investigation. A study investigating high myopia presenting to community healthcare clinics with the aim of compiling guidelines for assessment and subsequent referral found that 44% of the children had an ocular or systemic condition associated with myopia greater than 5 D (Logan et al 2004). The study highlights the fact that detection and prompt referral of these cases by community healthcare services may, in some cases, prolong vision and possibly life expectancy.

Predictor of future myopia

One of the most frequent questions asked by parents is whether their child is likely to become myopic. One of the best ways of predicting future myopia is based on the refractive error of the child at 9 years of age (US school grade 3). Those with +0.75 D (or more) hyperopia are less likely to become myopic (Zadnik et al 1999).

In order to predict those children at risk of abnormal refractive development and for any preventative care to be effective, optometrists must first understand the progression and consequences of refractive error as a function of age during postnatal development.

References

Adler D, Millodot M 2006 The possible effect of under-correction on myopia progression in children. Clinical and Experimental Optometry 89:315–321

Ainsworth J R, Marr J E 2000 Myopia in young children. Ophthalmic and Physiological Optics 20:S1–S2

Alsbirk P H 1979 Refraction in adult West Greenland Eskimos. Acta Ophthalmologica 57:84–95

Angle J, Wissmann, D A 1978 Age, reading and myopia. American Journal of Ophthalmic and Physiological Optics 55:302–308

Atkinson J, Braddick O, French J 1980 Infant astigmatism: its disappearance with age. Vision Research 20:891–893

Au Eong K G, Tay T H, Lim M K 1993 Education and myopia in 110,236 young Singaporean males. Singapore Medical Journal 34:489–492

Banks M S 1980 Infant refraction and accommodation. International Ophthalmology Clinics 20:205–232

Barnes M, Williams C, Lumb R et al and ALSPAC study team 2001 The prevalence of refractive errors in a UK birth cohort of children aged 7 years. Investigative Ophthalmology and Visual Science ARVO E-abstract 2096.

Brown N 1974 The change in lens curvature with age. Experimental Eye Research 19:1759–1766

Brown N P, Koretz, J F, Bron A J 1999 The development and maintenance of emmetropia. Eye 13:83–92

Bullimore M A, Jones L A, Moeschberger M L et al 2002 A retrospective study of myopia progression in adult contact lens wearers. Investigative Ophthalmology and Visual Science 43:2110–2113

Chang S W, Tsai I L, Hu F R et al 2001 The cornea in young myopic adults. British Journal of Ophthalmology 85:916–920

Chen, C-J, Cohen B H, Diamond E L 1985 Genetic and environmental effects on the development of myopia in Chinese twin children. Ophthalmic Paediatrics and Genetics 6:113–119

Chen C Y, Stankovich J, Scurrah K J et al 2007 Linkage replication of the MYP12 locus in common myopia. Investigative Ophthalmology and Visual Science 48:4433–4439

Chung K, Mohidin N, O'Leary D J 2002 Undercorrection of myopia enhances rather than inhibits myopia progression. Vision Research 42:2555–2559

Cook, R C, Glassock R E 1951 Refractive and ocular findings in the newborn. American Journal of Ophthalmology 34:1407–1413

Cordain L, Eaton S B, Miller B et al 2002 An evolutionary analysis of the aetiology and pathogenesis of juvenile-onset myopia. Acta Ophthalmologica Scandinavica 80:125–135

Curtin B J 1985 The myopias: basic science and clinical management. Harper & Row, Philadelphia

Dandona R, Dandona L, Srinivas M et al 2002 Refractive error in children in a rural population in India. Investigative Ophthalmology and Visual Science 43:615–622

Dirani M, Shekar S N, Baird P N 2008 The role of educational attainment in refraction: the genes in myopia (GEM) twin study. Investigative Ophthalmology and Visual Science 49:534–538

Dobson, V, Fulton A B, Manning K et al 1981. Cycloplegic refractions of premature infants. American Journal of Ophthalmology 91: 490–495

Edwards M H 1991 The refractive status of Hong Kong Chinese infants. Ophthalmic and Physiological Optics 11:297–303

Edwards M H 1998 Myopia: definitions, classifications and economic implications. In: Rosenfield M, Gilmartin B (eds) Myopia and nearwork. Butterworth-Heinemann, Oxford, pp 1–12

Edwards M H, Li R W H, Lam C S Y et al 2002 The Hong Kong progressive lens myopia control study: study design and main findings. Investigative Ophthalmology and Visual Science 43:2852–2858

Ehrlich D L, Anker S, Braddick O J 1994 On- and off-axis refractions of infants. Investigative Ophthalmology and Visual Science 35 (suppl):1806

Erickson P 1991 Optical components contributing to refractive anomalies. In: Grosvenor T, Flom M C (eds) Refractive anomalies – research and clinical implications. Butterworth-Heinemann, Boston, pp 199–218

Fan D S P, Lam D S C, Lam R F et al 2004 Prevalence, incidence and progression of myopia of school children in Hong Kong. Investigative Ophthalmology and Visual Science 45:1071–1075

Farbrother J E, Kirov G, Owen M J et al 2003 Linkage analysis of 18p, 12q and 17q high myopia loci in 51 uk families. 2003 Annual Meeting Abstract and Program Planner accessed at www.arvo.org Association for Research in Vision and Ophthalmology Abstract 4780

Fledelius H 1982 Ophthalmic changes from age of 10 to 18 years. A longitudinal study of sequels to low birth weight. IV. Ultrasound oculometry of vitreous and axial length. Acta Ophthalmologica 60:403–411

Friedman N E, Zadnik K, Mutti D O 1996 Quantifying corneal toricity from videokeratography with Fourier analysis. Journal of Refractive Surgery 12:108–113

Fulk G W, Cyert L A, Parker D E 2000 A randomised trial of the effect of single vision vs. bifocal lenses on myopia progression in children with esophoria. Optometry and Vision Science 77:395–401

Fulton A B, Dobson V, Salem D et al 1980 Cycloplegic refractions in infants and young children. American Journal of Ophthalmology 90:239–247

Garner L F, Kinnear R F, Klinger J D 1985 Prevalence of myopia in school children in Vanuatu. Acta Ophthalmologica Scandinavica 63:323–326

Garner L F, Yap M, Scott R 1992 Crystalline lens power in myopia. Optometry and Vision Science 69:863–865

Garner L F, Yap M K H, Kinnear R F et al 1995 Ocular dimensions and refraction in Tibetan children. Optometry and Vision Science 72:266–271

Gernet H 1981 Oculometric findings in myopia. In: Fledelius H C, Alsbirk P H, Goldschmidt E (eds) Doc Ophthal Proc Series. Dr W. Junk Publishers, The Hague, pp 28, 71–77

Gilmartin B 2004 Myopia: precedents for research in the twenty-first century. Clinical and Experimental Ophthalmology 32:305–324

Goh P P, Abqariyah Y, Pokharel G P et al 2005 Refractive error and visual impairment in school-age children in Gombak District, Malaysia. Ophthalmology 112:678–685

Goh W S H, Lam C S Y 1994 Changes in refractive trends and optical components of Hong Kong Chinese aged 19–39 years. Ophthalmic and Physiological Optics 14:378–382

Goldschmidt E 1981 The importance of heredity and environment in the etiology of low myopia. Acta Ophthalmologica 59:759–762

Goldschmidt E 2003 The mystery of myopia. Acta Ophthalmologica Scandinavica 81:431–436

Goss D A 1991 Childhood myopia. In: Grosvenor T, Flom, M C (eds) Refractive anomalies — research and clinical implications. Butterworth-Heinemann, Boston

Goss D A, Erickson P 1990 Effects of changes in anterior chamber depth on refractive error of the human eye. Vision Science 5:197–201

Goss D A, Winkler R L 1983 Progression of myopia in youth: age of cessation. American Journal of Ophthalmic and Physiological Optics 60:651–658

Goss D A, VanVeen H G, Rainey B B et al 1997 Ocular components measured by keratometry, phakometry, and ultrasonography in emmetropic and myopic optometry students. Optometry and Vision Science 74:489–495

Grosvenor T 1970 Refractive state, intelligence test scores, and academic ability. American Journal of Optometry and Archives of the American Academy of Optometry 64:482–498

Grosvenor T, Scott R 1993 Three-year changes in refraction and its components in youth-onset and early adult-onset myopia. Optometry and Vision Science 68:677–683

Guggenheim J A, Kirov G, Hodson S A 2000 The heritability of high myopia: a reanalysis of Goldschmidt's data. Journal of Medical Genetics 37:227–231

Gwiazda J, Scheiman M, Mohindra I et al 1984 Astigmatism in children: changes in axis and amount from birth to six years. Investigative Ophthalmology and Visual Science 25:88–92

Gwiazda J, Thorn F, Bauer J et al 1993 Myopic children show insufficient accommodative response to blur. Investigative Ophthalmology and Visual Science 34:690–694

Gwiazda J, Ong E, Held R et al 2000 Myopia and ambient night-time lighting. Nature 404:144

Gwiazda J E, Hyman L, Norton J J et al 2004 Accommodation and related risk factors associated with myopia progression and their interaction with treatment in COMET children. Investigative Ophthalmology and Visual Science 45:2143–2151

Hammond C J, Snieder H, Gilbert C E et al 2001 Genes and environment in refractive error: The Twin Eye Study. Investigative Ophthalmology and Visual Science 42:1232–1236

He M, Zeng J, Liu Y et al 2004 Refractive error and visual impairment in urban children in southern China. Investigative Ophthalmology and Visual Science 45:793–799

Hemenger R P, Garner L F and Ooi C S 1995 Change with age of the refractive index gradient of the human ocular lens. Investigative Ophthalmology and Visual Science 36:703–707

Hirsch M J 1959 The relationship between refractive state of the eye and intelligence test scores. American Journal of Optometry and Archives of the American Academy of Optometry 36:12–21

Hirsch M J, Weymouth F W 1991 Changes in optical elements: hypothesis for the genesis of refractive anomalies. In: Grosvenor T, Flom M C (eds) Refractive anomalies – research and clinical implications. Butterworth-Heinemann, Boston

Hung L-F, Crawford M L J, Smith E L 1995 Spectacle lenses alter eye growth and the refractive status of young monkeys. Nature Medicine 1:761–765

Inagaki Y, Tanaka M, Hirano A et al 1985 Rearranged automated keratometer for newborn infants and patients in the supine position. American Journal of Ophthalmology 99:664–666

Ip J M, Huynh S C, Kifley A et al 2007 Variation of the contribution from axial length and other oculometric parameters to refraction by age and ethnicity. Investigative Ophthalmology and Visual Science 48:4846–4853

Johnson G J 1988 Myopia in arctic regions. Acta Ophthalmologica Scandinavica 66:13–18

Jones L A, Mitchell G L, Mutti D O et al 2005. Comparison of ocular component growth curves among refractive error groups in children. Investigative Ophthalmology and Visual Science 46:2317–2327

Junghans B, Crewther S G, Kiely P et al 2002 The prevalence of hypermetropia and myopia amongst a large multicultural population of school children in Sydney. 9th International Conference on Myopia, Hong Kong and Guangzhou

Kendall J, Stayte M A, Wortham C 1989 Ocular defects in children from birth to 6 years of age. British Orthoptic Journal 46:3–6

Kinge B, Midelfart A, Jacobsen G et al 1999 Biometric changes in the eyes of Norwegian university students – a three-year longitudinal study. Acta Ophthalmologica Scandinavica 77:648–652

Kleinstein R N, Jones L A, Hullet S et al 2003 Refractive error and ethnicity in children. Archives of Ophthalmology 121:1141–1147

Koretz J F, Kaufman P L, Neider M W et al 1989 Accommodation and presbyopia in the human eye – aging of the anterior segment. Vision Research 29:1685–1692

Lam C S Y, Goh, W S H 1991 The incidence of refractive errors among school children in Hong Kong and its relationship with the optical components. Clinical and Experimental Optometry 74:97–103

Lam C S Y, Goh W S H, Tang Y K et al 1994 Changes in refractive trends and optical components of Hong Kong Chinese aged over 40 years. Ophthalmic and Physiological Optics 14:383–388

Lam C S Y, Goldschmidt E, Edwards M H 2002 Prevalence of myopia in local and international schools in Hong Kong. 9th International Conference on Myopia, Hong Kong and Guangzhou

Larsen J S 1971 The sagittal growth of the eye. I. Ultrasonic measurement of the depth of the anterior chamber form birth to puberty. Acta Ophthalmologica 49:239–262

Lin L L-K, Shih Y-F, Lee Y-C et al 1996a Changes in ocular refraction and its components among medical students – a 5-year longitudinal study. Optometry and Vision Science 73:495–498

Lin L L-K, Shih Y-F, Tsai C-B et al 1996b Epidemiological study of ocular refractions among school-children. Investigative Ophthalmology and Visual Science 37:S1002

Logan N S, Gilmartin B, Marr J E et al 2004 Community-based study of the association of high myopia in children with ocular and systemic disease. Optometry and Vision Science 81:11–13

Logan N S, Rudnicka A R, Shah P et al 2007 The epidemiology of refractive error in UK children: The Aston Eye Study methodology. Investigative Ophthalmology and Visual Science 48: ARVO E-abstract 4847

Lyhne N, Sjolie A K, Kyvik K O et al 2001 The importance of genes and environment for ocular refraction and its determiners: a population based study among 20–45 year old twins. British Journal of Ophthalmology 85:1470–1476

McBrien N A, Adams D W 1997 A longitudinal investigation of adult-onset and adult-progression of myopia in an occupational group. Investigative Ophthalmology and Visual Science 38:321–333

McBrien N A, Young T L, Pang C P et al 2009 Myopia: recent advances in molecular studies; prevalence, progression and risk factors; emmetropisation; therapies; optical links; peripheral refraction; sclera and ocular growth; signalling cascades; and animal models. Optometry and Vision Science 86:45–66

Marr J E, Halliwell-Ewen J, Fisher B et al 2001 Associations of high myopia in childhood. Eye 15:70–74

Matsumura H, Hirai H 1999 Prevalence of myopia and refractive changes in students from 3 to 17 years of age. Survey of Ophthalmology 44:S109–S115

Maul E, Barroso S, Munoz S R et al 2000 Refractive error study in children: results from La Florida, Chile. American Journal of Ophthalmology 129:445–454

Mayer D L, Hansen R M, Moore B D et al 2001 Cycloplegic refractions in healthy children aged 1 through 48 months. Archives of Ophthalmology 119:1625–1628

Mohney B G 2002 Axial myopia associated with dense vitreous haemorrhage of the neonate. Journal of the American Association of Paediatric Ophthalmology and Strabismus 6:348–353

Morgan I, Rose K 2005 How genetic is school myopia? Progress in Retinal and Eye Research 24:1–38

Morgan K S, Kennemer J C 1997 Off-axis photorefractive screening in children. Journal of Cataract and Refractive Surgery 23:423–428

Murthy G V S, Gupta S K, Ellwein L B et al 2002 Refractive error in children in an urban population in New Delhi. Investigative Ophthalmology and Visual Science 43:623–631

Mutti D O, Zadnik K 1995 The utility of three predictors of childhood myopia: a Bayesian analysis. Vision Research 35:1345–1352

Mutti D O, Zadnik K 1996 Is computer use a risk factor for myopia? Journal of the American Optometric Association 67:521–530

Mutti D O, Zadnik K, Adams A J 1996 The nature versus nurture debate goes on. Investigative Ophthalmology and Visual Science 37:952–957

Mutti D O, Zadnik K, Fusaro R E et al 1998 Optical and structural development of the crystalline lens in childhood. Investigative Ophthalmology and Visual Science 39:120–133

Mutti D O, Mitchell G L, Moeschberger M L et al 2002a Parental myopia, nearwork, school achievement and children's refractive error. Investigative Ophthalmology and Visual Science 43:3633–3640

Mutti D O, Semina E, Marazita M et al 2002b Genetic loci for pathological myopia are not associated with juvenile myopia. American Journal of Medical Genetics 112:355–360

Mutti D O, Mitchell G L, Jones L A et al 2005 Axial growth and changes in lenticular and corneal power during emmetropization in infants. Investigative Ophthalmology and Visual Science 46:3074–3080

Mutti D O, Hayes J R, Mitchell G L et al and Cleere Study Group 2007 Refractive error, axial length, and relative peripheral refractive error before and after the onset of myopia. Investigative Ophthalmology and Visual Science 48:2510–2519

Naidoo K S, Raghunandan A, Mashige K P et al 2003 Refractive error and visual impairment in African children in South Africa. Investigative Ophthalmology and Visual Science 44:3764–3770

Negrel A D, Maul E, Pokharel G P et al 2000 Refractive Error Study in Children: sampling and measurement methods for a multi-country survey. American Journal of Ophthalmology 129:421–426

Ojaimi E, Rose K A, Morgan I G et al 2005a Distribution of ocular biometric parameters and refraction in a population-based study of Australian children. Investigative Ophthalmology and Visual Science 46:2748–2754

Ojaimi E, Rose K A, Smith W et al 2005b Methods for a population-based study of myopia and other eye conditions in school children: The Sydney Myopia Study. Ophthalmic Epidemiology 12:59–69

O'Leary D J, Allen P M 2001 Facility of accommodation in myopia. Ophthalmic and Physiological Optics 21:352–355

Ong E, Grice K, Held R et al 1999 Effect of spectacle intervention on the progression of myopia in children. Optometry and Vision Science 76:363–369

Pacella R, McLellan J, Grice K et al 1999 Role of genetic factors in the etiology of juvenile-onset myopia based on a longitudinal study of refractive error. Optometry and Vision Science 76:381–386

Parssinen O, Lyyra A L 1993 Myopia and myopic progression among school children: a three-year follow-up study. Investigative Ophthalmology and Visual Science 34:2794–2802

Parssinen O, Hemminki E, Klemetti A 1989 Effect of spectacle use and accommodation on myopia progression: final results of a three-year randomised clinical trial among schoolchildren. British Journal of Ophthalmology 73:547–551

Pennie F C, Wood I C J, Olsen C et al 2001 A longitudinal study of the biometric and refractive changes in full-term infants during the first year of life. Vision Research 41:2799–2810

Pointer J S 2000 An optometric population is not the same as the general population. Optometry in Practice 1:92–96

Pointer J S 2001 A 6-year longitudinal optometric study of the refractive trend in school-aged children. Ophthalmic and Physiological Optics 21:361–367

Pokharel G P, Negrel A D, Munoz S R et al 2000 Refractive error study in children: results from Mechi Zone, Nepal. American Journal of Ophthalmology 129:436–444

Quek T P L, Chua C G, Chong C S et al 2004 Prevalence of refractive errors in teenage high school students in Singapore. Ophthalmic and Physiological Optics 24:47–55

Quinn G E, Shin C H, Maguire M G et al 1999 Myopia and ambient lighting at night. Nature 399:113–114

Robinson B E 1999 Factors associated with the prevalence of myopia in 6-year-olds. Optometry and Vision Science 76:266–271

Rose K, Younan C, Morgan I et al 2003 Prevalence of undetected ocular conditions in a pilot sample of school children. Clinical and Experimental Ophthalmology 31:237–240

Rosenfield M, Gilmartin B (eds) 1998 Myopia and nearwork. Butterworth-Heinemann, Oxford

Rosner M, Belkin M 1987 Intelligence, education and myopia in males. Archives of Ophthalmology 105:1508–1511

Saunders K J, Woodhouse J M, Westall C A 1995 Emmetropisation in human infancy: rate of change is related to initial refractive error. Vision Research 35:1325–1328

Saunders K J, McCulloch D L, Shepherd A J et al 2002 Emmetropisation following preterm birth. British Journal of Ophthalmology 86:1035–1040

Saw S M, Katz J, Schein O D et al 1996 Epidemiology of myopia. Epidemiology Review 18:175–187

Saw S-M, Carkeet A, Chia K-S et al 2002a Component dependent risk factors for ocular parameters in Singapore Chinese children. Ophthalmology 109:2065–2071

Saw S-M, Zhang M L, Hong R Z et al 2002b Nearwork activity, night lights and myopia in the Singapore-China study. Archives of Ophthalmology 120:620–624

Saw S M, Goh P P, Cheng A et al 2006 Ethnicity-specific prevalences of refractive errors vary in Asian children in neighbouring Malaysia and Singapore. British Journal of Ophthalmology 90:1230–1235

Scammon R E, Wilmer H A 1950 Growth of the components of the human eyeball II. Archives of Ophthalmology 43:620–637

Smith E L, Hung L F 1999 The role of optical defocus in regulating refractive development in infant monkeys. Vision Research 39:1415–1435

Sorsby A, Leary G A 1970 A longitudinal study of refraction and its components during growth. Medical Research Council Special Report Series 309

Sorsby A, Benjamin B, Davey J B et al 1957 Emmetropia and its aberrations. Medical Research Council Special Report Series 293

Sorsby A, Benjamin B, Sheridan M 1961 Refraction and its components during the growth of the eye from the age of three. Medical Research Council Special Report Series 301

Sperduto R D, Seigel D, Roberts J et al 1983 Prevalence of myopia in the United States. Archives of Ophthalmology 101:405–407

Stayte M, Reeves B, Wortham C 1993 Ocular and vision defects in preschool children. British Journal of Ophthalmology 77:228–232

Stone R A, Lin T, Desai D et al 1995 Photoperiod, early post-natal eye growth, and visual deprivation. Vision Research 35:1195–1202

Teasdale T W, Fuchs J, Goldschmidt E 1988 Degree of myopia in relation to intelligence and educational level. Lancet ii:1351–1354

Thorn F, Held R, Gwiazda J 2002 The dynamics of myopia progression onset and offset revealed by exponential growth functions fit to individual longitudinal refractive data. Investigative Ophthalmology and Visual Science ARVO E-abstract 2866

Villarreal G M, Ohlsson J, Cavazos H et al 2003 Prevalence of myopia among 12- to 13-year-old schoolchildren in northern Mexico. Optometry and Vision Science 80:369–373

Wallman J, Gottlieb M D, Rajaram V et al 1987 Local retinal regions control local growth and myopia. Science 237:73–77

Weale R A 1982 A biography of the eye. H K Lewis & Co Ltd, London

Wildsoet C F 1997 Active emmetropization – evidence for its existence and ramifications for clinical practice. Ophthalmic and Physiological Optics 17:279–290

Wildsoet C F 1998 Structural correlates of myopia. In: Rosenfield M, Gilmartin B (eds) Myopia and nearwork. Butterworth-Heinemann, Oxford, pp 31–56

Wildsoet C F, Schmid K L 2001 Emmetropisation in chicks uses optical vergence and relative distance clues to decode defocus. Vision Research 41:3197–3204

Wood I C J, Mutti D O, Zadnik K 1996 Crystalline lens parameters in infancy. Ophthalmic and Physiological Optics 16:310–317

Wu M M M, Edwards M H 1999 The effect of having myopic parents: an analysis of myopia in three generations. Optometry and Vision Science 76:387–392

Young F A, Baldwin W R, Box R A et al 1969 The transmission of refractive error within Eskimo families. American Journal of Optometry 46:676–685

Young F A, Leary G A, Baldwin W R et al 1970 Refractive errors, reading performance and school achievement among Eskimo children. American Journal of Optometry and Archives of the American Academy of Optometry 47:384–390

Young T L, Metlapally R, Shay A E 2007 Complex trait genetics of refractive error. Archives of Ophthalmology 125:38–48

Zadnik K, Mutti D O, Friedman N E et al 1993 Initial cross-sectional results from the Orinda longitudinal study of myopia. Optometry and Vision Science 70, 750–758

Zadnik K, Mutti D O, Friedman N E et al 1999 Ocular predictors of the onset of juvenile myopia. Investigative Ophthalmology and Visual Science 40:1936–1943

Zadnik K, Jones L A, Irvin B C et al 2000 Myopia and ambient night-time lighting. Nature 404:143–144

Zadnik K, Jones L A, Mitchell G L et al 2002 Baseline ocular component data from the Collaborative Longitudinal Evaluation of Ethnicity and Refractive Error (CLEERE) study. 9th International Conference on Myopia, Hong Kong and Guangzhou

Zadnik K, Manny R E, Yu J A et al 2003 Ocular component data in schoolchildren as a function of age and gender. Optometry and Vision Science 80:226–236

Zadnik K, Mitchell G L, Jones L A et al 2004 Factors associated with rapid myopia progression in school-aged children. Investigative Ophthalmology and Visual Science 45: ARVO E-Abstract 2306

Zhao J, Pan X, Sui R et al 2000 Refractive error study in children: results from Shunyi District, China. American Journal of Ophthalmology 129:427–435

CHAPTER **12**

Visual acuity and contrast sensitivity

Marc Lay · Elizabeth Wickware · Mark Rosenfield

Introduction

Visual acuity (VA) may be defined as the ability of the visual system to detect spatial changes. Clinically, it is usually assessed by asking the patient to detect the presence or absence of a target (detection acuity), to resolve a critical element of a stimulus pattern (resolution acuity) or to identify a particular symbol (recognition acuity). Assessment of VA is frequently the first test carried out following the case history. It is a simple procedure, but represents one of the most important pieces of information obtained during the examination, and if done carelessly or incorrectly will lead to mistakes, an unnecessarily prolonged examination and possibly an incorrect diagnosis. Thus, it is vital that this test be carried out with proper care and attention.

VA testing is conventionally performed at viewing distances of 6 m (20 ft) and 40 cm (16 in). These are the standard distances for the assessment of distance and near acuity, respectively. However, other test distances may also be used, based on the patient's vocational and avocational demands.

Detection acuity

In this acuity test, the patient is required to detect the presence or absence of a specific target. For example, a dot, symbol or grating might be presented on one side of a card or screen, with an equiluminant, blank area on the other side. The patient is asked to identify on which side of the card the stimulus lies (or in the case of infants, their eye movements are observed to see whether they fixate towards the direction of the stimulus; see **Fig. 28.4**). An example of a detection acuity test is shown in **Figure 12.1**. This procedure, when used with either sine- or square-wave gratings, is frequently combined with variations in target contrast to assess the contrast sensitivity function. Examples of contrast sensitivity tests appear later in this chapter.

Resolution acuity

Here, the patient is required to locate the critical element of a stimulus pattern, such as the orientation of the gap in a Landolt C optotype or the direction of the limbs in a Tumbling E. These two tests are shown in **Figure 12.2**. An advantage of this type of test is that it does not require prior knowledge, and therefore can be performed on children or patients who do not speak the same language as the practitioner, provided adequate instructions can be given so that patients understands what is being asked of them. A further advantage of Landolt C and Tumbling E optotypes is that each symbol in the line has the same level of difficulty. This is not the case for the conventional Snellen chart (see below), where some letters are more difficult to resolve under degraded conditions than others. Comparing Landolt Cs and Tumbling Es, Landolt Cs are slightly better since blurred Landolt C optotypes tend to look like circles irrespective of the position of the gap. However, when Tumbling Es are defocused, it is often possible to identify whether the limbs are positioned

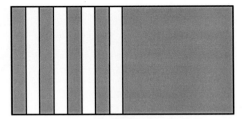

Figure 12.1 Example of a detection acuity test. One side of the card contains a stimulus, such as a square-wave grating as shown here, while the other side contains an equiluminant blank area. The patient is asked to identify which side of the target contains the grating. The spatial frequency (number of stripes per degree) is increased until the patient is no longer able to identify which side of the target contains the stimulus.

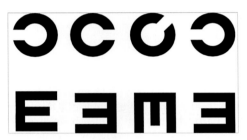

Figure 12.2 Example of Landolt C and Tumbling E optotypes. Presented using Test Chart 2000. (Picture reproduced with permission from Thomson Software Solutions.)

horizontally or vertically. This gives the patient a 50% chance of guessing the orientation correctly.

Recognition acuity

In this test, the patient is asked to identify a particular object, such as a letter, number or symbol. Clearly, this requires prior knowledge, since patients presented with a chart containing letters from an unfamiliar alphabet will be unable to complete the test even if they have excellent VA. In the case of the symbol or picture charts, which are sometimes used for paediatric patients (**Fig. 12.3**), identification of the pictures can be a particular problem. A child might be able to resolve the picture but be unable to name it (for instance, some older charts include a rotary dial telephone, which many children today have never seen). Nevertheless, the letter chart remains the most common method of quantifying VA in the clinical setting, namely in the form of the standard Snellen chart, which many people recognize and associate with optometry.

The Snellen fraction

The most common way to record VA is using the Snellen fraction, which is defined as:

Test distance/
Distance at which the letter subtends 5 minutes(min)of arc

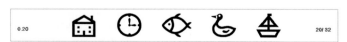

Figure 12.3 Example of paediatric symbol optotypes. Presented using Test Chart 2000. (Picture reproduced with permission from Thomson Software Solutions.)

A VA of 6/6 indicates that at a viewing distance of 6 m, the smallest letter that could be resolved subtended 5 minutes of arc at a distance of 6 m. Similarly, 6/12 indicates that at a viewing distance of 6 m, the smallest letter that could be resolved subtended 5 minutes of arc at a distance of 12 m. In the United States, the standard test distance (and therefore the numerator of the Snellen fraction) is 20 feet, and VA of 20/60 indicates that at a viewing distance of 20 feet, the smallest letter that could be resolved subtended 5 minutes of arc at a distance of 60 feet.

Angular subtense is an indirect measure of letter height. The bigger the letter, the greater the distance at which it will subtend 5 minutes of arc. This is illustrated in **Figure 12.4**. In this figure, the larger letter subtends 5 minutes of arc at a greater distance (y) than the smaller letter (x). By simple geometry, it can be shown that a letter that subtends 5 minutes of arc at 12 m (a 6/12 letter) is twice as big as a 6/6 letter. Similarly, a 6/60 letter is 10 times as big as a 6/6 letter. The Snellen fraction may also be recorded as its decimal equivalent. Therefore, VAs of 6/6, 6/24 and 6/60 could be recorded as decimal equivalent VAs of 1.0, 0.25 and 0.10, respectively.

Snellen optotypes were originally designed by Herman Snellen of Utrecht, Germany, in 1862 (Duke-Elder & Abrams 1970). Different styles are sometimes used (as shown in **Fig. 12.5**), but they are all based on a 5 × 5 or 5 × 4 matrix. Older charts often used letters with serifs, although these are less commonly found today.

Minimum angle of resolution

The minimum angle of resolution (MAR) is the angular size of the critical detail that must be resolved for the patient to be able to identify the optotype correctly. In the case of a Landolt C, it is the width of the gap in the ring. For example, at a viewing distance of 6 m, a 6/6 letter subtends 5 minutes of arc. Since the gap between the limbs of a Snellen letter is one-fifth of the letter height, this gap will subtend one minute of arc and the MAR is 1 minute. Similarly, a 6/12 letter subtends 5 minutes of arc at 12 m. Therefore, at a viewing distance of 6 m, the letter will subtend 10 minutes of arc, and the MAR is 2 minutes. The MAR may also be calculated as the reciprocal of the Snellen fraction. For a 6/30 letter, MAR = 30/6 = 5 minutes.

Although the Snellen fraction remains the most common method of recording VA, it has several significant problems, particularly when the chart is not located at the standard distance of 6 m (20 ft). In this situation, the letter size must be adjusted to give the appropriate decimal equivalent. For example, if one is using a 4.5 m viewing distance, then the numerator of the Snellen fraction should be 4.5 m. In order

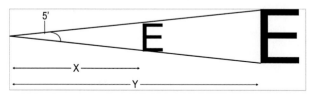

Figure 12.4 The smaller letter E subtends 5 minutes arc at x metres. The larger letter E subtends 5 minutes arc at y metres. Therefore, the distance at which the letter subtends 5 minutes reflects the size of the letter. The larger the distance, the taller the letter.

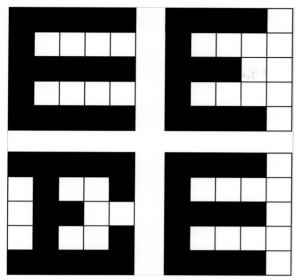

Figure 12.5 Examples of different optotype styles. The top left is a sans serif letter formed on a 5 × 5 grid. The top right letter is a sans serif letter formed on a 5 × 4 grid, with the middle limb shorter than the other two. The bottom left letter is a serif E constructed on a 5 × 5 grid. The bottom right letter is a sans-serif letter formed on a 5 × 4 grid, with the middle limb the same length as the other two.

to achieve a decimal equivalent of 1.0, the letter should subtend 5 minutes of arc at 4.5 m. In the case of a projected or computerized chart, the vertical height of the letter is adjusted to ensure that the letter does indeed subtend 5 minutes at 4.5 m. Using the definition of the Snellen fraction stated above, where the numerator is the test distance, this letter should now be referred to as a 4.5/4.5 letter (or a 1.0 decimal equivalent). However, for convenience in the clinical setting, this letter is usually called a 6/6 letter, even though the viewing distance is not 6 m.

The advantage of designating this optotype as 6/6 is to simplify the comparison of acuities on successive visits. For example, if the patient has 4.5/13.5 acuity on the first visit and 5.5/16.5 acuity on the second visit, then it is not immediately obvious whether the VA has got better, worse or stayed the same. By referring to the acuity as 6/18 on both visits, it is clear that no change has occurred. It would be more accurate to say that the patient has 0.33 decimal equivalent visual acuity on both occasions.

There is an exception to retaining 6 m (or 20 ft) as the numerator, and this is when a patient is unable to resolve the largest letter on the chart. In this case, the viewing distance, meaning the distance between the patient and the chart, must be reduced. For example, if a computerized chart is calibrated for a viewing distance of 4.0 m, and the patient can just identify the letter denoted 6/24 (more accurately a 0.25 decimal equivalent optotype) at a viewing distance of 2.0 m, then the VA is recorded as 2/16. Returning to the definition of the Snellen fraction, we can see why this was recorded as such. The denominator reflects the actual distance at which the letter subtends 5 minutes of arc, so the so-called '6/24' letter is actually a 4/16 letter, subtending 5 minutes of arc at 16 m. The numerator indicates that a 2 m viewing distance was used instead of the 4 m distance the letter was calibrated for. Thus, the VA was 2/16.

Only printed charts can be moved toward the patient, so when projected or computerized charts are used, it is necessary to have the patient approach the chart. Care must be taken with older patients, who may need assistance when getting out of the examination chair. Of course, all patients with poor VA must be helped to ensure that they do not trip or fall when moving towards the chart. Therefore, moving a printed chart towards the patient is more convenient. Calculating the VA is also simpler when using a printed chart, since only the numerator needs to be changed. For example, when using a printed chart which is calibrated for a viewing distance of 6 m, if the patient can first identify the 6/60 optotype at a distance of 3.5 m, then their VA is simply 3.5/60.

A further problem with the Snellen system occurs when the patient is unable to read all of the letters on a particular line. Standard practice is for VA to be recorded as the smallest line for which the patient is able to read at least half the letters. Any errors are indicated by a minus superscript, while additional letters which are identified correctly on the subsequent line are shown by a plus superscript. For example:

$6/12^{+1}$ indicates that the patient correctly read at least half of the letters on the 6/12 line and one extra letter on the 6/9 line.

$6/6^{-2}$ indicates that the patient correctly read all but two of the letters on the 6/6 line.

6/18 indicates that the patient was able to read all of the 6/18 line correctly, but could not correctly identify any of the letters on the subsequent line.

A significant problem with this procedure is that on the standard Snellen chart, the number of letters on each line increases as the patient progresses down the chart. Therefore, if the line contains two letters, then the patient only has to identify one of these correctly to receive credit for that line. However, if the line contains six letters, then at least three must be resolved correctly for the patient to receive credit. In addition to this inequality, it is frequently unclear how to deal with the superscripts, particularly if statistical analysis of the findings is required. Further, some errors are simply ignored. For example, if a patient identifies five out of the six letters correctly on the 6/9 line, and all of the letters but one on the 6/6 line, then their VA is recorded as $6/6^{-1}$, and the error of the 6/9 line is not accounted for.

To overcome many of these problems, charts using the logMAR principle have now been widely adopted as a superior method of quantifying VA (Bailey 2006). In logMAR charts, every line has the same number of letters, and it is straightforward to quantify an acuity score which accounts for every letter on the chart.

The logMAR chart expresses VA as the logarithm of the MAR. For example, a 6/60 letter has a MAR = 10 and logMAR = 1.0. Similarly, if logMAR = 0.0, MAR = 1.0, which is equivalent to a 6/6 letter. A negative logMAR value indicates letters smaller than 6/6. For example, if logMAR = −0.1, then MAR = 0.794, and at a viewing distance of 6 m, VA ≈6/4.8.

Each line on a logMAR chart contains five letters, and lines are generally denoted from 1.0 to −0.3 in 0.1 steps. The space between the letters is equal to the letter width on that particular line, while the vertical space between each

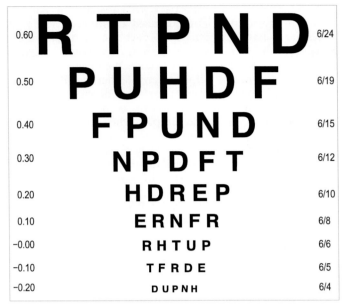

logMAR		Snellen
0.60	R T P N D	6/24
0.50	P U H D F	6/19
0.40	F P U N D	6/15
0.30	N P D F T	6/12
0.20	H D R E P	6/10
0.10	E R N F R	6/8
−0.00	R H T U P	6/6
−0.10	T F R D E	6/5
−0.20	D U P N H	6/4

Figure 12.6 Example of a logMAR chart. The numbers on the left-hand side indicate the logMAR units, while the numbers on the right show the equivalent expressed as a Snellen fraction. Presented using Test Chart 2000. (Picture reproduced with permission from Thomson Software Solutions.)

line is equal to the height of the letters on the lower line. Therefore, the space between the 0.7 and 0.6 lines is equal to the height of a 0.6 logMAR letter. A photograph of a log-MAR chart is shown in **Figure 12.6**. Since correctly identifying the five letters on each line corresponds to a change in logMAR VA of −0.1, each letter represents a change of −0.1/5 = −0.02. Thus, if the patient is able to read all of the 0.8 line but no further, their logMAR VA is 0.8. If they can read all of the 0.8 line and two letters on the 0.7 line, then their logMAR acuity is 0.76. If they can read all of the 0.8 line, two letters on the 0.7 line and two letters on the 0.6 line, then their logMAR VA is 0.72, and 0.02 is subtracted from their score for each letter read correctly, irrespective of the position of that letter on the chart.

As noted previously, letters are not equally difficult to resolve when viewed under degraded stimulus conditions. For example, Hartridge and Owens (1922) ranked letters in order of increasing difficulty and observed that that L, A, J and E were the easiest to identify, while C, B, O, R and S were the hardest. Bennett and Rabbetts (1989) stated that while one could argue that all letters used should have similar legibility, it could also be contended that every line should either contain one of the more difficult letters, or a pair that are easily confused, such as C and G or F and P. Letters that are commonly used on tests are the Sloan series (Sloan 1959), which use the following letters based on a 5 × 5 grid: C, D, H, K, N, O, R, S, V and Z (Bailey 2006). Additionally, the British Standard for VA optotypes (BS 4274–1:2003) listed 12 sans serif letters to be formed on a 5 × 5 grid. The following letters were recommended: C, D, E, F, H, K, N, P, R, U, V and Z. Specific angles and curvatures are recommended in this standard.

Other charts are also necessary when working with paediatric and special populations, and these are discussed further in Chapter 28.

Near visual acuity

This should always be tested at a standard test distance; typically 40 cm. If the patient habitually performs near tasks at other distances, e.g. viewing a computer monitor, then it is valuable to assess their acuity at these other distances as well. However, by always testing at 40 cm, this facilitates the comparison of acuities at subsequent visits. If testing at a distance other than 40 cm, it is essential to record the testing distance accurately.

Near VA should be recorded under good illumination, i.e. with the overhead lamp lit and directed onto the near text. This is particularly important for elderly patients because their optical media do not transmit light as well as younger subjects, resulting in reduced retinal illumination. Five methods are most commonly used to quantify near VA, namely Snellen, logMAR, Jaeger, M and N notations.

1. *Snellen chart*: This uses the same principles as the distance chart. The standard test distance is 40 cm (16 in). However, for standardization of recording, numerators of either 6 or 20 are conventionally used, even though this does not correspond to the test distance. Thus, a near VA of 20/40 at a test distance of 40 cm (16 in) should more accurately be described as 40/80 or 16/32. An alternative solution would be to describe this as a 0.50 decimal equivalent at 40 cm, or as 0.40/0.8 M.

2. *LogMAR chart*: In addition to charts using optotypes which follow the same principles adopted for distance logMAR charts, the Bailey–Lovie Word Reading chart **(Fig. 12.7)** contains unrelated words printed using lower-case Times Roman font (Bailey & Lovie 1980). The use of unrelated words means the patient cannot guess based on the context of the sentence. Although charts that require the reading of sentences are more natural, unrelated word reading charts test the ability to see rather than the ability to read (Bailey 2006).

3. *Jaeger Chart*: Here, letters vary in size from around 0.5 mm to 19.5 mm. Twenty different optotype sizes are used, typically denoted from J1 (the smallest) to J20 (the largest). Since the dimensions of these letters are not standardized, these charts are of limited value.

4. *M notation*: The M number specifies the distance in metres at which the letter subtends 5 minutes of arc. Thus, the M number corresponds to the denominator of the Snellen

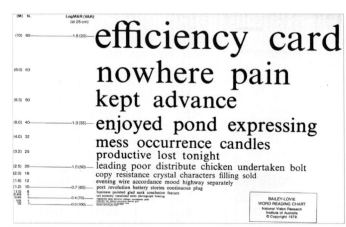

Figure 12.7 The Bailey–Lovie Word Reading chart.

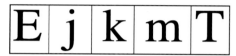

Figure 12.8 Example of the N (point size) acuity system. N refers to the height of the 'block' on which the letter is constructed. For example, if these are N10 letters, then the block or square is 10/72 inches high. A lower-case letter which has neither ascenders nor descenders (e.g. the letter m), is approximately half the size of the block, i.e. 5/72 inches high.

fraction. For example, when testing at 0.40 m, if the smallest type which can be read is 0.5 M, then VA = 0.40/0.50.

5. *N notation*: This corresponds to the point size, with one point being 1/72 of an inch. The smallest size used when measuring near visual acuity is generally N5, i.e. 5/72 inches high. Point size is widely used in word processing (e.g. 12 point) and in the printing industry. Technically, the point (or N) size indicates the height of the block on which the letter is mounted, and does not reflect the height of the individual letter. For example, if the letters in **Figure 12.8** represent 10 point (or N10) letters, then each of the rectangles or blocks which surround the letters will be 10/72 inches high. It can be seen from the diagram that the height of the individual letters varies depending on whether the letter has 'ascenders' as in the letter k, or 'descenders' as in the letter j. In the case of the smaller lower-case letters, e.g. a, c, e, m, n, o, r, s, u, v, w, x and z, the height of the letter is generally about half the height of the block. Thus, an 8 point letter 'c' is actually about 4/72 inches high.

Size of newspaper print

One of the most common complaints expressed by patients upon arriving for an eye examination is difficulty reading newspaper print. In considering what level of VA is required to read newspaper text comfortably, 1M acuity is generally recommended (Tinker & Paterson 1944). Assuming a viewing distance of 40 cm, this would be equivalent to 20/50 or N8.2. More recently, DeMarco and Massof (1997) noted that the size of newspaper print was extremely variable. For example, they observed that stock market listings, obituaries and front page columns averaged 0.78 M, 0.86 M and 1.18 M, respectively. Indeed, correcting a patient to 1M would not allow them to read half of the sections in 75% of the newspapers examined. Accordingly, the authors suggested that in order to be able to read all of the sections in the newspaper, patients should be able to read 0.65 M print. At a viewing distance of 40 cm, this is equivalent to visual acuity of 6/9.75 (20/32.5) or N5.4. Given that the contrast of newspaper print is significantly poorer than the high-contrast charts generally used in clinical measurement of near VA, even better VA than these values stated above may often be necessary.

Clinical procedure for measuring visual acuity

Visual acuity should be measured both without and with the habitual refractive correction. The former is sometimes referred to as a measurement of 'vision' while the term VA may be restricted to the value obtained through the optimum refractive correction. However, many practitioners simply refer to these values as uncorrected and corrected VA. Acuities should be recorded both monocularly and binocularly. It is essential to ensure that during the measurement of monocular VA, the eye not being tested is fully occluded. Occluding patients with a hand (whether the patient's or the practitioner's) is inadequate since they might peek between the fingers. An opaque black occluder is most satisfactory. It is also important to check that patients are not partially closing their viewing eye (squinting), since this might improve their VA by producing a pinhole effect. It is critical that practitioners always observe the patient (rather than the chart) during VA measurement. If practitioners are either unfamiliar with the chart (or are unable to resolve it themselves – a common problem!), they should make a 'cheat sheet' to keep on hand.

British Standard BS-4274-1, 2003 specifies that the luminance of the chart presented shall be uniform (the variation across the chart should not exceed 20%) and not less than 120 cd/m². However, both Bennett and Rabbetts (1989) and Bailey (2006) noted that a test chart luminance between 80 and 320 cd/m² may be reasonable and practical.

While using a projector, computerized, or internally illuminated acuity chart, the room should be dimly illuminated. However, if a printed chart is being used, then the chart must be evenly and adequately illuminated. Specifically, the room lights should be left on and some local lighting of the chart itself may also be required. Care should be taken to ensure that shadows do not fall across the chart. In all cases, any glare sources within the patient's field of view should be eliminated.

Usually the uncorrected VA is measured first. Since corrected VA is likely to be better than uncorrected, recording uncorrected VA first decreases the likelihood of the patient memorizing the chart. Alternatively, some practitioners suggest that the patient be examined in the condition in which they entered the test room. Thus, if the patient enters the room without wearing any correction, then this may represent the patient's habitual status. An advantage of computerized charts is that an almost infinite number of charts are available, and letters can be randomized, so that memorization of the chart is no longer an issue.

For both corrected and uncorrected VA, the patient is asked to read the smallest line that they can see clearly. However, some patients are confused by these instructions, and take them as a direction to read the bottom line on the chart, something they may be unable to do. For these patients it may be easier to ask them to read the whole chart starting from the top. Although slower, this latter method promotes patient confidence, and reinforces to the patient that they are performing the test correctly. Alternatively, individual lines may be isolated, and the patient asked to read them. Isolating lines is particularly useful when testing smaller letters, where any difficulty can cause patients to lose their place on the chart.

In an optometric examination, it is conventional to examine the patient's right eye first, followed by the left eye. Always encourage the patient to guess during the test. In addition, when patients say that they cannot read any further, always suggest that they 'try the next line'. Some patients are embarrassed by making mistakes, yet can frequently read beyond their initial stopping position. It is quite common for patients to be referred from screening programmes due to a finding of reduced VA. However, if patients are given a little extra time and encouragement during the test, they are often found to have significantly better VA than the vision screening suggested.

If patients are unable to resolve the largest letter on the chart at the standard viewing distance, then this distance should be reduced as described earlier. Some practitioners advocate determining whether the patient can count the number of fingers being displayed by the examiner at a particular distance. This is recorded as finger counting, e.g. finger counting at 1 m. However, if patients are able to count fingers, they should be able to resolve a Snellen letter at some distance. This is preferable to finger counting, since it is both more standardized and reproducible (see p 478).

If patients are unable to identify the largest letter at any distance, then they should be asked to determine whether the examiner's hands are stationary or moving. If they can successfully do so, this is recorded as *hand motion (HM)* at the test distance, e.g. HM at 1 m. If the patient is unable to detect hand motion, then hold a light source, e.g. a transilluminator or penlight, in various areas of the visual field and ask the patients to determine the direction of the light source. Take particular care to ensure that the non-tested eye is fully occluded so that no light can enter that eye. Remember that patients may have visual loss in only one area of their visual field, e.g. superior, inferior, nasal. If patients are able to identify correctly the position of the light, this is recorded as *light projection (LPROJ)*. If patients cannot detect light projection, investigate whether they can determine whether the light is on or off. If successful, this is recorded as *light perception (LP)*. If not, this is recorded as *no light perception (NLP)*. Finally, VA should never be recorded as <6/60. In this case, patients could either have 4/60 acuity or NLP. Clearly, there is a huge difference between these two possibilities, though either could be true if <6/60 is all that is recorded.

Effect of blur on visual acuity

The most common reason why patients present with reduced VA is uncorrected refractive error. Thus, an understanding of how refractive error affects VA is important for the practitioner. In the optically ideal situation, an object consisting of a point source would be imaged precisely on the retina. However, in many patients the image is formed either in front of or behind the retina (see Ch. 11). In either of these cases, a blurred patch of light (or blur circle) will be formed on the retina (**Fig. 12.9A**).

The amount of refractive error will change the distance between the retina and the point conjugate with the object of regard, and accordingly the diameter of the retinal blur circle. This is illustrated in **Figures 12.9A** and **12.9B**. The patient's ability to resolve small objects varies with the size of the retinal blur circle. Consider the situation where a patient is asked to view two small objects placed close together. In **Figure 12.10A**, the two objects are imaged close to the retina, so small blur circles are produced. Since the circles do not overlap, the patient is able to identify that two distinct objects are present. However, in **Figure 12.10b**, the images of the two objects lie further away from the retina, resulting in larger and overlapping blur circles. The patient would not be able to distinguish the two separate objects. If the two objects shown in **Figure 12.10B** were not point sources, but directly opposing

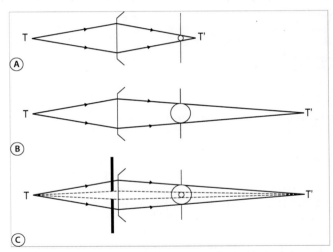

Figure 12.9 The image (T') of an object (T) is focused behind the retina, resulting in a retinal blur circle whose diameter is related to the distance from the image to the retina. **(A)** A small degree of refractive error resulting in a small blur circle, **(B)** A greater degree of refractive error and larger blur circle. **(C)** A pinhole aperture has been introduced, which allows only those rays lying within the dashed lines to pass through. This reduces the blur circle diameter, resulting in improved visual resolution.

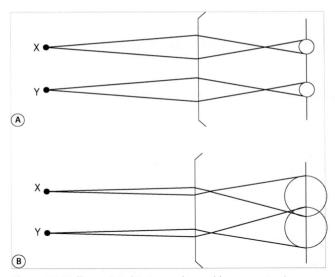

Figure 12.10 Two point objects are observed by an ametropic eye, resulting in retinal blur circles. **(A)** The degree of refractive error is small, so the blur circles do not overlap and the observer is able to resolve the space between the two objects. **(B)** The degree of refractive error is larger, so the blur circles overlap and the observer will not be able to resolve the space between the two objects.

points in the gap between the limbs of a letter E or F, then the patient would be unable to resolve the gap, and therefore could not identify the letter.

The diameter of the retinal blur circle will also vary with pupil size, as shown in **Figure 12.9C**. Introduction of a pinhole aperture reduces the diameter of the retinal blur circle, resulting in a significant improvement in visual acuity. It should also be noted that the pinhole has no effect on the degree of refractive error. The emergent rays have the same vergence as they would if the pinhole aperture were absent. Manufacturers of pinhole glasses have claimed that their devices will 'cure' refractive error. While they will produce improved VA, the degree of ametropia remains unchanged.

The pinhole aperture is an extremely important clinical test. In any situation where a patient's VA does not reach the expected level, it should be re-measured through a pinhole. If acuity improves, this indicates that the loss of vision is refractive and can be improved with correcting lenses. However, if the vision does not improve through a pinhole, then the visual loss is due to non-refractive causes, such as amblyopia or ocular disease. It should also be noted that in a patient with good acuity initially, the pinhole aperture may actually worsen the VA due to the reduction in the amount of light reaching the retina.

Effect of age on visual acuity

In a review of the effect of age on VA, Elliott et al (1995) noted that mean logMAR VA in normal, healthy eyes improved from −0.13 in 18- to 24-year-old subjects to −0.16 in 25- to 29-year-olds, and then gradually declined with age, reaching a mean value of −0.02 in subjects over 75 years of age. The mean values are shown in **Table 12.1**. It is worthy of note that for all ages tested, mean VA was better than 6/6 (20/20). Accordingly, Elliott et al observed that 6/6 (20/20) does not represent normal VA in a healthy eye. This commonly held assumption is actually based on a calculation error (Velasco e Cruz 1990).

In the nineteenth century, Helmholtz reported that the normal minimum separable threshold was approximately 1 minute of arc (Brown 1979). This value was subsequently adopted by Snellen when constructing his acuity chart. However, in calculating the minimum resolution, Helmholtz used a grating target composed of black wires separated by a space equivalent to the width of the wire. The minimum resolvable visual angle was wrongly assumed to be the sum of the width of two bars, rather than the space between the bars. Indeed, Helmholtz found that good

eyes were able to resolve the space between the bars when the space subtended 0.5 minutes of arc (equivalent to 6/3), and Tscherning (1898; cited by Velasco e Cruz 1990) concluded that Snellen's normal acuity was half that found by Helmholtz. Elliott et al suggested that possible reasons why the myth of 6/6 representing normal VA persists include the manufacture of charts with bottom lines of only 6/6 or 6/5, or the relatively low luminance and contrast provided by projection charts such as those favoured in North America.

Contrast sensitivity testing

Though crucial for assessing visual function, clinical measurements of VA do not provide a comprehensive picture of how a patient will perform during real-world tasks. Our environment contains vast amounts of information, including a wide spectrum of contrasts and spatial frequencies. Accordingly, testing a patient's ability to resolve only small, high-contrast targets does not provide the best assessment of visual performance in the natural environment.

The least amount of contrast required to make a target visible is defined as the contrast threshold, and the reciprocal of that threshold is contrast sensitivity (CS). There are two standard methods of calculating contrast for a given target. Early contrast tests utilized the Weber contrast function:

$$\text{Contrast} = (L_t - L_b)/L_b$$

(where L_{t} and L_{b} represent the luminance of the target and background, respectively).

However, since the development of sine-wave contrast sensitivity tests, the Michelson contrast equation is more commonly chosen:

$$\text{Michelson contrast} = (L_{max} - L_{min})/(L_{max} + L_{min})$$

(where L_{max} and L_{min} represent the maximum and minimum luminance of the grating, respectively).

Table 12.1 Mean visual acuity (VA) for 223 subjects with normal, healthy eyes from 18 to 80 years of age in consecutive 5-year periods

Age range (years)	Mean VA (logMAR)	Mean Snellen denominator (6/x)	Mean Snellen denominator (20/x)
18–24	−0.13	4.5	14.8
25–29	−0.16	4.2	13.8
30–34	−0.15	4.2	14.2
35–39	−0.14	4.3	14.5
40–44	−0.13	4.4	14.8
45–49	−0.12	4.6	15.2
50–54	−0.10	4.8	15.9
55–59	−0.10	4.8	15.9
60–64	−0.07	5.1	17.0
65–69	−0.05	5.3	17.8
70–74	−0.04	5.5	18.2
75+	−0.02	5.7	19.1

Data are shown in logMAR units, as the value of the denominator when expressed in metric units (using 6 m as the numerator), and as the value of the denominator when expressed in imperial units (using 20 feet as the numerator).
Data reproduced with permission from Elliott et al 1995.

The sine-wave grating which is most commonly used as a test stimulus is a periodic function characterized by its amplitude (or luminance) and spatial frequency, i.e. the number of cycles per unit angular subtense, usually expressed as cycles per degree (cpd). Therefore, at each spatial frequency, varying the stimulus amplitude until the threshold for detection is reached will provide a measure of the patient's CS. If this is repeated over a wide range of spatial frequencies, the contrast sensitivity function (CSF) is determined. This function is analogous to the modulation transfer function of optical systems.

Low-contrast optotypes were first utilized clinically by Bjerrum in 1884. The original tests incorporated a Snellen chart design with letters printed in varying grey tones. In 1918, George Young developed the first commercially available light-difference threshold (i.e. CS) test, comprising a series of ink spots of multiple dilutions (Robson 1993). Subsequently, Schade (1956) measured the human CSF by determining contrast thresholds for perceiving sine waves at various spatial frequencies (Robson 1993). Research in the area of CS was advanced immensely by the work of Campbell and Robson in the 1960s. Their findings described the CSF as a series of independent channels, each tuned (i.e. most sensitive) to different spatial frequencies. The neurophysiology is composed of centre–surround-oriented ganglion cells in the retina, and the composition and size of their receptive fields dictates the spatial frequencies that are encoded. Stimulation in the centre of a typical receptive field increases the cell's response, while stimulating the surround will decrease cell activity. A smaller receptive field would be best at detecting higher spatial frequencies, whereas a larger receptive field would better identify lower spatial frequencies. While there are contributions from both the magnocellular and parvocellular pathways, there are still unanswered questions regarding the specific physiological mechanisms involved. However, the discussion here will focus on the clinical applications of CS testing, and which tests are most relevant for diagnostic purposes.

As mentioned previously, CSF testing procedures assess visual performance using a wider range of stimuli than is required to quantify VA. Many investigations have confirmed that measuring CS consecutively over time is a reliable way to detect changes in the visual pathway, even when VA remains constant (Järvinen & Hyvärinen 1997). For example, a patient presenting with 6/6 acuity may still report difficulty with some visual tasks. Though seemingly paradoxical, in some disease conditions such as multiple sclerosis, the ability to distinguish lower spatial frequencies can be lost while VA remains unaffected. In addition, CS tests can be sufficiently sensitive to detect subtle changes in patients with various abnormal conditions (Bansback et al 2007). Sisto et al (2005) showed that CS is the most sensitive test for determining visual pathway involvement in multiple sclerosis. The CSF has also been used to examine visual performance following cataract surgery (Walker et al 2006). It is valuable for assessing how the patient will function in their everyday environment, and has been shown to be a better predictor of both falls in older patients (Lord 2006) and driving recognition performance (Wood & Owens 2005) than VA.

To understand these findings, it is important to remember that VA tests high spatial frequencies at high contrast only, despite the fact that many daily tasks require the perception of low spatial frequency information at a variety of contrast levels. When examining the light-adapted (or photopic) contrast sensitivity function (**Fig. 12.11**), theoretical VA can be predicted by extrapolating the CSF curve to determine its x-axis intercept (shown as the grating acuity limit in **Fig. 12.11**), which would represent 100% contrast. However, while this portion of the curve could fall within the normal range, other regions, such as the lower spatial frequency function, may still be abnormal.

While there are no strict boundaries, Regan (1991) denoted three types of CS loss. A type I CS loss was defined as reduced sensitivity to high spatial frequencies only, while low spatial frequency perception is unaffected. This attenuation of high spatial frequencies occurs most commonly as a result of retinal defocus, as found in patients with uncorrected refractive error. A type II CS loss indicates decreased sensitivity across all spatial frequencies. This may be produced by light scattering (e.g. due to cataract or other media opacities) or amblyopia. The final category, type III CS loss, is reduced sensitivity at low spatial frequencies (approximately 2 cpd) only. Individuals with type III loss will have normal VA.

The clinical tests described in the remainder of this chapter provide a more comprehensive picture of a patient's visual function than can be obtained by looking at VA alone. Important factors to note about each test include the type of stimuli presented (e.g. gratings or letters), the number of choices, flexibility (computer versus hard copy), and repeatability. Regarding stimulus type, gratings are standardized stimuli which can be used to assess CS at specific spatial frequencies. Letters may also be used to assess CS, but different letters of the same size contain a wide spectrum of spatial frequencies. While approximations can be made of the spatial frequency for a letter of a given size, it is difficult to identify the exact spatial frequency being tested since a letter can contain a band of spatial frequencies. This is unlike a sine wave, which comprises a single spatial frequency.

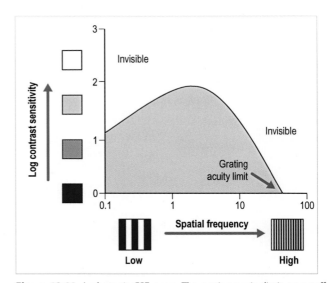

Figure 12.11 A photopic CSF curve. The grating acuity limit, or cutoff frequency, indicated is the highest spatial frequency grating that can be detected at maximum contrast. (Reproduced with permission from Elliott 2006.)

Pelli–Robson test

One of the most widely utilized clinical CS tests is the Pelli–Robson Contrast Sensitivity chart (Haag-Streit USA, Mason, OH) (**Fig. 12.12**). The 86 × 63 cm chart should be viewed at a distance of 1 m. The manufacturer recommends an external illumination of 85 cd/m². The test consists of triplets of Sloan letters (each subtending 2.8° at 1 m, or a Snellen equivalent of approximately 6/200). Each group of three letters has 0.15 log units (Weber contrast rating) less contrast than the preceding set. There are two sets of triplets per line and a total of eight lines (Pelli et al 1988). Contrast levels range from 100% (0.00 log units) to 0.56% (−2.25 log units). While performing the test, the patient is asked to identify the letters. Although only 10 Sloan letters are used, any letter of the alphabet is a possible answer for a naive patient, thereby making this a 26-alternative forced-choice test. Accordingly, there is a low probability of a risk-taking patient achieving a false-positive.

Several studies have verified that the Pelli–Robson CS chart has good repeatability (Elliott & Bullimore 1993). Due to the large angular subtense of the letters, this test is useful for identifying low spatial frequency loss. The large target size makes the Pelli–Robson chart an effective tool even when moderate uncorrected refractive error is present. Higher spatial frequencies can also be tested by increasing the test distance. With respect to lighting conditions, Cox et al (1999) determined that the surround luminance has minimal effect on CS measurements with letter charts. However, Cox et al also stated that sine-wave gratings (discussed later), especially computer-generated gratings, 'may have their measurements affected by inappropriately lit task surrounds'. Therefore, while environmental conditions are of concern while performing any clinical test, sine-wave CS tests are especially sensitive to surround luminance.

Although the Pelli–Robson Chart utilizes only one letter size, the designers of the test stated that the information obtained from both traditional high-contrast VA measurements and the Pelli–Robson CS test would provide 'as much information on a subject's CS as would be clinically useful' (Pelli et al 1988).

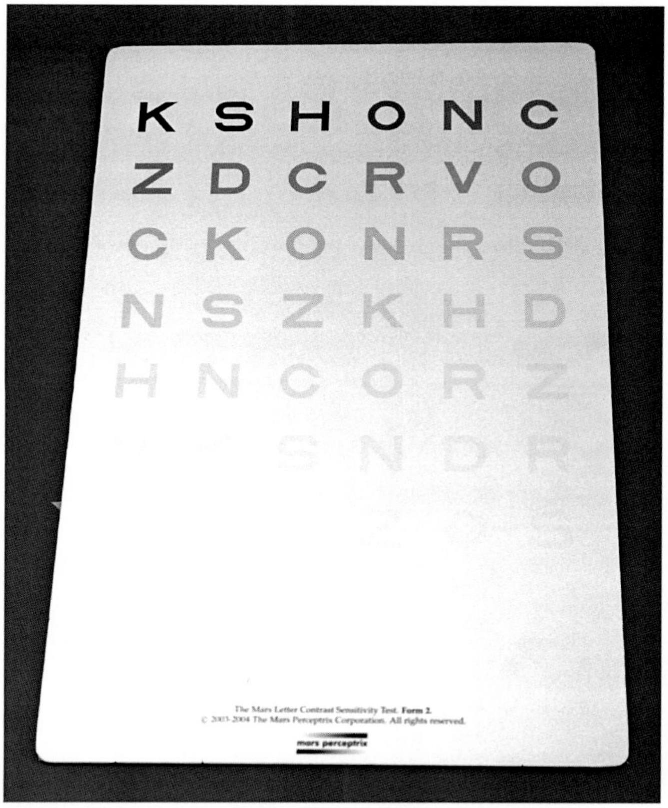

Melbourne Edge Test

The Melbourne Edge Test (National Vision Research Institute, Melbourne, Australia) uses edge detection to measure CS (**Fig. 12.13**). The patient views 20 bisected, 25 mm diameter circular patches of decreasing contrast (from 5 to 24 dB). Each circle is divided by an edge that can be oriented in one of four possible directions (vertical, horizontal and two oblique orientations). Therefore, this is a four- alternate forced-choice test for determining the peak of the CSF (Wolffsohn et al 2005). This peak normally occurs between 2 and 6 cpd, with a rapid decrease in sensitivity at higher spatial frequencies. The peak of the CS function has been shown to be a reliable predictor of increased likelihood of falls and other common household injuries. Wolffsohn also noted that the backlit version of the Melbourne Edge Test is more repeatable, and the contrast is less affected by external light sources, when compared with the externally lit version. The Melbourne Edge Test provides a reliable method for tracking CS, and normative values have been established for different age groups (Eperjesi et al 2004).

An advantage of this test is that it is independent of VA. By using edge detection rather than the resolution of letters or symbols, the test can be performed by low-vision

Figure 12.12 The Pelli–Robson contrast sensitivity chart.

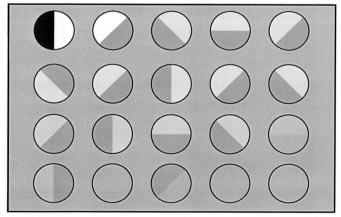

Figure 12.13 The Melbourne Edge contrast sensitivity chart. The patient is asked to indicate whether the edge is oriented horizontally, vertically or obliquely.

patients. However, this test does not allow the construction of a CS curve, since it does not test at different spatial frequencies.

Vistech chart

The Vistech chart (Vision Sciences Research Corporation, San Ramon, CA) provides an assessment of the complete CS function at multiple (1.5, 3, 6, 12 and 18 cpd) spatial frequencies. This chart uses sine-wave gratings at three orientations (**Fig. 12.14**). The standard test distance is 3 m, but the manufacturer has also published normal values for a 1 m test distance. A light meter is provided with the system, which is helpful since varying illumination levels may affect CS measurements. The effects of lighting are particularly important when using a sine-wave stimulus. Excessive external light levels can render a low-contrast target undetectable for a normal patient and would reduce the accuracy of any measurements obtained. Pesudovs et al (2004) also reported that the repeatability of the Vistech test is lower when compared with updated versions of the device. Additionally, the contrast step size of the Vistech chart is not constant (average of 0.25 log units), and the overall step size is larger than most CS tests. A smaller contrast step size is likely to increase the repeatability of CS and VA measurements (Pesudovs et al 2004).

Functional Acuity Contrast Test

The newer version of the Vistech, the Functional Acuity Contrast Test (FACT), contains significant modifications that improve upon the original Vistech chart. The FACT (Vision Sciences Research Corporation, San Ramon, CA) uses similar stimuli to the Vistech chart, but with a constant contrast step size of 0.15 log units. This smaller step provides better resolution when determining CS changes. This will decrease the variability between measurements. Five spatial frequencies are examined at nine contrast levels. The gratings are oriented in one of three positions: up, left, or right. The patient reads across each row and continues until the contrast is below threshold. The modifications adopted in this

test serve to increase retest agreement, and the test still assesses the CS over a wide range of spatial frequencies. The distance test is performed at 10 feet. A near version of the FACT test is also available for testing at 18 inches.

VectorVision charts

The CSV-1000E contrast sensitivity chart (VectorVision, Grenville, OH), uses a sine-wave stimulus similar to the FACT chart (**Fig. 12.15**). Unlike the previously mentioned tests, it is a retro-illuminated transparent chart. There are four rows of gratings having frequencies of 3, 6, 12 and 18 cpd at the recommended 2.5 m test distance. The contrast levels tested range from 0.7 to 2.29 log units. This test is a clinically reliable diagnostic tool for assessing patients undergoing treatment for glaucoma (Pomerance & Evans 1994). An additional test produced by the same manufacturer is the CSV-1000RS, which is recommended for screening refractive surgery patients. The test assesses Early Treatment of Diabetic Retinopathy Study (ETDRS) high-contrast logMAR acuity from −0.30 to 0.70 (Snellen equivalent: 6/3 to 6/30) and includes one row of sine-wave gratings having a spatial frequency of 12 cpd. However, the CSV-1000RS test does not examine CS at either end of the spatial frequency range. The manufacturer recommends that if a deficit is found with this screening instrument, then the patient should be tested further with the CSV-1000E.

Mars test

A newer CS test, which is similar in format to the Pelli–Robson, is the Mars Letter CS Test (see **Fig. 31.13**). This has the advantage of being relatively small (23 × 35.5 cm). The test ranges from 91% to 1.2% contrast, and each letter is 0.04 log units lower in contrast than the preceding letter. The chart is designed for a test distance of 0.5 m, and at this distance each letter subtends two degrees (Snellen equivalent =

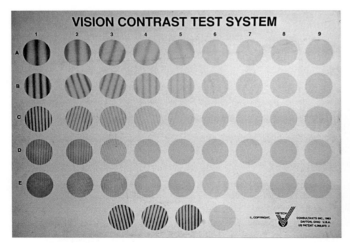

Figure 12.14 The Vistech VCTS chart.

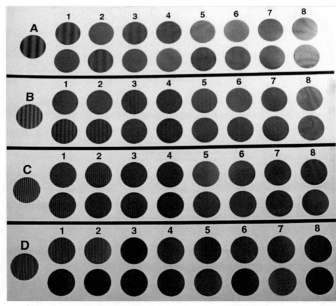

Figure 12.15 The CSV-1000 contrast sensitivity test.

6/144). The Mars test shows excellent agreement with the Pelli–Robson test, and they have similar levels of repeatability (Dougherty et al 2005). There is a possible concern that the Mars test would not be ideal for low-vision patients, due to the smaller angular subtense of the letters when compared with the Pelli–Robson test. However, Dougherty et al demonstrated that the Mars test actually exhibits better repeatability with low-vision subjects when compared with the Pelli–Robson chart.

Lea Test

When examining children or other patients who cannot communicate verbally, the Lea Test (Lea-Test, Helsinki, Finland) provides a series of CS tests using both Lea symbols (symbols of constant size (10M) but decreasing contrast) and gratings (see Ch. 28). The gratings comprise three spatial frequencies (0.5 c/cm, 2 c/cm and 8 c/cm) at three contrast levels (100%, 10% and 2.5%). This test has been validated against the Pelli–Robson test (Leat and Wegmann 2004). Lea-Test also manufactures a low-contrast (2.5%) chart which is designed to be used with the ETDRS light box. This has the advantage of standardizing the illumination level.

Computerized testing

Computerized CS tests can be set to display a range of spatial frequencies at almost any contrast level. These tests are not limited to what is printed on a chart, and can be modified based on the specific situation (e.g. when examining a low-vision patient). However, there is no standard testing protocol for many of the computerized tests that are available.

Test Chart 2000 (Thomson Software Solutions, London, UK) includes a computerized CS test designed for a 1 m test distance. The letters are presented as triplets of decreasing contrast, similar to the Pelli–Robson chart. Each line only has one triplet, unlike the two printed on each line of the Pelli–Robson chart. Interestingly, Thayaparan et al (2007) found Test Chart to be less repeatable than the Pelli–Robson chart. The authors suggested that this may have been due to the monitor rather than the software design, since the monitor can affect the contrast rendering on the screen. They suggested a cathode ray tube monitor should be used for a more accurate contrast output.

The Optec® 6500 CS Tester (Vision Sciences Research Corporation, San Ramon, CA) presents the FACT test in a computerized unit. The unit is enclosed so that light levels can be standardized, and there are both daytime (85 cd/m^2) and night time (3.0 cd/m^2) illumination options.

Low-contrast visual acuity charts

While low-contrast VA tests can provide valuable information, low-contrast VA testing should not be considered equivalent to CS testing, since the effect of spatial frequency is not tested systematically. Nevertheless, there are numerous examples of both printed and computerized charts which allow the patient's acuity to be assessed over a range of contrast levels at both distance and near. For example, Precision Vision (Precision Vision, La Salle, IL) produce distance logMAR acuity charts ranging in contrast from 1.25% to 25% for testing at 4 m. Similarly, the computer-based Test Chart 2000 acuity system (see above) can be used to present either Snellen or logMAR charts (including isolated optotypes) at any contrast level. Two examples of near tests are the SKILL low-contrast VA test and the Colenbrander Mixed Contrast Card.

The Smith-Kettlewell Institute Low Luminance (SKILL) VA test (Smith-Kettlewell Eye Research Institute, San Francisco, CA) is designed for a 40 cm working distance and contains logMAR charts on both sides of the card. One side has a high-contrast (>90%) black-on-white letter chart ranging from 12.5 M to 0.4 M, while the other side is a low-contrast (14%) chart of black letters on a dark grey background. The darker background is designed to simulate lower luminance conditions. The SKILL score is taken as the difference in performance on the low-contrast versus the high-contrast side (Haegerstrom-Portnoy et al 1997).

The Colenbrander Mixed Contrast Card (Precision Vision, La Salle, IL) provides a CS test similar to the SKILL test. This test includes both high and 10% contrast text forming sentences at a 4th grade reading level. The acuity ranges from 6.3 M to 0.32 M, and the test is designed for a 40 cm viewing distance. The ability to have the whole test printed on a handheld card is also convenient in a clinical setting.

All of the previously discussed tests have their own specific applications, as well as individual strengths and weaknesses. For example, if a practitioner wishes to assess CS at a range of spatial frequencies with one diagnostic tool, the Vistech chart would be more appropriate than the Pelli–Robson chart. In addition, there have been studies which have determined strong correlations between CS and functional ability. Therefore, for a patient with difficulty reading, certain tests (e.g. Pelli–Robson) may be more applicable to determine the effect of CS on reading rate (Leat & Woo 1997).

Measurement procedures

All of the tests discussed determine the contrast threshold using one of three basic procedures: ascending limits, descending limits or the staircase method. Each method has distinct advantages and disadvantages. With the ascending limits procedure, stimuli are presented initially at a subthreshold level. Target intensity is increased in a stepwise fashion until a positive response is obtained, so that the patient is now able to resolve or identify the stimulus. The point at which the response changes from negative to positive corresponds with the patient's contrast threshold. However, when testing an untrained patient, it is important that they understand the stimulus characteristic being sought. Otherwise, the patient may fail to identify the critical information, such as the presence of an edge in the Melbourne Edge Test, or the direction of the grating in the FACT test.

The method of descending limits begins with a superthreshold contrast level that is easily detected by the patient. Stimulus intensity is decreased until a 'not seen' response is obtained. A common example of this method is with clinical VA measurement. The higher contrast levels (or larger

MAR in VA testing) allow the patient to become accustomed to the testing scenario.

The final category of threshold determination, the staircase method, is essentially a mixture of the ascending and descending limit methods. This procedure typically begins with the stimulus contrast at a level below threshold, and contrast is increased until a change in response (from non-seeing to seeing) is recorded. Contrast is decreased subsequently until the target is no longer visible (or identifiable). Each change in response (or reversal) is found multiple times. The stimulus values at each reversal are averaged to obtain the mean sensitivity. This is useful since the method of descending limits tends to underestimate the patient's threshold, while ascending limits will overestimate the value. Accordingly, the average of these two procedures should result in a more accurate finding of the patient's contrast threshold.

Practitioners should be aware that regardless of the test utilized, the results may be modified by the specific criterion adopted by the patient during the testing procedure. Therefore, instructions and testing protocols should be standardized to ensure that variations in the CSF reflect actual changes in vision rather than fluctuations in the patient's criterion for judging the visibility of the stimulus.

Summary

Visual acuity (VA) and contrast sensitivity function (CSF) are among the most important procedures within the optometric examination for quantifying a patient's visual resolution. It is hoped that the patient's performance in these clinical tests will reflect their ability to carry out tasks in the naturalistic visual environment. If clinical examination is restricted to a narrow range of test parameters, such as testing with only small, high-contrast stimuli under optimal illumination, then the results will not correlate with real-world visual performance. By using a variety of testing conditions, together with other procedures such as central and peripheral visual fields (see Ch. 20) and colour vision assessment (see Ch. 19), one can gain a better estimate of the patient's visual ability in the real world.

References

Bailey I L 2006 Visual acuity. In: Benjamin W J (ed.) Borish's clinical refraction, 2nd edn. Butterworth-Heinemann, St Louis, pp 217–246

Bailey I L, Lovie J E 1980 The design and use of a new near-vision chart. American Journal of Optometry and Physiological Optics 57:378–387

Bansback N, Czoski-Murray C, Carlton J et al 2007 Determinants of health related quality of life and health state utility in patients with age related macular degeneration: the association of contrast sensitivity and visual acuity. Quality of Life Research 16:533–543

Bennett A G, Rabbetts R B 1989 Clinical visual optics, 2nd edn. Butterworths, London, p 23–72

British Standard BS 4274–1:2003 Visual acuity test types. Test charts for clinical determination of distance visual acuity. Specification. BSI, London

Brown J L 1979 Visual acuity and form discrimination. In: Records R E (ed.) Physiology of the human eye and visual system. Harper & Row, Hagerstown, pp 390–418

Cox M J, Norman J H, Norman P 1999 The effect of surround luminance on measurements of contrast sensitivity. Ophthalmic and Physiological Optics 19:401–414

DeMarco L M, Massof R W 1997 Distributions of print sizes in U.S. newspapers. Journal of Visual Impairment and Blindness. 91:9–13

Dougherty B E, Flom R E, Bullimore M A 2005 An evaluation of the Mars Letter Contrast Sensitivity Test. Optometry and Vision Science 82:970–975

Duke-Elder S, Abrams D 1970 System of ophthalmology, vol V. Ophthalmic Optics and Refraction. C V Mosby, St Louis, pp 420–429

Elliott D B 2006 Contrast sensitivity and glare testing. In: Benjamin W J (ed.) Borish's clinical refraction, 2nd edn. Butterworth-Heinemann, St Louis, pp 247–288

Elliott D B, Bullimore M A 1993 Assessing the reliability, discriminative ability, and validity of disability glare tests. Investigative Ophthalmology and Visual Science 34:108–119

Elliott D B, Yang K C H, Whitaker D 1995 Visual acuity changes throughout adulthood in normal, healthy eyes: Seeing beyond 6/6. Optometry and Vision Science 72:186–191

Eperjesi F, Wolffsohn J, Bowden J et al 2004 Normative contrast sensitivity values for the back-lit Melbourne Edge Test and the effect of visual impairment. Ophthalmic and Physiological Optics 24:600–606

Haegerstrom-Portnoy G, Brabyn J, Schneck M E et al 1997 The SKILL card. An acuity test of reduced luminance and contrast. Investigative Ophthalmology and Visual Science 38:207–218

Hartridge H, Owens H B 1922 Test types. British Journal of Ophthalmology 6:543–549

Järvinen P, Hyvärinen L 1997 Contrast sensitivity measurement in evaluations of visual symptoms caused by exposure to triethylamine. Occupational and Environmental Medicine 54:483–486

Leat S J, Wegmann D 2004 Clinical testing of contrast sensitivity in children: age-related norms and validity. Optometry and Vision Science 81:245–254

Leat S J, Woo G C 1997 The validity of current clinical tests of contrast sensitivity and their ability to predict reading speed in low vision. Eye 11(6):893–899

Lord S R 2006 Visual risk factors for falls in older people. Age and Ageing 35(Suppl 2):ii42–ii45

Pelli D G, Robson J G, Wilkins A J 1988 The design of a new letter chart for measuring contrast sensitivity. Clinical Vision Science 2:187–199

Pesudovs K, Hazel C A, Doran R M et al 2004 The usefulness of Vistech and FACT contrast sensitivity charts for cataract and refractive surgery outcomes research. British Journal Ophthalmology 88:11–16

Pomerance G N, Evans D W 1994 Test-retest reliability of the CSV-1000 contrast test and its relationship to glaucoma therapy. Investigative Ophthalmology and Visual Science 35:3357–3361

Regan D 1991 The Charles F. Prentice Award Lecture 1991: Specific Tests and Specific Blindnesses: Keys, Locks, and Parallel Processing. Optometry and Vision Science 68:489–512

Robson J G 1993 Contrast sensitivity: one hundred years of clinical measurement. In: Shapley R, Lam D M-K (eds) Contrast sensitivity. MIT Press, Cambridge, pp 254–265

Schade O H 1956 Optical and photoelectric analog of the eye. Journal of the Optical Society of America 46:721–739

Sisto D, Trojano M, Vetrugno M et al 2005 Subclinical visual involvement in multiple sclerosis: a study by MRI, VEPs, frequency-doubling perimetry, standard perimetry, and contrast sensitivity. Investigative Ophthalmology and Visual Science 46:1264–1268

Sloan L L 1959 New test charts for the measurement of visual acuity at far and near distances. American Journal of Ophthalmology 48:807–813

Thayaparan K, Crossland M D, Rubin G S 2007 Clinical assessment of two new contrast sensitivity charts. British Journal of Ophthalmology 91:749–752

Tinker M A, Paterson D G 1944 Wartime changes in newspaper body type. Journalism Quarterly 21:7–11

Velasco e Cruz, A A 1990 Historical roots of 20/20 as a (wrong) standard value of normal visual acuity. Optometry and Vision Science 67:661

Walker J G, Anstey K J, Hennessy M P et al 2006 The impact of cataract surgery on visual functioning, vision-related disability and psychological distress: a randomized controlled trial. Clinical and Experimental Ophthalmology 34:734–742

Wolffsohn J S, Eperjesi F, Napper G 2005 Evaluation of Melbourne Edge Test contrast sensitivity measures in the visually impaired. Ophthalmic and Physiological Optics 25:371–374

Wood J M, Owens D A 2005 Standard measures of visual acuity do not predict drivers' recognition performance under day or night conditions. Optometry and Vision Science 82:698–705

CHAPTER 13

Objective refraction

David A Atchison

Introduction

Techniques for determining the refractive error of the eye can be divided into three groups: subjective, objective or methods that may be subjective or objective. Subjective methods require considerable patient involvement, with the patient making judgements about the correct focus. Usually, this involves them reporting which of two views of a target, seen through different lens combinations, is superior. This process is repeated in a systematic manner to obtain the patient's refraction. Subjective refraction is addressed in Chapter 14.

Objective methods require much less patient involvement than subjective refraction, with the patient usually being required merely to keep their eyes open and look at a target. Objective refraction techniques rely upon some of the radiation incident upon the patient's fundus being reflected diffusely. Objective methods involve the examiner to different extents. One class of objective techniques involves visual (manual) instruments, in which the examiner makes the judgement of correct defocus. Another class of objective testing uses automatic instruments, in which an electronic detector makes the decision about the correct focus or error of focus and the examiner's role is reduced to aligning the instrument's optical axis with the patient's eye. Automated instruments have largely replaced manual instruments with one major exception, namely retinoscopy. This continues to be an important technique and is covered in detail in the next section.

Although a subjective refraction by a competent examiner remains the 'gold standard' for prescribing correcting lenses, objective refraction is playing an increasingly important role. It is particularly important when subjective refraction is difficult because of limited cooperation by the patient or when screening large numbers of patients. Wavefront-sensing instruments have added a new dimension to objective refraction by providing information on the higher-order aberrations.

This chapter will cover many of the important objective techniques. Because instruments change rapidly, and techniques come in and out of favour, the emphasis will be on principles of refraction rather than describing particular instruments.

Retinoscopy

Introduction

Retinoscopy was introduced by Cuignet in the 1870s. This is the term most commonly used in English-speaking countries, although it is also known by other names including skiascopy, skiametry, umbrascopy, and pupilloscopy.

In retinoscopy, the fundus (retina) acts as a screen over which a patch of light is moved. The examiner observes the shape and movement of the reflected light within the patient's pupil through a retinoscope. The appearance of this reflected light is referred to as the 'reflex'. Based upon the direction and speed of the reflex, lenses are placed in front of the patient's eye until the speed of movement of the reflex is infinitely quick – this is called the point of 'reversal' or 'neutralization'.

Now the fundus of the patient's eye is focused at (or conjugate with) the sighthole of the retinoscope and as the light patch moves over the patient's fundus there is almost instantaneous cutoff of the return beam as it reaches the edge of the sighthole.

Retinoscopes are relatively simple optical instruments. They have four components: a light source, a lens that can be moved to vary the position of the image of the light source (the 'immediate' source), a mirror which is semi-reflecting or has a hole in it so that the examiner can view the patient's eye along the direction of the light beam entering the patient's eye, and a sighthole. Usually the mirror is plane, but in early instruments it was often concave. The shape of the mirror will affect the direction and speed of movement. In what follows, the mirror will be assumed to be flat. In some instruments, the light source rather than the lens can be moved.

If the mirror has a hole, this forms the effective sighthole (**Fig. 13.1**) and a patch corresponding with the sighthole will appear in the reflex, which may be apparent close to neutralization (Rabbetts 2007). However, this is unlikely to cause significant difficulties to the examiner. The sighthole size is usually about 1.5 mm to 2 mm in diameter. The precision of reversal may be improved by using a smaller sighthole, provided the reduction in light reaching the examiner's eye is not a problem. A sighthole of variable dimensions is available in some instruments.

There are two main types of retinoscope. The spot retinoscope has a light bulb with a small coiled filament. Some spot retinoscopes have restricted focusing ranges so that the beam of light entering the patient's eye is always divergent (i.e. the immediate source is always behind the instrument, as in **Figure 13.1**). The streak retinoscope has either an uncoiled linear filament light bulb or a slit aperture painted on the bulb, and these produce a 'streak' of light. Some retinoscopes can change from one type to the other merely by a change of light bulb, and this does not affect the focusing range.

Either the source or a slit aperture near the lens can rotate. In operation, the streak is orientated to lie at right angles to the direction of movement of the instrument. Although the spot retinoscope may be easier to use initially compared with the streak retinoscope, the streak retinoscope is potentially more accurate in determining the axis of high cylinders.

Principles of retinoscopy

In the operation of the retinoscope, the instrument is tilted by the examiner so that a light beam scans across a particular meridian of the patient's pupil. The instrument is then tilted in the opposite direction, and the examiner continues this to-and-fro movement, whilst observing the shape and movement of the reflex. The reflex will move in the same direction as the instrument when examining eyes with hyperopia, emmetropia and 'low' myopia (i.e. myopia less than the dioptric equivalent of the working distance; see next section). This is referred to as 'with' movement. The reflex will move in the opposite direction to the instrument for higher degrees of myopia, and this is referred to as 'against' movement. The closer the patient's far point lies to the retinoscope sighthole, the faster the speed of the reflex.

Elaboration will now be given for the reflex movements in the different spherical ametropias. **Figure 13.2A** shows the retinoscope, represented by its mirror, in front of a low myopic eye. The light reflected from R on the patient's fundus converges as it leaves the eye towards R' (the far point of the eye) behind the sighthole. Because all of the light travels through the sighthole, the pupil appears to be fully illuminated. The reflex colour is usually red or orange, but this depends on the colour of the retinoscope beam and reflection properties of the fundus.

In **Figure 13.2B**, the retinoscope is tilted upwards. The light reaching the patient's fundus is also directed upwards and the light leaving the patient's eye is directed downwards. Some of the reflected light leaving the patient's eye at the bottom of the pupil is vignetted (cut off) by the edge of the sighthole. This part of the pupil appears dark, as shown on the left of the diagram. As the tilting of the mirror continues, the dark region will increase in size. This is interpreted by the examiner as the reflex moving across the pupil in the same direction as the retinoscope is tilted, that is, there is a 'with' movement. If the retinoscope is then tilted

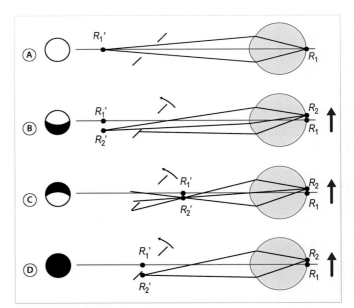

Figure 13.2 Principle of reflex movement. **(A)** Reflex in a low myopic eye. **(B)** Effect of tilt on the reflex formation for a low myopic eye. **(C)** Effect of tilt on the reflex formation for a moderate myopic eye. **(D)** Effect of tilt on reflex formation at reversal.

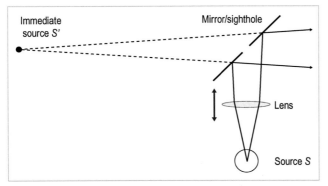

Figure 13.1 The optical components of a retinoscope.

downwards, all other movements swap direction, so the appearance of with movement continues.

The situation just described for low myopia also explains with movement for a hyperope, but here the light leaving the patient's eye diverges as if it came from R' (the far point) behind the patient's eye.

Let us now consider a myope of higher degree, in which R' lies between the patient's eye and the retinoscope (**Fig. 13.2C**). When the retinoscope is tilted upwards, the light emerging from the top of the patient's pupil is vignetted at the sighthole, and so the top of the patient's pupil appears dark to the examiner. This is interpreted as the reflex moving in the opposite direction to the retinoscope movement, i.e. an 'against' movement of the reflex.

Reversal (or neutralization) occurs when the far point of the eye coincides with the retinoscope sighthole (**Fig. 13.2D**). Depending on the degree to which the retinoscope is tilted, vignetting is either zero or total. In other words, as R' scans across the sighthole, the pupil appears either completely illuminated or completely dark. In practice, reversal is not as distinct as shown here because of the finite size of the fundus patch, the light not reflecting from a distinct fundal site, and the influence of higher-order aberrations.

Correction for spherical refractions

In spherical hyperopia, the resulting with movement is neutralized with positive lenses placed in front of the eye, which are generally mounted in a trial frame or phoropter (refractor head). The speed of the reflex helps determine subsequent lens power selection, with a slow speed indicating that higher lens powers are needed. Lens selection is varied until reversal is reached. As reversal approaches, the reflex becomes brighter and wider. Reversal takes some experience to appreciate. To check it has been correctly identified, the examiner can do two things. The first is 'bracketing' whereby the examiner determines which lenses are required to give just noticeable with and against movements, and then reversal is taken as the midpoint. Alternatively, the examiner can move towards and away from the patient over a few centimetres while continuing to pivot the retinoscope. If reversal has indeed been achieved, then if the examiner moves towards the patient, the far point will lie behind the sighthole, and a fast with movement will be observed. If the examiner then moves away from the patient so that the far point lies in front of the sighthole, a fast against movement of the reflex becomes apparent.

Following reversal, a negative lens whose power corresponds with the reciprocal of the 'working distance' between the retinoscope and the patient's eye must be added so that the refraction is referenced to optical infinity rather than the position of the retinoscope. For example, if reversal is obtained with +3.50 DS at a 67 cm working distance, the patient's correction is +3.50 DS − 1/(0.67 m) = + 3.50 DS − 1.50 DS = +2.00 DS.

Other than the towards/away procedure described above to confirm reversal, it is important to maintain a constant working distance during retinoscopy, The working distance will mainly depend on the comfort of the examiner. Working distances of 50 cm and 67 cm are most commonly used, as these correspond to 2.00 DS and 1.50 DS, respectively. Working distances less than 50 cm are not favoured because a slight error in working distance may lead to appreciable errors in refraction. For example, a 5 cm error at a working distance of 40 cm may change the result by nearly 0.37 DS, while the same error at a working distance of 67 cm will change the finding by less than 0.12 DS.

For myopia, reversal occurs without the need for lenses when the myopia is equivalent to the working distance in dioptres. For example, reversal occurs at 67 cm when examining a 1.50 D myopic patient. For low myopia, with movement will be seen, requiring positive-powered lenses for reversal. For example, if reversal is obtained with +0.50 DS at 67 cm working distance, the patient's correction is +0.50 DS − 1/(0.67 m) = +0.50 DS − 1.50 DS = −1.00 DS.

For higher amounts of myopia than the working distance equivalent, the examiner initially sees against movement. This must be neutralized with a negative lens. After confirming reversal, the working distance power is added. For example, if reversal is obtained with −2.00 DS at 67 cm working distance, the patient's correction is −2.00 DS − 1/(0.67 m) = −2.00 DS − 1.50 DS = −3.50 DS.

As an alternative to correcting for the working distance by adding negative lens power, a positive working distance lens can be added to the trial frame or phoropter and then ignored in the subsequent analysis. For 50 cm and 67 cm working distances, the working distance lens powers are +2.00 DS and +1.50 DS, respectively.

Correction when astigmatism is present

When an eye has astigmatism, meridians of maximum and minimum ocular power will exist. These are referred to as the principal meridians, and each must be identified and corrected. Reversal can be achieved with two spherical lenses, one for each principal meridian, or with a combination of spherical and cylindrical lenses. The second method is preferable, but the beginner may find the first method helpful when first correcting astigmatism. A later section will describe how to identify the orientation of the principal meridians, but for the present we will assume that these are known.

For the first method, reversal is obtained with spherical lenses for each principal meridian separately. A correction is then made for the working distance, and the result converted to sphere, cylinder and axis format.

For the second method, either negative- or positive-power cylinders may be used. It is more common in optometric practice to use negative cylinders, and these are generally preferred because they allow better control of accommodation when one or both principal meridians are hyperopic. Reversal is obtained first for the principal meridian having the slower with or quicker against movement (this is the more hyperopic or less myopic meridian) using a spherical lens. This leaves the eye myopic along the other principal meridian, and against movement will be seen here. Negative cylinders are added, with their axes along the first corrected meridian, to obtain reversal along the second meridian. Correction is then made for the working distance. Note that if positive cylinders are used, the principal meridian having the quicker with or slower against movement is corrected first, and positive cylinders are used with their axes along this meridian.

Example 13.1

An eye requires the correction +2.50 / −3.00 × 30; working distance 67 cm. Describe the results at the steps involved in retinoscopy.

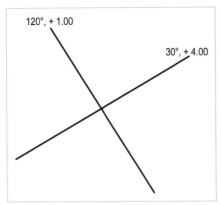

Figure 13.3 Powers along the principal meridians in Example 13.1: first method before an allowance is made for working distance.

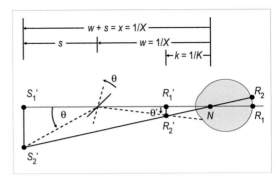

Figure 13.4 Deriving the relative speed and direction of reflex movement. N is the nodal point of the patient's eye.

Using the first method:

Both principal meridians 30° and 120° have with movement

Along 30°, reversal is obtained with +4.00 DS (Fig. 13.3)

Along 120°, reversal is obtained with +1.00 DS (Fig. 13.3)

Result in negative cylinder form is +4.00 / −3.00 × 30

Add −1.50 D sphere for the working distance to give +2.50 / −3.00 × 30.

Using the second method:

Both principal meridians 30° and 120° show with movement

The slower with movement is obtained along 30°: reversal is obtained with +4.00 DS

Against movement is then seen along the 120° meridian

Reversal along 120° is achieved with a −3.00 cylinder axis 30

Therefore, the neutralizing lenses in negative cylinder form are +4.00 / −3.00 × 30

Add −1.50 D sphere for the working distance to give +2.50 / −3.00 × 30.

Relative speed and direction of reflex movement

In the subsequent ray diagrams, distances and their reciprocals to the left of the reference plane are taken as negative and small angle approximations are used. The distance from the patient's eye to the retinoscopic mirror/sighthole is the working distance w and the distance from the eye's nodal point to the far point is k.

In **Figure 13.4** the far point is shown between the patient's eye and the retinoscope mirror. The immediate source is at S_1', a distance s from the mirror. Tilting the retinoscope by angle θ moves S_1' to S_2' by distance $S_1'S_2' = \theta s$ as the illuminated portion of the patient's fundus moves from R_1 to R_2. The far point of the patient's eye moves from R_1' to R_2'.

From similar triangles $S_1'NS_2'$ and $R_1'NR_2'$

$$R_1R_2/k = S_1'S_2'/(w + s)$$

or

$$R_1R_2 = \theta sk/(w + s).$$

Relative to the mirror, the far point has moved by angle θ', which is also the angle that the reflex has moved across the pupil relative to the mirror. The angle is given by

$$\theta' = R_1R_2/(k - w) = \theta sk/[(w + s)(k - w)].$$

The ratio of the angular velocity of the reflex to the angular velocity of the mirror tilt is given by

$$\theta'/\theta = sk/[(w + s)(k - w)].$$

Several substitutions can be made into this equation: k replacing $1/K$, where K is the refractive error, w replacing $1/W$, and s replacing $1/X - 1/W$, where X is the vergence of immediate source from the patient's eye. This gives

$$\frac{\theta'}{\theta} = \frac{W}{W - K} \frac{W - X}{W} = \frac{W - X}{W - K} \tag{13.1}$$

Equation (13.1) contains two factors: the 'refraction' factor and the 'retinoscopy' factor. **Figure 13.5** shows the refraction factor $W/(W - K)$ as a function of K when W is kept fixed at −1.50 D. In the usual set-up of the retinoscope with a diverging beam, positive values of the refraction factor correspond to with movement and negative values correspond to against movement. The refraction factor

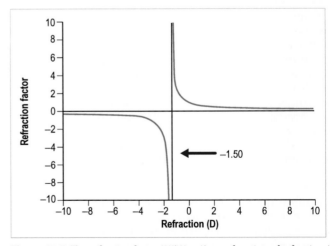

Figure 13.5 The refractive factor $W/(W − K)$ as a function of refraction K for a working distance of 67 cm ($W = -1.50$ D). Note that the refraction is actually the residual refraction as lenses are placed in front of the patient's eye.

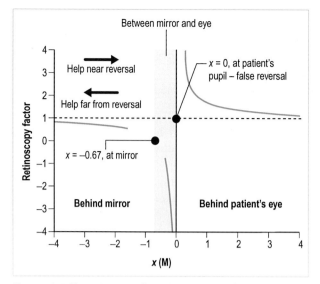

Figure 13.6 The retinoscopic factor ($W − X$)$/W$ as a function of distance x of the immediate source from the patient's eye for a working distance of 67 cm ($W = −1.50$ D). Direction of movement is reversed for the shaded region, corresponding to the immediate source being between the patient's eye and the mirror. There is a gap in the curve between $x = −1.6$ and $−0.4$ m because, due to physical limitations, the immediate source cannot reach the position of the mirror.

approaches infinity as K approaches W. This corresponds to reversal.

The retinoscopy factor in Equation (13.1) is ($W − X$)$/W$. **Figure 13.6** shows the retinoscopy factor as a function of x, where $x = 1/X$, when W is kept fixed at $−1.50$ D. If the immediate source is behind the mirror, X is negative. For some spot retinoscopes x (and X) is restricted to negative values, because the limited range of distances between the light source and the retinoscope lens means that the light leaving the retinoscope is always diverging. The retinoscopy factor is positive when the immediate source S is behind the mirror or behind the patient's eye (all positive x values), but it is negative when the immediate source is between the patient's eye and the retinoscope (shaded region in **Fig. 13.6**). For these positions of the immediate source, corresponding to very convergent settings of the streak retinoscope, the reflex direction is opposite from that which usually occurs.

If the immediate source is at the patient's pupillary plane, for which $x = 0$ and X is infinite, the retinoscopy factor and the reflex speed are infinite. Retinoscopy appears to be at reversal, but this is independent of refractive state and so is referred to as *false reversal*.

To avoid confusion, convergent settings of the retinoscope should be avoided so as to prevent the opposite direction of the reflex movement or false reversal from occurring. For the majority of retinoscopes, this can be ensured by having the sleeve of the retinoscope all or most of the way *down*. As mentioned earlier, there are some instruments (e.g. the Copeland retinoscope) for which the source is moved relative to the lens and in these instruments the sleeve is placed all or most of the way *up*.

Having said this, a skilled retinoscopist may deliberately manipulate the sleeve position. High refractions give low refraction factors and slow reflex movements, which may be hard to detect. The speed can be increased by increasing

the retinoscopic factor, which means the beam diverges as little as possible (see **Fig. 13.6**). This is achieved by moving the sleeve upwards to a certain extent. This will narrow the band of light from the retinoscope on the face but widen the reflex. The same retinoscopist may make reversal more definite through reducing the retinoscopic factor by placing the sleeve all the way down, in which case the band on the face is wide and the reflex is narrow.

The retinoscopy equation is applicable for spherical ametropia or for the principal meridians of astigmatic eyes. The situation is more complicated if scanning is done along orientations other than the principal meridians of astigmatic eyes. This is shown in **Figure 13.7A**. The direction of reflex movement can be determined. The components of the beam along the principal meridians are calculated. The components are multiplied by the appropriate θ'/θ for each principal meridian, and the effects are combined to find the direction and speed of reflex movement. The direction of movement of the illuminated streak and reflex are on the same side of the principal meridian when both principal meridians are myopic or hyperopic relative to the retinoscope. They are on opposite sides when one meridian is myopic and the other is hyperopic relative to the retinoscope, which is the situation shown in **Figure 13.7A**. A fuller account of this is given by Rabbetts (2007).

Although the reflex movement is interpreted to be perpendicular to the orientation of the reflex in streak retinoscopy (as in **Fig. 13.7A**), the true direction of movement is usually at some other angle. This can be conveniently ignored, but for the interested reader further details are provided by Rabbetts (2007) and by Smith and Haymes (2003).

Method for retinoscopy

Some of the procedures in retinoscopy will now be described. Firstly, the room lights are usually turned off or dimmed to encourage a reasonable degree of pupil dilation and reduce reflections from lens surfaces. The examiner is positioned at an appropriate working distance, such as

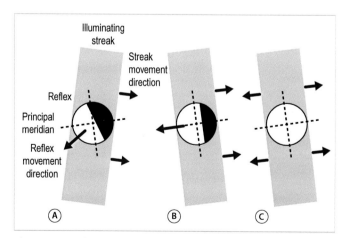

Figure 13.7 Reflex appearances in streak retinoscopy. **(A)** The illuminating streak is not parallel nor perpendicular to the principal meridians as there is a break in alignment between the illuminating streak and the reflex. Note that the streak is always moved at right angles to its orientation. The reflex shows against movement. **(B)** The illuminating streak is rotated so that it and the reflex are aligned and parallel to one of the principal meridians. The reflex continues to show against movement. **(C)** At reversal, the reflex has expanded to fill the pupil.

50 cm or 67 cm, and at the patient's eye level. Except for the deliberate use of the towards/away procedure, the selected working distance should be maintained during the procedure. Both of the examiner's eyes should be kept open. The examiner can choose to use a working distance lens in a trial frame or phoropter to compensate for the distance (e.g.+1.50 DS for 67 cm). If so, this is ignored when determining the correction at the end (see Example 13.2, below).

The patient is asked to fixate a distant object with the eye not under examination. The target may be a muscle light, a row of letters or a duochrome chart. Other, age-appropriate targets may be used when examining children (see Ch. 28). Usually, the eye not being examined is kept 'fogged' or myopic with additional positive lenses in an effort to relax accommodation. The examiner observes as close to the patient's line of sight as possible without obscuring the view of the fixation target. When examining the patient's right eye, the examiner holds the retinoscope with the right hand and looks through the right eye. The reverse is the case when examining the patient's left eye. As for direct ophthalmoscopy, use of the non-dominant eye and/or hand may require perseverance.

Reversal in streak retinoscopy

With streak retinoscopy, the light source is drawn out into a streak. The reflex moves with or against the direction of instrument motion. Initially, the examiner may scan along the 180°, 90°, 45° and 135° meridians to get an idea of the refractive error. The streak is always orientated at right angles to the meridian being scanned. If the speed of reflex movement is similar for all meridians and the streak and reflex remain in alignment, there is negligible astigmatism. Usually, some degree of astigmatism is present, and the examiner should identify the first principal meridian to neutralize (namely, the more hyperopic or less myopic principal meridian). If the refraction is high but the astigmatism is relatively low, it may not initially be obvious which is the more hyperopic meridian, but as reversal is approached this should become apparent. To identify the principal meridian, the illuminating streak and the reflex must be parallel and the reflex must have good definition. If there is a break in alignment (**Fig. 13.7A**), the streak must be rotated until alignment is achieved (**Fig. 13.7B**). Reversal is then achieved as described previously (**Fig. 13.7C**).

After achieving reversal along the first principal meridian, the streak is rotated through 90°. If the first meridian was correctly identified, a sharply defined reflex will be seen moving parallel to the direction of instrument motion. If the reflex is not clearly defined and a break in alignment is observed, then the axis estimate is incorrect. If the first meridian was correctly identified as the more hyperopic (or less myopic), then the second meridian will show against movement. Negative cylinders are introduced with their axes along the previously neutralized meridian, and reversal is obtained along the second meridian.

Should an error be made in the selection of the principal meridians, this may become obvious by the break in streak illumination and reflex alignment when cylinders are placed in front of the eye. As the orientation of the illuminating streak is altered to correct this, so too is the axis of any cylindrical lens. The correct axis may be determined by 'straddling', in which the illuminating streak is rotated by 45° in both directions relative to the axis. The speed

and alignment of the reflex are compared for these meridians, and the cylinder axis is adjusted until the appearances are similar.

Example 13.2

This is an example of the procedure in streak retinoscopy for the correction +2.50 / −3.00 × 30 at a working distance of 67 cm. It is an elaboration of the second method used in Example 13.1 (above). It will be demonstrated both with and without a working distance lens correction. It omits details of patient instructions, target appearance, and dealing with the non-tested eye.

Method without a working distance lens:

Step 1. Identify the principal meridians.
No breaks in alignment between the reflex and streak occur when the streak is orientated at 120° and moves along the 30° meridian, or when the streak is orientated at 30° and moves along the 120° meridian. Hence, the principal meridians are 30° and 120°.

Step 2. Choose which principal meridian to investigate first.
With movement is seen for both principal meridians, but is slower along 30° than along 120° degrees because the 30° meridian is more hyperopic. Hence, find reversal along 30° first.

Step 3. Obtain reversal along the first principal meridian using spheres.
The streak is orientated at 120° and moved along 30° (**Fig. 13.8A**). +4.00 DS is required.

Step 4. Neutralize along second principal meridian.
Leave the spherical correcting lens in place. Rotate the streak by 90° to 30° and find reversal along the 120° meridian (**Fig. 13.8B**). Correct with negative cylinders, axis aligned with first principal meridian, i.e. 30°. −3.00 DC × 30 is required.

Step 5. Add working distance correction to sphere: +4.00 − 1.50 = +2.50 DS.
Result is +2.50/−3.00 × 30.

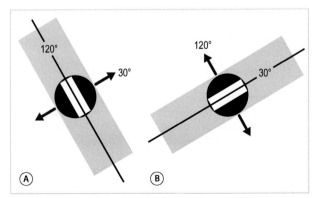

Figure 13.8 Example 13.2: no working distance lens. **(A)** The streak is orientated at 120° and moved along 30° (first principal meridian). **(B)** The streak is orientated at 30° and moved along 120° (second principal meridian).

*Method with working distance lens
(67 cm working distance)*

Step 1. Introduce a +1.50 DS in the phoropter or trial frame.

This is ignored in subsequent steps (although it must be removed when measuring distance visual acuity or during the subjective refraction).

Step2. Identify principal meridians (as per Step 1, method for no working distance lens shown above).

Step 3. Choose the principal meridian to investigate first.

With movement is seen along 30° and against movement is seen along 120° degrees. Hence, find reversal along 30° first.

Step 4. Obtain reversal along the first principal meridian using spheres.

The streak is orientated at 120° and moved along 30°. +2.50 DS is required.

Step 5. Neutralize along second principal meridian (as per Step 4, method for no working distance lens shown above). −3.00 DC × 30 required.
Result is +2.50/−3.00 × 30.

Reversal in spot retinoscopy

The light source of a spot retinoscope is circular. This produces a circular reflex for spherical refractions, and an elliptical reflex when astigmatism is present. The principal meridians are determined by altering the direction of the retinoscope until the reflex moves parallel to the illuminating spot on the face. Except for not rotating the light source, the procedure is similar to that used in streak retinoscopy. **Figure 13.9A** shows against movement but with the reflex not moving parallel to the direction of retinoscope movement; **Figure 13.9B** shows against movement when the two directions are exactly opposite and therefore coincident with a principal meridian; and **Figure 13.9C** shows the appearance at reversal.

Other factors and problems in retinoscopy

Accommodation (see Chapter 15)

As for other methods of refraction, it is important to relax accommodation in young subjects, otherwise myopia may be overestimated and hyperopia may be underestimated or missed.

During refraction, variation in accommodation may be noted by variations in the speed and brightness of the reflex and by fluctuations in pupil size. Remedies include using positive lenses in front of the non-tested eye to relax accommodation (fogging), using a blue target (because of chromatic aberrations, eyes are more myopic in blue than at other wavelengths and therefore this is another form of fogging) and asking the patient to imagine that the target is a long distance away. The most common method is to use fogging lenses, but care must be taken not to make the target appear too blurred as young patients may increase accommodation to a 'resting state' or tonic level. This can be avoided by using large letters (e.g. 6/60 optotypes) as a target so that some detail can be discerned. Ward and Charman (1987) indicated that this limit of fogging is about 2.0 D, but Chiu et al (1997) found that fogging could be as high as 5 D in young myopic subjects without any significant changes in refractive error. The level of fogging is based on any knowledge of the patient's ametropia, and may be varied during the procedure, such as when latent hyperopia is suspected.

Obliquity

Retinoscopy is usually performed slightly temporal to the patient's line of sight. This off-axis error may affect the result. However, to minimize this effect, it is recommended that the obliquity be no more than 5°, although even at this angle a difference of up to 0.50 D may be found, when compared with the on-axis refractive error (Atchison et al 2006).

Chromatic aberration

The eye is more powerful at shorter wavelengths, and the corresponding variation in ocular refraction amounts to 2 D across the visible spectrum (Atchison & Smith 2000). The spectral distribution of the light source and the spectral distribution of light reflected from the fundus will have some influence on refractive error, with Charman (1975) estimating that these could cause a change of up to 0.2 D of hyperopia in retinoscopy, when compared with subjective results.

Site of reflection

The longer the wavelength, the deeper the penetration of light into the retina and choroid before reflection occurs, and to some extent this counteracts the influence of chromatic aberration and spectral distribution of the reflected light. Millodot and O'Leary (Millodot & O'Leary 1978; O'Leary & Millodot 1978) found differences in retinoscopy and subjective refraction as a function of age, with young subjects having more hyperopic refractions with retinoscopy than with subjective refraction. To explain this, they suggested that the main reflection layers are the vitreous–retinal interface and a layer

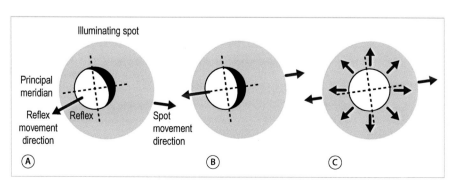

Figure 13.9 Reflex appearances in spot retinoscopy. **(A)** The illuminating spot is moved at an angle to the principal meridian as the illuminating spot and the reflex move in different directions. The reflex shows against movement. **(B)** The illuminating spot is moved so that its movement and the reflex movement are parallel to one of the principal meridians. The reflex continues to show against movement. **(C)** At reversal, the reflex expands to fill the pupil.

near the pigment epithelium, with an age-related change in refractive index being responsible for most of the reflection occurring at the vitreous–retinal interface in young people, and for most of the reflection occurring at the deeper layer in older individuals. This is an important issue in objective refractors (see later in this chapter). It is because of the variation in the site of reflection that the term 'fundus' has been used in much of this chapter rather than 'retina'.

Amblyopia and strabismus

In amblyopia, one eye has poor vision even when corrected, and the vision in this eye may be suppressed under binocular viewing conditions. If, during retinoscopy, the fixating eye is the amblyopic eye, it may not see the fixation target and the examiner may have to move further to the temporal side of the tested eye so that it can see the fixation target, although this increases the angle of obliquity.

In the case of a patient with strabismus, only one of the eyes will be fixating the object of regard (see Ch. 16). This presents a challenge to the examiner in retinoscopy, as we usually assume that the non-tested eye is fixating on the target and that any deviation of the tested eye is small. The examiner may ask the patient to alter gaze to another fixation target so that the tested eye is better positioned, or may move to be aligned better with the tested eye. Where eccentric fixation is present with strabismus, the examiner must decide whether to refract the fovea or the eccentric fixating point on the fundus.

Pupils and aberrations

Small pupils may also present a problem, particularly if the reflex is dull because of media opacities. Raising the instrument sleeve helps by decreasing the width of the beam and increasing the brightness of the reflex.

Large pupils may also be a problem as there is no longer a sharp reversal because of higher-order aberrations. In particular, the reflex may move at different speeds across the central and peripheral parts of the pupils. With positive spherical aberration, where the power associated with the peripheral pupil is greater than that found centrally, the peripheral pupil may exhibit against motion while the central pupil shows with movement. It is best to concentrate on the central pupil area only, which can be helped by using small scans across the pupil, or by increasing the ambient illumination to produce some pupillary constriction. Alternatively, a 3–4 mm diameter aperture placed in a well-centred trial frame may also help.

When other aberrations are also significant, such as media irregularities (as found in keratoconus), unusual reflexes such as a split (or scissors) reflex may occur. Here, two regions of the pupil appear illuminated and move towards or away from each other, giving an opening and closing effect similar to the action of a pair of scissors. This is probably produced by coma aberration (Roorda & Bobier 1996). These reflexes are difficult to interpret, but the examiner should concentrate as much as possible on the centre of the pupil.

Media opacities

Opacities of the cornea and lens can make retinoscopy difficult. Reducing the working distance may help, as this provides an increase in brightness and the examiner may find a clearer area to examine. Either this shorter working distance can be retained or the normal distance can be resumed once the examiner feels more confident about interpreting the reflex movement.

Anomalous 'with' movement in myopia

Anomalous with movement can occur in moderate degrees of myopia (Howland 1978; Mutti 2004). This occurs when the retinoscope beam entering the eye is not fully limited by the pupil, that is, when an edge of the entering beam is within the pupil. The anomaly increases as both pupil size and myopia increase. This can be particularly confusing for students refracting model eyes that have large apertures. Having the sleeve all the way down will reduce the chances of this being noticed, as will restricting the scan across the pupil. The edge of the entering beam may also fall within the pupil in hyperopia, but as this makes the reflex easier to see and the with motion is in the correct direction, it is not a significant problem.

Other retinoscopic techniques

The technique described above is conventional static retinoscopy, but there are many other variants of retinoscopy. Three of these are described briefly below.

Modindra near retinoscopy (see Chapter 28)

Mohindra (Mohindra 1975, 1977a,b; Mohindra & Molinari 1979) developed this technique for use with infants without the need for cycloplegia, but it can be extended to other young patients. Retinoscopy is conducted in a dark room so that the retinoscope is the only light source and it is likely that a child will look at it, particularly if encouraged with occasional interesting sounds from the examiner. The usual working distance is 50 cm, but no working distance lens is used. On the basis that there is likely to be a lag of accommodation to the retinoscope of approximately 0.75 D, 1.25 DS is deducted from the retinoscopy result. Mohindra claimed that the retinoscope beam is a poor stimulus to blur-driven accommodation, and that the technique in children correlates well with cycloplegic and subjective refraction.

Dynamic retinoscopy

The fundamental principles of dynamic retinoscopy were laid down at the start of the twentieth century by Cross, although his ideas have been since extended and developed. This is a controversial technique with many adherents, but is believed to be useless by others. It is used to investigate the relationship between accommodation and convergence, and represents the refractive state when the eyes are focused on a near target. A number of techniques for performing this procedure are described in Chapter 15.

Estimation techniques

Copeland pioneered the use of retinoscopy without the need for trial lenses. This involves testing the speed and direction of reflex at meridians other than the principal meridians (straddling), as mentioned previously, minimizing the width of the streak reflex, and altering sleeve height as the streak is rotated to examine different meridians (spiralling). The retinoscope must be held with both hands to perform the latter technique. Further description is given by Corboy et al (2003).

Concluding remarks about retinoscopy

Retinoscopy is an important skill for the clinician to master. It provides a starting point for a subjective refraction, but can also detect anomalies such as keratoconus and other corneal changes, poor accommodative function, and media opacities rapidly. It has considerable value in many aspects of optometric practice such as binocular vision and contact lens practice. Although its role as an objective optometer can be taken over by automated refractors, these do not work satisfactorily on a considerable number of patients.

Objective optometers

Optometers are a class of instruments for determining the refractive error of the eye. These can be both subjective and objective in nature. Objective optometers can be divided into visual (manual) optometers and automated optometers. The former use visible radiation and the decisions are made by the examiner, whereas the latter nearly always use near-infra-red radiation and the role of the examiner is reduced to that of alignment and initiating the measurement. Instruments are now overwhelmingly of the latter type and so only limited mention will be given to the former.

Badal optometer

Many sophisticated optometers incorporate a Badal optometer. At its simplest, this consists of a target and a positive lens placed at its focal distance from the eye (**Fig. 13.10**). The lens is referred to as a Badal lens. The principle associated with this optometer, the Badal principle, is that the angular subtense of the image of the target in the lens is unaffected by target position. Formally

$$\alpha = hF \qquad (13.2)$$

where α is angular subtense, h is target size and F is lens power. Two other consequences of this arrangement are that the target luminance is not affected by the position of the target and that refraction R_x is linearly related to target position. Formally the latter is given by

$$R_x = -F - F^2 l \qquad (13.3)$$

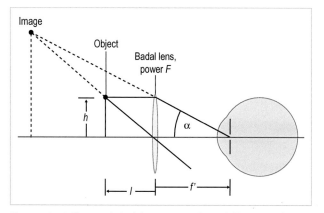

Figure 13.10 The simple Badal optometer. The Badal lens has a focal length f' and a power F. The entrance pupil of the eye is at the second focal point of the Badal lens. The object of height h is a distance l from the Badal lens. The image subtends an angle $\alpha = h/f' = hF$ at the eye.

where l is the (negative) distance of the target from the first principal plane of the lens. This relationship can be also expressed as

$$\Delta R_x / \Delta l = -F^2 \qquad (13.4)$$

where $\triangle R_x$ and $\triangle l$ are changes in refraction and target position, respectively. For example, if $F = 10$ D and 14.1 D, then Equation (13.4) shows that the refraction changes by 1 D and 2 D, respectively, for every 0.01 m movement in target position.

The reference point of the eye can vary between instruments, but the ideal location is the entrance pupil approximately 3 mm inside the eye, because then the consistency of angular size occurs not only when the target is in focus, but also when it is blurred. However, for the image-size principle (page 203), the focal point of the Badal lens is near the anterior focal point of the eye. Most instruments include a camera or alignment system to help maintain the required distance of the optometer from the eye.

The simple Badal optometer just described may not be satisfactory because of problems with eye range and eye clearance. These may be addressed by the use of auxiliary lenses or lens systems. A few of these are described by Atchison and Smith (2000).

Relay systems

Since optometers must incorporate alignment, fixation, stimulus and imaging systems, relay systems often must be used. A simple relay system consists of two lenses separated by twice the sum of their focal lengths, which presents a magnification which is the negative ratio of their powers. Combined with relay systems is the concept of 'remote' refraction, in which the refraction does not take place immediately in front of the eye as occurs for lenses in a trial frame or phoropter (refractor head). This was taken to extreme lengths in the Humphrey Vision Analyser, a discontinued subjective refraction instrument, in which targets were projected into the eye through a concave mirror 3 m away (Alvarez 1978).

Pupil region used for measurement and higher-order aberrations

Because of ocular aberrations, not all parts of a patient's pupil correspond to the same refractive power. The refraction obtained with an automated optometer should be similar to the 'gold standard' of subjective refraction, although it must be acknowledged that this varies between types of subjective refraction, between examiners (inter-observer variability) and within an examiner (intra-observer variability). An objective refraction coinciding with part of the pupil may not give the result favoured by a subject looking through the whole pupil. Ideally, the refraction should involve parts of the pupil reasonably close to the axis (say within 3 mm diameter) so that it is not unduly affected by aberrations and can be determined accurately for small pupils. However, sampling only a small part of the pupil may result in the instrument having a large depth of focus and poor precision when assessing refractive error.

The instruments that determine higher-order aberrations sample over the whole pupil or at least a high proportion of a large pupil. Various methods can be used to determine the refractive error from these aberrations. To give some background to this, the new terminology used with these 'aberrometers' must be explained. The wave aberration of

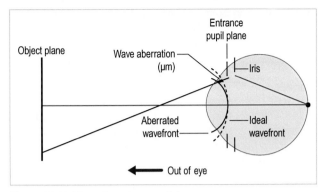

Figure 13.11 Wave aberration out of the eye.

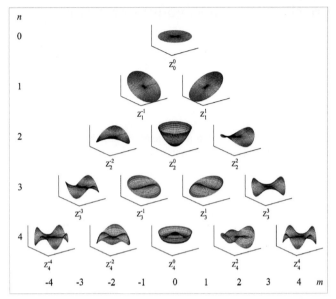

Figure 13.12 The set of Zernike aberration polynomials up to the fourth order. This is a three-dimensional representation in which the height of the aberration is shown as a function of pupil position. (Reproduced from Atchison (2004) with permission from the editor of Clinical and Experimental Optometry.)

an optical system is the departure of the wavefront from an ideal wavefront, measured at a convenient location. For the eye, because the back of the eye is not accessible, it is given for the wavefront exiting the eye and usually referenced to the entrance pupil of the eye or to the corneal plane (**Fig. 13.11**). Wave aberrations of the eye are very small, and are measured in units of micrometres. These aberrations are usually described as a system of Zernike aberration polynomials, with each Zernike polynomial having a shape dependent on the relative distance from the centre of the pupil and the meridian in the pupil. Each polynomial is multiplied by a coefficient, which is a measure of how important that particular polynomial is to the aberrations of the eye. Zernike polynomials are based on a 'unit' pupil, which means that the coefficients change according to the pupil size of interest.

In the Zernike aberration polynomial system adopted by the American National Standards Institute (2004), the meridians are measured as anticlockwise angles from the right-hand side as we look at a patient's eye and a wave aberration is considered to be positive if it is ahead of the ideal wavefront. There is a system for numbering the Zernike aberration polynomials, which is $Z(n, m)$ or Z_n^m where n is the highest power of radial dependence and m is the dependence on the meridian (**Fig. 13.12**). Further details about the Zernike polynomial system can be found in a number of references (e.g. Atchison 2004)

The conventional way of considering optical defects of the eye has been as refractive and higher-order aberrations, but with the use of the Zernike system this is becoming less useful, and now we usually refer to second-order aberrations and higher-order aberrations (third-, fourth-order, etc.). Zero-order and first-order aberrations do not affect monochromatic image quality and are often ignored. Second-order wave aberration coefficients can be converted into longitudinal aberrations, or refractions, using the formulae

$$M = -4\sqrt{3}c_2^0/R^2 \tag{13.5}$$

$$J_{180} = -2\sqrt{6}c_2^2/R^2 \tag{13.6}$$

$$J_{45} = -2\sqrt{6}c_2^{-2}/R^2 \tag{13.7}$$

with M being the mean spherical equivalent refraction, J_{180} (or J_0) being a Jackson cross-cylinder with powers of equal magnitude but opposite sign along $90°$ and $180°$ meridians, and J_{45} being a cross-cylinder with powers of equal magnitude but opposite sign along $45°$ and $135°$ meridians. The Zernike coefficients for defocus, astigmatism and oblique astigmatism are c_2^0, c_2^2 and c_2^{-2}, respectively, and R is the pupil

semi-diameter. Negative signs on the right-hand sides of the equations are necessary to convert from an error into a correction.

Conversion to conventional sphero-cylinder form $S/C \times \alpha$ with a negative cylinder is given by

$$C = -2\sqrt{(J_{180}^2 + J_{45}^2)} \tag{13.8}$$

$$S = M - C/2 \tag{13.9}$$

$$\alpha = [\tan^{-1}(J_{45}/J_{180})]/2 \tag{13.10}$$

Some rules are needed to ensure that the axis comes out correctly. If J_{180} is 0, there will be an indeterminate result. In this case, if $J_{45} < 0$, $\alpha = 135°$, and if $J_{45} \geq 0$, $\alpha = 45°$. To keep α within the clinical conventional range of $0–180°$, the following equations must be applied:
If $J_{180} < 0$

$$\alpha = \alpha + 90° \tag{13.10a}$$

If $J_{180} \geq 0$ and $J_{45} \leq 0$

$$\alpha = \alpha + 180° \tag{13.10b}$$

Refractions based on Equations (13.5) to (13.7) minimize the root-mean-squared wave aberration (which is the standard deviation of the wave aberration about its mean level across the pupil), but this does not necessarily correspond to a satisfactory subjective refraction as it places large emphasis on the outer parts of the pupil. To place more emphasis on the central parts of the pupil, Equations (13.5) to (13.7) can be modified by including even-order, higher-order spherical aberration and astigmatic terms to give:

$$M = -(4\sqrt{3}c_2^0 - 12\sqrt{5}c_4^0 + 24\sqrt{7}c_6^0 - 40\sqrt{9}c_8^0 \\ +60\sqrt{11}c_{10}^0 - \ldots)/R^2 \tag{13.11}$$

$$J_{180} = -(2\sqrt{6}c_2^2 - 6\sqrt{10}c_4^2 + 12\sqrt{14}c_6^2 - 20\sqrt{18}c_8^2 \\ +30\sqrt{22}c_{10}^2 - \ldots)/R^2 \tag{13.12}$$

$$J_{45} = -(2\sqrt{6}c_2^{-2} - 6\sqrt{10}c_4^{-2} + 12\sqrt{14}c_6^{-2} - 20\sqrt{18}c_8^{-2} \\ +30\sqrt{22}c_{10}^{-2} - \ldots)/R^2 \tag{13.13}$$

In theory, as the number of terms is increased the refraction approaches the paraxial refraction, which is that occurring for very small pupils. However, practically it is a good idea to truncate the equations after the fourth- or the sixth-order terms as instrument noise can lead to inaccuracies in the higher-order coefficients that distort the refraction.

Example 13.3

The aberrations coefficients for a post-LASIK patient with a 6 mm diameter pupil are $C_2^0 = 1.356$ µm, $C_2^{-2} = -0.034$ µm, $C_2^2 = -0.456$ µm, $C_4^0 = 0.357$ µm, $C_4^{-2} = -0.017$ µm, and $C_4^2 = 0.053$ µm. What are the refractions based on (1) second-order coefficients only, and (2) on both second- and fourth-order coefficients?

The refraction can be determined in dioptres by converting the pupil semi-diameter (3 mm) and the aberration coefficient into the unit of metres. However, when these are in millimetres and micrometres, respectively, this is not necessary.

For (1), applying Equations (13.5) to (13.7) gives $M = -1.044$ D, $J_{180} = 0.248$ D, and $J_{45} = 0.016$ D. Equations (13.8) to (13.10b) give $C = -0.50$ D, $S = -0.79$ D, and $\alpha = 2°$. The refraction in conventional notation is thus $-0.79 \, / -0.50 \times 2$.

For (2), applying Equations (13.11) to (13.13) gives $M = -0.021$ D, $J_{180} = 0.360$ D, and $J_{45} = -0.017$ D. Equations (13.8) to (13.10b) give $C = -0.72$ D, $S = +0.38$ D, and $\alpha = 179°$. The refraction in conventional notation is thus $+0.38 \, / -0.72 \times 179$.

An alternative to estimating refraction from a combination of aberration coefficients is to find the refraction that optimizes aberration-based 'image quality metrics' such as the Strehl intensity ratio. The Strehl intensity ratio is the ratio of the peak value of the point spread function to the peak of the diffraction-limited point spread function. This can be modified by the contrast sensitivity of the retina and brain to give the 'visual' Strehl ratio. Some of these metrics seem to provide better estimations of subjective refraction than does the paraxial refraction criterion (Guirao & Williams 2002; Cheng et al 2003, 2004; Marsack et al 2004; Thibos et al 2004). Thibos et al (2006) discussed incorporating chromatic aberration effects in image quality metrics.

Aberrations should be referenced to the pupil centre as this is the best reference point for aberrations. However, this changes with accommodation and illumination, and this is an issue when comparing aberrations at different pupil sizes (Walsh 1988; Wilson et al 1992; Yang et al 2002) or when using wavefront-guided corneal refractive surgery following measurement with pharmacologically dilated pupils. Some instruments align with the corneal reflection (first Purkinje image) and at least one instrument uses the visual axis, i.e. a line passing from the fixation object to the fovea through a position in the pupil that has no transverse chromatic aberration.

Wavelength and site of reflection

The issues of wavelength and site of reflection have been discussed in the context of retinoscopy. These are even more important issues for automated instruments which use near-infrared radiation in the approximate range of 800–900 nm. The advantages to using near-infrared instead of visible radiation are: comfort, because the eye is not sensitive to infrared radiation; the radiation cannot influence accommodation; pupil dilation is usually not required, because pupillary responses are not sensitive to infrared; and fundus reflectance is much higher than in visible radiation. There is a hyperopic shift in refraction because of the longitudinal chromatic aberration of the eye, amounting to approximately 0.75 D (depending on the reference wavelength). Infrared radiations penetrate deeper into the fundus than visible wavelengths, which would suggest a partially balancing myopic shift in refraction. However, some researchers consider that the waveguide properties of photoreceptors ensure that the effective site of most of the fundus reflection is the outer limiting membrane of the eye (Williams et al 1994; López-Gil & Artal 1997). A calibration correction must be made to the results so that the refraction is relevant to visible wavelengths and therefore to vision.

Except for the defocus term, aberrations seem to change little with wavelength (López-Gil & Howland 1999; Marcos et al 1999; Llorente et al 2003; Fernández et al 2005).

Instrument myopia

Optometers may record more myopic (or less hyperopic) findings compared with subjective refraction. This is attributed to the awareness that the target is actually close by and is referred to as instrument or proximal myopia. This is a particular problem with manual optometers as the patient can see the target and there is no incentive to relax accommodation. In automated optometers, the measuring radiation is either not visible or is barely visible, and an auxiliary fixation target is required. Attempts are made to relax accommodation by keeping this target 'fogged' during refraction. One recent study indicated that modern wavefront analysers do not succeed in eliminating instrument myopia (Cervino et al 2006), but the adequacy of calibration for the issues of wavelength and site of reflection should be taken into account in such analyses. A similar concern is associated with using wavefront analysers to determine accommodation response in the presence of higher aberrations.

Reference plane

Objective refractors are usually referenced to the corneal plane, but refractive errors can be obtained at various spectacle vertex distances by an effectivity equation, and most optometers allow the examiner to select one of a range of vertex distances.

Alignment

Many instruments rely on the examiner for alignment and initiating measurement. However, others, including some hand-held instruments, have added sophistication where the measurement is automatically initiated once the examiner aligns the instrument to the eye, and some have active alignment mechanisms that take over once the instrument is approximately aligned by the examiner.

Reducing corneal and other reflections

Unwanted reflections occur in optometers and contribute to 'noise' and therefore affect accuracy. These include reflection from the anterior cornea, the vitreous–retina boundary and from the optometer lenses. Most optometers include measures to reduce these. These include having as few optical elements as possible that are common to both the illumination and detection pathways, anti-reflection surface treatments, tilting surfaces, having polarized radiation together with polarizing filters, and placing small stops where they block much of the (out-of-focus) reflections while passing most of the desirable radiation.

Accuracy and reliability

It is not possible to know the absolute accuracy (validity) of a particular optometer for assessing refraction. Instruments can be compared with model eyes whose optical properties may be well known, but for some instruments the reflecting characteristics of the imaging surface affect the results, while model eyes do not possess some of the variables of real eyes such as accommodation and varying depth of penetration before reflection. The best that can be achieved is to compare the results with those obtained using subjective refraction as a gold standard.

Reliability, or the ability for an instrument to give repeatable measurements, can be more easily determined than accuracy. It is usually given in terms of intra- or inter-examiner repeatability, and can be expressed as the 95% limits of agreement or as the percentage agreement for a particular difference in refraction. As an example for a single examiner, the percentage of occasions in which measures of spherical equivalent might agree to within ± 0.25 D is 60%, together with the 95% limits of agreement (within approximately two standard deviations of the mean difference) being ± 0.59 D.

Many studies of accuracy and reliability consider sphere S, cylinder C and axis α of refraction separately. However, these are interdependent quantities and it is better to consider spherical equivalent M and the two Jackson cross-cylindrical components J_{180} and J_{45} (see Ch. 14 regarding Jackson cross-cylinders). From Equations (13.8) to (13.10), the required conversions into these quantities are

$$M = S + C/2 \tag{13.14}$$

$$J_{180} = -(C/2)\cos 2\alpha \tag{13.15}$$

$$J_{45} = -(C/2)\sin 2\alpha \tag{13.16}$$

Example 13.4

What are the M, J_{180} and J_{45} components of the prescriptions (1) $+3.00 / -1.00 \times 60$, and (2) $+3.00 / -1.00 \times 45$?

(1) $M = +3.00 + -1.00/2 = 2.50$ D; $J_{180} = -(-1.00/2)$
$\cos(2 \times 60°) = +0.50\cos(120°) = -0.25$ D; $J_{45} = -(-1.00/2)\sin(2 \times 60°) = +0.50\sin(120°) = +0.433$ D.

(2) $M = +3.00 + -1.00/2 = 2.50$ D; $J_{180} = -(-1.00/2)$
$\cos(2 \times 45°) = 0.00$ D; $J_{45} = -(-1.00/2)\sin(2 \times 45°) = +0.50\sin(45°) = +0.50$ D.

A useful technique to compare two measurements is the difference in dioptric strengths ΔS given by

$$\Delta S = \sqrt{(\Delta M^2 + \Delta J_{180}^2 + \Delta J_{45}^2)} \tag{13.17}$$

where ΔM, ΔJ_{180} and ΔJ_{45} are the component differences of the two measurements.

Accuracy and reliability are best plotted using Bland–Altmann diagrams (Bland & Altmann 1986), in which

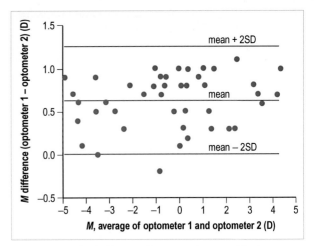

Figure 13.13 Bland–Altmann plot comparing two objective optometers. For a group of patients, differences between spherical equivalent measurements are compared with averages of the measurements. The lines show the mean difference and the 95% limits of agreement between the optometers. There is a systematic difference between the two optometers, with optometer 1 giving more positive/less negative measurements than optometer 2.

differences between two measurements are plotted against the means of the two measures. This readily shows differences between the two measurements, together with any trends in the differences as a function of refractive error (**Fig. 13.13**).

Goss and Grosvenor (1996) summarized a number of non-cycloplegic refraction studies of reliability up to the mid-1990s, and found that objective autorefractors and subjective refraction had similar reliability. They found also that some autorefractors had a positive bias compared with subjective refraction, while others had a negative bias. Accuracy and repeatability in any study will be affected by population characteristics, with some important variables including refraction range, contact lens wear, media clarity, refractive surgery and age (Winn et al 1996).

The practitioner should, of course, be mindful of conditions that may produce invalid results, including refractions outside the range of an instrument, accommodative abnormalities, small pupils, and scattering and absorption in cloudy media.

Principles and terms for types of optometers

Principles upon which optometers are based include parallax, Scheiner, split-image/vernier alignment, retinoscopic, best-focus, knife-edge, ray-deflection, and image-size. More than one principle is applied in many optometers. Sometimes it is convenient to describe these principles as used subjectively and, as applicable, this will be done here.

Other terms can be used to describe types of optometers. Some optometers are referred to as 'into-the-eye' instruments as the quality of the fundus image is important. A good example of this is the laser ray-tracing technique (page 204). Other optometers are referred to as 'out-of-the eye' instruments as the fundus acts merely as a secondary radiation source, e.g. the Hartmann–Shack sensing aberroscope (page 205). Some optometers are referred to as 'sequential' as measurements are required in succession, such as when refraction is measured in one principal meridian before the other principal meridian or when different pupil positions are used in succession, while others are referred to as simultaneous because all measurements are made at the same time. Some instruments are referred to as 'nulling' as active optical elements respond to signals from detectors to make the fundus conjugate with the detector or at some other suitable position, while others are referred to as 'non-nulling' or 'open-loop' because this is not done. Finally, instruments that measure higher-order aberrations as well as perform basic refraction are referred to as 'aberrometers'. A description of different optometers using these terms is given in **Table 13.1**.

The emphasis in the following sections is on how principles are applied, rather than a description of the construction and operation of particular instruments. For details of these instruments, useful texts are those of Henson (1996), Rabbetts (2007) and Campbell et al (2006). Campbell et al (2006) has the most detail, including advantages and disadvantages of various instruments and how they overcome problems such as corneal reflections. Henson includes some excellent three-dimensional diagrams.

Parallax principle

The image S_2' of an off-axis intermediate source S_1' is formed near the edge of the patient's pupil (**Fig. 13.14**). The target T casts a shadow T_1' on the fundus. By viewing at an angle to the illumination, the examiner sees a parallax displacement of T and the real image T_2' of T_1' (**Fig. 13.14**, top). T is moved longitudinally, which causes transverse movement in T_1' and T_2', that is, T_2' moves in parallax as T is moved back and forth. When T is conjugate with the fundus, the fundus image T_1' is on the optical axis and T_2' coincides with T (**Fig. 13.14**, bottom).

To the author's knowledge, the parallax principle is not being applied in any current optometers.

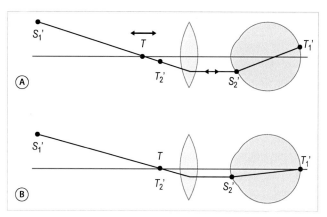

Figure 13.14 Parallax optometer. **(A)** Target T is not conjugate with its fundus image at T_1'. T_2' is displaced laterally relative to T. **(B)** Target T has been moved longitudinally to be conjugate with T_1'. T_2' is aligned with T.

Split-image/vernier alignment principle

In split-image/vernier alignment a target has a straight edge that can be split into two. Refractive error causes the two parts of the fundus image to be misaligned and this is seen either by the patient (when the instrument is used subjectively) or by the examiner on reflection from the fundus when the instrument is used objectively (**Fig. 13.15**). The straight edge is at right angles to the misalignment. When the eye is focused correctly for the target, its two halves are seen in alignment (or in coincidence). Usually, this method is combined with the Scheiner principle (see below), which ensures that radiation from the two halves of the target pass into the eye through different pupil regions. A bonus of using the Scheiner principle is that reflected radiation from the cornea is angled away from the detection system of the instrument.

Table 13.1 Descriptors for application of optometer principles

Principle	Manual/ automated	Into-/out-of- the-eye	Sequential/ simultaneous	Nulling/ non-nulling	Aberrometers using principle
Parallax	Manual	Into	Sequential	Nulling	None
Split-image	Manual	Into	Sequential	Nulling	None
Scheiner	Automated	Into	Sequential	Nulling	None
Retinoscopic	Automated	Out	Sequential	Can be either	Yes
Best-focus	Automated	Into	Can be either	Nulling	None
Knife-edge	Automated	Into	Simultaneous	Nulling	None
Image-size	Automated	Into (in part)	Simultaneous	Partial nulling	None
Ray deflection	Automated				Yes
optometer		Out	Simultaneous	Non-nulling	
laser ray-tracing		Into	Sequential	Partial nulling	
Tscherning		Into	Simultaneous	Partial nulling	
Hartmann–Shack		Out	Simultaneous	Partial nulling	
Photorefraction	Automated	Out	Sequential *	Non-nulling	None

* With recent developments in video-retinoscopy, simultaneous measurement is possible.

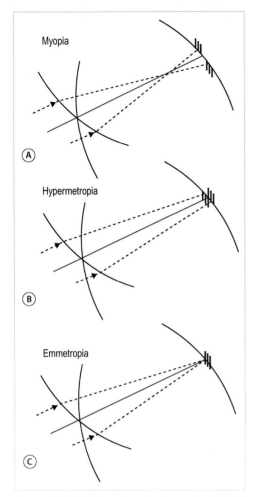

Figure 13.15 Split-image/vernier alignment principle. The two parts of a target with three lines are imaged onto the retina through different parts of the pupil. The retinal appearance is shown for collimated light entering the eye in **(A)** myopia, **(B)** hyperopia, and **(C)** emmetropia. The two parts of the target are misaligned in myopia and hyperopia, but not in emmetropia.

To deal with astigmatism, there is a second portion of the target at right angles to the first. This is also split into two parts. When the alignment of the target does not coincide with a principal meridian of the eye, the two halves of the secondary target will be misaligned, and the instrument must be rotated so that the image is aligned along one of the principal meridians before refraction measurements can be made (**Fig. 13.16**).

The split-image/vernier alignment principle works well because the eye is very sensitive to vernier misalignment. It has been applied in a number of manual as well as subjective optometers, but not in automated optometers. An instrument using this principle is the Coincidence Refractometer (Carl Zeiss), formerly known as the Hartinger optometer.

Scheiner principle

This can be understood with reference to **Figure 13.17**. A mask containing two small holes (the Scheiner disk) is placed near the patient's eye. For a point object at the focal plane of a positive lens and for a defocused eye, the thin beams passing through the two holes intersect the retina at two locations and the patient will see a diplopic image. The situation in **Figure 13.17A** is referred to as uncrossed diplopia because,

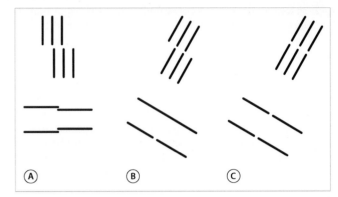

Figure 13.16 Appearance of the full target in an optometer using the split-image/vernier alignment principle. **(A)** The optometer has refraction and astigmatic axis errors relative to those of the eye. **(B)** The target has been rotated to match the astigmatic axis of the eye. **(C)** The target has been moved to match the refraction of the eye along one meridian.

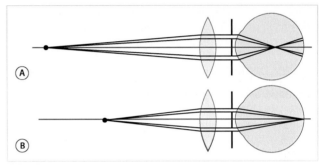

Figure 13.17 Imagery of a point object for a myope using a simple Scheiner disk optometer. **(A)** Object at focal point of lens gives a doubled image. **(B)** Moving the object closer to the eye removes the doubling.

although the beams cross, the patient interprets the beam passing through the top hole as being above the beam passing through the bottom hole (due to retinal inversion). In the simple optometer in **Figure 13.17**, the target position required to remove the doubling determines the refractive error (**Fig. 13.17B**). In the presence of astigmatism, doubling cannot be removed unless the Scheiner disk is rotated so that the pinhole axis coincides with one of the principal meridians.

The Scheiner principle has been incorporated in several automated optometers using nulling techniques. In one configuration, the target is a moveable aperture and infrared light-emitting diodes replacing the pinholes are imaged at the patient's pupil (**Fig. 13.18**). If the aperture is not

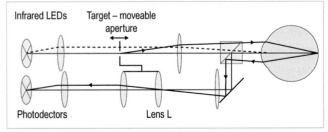

Figure 13.18 Application of the Scheiner principle for a myopic eye in an automated optometer. The LED sources are conjugate with the pupil of the eye. The lens assembly on the outward path moves in conjunction with the target. The aperture target moves to be conjugate with the fundus, at which point the lens L and the photodetectors are also conjugate with the retina. See text for further details. (Based on Figure 18.4 of Rabbetts 2007.)

conjugate with the fundus, there are two blurred images corresponding to the path of radiation from each of the sources. The sources are flashed alternatively. Image movement is detected on reflection out of the eye by a set of photodetectors. If the sources are aligned along a principal meridian of the eye, the target can be moved until no movement is detected. However, if the sources are not so aligned the movement cannot be eliminated. To help with astigmatism, there are two additional light-emitting diodes aligned perpendicularly to the first pair and which alternate at a different frequency. Also, there are two pairs of photodetectors that are aligned with the meridians of the sources. When the sources and detectors are not aligned along the principal meridians of the eye, the meridians along which the images fall will not coincide with those of the source/detectors meridians. The instrument can recognize this, and the sources and photodetectors are rotated to identify the principal meridians and make measurements along them.

Current automated instruments using the Scheiner principle include the ARK-900 (Nidek) and BAR 8 (Grand Seiko).

Retinoscopic principle

This principle has been employed by a number of automated optometers, including the first commercial autorefractor, the Bausch and Lomb Ophthalmetron (Knoll & Mohrman 1972). The basic principle is shown in **Figure 13.19**. An illuminating streak is scanned across a small region of the fundus. Unlike retinoscopy, in which the streak is scanned forwards and backwards, at the end of its path the streak disappears to be replaced by another streak traversing the same path. The streak is produced by having the illuminating beam pass through a rotating drum (or chopper drum) that has slits in it. The outgoing pathway has an aperture which has a similar function to the sighthole in retinoscopy. It is conjugate with the fundus in emmetropia, in front of the fundus in myopia and 'behind' the fundus in hyperopia. The photodetectors of the outgoing beam are conjugate with, or near, the cornea. The direction of movement of radiation across the detectors can be understood by treating the conjugate point as a virtual aperture and considering the path of radiation through it and to the cornea. In the top of **Figure 13.19** for a myopic eye, at the beginning of the scan the radiation from the top of the fundus that passes through the aperture also passes though the bottom of the pupil and cornea. As the scan continues the radiation passing the cornea moves upwards ('against' movement) and at the end of the scan passes only through the top of the cornea. The bottom of **Figure 13.19** shows the situation for a hyperopic eye and 'with' movement. At the detector plane, there are time differences between stimulation of the detectors.

From this point, there are differences between the operation of different instruments. In the Ophthalmetron, the detector assembly moves along its axis to eliminate the time difference between the two detectors, so that the detector position measures the refraction. At the same time, the ingoing and outgoing systems rotate to determine the refraction in all meridians. This can be described as 'nulling' with respect to the detector movement and 'open loop' with respect to the meridional investigation. In other instruments the time differences can be converted into a refractive error;

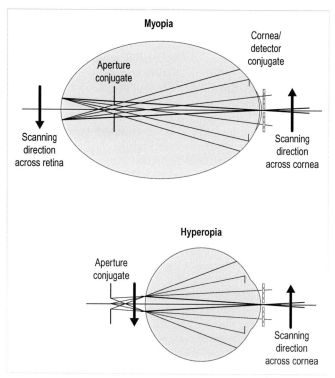

Figure 13.19 Retinoscopic principle. An incoming beam passes through a chopper drum (not shown) and scans across the retina. For a myopic eye **(top)**, the aperture of the system is conjugate with a point in front of the retina. The outgoing beam passes to the detectors, which are conjugate with the cornea. As the retina is scanned from top to bottom, the radiation reaching the detectors passes across the cornea from bottom to top. For a hyperopic eye **(bottom)**, the aperture of the system is conjugate with a point behind the retina, and the radiation reaching the detectors passes across the cornea from top to bottom. The time displacement and the order in which detectors are stimulated determine aberrations for this meridian of the eyes.

essentially, this is like measuring the retinoscopic reflex speed and it is 'open looped'. Rather than both the ingoing and outgoing systems rotating, one instrument has only one rotating element, namely a Pechan prism (Campbell et al 2006) that is common to both systems. This particular instrument has four detectors arranged in an annulus, with one pair of detectors giving the primary information about refraction and a pair at 90° to the first pair giving meridional information. This works because when the first pair is not aligned along a principal meridian, there is a time difference for the second pair. Only a few meridians need to be assessed with this instrument. A further design eliminates the prism and uses oblique slits in the chopper drum and additional computer processing of the time difference data.

The retinoscopic principle has been used in the Nidek OPD-Scan aberrometer (MacRae & Fujieda 2001; Hieda & Kinoshita 2003; Buscemi 2004). Both ingoing and outgoing systems rotate. Rather than a pair of detectors, there are eight detectors, four on either side of the optical axis (see **Fig. 13.19**), together with an additional reference pair of detectors perpendicular to them. The time at which peak-intensity radiation strikes each detector is compared with that for the reference detectors, and this time difference is converted into a longitudinal aberration. Measurement time takes place in less than half a second, measurements are taken for up to 1440 pupil positions (360 angles × 4 radial positions), and there is an extremely high dynamic range of up to ±20 D. Measurements are restricted to 6 mm diameter. Interpolation is required between the pupil positions corresponding with the detectors (and in the approximately 2.0 mm diameter pupil centre). To determine refractive error, an elliptical fit is made to the longitudinal aberrations corresponding with an annulus of positions in the pupil. As measurement at any pupil position is in a radial direction only, no information is collected about findings at right angles to these points, and there must be doubts about the accuracy of the higher-order aberration results (Atchison 2006).

Current automated instruments using the retinoscopic principle include the NR 5500 (Nikon) and OPD-Scan (Nidek).

Best-focus principle

This is similar to the perception of blur that a patient is asked to detect during a subjective refraction. It is also referred to as the grating focus principle as the target is a square-wave grating consisting of light and dark bars. As for the retinoscopic technique, this can be produced by a chopper drum (**Fig. 13.20**). In the discontinued Coherent Dioptron, the grating is imaged into the eye, and re-imaged onto a photodetector behind a square-wave grating mask. The spatial frequency of the mask and the aerial image are matched. The signal from the photodetector modulates as the target is moved transversely. The signal modulation is monitored as a lens, common to input and output paths, moving along the optical axis. Maximum modulation occurs when the aerial image is focused at the mask; this corresponds to the object being focused at the fundus. The refraction is determined by the lens position corresponding to the maximum modulation. Measurements are made in a number of meridians of grating/mask orientation, and the results are combined to determine the full refraction.

Another discontinued instrument, the Canon Autoref R-1, used a target consisting of three gratings targets orientated at 120° to each other in a triangular pattern, with a similar arrangement for their corresponding masks and aerial images (Matsumura et al 1983). Rather than a single optometer lens assembly moving to maximize modulation for each meridian in turn, separate assemblies in each of the input and output paths move synchronously and continuously through a large

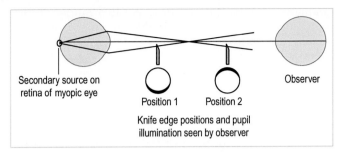

Figure 13.21 Knife-edge principle. When the knife edge is between the eye and the far point of a myopic eye (position 1), the light which passes through the lower part of the pupil is vignetted and this appears dark to an observer. When the knife edge is between the far point and the observer (position 2), the light which passes through the upper part of the pupil is vignetted and this appears dark to an observer.

range of longitudinal positions. The time at which the maximum signal occurs for each meridian determines the optimum lens assembly position, and hence refractive error, for that orientation. The full refraction is obtained by combining results for all three orientations.

To the author's knowledge, the best-focus principle is not being applied in any current optometers.

Knife-edge principle

The knife-edge principle has been adapted from the Foucault knife-edge test that analyses the aberrations in an optical system. A sharp edge is passed across the beam in the vicinity of the image of a point source. As applied to the eye (**Fig. 13.21**), if the retina is conjugate with a point beyond the edge (relative hyperopia), as the edge is moved upwards the light passing through the bottom part of the pupil is vignetted for an observer viewing from the opposite side of the knife edge. Thus, this part of the pupil appears dark. The opposite situation occurs in relative myopia, and if the retina is conjugate with the edge (and ignoring higher-order aberrations) the whole pupil appears to go dark uniformly.

This is a reasonable description of what is observed in retinoscopy, but with the sighthole taking the place of the knife edge, the fundus 'source' being a patch rather than a point, and with this source moving instead of the sighthole. Thus, the retinoscopic principle is really the knife-edge principle.

The knife-edge principle has been applied in a sophisticated manner in the Humphrey Instruments series of automated refractors (e.g. HARK 599). Four infrared bar sources act as knife edges and form a hollow cross (**Fig. 13.22**). The ingoing and outgoing paths are identical, except for a detector imaging lens and a four-photodetector assembly placed behind the sources and conjugate with the pupil. Variable refracting elements common to the ingoing and outgoing paths are manipulated to ensure that the radiation reflected from the retina is even across the photodetectors. In theory, this would mean that the dark hollow part of the cross would be imaged between the bar sources and no radiation would pass to the detectors. However, the fundus image is effectively larger than it would be if the fundus was an infinitely thin diffuse reflector.

Spherical power is manipulated by varying the length of a folded optical path. Cylindrical power is varied by two Stokes lenses, conjugate with the eye, and with one having 90°/180° axis and the other having 45°/135° axis. A Stokes lens consists

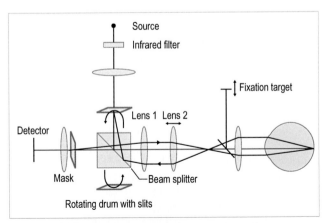

Figure 13.20 Best-focus principle. Most of the optical path is common to ingoing and outgoing pathways. Lens 2 moves so that the pathways are collimated between lenses 1 and 2. The mask is conjugate with the rotating drum. Other details are explained in the text.

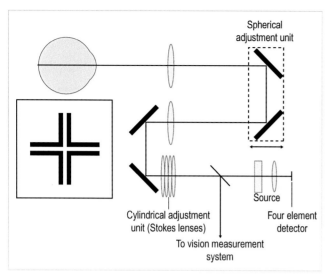

Figure 13.22 Application of knife-edge principle in Humphrey autorefractors. The inset shows the illuminated hollow cross source. See text for further details.

of two cylinders of equal and opposite power that are rotated in opposite directions to produce variable cylinder power but always zero spherical equivalent power. The resulting powers can be converted into conventional refraction using Equations (13.08) to (13.10b) and (13.14) to (13.16).

This arrangement has interesting features, such as the commonality of ingoing and outgoing pathways. Because the correction is in place at the end of measurement, subsequent visual testing is possible.

Image-size principle

The construction of optometers using this principle ensures that the angular retinal image size of an annular target depends upon the degree of ametropia. This is re-imaged onto a CCD camera. Analysis of the shape and dimensions of the final image determines the refraction. An LED source, a collimating lens and a ring mask target move together and in conjunction with a lens in the detection system (**Fig. 13.23**). This movement is controlled through the quality of the image on the camera. The LED is imaged to the anterior focal point of the eye, the ring mask is imaged to the retina and another fixed ring mask imaged to the pupil. A Badal lens has its focal

point at a position approximately conjugate with the anterior focal point of eye, unlike the usual situation where the focal point is at (or conjugate to) a point in the eye such as the entrance pupil. On the outgoing pathway, another Badal lens has its focal point approximately conjugate with the nodal point of the eye to ensure that image size at the CCD camera is directly related to angles within the eye. Instrument calibration is required to interpret the sizes of images. This is a partial nulling technique, as the image does not need to be accurately focused at the retina.

Current automated instruments using the image-size principle include the WR 5100K (Grand Seiko) and RM-A7000 (Topcon).

Ray-deflection principle

In this principle, the angle of a thin beam is compared to its ideal angle, with the difference referred to as the angle of deflection. For example, for an unaberrated emmetropic eye, rays from a point on the fundus leaving the eye are parallel to each other, but for myopic eyes the rays are deflected towards the optical axis (**Fig. 13.24**). With knowledge about the positions of rays in the pupil, angles of deflection can be converted into refractive error. In automated refractors, the principle is usually combined with the Scheiner principle to isolate two small regions of the pupil.

If rays passing through many positions in the pupil are examined rather than only a few points, we refer to the deflection angles as transverse ray aberrations and it is possible to use these to determine higher-order aberrations of the eye. Most types of aberrometers apply the ray-deflection principle. A subjective equivalent to the laser ray-tracing

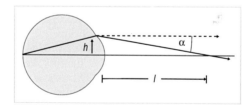

Figure 13.24 Ray-deflection principle. For an unaberrated emmetropic eye, rays from the retina exit the eye parallel to the optical axis (*dotted line*). For a myopic eye, a ray at a height h in the pupil is deflected by angle α. Refraction of this eye is given by $\alpha/h = -1/l$.

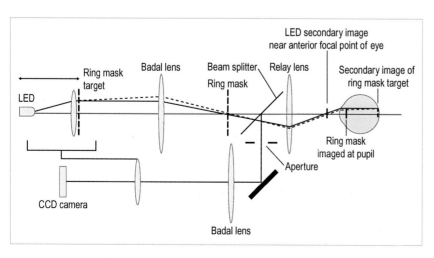

Figure 13.23 Image-size principle. See text for details. (Based upon Figure 18.9 of Rabbetts 2007.)

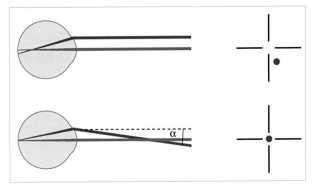

Figure 13.25 Application of the ray-deflection principle in a subjective aberrometer. If there is aberration corresponding to a particular peripheral pupil position, the target spot appears displaced from the reference position **(top)**. The subject must alter the orientation of the incoming beam so that the spot will appear to be at the reference position; now the beam orientation is a measure of transverse aberration **(bottom)**.

technique (see below) has been developed, in which two narrow beams are seen by the subject at one time, one of which passes through the centre of the pupil and the other through one of many peripheral pupil locations **(Fig. 13.25)**. The patient changes the angle of the second beam so that they appear to coincide; the angle of the beam gives the transverse ray aberration for the pupil position (Carr et al 2004).

An automated optometer using the ray-deflection principle is the R-30 (Canon).

Laser ray-tracing

This is an into-the-eye, sequential method of measuring low- and higher-order aberrations (Navarro & Losada 1997). A narrow laser beam is directed into the eye. Two scanning mirrors combine to pass this through a sequence of several pupil positions **(Fig. 13.26)**. For each position, the fundal image acts as a secondary source to pass light back through the whole pupil and onto a CCD array. Since the fundal images corresponding with the different pupil positions will differ in location because of aberrations, the final images will also vary in their locations. However, all should be similar in appearance. Image centroids are compared with those of the reference image, corresponding to the pupil centre, to give transverse aberrations. Wave aberrations can be derived from the transverse aberrations, and refractive error can be determined using Equations (13.6) to (13.14). With improvements in technology, many measurements can be taken within a second. Considerable

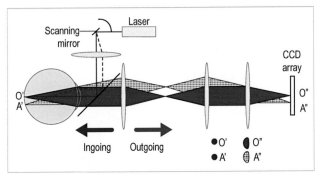

Figure 13.26 Laser ray-tracing. See text for details.

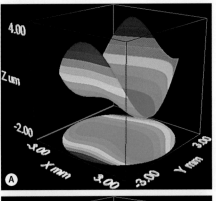

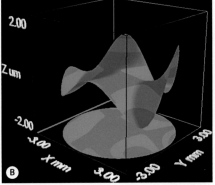

Figure 13.27 Three-dimensional representation of the wave aberration of a patient following refractive surgery. Map **(A)** includes aberrations of second and higher orders, but map **(B)** includes only the higher-order aberrations.

computation is required and eye movements may potentially affect the results. The technique can measure a wide range of refractive errors and aberrations (large dynamic range). Unlike 'simultaneous' aberration techniques, it does not suffer from the possibility that centroids corresponding to different pupil locations can be confused.

For other aberrometers using the ray-deflection principle, transverse aberrations across the pupil are combined to determine the eye's wavefront aberration **(Fig. 13.27)**.

An instrument using laser ray-tracing is the Tracey aberrometer (Tracey Technologies).

Tscherning aberrometry

The time taken for the laser ray-tracing technique could be reduced by measuring the fundus locations of several beams simultaneously, but on re-imaging it would not be possible to distinguish between the different intersections (because of the small differences) nor the pupil positions to which they correspond. This problem is overcome in the Tscherning aberrometer technique by using a defocusing lens in front of the eye to spread the image across the fundus (Mierdel et al 2001; Mrochen et al 2004). A grid mask in front of the eye passes radiation only through selected pupil positions, and the fundal image is re-imaged through the whole pupil **(Fig. 13.28)**. If auxiliary optics are provided in front of the eye to correct most of the defocus, and provided higher-order aberrations are not extreme, it will be obvious which image point coincides with each pupil position. Transverse aberrations are determined by comparing image positions with those from a reference schematic eye, which may induce some error because real eyes will

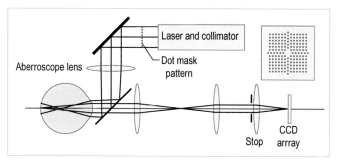

Figure 13.28 Tscherning aberrometer. The inset shows the appearance of the retinal image for a perfect eye in the Wavefront Analyzer. See text for further details.

have different paraxial image sizes. The transverse aberrations across the pupil are combined to determine the eye's wavefront aberration.

One Tscherning aberrometer is the Wavefront Analyzer (Wavelight Laser Technologies).

Hartmann–Shack aberrometry

The Hartmann–Shack technique was adapted from astronomy for vision science in the 1990s (Liang et al 1994; Liang & Williams 1997) and is currently the most popular technique used for commercial aberrometers. A narrow beam from a point radiation source is passed into the eye, and the light reflected from the fundus travels through an optical system to a 'Hartmann–Shack sensor' (or 'wavefront sensor') consisting of an array of micro-lenses and a CCD camera array (**Fig. 13.29**). The micro-lens array is conjugate with the pupil, and its own focal plane is at the camera array. Each micro-lens isolates a narrow beam passing through a small area of the pupil. Depending on the pupil size, magnification between

the pupil and the array sampling density, up to several hundred pupil positions may be sampled. For a perfect eye, the wavefront arriving at the sensor is a plane wave. However, this is not the case for an eye having aberrations. The transverse ray aberration (slope of the wavefront) associated with each micro-lens can be determined from the departure of its corresponding image from the ideal position.

It may take only a few milliseconds to capture an image. Because of this, fluctuations in aberrations over the order of seconds can be followed and the Hartmann–Shack aberrometer can form part of an adaptive optics system to correct ocular aberrations of the eye (Liang et al 1997). Software algorithms can determine the pupil centre accurately even if pupil centration is not precise. Because of the simultaneous nature of measurement at many pupil locations, images may overlap with high levels of defocus or aberrations. Thus, the technique has a limited dynamic range, depending on the focal length and sampling density of the Hartmann–Shack sensor and software algorithms. Auxiliary moving optics are required on the imaging path to correct most of the defocus.

Current Hartmann–Shack instruments include the COAS (Wavefront Sciences), WaveScan (VISX), Zywave (Bausch and Lomb) and LadarWave (Alcon).

Photorefraction (see Chapter 28)

This was pioneered by Howland and Howland (1974), and uses photography of the eyes for determining refractive error. Its main application is the screening of infants and young children as it requires only minimal attention on the part of the patient. It is useful in the detection of anisometropia and strabismus. In essence, a flash photograph is taken of both eyes together, with the flash source near the camera. Size and

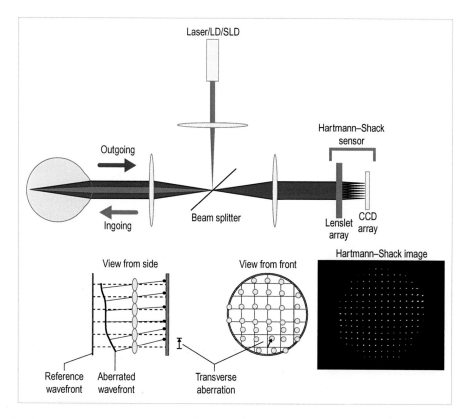

Figure 13.29 Hartmann–Shack aberrometer. The top part shows the basic setup, the bottom-left part shows transverse aberrations and the bottom-right part shows an image of an eye. (Based on Figure 3 of Atchison 2005.)

location of the fundus reflection as seen in the pupil by the camera determines refraction. There are three forms: orthogonal, isotropic and eccentric. The first two of these are applications of the image size principle, while the third is an application of the retinoscopic principle.

The original form of photorefraction is orthogonal photorefraction (see Howland et al 1983). The camera lens is focused at the patient's eyes. A small flash source of light is mounted centrally in front of the camera lens. The light returning from the fundus to the camera lens (the point spread image) falls on four cylindrical lenses arranged radially around the source at 90° intervals. If the eye is focused at the source, the light leaving the eye returns to the source and the pupil appears dark because the light cannot pass into the camera. Otherwise, the image on the camera plane is a cross. The length of the cross arms is proportional to the sizes of the point spread image, which in turn is proportional to the refractive error relative to the camera. Two meridians are measured simultaneously. Photographs are taken with the lens elements at 90°/180°, at 45°/135° and with them removed. The first two are taken to give reasonable information about astigmatism and the third is taken to measure pupil size. The latter is important, as the image size is proportional to pupil size.

The simplest form of photorefraction is isotropic photorefraction (Howland et al 1983). Again, a small flash source of light is mounted centrally in front of the camera lens, but the cylindrical lenses are not present (Fig. 13.30). If the eye is not focused at the source, a circle of light is formed at the retina for spherical refractions while an ellipse is formed in astigmatic eyes. The size and shape of the image depend upon the refractive error relative to the source. Howland and colleagues took photographs with the camera focused both in front of and behind the patient's pupil plane by 0.5 D to overcome ambiguity in the sign of refraction of a single image, together with a photograph with the camera focused at the pupil in order to measure pupil size. Using geometrical optics, refraction is determined from the camera image sizes, the pupil size and dimensions of the camera set-up.

The range of refractive errors that can be measured by orthogonal and isotropic photorefraction is limited. Eccentric photorefraction, which is similar to retinoscopy and is sometimes called photoretinoscopy, can measure large errors (Bobier & Braddick 1985; Howland 1985; Crewther et al 1987). It uses an eccentric point source, which may be provided effectively by masking part of the camera, when

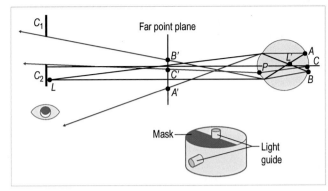

Figure 13.31 Eccentric photorefraction with a myopic eye. The bottom part of pupil (on same side as light source) is illuminated. L is the eccentric light source; L' is the image of image source in eye; C_1 and C_2 are edges of camera aperture; ACB is the blurred image on retina; $A'C'B'$ is the image of fundus reflex; and the path $CPC'C_2$ is the ray path corresponding to the top edge of the illuminated crescent in the pupil. The bottom half of the figure show the appearance of a photoretinoscope placed on a camera. (Based on Figures 18.50 and 18.52 of Campbell et al 2006.)

using the small centred light used for isotropic photorefraction, and with the part of the mask closest to the source, forming a 'knife edge'. This is similar to retinoscopy, but with the sighthole moving rather than the light beam moving across it. The camera vignets some of the light returning from the fundus, leaving a meniscus-shaped image. For myopia relative to the light source, the image is on the same side of the pupil as the source; in relative hyperopia the image is on the opposite side (**Fig. 13.31**). Refraction is determined from the placement of the camera, source and patient. To consider astigmatism, different meridians are investigated.

The photoretinoscopic technique has developed into video-retinoscopy using rows of infrared LEDs within the mask. Rows can be illuminated sequentially, and the rate of movement of the detected crescent measured to determine refraction. A more recent development is to have all the LEDs on simultaneously, and to measure the slope of image intensity at right angles to the edge of the mask; the slope is linearly related to the refractive error for a considerable range. In the most sophisticated developments, there are six sets of knife edges and LEDs to give multimeridional refraction. Accommodation, pupil size and gaze direction can be monitored across time, which makes such devices useful in research applications such as accommodation dynamics (e.g. Kasthurirangan et al 2003).

Current photoretinoscopy instruments include the Power-Ref II and Plusoptix S04, both manufactured by Plusoptix.

Conclusion

Objective refraction has existed since the late nineteenth century when retinoscopy was first developed. Since then there has been steady progress, with automated instruments now supplanting manual instrumentation. Automated optometers are likely to be supplanted soon by the aberrometers that give information about fine levels of optical defects within eyes, and hence improve retinal image quality and visual performance through their contribution to

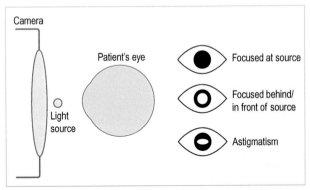

Figure 13.30 Isotropic photorefraction, showing camera images in spherical ametropia and when astigmatism is present.

wavefront-guided surgery, and the design of contact and intraocular lenses. At present, there is considerable effort going into making the results with such instruments closer to subjective refraction. In the near future, subjective refraction itself may perhaps become redundant.

References

Alvarez L W 1978 Development of variable-focus lenses and a new refractor. Journal of the American Optometric Association 49(1): 24–29

American National Standards Institute 2004 American National Standard for Ophthalmics – Methods for reporting optical aberrations of the eye. ANSI Z80.28–2004

Atchison D A 2004 Recent advances in representation of monochromatic aberrations of human eyes. Clinical and Experimental Optometry 87(3):138–148

Atchison D A 2005 Recent advances in measurement of monochromatic aberrations of human eyes. Clinical and Experimental Optometry 88(1):5–27

Atchison D A 2006 The skew ray issue in ocular aberration measurement. Optometry and Vision Science 8(6):396–398

Atchison D A, Smith G 2000 Optics of the human eye. Butterworth-Heinemann, Oxford, pp 68–70, 184

Atchison D A, Lucas S D, Ashman R et al 2006 Refraction and aberration across the horizontal central 10° of the visual field. Optometry and Vision Science 83(4):213–221

Bland J M, Altman D G 1986 Statistical methods for assessing agreement between two methods of clinical measurement. Lancet 1 (8476):307–310

Bobier W R, Braddick O J 1985 Eccentric photorefraction: optical analysis and empirical measures. American Journal of Optometry and Physiological Optics 62(9):614–620

Buscemi P M 2004 Retinoscope double pass aberrometry: principles and application of the Nidek OPD-Scan, Chapter 19. In: Krueger R R, Applegate R A, MacRae S M (eds) Wavefront customized visual corrections: the quest for super vision II. Slack, Thorofare NJ, pp 149–153

Campbell C E, Benjamin W J, Howland H C 2006 Objective refraction: retinoscopy, autorefraction, and photorefraction, Chapter 18. In: Benjamin W J (ed.) Borish's Clinical Refraction, 2nd edn. Butterworth-Heinemann, Oxford, pp 682–764

Carr J D, Lichter H, Garcia J et al 2004 Spatially resolved refractometry: principles and application of the Emory Vision InterWave aberrometer, Chapter 20. In: Krueger R R, Applegate R A, MacRae S M (eds) Wavefront customized visual corrections: the quest for super vision II. Slack, Thorofare NJ, pp 155–160

Cervino A, Hosking S L, Rai G K et al 2006 Wavefront analysers induce instrument myopia. Journal of Refractive Surgery 22(8):795–803

Charman W N 1975 Some sources of discrepancy between static retinoscopy and subjective refraction. British Journal of Physiological Optics 30(4):108–118

Cheng X, Thibos L N, Bradley A 2003 Estimating visual quality from wavefront aberration measurements. Journal of Refractive Surgery 19(5):S579–S584

Cheng X, Bradley A, Thibos L N 2004 Predicting subjective judgment of best focus with objective image quality metrics. Journal of Vision 4(4):310–321

Chiu N N, Rosenfield M, Wong L C 1997 Effect of contralateral fog during refractive assessment. Journal of the American Optometric Association 68(5):305–308

Corboy J M, Narath D, Stone R et al 2003 The retinoscopy book: an introductory manual for eye care professionals, 5th edn. Slack, Thorofare NJ

Crewther D P, McCarthy A, Roper J et al 1987 An analysis of eccentric photorefraction. Clinical and Experimental Optometry 70(1):2–7

Fernández E J, Unterhuber A, Prieto P M et al 2005 Ocular aberrations as a function of wavelength in the near infrared measured with a femtosecond laser. Optics Express 13(2):400–409

Goss D A, Grosvenor T 1996 Reliability of refraction: a literature review. Journal of the American Optometric Association 67(10):619–630

Guirao A, Williams D R 2002 A method to predict refractive errors from wave aberration data. Optometry and Vision Science 80(1):36–42

Henson D B 1996 Optometers, Chapter 8. In: Optometric instrumentation, 2nd edn. Butterworth-Heinemann, Oxford, pp 162–198

Hieda O, Kinoshita S 2003 Measuring of ocular wavefront aberration in large pupils. Seminars in Ophthalmology 18(1):35–40

Howland H C 1978 Retinoscopy of infants at a distance: limits of normal and anomalous reflexes. Vision Research 18(5):597–599

Howland H 1985 Optics of photoretinoscopy: results from ray tracing. American Journal of Optometry and Physiological Optics 62(9):621–625

Howland H C, Howland B 1974 Photorefraction: a technique for the study of refractive state at a distance. Journal of the Optical Society of America 64(2):240–249

Howland H C, Braddick O, Atkinson J et al 1983 Optics of photorefraction: orthogonal and isotropic methods. Journal of the Optical Society of America 73(12):1701–1708

Kasthurirangan S, Vilupuru A S, Glasser A 2003 Amplitude dependent accommodative dynamics in humans. Vision Research 43 (27):2945–2956

Knoll H A, Mohrman R 1972 The Ophthalmetron, principles and operation. American Journal of Optometry and Archives of American Academy of Optometry 49(2):122–128

Liang J, Williams D R 1997 Aberrations and retinal image quality of the normal human eye. Journal of the Optical Society of America A 14(11):2873–2883

Liang J, Grimm B, Goelz S et al 1994 Objective measurement of wave aberrations of the human eye with the use of a Hartmann-Shack wave-front sensor. Journal of the Optical Society of America A 11(7):1949–1957

Liang J, Williams D R, Miller D T 1997 Supernormal vision and high-resolution retinal imaging through adaptive optics. Journal of the Optical Society of America A 14(11):2884–2892

Llorente L, Diaz-Santana L, Lara-Saucedo D et al 2003 Aberrations of the human eye in visible and near infrared illumination. Optometry and Vision Science 80(1):26–35

López-Gil N, Artal P 1997 Comparison of double-pass estimates of the retinal-image quality obtained with green and near-infrared light. Journal of the Optical Society of America A 14(5):961–971

López-Gil N, Howland H C 1999 Measurement of the eye's near infrared wave-front aberration using the objective crossed-cylinder aberroscope technique. Vision Research 39(12):2031–2037

MacRae S M, Fujieda M 2001 Slit skiascopic-guided ablation using the Nidek laser. Journal of Refractive Surgery 16(5):S576–S580

Marcos S, Burns S A, Moreno-Barriuso E et al 1999 A new approach to the study of ocular chromatic aberrations. Vision Research 39(26):4309–4323

Marsack J D, Thibos L N, Applegate R A 2004 Metrics of optical quality derived from wave aberrations predict visual performance. Journal of Vision 4(4):322–328

Matsumura S, Maruyama S, Ishikawa R et al 1983 The design of an open view autorefractometer. In: Breinen G M, Siegel I M (eds) Advances in diagnostic visual optics. Springer, Berlin, pp 36–42

Mierdel P, Kaemmerer M, Mrochen M et al 2001 Ocular optical aberrometer for clinical use. Journal of Biomedical Optics 6(2):200–204

Millodot M, O'Leary D 1978 The discrepancy between retinoscopic and subjective measurements: effects of age. American Journal of Optometry and Physiological Optics 55(5):309–316

Mohindra I 1975 A technique for infant refraction. American Journal of Optometry and Physiological Optics 52(12):867–870

Mohindra I 1977a Comparison of 'near retinoscopy' and subjective refraction in adults. American Journal of Optometry and Physiological Optics 54(5):319–322

Mohindra I 1977b A non-cycloplegic refraction technique for infants and young children. Journal of the American Optometric Association 48(4):518–523

Mohindra I, Molinari J F 1979 Near retinoscopy and cycloplegic retinoscopy in early primary grade school children. American Journal of Optometry and Physiological Optics 56(1):34–38

Mrochen M, Jankov M, Iseli H P et al 2004 Retinal imaging aberrometry: principles and application of the Tscherning aberrometer, Chapter 17. In: Krueger R R, Applegate R A, MacRae S M (eds) Wavefront customized visual corrections: the quest for super vision II. Slack, Thorofare NJ, pp 137–143

Mutti D O 2004 Sources of normal and anomalous motion in retinoscopy. Optometry and Vision Science 81(9):663–672

Navarro R, Losada M A 1997 Aberrations and relative efficiency of light pencils in the living human eye. Optometry and Vision Science 74(7):540–547

O'Leary D, Millodot M 1978 The discrepancy between retinoscopic and subjective refraction: effect of light polarisation. American Journal of Optometry and Physiological Optics 55(8):553–556

Rabbetts R B 2007 Chapters 17 and 18. In: Bennett and Rabbetts' clinical visual optics, 4th edn. Butterworth-Heinemann, Oxford, pp 345–383

Roorda A, Bobier W R 1996 Geometrical technique to determine the influence of monochromatic aberrations on retinoscopy. Journal of the Optical Society of America A 13(1):3–11

Smith G, Haymes S 2003 The retinoscopy pupil reflex in the presence of astigmatism. Ophthalmic and Physiological Optics 23(4):295–305

Thibos L N, Hong X, Bradley A et al 2004 Accuracy and precision of objective refraction from wavefront aberrations. Journal of Vision 4(4):329–351

Thibos L N, Himebaugh N L, Coe C D 2006 Wavefront refraction, Chapter 19. In: Benjamin W J (ed.) Borish's clinical refraction, 2nd edn. Butterworth-Heinemann, Oxford, pp 765–789

Walsh G 1988 The effect of mydriasis on pupillary centration of the human eye. Ophthalmic and Physiological Optics 8(2):178–182

Ward P A, Charman W N 1987 An objective assessment of the effect of fogging on accommodation. American Journal of Optometry and Physiological Optics 64(10):762–767

Williams D R, Brainard D H, McMahon M J et al 1994 Double-pass and inteferometric measures of the optical quality of the eye. Journal of the Optical Society of America A 11(12):3123–3135

Wilson M A, Campbell M C W, Simonet P 1992 Change of pupil centration with change of illumination and pupil size. Optometry and Vision Science 69(2):129–136

Winn B, Pugh J R, Strang N C et al 1996 Medical Devices Agency Evaluation Report MDA/96/36: Autorefractors. Cited by Strang N C, Gray L S, Winn B et al 1998 Clinical evaluation of patient tolerance to autorefractor prescriptions. Clinical and Experimental Optometry 81(3):112–118

Yang Y, Thompson K, Burns S A 2002 Pupil location under mesopic, photopic, and pharmacologically dilated conditions. Investigative Ophthalmology and Visual Science 43(7):2508–2512

CHAPTER 14

Subjective refraction

Mark Rosenfield

Introduction

In optometry, the term refraction is used not only to refer to the change in the vergence of light that occurs at a boundary separating media having different indices of refraction, but also to the determination of the lens which corrects the patient's refractive error. In subjective refraction, the patient, while viewing a specific target, is asked to evaluate different lenses by indicating which lens makes the object of regard appear clearer. Typically, either a phoropter or trial frame is used to facilitate the placement of lenses in front of the patient. Obviously, good communication between the patient and examiner is critical; otherwise the patient will not comprehend what is being asked of them. In fact, subjective refraction may be impossible in some circumstances, such as where the patient does not speak the same language as the clinician (and an interpreter is not present) or when the patient is unable to respond to the questions asked (e.g. infants and very young children). In these situations, only objective examination may be possible.

Subjective refraction is the part of the refractive examination with which patients are most familiar. While it is not uncommon for a patient to report that, to their knowledge, certain techniques (even those as routine as retinoscopy) have not been performed on them before, almost all experienced patients are familiar with the standard question: 'Which lens is better, number 1 or number 2?' The goal of subjective refraction is to develop and refine a prescription through which the patient can see comfortably. The practitioner must remember that although the eye represents an optical system, this cannot be considered in isolation. The patient's perception of the object of regard develops after both neural processing and mental comparison with their prior visual experience. Therefore, a patient may prefer a refractive correction which differs from that obtained by an objective procedure (see Ch. 13), even when the latter has been measured accurately. The patient's current refractive prescription may also play a role in their choice of lenses. For example, a patient who has previously worn a spherical correcting lens will often reject any cylindrical correction, even when it is clear from the objective findings that astigmatism is present in that eye.

The level of blur perception can also be assessed during the subjective examination. For example, while some patients are extremely sensitive to small changes in lens power or cylinder axis orientation, others will fail to notice a relatively large change in these parameters. While this should not be taken as an excuse to perform a sloppy examination, it does provide a guide for the clinician as to the patient's degree of tolerance to relatively small changes in refractive correction. Finally, subjective refraction may be the only way of determining the refractive error in those patients where objective examination is impossible, such as those with very small pupils or media opacities.

In most cases, the subjective examination follows these four steps:

1. initial sphere check
2. cylinder axis refinement
3. cylinder power refinement
4. second sphere check.

These steps are usually carried out after objective refraction, i.e. retinoscopy or autorefraction. For those occasions where objective examination cannot be performed as noted above, an 'independent subjective refraction' must be undertaken.

Initial sphere check

The goals of this phase of the examination are to minimize the patient's accommodative response, and to achieve the appropriate starting point for assessing the astigmatic correction. Control of accommodation is a critical element of the subjective examination (Michaels 1985). The desired end point of the subjective procedure is to position the patient's far point close to optical infinity. The far point is defined as the point conjugate with the retina in the absence of accommodation. However, since zero accommodation is almost never achieved in a pre-presbyopic patient, it would be more accurate to define the far point as existing under conditions of minimal accommodation (Rosenfield 2006). Minimal accommodation can be achieved by the use of a cycloplegic pharmacological agent to paralyse the ciliary muscle (see Ch. 7). More commonly, 'fogging techniques' are employed to attenuate the accommodative response. To 'fog', lenses are introduced to make the patient effectively myopic, with the image of a distant object lying anterior to the retina, thereby ensuring that only minimal accommodation should occur.

At this stage of the examination, the practitioner is seeking to determine the maximum plus (or minimum minus) spherical lens which provides the patient with the best visual acuity (VA). This lens is known as the 'best sphere'. The procedure should begin with the patient 'fogged' or rendered myopic to ensure minimum accommodation. If retinoscopy has already been carried out, the patient will usually be fogged by either 1.50 or 2.00 D, depending on whether a working distance of 67 cm or 50 cm, respectively, was used (see Ch. 13). While one could now start reducing the fogging lens in 0.25 DS steps from the retinoscopy finding, it is more efficient to remove approximately half of the working distance immediately, and then continue to reduce fog by adding minus spheres in 0.25 DS steps. The patient's acuity should be checked after each step.

For example, if retinoscopy is being performed at a working distance of 67 cm, and a neutral reflex is observed through a −3.50 DS, then −0.75 DS (half the working distance) can be added immediately to the neutralizing lens. The patient should still be fogged, which will minimize accommodation, when viewing through the −4.25 DS. Additional −0.25 spherical lenses can then be added to the −4.25 DS, until further minus lens power does not produce any improvement in acuity. Once the optimum acuity has been achieved, the image of the distant object will fall on the retina. Any more minus lens power will move the image of the distant object behind the retina, and a pre-presbyopic patient could accommodate to move this image forward onto the retina, thereby maintaining optimal VA. Indeed, the minification of the optotypes that occurs with excessive minus lens power and accommodation may appear to improve target contrast (Mutti & Zadnik 1997), so caution must be exercised to ensure that the additional minus lens power does indeed improve VA. A true improvement in VA is discerned when the patient can either resolve more letters, or at least can read them more easily.

When an independent subjective refraction is being performed, i.e. not following objective testing, the first step is to ensure that the patient is fogged to minimize accommodation. If the patient's acuity is better than 6/15 (20/50), plus spheres should be added in 0.25 DS steps until the patient's VA is reduced to 6/15 (20/50). At that point the patient will be fogged, with a minimal accommodative response, and the sphere can be checked as described above. However, if the VA is worse than 6/15 (20/50), then the practitioner should first determine whether myopia or hyperopia is present. This can be ascertained by adding a +1.00 DS and rechecking the VA. If the +1.00 DS improves VA, then the patient is hyperopic, and the practitioner should continue to add plus, past the point of best VA, continuing as the acuity starts to deteriorate. Fog the patient (i.e. add excessive plus lens power) until the acuity is around 6/15 (20/50). If +1.00 DS reduces the acuity, then the patient is probably myopic, so add minus spheres until the VA just reaches 6/15 (20/50). Finally, reduce the plus sphere (or add minus spheres) in 0.25 D steps, checking acuity at each step, until the maximum plus (or minimum minus) lens that gives the best VA has been determined.

Cylinder refinement

After the best sphere has been determined, the second stage of the examination is to check the astigmatic correction. This can be divided into two stages, firstly checking the cylinder axis, and secondly checking the cylinder power. The axis must be checked first to ensure that cylindrical lenses are introduced at the appropriate orientation. Assuming the use of minus cylinders, the correctly orientated cylindrical lens will move the front focal line backwards until it coincides with the back focal line, and the interval of Sturm will be eliminated. If the cylinder is introduced at an incorrect axis, either the back focal line will be moved backwards (if the cylinder axis was introduced 90° away from its proper orientation) or both focal lines will move posteriorly. In either event, the interval between the focal lines will remain, and the patient's astigmatism will not be fully corrected. In the case of plus cylinders, a cylinder at the appropriate axis will move the back focal line forward, while having no effect on the position of the front focal line.

With the best sphere in place, if uncorrected astigmatism is still present, then it is generally assumed that the circle of least confusion (COLC), i.e. the dioptric midpoint between the anterior and posterior focal lines, is positioned on or close to the retina. This assumption is based on the premise that with uncorrected astigmatism, best VA will be reached when the COLC is located on the retina. However, the justification for this assumption is limited, and there is objective evidence to suggest that optimum acuity will vary depending upon the choice of target adopted. For example, Williamson-Noble (1943) observed that the resolution of letters having vertical components (e.g. uppercase U, F and N) was better with 1.00 D of uncorrected with-the-rule, simple myopic astigmatism (with the vertical focal line on or close to the retina), compared with 1.00 D of compound astigmatism where the COLC was on the retina. Accordingly, it has been proposed that circular targets, such as Landolt Cs or Verheoff circles might be better for maintaining the COLC on the retina. In contrast, Borish and Benjamin (2006) suggested that circular targets 'do not allow easy communication between the examiner and patient', although no rationale was provided for this statement. However, Borish and Benjamin suggested that an isolated row of letters, which presumably would contain a wide variety of spatially orientated letter components, should be used as the target.

Cylinder refinement is most commonly carried out using either the Jackson Cross Cylinder (JCC) or the Fan Chart (FC). A less commonly performed procedure, the Stenopaeic Slit, will also be discussed.

Cylinder axis refinement using the JCC

The JCC consists of plus and minus cylinders of equal magnitude, oriented with their axes 90° apart. In 1887, Edward Jackson described the use of a fixed-power Stokes lens to determine the cylinder power necessary to correct astigmatism. In a subsequent paper, he indicated that this lens could also be used to obtain the correcting cylinder axis (Jackson 1907). An example of a hand-held JCC is shown in **Figure 14.1**. The most commonly used powers are ±0.25 D, ±0.37 D, ±0.50 D and ±1.00 D, although the latter is generally only used with low-vision patients. In the United States, the convention is for the minus axis to be marked with red dots and the plus axis to be marked with white dots. However, in the United Kingdom, the opposite colour convention exists, with the minus axis generally marked in white. Using a higher-powered JCC increases the magnitude of the difference between the appearances of the two presentations, but may also reduce the level of precision that can be achieved in the final result. Accordingly, the lowest-power JCC which still allows the patient to choose between the two presentations should be selected.

For axis refinement, the JCC is positioned so that its axes lie 45° away from the cylinder axis that has been determined by objective refraction (most commonly by retinoscopy). Consider the following example: following retinoscopy and the first sphere check, the following lenses are positioned before the eye: +3.00 −1.50 × 75. Accordingly, the JCC will be introduced with the axes at (75+45) = 120° and (75−45) = 30°. On almost all modern phoropters, the JCC is mechanically linked to the correcting cylinder so that the axis position can readily be achieved by either lining up the 'A' (for axis) markings or, more commonly, the JCC thumbwheels with the correcting cylinder axis. In the case of a hand-held JCC, the lens is usually oriented so that if the handle of the JCC is placed in line with the correcting cylinder axis, then the JCC is aligned appropriately for axis refinement. These JCC positions (in a phoropter) are illustrated in **Figure 14.2**.

The patient should be instructed to view a distant object. Commonly used targets include: (1) a line of letters corresponding to one line larger than the best acuity achieved

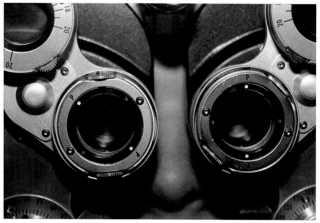

Figure 14.2 Example of JCCs used in a phoropter. For both the right and left eyes, a cylinder axis of 90° was found on retinoscopy. The JCC introduced in front of the right eye is in the axis position, with the thumbwheels coincident with the 90° cylinder axis determined by retinoscopy. The plus (white dots) and minus (red dots) cylinder axes lie at 90° ±45, i.e. 135° and 45°. The JCC introduced in front of the left eye is shown in the power position, with the 'P' markings corresponding with the 90° cylinder axis determined by retinoscopy. The plus (white dots) and minus (red dots) cylinder axes lie at 90° and 180°, respectively.

at this stage of the examination, (2) a line of letters corresponding to two lines larger than the best acuity achieved at this stage of the examination or (3) a circular target such as a line of Landolt Cs or Verheoff circles (**Fig. 14.3**). Circular targets may be advantageous if the COLC is not positioned on the retina during the procedure, as will be discussed later.

The patient views the target consecutively through the JCC oriented in each of the two positions described above, and is asked to indicate whether one presentation 'appears clearer or darker than the other'. It may be advantageous to inform the patient that both images will be slightly blurred (otherwise the patient will often point this out to you, rather than answering the actual question!). Most practitioners describe the two JCC positions by number, e.g. 'better with lens 1 or lens 2'. If this is done, then at subsequent presentations it can aid communication if different numbers are used, i.e. lens 3 or lens 4. This makes it clear to the patient that you are showing them a different lens condition, rather than repeating the previous presentation.

Assuming the use of minus cylinders, the correcting cylinder axis should be rotated towards the preferred position of the JCC minus axis (if plus cylinders are being used, then

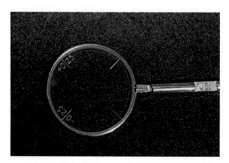

Figure 14.1 A ±0.25 D hand-held Jackson Cross Cylinder (JCC) The numbers indicate the plus and minus cylinder axes.

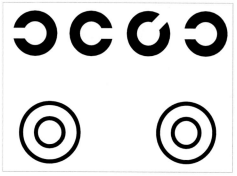

Figure 14.3 Example of Landolt Cs **(top)** and Verhoeff circles **(bottom)**. Each of these is an effective target for the JCC procedure as the circular shape will help to maintain the circle of least confusion (COLC) on the retina.

the correcting cylinder axis should be rotated towards the preferred position of the JCC plus axis). Using the example described above, the lenses present after retinoscopy and the first sphere check are $+3.00 -1.50 \times 75$. Accordingly, the JCC will be introduced with the axes at 30° and 120°. If the patient indicates that the target appears clearer when the JCC minus axis lies along 30°, then the correcting cylinder axis is rotated away from 75° towards 30°. Del Priore and Guyton (1986) suggested that the degree of rotation should be related to the power of the correcting cylinder, with smaller amounts of rotation being required with larger cylinder powers. For example, they suggested that the initial rotation for a 0.50 D, 1.00 D and 3.00 D cylinder should be 15°, 5° and 2°, respectively. However, if a bracketing technique is adopted, then the size of the initial rotation does not matter. Ten degrees is often a useful starting value, since it allows easy bracketing of the axis direction. Therefore, using the previous example, the correcting cylinder will be rotated from 75° to 65°. The JCC is presented again, now aligned with its axes at $65° \pm 45$ (i.e. 20° and 110°), and the patient asked which presentation is preferred. This process continues until either the patient reports no difference between the two presentations, or the patient's responses move the setting back and forth within a narrow range of axis locations. In this event, select the axis in the middle of this range. For an example of a JCC axis procedure, see **Table 14.1**.

During axis refinement using the JCC, the patient is actually viewing the resultant of a series of obliquely crossed cylinders. Cylinders are said to be obliquely crossed when their axes are neither parallel nor perpendicular to one another. The resultant of a pair of obliquely crossed cylinders can be determined either algebraically or graphically (Jalie 1980; Stoner et al 2005). Consider the initial step in **Table 14.1**. The lenses present after retinoscopy and the initial sphere refinement are $+3.00 -1.50 \times 75$. If the actual refractive correction for this eye is $+3.25 -2.00 \times 60$, then an obliquely crossed cylinder exists. It can be determined that with the lenses present, an additional $+0.52 -1.03 \times 37$ is required to correct the resultant error, or make the eye emmetropic. As shown in **Table 14.1**, a JCC is now introduced, having its minus cylinder axis at either 30° (position 1) or 120° (position 2). If the power of the JCC is ±0.50, then the resultant of the eye, JCC and the $+3.00 - 1.50 \times 75$ lenses can be calculated. For positions 1 and 2, an additional $+0.12 -0.25 \times 75$ and $+1.00 -2.00 \times 34$, respectively, will be required to correct the eye fully. In

both cases the COLC will lie on the retina, but since the diameter of the blur circle is smaller with position 1 (due to the smaller amount of uncorrected astigmatism), the patient should report that position 1 is clearer. This information can then be used to determine the direction in which the correcting cylinder axis should be rotated.

Cylinder power refinement using the JCC

After the cylinder axis has been confirmed, the cylinder power can be checked by rotating the JCC so that its plus and minus axes lie parallel and perpendicular to the axis of the correcting cylinder. With the COLC on the retina, these two options will either increase or decrease the magnitude of uncorrected astigmatism, while still keeping the COLC on the retina. On most phoropters, this is achieved by lining up the 'P' (for power) markings with the correcting cylinder axis. When the JCC is flipped, either the plus or minus axis will line up with the axis of the correcting cylinder (see **Fig. 14.2**). If the patient prefers the position with the JCC minus axis parallel to the correcting cylinder axis, then the minus cylinder power should be increased. If the patient prefers the position with the JCC plus axis parallel to the correcting cylinder axis, then the minus cylinder power should be decreased.

Consider the example shown in **Table 14.1**. After axis refinement has been completed, the lenses present before the eye are: $+3.00 -1.50 \times 60$. If the actual refractive correction for this eye is $+3.25 -2.00 \times 60$, then 0.50 D of uncorrected astigmatism remains. If a ±0.50 D JCC is now introduced, firstly with the minus axis at 60° (position 1) and then with the minus axis at 150° (position 2), it can be calculated that position 1 will leave the patient with 0.50 D of uncorrected astigmatism, whereas position 2 will leave 1.50 D of astigmatism. With the COLC on the retina in both cases, the diameter of the blur circle will be significantly smaller when looking through the JCC in position 1 (minus axis at 60°), thereby indicating that the power of the minus correcting cylinder should be increased.

However, increasing the power of the minus correcting cylinder will also move the position of the COLC. In the example shown in the previous paragraph, before the JCC was introduced, one of the principal meridia was 0.25 D myopic and the other was 0.25 D hyperopic. If the lenses are now changed to $+3.00 -1.75 \times 60$ as indicated by the findings of the JCC power procedure, one meridian will

Table 14.1 Example of cylinder axis refinement using the JCC. The correcting cylinder axis is rotated in the direction of the preferred orientation of the JCC minus cylinder axis

Lenses present	JCC presentation	JCC presentation
$+3.00 -1.50 \times 75$	Minus axis 30 (position 1)	Minus axis 120 (position 2)
Patient prefers position 1. Move correcting cylinder axis from 75 to 65		
$+3.00 -1.50 \times 65$	Minus axis 20 (position 3)	Minus axis 110 (position 4)
Patient prefers position 3. Move correcting cylinder axis from 65 to 55.		
$+3.00 -1.50 \times 55$	Minus axis 10 (position 5)	Minus axis 100 (position 6)
Patient prefers position 6. Move correcting cylinder axis from 55 to 60		
$+3.00 -1.50 \times 60$	Minus axis 15 (position 7)	Minus axis 105 (position 8)
Patient reports no difference between positions 7 and 8. Therefore cylinder axis endpoint is 60°.		

become 0.25 D hyperopic while the other will be fully corrected. Accordingly, the COLC will lie 0.12 D behind the retina. Since the procedure is based upon maintaining the COLC on the retina, so that the patient is comparing different-sized blur circles (and not different-shaped blurred retinal images), theoretically a +0.12 sphere should be added to move the COLC back onto the retina. This would change the correcting lenses to $+3.12 -1.75 \times 60$. However, in practice, the sphere is only changed when the cylinder power is altered by at least ±0.50 D, thereby shifting the COLC 0.25 D away from the retina. The general rule is that when the power of the correcting cylinder is changed by xD, the sphere should be altered by $-x/2D$, or half the amount of change in the opposite direction. For example, if the power of the correcting cylinder was changed from -1.25 D to -0.75 D (0.50 D less minus power), then the power of the sphere should be changed by -0.25 D. This will keep the COLC on the retina throughout the JCC procedure.

The end point for cylinder power refinement is reached when either the patient reports no difference between the two presentations, or the patient's responses move the setting back and forth within a narrow range of powers. In this event, select the cylinder power in the middle of this range.

JCC procedure when no astigmatism is observed objectively, or as part of an independent subjective refraction

If an independent subjective refraction is being performed, i.e. when objective testing cannot be carried out, or alternatively in the case where no astigmatism is observed during the objective examination, then the practitioner must first determine whether any astigmatism is present. This can be assessed from the level of VA that is achieved through the best sphere lenses. **Table 14.2** shows the average level of VA that can be expected for a purely spherical refractive error, or where astigmatism is present but the COLC is on the retina.

Two procedures have been suggested for determining whether any astigmatism is present. For both, the initial step is to find the best sphere, as described previously, which should place the COLC on or close to the retina. For the first technique, described both by Bennett and Rabbetts (1989)

and Borish and Benjamin (2006), a JCC is introduced over the best sphere with the axes at 45° and 135°. The JCC is flipped and the patient asked which position is 'clearer and darker'. If the patient indicates a preference, then their correcting cylinder axis is closer to the preferred JCC axis position. This procedure is then repeated with the JCC axes at 90° and 180°. For example, a patient who reports that the target appears clearer when the minus axis of the JCC is first at 45° and then at 180° will have a minus correcting cylinder axis that lies between these two orientations, i.e. between 45° and 180°. Accordingly, a cylinder whose power can be estimated from **Table 14.2** (based on the VA through the best sphere) should be introduced at axis 22.5°, and the cylinder axis refined further based on the technique described previously. Finally, after axis refinement, the power of the cylinder should be verified as indicated above. In the case of a patient who prefers a spherical refractive correction, they will indicate no difference between the JCC with axes at 45° and 135°, and similarly no difference between the JCC with axes at 90° and 180°.

An alternative and possibly superior technique was described by Polasky (1991). Here, a -0.25 D cylinder axis 45° is introduced over the best sphere. A JCC is placed over this 0.25 D cylinder in the *power* position (i.e. with its axes at 45° and 135°) and then flipped. If the patient prefers the plus JCC axis along 45° (i.e. rejects the -0.25 D cylinder), then the procedure is repeated with the cylinder axis rotated to 90°, 135° and 180°. The patient should reject the cylinder (i.e. indicate that they prefer the plus axis of the JCC) in all these positions. Only if the patient rejects the cylinder in all four orientations can it be assumed that they have a spherical refractive error. If the patient does not reject the cylinder in one orientation, i.e. they either prefer the minus JCC axis parallel to the -0.25 D cylinder axis, or alternatively report no difference between the two positions, then the JCC should be switched to the *axis* mode (with the 0.25 D cylinder in the preferred orientation) and axis refinement continued as described previously. For example, after best sphere determination, a $+2.25$ DS is present. A -0.25 D cylinder axis 45° is introduced before the eye with the JCC in the power position over this cylinder. If the patient prefers the JCC with the minus cylinder axis along 45°, then the -0.25 cylinder axis 45° is left in place, the JCC switched to axis position (with the axis at 45° ± 45°) and cylinder axis refinement carried out as described previously.

With the second procedure, a patient having a spherical refractive error should make an affirmative response to indicate that they prefer the plus JCC cylinder axis over the introduced -0.25 D cylinder. They will do this for all four presentations, i.e. with the 0.25 D cylinder at axis 45°, 90°, 135° and 180°. In contrast, for the first technique, a patient with a spherical error will indicate no difference between the JCC with minus axis at 45° or 135°, and subsequently between 90° and 180°. The requirement of a positive response may make the second procedure superior for the clinician.

JCC: other issues

As with all aspects of subjective refraction, the quality of the instructions to the patient is critical. Instructions must be simple, straightforward and avoid the use of technical terminology. With regard to the JCC procedure, it is important to emphasize to the patient that they are choosing the better of two blurry images. Frequently, a patient will report that neither presentation is particularly clear, but reminding the

Table 14.2 Expected level of visual acuity as a function of refractive state

Vision	Spherical ametropia (D) (myopia or absolute hyperopia)	Astigmatism (D) with the COLC on or close to the retina
6/6 (20/20)	Small	Small
6/9 (20/30)	0.50	1.00
6/12 (20/40)	0.75	1.50
6/18 (20/60)	1.00	2.00
6/24 (20/80)	1.50	3.00
6/36 (20/120)	2.00	4.00
6/60 (20/200)	2.00 to 3.00	high

Reproduced with permission from Bennett and Rabbetts (1989).

patient that these are just intermediate steps will generally reassure them, particularly as they should observe an improvement in target clarity during the course of the procedure. Further, it is important to give the patient sufficient time to observe the first presentation before the JCC is flipped. Often, inexperienced students will show the first JCC position very briefly before flipping the lens. Thus, the patient will get plenty of time to view the second presentation, but very little time for the first. This will result in the patient either having to ask for the two presentations to be repeated, thereby prolonging the procedure, or making an incorrect response based on what they saw of the first presentation.

One criticism of the JCC procedure is that it requires the patient to remember the appearance of the first target presentation while viewing the second one. For the majority of patients, this is not a problem, but LeVine (1990) suggested that patients with Alzheimer's disease or similar disorders may have difficulty remembering the appearance of the first image. A number of devices have been proposed to overcome this problem by allowing simultaneous viewing of the two JCC presentations. These include the use of mirrors (Simultan test; Biessels 1967), biprisms (AutoCross test; Matsuura 1961) and prisms with divided lenses (LeVine 1990) to create simultaneous presentations. Recently, Marco Instruments (Jacksonville, Florida) offered a phoropter which includes a split-image device to allow simultaneous viewing of the two JCC presentations (Borish & Benjamin 2006).

As noted previously, the use of rectilinear targets may not be optimal for maintaining the COLC on the retina. Indeed, if the COLC is away from the retina, this might result in the patient making an incorrect selection during the JCC procedure, particularly if the orientation of the focal lines is close to the horizontal and vertical meridia. Consider an eye which has 0.50 D of uncorrected astigmatism, with the back focal line being 0.25 D myopic and the front focal line being 0.75 D myopic. If a ±0.25 D JCC is now introduced in the power position, one JCC position will leave the patient with 0.50 D of spherical myopia, whereas the alternative presentation will create 1.00 D of uncorrected astigmatism, with the back focal line on the retina. If a rectilinear target is used, such as a letter E, F, H or L, then the patient might choose the latter presentation, which actually increases the magnitude of astigmatism but results in one element of the target being focused on the retina. This is consistent with the observations of Williamson-Noble (1943). Indeed, Bannon and Walsh (1945) stated that for the recognition of letters, the vertical strokes are most important, so a patient may prefer a lens that makes the vertical strokes clear. They suggested that when using a JCC with letter targets, one is likely to determine more against-the-rule astigmatism. However, if a circular target is used, the patient will be more likely to choose the presentation that results in a smaller degree of astigmatism.

In order to maintain the COLC on the retina, it has been suggested that when working with a pre-presbyopic patient, the spherical portion of the refractive correction should be over-minused (or under-plused), so that the patient is left hyperopic. The presumption is that the patient will then accommodate to place the COLC on the retina (Borish & Benjamin 2006). However, there is little objective evidence to support this proposal. For example, Portello et al (2001) used an infrared optometer to measure the accommodative response in subjects with uncorrected astigmatism. A range of fixation targets was used, including a starburst, Verhoeff circles, a row of letters and an orthogonal line target. The latter is conventionally used for the dynamic cross cylinder procedure to assess accommodation (see Fig. 15.5) (Rosenfield 1997). The results demonstrated that subjects generally exerted the minimum accommodation necessary to place the anterior focal line within the depth of focus of the eye. However, under none of the conditions tested was the COLC positioned on or close to the retina. Furthermore, Loo and Jacobs (1994) reported that the accuracy of the spherical refraction did not produce any significant change in the precision of JCC axis determination, irrespective of whether the patient had up to 0.75 D of myopia or hyperopia. Accordingly, there seems little justification for modifying the spherical component away from the previously found best sphere before starting the JCC procedure.

A disadvantage when using a phoropter is that it is somewhat inconvenient to change the power of the JCC. This is much easier when hand-held JCCs are used. However, it is possible to hold a hand-held JCC over the phoropter to overcome this difficulty. In considering the most appropriate JCC power to use, O'Leary (1988) noted that when large amounts of uncorrected astigmatism are present, confusing answers may sometimes arise if a low-powered JCC (e.g. ±0.25 D) is used. For example, if 1 D of uncorrected astigmatism is present when starting the axis refinement procedure, and the cylinder lies 10° away from the correct axis, then the resultant astigmatism when a ±0.25 D JCC is presented in the two alternative positions is 1.96 D and 2.57 D, respectively, a difference of 0.61 D. However, for the same situation when a ±0.50 D JCC is used, the resultant astigmatism for the two JCC positions will be 1.80 D and 2.95 D, respectively, a difference of 1.15 D. Accordingly, the higher JCC power will make it easier for the patient to differentiate between the two positions. This is particularly important when the patient has reduced VA. During the course of the procedure as the VA improves, the practitioner can switch to a lower-powered JCC. When only small axis and power errors are present, the appearance of the 'better' position will become increasing blurred as the JCC power is increased (O'Leary 1988). Under these conditions, a low-powered JCC (±0.25) should be used.

When using hand-held JCCs, it can be difficult to ensure that they are oriented appropriately. When refining the cylinder axis, the JCC axes should be oriented 45° away from the correcting cylinder axis. This is generally achieved by holding the handle of the JCC parallel to the correcting cylinder axis. However, if a small axis error is present (<10°), axis refinement using the JCC should still be successful even if the JCC is held up to 20° away from the correct orientation. If a larger axis error is present after retinoscopy, greater care will be needed to ensure correct placement of the JCC, otherwise the difference between the resultants when the JCC is presented in the two orientations will be diminished.

Cylinder axis refinement using the Fan Chart (FC)

Since the first description of astigmatism by Sir Isaac Newton in the seventeenth century (Shapiro 1984), numerous testing methods have been developed for determining the astigmatic error. However, for the subjective assessment of astigmatism, the JCC is the most widely used procedure in contemporary clinical optometric practice. Other subjective astigmatic tests, such as the FC (also known as the astigmatic dial), are less commonly used in today's clinical environment. The most probable explanation is that the JCC is easier to perform for both the practitioner and patient. However, the FC still provides a useful alternative in situations when the JCC is not successful. Indeed, Borish and Benjamin (2006) stated that no single subjective test will work in all situations, and the practitioner must have a viable alternative procedure for a given patient when the JCC fails to yield accurate results. The FC is particularly good for patients with short-term memory problems since all the choices are displayed simultaneously, and also represents the fastest way of confirming the absence of astigmatism subjectively.

While early references to fan-shaped figures were made by Purkinje (1819–1823: cited by Duke-Elder & Abrams 1970), the extensive work of John Green (1868, 1878) described 26 forms of astigmatic charts, some of which are similar to the modern form. Indeed, in his 1878 paper, Green described being able to rotate the chart into any desired position. The use of rotating arrows, dials, blocks and charts was also elaborated in later papers (e.g. Maddox 1921; Verhoeff 1923; Raubitschek 1952).

As with the JCC procedure, the first step after the objective refraction (retinoscopy or autorefraction) is the initial sphere check. This is presumed to place the COLC on the retina. However, before determining the cylinder axis using the FC, the sphere should be modified to move the back (or posterior) focal line onto the retina. This is achieved by estimating the amount of astigmatism that remains uncorrected after the best sphere has been found. With the best sphere in place, distance VA is measured through these lenses, and the magnitude of uncorrected astigmatism can be estimated using **Table 14.2**. Thus, a patient with 6/9 (20/30) acuity through the initial best sphere is presumed to have 1 D of uncorrected astigmatism. Plus sphere is added, corresponding to *half the estimated uncorrected astigmatism*. Using the example described above where the VA through the best sphere is 6/9 (20/30), +0.50 DS would be added to the best sphere. This will move the back focal line onto the retina as shown in **Figure 14.4**. An alternative procedure for fogging the patient is to add an excessive amount of plus sphere power to degrade the VA so that the lines on the FC are barely visible, and then to reduce the plus sphere until one line on the chart can just be resolved.

Examples of different forms of this test are shown in **Figure 14.5**. With the back focal line on or close to the retina, any correcting cylinder should be removed, and the patient's attention turned to the fan chart, clock dial or other astigmatic chart being used. If cylinder at an incorrect axis is left before the eye when performing the FC procedure, then the patient will indicate the cylinder axis that corrects the resultant of their eye and this incorrect cylinder.

With the back focal line on or close to the retina and any cylindrical lenses removed, the orientation of the clearest line on the fan chart now corresponds with the *orientation of the focal line nearest the retina from the patient's viewpoint*. Consider the situation where following the initial sphere

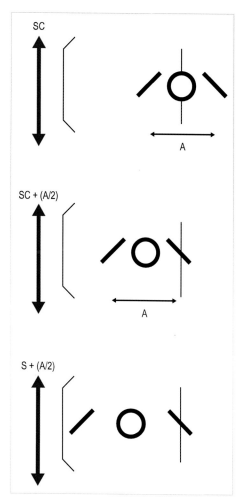

Figure 14.4 Position of the front and back focal lines before starting the fan chart (FC) procedure. After determining the initial best sphere, the circle of least confusion is assumed to be on or close to the retina **(top)**. SC represents the sphere and cylinder lenses present after the initial sphere check. 'A' dioptres of uncorrected astigmatism are present. Plus sphere equal to A/2 dioptres should then be added to the initial best sphere (SC), which will move both focal lines forward, so that the back focal line now lies on the retina **(middle)**. Finally, the cylindrical lenses found during retinoscopy are removed, thereby increasing the astigmatic interval **(bottom)**. The patient is now ready to view the FC for axis determination.

refinement the eye requires an additional $-1.00\,DC \times 60$ to be corrected. Thus, the back focal line (the 150° focal line) will lie on the retina, while the 60° focal line lies 1 D in front of the retina. It should be noted that the orientation of the focal lines as described above is based on the practitioner viewing the patient using standard axis terminology (Stoner et al 2005). However, when the patient is viewing the FC, the orientation of the lines on the chart from their perspective will be 180° away from that of the practitioner. In this example, the focal line nearest the retina is oriented along 150° for the practitioner facing the patient. However, for the patient viewing the fan chart (sitting opposite the practitioner), the orientation of this focal line from their viewpoint will be $(180-150) = 30°$, and the clearest line on the chart will correspond with this orientation. Further examples are shown in **Table 14.3**.

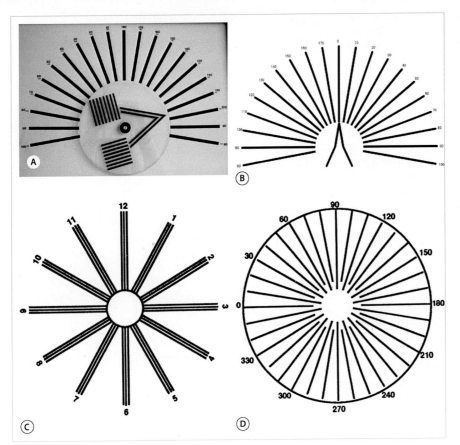

Figure 14.5 Examples of fan charts. **(A)** A classic 'Fan and Block' chart. The outside fan chart is used to determine the correcting cylinder axis. The Maddox arrow in the centre allows the axis to be refined more precisely, while the two blocks of lines adjacent to the arrow are used to determine the cylinder power. **(B)** Another fan chart with a modified arrow, taken from the computerized Test Chart program (Thomson Software Solutions, London, UK). The numbers around the outside indicate the negative correcting cylinder axis. **(C)** A clock dial and **(D)** the Lancaster–Regan sunburst dial. (**C** and **D** are reproduced with permission from Borish and Benjamin 2006.)

Table 14.3 Orientation of the clearest line on a fan chart (FC). This will correspond to the orientation of the focal line nearest the retina from the patient's perspective

Least ametropic meridian (°)	Orientation of focal line nearest the retina from the practitioner's perspective (°)	Orientation of focal line nearest the retina from the patient's perspective (°)
15	105	75
30	120	60
45	135	45
60	150	30
75	165	15
90	180	180
120	30	150
135	45	135
150	60	120
180	90	90

Since FCs contain a limited number of lines, the degree of precision with which the correcting cylinder axis can be assessed is limited. For example, clock dials (see **Fig. 14.5C**) have lines positioned at 30° intervals, and accordingly, the cylinder axis can only be measured within ±15°. Other fan charts have lines at 10° intervals, which is clearly advantageous. Nevertheless, once the approximate correcting cylinder axis has been determined using an FC or clock dial, rotating arrows or dials can then be used to determine the axis more precisely.

Examples of rotating arrows are shown in **Figure 14.5A** and **B** and **Figure 14.6**. Based on the FC finding, the arrow is pointed towards the orientation of the clearest line indicated by the patient. The patient is asked whether the two sides of the arrow appear equally clear and dark, or whether one side seems clearer and darker than the other. If the patient reports that one side of the arrow is darker, then the arrowhead is rotated *away from the clearer side*, until the patient reports that the two sides appear equal. Once this position of equality has been achieved, the direction of the arrowhead axis corresponds with the orientation of the focal line nearest the retina from the patient's viewpoint. Most charts include a scale which indicates the correcting cylinder axis corresponding with the preferred direction of the arrow. These rotating arrow charts allow the axis of astigmatism to be determined very precisely, often within ±2.5°.

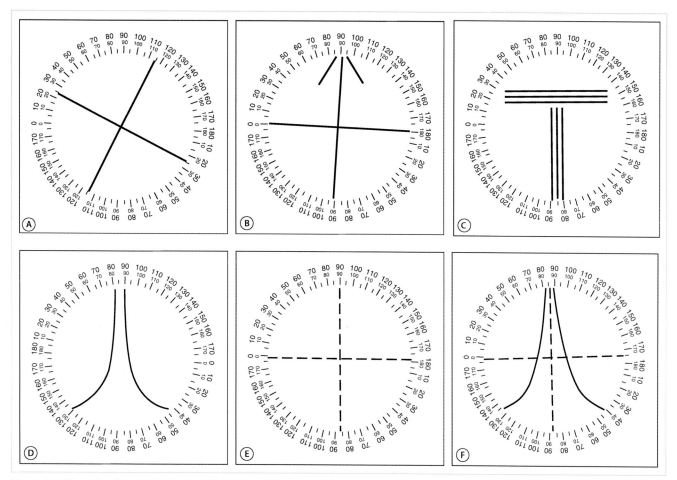

Figure 14.6 Examples of rotating astigmatic dials: **(A)** rotating cross; **(B)** Lebensohn astigmometer; **(C)** rotating T-chart; **(D)** Raubitschek arrow; **(E)** Robinson–Cohen cross; **(F)** combination of Raubitschek paraboline arrow and dashed cross. The arrow or paraboline charts shown in b, d and f are used to refine the cylinder axis, while the cross or T-charts in a, b, c, e and f are used to determine the cylinder power. (Reproduced with permission from Michaels 1985.)

Cylinder power refinement using the fan chart (FC)

Once the cylinder axis has been found, the power of the correcting cylinder can be determined. This is achieved by introducing minus cylinder power to move the front focal line posteriorly until all the lines on the FC appear equally clear and dark. However, by giving the patient up to 24 lines to compare, it can be difficult for them to determine when all the lines have similar appearances. The task can be made easier by displaying only two targets, one of which will be clear (corresponding to the focal line on or close to the retina) and the other blurred (corresponding to the myopic focal line), and then adding minus cylinder power until these two lines appear equally clear and dark. These two lines are generally displayed in the form of a letter T, a cross, or two squares of lines otherwise known as blocks (see **Figs 14.5A** and **14.6**). In all cases, the chart is rotated until the orientation of one of the targets corresponds with the direction of the clearest line on the FC.

When the patient reports that the two orthogonal targets are equally clear and dark, either all of their astigmatism has been corrected or, alternatively, uncorrected astigmatism is still present and the COLC lies on the retina. To determine which of these two situations exists, simply add an additional +0.50 DS to the lenses already present and ask the patient to view the appearance of the chart used for cylinder power determination (T, cross or blocks) again. The plus sphere will move both focal lines anteriorly. If the astigmatism has been fully corrected, then both focal lines will be equidistant from the retina, and the patient will report that the two rectilinear targets appear equally blurred. However, if uncorrected astigmatism is still present, then with the additional +0.50 DS, one focal line will now be closer to the retina than the other, and the patient will report that one target is clearer or darker. This is illustrated in **Figure 14.7**. If it is determined that uncorrected astigmatism is still present, then leave the additional +0.50 DS in place (to provide additional fog and better control of accommodation), rebalance the cross, T-chart or blocks, and finally add an additional +0.50 DS to check that the astigmatism is now corrected.

Comparison of the JCC and FC procedures

As noted previously, the JCC is the most frequently used procedure to confirm the axis and magnitude of astigmatism subjectively. The JCC may be preferred over the FC because it is easier for the practitioner to perform, the instructions to the patient are simpler and the technique takes less time to complete. However, as Borish and Benjamin (2006)

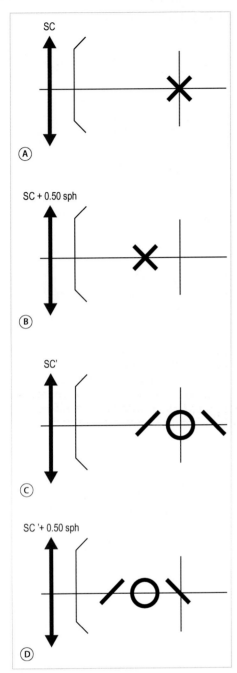

Figure 14.7 A +0.50 test should be performed after the FC to confirm that all of the astigmatism has been corrected. **(A)** Following the FC procedure, the astigmatism has been corrected by the sphero-cylindrical combination SC so that the two focal lines are coincident. If a +0.50 DS is now introduced, both focal lines will move forward, but will remain equidistant from the retina. **(B)**. If the patient views an FC, blocks or T-chart with the additional +0.50 DS present, they will report that all the lines remain equally clear (or more precisely, equally blurred). However, if following completion of the FC procedure uncorrected astigmatism is present, with the COLC on the retina, a patient viewing an FC would also report that all the lines appear equally clear. **(C)** This condition is identified when an additional +0.50 DS is introduced, both focal lines move forward and the patient will report that one set of lines on the FC, blocks or T-chart is clearer than the other. **(D)** The orientation of the clearer lines will correspond to the orientation of the back focal line from the patient's viewpoint.

observed, no single test will work in all situations, and the practitioner should be able to carry out an alternative procedure should the JCC fail to give accurate results on a given patient. Indeed, there are some situations where the FC may be superior to the JCC technique. For example, when confirming the presence of a spherical refractive error, this may be done more quickly with the FC. The patient will indicate that all the lines on the FC appear equally clear and dark. If the equality remains when an additional +0.50 DS is added (to check that the COLC does not lie on the retina), then the astigmatic confirmation is completed, and the practitioner can move on to the second sphere check. The FC is also quicker than the JCC for determining the astigmatic axis in patients where objective refraction is impossible, such as those with very small pupils or media opacities. One other advantage of the FC over the JCC which may be particularly significant for the eye care practitioner is that it is a very effective way of refracting oneself!

The instructions that must be given to the patient during the FC procedure are somewhat more complex than the simple JCC question: 'Which is better, lens 1 or lens 2?' However, with practice, these can be made fairly simple, such as: 'Do you see the lines that go around like a fan? Do they all look equally clear and dark or does one line look clearer and darker than the others?' Difficulty can arise when the patient is asked to indicate the orientation of the clearest line. If an arrow or other movable marker is present on the chart, then this will make communication easier (note, if an indirect chart is being used, i.e. one viewed via a plane mirror, then the practitioner can simply reach up and point to the chart with their hand, without having to move away from the chair side). Otherwise, the clock face can be used, such as having the patient state at which hour the clearest line lies (e.g. 2 o'clock). The use of an arrow or paraboline to refine the cylinder axis, and either a cross, T-chart or blocks to confirm the cylinder power, makes the instructions simpler, as it becomes a two-alternative question, similar to that used with the JCC.

Another reason why the JCC may be preferred over the FC is that the latter requires an additional chart (or charts), whereas the JCC can be performed with a simple Snellen chart. However, with the increased use of computerized charts presented on flat-panel video monitors, this disadvantage may cease to be relevant.

The JCC technique can be performed using either plus or minus cylinders, although minus cylinders are preferred during the entire refraction procedure since they permit better control of accommodation. This is particularly true during retinoscopy, where the use of plus cylinders requires the practitioner to leave with motion prior to introducing the cylinder, with the risk that this meridian may be hyperopic and therefore could induce accommodation. In contrast, the FC procedure should only be undertaken with minus cylinders on a patient with active accommodation. If one was to perform the procedure with plus cylinders, this would necessitate the front focal line being positioned on the retina with the back focal line behind the retina. Under these circumstances, many patients would accommodate to position the COLC on or close to the retina.

As noted previously, before starting the FC chart procedure with minus cylinders, the patient must be fogged, so that the back focal line is positioned on or slightly in front of the retina. This differs from the JCC, which requires the COLC on the retina. While the FC does require an extra step to ensure fogging, this also has the advantage of ensuring that the patient's accommodation is controlled. With the JCC, one focal line is positioned behind the retina, and depending on the orientation of that back focal line and the particular target being viewed, the patient may exert some accommodation during the procedure. If this accommodation is maintained, then the final result will not reflect the true refractive error present under conditions of minimal accommodation.

Finally, when considering the accuracy of the two procedures, both Ong et al (1974) and Rappon and Rosenfield (1999) reported no significant difference between the JCC and FC (when used in conjunction with a paraboline arrow) to determine an astigmatic error. Interestingly, Polasky (1991) suggested that the sensitivity of the JCC procedure is reduced in patients with acuities between 6/9 (20/30) and 6/15 (20/50), and the test may not work in patients having VA of 6/18 (20/60) or worse. The author's personal experience is that the JCC can be effective in these patients, but is more successful when higher-powered cross-cylinders (e.g. ±0.50 or ±1.00 D) are used. Polasky also stated that the FC may be more successful than the JCC for patients with long-standing uncorrected astigmatism.

It is clear that the practitioner should be comfortable carrying out either of these two procedures. As noted earlier, there is no subjective test yet devised that will work on 'every patient, every time', and therefore it is critical to have a back-up technique when the initial test is unsuccessful. There are some patients where neither the JCC nor the FC is effective, and another method must be employed to determine the astigmatic error subjectively, such as the stenopaeic slit.

The stenopaeic slit

This is an opaque disc containing a central slit aperture of about 1 mm in width (**Fig. 14.8**). It will reduce the effective pupil diameter in the meridian perpendicular to the slit. Although it is not found in most phoropters, it is a standard accessory in almost all trial sets. Stenopaeic slit refraction is usually attempted when retinoscopy and more conventional subjective refractive techniques, i.e. JCC and FC, fail to provide satisfactory results. The slit may be used to locate the principal meridia of an astigmatic eye. The slit is rotated until the patient reports the orientation that gives the best VA. This will occur when the slit is perpendicular to one of the principal meridia. Consider an eye with simple myopic astigmatism, where the horizontal focal line (H) is on the retina (therefore negative correcting cylinder axis = 90°). If the slit is placed horizontally, it will reduce the width of the vertical ray bundle, thereby limiting the size of the vertical focal line, as shown in **Figure 14.9**.

Since the clearest image will be observed when the smallest diameter blur circle/ellipse coincides with the retina, the patient will report the best vision when the attenuated vertical focal line lies at the retinal plane, i.e. when the horizontal meridian is corrected. Accordingly, plus and minus spheres are introduced until the best sphere (maximum plus or minimum minus sphere that gives the optimum VA) is determined while looking through the slit. If the slit is then rotated through 90°, i.e. placed vertically, the target will now be clearest when the horizontal focal line is on the retina, i.e. when the vertical meridian is corrected. Thus, the best sphere is determined again while the patient is looking though the slit oriented at this second meridian. This technique can be very useful in low-vision patients when other techniques to determine the astigmatic axis are unsuccessful. Indeed, patients can create their own stenopaeic slit by partially closing their eyelids.

When rotating the slit initially to determine the orientation of the principal meridian, care must be taken to ensure that the COLC does not already lie on the retina. Should that be the case, then the patient would report that slit rotation fails to change the appearance of the target, and the examiner might assume incorrectly that no astigmatic error exists. In order to ensure that the COLC does not coincide with the retina, the initial best sphere is determined before the slit is introduced (which is presumed to place the COLC on the retina), and an additional +0.75 DS should then be added to move the COLC forward of the retina. This procedure is outlined below.

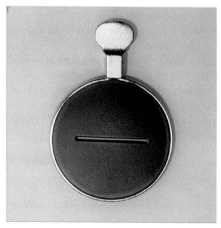

Figure 14.8 A stenopaeic slit oriented horizontally.

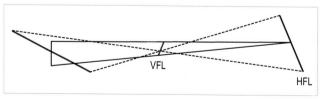

Figure 14.9 If a stenopaeic slit is introduced with the slit horizontal, then the horizontal ray bundle will pass normally whereas the width of the vertical ray bundle will be restricted. As shown, this produces a normal-sized horizontal focal line (HFL), but a small vertical focal line (VFL). Since the clearest image will be observed by the patient when the smallest diameter blur circle/ellipse coincides with the retina, the patient will report the best vision when this attenuated vertical focal line lies at the retinal plane, i.e. when the horizontal meridian is corrected.

Stenopaeic slit procedure

1. Occlude the left eye.
2. Find the best sphere (maximum plus or minimum minus sphere that gives the optimum VA) for the right eye while the patient is viewing an acuity chart.
3. Add an additional +0.75 DS to this best sphere. This will introduce a small amount of fog and move the COLC in front of the retina.
4. Introduce the stenopaeic slit and rotate it to find the position that gives the best VA. It may be easier to have the patient rotate the slit by turning the appropriate knob on the trial frame. Note the orientation of the slit. With the slit in this position, add plus or minus spherical lenses in front of the slit (and previous best sphere lenses) to determine the most positive (or least negative) sphere that gives the optimum VA for that slit orientation.
5. Now rotate the slit through 90° and again add plus or minus spherical lenses to determine the most plus (or least minus) sphere that gives the optimum VA.
6. The two powers determined indicate the refractive correction required in their respective meridia.

For example, the patient initially reports that they achieve best vision with the slit oriented along 45°. The best sphere achieved with the stenopaeic slit oriented along 45° is +3.00 DS. The slit is then rotated through 90°, and the best sphere achieved with the stenopaeic slit oriented along 135° is −2.00 DS. Based on this information, the refractive correction for this eye will be +3.00 −5.00 × 45. If necessary, this refractive correction can then be refined subsequently using the JCC procedure.

An alternative method of using the stenopaeic slit was described by Bennett (1960). Rather than determining the principal meridian, the best spheres can be found with the slit oriented along 45°, 90° and 180°. A series of equations were provided to convert the findings into the conventional sphere, cylinder and axis format (Rosenfield & Portello 1996).

Second sphere check

Once cylinder refinement has been completed, the final step in the monocular subjective refraction is to check the sphere power a second time. The procedure is similar to the first sphere check. It is necessary to recheck the sphere power again because of changes in either the cylinder axis or power that may have been introduced during the cylinder refinement. Accordingly, the patient is fogged, typically by approximately 0.75 D to ensure accommodation is controlled adequately, and then the fog is reduced by adding minus spheres, typically in 0.25 D steps, until the maximum plus (or minimum minus) lens that gives the optimum VA is obtained.

Hyperfocal distance refraction

It might be considered that the goal at the end of the second sphere check is to leave the patient emmetropic, i.e. having their far point at optical infinity. However, while giving the patient good distance VA, this will fail to provide the patient with the largest range of clear vision possible without needing to accommodate. It is preferable to perform a

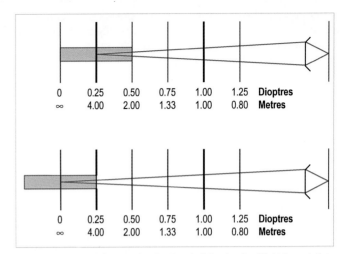

Figure 14.10 By definition, the distal end of the depth of field lies at infinity in a hyperfocal distance refraction. If the total depth of field of the eye is ±0.25 D (represented by the shaded area), then the range of clear vision without accommodating under these conditions will be 0.25 D ± 0.25, i.e. from 0 to 0.50 D, or from infinity to a point 2 m away from the eye **(upper)**. However, if the patient is made perfectly emmetropic, so that the point conjugate with the retina lies at optical infinity **(lower)**, then the range of clear vision without accommodation will be 0 D ± 0.25, i.e. from 0 to 0.25 D, or from infinity to a point 4 m away from the eye.

hyperfocal distance refraction, which places the distal end of the depth of field at optical infinity.

The depth of field is the range of object distances (expressed in dioptres) within which the VA does not deteriorate (Bennett & Rabbetts 1989). The magnitude of the depth of field varies with pupil size, VA and the form of the target, but is generally of the order of ±0.20 to 0.40 D (Campbell 1957; Atchison et al 1997; Rosenfield & Abraham-Cohen 1999).

Consider an example where the depth of field is ±0.25 D. If a hyperfocal distance refraction is performed, with the distal end of the depth of field at optical infinity, then the proximal end will lie 0.50 D away from the eye, and the patient will have clear vision (without needing to accommodate) from a point 2 m away from their eye out to optical infinity. This is illustrated in **Figure 14.10** (upper figure). If the same patient was made emmetropic, i.e. having the far point at infinity, then their range of clear vision without accommodation would be from a point 4 m away from their eye out to optical infinity (see **Fig. 14.10**, lower figure). Thus, if an object is placed 2.5 m in front of the eye, the patient with the hyperfocal refraction will be able to see this clearly without accommodating, whereas the emmetropic patient would have to accommodate to see it clearly. The hyperfocal distance refraction allows the maximum range of clear vision without accommodation.

Procedure for performing a hyperfocal distance refraction

If the acuity chart is presumed to be at optical infinity (generally considered to be a viewing distance of at least 6 m), this is simply a matter of ensuring that the goal of the second sphere check is to obtain the maximum plus (or minimum minus) spherical lens that provides the optimum VA. As shown in **Figure 14.11**, as the fog is reduced, this end point will be achieved when the distal end of the

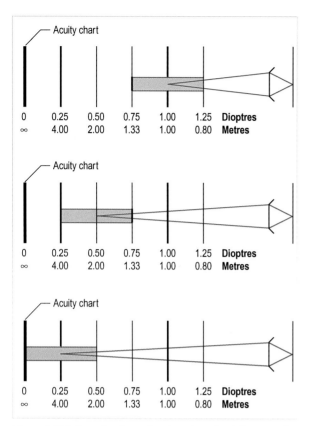

Figure 14.11 Procedure for performing a hyperfocal distance refraction in a room where the chart to be considered to be at optical infinity (viewing distance =6 m). The shaded area represents the depth of focus, which is assumed to be ±0.25 D. After the cylinder has been refined, the patient is fogged so that the depth of field lies in front of the eye **(top)**. As the degree of fog is reduced, the patient's VA will improve, but they will not reach their optimal VA as the chart does not lie within the depth of field **(middle)**. However, the distal edge of the depth of field will coincide with the chart when the concept of maximum plus (or minimum minus) sphere to give the best VA is used **(bottom)**. Adding more minus (or less plus) sphere will move the depth of field away from the eye, but does not improve distance VA since the chart remains within the depth of field.

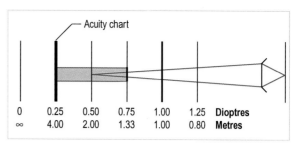

Figure 14.12 Procedure for performing a hyperfocal distance refraction in a room where the chart to be considered to be closer than optical infinity (<6 m). For example, if the chart lies 4 m away from the patient, then a maximum plus to best VA refraction will place the distal end of the depth of field at the chart (see also **Fig. 14.11**, bottom). Accordingly, an additional −0.25 DS should be added to the best sphere to achieve a hyperfocal distance refraction. The shaded area represents the depth of focus, which is assumed to be ±0.25 D.

depth of field coincides with the acuity chart, and therefore lies at optical infinity.

However, if the acuity chart is positioned at a closer distance, then the maximum plus sphere that provides optimum VA will not represent a hyperfocal condition. If the chart is positioned 4 m away from the patient, then the best sphere will place the distal end of the depth of field at 4 m (0.25 D), as shown in **Figure 14.12**. Accordingly, an additional −0.25 DS must be added to this finding to produce a hyperfocal distance refraction. For example, when working in a 4 m room, the lenses that provide maximum plus for best VA are: +3.00 −1.00 × 90. Therefore, +2.75 −1.00 × 90 would provide a hyperfocal distance refraction, thereby giving the patient optimal distance VA and the maximum linear range of clear vision without accommodation.

Check tests

After the second sphere check has been completed, it is useful to perform a 'check test' to verify that the patient has not been overcorrected. This is especially important for myopic patients, where the addition of extra minus lens power will stimulate an accommodative response. This accommodation can cause the letters to appear smaller and darker, which the patient may confuse as being clearer (due to the increased contrast). The practitioner must take care to ensure that extra minus sphere power actually improves VA (i.e. the patient is either able to read more letters correctly, or alternatively can read them more easily), rather than just make the letters look darker.

Three check tests will be described; normally only one or at most two would be performed on a given eye. The three tests are the duochrome, +0.50 and +1.00 check tests.

Duochrome test (or bichrome test)

The clinical duochrome (or bichrome) test utilizes the chromatic aberration of the human eye (Bedford & Wyszecki 1957; Charman & Jennings 1976) to determine the presence of spherical ametropia. For an emmetropic eye, light having a wavelength around 570 nm will be focused accurately on the retina, while wavelengths shorter and longer than 570 nm will be focused in front of and behind the retina, respectively (Bennett & Rabbetts 1989). The British Standard on duochrome filters (BS 3668: 1963) recommends a green filter having a peak luminosity of approximately 535 nm and a red filter of approximately 620 nm. These wavelengths provide red and green foci that are located approximately 0.25 D on either side of the retina (Bennett 1963). Accordingly, an emmetropic subject viewing a distant duochrome chart should observe objects on the red and green backgrounds equally clearly. However, uncorrected myopic observers will indicate increased contrast and clarity for the targets on the red background, while uncorrected hyperopes may indicate a preference for the targets on the green background, depending on their state of accommodation.

The duochrome test should be carried out under reduced illumination to avoid saturating the coloured targets. However, it is not necessary to conduct the test in an otherwise completely dark room (Rosenfield et al 1995). It is preferable to have the same targets on the red and green backgrounds; otherwise, the patient may express a preference for one side which may relate to the appearance and/or clarity of one particular optotype versus another. If the patient indicates that the target on the red background is clearer, additional minus spheres are added until the targets on the two sides become equally clear and dark. Conversely, if the patient states that the target on the green background is clearer, additional plus sphere should be added until the position of equality is achieved.

There are some patients on whom this test does not appear to work. Irrespective of the lenses before the eye, they continue to indicate that the targets on one side remain clearer or darker (e.g. on the red background). It is not apparent why this should be the case. Furthermore, the duochrome test should only be used as a check in confirming the spherical power. Even if the test indicates that a patient requires additional lens power (e.g. an additional −0.50 DS) to achieve equality, the determination of the final result should still be the maximum plus (or minimum minus lens) that provides the optimum VA.

+0.50 check test

The principle underlying this test is that the addition of a +0.50 DS should make the patient 0.50 D myopic if the patient is fully corrected after the second sphere check. This should produce a significant and easily noticeable decrease in target clarity. Accordingly, after the second sphere check has been completed, an additional +0.50 DS is introduced while the patient views the lowest line of letters that can be clearly seen at this stage of the examination. Following the addition of the +0.50 DS, the patient should have no hesitation in reporting that their vision has got worse. In the event that the patient either reports no difference or even a slight improvement in their vision following the introduction of the +0.50 DS, or is unsure about any change in target clarity after +0.50 DS is introduced, this indicates that the patient has been overminused. Accordingly, the patient should be refogged and the sphere power rechecked.

+1.00 check test

This is similar in principle to the +0.50 test described above, in that the addition of a +1.00 DS should make the patient 1.00 D myopic if they were fully corrected after the second sphere check. Once the second sphere check has been completed, an additional +1.00 DS is introduced and the VA re-measured. As noted in **Table 14.2**, the expected VA should now be around 6/18 (20/60) ± 1 line. If the acuity through +1.00 DS is markedly different, particularly if it is better than expected, then the patient has probably been overminused. The eye should be refogged and the sphere power rechecked.

Binocular balancing (also referred to as spherical equalization)

Once the monocular subjective refraction has been completed on each eye, the final stage of the distance subjective examination is to perform binocular balancing. The aim of this procedure is to ensure that when viewing a near target through the determined prescription, the accommodative stimulus is equal in each eye. Up to this point, the subjective examination has been performed monocularly. However, the ultimate goal is to provide a refractive correction which can be worn comfortably under binocular-associated viewing conditions. Since both eye position and the accommodative response can change when switching between monocular and binocular viewing in some patients, it is

important that the refractive state of the two eyes be determined during closed-loop binocular viewing.

It should also be noted that having a balanced prescription does not mean the patient is corrected appropriately. For example, if both eyes are left with 0.50 D of hyperopia, this is still a balanced prescription, since the accommodative stimulus will be equal when viewing a near object positioned in the patient's midline. There are five principle methods used in binocular balancing, namely:

1. successive alternate occlusion
2. vertical prism dissociation
3. Humphriss method
4. Polaroid/vectograph
5. Septum/Turville's infinity balance (TIB)

Successive alternate occlusion

In this technique, an equal amount of dioptric fog is introduced before each eye, and the effect of that fog on the patient's VA is compared between the two eyes. It is important to note that what is being compared here is the effect of the fogging lenses. However, the goal of binocular balancing is not to provide equal VA in the two eyes. Indeed, if a patient had best corrected VA in their right and left eyes of 6/6 (20/20) and 6/12 (20/40), respectively, then the only way to provide balanced acuities would be to reduce the resolution of the right eye to 6/12 (20/40). Obviously, this would not be to the advantage of the patient!

When performing successive alternate occlusion, each eye is fogged by an equal amount (typically +0.75 or +1.00 D) and the patient is directed to view a line of letters which can be resolved by both eyes through the fogging lenses (usually around 6/15 (20/50)). A paddle occluder is used to cover first one eye and then the other, and the patient is asked to report whether the image seen by one eye is clearer, or if they appear equally blurred. The patient should be reassured that both images are blurry, and this is not their final prescription. Communication can be facilitated by the use of numbers, so that the practitioner will describe the image seen by the right eye as image number 1, and that viewed by the left eye as image number 2. If the patient indicates that one eye is clearer, add +0.25 DS to that eye and repeat the procedure until the patient reports that both eyes are equally blurred. If the patient states immediately that both eyes appear equally blurred, add an additional +0.25 DS to one eye, whereupon the patient should indicate that this eye is now worse than the fellow eye. This will verify that the test is being performed correctly, and that the patient understands what is being asked. Once the eyes are equally fogged, add minus spheres *binocularly* in −0.25 DS steps until the maximum plus sphere which gives the optimum VA is achieved. Finally, a binocular check test, similar to those described following the monocular second sphere check, can be performed to verify that the patient has not been given excessive minus sphere power (or insufficient plus sphere power).

Unfortunately, the patient is always dissociated during this procedure. The goal of binocular balancing is to check the spherical component of the refractive correction under binocular viewing conditions. However, with this particular technique the patient always has one eye occluded. Accordingly, it is unlikely to provide any additional information beyond that already found in the monocular subjective examination.

Vertical prism dissociation

This procedure is very similar to the successive alternate occlusion technique described above. Again, equal amounts of fog are introduced before each eye, and the patient is asked to indicate whether the image seen by one eye is clearer than the other, or if they appear equally blurred. Rather than using an occluder to isolate the two images, the patient is dissociated by the introduction of vertical prism. Most commonly, 4Δ base-up is placed before one eye, and 4Δ base-down before the fellow eye. When viewing through the prisms (and the fogging lenses), the patient should experience vertical diplopia, and they are asked to indicate whether the top or bottom image is clearer. Additional plus spheres are added to the eye seeing the clearer image, until both eyes are fogged equally. Finally, once equal blur has been achieved, minus spheres are added binocularly in −0.25 D steps until the maximum plus sphere which gives the optimum VA is reached. Binocular sphere check tests are again performed to verify the refractive correction.

The criticism of the successive alternate occlusion procedure, namely that it only tests the patient under dissociated viewing conditions, is equally valid here. Indeed, Borish and Benjamin (2006) observed that equalization of blur using either of these two techniques often does not result in equalization of accommodation, i.e. it fails to provide a balanced prescription.

Humphriss method

Humphriss (Humphriss & Woodruff 1962; Humphriss 1988) noted that if one eye is fogged by +0.75 or +1.00 DS, then foveal vision will be suspended in that eye. However, the parafoveal and outer areas of the retina are unaffected, thereby providing a binocular lock for fusion. Millodot (1972) suggested that an area of approximately 2–3° in diameter would be affected by 0.75 D of fog. Humphriss claimed that this central inhibition will have little or no effect on binocular vision, and he described this as a psychological septum.

Humphriss (1988) described a procedure which he specifically stated was not a balancing technique, but rather 'measures the point at which a patient begins to accommodate for each eye separately, under conditions of normal binocular vision'. Since this procedure allows the two eyes to be placed under similar accommodative states, i.e. having equal accommodative stimuli for each eye, this will provide a balanced prescription. Humphriss described the technique using letter targets, although it may also be carried out with the duochrome test, as described below.

While viewing a letter target (around 6/12 or 20/40), one eye is fogged by +0.75 or +1.00 D. A +0.25 DS is introduced over the monocular findings before the unfogged eye for a full second, and then replaced by a −0.25 DS. The patient is asked which of the two lenses appears clearer. If the patient is not accommodating, then they should immediately respond that the target is clearer with the minus lens. If the patient gives one of three responses, either that (1) the plus lens is clearer, (2) that there is no difference between the two lenses or (3) that the minus lens is clearer, but it makes the letters smaller or blacker, then it can be assumed that the patient is accommodating. With any of these three answers, additional plus sphere should be added and the test repeated until the patient has no hesitation in responding that the −0.25 DS is preferred.

However, the Humphriss balancing procedure may be performed more easily when using the duochrome chart. This duochrome procedure (with monocular fog) produces significantly less disruption to binocular vision than either the successive alternate occlusion or vertical prism dissociation techniques. One eye is fogged by either +0.75 or +1.00 D and the patient directed to view a duochrome chart. Using this chart, an end point is reached on the unfogged eye (such as initially clearer on red but requires −0.25 DS to achieve equality). The fog is then transferred to the fellow eye and the same end point should be sought in the second unfogged eye. In order to balance the two eyes, it is immaterial whether the initial response to the duochrome is red, green or equal, provided it is the same for both eyes, and the same lens power is required to achieve reversal. For example, if the right eye is left with the green target clearer and an additional +0.50 DS being required to produce reversal, then the same end point should be obtained in the left eye to produce a balanced prescription. An example of a Humphriss balancing procedure is shown in **Table 14.4**.

A significant advantage of the Humphriss procedure is that the patient is not being asked to compare the clarity of the images seen by the two eyes. Rather, the patient is viewing the duochrome chart and each eye is tested separately (with the non-tested eye being fogged). This is the method of choice when balancing a patient who has a significant difference in acuity between the two eyes. However,

Table 14.4 Example of a Humphriss balancing procedure

	OD	OS
	+1.50 (Red)	FOGGED
	+1.25 (Red)	FOGGED
	+1.00 (Equal)	FOGGED
	+0.75 (Green)	FOGGED
	+0.50 (Green)	FOGGED
	FOGGED	+3.00 (Green)
	FOGGED	+3.25 (Green)
	FOGGED	+3.50 (Equal)
	FOGGED	+3.75 (Red)
	FOGGED	+4.00 (Red)
Then for each eye:	**OD**	**OS**
(i) Equal response	+1.00	+3.50
(ii) First/last red*	+1.25	+3.75
(iii) First/last green*	+0.75	+3.25
(iv) Second/second last red*	+1.50	+4.00
(v) Second/second last green*	+0.50	+3.00

*First red indicates the first red response after equal. Last red indicates the last red response before obtaining an equal response. Second red indicates the second red response after obtaining an equal response. Second last red indicates the second last red response before obtaining an equal response. Thus, any similar combination will give a balanced prescription, e.g. both eyes first red, both eyes second last green, both eyes neutral, etc.
OD = right eye; OS = left eye.

care must be taken to ensure that sufficient fog is introduced to transfer attention to the unfogged eye when working on the eye with poorer acuity. On some occasions, more than 1.00 D of fog may be required to ensure that the responses relate to the non-fogged eye.

Once the two eyes are balanced, fog both eyes by +1.00 DS and slowly reduce the fog binocularly in −0.25 D steps until the patient has the maximum plus (or minimum minus) sphere which provides the optimum VA.

Polaroid/vectograph

This technique uses crossed polaroid filters to produce partial dissociation of the two eyes (Rosenberg & Sherman 1965; Grolman 1966). The vectograph projector slide includes both polarized and non-polarized letters and targets (**Fig. 14.13**). When viewed through cross-polarized filters, some parts of the target are seen by either the right or left eye only. The non-polarized stimuli are seen by both eyes, providing a fusion lock. This test can be used for binocular balancing by introducing an equal amount of fog before each eye, and asking the patient to compare the clarity of the monocularly viewed letters. If the patient indicates that the image seen by one eye is clearer (or more precisely is less blurred), then additional plus spheres are added to that eye until both eyes are fogged equally. As the letters used for binocular balancing generally range between 6/12 (20/40) and 6/7.5 (20/25), only 0.50 D of fog should be introduced, otherwise the patient will not be able to resolve the targets.

This technique has the advantage of providing minimal disruption of binocular vision. The non-polarized targets require an accurate fusional vergence response in order to maintain binocular single vision. A frequent criticism of this procedure is that the chart appears to have very low contrast when viewed by the practitioner without the cross-polarized filters. However, Borish and Benjamin (2006) pointed out that polarization reduces the amount of light reflected from the letters by about 50%. When viewed through a filter, the light reflected from the letters is blocked, but 50% of the light from the background is transmitted. Thus, the letters appear as black letters on a grey-white background. If the light is polarized in the same direction as the analyser, then light reflected from both the letters and background will be transmitted equally, resulting in an even light field. The chart contrast is approximately 75% when the letters are viewed through the filter. Accordingly, the patient's view of the chart through the filters has much higher contrast than the practitioner's viewpoint.

Additionally, some charts are available with polarized duochrome tests. When viewed through the cross-polarized filters, only one target on each coloured background will be visible to the right and left eyes, respectively, as illustrated in **Figure 14.14**. The goal is to achieve equivalent responses from the two eyes. The actual response is immaterial as far as the balancing procedure is concerned, as long as it is the same in both eyes. Thus, a patient could respond that the targets on the red and green backgrounds appear equally clear, or they could indicate that the target on the green background is initially clearer but with the addition of a +0.25 DS the two targets now appear equal. The goal is to obtain the same end point in both eyes. An advantage of the polarized duochrome technique is that the use of fogging lenses is not required, and therefore there is minimal disruption to the habitual accommodative and vergence responses.

Septum techniques/Turville's infinity balance

This procedure uses an occluder or septum to separate the visual fields of the two eyes (Morgan 1960). Accordingly, two areas of the acuity chart are only visible to the right and left eyes, respectively, while the remainder of the chart can be seen by both eyes (**Fig. 14.15**). The binocular areas serve to maintain binocular single vision. As with the Polaroid procedure with letters described above, an equal amount of fog is introduced before each eye, and the patient is asked to compare the clarity of letters seen by either the right or left eye. If the patient indicates that the image seen by one eye is clearer (or more precisely is less blurred), then additional plus spheres are added to that eye until both eyes are fogged equally.

As an alternative to comparing the appearance of letters under fog, this test can also be performed using a duochrome chart which has two targets on both the red and green backgrounds. Correct placement of the septum will ensure that only one target on each coloured background will be visible to the right and left eyes, respectively. The procedure is then carried out in the same way as the polarized duochrome target (see above), with the goal being to obtain equivalent duochrome responses from the two eyes.

The septum is rarely used with charts that are viewed directly, since the septum must be placed approximately midway between the patient and the chart. Once it is positioned correctly in the middle of the examination room, it is almost inevitable that once the room lights are turned off, the practitioner will then walk into the septum! However, this technique is more convenient when used with an indirect chart, i.e. one that is viewed via a plane mirror, since the septum can simply be hung on the mirror.

Comparison of binocular balancing procedures

It should be emphasized that the goal of binocular balancing is to provide a refractive correction which can be worn comfortably under binocular-associated viewing conditions. Since most of the subjective procedure is performed monocularly, this technique is added to compensate for any differences in either accommodation or vergence that may occur when the patient switches to binocular observation. Ideally, there should be minimal disruption to binocularity during the procedure, so that the patient can maintain their habitual accommodative and vergence responses.

It was noted earlier that the two eyes are entirely dissociated (i.e. presented with non-fusible targets) during both the successive alternate occlusion and vertical prism dissociation techniques. Suspension of binocular vision will stimulate dissipation of fusional vergence, which could also lead to a change in the accommodation response. One would therefore predict little change between the findings obtained by these two procedures, and the refractive state measured under monocular viewing. That is generally the case, and Michaels (1985) noted that differences seldom exceed 0.25 to 0.50 D.

The Humphriss, Polaroid and septum (TIB) procedures all contain fusible stimuli, and therefore would be predicted to maintain a higher level of binocularity. In particular, the use of either the Polaroid or TIB procedures with a duochrome target should minimize the degradation of binocular vision, since no fogging lenses are required. However, in a

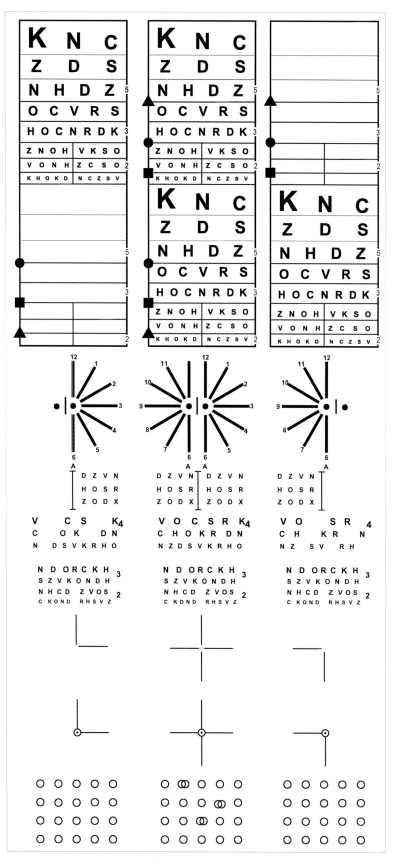

Figure 14.13 Diagram depicting Grolman's vectographic slide. The central image represents the actual slide, whereas the images to each side indicate the portions seen by each eye. The slide is constructed so that when one eye is viewing its chart, some symbols and borders are visible to the eye not being tested to ensure binocular fusion. (Reproduced with permission from Borish & Benjamin 2006.)

comparison of binocular balancing techniques in 25 patients having normal binocular vision, West and Somers (1984) reported no significant difference between the procedures, which included Polaroid vectograph and vertical prism dissociation. These authors noted that while all methods may work satisfactorily for normal patients, this conclusion may not be valid in patients with reduced binocularity. Indeed, Portello et al (2000) observed that when esophoria was

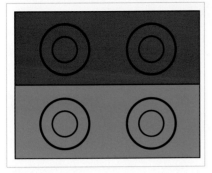

Figure 14.14 Example of a polarized duochrome. When viewed through cross-polarized filters, the left-hand circles on the red and green backgrounds, respectively, are seen by only one eye, while the right-hand circles on the two coloured backgrounds are only seen by the fellow eye.

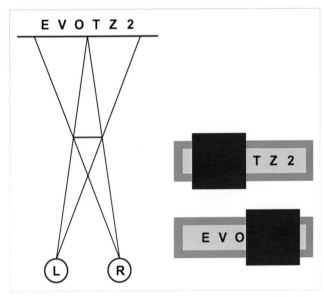

Figure 14.15 A Turville infinity balance (TIB). A septum is introduced halfway between the patient and the chart, so that the right eye can see only the right-hand side of the chart, while the left eye can only see the left side of the chart. The top and bottom right-hand figures illustrate what is seen by the right and left eyes, respectively. It is useful to allow a binocular fusion lock by having some letters or details (e.g. the chart border) that can be viewed by both eyes.

induced by the introduction of base-in prism, the Humphriss procedure measured approximately 0.25 D less myopia, when compared with either vertical prism dissociation or successive alternate occlusion. They attributed this difference to the reduction in fusional vergence required to compensate for the heterophoria. Accordingly, when performing binocular balancing on patients with heterophoria, techniques should be used which maintain ocular alignment by assessing ametropia under associated viewing conditions.

Binocular subjective refraction

It is possible to do the entire subjective examination binocularly, thereby eliminating the need for binocular balancing. This procedure may be carried out using a modification of the Humphriss procedure, i.e. with the non-tested eye being

fogged rather than occluded, or using either a septum or Polaroid technique to create monocular targets during closed-loop binocular viewing.

In addition to a reduction in the duration of the examination, this technique will have significant benefit for patients whose accommodative state differs between monocular and binocular viewing. Amos (1990, 1991) described three clinical indications for binocular refraction, namely refractive, VA and ocular motility considerations. Bennett and Rabbetts (1989) stated that for patients with good binocular vision, binocular refraction is advantageous because the fixed convergence required to view the test chart helps to stabilize the accommodative response. Additionally, Amos (1991) noted that binocular viewing encourages greater relaxation of accommodation in patients with hyperopic anisometropia.

Binocular refraction may also be of benefit in patients with nystagmus (whose magnitude is generally smaller during binocular viewing) and patients with significant vertical and cyclo-deviations. In these patients, the orientation of the correcting cylinder axis may change during binocular fixation, when compared with the monocular findings.

Summary

Even with the expanding scope of practice of optometry, subjective refraction remains a key element of the eye examination. Indeed, a recent survey of optometrists in a wide range of practice environments within the United States revealed that the correction of refractive error and binocular vision anomalies still comprise by far the largest part of contemporary clinical practice. More than 50% of the diagnoses recorded were refractive in nature (Soroka et al 2006). With objective refraction becoming increasingly automated, one could argue that there is an even greater need for a high-quality subjective examination, to ensure that a refractive correction has been achieved which leaves the patient comfortable and satisfies their visual requirements.

Several studies have examined the repeatability of subjective refraction, and most have concluded that a change in refractive error of ±0.50 D should be adopted as the minimum significant shift in refractive status (Kratz & Flom 1977; Rosenfield & Chiu 1995; Bullimore et al 1998). While Bullimore et al (1998) reported that automated refraction was more repeatable than subjective refraction, in an additional study (Bullimore et al 1996) they compared patients' acceptance of spectacle prescriptions determined by either autorefractor or subjective refraction. Two pairs of spectacles were made up with each refractive correction, and the patients (n=195) wore the two prescriptions in a double-masked, cross-over design, with each pair being worn for at least 3 weeks. When asked which pair they would prefer to keep, 100 patients (51%) preferred those determined by subjective refraction, 56 (29%) preferred the autorefractor finding, and the remainder (39 patients, 20%) considered both pairs equally acceptable. The authors concluded that overall patient acceptance and satisfaction was better for prescriptions determined by subjective refraction.

The subjective refraction also allows the practitioner to engage in a dialogue with the patient. This part of the examination, along with the case history (see Ch. 26), provides an opportunity for patients to express their opinions concerning the quality of their visual performance. As more clinical testing becomes automated and specialized, patients can sometimes feel that they are simply progressing from one machine to another, and lack confidence that the final prescription will satisfy their requirements. By allowing patients to participate in the subjective process, the optometrist has an opportunity to ensure that the patients' visual needs are being met, and that the final result will be satisfactory in providing comfortable vision.

Acknowledgement

I would like to thank Elizabeth Wickware for her comments on an earlier version of this manuscript and Sylvia Chun for preparing many of the figures in this chapter.

References

Amos J F 1990 Binocular refraction: when is it clinically advantageous? Clinical Eye and Vision Care 2:79–81

Amos J F 1991 Binocular subjective refraction. In: Eskridge J B, Amos J F, Bartlett J D (eds) Clinical procedures in optometry. Lippincott, Philadelphia, pp 189–193

Atchison D A, Charman W N, Woods R L 1997 Subjective depth-of-focus of the eye. Optometry and Vision Science 74:511–520

Bannon R E, Walsh R 1945 On astigmatism. Part III – Subjective tests. American Journal of Optometry and Archives of American Academy of Optometry 22:210–218

Bedford R E, Wyszecki G 1957 Axial chromatic aberration of the human eye. Journal of the Optical Society of America 47:564–565

Bennett A G 1960 Refraction by automation? Optician 139:5–9

Bennett A G 1963 The theory of bichromatic tests. Optician 146:291–296

Bennett A G, Rabbetts R B 1989 Clinical visual optics, 2nd edn. Butterworths, London

Biessels W J 1967 The cross-cylinder simultan test. Journal of the American Optometric Association 38:473–476

Borish I M, Benjamin W J 2006 Monocular and binocular subjective refraction. In: Benjamin W J (ed.) Borish's clinical refraction, 2nd edn. Butterworth-Heinemann, St Louis, pp 790–872

British Standard 3668: 1963 Red and green filters used in ophthalmic dichromatic and dissociation tests. British Standards Institute, London, pp 4–6

Bullimore M A, Adams C W, Fusaro R E et al 1996 Patient acceptance of auto-refractor and clinician prescriptions: a randomized clinical trial. Visual Science and its Applications. Technical Digest Series, vol 1. Optical Society of America, Washington DC, pp 194–197

Bullimore M A, Fusaro R E, Adams C W 1998 The repeatability of automated and clinician refraction. Optometry and Vision Science 75:617–622

Campbell F W 1957 The depth of field of the human eye. Optica Acta 4:157–164

Charman W N, Jennings J A M 1976 Objective measurements of the longitudinal chromatic aberration of the human eye. Vision Research 16:999–1005

Del Priore L V, Guyton D L 1986 The Jackson cross cylinder. A reappraisal. Ophthalmology 93:1461–1465

Duke-Elder S, Abrams D 1970 System of ophthalmology, vol. V. Ophthalmic Optics and Refraction. CV Mosby, St Louis, pp 439–443

Green J 1868 On a new system of tests for the detection and measurement of astigmatism, with an analysis of sixty-four cases of refractive anomalies observed by the aid of this method. Transactions of the American Ophthalmological Society 1:131–144

Green J 1878 On some improvements in instruments and appliances for diagnosis. Transactions of the American Ophthalmological Society 2:467–488

Grolman B E 1966 Binocular refraction – a new system. New England Journal of Optometry 17:118–130

Humphriss D 1988 Binocular refraction. In: Edwards K, Llewellyn R (eds) Optometry. Butterworths, London, pp 140–149

Humphriss D, Woodruff E W 1962 Refraction by immediate contrast. British Journal of Physiological Optics 19:15–20

Jackson E 1887 Trial set of small lenses and a modified trial-frame. Transactions of the American Ophthalmological Society 4:595–598

Jackson E 1907 The astigmic lens (cross cylinder) to determine the amount and principal meridians of astigmia. Ophthalmic Record 16:378–383

Jalie M 1980 The principles of ophthalmic lenses, 3rd edn. Association of Dispensing Opticians, London, pp 287–294

Kratz L D, Flom M C 1977 The Humphrey Vision Analyzer: reliability and validity of refractive-error measures. American Journal of Optometry and Physiological Optics 54:653–659

LeVine M L 1990 Monocular simultaneous refraction. Journal of the American Optometric Association 61:745–748

Loo A, Jacobs R J 1994 Jackson crossed cylinder axis test. Paper presented at Academy Europe '94, Amsterdam, The Netherlands. American Academy of Optometry, pp 208

Maddox E E 1921 Some new tests for astigmatism. American Journal of Ophthalmology 4:571–572

Matsuura T T 1961 The Matsuura AutoCross. Optometric Weekly 52:2153–2156

Michaels D D 1985 Visual optics and refraction: a clinical approach, 3rd edn. CV Mosby, St Louis

Millodot M 1972 Variation of visual acuity in the central region of the retina. British Journal of Physiological Optics 27:24–28

Morgan M W 1960 The Turville infinity binocular balance test. Journal of the American Optometric Association 31:447–450

Mutti D O, Zadnik K 1997 Refractive error. In: Zadnik K (ed.) The ocular examination. WB Saunders, Philadelphia, pp 51–86

O'Leary D 1988 Subjective refraction. In: Edwards K, Llewellyn R (eds) Optometry. Butterworths, London, pp 111–139

Ong J, Shanks F, McConnell W 1974 Validity of four current subjective tests of astigmatism. American Journal of Optometry and Physiological Optics 51:587–592

Polasky M 1991 Monocular subjective refraction. In: Eskridge J B, Amos J F, Bartlett J D (eds) Clinical procedures in optometry. Lippincott, Philadelphia, pp 174–193

Portello J K, George S, Rosenfield M et al 2000 Heterophoria and binocular balancing. Optometry and Vision Science (supplement) 77:186

Portello J K, Hong S E, Rosenfield M 2001 Accommodation to astigmatic stimuli. Optometry and Vision Science (supplement) 78:91

Rappon J M, Rosenfield M 1999 A new technique for the subjective assessment of astigmatism. Optometry and Vision Science (supplement) 76:184

Raubitschek E 1952 The Raubitschek arrow test for astigmatism. American Journal of Ophthalmology 35:1334–1339

Rosenberg S, Sherman A 1965 Vectographic project-o-chart slides. Journal of the American Optometric Association 39:1002–1006

Rosenfield M 1997 Accommodation. In: Zadnik K (ed.) The ocular examination. Measurement and findings. Saunders, Philadelphia, pp 87–121

Rosenfield M 2006 Refractive status of the eye. In: Benjamin W J (ed.) Borish's clinical refraction, 2nd edn. Butterworth-Heinemann, St Louis, pp 3–34

Rosenfield M, Abraham-Cohen J A 1999 Blur sensitivity in myopes. Optometry and Vision Science 76:303–307

Rosenfield M, Chiu N N 1995 Repeatability of subjective and objective refraction. Optometry and Vision Science 72:577–579

Rosenfield M, Portello J K 1996 Multi-meridional keratometry. Ophthalmic and Physiological Optics 16:83–85

Rosenfield M, Aggarwala K R, Raul C et al 1995 Do changes in pupil size and ambient illumination affect the duochrome test? Journal of the American Optometric Association 66:87–90

Shapiro A E (ed.) 1984 The optical papers of Isaac Newton, vol. 1. The Optical Lectures 1670–1672, Cambridge University Press, Cambridge, pp 212–215

Soroka M, Krumholz D, Bennett A, National Board of Examiners Domain Task Force 2006 The practice of optometry: National Board of Examiners in Optometry survey of optometric patients. Optometry 77:427–437

Stoner E D, Perkins P, Ferguson R 2005 Optical formulas tutorial, 2nd edn. Elsevier, St Louis

Verhoeff F H 1923 The 'V' test for astigmatism, and astigmatic charts in general. American Journal of Ophthalmology 6:908–910

West D, Somers W W 1984 Binocular balance validity: a comparison of five common subjective techniques. Ophthalmic and Physiological Optics 4:155–159

Williamson-Noble F A 1943 A possible fallacy in the use of the cross-cylinder. British Journal of Ophthalmology 27:1–12

CHAPTER 15

Clinical assessment of accommodation

Mark Rosenfield

Introduction

Accommodation refers to a temporary change in the refractive power of the crystalline lens resulting from contraction of the ciliary muscle, thereby altering the location of the point in space optically conjugate with the retina (Rosenfield 1997). This change in the refractive power enables the eye to change focus from a distant target to a closer object of regard. Accommodation is quantified in dioptres (D), and in the case of an emmetropic patient, the accommodative stimulus when viewing a near object is simply the reciprocal of the target distance in metres. Therefore, when viewing an object at a distance of 25 cm, the accommodative stimulus is $1/0.25 = 4.0$ D.

Clinically, the two primary tests of accommodation are the amplitude of accommodation, which is an assessment of the patient's maximum accommodative ability, and measurement of the accommodative response for a specific stimulus demand. Patients with reduced accommodative ability (most commonly due to presbyopia) will require a corrective lens to enable them to see clearly at near, and this chapter will discuss the determination of the appropriate lens power for this condition. Other clinical tests examine the interaction of the accommodation and vergence systems, including assessment of relative accommodation and accommodative facility, as well as quantifying the cross-link ratios between these two functions, i.e. accommodative convergence to accommodation (AC/A) and convergent accommodation to convergence (CA/C). Assessment of the AC/A ratio is discussed in Chapter 16 while measurement of the CA/C ratio is not a standard clinical procedure at the present time. However, techniques for measurement of the latter ratio have been described previously (Wick & Currie 1991; Bruce et al 1995; Rosenfield et al 1995).

Amplitude of accommodation

Definitions

- The *far point* of accommodation is the point conjugate with the retina when accommodation is fully relaxed.
- The *near point* of accommodation is the point conjugate with the retina when accommodation is fully exerted.
- The *amplitude* of accommodation is the dioptric distance between the far point and the near point of accommodation.

Accordingly, the amplitude may be calculated as the dioptric value of the far point minus the near point. If the far point of accommodation is located at optical infinity, i.e. 0 D, then the amplitude of accommodation will simply be equal to the near point of accommodation, or the reciprocal of the closest distance (in metres) at which distinct vision can be obtained. When measuring this parameter clinically, it is simplest to measure the near point after the subject's refractive error has been fully corrected, thereby placing the far point at or close to 0 D.

There are three main procedures for measuring the amplitude of accommodation in the clinical setting, namely: (1) the push-up (and/or push-down) technique; (2) the minus lens technique and (3) using dynamic retinoscopy or other objective or subjective optometers.

Push-up technique

This procedure seeks to locate the near point of accommodation, i.e. the closest distance at which the target still appears in focus. In practice, such an end point is difficult to identity consistently. Accordingly, rather than attempt to determine this last point of clear vision, it is conventional to move the target towards the patient until they observe the first, slight, sustained blur. While the target location corresponding with this first blur will be marginally closer to the patient than the true near point, the difference is extremely small and, perhaps more importantly, this end point can be demonstrated consistently in most patients.

A diagrammatic representation of this procedure is shown in **Figure 15.1**. The accommodative stimulus is increased steadily in a ramp-like fashion, and in a normal, pre-presbyopic individual, the subject will make an appropriate increase in the accommodative response. It should be noted from **Figure 15.1** that with the exception of a single stimulus level, the accommodative response is never actually equal to the stimulus; for low dioptric (i.e. distant) targets the response generally exceeds the stimulus (usually referred to as a lead of accommodation) while for higher dioptric (i.e. near) objects of regard the response is typically less than the stimulus (lag of accommodation). The depth of focus of the eye allows the subject to maintain a clear image of the object despite these errors in accommodation.

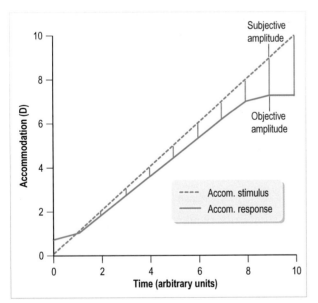

Figure 15.1 Diagrammatic illustration of the push-up amplitude of accommodation procedure. The solid line indicates the accommodative response to the steadily increasing accommodative stimulus (*broken line*) plotted with respect to time. The end point (i.e. the report of the first, slight, sustained blur) of this test will occur when the separation between the accommodative stimulus and response (shown by the vertical lines) exceeds one-half of the depth of focus of the eye. The objective amplitude represents the maximum, objectively measured accommodative response (not usually measured during this procedure) while the subjective amplitude is the accommodative stimulus that produces this maximum response.

Examination of **Figure 15.1** indicates that the subject will report the first slight blur when the difference between the accommodative stimulus and response exceeds one half of the depth of focus of the eye, typically around 0.4 D (Campbell 1957; Atchison et al 1997; Wang & Ciuffreda 2006). It will also be apparent from this figure that different measurements of the amplitude will be recorded depending upon whether the accommodative stimulus or the actual accommodative response is being measured.

Clinical procedure

The patient observes a finely detailed test object (see later discussion on optimum target size) which is advanced toward the eye until the detail 'just begins to blur and remains blurred', i.e. the first slight, sustained blur. The patient should always be encouraged to try to clear the target when they first report blur, since the aim is to achieve the maximum accommodative response. The reciprocal of the distance from the target at this position of first slight, sustained blur to the spectacle plane (in metres) represents the near point of accommodation (in dioptres). The push-up amplitude is typically measured both monocularly and binocularly. The latter reflects the maximum accommodation possible when converging accurately on a near target.

Push-down amplitude of accommodation

In the push-down procedure, the target is advanced a little beyond this point of the first sustained blur (i.e. closer than the near point), and then moved away from the patient until the target 'just becomes absolutely clear'. This procedure attempts to obtain a more accurate determination of the near point, i.e. the closest distance at which the target remains clear, rather than the first slight blur. In a comparison of amplitudes determined using both the push-up and push-down techniques, Fitch (1971) reported higher amplitudes of accommodation using the push-up procedure, which were statistically significant in subjects over 40 years of age. More recently, Woehrle et al (1997) observed no significant difference between findings obtained using the push-up and push-down procedures in 25 subjects between 10 and 40 years of age. While the mean difference between the two techniques was only 0.05 D, the standard deviation of the differences was 1.86 D with a range from +3.63 D to −3.36 D. It should also be noted that the end point used by Woehrle et al required the subject to identify an isolated Snellen letter correctly. This could have been satisfied while the target was still somewhat blurry, and therefore may not match the push-up end point of minimal blur.

A useful compromise might be to take the mean of the push-up and push-down findings (Coates 1955). This averaged measurement may provide a more accurate assessment of the near point of accommodation since it will encompass the slight overestimate of the near point during the push-up procedure and the possible small underestimate occurring with the push-down technique.

An additional factor to consider is whether the subject or operator moves the target. Fitch (1971) demonstrated that when the subject was allowed to grasp the target, this resulted in a significant increase in the amplitude of accommodation in all subjects under 50 years of age. It would seem likely that this resulted from the effect of enhanced cues to proximally induced accommodation (Rosenfield & Gilmartin 1990).

Minus lens technique

In this procedure, the target remains at a fixed position (typically 40 cm; corresponding to a stimulus of 2.50 D), and minus lenses are introduced to move the location of the optical image of this target. This is illustrated in **Figure 15.2**. Lenses are typically introduced in 0.25 D steps until the patient reports the first noticeable, sustained blur that cannot be cleared by further conscious effort. The total amplitude is equal to the amount of minus lens power introduced, plus the 2.50 D required to focus initially on the target. This should be carried out for each eye individually. However, it is not performed binocularly as this would be testing positive relative accommodation (PRA), as described in a later section of this chapter.

Differences between minus lens and push-up findings

During testing with the minus lens technique, the target remains fixed and accordingly the psychological proximal stimulus to accommodation remains relatively constant. However, the target minification resulting from the minus lenses will make the target appear smaller. This change in image size will make the patient more sensitive to identifying the first noticeable blur, and therefore they are likely to report the test end point earlier. This is discussed in the later section on target size. Both the size effect and reduced proximal stimulus will account for the lower amplitude of accommodation generally observed with the minus lens procedure, when compared with the push-up technique (Wold 1967; Hokoda & Ciuffreda 1982).

Optometers

The amplitude of accommodation may also be measured using any type of optometer, i.e. an instrument that measures the actual accommodative response. Since both the push-up/push-down and minus lens techniques measure the stimulus level that corresponds with this maximum response, one would expect that any procedure that actually measures the accommodative response would demonstrate a lower amplitude when compared with the subjective findings (see **Fig. 15.1**).

Objective measurements may be particularly useful for patients who are unable to cooperate with the subjective procedure for any reason, such as an inability to report the

Table 15.1 Assessment of the amplitude of accommodation using dynamic retinoscopy

Distance of target from patient	Distance of the retinoscope from the patient when a neutral reflex is observed
40 cm (AS=2.50 D)	50 cm (AR=2.00 D)
25 cm (AS=4.00 D)	33 cm (AR=3.00 D)
20 cm (AS=5.00 D)	25 cm (AR=4.00 D)
17 cm (AS=6.00 D)	20 cm (AR=5.00 D)
14 cm (AS=7.00 D)	20 cm (AR=5.00 D)
13.5 cm (AS=8.00 D)	20 cm (AR=5.00 D)

For each target distance, the accommodative response (AR) is determined by finding the position of the point conjugate with the retina. Eventually, a point will be reached where further increases in the accommodative stimulus (AS) are not accompanied by an increase in the AR. In the example given above, the objective amplitude of accommodation (or maximum AR) is 5.00 D.

required end point. In addition, it will provide a veridical measurement of the maximum accommodative response. The most common technique used in the clinical setting to assess the objective amplitude is Cross–Nott dynamic retinoscopy (see p 235). The accommodative response is measured for a series of increasing stimulus levels until the maximum response is achieved. This maximum response corresponds to the objective amplitude. An example of a typical series of measurements is provided in **Table 15.1**. Woodhouse et al (1993) used this technique to measure the amplitude of accommodation in a group of children with Down's syndrome (see Chs 28 and 32). However, any optometer, such as an autorefractor, may be used to determine the objective amplitude, providing an adequate range of stimuli can be introduced.

Factors affecting the amplitude of accommodation

The magnitude of this parameter is affected by a number of factors, such as whether the test is performed monocularly or binocularly, gaze angle, underlying refractive error and the patient's racial characteristics. These topics were reviewed by Rosenfield (1997). Two additional factors which will be discussed here are the size of the target and the patient's age.

Effect of target size

Somers and Ford (1983) noted that when observing larger targets, the borders of the image are further apart and there is less overlap of their blur distributions. Thus, the use of larger optotypes when measuring the amplitude of accommodation may produce a delay in the patient first appreciating the presence of blur, resulting in an erroneously elevated amplitude of accommodation. This was confirmed by Rosenfield and Cohen (1995), who measured the subjective push-up amplitude of accommodation using Snellen optotypes ranging in size from 6/6 to 6/30. The mean values of amplitude of accommodation for the five target sizes are illustrated in **Figure 15.3**, and it is apparent that variations in target size do indeed produce significant changes in the subjective amplitude of accommodation.

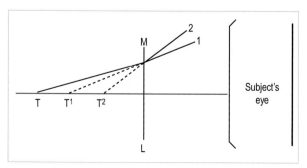

Figure 15.2 Measurement of the amplitude of accommodation using the minus lens procedure. As minus lenses (ML) of increasing power are introduced before the eye, light rays from the near target (T) are increasingly diverged to produce images of T at T^1 and T^2. The increasing proximity of these images increases the stimulus to accommodation.

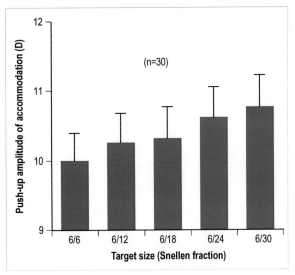

Figure 15.3 Mean push-up amplitude of accommodation recorded when viewing Snellen optotypes of varying sizes. All Snellen fractions are referenced to 40 cm. Error bars indicate 1 SEM. (Figure reproduced with permission from Rosenfield & Cohen 1995.)

Table 15.2 Amplitude of accommodation (D) as a function of age

Age (years)	Donders	Duane
10	14	11
15	12	10.25
20	10	9.5
25	8.5	8.5
30	7	7.5
35	5.5	6.5
40	4.5	5.5
45	3.5	3.5
50	2.5	
55	1.75	
60	1	1.25
65	0.5	
70	0.25	1
75	0	

Data from the classic studies of Donders (1864) and Duane (1912).

While a small target represents the most suitable stimulus for the push-up procedure, caution must be exercised when proposing an appropriate stimulus size due to the age-related recession of the near point. Since a 6/6 letter on a chart calibrated for a viewing distance of 40 cm will subtend 5 minutes of arc at 40 cm and 20 minutes of arc at 10 cm, it is apparent that the same target should not be used on patients with amplitudes of 2.5 D and 10.0 D, respectively. Berens and Fonda (1950) proposed that the amplitude of accommodation should be measured using a target which subtends an angle of no more than 5 minutes of arc at the individual's near point. For patients under 30 years of age, they recommended a letter that subtended 5 minutes of arc at a distance of 20 cm (physical height of this letter = 0.29 mm). However, it is evident that this target will subtend 10 minutes of arc when located at the near point of a patient having a 10 D amplitude of accommodation. An alternative and perhaps more practical target would be the use of a series of fine lines, perhaps in the shape of a cross, which could be photographically reduced (Berens & Fonda 1950). However, such a target might still be difficult to manufacture commercially.

Effect of age on amplitude of accommodation

The decline in the amplitude of accommodation with age has been well documented, with the classic studies of Donders (1864) and Duane (1912) being most commonly cited. Both workers reported a decline in amplitude at a rate of approximately 0.3 D per year. These findings are shown in **Table 15.2**.

Hofstetter (1944) proposed three equations to represent the minimum, mean and maximum expected amplitudes, namely:

- Minimum amplitude = 15 − 0.25 * age in years
- Mean amplitude = 18.5 − 0.3 * age in years
- Maximum amplitude = 25 − 0.4 * age in years

These equations may be more useful in the clinical setting than the classic tables, since they allow the practitioner to determine the range of normal values for a given age.

Assessment of the accommodative response

The assessment of the accommodative response to a range of stimuli is an important part of the clinical optometric examination. Measurement of the amplitude only provides information with regard to the maximum potential accommodative response, rather than the actual response to a submaximal stimulus. Patients' symptoms frequently relate to near-visual activities, and inappropriate responses, whether under- or over-accommodation relative to the plane of the object of regard are a frequent cause of asthenopia (Birnbaum 1993). Accordingly, it is essential for the clinician to determine the actual accommodative response to the specific stimulus demand for which the patient is reporting difficulty. Furthermore, in some cases a more complete examination of a range of responses may be appropriate, and this can be achieved by plotting an accommodative stimulus–response curve (Morgan 1944; Ciuffreda & Kenyon 1983). An example of such a plot is illustrated in **Figure 15.4**. Only for a single stimulus level (the so-called crossover point) are the accommodative stimulus and response equal.

While the plot illustrated in **Figure 15.4** represents an average finding, patients presenting with symptoms relating to near-visual activities may exhibit different results. For example, some patients may show a tendency to overaccommodate for near targets (Birnbaum 1993), rather than exhibiting the more typical lag of accommodation (Morgan 1944; Heath 1956; Charman 1982; Ciuffreda & Kenyon 1983). While the object of regard will remain clear as long as the accommodative error does not exceed the depth of focus of the eye, such a patient may still experience symptoms, possibly due to the effect of excessive accommodative convergence. An excessive lag or underaccommodation relative to the accommodative stimulus may also produce

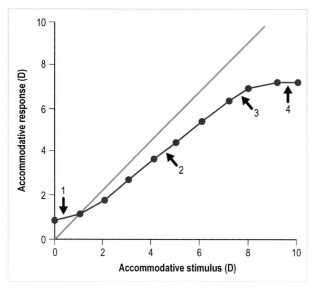

Figure 15.4 Static accommodative stimulus–response curve for a normal subject. 1 = initial non-linear region, 2 = linear region, 3 = transitional soft saturation region, 4 = hard saturation presbyopic region. The diagonal line represents the unit ratio (or 1:1) line. (Figure redrawn with permission from Ciuffreda and Kenyon 1983.)

asthenopia. This is most typically found in early presbyopes, but may also be associated with both systemic and ocular pathological conditions (Hofstetter 1942; Ciuffreda 1991).

A number of techniques are available to the clinician for the assessment of the near accommodative response and these will be discussed below.

Dynamic cross-cylinder

In this test, subjects view a pattern of intersecting horizontal and vertical lines through a cross-cylinder (typically ±0.50 D) to create mixed astigmatism, with the horizontal and vertical lines theoretically equidistant in front of and behind the retina (**Fig. 15.5**). The cross-cylinder is usually introduced before the eye with the negative cylinder axis vertical. This will produce a myopic horizontal focal line and a hyperopic vertical focal line. The patient is directed to view the rectilinear target through the cross-cylinder and asked to indicate whether the vertical or horizontal lines appear clearer.

If the patient is accommodating exactly in the plane of the target (**Fig. 15.5A**), then after introduction of the cross-cylinder, the circle of least confusion will lie on the retina and the patient will report that both sets of lines (horizontal and vertical) are equally clear (or more accurately, equally

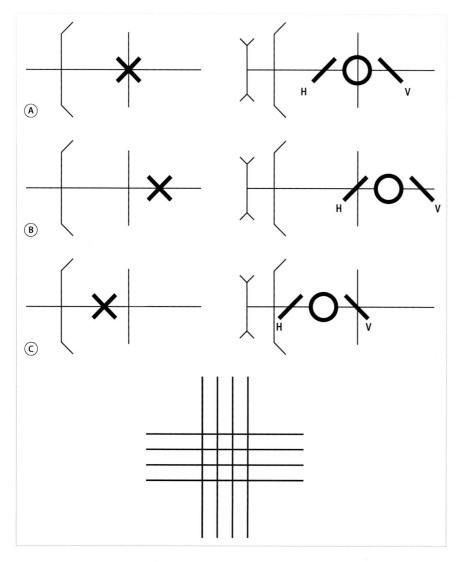

Figure 15.5 Effect of introducing a cross-cylinder (negative axis vertical) in patients exhibiting accurate accommodative responses, i.e. response equals stimulus (**A**), a lag of accommodation, i.e. stimulus exceeds the response (**B**) and a lead of accommodation, i.e. response exceeds the stimulus (**C**). In each case, the left-hand figure represents the position of the focal lines conjugate with the object of regard before the cross-cylinder is introduced, while the right-hand figure shows the position of the horizontal (H) and vertical (V) focal lines after the cross-cylinder lens is introduced. The rectilinear target typically used for this procedure is illustrated in the lower part of this figure.

blurred). However, if the patient was initially underaccommodating for the target, i.e. a lag of accommodation was present (**Fig. 15.5B**), then following the introduction of the cross-cylinder the patient should report that the horizontal lines are clearer since the horizontal focal line is closer to the retina. Alternatively, if the patient was initially overaccommodating for the target (a lead of accommodation), then following the introduction of the cross-cylinder, the patient should report that the vertical lines are clearer (**Fig. 15.5C**). In the case of a lag of accommodation (horizontal lines clearer), positive spherical lenses are introduced until both sets of lines appear equally clear; for a lead of accommodation (vertical lines clearer), minus spheres are introduced. The lens power required to make the two sets of lines appear equally clear provides a measure of the accommodative error. For example, if the patient is viewing a target at 40 cm (accommodative stimulus = 2.50 D) and requires a +0.50 DS lens to equalize the two sets of lines, then a 0.50 D lag of accommodation is present and the initial accommodative response was 2.00 D.

This test is usually performed under dim illumination in order to minimize the depth of focus of the eye by achieving the largest pupillary diameter. However, sufficient illumination must be provided to allow the patient to see the target clearly. This low level of ambient illumination departs from the more typically recommended luminance levels for the performance of near-vision tasks. The procedure may be carried out under both monocular and binocular fused conditions. The former will primarily assess the blur-driven accommodative response, although there may also be a significant contribution from proximally induced accommodation. Under binocular fused conditions (the most naturalistic viewing environment), blur-driven, proximal and convergent accommodation will be stimulated.

There are a number of significant problems with the dynamic cross-cylinder test which make it of limited value in pre-presbyopic patients with active accommodation. For example, it is assumed that a patient who accommodates accurately to a more conventional target will produce an accommodative response to the dioptrically conflicting, rectilinear target that lies exactly midway between the two foci (i.e. places the circle of least confusion (COLC) on the retina; see **Fig. 15.5A**). However, there is little evidence to support this proposal. For example, Portello et al (2001) used an infrared optometer to measure the accommodative response in subjects with uncorrected astigmatism. The authors demonstrated that subjects generally exerted the minimum accommodation necessary to place the anterior focal line within the depth of focus of the eye. However, under none of the conditions tested was the COLC positioned on or close to the retina.

Thus, the assumption that the subject will accommodate to place the circle of least confusion on the retina seems unfounded. Indeed, the rectilinear targets used are not conducive to maintaining the circle of least confusion on the retina due to their horizontal and vertical orientations (Williamson-Noble 1943). Additionally, it is questionable whether subjects would prefer to maintain the two sets of lines equally blurred by placing the circle of least confusion on the retina, or whether they would alter their accommodative response to improve the clarity of one set of lines. This latter situation is frequently found in young patients, who will often indicate that first the vertical lines are clearer, now the horizontal, now the vertical, etc.

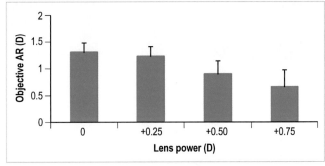

Figure 15.6 Mean objective measurement of the accommodative response while performing a binocular fused, dynamic cross-cylinder test under standard clinical conditions in eight patients who all exhibited a lag of accommodative to the 2.50 D stimulus. As plus lenses were introduced per the standard clinical procedure, a significant decline in the accommodative response was observed. (Data from Benzoni et al 2006.)

The observation that the accommodative response changes following the introduction of lenses provides an additional difficulty with this test. If a lag of accommodation is observed, plus lenses are introduced to obtain the required end point. However, in a young patient with active accommodation, the introduction of additional plus power will stimulate a reduction in the blur-driven accommodative response. Several studies (Fry 1940; Goodson & Afanador 1974; Benzoni et al 2006) have verified that this is indeed the case (**Fig. 15.6**). If the reduction in accommodation is equal to the magnitude of the plus lens, then the subjective response to the test will remain unchanged.

In a recent investigation, Benzoni et al (2006) observed a significant difference in the accommodative response to a 2.50 D stimulus measured using the subjective dynamic cross-cylinder test, when compared with an objective, infrared optometer. The mean accommodative responses for these two measurement techniques in 25 subjects were 1.68 and 2.35 D, respectively. Further, of the 10 subjects who exhibited a lead of accommodation with the subjective procedure, only one had a lead (response >2.50 D) when measured objectively. The authors concluded that this test should only be used to quantify the power of a near-vision addition in a presbyopic patient.

Near duochrome

The duochrome (bichrome) test (O'Connor Davies 1957; Bennett 1963) utilizes the chromatic aberration of the human eye (Bedford & Wyszecki 1957; Charman & Jennings 1976) to determine the locus of the point conjugate with the retina. The test is performed in a similar manner to the distance test, i.e. minus lenses are introduced if the subject indicates that the target on the red background appears clearer or darker, or plus lenses if a green preference is indicated, until equality is achieved. However, it has been suggested that the standard red and green filters may not be appropriate for near-vision testing. Several investigators (Ivanoff 1953; Jenkins 1963; Millodot & Sivak 1973) have demonstrated that the wavelength conjugate with the retina changes from ≈600 nm during distance fixation to ≈530 nm when observing a target at a viewing distance of 40 cm. Therefore, Wilmut (1958) proposed that blue (peak wavelength ≈495 nm) and yellow (peak wavelength ≈575 nm) filters should be used for near-vision testing to account for this change in the location of the chromatic interval. However, Rosenfield et al (1996) compared the subjective responses to both red–green and blue–yellow near duochrome tests with objective measures of accommodation obtained using an infrared optometer. They noted that 4 and 9 of the 20 subjects were unable to provide useful subjective responses with the red–green and blue–yellow tests, respectively. Further, the response measured subjectively with the blue–yellow test was significantly greater than the objective measurement, whereas no significant difference was recorded between the red–green response and the objective findings. Accordingly, they concluded that the blue–yellow near duochrome did not provide an accurate assessment of the accommodative response.

Probably the major reason why the red–green duochrome test has not been used more widely for near examinations is the shortage of suitable near tests, particularly in the United States. However, units are commercially available, for example the near-point analysis test produced by the Bernell Corporation (Mishawaka, IN), which also includes both suppression and associated phoria tests.

Dynamic retinoscopy

The principle of both static (i.e with minimal accommodation) and dynamic (with a stimulated accommodative response) retinoscopy is that a neutral reflex is observed when the point conjugate with the retina coincides with the retinoscope sighthole (see Ch. 13). Consider a fully corrected patient viewing a target at a distance of 33 cm. If the patient exerts an accommodative response of 2.50 D, the point conjugate with the retina will lie 40 cm in front of the principal point of the eye. Thus, a retinoscopist working at 67 cm, 40 cm or 33 cm will observe against, neutral or with movement, respectively.

A number of variations on this procedure exist and these are detailed below.

Cross–Nott technique

This technique, initially devised by Cross (1911) and subsequently refined by Nott (1925, 1926), does not require the use of supplementary lenses. The patient wears their full distance refractive correction, and is directed to view a near target. If with movement is seen (reflecting the typical lag of accommodation), then the retinoscopist adjusts the working distance away from the patient, while the fixation target remains stationary. The reciprocal of the retinoscopy working distance (in metres) at which a neutral reflex is observed indicates the magnitude of the accommodative response.

Sheard's technique

Sheard (1929) was one of the earliest workers to note that a lag of accommodation to a near target is the most common finding. He indicated that this lag could be measured by placing a target which is attached to the retinoscope mirror at the patient's usual reading distance, and performing retinoscopy through the distance refractive correction. Appropriate spherical lenses are added until a neutral reflex is observed. Sheard stated that the lag of accommodation is given by the lens power which provides 'the first indications

of a neutral shadow'. He pointed out that a range of neutrality is typically observed, and that this range reflects the magnitude of negative relative accommodation (NRA).

Monocular estimate method retinoscopy

It was noted previously that the introduction of plus lenses during the course of an accommodation measurement procedure may influence the accommodative response (see **Fig. 15.6**). The monocular estimate method (MEM) retinoscopy procedure attempts to overcome this difficulty by interposing the lenses very briefly (Haynes 1960; Valenti 1990) so that the subject does not have time to respond to the change in accommodative stimulus (Locke & Somers 1989). Rouse et al (1982) observed a high correlation between measurements of the accommodative response obtained using MEM retinoscopy and a vernier optometer. However, they also observed that the response determined using MEM retinoscopy was approximately 10% less than that measured with the optometer. This suggests that the introduction of the plus lenses does produce some relaxation of accommodation. Since the reaction time of accommodation is typically around 350 ms (Campbell & Westheimer 1960; Hogan & Gilmartin 1984), it is essential that a lens be present for an interval shorter than this reaction time. This proposal was supported by Birnbaum (1993), who noted that the lens must be in front of the eye for no longer than one-fifth of a second. The degree of skill required to interpose a lens, assess the direction of the reflex and remove the lens in under 200 ms would seem to be extremely high. Interestingly, both Locke and Somers (1989) and Jackson and Goss (1991) observed no significant difference between dynamic retinoscopy measurements obtained using the MEM and Sheard techniques. These equivalent results indicate that attempting to interpose the lenses for a period shorter than the typical accommodative response time ($\approx$350 ms) is either unnecessary or practically impossible.

Autorefractors

Any commercial infrared autorefractor may be used to assess the accommodative response providing it allows near stimuli to be presented. These instruments are objective, take measurements extremely quickly (typically in less than 0.2 s) and are relatively easy to operate. Ideally, a range of near dioptric stimuli should be available. Two such instruments which have been widely used for research purposes are the Canon Autoref R-1 (McBrien & Millodot 1985) and the newer Grand Seiko WAM 5500 autorefractors (Chat & Edwards 2001; Mallen et al 2001). The former instrument is no longer manufactured, but both of these devices have a wide-open field of view, which allows presentation of near targets at a wide range of physical viewing distances.

Positive and negative relative accommodation

Positive and negative relative accommodation (PRA and NRA) represents changes in accommodation that can be elicited while the stimulus for vergence is held constant. These parameters are measured clinically by introducing increasing minus (for PRA) or plus (for NRA) lenses while the patient views a near target, typically located at a viewing distance of 40 cm (2.50 D). The end point is taken when the patient reports the first slight, sustained blur. As with the amplitude of accommodation, the patient should always be encouraged to try to clear the target, and, particularly when introducing minus lenses (i.e. PRA), care must be taken to allow the patient adequate time to clear the image, especially at the higher accommodative stimulus levels. The amount of additional spherical power which has been added to the distance correction represents the magnitude of relative accommodation.

Measurements of relative accommodation do not test the accommodation system in isolation, but rather examine the interaction between accommodation and vergence. The component changes which occur during PRA and NRA testing are shown in **Figure 15.7**. In PRA, the minus lenses increase the demand for blur-driven accommodation. This change is accompanied by an increase in accommodative convergence (AC). However, this increased vergence response will place the images on non-corresponding retinal points, with resultant diplopia unless compensated by a reduction in the output of disparity vergence (i.e. disparity divergence). This divergence response will lead to decreased convergent accommodation (CA) due to the convergent accommodation to convergence, or CA/C, ratio. This reduction in CA must be compensated for to prevent the target becoming blurred,

and this will occur via an increase in blur-driven accommodation. This latter change will cause the cycle to begin repeating itself, and this will continue until an equilibrium position is reached, with the accommodation and vergence responses allowing the target to be seen as both clear and single. Accordingly, it is an oversimplification to state simply that PRA requires an increase in accommodation without any accompanying change in vergence. While the latter approximates the ultimate changes in the aggregate accommodation and vergence responses, the statement fails to specify the changes in component contributions from both oculomotor systems that must occur during this test.

The expected findings in pre-presbyopic patients for PRA and NRA are around −3.00 D and +2.00 D, respectively. If higher readings are observed, then a suppression check should be introduced to verify that the patient is indeed viewing with both eyes. Examples of appropriate suppression checks are described in the next section, which describes the testing of accommodative facility. A high NRA value (>2.00 D) suggests an initial accommodative response greater than the expected value for the 2.50 D stimulus. This might result from a lead of accommodation or an error in the patient's refractive correction. If hyperopia is present, such as latent hyperopia or as a result of a myopic patient being overcorrected, then an increased accommodative response will usually occur in a young patient. This elevated response allows greater potential for relaxation of blur-driven accommodation, resulting in an increased NRA value.

A reduced PRA finding may develop from either difficulty in increasing blur-driven accommodation (e.g. due to accommodative insufficiency or presbyopia) or decreasing disparity vergence (e.g. convergence excess). Conversely, reduced NRA may result from difficulty in decreasing blur-driven accommodation (e.g. due to accommodative excess) or increasing disparity vergence (e.g. convergence insufficiency) (Scheiman & Wick 1994).

Accommodative facility

This test examines the ability to make rapid step changes in accommodation. The test is most frequently performed using 'flipper' lenses under either monocular or binocular conditions. The patient views a line of fine print (typically 6/9 letters) at a distance of 40 cm (accommodative stimulus = 2.50 D) through their distance refractive correction. This correction should be either in the form of the patient's own spectacles (or contact lenses) or alternatively set up in a trial frame. Most commonly, ±2.00 D lenses are introduced alternatively before the viewing eye (as shown in **Fig. 15.8**) and the patient required to indicate when the target becomes 'absolutely clear'. At this point the alternative lens is flipped in front of the eye as rapidly as possible. These conditions provide accommodative stimuli of 0.50 and 4.50 D. The result is quantified in terms of the number of cycles (i.e. clearing both the plus and minus lenses) completed in 60 s. The full 1 minute test period should always be performed to check for variations due to fatigue of accommodation (Griffin 1988). However, care must be taken to note whether any asymmetry exists between the time taken to clear the plus and minus lenses.

While these are the most commonly used stimulus levels, other values may be adopted if desired, e.g. the use of

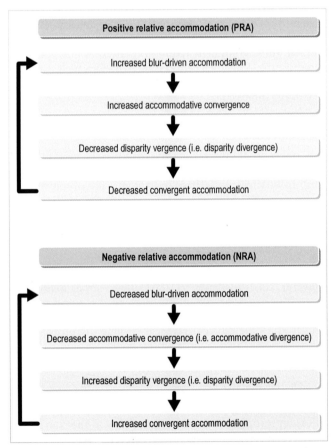

Figure 15.7 Component changes in accommodation and vergence that take place during the assessment of positive and negative relative accommodation (PRA and NRA).

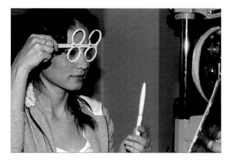

Figure 15.8 Binocular accommodative facility being performed on a patient. The patient is viewing a target at a distance of 40 cm through flippers containing ±2.00 lenses. Once the patient reports that the target appears clear, then the flipper is switched to the alternate pair of lenses. A pen is held halfway between the patient and the target to serve as a suppression check. The pen tip should be seen in physiological diplopia throughout the procedure.

±1.00 D lenses or an alternative working distance. When tested monocularly, the procedure tests the patient's ability to vary the blur-driven accommodative response rapidly. However, during binocular testing, the patient's ability to increase and decrease accommodation while maintaining an appropriate vergence response is assessed. Accordingly, this test examines the patient's ability to change PRA and NRA rapidly. For binocular testing, suppression checks should always used, e.g. using either polarized filters and targets, or more simply by introducing an additional target such as a pencil in the midline halfway between the observer and the object of regard. The patient should ensure that this supplementary stimulus is seen in physiological diplopia, and is instructed to report if it becomes single at any time during the test. Both Burge (1979) and Griffin (1988) noted significantly elevated binocular findings when a suppression check was not used.

Several investigators (Hennessy et al 1984; Zellers et al 1984; Levine et al 1985; McKenzie et al 1987) have suggested clinical pass criteria of 11 cycles per minute (cpm) for monocular testing and 8 cpm for binocular assessment, since approximately 67% of young patients would be predicted to achieve these norms. However, Daum (1991) pointed out that since values of accommodative facility are not normally distributed, this statistical assumption may not be valid. Hoffman and Rouse (1980) also noted that a difference of more than 2 cpm between the two eyes (during monocular testing) should be regarded as a possible indicator of accommodative difficulties when accompanied by near-visual symptoms. Scheiman et al (1988) examined accommodative facility in children between 6 and 12 years of age using ±2.00 D flippers and reported that facility rates were considerably lower than those found in young adults. Using a passing criterion of 1 standard deviation below the mean (Hennessy et al 1984), Scheiman et al proposed that the monocular pass rates for 6-, 7- and 8–12-year-old children should be at least 3.0, 4.5 and 5.0 cpm, respectively. The authors also noted that the binocular pass rates were extremely low (between 0.5 and 2.5 cpm for these age groups), and therefore they suggested that the value of the binocular accommodative facility test in children was questionable.

In a comparison of accommodative facility findings in patients with and without near-vision symptoms, Hennessy et al (1984) reported significantly lower facility rates (for both monocular and binocular testing) in the symptomatic group. While Levine et al (1985) did not observe this lower mean rate, they noted greater variability in facility rates when symptomatic subjects were tested repeatedly, in comparison with asymptomatic patients. Additionally, Bobier and Sivak (1983) noted that increased accommodative facility following vision training was associated with an improvement in the dynamically measured temporal characteristics (latency, movement time, response time) of the accommodative response. These findings indicate that clinical accommodative facility testing is a valuable tool when screening patients for accommodative dysfunction.

Assessment and correction of presbyopia

Presbyopia refers to the decline in accommodative responsivity with age (**Fig. 15.9**). Although this typically does not present clinical difficulties until individuals reach their early forties, Donders (1864) noted that the loss of amplitude actually begins around (or even slightly before) puberty (see **Table 15.2**). Presbyopia may be corrected by using supplementary convex lenses (in addition to any correction for distance refractive error) to allow diverging rays from a near object of regard to be focused upon the retina.

Seven standard clinical techniques are available for determining the appropriate near-vision addition namely:

- dynamic cross-cylinder
- plus build up
- add based on patient's age
- proportion of amplitude
- dynamic retinoscopy

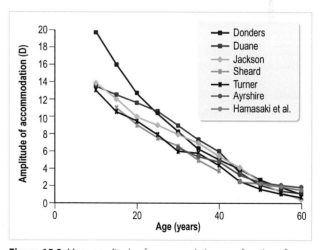

Figure 15.9 Mean amplitude of accommodation as a function of age. Values are taken from the investigations of Donders (1864), Duane (1912), Jackson (1900), Sheard (1920), Turner (1958), the Ayrshire Study Circle (1964) and Hamasaki et al (1956). All data were collected under monocular viewing conditions with the exception of the study by Jackson, who obtained binocular measurements. It should be noted that with the exception of the results of Donders for the 10–20-year-old subjects, all the remaining data show relatively limited variation.

- NRA/PRA balance
- near duochrome.

The first three techniques represent the most commonly used clinical procedures. However, whichever technique is adopted, it is essential that a careful history is taken to determine the patient's visual requirements. For example, the patient should be questioned in detail about their visual activities both during and outside their work time. Since computer use is now almost universal, all patients should be questioned about this activity, particularly with regard to the monitor viewing distance, gaze angle and whether concurrent viewing of hard copy material is required. Special requirements such as musical instrument playing or machine operation should also be considered. A common error is to assume falsely that patients perform all (or any) of their near work at 40 cm. It should be noted that each of the techniques described below represents only the first step in determining the appropriate near addition. The patient's actual reading performance through the add must always be checked. Both the level of visual acuity and the range of clear vision through the add should be examined. Increasing the near addition both decreases the available range of clear vision and moves it closer to the patient. For example, in an absolute presbyope (assuming a depth of focus of ±0.40 D), the range of clear vision through a +2.00 D add will be 20.9 cm, i.e. 41.6–62.5 cm, whereas through a +3.00 D add it will only be 9.0 cm, i.e. 29.4–38.4 cm. It is valuable to record the range of clear vision for a particular lens, e.g. *ADD +2.00, 6/6, range 22–41 cm*. One should try to ensure that the patient's preferred (or required) working distance lies in the middle of the range. If practical, the patient should be encouraged to bring their particular near-visual material into the consulting room (e.g. music, sewing, unusual-sized text, inspection material) and the add assessed using a trial frame while viewing this material.

Dynamic cross-cylinder

This test will provide an indication of the accommodative error. It should be noted that many of the difficulties associated with this test in younger patients (e.g. large fluctuations of accommodation; see p 234) disappear in the presbyopic individual. If the patient cannot initially see the target clearly, then sufficient plus power is introduced until the lines can be recognized. The binocular fused measurement is generally used as the tentative near addition, although monocular findings may be recorded, particularly if the binocular balance is in doubt. The binocular value is sometimes lower than the monocular findings, due to the introduction of convergent accommodation under binocular viewing conditions.

Plus build up

Plus spherical power is added to the distance refraction (in 0.25 DS steps) until the patient is able to achieve their optimum near visual acuity at the appropriate working distance. The minimum plus power that gives clear vision at the required distances places the proximal end of the depth of field coincident with the object of regard. Thus, additional plus power (typically an additional +0.25 sphere) will be needed to place the preferred reading position in the centre of the range of clear vision. This test is generally performed binocularly, but again may be done monocularly, particularly if the binocular balance (see Ch. 14) is in doubt.

Add based on patient's age

The tentative add may simply be based on the patient's age. However, the required addition may need to be adjusted appropriately due to variations in the required working distance or if the amplitude of accommodation differs significantly from the average for the patient's age. In a study of patients returning to an optometric clinic with unsatisfactory presbyopic adds, Hanlon et al (1987) observed that age-expected powers produced the fewest number of errors while the binocular dynamic cross-cylinder procedure produced the highest number of returning patients. Pointer (1995) reviewed cross-sectional clinical data in 600 Caucasian patients and noted that female patients generally required a higher add than the equivalent-aged males. Additionally, he found that the rate of increase of the required add with age was steeper between 41 and 55 years of age, but slowed significantly between 55 and 80 years of age. Similar findings were also reported by Blystone (1999), who noted that, between 40 and 50 years of age, on average the required add increased by 0.12 D/year, whereas after 50 years of age, the rate of increase was only 0.03 D/year. Typical near adds for a population of Western European origin are shown in **Table 15.3**. Other ethnic groups may require different values, depending on the age-related loss of accommodative ability for that population.

Proportion of amplitude

A rule of thumb is that the patient should be able to sustain one-half of their accommodative amplitude. Accordingly, the near add corresponds to the difference between the required working distance (in dioptres) and one-half of their amplitude.

For example, if a patient has an amplitude of accommodation of 3 D and requires a working distance of 40 cm, then the required add is equal to (2.50 – 1.50) = +1.00 D. However, some practitioners advocate that this rule should indicate that a patient can maintain 67% of their amplitude rather than 50%.

Table 15.3 Expected near-vision addition (add) as a function of age for patients of Western European origin

Age (yrs)	Add (D)
40	0
45	+1.00
48	+1.25
50	+1.50
52	+1.75
55	+2.00
60	+2.25
65	+2.50

Patients having other ethnic backgrounds may require a different add.

Dynamic retinoscopy

Dynamic retinoscopy can be used to determine the accommodative response for a given stimulus (see earlier section). Plus lenses are introduced over the distance prescription while the patient views a near target at their preferred working distance until an appropriate response is obtained. It is usual to leave the patient with a small (0.25–0.50 DS) lag of accommodation to take advantage of the depth of field of the eye. This allows the practitioner to prescribe the lowest possible add, thereby giving the patient the widest range of clear vision.

NRA/PRA balance

Having determined a tentative add using one of the techniques described above, negative relative accommodation (NRA) and positive relative accommodation (PRA) are measured through this preliminary add. The add is then modified so that equal values of PRA and NRA are obtained.

For example, a preliminary add of + 1.00 is determined on an emmetropic patient. Through this add, the NRA and PRA are measured. If the patient reports first slight, sustained blur or NRA through a +2.00 add (i.e. NRA = + 1.00 D) and first blur or PRA through a +0.50 D add (i.e. PRA = −0.50 D), then the near correction should be modified to lie in the middle of the PRA–NRA range, i.e. +1.25 D. Through this lens the patient will have PRA = NRA = 0.75 D.

The concept of balancing PRA and NRA findings when determining a near-vision addition is analogous to Percival's middle third technique for prescribing prism (see Ch. 16), i.e. to provide maximum flexibility between the two oculomotor components.

Near duochrome

This test may be performed at near using a near duochrome unit placed at the appropriate working distance. The principles of the test are the same as for the distance test. Appropriate lenses are added until a 'balance point' is achieved.

Summary

Assessment of accommodation is a critical part of the optometric examination. Haine (2006) observed that blurred vision at near is the most common complaint amongst adult patients presenting in ophthalmic private practice. Providing the patient with comfortable, clear and single vision at their required viewing distance(s) will enable them to complete their habitual occupational and recreational tasks safely and satisfactorily.

Source notes

This chapter is based on: Rosenfield M 1997 Accommodation In: Zadnik K (ed.) The ocular examination. Measurement and findings. WB Saunders, Philadelphia, pp 87–121.

References

Atchison D A, Charman W N, Woods R L 1997 Subjective depth-of-focus of the eye. Optometry and Vision Science 74:511–520

Ayrshire Study Circle 1964 An investigation into accommodation. British Journal of Physiological Optics 21:31–35

Bedford R E, Wyszecki G 1957 Axial chromatic aberration of the human eye. Journal of the Optical Society of America 47:564–566

Bennett A G 1963 The theory of bichromatic tests. Optician 146:291–296

Benzoni J A, Rosenfield M, Collier J et al 2006 Does the dynamic cross cylinder test measure the accommodative response accurately? Optometry and Vision Science 83:E-060030

Berens C, Fonda G 1950 A Spanish-English accommodation and near-test card using photoreduced type. American Journal of Ophthalmology 33:1788–1792

Birnbaum M H 1993 Optometric management of nearpoint vision disorders. Butterworth-Heinemann, Boston, pp 53–71

Blystone P A 1999 Relationship between age and presbyopic addition using a sample of 3,645 examinations from a single private practice. Journal of the American Optometric Association 70:505–508

Bobier W R, Sivak J G 1983 Orthoptic treatment of subjects showing slow accommodative responses. American Journal of Optometry and Physiological Optics 60:678–687

Bruce A S, Atchison D A, Bhoola H 1995 Accommodation-convergence relationships and age. Investigative Ophthalmology and Visual Science 36:406–413

Burge S 1979 Suppression during binocular accommodative rock. Optometric Monthly 70:867–880

Campbell F W 1957 The depth of field of the human eye. Optica Acta 4:157–164

Campbell F W, Westheimer G 1960 Dynamics of the accommodation response of the human eye. Journal of Physiology (London) 151:285–295

Charman W N 1982 The accommodative resting point and refractive error. Ophthalmic Optician 21:469–473

Charman W N, Jennings J A M 1976 Objective measurements of the longitudinal chromatic aberration of the human eye. Vision Research 16:999–1005

Chat S W S, Edwards M H 2001 Clinical evaluation of the Shin-Nippon SRW-5000 autorefractor in children. Ophthalmic Physiological Optics 21:87–100

Ciuffreda K J 1991 Accommodation and its anomalies. In: Charman W N (ed.) Vision and visual dysfunction, vol 1. Visual optics and instrumentation. CRC Press, Boca Raton, FL, pp 231–279

Ciuffreda K J, Kenyon R V 1983 Accommodative vergence and accommodation in normals, amblyopes and strabismics. In: Schor C M, Ciuffreda K J (eds) Vergence eye movements: basic and clinical aspects. Butterworths, Boston, pp 101–173

Coates W R 1955 Amplitudes of accommodation in South Africa. British Journal of Physiological Optics 12:76–81, 86

Cross A J 1911 Dynamic skiametry in theory and practice. A J Cross Optical Co., New York

Daum K M 1991 Accommodative facility. In: Eskridge J B, Amos J F, Bartlett J D (eds) Clinical procedures in optometry. Lippincott, Philadelphia, pp 687–697

Donders F C 1864 On the anomalies of accommodation and refraction of the eye (translated by W D Moore). The New Sydenham Society, London

Duane A 1912 Normal values of the accommodation at all ages. Journal of the American Medical Association 59:1010–1013

Fitch R C 1971 Procedural effects on the manifest human amplitude of accommodation. American Journal of Optometry and Archives of the American Academy of Optometry 48:918–926

Fry G A 1940 Significance of fused cross cylinder test. Optometric Weekly 31:16–19

Goodson R A, Afanador A J 1974 The accommodative response to the near point crossed cylinder test. Optometric Weekly 65:1138–1140

Griffin J R 1988 Binocular anomalies. In: Procedures for vision therapy, 2nd edn. Professional Press, New York

Haine C L 2006 The ophthalmic case historian. In: Benjamin W J (ed.) Borish's clinical refraction, 2nd edn. Butterworth-Heinemann, St Louis, pp 195–216

Hamasaki D, Ong J, Marg E 1956 The amplitude of accommodation in presbyopia. American Journal of Optometry and Archives of the American Academy of Optometry 33:3–14

Hanlon S D, Nakabayashi J, Shigezawa G 1987 A critical view of presbyopic add determination. Journal of the American Optometric Association 58:468–472

Haynes H M 1960 Clinical observations with dynamic retinoscopy. Optometric Weekly 51:2243–2246, 2306–2309

Heath G G 1956 Components of accommodation. American Journal of Optometry and Archives of the American Academy of Optometry 33:569–579

Hennessy D, Iosue R A, Rouse M W 1984 Relation of symptoms to accommodative infacility of school-aged children. American Journal of Optometry and Physiological Optics 61:177–183

Hoffman L, Rouse M 1980 Referral recommendations for binocular function and/or developmental perceptual deficiencies. Journal of the American Optometric Association 51:119–125

Hofstetter H W 1942 Factors involved in low amplitude cases. American Journal of Optometry and Archives of the American Academy of Optometry 19:279–289

Hofstetter H W 1944 A comparison of Duane's and Donders' table of the amplitude of accommodation. American Journal of Optometry and Archives of the American Academy of Optometry 21:345–363

Hogan R E, Gilmartin B 1984 The choice of laser speckle exposure duration in the measurement of tonic accommodation. Ophthalmic Physiological Optics 4:365–368

Hokoda S C, Ciuffreda K J 1982 Measurement of accommodation amplitude in amblyopia. Ophthalmic and Physiological Optics 2:205–212

Ivanoff A 1953 Les Aberrations de l'Oeil. Leur role dans l'accommodation. Éditions de la revue d'optique théorique et instrumentale, Paris

Jackson E 1900 A manual of the diagnosis and treatment of the diseases of the eye. W B Saunders, Philadelphia, p 126

Jackson T W, Goss D A 1991 Variation and correlation of clinical tests of accommodative function in a sample of school-age children. Journal of the American Optometric Association 62:857–866

Jenkins T C A 1963 Aberrations of the eye and their effects on vision. Part II. British Journal of Physiological Optics 20:161–201

Levine S, Ciuffreda K J, Selenow A et al 1985 Clinical assessment of accommodative facility in symptomatic and asymptomatic individuals. Journal of the American Optometric Association 56:286–290

Locke L C, Somers W 1989 A comparison study of dynamic retinoscopy techniques. Optometry and Vision Science 66:540–544

McBrien N A, Millodot M 1985 Clinical evaluation of the Canon Autoref R-1. American Journal of Optometry and Physiological Optics 62:786–792

McKenzie K M, Kerr S R, Rouse M W et al 1987 Study of accommodative facility testing reliability. American Journal of Optometry and Physiological Optics 64:186–194

Mallen E A H, Wolffsohn J S, Gilmartin B et al 2001 Clinical evaluation of the Shin-Nippon SRW-5000 autorefractor in adults. Ophthalmic Physiological Optics 21:101–107

Millodot M, Sivak J 1973 Influence of accommodation on the chromatic aberration of the eye. British Journal of Physiological Optics 28:169–174

Morgan M W 1944 Accommodation and its relationship to convergence. American Journal of Optometry and Archives of the American Academy of Optometry 21:183–195

Nott I S 1925 Dynamic skiametry, accommodation and convergence. American Journal of Physiological Optics 6:490–503

Nott I S 1926 Dynamic skiametry. Accommodative convergence and fusion convergence. American Journal of Physiological Optics 7:366–374

O'Connor Davies P H 1957 A critical analysis of bichromatic tests used in clinical refraction. British Journal of Physiological Optics 14:170–182, 213

Pointer J S 1995 Broken down by age and sex. The optical correction of presbyopia revisited. Ophthalmic Physiological Optics 15:439–443

Portello J K, Hong S E, Rosenfield M 2001 Accommodation to astigmatic stimuli. Optometry and Vision Science (suppl)78:91

Rosenfield M 1997 Accommodation. In: Zadnik K (ed.) The ocular examination. Measurement and findings. W B Saunders, Philadelphia, pp 87–121

Rosenfield M, Cohen A S 1995 Push-up amplitude of accommodation and letter size. Ophthalmic and Physiological Optics 15:231–232

Rosenfield M, Gilmartin B 1990 Effect of target proximity on the open-loop accommodative response. Optometry and Vision Science 67:74–79

Rosenfield M, Ciuffreda K J, Chen H W 1995 Effect of age on the interaction between the AC/A and CA/C ratios. Ophthalmic Physiological Optics 15:451–455

Rosenfield M, Portello J K, Blustein G H 1996 Comparison of clinical techniques to assess the near accommodative response. Optometry and Vision Science 73:382–388

Rouse M W, London R, Allen D C 1982 An evaluation of the monocular estimate method of dynamic retinoscopy. American Journal of Optometry and Physiological Optics 59:234–239

Scheiman M, Wick B 1994 Clinical management of binocular vision. Lippincott, Philadelphia

Scheiman M, Herzberg H, Frantz K et al 1988 Normative study of accommodative facility in elementary schoolchildren. American Journal of Optometry and Physiological Optics 65:127–134

Sheard C 1920 Dynamic skiametry and methods of testing the accommodation and convergence of the eyes. Cleveland Press, Chicago

Sheard C 1929 Dynamic skiametry. American Journal of Optometry 6:609–623

Somers W W, Ford C A 1983 Effect of relative distance magnification on the monocular amplitude of accommodation. American Journal of Optometry and Physiological Optics 60:920–924

Turner M J 1958 Observations on the normal subjective amplitude of accommodation. British Journal of Physiological Optics 14:59–64

Valenti C A 1990 The full scope of retinoscopy. Optometric Extension Program. Santa Ana, CA

Wang B, Ciuffreda K J 2006 Depth-of-focus of the human eye: theory and clinical implications. Survey of Ophthalmology 51:75–85

Wick B, Currie D 1991 Convergence accommodation: laboratory and clinical evaluation. Optometry and Vision Science 68:226–231

Williamson-Noble F A 1943 A possible fallacy in the use of the cross-cylinder. British Journal of Ophthalmology 27:1–12

Wilmut E B 1958 Chromatic selectivity of the eye in near vision. Optician 135:185–187

Woehrle M B, Peters R J, Frantz K A 1997 Accommodative amplitude determination: Can we substitute the pull-away for the push-up method? Journal of Optometric Vision Development 28:246–249

Wold R M 1967 The spectacle amplitude of accommodation of children aged six to ten. American Journal of Optometry and Archives of the American Academy of Optometry 44:642–664

Woodhouse J M, Meades J S, Leat S J 1993 Reduced accommodation in children with Down syndrome. Investigative Ophthalmology and Visual Science 34:2382–2387

Zellers J A, Alpert T L, Rouse M W 1984 A review of the literature and a normative study of accommodative facility. Journal of the American Optometric Association 55:31–37

CHAPTER 16

Binocular vision assessment

Bruce J W Evans

Introduction

Binocular vision anomalies are often detected, diagnosed, and treated during an optometric eye examination, so a binocular vision assessment is an important part of this examination. This chapter will first deal with the detection of binocular vision anomalies and then will consider the diagnosis. Although this chapter is entitled 'Binocular vision assessment', brief comments will be included on the main methods of managing binocular vision anomalies in primary eye care practice.

Detection of binocular vision anomalies

Symptoms

Typically, the first clue that a binocular vision anomaly may be present is the reporting of one or more symptoms. The significance of symptoms is dependent on many factors, including the age of the patient.

Many of the symptoms listed in **Table 16.1** are non-specific. For example, blurred vision when reading could be caused by a binocular vision anomaly such as a decompensated heterophoria or convergence insufficiency, or by other conditions including refractive errors, accommodative anomalies, visual stress (described at the end of this chapter), tear film dysfunction, or ocular pathology. Further clinical tests are required to confirm the presence of binocular vision anomalies, as described below. As data are gathered from relevant tests, the clinician will develop a diagnosis. Common diagnoses are summarized in the next main section of this chapter.

Visual acuity

Reduced visual acuity in one eye that is not immediately resolved with refractive correction or explained by ocular pathology is suggestive of amblyopia. The two most common causes of amblyopia are anisometropia and strabismus, and the detection of these conditions is described in more detail below. Strabismic amblyopia is best detected using crowded optotypes. With modern computerized letter charts, it is quite easy to obtain a variety of optotypes appropriate for patients of different ages, and to place these in a 'crowding box', which creates a simple yet crowded visual acuity task (**Fig. 16.1**).

Usually, binocular visual acuity is a little better than the best monocular acuity. If binocular visual acuity is worse than the best monocular finding, then this can be a sign of decompensated heterophoria (Jenkins et al 1994, 1995).

Cover test

The cover test is the most important binocular vision test. Typically, the cover test is carried out using an isolated letter from the line above the poorer eye's visual acuity as a target. Only if the visual acuity is worse than 6/60 should a muscle light be used for fixation.

Table 16.1 Symptoms suggestive of common binocular vision anomalies

Symptom	Details to be obtained	Suggestive of
Reports of a turning eye (e.g. by parents in young children)	When did it start? How often does it happen? Are there any precipitating factors? How is the general health? How long does it last for? Is it getting worse?	Strabismus Decompensating heterophoria Hyperopia Incomitancy
Diplopia	When did it start? How often does it happen? Are there any precipitating factors? How is the general health? How long does it last for? Is it getting worse? Are the double images predominantly side by side or one beneath the other?	Strabismus Decompensating heterophoria Convergence insufficiency Incomitancy (varies with gaze)
Blurred vision in one eye	When was it first noticed? Would it have been detected before (e.g. at previous eye care)?	Amblyopia Anisometropia Change in refractive error
Tired/sore/aching eyes or headaches	When did it start? Are there any precipitating factors (e.g. visual tasks)	Convergence insufficiency Decompensating heterophoria Visual stress
Visual perceptual distortions on viewing text (text blurring/ moving or other distortions)	Is it just with text (more likely to be visual stress)? How soon after starting reading? Does the patient close or cover one eye?	Visual stress Convergence insufficiency Decompensating heterophoria

Unfortunately, there are no hard and fast rules with symptoms and the information in this table can only give a general guide.

The patient's history or previous records might lead the practitioner to suspect that strabismus may be present. If so, the deviated eye is typically the one with the poorer acuity. Accordingly, the other eye should be covered first. This first cover test is the 'purest' binocular vision test of all, since before the cover is applied the patient has their habitual visual status and is viewing the target in a completely natural way. The eyes should be watched as the cover approaches since, if a dissociated vertical deviation (Evans 2007a) is present, the eye that the occluder is approaching may move before the cover actually reaches the eye.

As the cover moves over one eye the practitioner should watch the uncovered eye. It is the behaviour of the uncovered eye that reveals whether the patient has strabismus (also referred to as heterotropia). For example, as the left eye is covered, the practitioner should watch the right eye. If the right eye moves, then this indicates that strabismus is present. The direction and amplitude of the movement should be estimated. If the uncovered eye moves outwards, this indicates the presence of a convergent strabismus, or esotropia (ET or SOT). Similarly, an inward movement of the deviated eye indicates exotropia (XT or XOT), while downward and upward movements of the non-occluded eye indicate hyper- and hypotropia, respectively. The cover is then slowly removed from the eye that has been occluded, and this eye is observed to see if a movement occurs as the eye takes up fixation, signifying heterophoria. The same directions of movement for heterotropia also describe heterophorias, i.e. outward and inward movements indicate esophoria (EP or SOP) and exophoria (XP or XOP), respectively; a downward movement indicates hyperphoria (HP) although a hypophoria is usually described as a hyperphoria of the other eye. To summarize, if there is a movement of the unoccluded eye, then strabismus is indicated. If there is no such movement, but there is a movement of the occluded eye upon removal of the cover, then heterophoria is present.

The amplitude of movement should always be estimated in prism diopters and practitioners can use the following technique to regularly 'calibrate' their estimations. On a typical Snellen chart (but not a logMAR chart) the distance from the first to the last letter of the 6/12 line is generally about 12 cm (although this should be measured to check the distance). If this is the case and the chart viewing distance is 6 m, then when the patient changes fixation between the first and last letters on the line, the eyes will make a saccade of 2Δ. Similarly, if a patient looks between two markings on the wall near the letter chart (at a viewing distance of 6 m) that are 24 cm apart, then the eyes are moving by 4Δ. The amplitude of eye movements on this task can be compared with the magnitude of movement seen during the cover test. At near, this type of comparison is even easier by using a centimetre ruler held at ⅓ m from the patient. If the patient looks from the

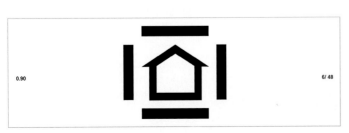

0.90   6/48

Fig. 16.1 Lea symbol in crowding box for testing visual acuity in young children, presented using Test Chart 2000. (Reproduced with permission from David Thomson and Lea Hyvarinen.)

1 cm mark to the 2 cm mark, the eyes are moving by 1 cm which, at ⅓ m, equates to 3Δ.

Alternatively, hand-held prisms (usually in the form of a prism bar) can also be used to neutralize the observed movement. This is generally performed when quantifying the movement observed with the alternating cover test (see below). Sufficient prism is introduced to reverse the movement (e.g. changing an eso into an exo deviation), and then the prism reduced to find the minimum prism which produces no observable movement on the cover test. This is especially useful in large angles where accurate estimation of the size of eye movements becomes difficult.

In heterophoria, the quality of the recovery movement should also be recorded. This gives an objective indication of how well the patient is able to compensate for the heterophoria (Evans 2007a). A higher grading in **Table 16.2** is more likely to be associated with decompensation and thus more likely to require treatment (Evans 2007a).

The description above is of one form of the cover test: the *cover/uncover (or unilateral cover) test*. This is useful for detecting strabismus, for estimating the magnitude of the deviation under normal viewing conditions, and for evaluating the recovery movement in heterophoria (see **Table 16.2**). But it is also valuable to know how much the angle increases ('builds') as the patient is dissociated for longer by repeated covering. So, after the cover/uncover test it is advisable to alternate the cover from one eye to the other for about six further covers to see how the angle changes. At the end of this *alternating cover test* as the cover is removed then the recovery movement can be observed again to estimate the effect of repeated covering on the recovery (see **Table 16.2**). A cover/uncover test is then performed once more on the other eye to assess any change in the recovery movement of this eye.

A great deal of information can be gleaned from the cover test (Evans 2007a). With practice, cover testing is nearly always possible, even with infants (see Ch. 28). In some patients, an eye is deviated before the test (strabismus) or becomes deviated during the test and is very slow to take up fixation. So, when the dominant eye is covered there may be no apparent movement, even though the uncovered eye is not fixating the target. A movement of the deviated eye can sometimes be elicited by asking the patient to 'look directly' at the target, or by moving the fixation target or the head a little.

Ocular motility

The ocular motility test is important for detecting incomitant deviations. To gain maximum information from this test, a thorough knowledge of the anatomy and physiology of the extraocular muscles is essential. The best target is a point light source, which should be bright enough to allow the corneal reflexes to be clearly seen, but not so bright as to cause lid closure. For infants, any target that will catch their attention should be used. The target should be held at about 50 cm from the patient and should be moved in an arc. It is easier to observe the eye movements in extreme gaze if no spectacles are worn, but if there is an accommodative strabismus then spectacles should be worn, or ideally the test repeated with and without spectacles.

There are really three different tests that can be carried out during the ocular motility test: the basic objective motility test, the motility test with cover testing in peripheral gaze, and the motility test with an analysis of reports of diplopia in peripheral gaze. With incomitant patients the situation can be made simpler by performing the test three times to gather these three sets of information. The first of these three tests, the basic objective ocular motility test (Evans 2005a), is described first.

For each test, the patient should be instructed to keep their head still, and to follow the light with their eyes. It is also useful to have them report if the target ever becomes *double* (see below) *or uncomfortable to look at* any time during the procedure. Either of these symptoms may indicate a muscle restriction. The smoothness, accuracy and extent of the eye movements should be observed. Various authors have preferences for different patterns of movement of the target. The star or H-pattern (**Fig. 16.2**) is often used, but other patterns have been recommended and each has its own merits.

The straight up and down (in the midline) positions are also tested to look for an A or V syndrome. The basic objective motility test is performed whilst watching the reflection of the light in the corneae to detect any marked underactions or over-actions. Any over- or under-actions can be graded from 'just detectable' to 'no movement in the direction of gaze that is being tested'. Throughout the test, the corneal light reflexes are observed. If one eye's reflex disappears, then either the light is misaligned or the patient's view of the light has been obscured (e.g. by their nose). This means that the light has been moved too far: the test should be carried out within the binocular field. If any abnormality is observed with the usual test when the patient is viewing with both eyes, then each eye is occluded and the eyes are tested monocularly.

If a marked deviation is present, this may be revealed by the basic ocular motility test. However, this method relies on an observation of corneal reflexes and eye position, and this is a coarse method of assessing ocular alignment. The cover test is a more accurate procedure and can be carried

Table 16.2 A grading system that can be used to gauge cover test recovery in heterophoria

Grade	Description
1	Rapid and smooth
2	Slightly slow/jerky
3	Definitely slow/jerky but not breaking down
4	Slow/jerky and breaks down with repeat covering, or only recovers after a blink
5	Breaks down readily, after 1–3 covers

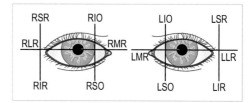

Fig. 16.2 The H-motility pattern, showing the muscles that are being predominantly assessed in each eye in each position of gaze. RSR, right superior rectus; RIO, right inferior oblique; RLR, right lateral rectus; RIR, right inferior rectus; RSO, right superior oblique; RMR, right medial rectus; and similarly for the left eye. When testing the vertical recti and oblique muscles, the eye should be abducted 23° and adducted 55°, respectively.

out during ocular motility testing. Cover testing in peripheral gaze is extremely useful and, like the basic ocular motility test, provides objective data. It requires practice, but is well worth the time that it takes to become skilled at this test. It is important to make sure that the cover is held over the line of sight, considering the position of the target.

An even more sensitive way of detecting incomitancy is to use the patient's own visual system to provide feedback on ocular alignment by asking the patient about diplopia to estimate the subjective angle in different positions of gaze. This is made easier by the use of red and green goggles. Although this can be informative with some patients, with others it can be a source of considerable confusion. Patients may become dissociated as the test progresses, may be confused about diplopia, or may suppress in certain positions of gaze. If the data obtained with this approach conflict with those obtained with the basic objective motility test or with cover testing in peripheral gaze, then these other two approaches should be given most weight.

Although most binocular vision anomalies are detected from symptoms and/or the tests already described in this section, some require other binocular tests. Many of these are described in the next section. In particular, microtropia and vertical strabismus are difficult to detect by cover testing, but both would be likely to cause reduced stereoacuity and an abnormal result on tests of foveal suppression. Foveal suppression can be detected using the polarized letters on the near Mallett unit.

Stereopsis

Stereopsis may be defined as the binocular perception of depth based upon retinal disparity. This results from the brain being presented with two slightly dissimilar retinal images. For stereopsis to be manifest, the images must be imaged on non-corresponding retinal points, with the disparity not exceeding Panum's fusional area. Clinical assessment of stereopsis is valuable because it indicates the level of binocularity. It can be used to aid in the detection of binocular anomalies as well as monitoring the success of therapy to treat these conditions.

Tests of stereoacuity can be classified into those that use true random dot stimuli (e.g. the TNO test and the random dot subtest of the Randot test) and contoured tests (e.g. the Titmus Wirt circles test and the circles subtest of the Randot test). With random dot tests, there are few monocular cues, and therefore a good performance in these tests indicates the absence of constant strabismus. With contoured tests, stereopsis is measured by presenting disparate targets and determining whether they are perceived in depth. The degree of retinal disparity can be varied to quantify the threshold of stereopsis (i.e. stereoacuity). Patients with small-angle constant strabismus often appear to exhibit stereoacuity on contoured tests, but these patients and those with decompensated heterophoria are unlikely to obtain the highest scores. Each test has its own methods and norms, and it is important that practitioners familiarize themselves with the particular test(s) that they use. Patients are often reluctant to give a response unless they are certain, and it is advisable for the practitioner to encourage the patient to 'guess', typically taking the last result before an error is made as the threshold. For a review of commercially available clinical stereopsis tests, see Cooper (1991).

Cyclodeviations

Subtle incomitant deviations can also be difficult to detect, particularly superior oblique palsies (see below). One reason for this is that the primary action of the superior oblique muscle is intorsion, and yet cyclotorsion is often not assessed. Probably the best test of cyclotorsion is the double Maddox rod test (Evans 2007a), but other tests include the Maddox wing test and asking about any tipping of the Nonius markers in the Mallett fixation disparity test. These tests are described in more detail in the next section.

Diagnosis and management of binocular vision anomalies

Decompensated heterophoria

Diagnosis

In any busy clinic, an optometrist will see many patients with heterophoria. This is a normal finding, and heterophoria only requires treatment if it is decompensated. A decompensated heterophoria occurs when the vergence system fails to compensate adequately with fusional (or disparity) vergence for a heterophoria, typically causing symptoms and/or an intermittent strabismus.

If a previously compensated heterophoria has become decompensated, then the practitioner needs to consider why this occurred. A number of factors could explain this, including changes in working conditions (e.g. more near work when school exams approach), changing visual status (e.g. visual loss from pathology such as cataract or retinal pathology), debility (e.g. tiredness or illness), or emotional stress. The practitioner needs to take a holistic approach.

The symptoms of decompensated heterophoria can be divided into three categories (Evans 2007a): visual (blur, diplopia, distorted vision), binocular factors (difficulty with stereopsis, monocular comfort, difficulty changing focus) and asthenopia (headache, aching eyes, sore eyes). These symptoms are non-specific: they can result from conditions other than decompensated heterophoria. The practitioner therefore needs to carry out clinical tests to make a differential diagnosis and the key clinical tests in the diagnosis of decompensated heterophoria will now be summarized.

In decompensated heterophoria the cover test recovery movement is typically poor. Specifically, as the eye that has deviated behind the cover regains fixation, its movement to regain alignment may be hesitant, slow, faltering, or inaccurate. In people who are too young, intellectually impaired, or uncooperative to give subjective results, the cover test may be the only method of determining whether a heterophoria is decompensated. A grading system for quantifying cover test recovery is summarized in **Table 16.2** (Evans 2007a).

Studies have found that for near heterophoria the aligning prism measured with the near Mallett unit is the best single subjective test for detecting symptomatic heterophoria (Jenkins et al 1989; Yekta et al 1989; Pickwell et al 1991; Karania & Evans 2006). This instrument detects fixation disparity, yet in an environment that simulates normal reading conditions. In particular, the instrument has both peripheral and, more importantly, foveal fusion locks **(Fig. 16.3)**. It is only the green strips in **Figure 16.3** that are seen monocularly,

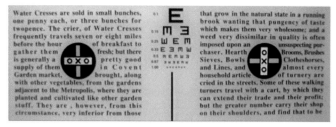

Fig. 16.3 The Mallett near-vision-unit fixation disparity test. The test for investigating horizontal deviation is shown on the left and that for assessing vertical deviation is on the right.

when wearing appropriately polarized filters, and which are therefore indicators for any fixation disparity. The patient is asked to look at the central X and to report any misalignment, however subtle. Any misalignment or movement (Karania & Evans 2006) of one or both strips indicates that under naturalistic viewing conditions the visual axes do not maintain perfect alignment. This in turn indicates that the patient may be having trouble compensating for their heterophoria. If symptoms are present, then treatment or correction is indicated.

The Mallett fixation disparity test does not measure fixation disparity, but rather the aligning prism (also termed associated heterophoria) or aligning sphere, i.e. the prism or sphere that eliminates any fixation disparity. Recent research has demonstrated that higher degrees of aligning prism are associated with more severe symptoms (**Fig. 16.4**; Karania & Evans 2006). Usually, the aligning prism or aligning sphere that eliminates the fixation disparity with the Mallett unit is likely to correct any symptoms. Indeed, randomized, controlled trials have found that the aligning prism based on the Mallett unit can significantly improve symptoms (Payne et al 1974) and reading performance (O'Leary & Evans 2006). The aligning prism will, of course, be much smaller than the dissociated heterophoria, because the Mallett unit

is designed to detect only that component of the heterophoria for which the patient is unable to compensate. The Mallett fixation disparity test is not infallible, and the practitioner should become suspicious if the instrument indicates a very large prism or sphere when the deviation is quite small or the fusional reserves are good (see below). Decompensated heterophoria can be treated with eye exercises or corrected with prisms or spheres (see later section).

Fusional reserves (vergence ranges)

In most cases, symptoms, cover test recovery, and the Mallett fixation disparity test are the only tests that are necessary to determine whether a heterophoria is compensated. Sometimes, these 'core tests' may give equivocal or contradictory results and additional data are required for diagnosis. In these cases, it is useful to measure the fusional reserves (also termed vergence ranges), which are also helpful for measuring the effect of treatment. The fusional reserves can be measured at any working distance, but their measurement is most relevant at the distance(s) at which the heterophoria may be decompensated. Fusional reserves are typically measured with a prism bar (**Fig. 16.5**) or with the rotary prisms in the phoropter, and the fusional reserve that opposes the heterophoria should be measured first (Rosenfield et al 1995). For example, in exophoria the convergent reserve is measured first, using base-out prisms (to force the patient to converge). The patient is asked to fixate a detailed (accommodative) isolated target, one line above the acuity of the worse eye and the prism bar is held in front of one eye, starting with the weakest prism strength (**Fig. 16.5**). The prisms should be changed at the rate of about $1-2\Delta$ per second (Evans 2007a) and the patient should be asked to report if/when the target blurs (blur point), and becomes diplopic (break point). The patient's eyes are observed to confirm the break point (when vergence ceases) and then the prism is reduced until recovery (single vision and ocular alignment) occurs. The other fusional reserve is then measured.

Positive and negative fusional reserves may also be termed positive and negative relative vergence (PRV and

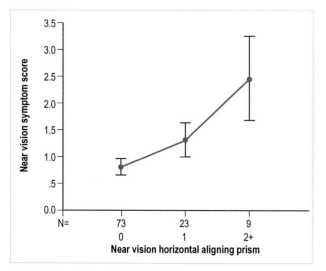

Fig. 16.4 Graph showing the relationship between the severity of symptoms and the degree of horizontal aligning prism (prism diopters) at near. The error bars represent the standard error of the mean (SEM). The number of participants (N; shown above scale for horizontal axis) is small for higher degrees of aligning prism and this may explain why the SEM increases. (Reproduced with permission from Karania & Evans 2006.)

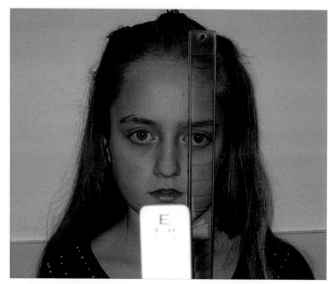

Fig. 16.5 Fusional reserves measured with a prism bar.

NRV), since these tests require the patient to adjust their vergence response while keeping the accommodative response constant. These tests are analogous to the measurements of positive and negative relative accommodation (PRA and NRA), which are discussed in Chapter 15. In considering the component changes shown in **Figure 15.7**, it is apparent that binocular single vision will be lost when either the patient is no longer able to change disparity vergence in the appropriate direction or they can change their vergence response but must make a corresponding change in blur-driven accommodation to accompany it. The former will result in the target becoming double, while the latter will result in the target becoming blurred.

When testing the vertical reserves, either base-up or base-down prism is introduced before one eye. Since base-up prism before the right eye stimulates a downward movement, this test is also referred to as right infravergence (RI). Similarly, base-down prism before the right eye will stimulate right supravergence (RS). Since vertical eye movements are being tested, there is no accommodative component involved and, accordingly, the patient should not be asked about a blur point when testing the vertical reserves. Expected findings for horizontal and vertical reserves are shown in **Table 16.3**.

The fusional reserves can assess two criteria that were classically used to evaluate heterophoria (Evans 2007a). Sheard's criterion is useful in exophoria and states that the fusional reserve (to blur point, or if no blur point then to break point) that opposes the heterophoria should be at least twice the heterophoria. For example, if a patient has a near exophoria of 8Δ (e.g. by cover testing) then Sheard predicts that the convergent fusional reserve should be at least 16Δ to avoid symptoms. Percival's criterion is useful in esophoria and says, in essence, that the fusional reserves should be balanced so that the larger one is less than twice the smaller one. For example, if a patient has a convergent fusional reserve at distance of 20Δ to blur point, then a divergent reserve (to blur point) of 11Δ would pass Percival's criterion, but 9Δ would fail.

Table 16.3 Expected findings for fusional reserve (or vergence range) testing (from Morgan 1944)

Values are given in the format: blur/break/recovery. The X value for distance base-in range indicates that the patient did not report a blur finding, but rather saw the target become double before it blurred. This is the normal finding for this particular condition, as there should be a

testing the vertical ranges, only break and recovery are determined.

Viewing distance (m)	Prism base direction	Findings
6	Base-out	9/19/10
6	Base-in	X/7/4
0.40	Base-out	17/21/11
0.40	Base-in	13/21/13
6	Base-up or base-down	3.5/2
0.40	Base-up or base-down	3.5/2

Dissociated heterophoria

The size of the deviation in heterophoria is a poor predictor of whether it is compensated. This is why most emphasis in this chapter is given to the cover test, as a method of detecting, quantifying, and assessing the recovery of a heterophoria. The Mallett fixation disparity test is also emphasized since this is reasonably sensitive and specific at determining whether heterophoria is compensated (Jenkins et al 1989; Yekta et al 1989). But there are occasions when it is useful to quantify the angle of the heterophoria, particularly for monitoring vertical deviations, which can be difficult to detect with cover testing.

Dissociation tests are useful for this purpose and work by presenting each eye with dissimilar (non-fusible) targets. Thus, separate images are created for the right and left eyes, and the patient is asked about the relative position of the image seen by one eye, compared with the image seen by the fellow eye. For distance testing, the most commonly used tests are the Maddox rod, Modified Thorington and Von Graefe tests. In the Maddox rod (or groove) test, one eye views a spotlight (also termed a muscle light) through a (usually) red lens with deep grooves ground into the lens, which distorts the light into a line. For testing horizontal deviations, the Maddox rod is introduced with the grooves horizontal, so that the patient will see a vertical line (also called a streak). The other eye sees the spotlight and the patient is asked for the relative position of the line with respect to the spot. In cases of esophoria, the images will be seen in uncrossed diplopia, with the right eye's target on the right-hand side of the left eye's target. For exophoria, the images will appear in crossed diplopia, with the right eye's target on the left. This can easily be remembered by noting that 'eXo' contains a cross in the middle of it. When testing vertical deviations, the Maddox rod is introduced with the grooves vertical, so that the patient sees a horizontal streak. For right hyper and left hyper deviations, the right eye's image will appear below and above the left eye's image, respectively. Once the direction of deviation has been determined, prisms can be introduced before one or both eyes, until the line or streak appears to be passing through the light. The amount of prism required to bring the images into alignment is a measure of the dissociated deviation.

A useful variation of the test is to use two Maddox rods, one before each eye and preferably of the same colour (Simons et al 1994) with their axes vertical so that two horizontal lines are seen. If they are separated, then there is a vertical deviation and if one appears tipped then there is a cyclodeviation. The eye whose image is tipped is usually the eye with a palsied cyclovertical muscle.

The modified Thorington test (**Fig. 16.6**) uses a Maddox rod over one eye whilst the patient views a light that is shone through a small central hole in a card. The card includes horizontal and vertical rows of numbers, calibrated in prism dioptres for the appropriate distance. This method has shown excellent repeatability and, as with other dissociated tests, the best results are obtained with a trial frame rather than a phoropter (Casillas & Rosenfield 2006).

The Von Graefe test uses dissociating prisms to create diplopic images. The patient views a single isolated letter, one line larger than the VA of the worse eye, and a 6Δ base-up prism is introduced before one eye. This will create vertical

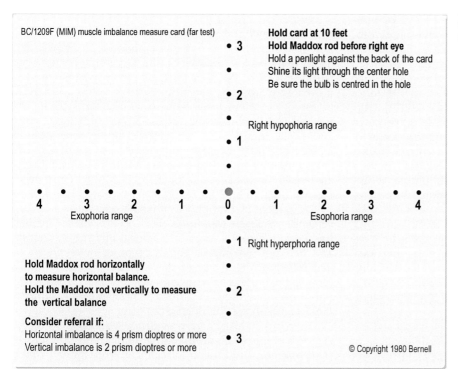

BC/1209F (MIM) muscle imbalance measure card (far test)

Hold card at 10 feet
Hold Maddox rod before right eye
Hold a penlight against the back of the card
Shine its light through the center hole
Be sure the bulb is centred in the hole

Right hypophoria range

4   3   2   1   0   1   2   3   4
Exophoria range   Esophoria range

Right hyperphoria range

Hold Maddox rod horizontally
to measure horizontal balance.
Hold the Maddox rod vertically to measure
the vertical balance

Consider referral if:
Horizontal imbalance is 4 prism dioptres or more
Vertical imbalance is 2 prism dioptres or more

© Copyright 1980 Bernell

Fig. 16.6 The distance Modified Thorington test (Bernell Corp., Mishawaka, IN).

diplopia, and the patient is asked about the relative position of one eye's image with respect to the fellow eye's image. Again, patients with eso- and exo-deviations will see the images in uncrossed and crossed diplopia, respectively. Once the direction of deviation has been determined, prism is introduced (usually in front of the eye that does not have the vertical dissociating prism in place) until the images appear one directly beneath the other. It is useful to take two readings, adjusting the prism power in opposite directions (i.e. from base-out to base-in, and from base-in to base-out) and average these. For assessment of the vertical deviation, base-in dissociating prism is introduced to produce horizontal diplopia. For distance viewing, 12Δ base-in prism is usually sufficient to create diplopia, although larger amounts of prism are often required at near. Again, the patient is asked if one image is higher than the other, and, if so, appropriate vertical prism is introduced until the images are lined up 'side by side'. Several investigations have determined that the repeatability of the Von Graefe test is significantly poorer than the Modified Thorington procedure (e.g. Morris 1960; Rainey et al 1998; Casillas & Rosenfield 2006).

When testing pre-presbyopic patients at near, the test targets should control accommodation, and the Maddox wing is a suitable dissociation test. Usually, the horizontal deviation is measured first and the instrument uses a septum so that one eye sees a scale and the other eye an arrow. The number on the scale to which the arrow points indicates the horizontal deviation. This instrument is also well suited to measuring the AC/A ratio, which describes the effect of accommodation on vergence. For example, an emmetropic patient gives a result for the horizontal heterophoria of 8Δ esophoria. The practitioner wants to determine what effect plus lenses will have on this deviation and places a pair of +2.00 DS lenses in the Maddox wing instrument.

The patient now reports that the arrow points to 0. The accommodative stimulus was reduced by 2 D, and the vergence angle has changed by 8Δ. So, the AC/A ratio is 8/2 = 4Δ/D. The Maddox wing test also has scales for measuring the vertical heterophoria and cyclophoria. These aspects of the test are particularly useful because cyclovertical deviations are difficult to detect on cover testing, but can be suggestive of incomitant deviations (see below).

The Modified Thorington and Von Graefe techniques may also be used to measure the dissociated deviation at near. Similar procedures are carried out to those for distance measurement. It is frequently quoted in the literature that the Maddox rod test should not be used to measure horizontal deviations at near because the light represents an inadequate stimulus to accommodation. However, Casillas & Rosenfield (2006) reported that the Maddox rod technique had a high level of repeatability for near testing, particularly when used with a trial frame.

There are many other types of dissociation test, which will not be described in detail here. These include Scobee's test (found on some projector charts), where red/green filters are used so that one eye sees a red cross and the other two green circles, and various haploscopic devices (e.g. synoptophore). It is important to note that none of the dissociation tests described above will differentiate between heterotropia and heterophoria since they only assess the deviation under dissociated viewing conditions. Only the unilateral cover test (or cover/uncover test) will indicate which of the two types of oculomotor deviation is present.

The type of heterophoria and the distance at which it is present or problematic can be important. A cyclovertical deviation is unusual and is suggestive of an incomitant deviation, typically a superior oblique palsy (discussed below in the section on incomitancy). An eso-deviation at distance or near should cause the practitioner to suspect hyperopia and in young patients a cycloplegic refraction would be indicated. An exo-deviation at near is common and can decompensate for any of the reasons listed earlier in this section, and may be linked to convergence insufficiency (see below). Although the Mallett fixation disparity test works well for detecting symptomatic heterophoria at near, it does not work so well for distance vision (Evans 2007a). This may be explained by the different nature of decompensated heterophoria at distance. The most common form of decompensating distance deviation is divergence excess exo-deviation. Patients with this condition may have a well-compensated exophoria or even orthophoria at distance for much of the time, but on occasions the heterophoria spontaneously breaks down into a large-angle exotropia. The patient is typically asymptomatic since they suppress the deviating eye. These cases can often be diagnosed from symptoms alone, and the clinical findings may be normal at the time of testing. In some cases the deviation is only apparent when the patient is looking in the far distance, at objects much further away than a 6 m letter chart.

Near point of convergence

Convergence insufficiency (CI) and decompensated exophoria at near are common conditions that often (but not always) occur together. Convergence insufficiency is, quite literally, a remote near point of convergence (NPC). This is measured by bringing a target in towards the eyes until the patient reports diplopia (subjective break point) or one eye is seen to stop converging, i.e. turn outwards (objective break point). The distance of the target from the eye is the near point of convergence. For pre-presbyopes, an accommodative (detailed) target should be used, although the patient should be encouraged to keep watching the target even after it has become blurred. The normal range of convergence is typically given as 6–10 cm (Hayes et al 1998), but an acceptable near point of convergence depends on the distance at which a person wishes to view near targets.

A pass/fail criterion of 6 cm might be appropriate for a child with short arms, and exceptionally 10 cm for an adult whose only near work is on a computer monitor at 50 cm. It is also useful to measure the recovery value. Once diplopia has been reported (or one eye seen to move outwards), the target is moved away from the patient until single vision is achieved, or the deviated eye turns back in to take up fixation. The recovery value should be around 7 cm (Scheiman et al 2003). The near point of convergence should be considered in the context of the near point of accommodation: it has been suggested that symptoms in convergence insufficiency are largely the result of accompanying accommodative insufficiency (Marran et al 2006).

Decompensated exophoria at near is also known as convergence weakness exophoria. This occurs when a patient has a decompensated exophoria at near but not at distance, and it is not uncommon for this type of heterophoria to decompensate. This may or may not be associated with a remote near point of convergence. The precise diagnosis (CI or decompensated exophoria at near or both) is important because this will influence the most appropriate type of eye exercises. Whilst there is evidence that a battery of eye exercises is more helpful than just simple push-up exercises (Convergence Insufficiency Treatment Trial Study Group 2008), it would seem intuitively sensible to concentrate therapy on the main weakness. In an individual case the practitioner can determine whether it is the near point of convergence or the convergent fusional reserve that requires the greatest emphasis during treatment.

Management

The main approaches to the management of decompensated heterophoria are summarized in **Table 16.4**. It is beyond the scope of this chapter to describe management in detail, but some general guidance will now be given.

In any young person with decompensated esophoria, latent hyperopia should be suspected. A cycloplegic

Table 16.4 Summary of the main approaches to the treatment of decompensated heterophoria

Management	Advantages	Disadvantages	Indicated for:	Contra-indicated for:
Eye exercises	May avoid the need for spectacles	Requires time & effort from patient & practitioner	Convergence insufficiency. Decompensated near exophoria. Esophoria (harder than exophoria)	Cyclovertical deviations
Refractive correction	If a refractive error is the cause of decompensation, then refractive correction is the proper treatment	Requires spectacle or contact lens wear or refractive surgery	Decompensated esophoria from latent hyperopia. Decompensated exophoria from onset of myopia	Other types of decompensated heterophoria (but refractive modification may be appropriate)
Refractive modification	The refractive modification is gradually reduced, so the 'exercises glasses' are a treatment. Requires no effort from patient	Requires spectacle wear, fairly frequent check-ups & changes of spectacles (e.g. every 3 months)	Decompensated near esophoria (multifocals). Decompensated exophoria ('negative add')	Older patients. Decompensated distance esophoria. Cyclovertical deviations
Prismatic correction	Simple approach. Helpful temporarily if too busy for exercises	Possible (but unlikely; North & Henson 1992) that patient will adapt to prism	Decompensated hyperphoria, esophoria, exophoria	Decompensated cyclophoria
Surgery	Can be helpful in rare cases that do not respond to other forms of management, but best considered as 'last resort'	Surgery may lack the accuracy for subtle degrees of decompensated heterophoria	Large-angle exophoria. Large-angle esophoria where no hyperopia. Cyclovertical incomitancies	Subtle deviations Cases that can be treated with other, less invasive, approaches

refraction is usually required and if significant hyperopia is found then refractive correction is indicated.

Decompensated exophoria commonly occurs at near and this generally responds well to eye exercises. A battery of exercises is more successful than simple push-up exercises (Convergence Insufficiency Treatment Trial Study Group 2008), although quite sophisticated therapy can be prescribed in a package designed for home use (Evans 2000).

Refractive modification is an underused approach to treatment, and is particularly suitable for the cases listed in **Table 16.4** when the patient is of a suitable age and is not keen on eye exercises. Surgery is only very rarely needed for heterophoria.

Strabismus

For the primary care optometrist, the approach that needs to be taken in dealing with strabismus will vary with the age of the patient and with the interval since the strabismus first developed. This section will deal with four combinations of these factors.

Adults with long-standing strabismus

Most cases of strabismus that are encountered in optometric practice are adults where the history indicates that the strabismus has been present since early childhood. These patients generally have no symptoms from their strabismus because they have sensory adaptations (harmonious abnormal retinal correspondence and/or suppression) that developed at the time of onset of the strabismus (Evans 2007a). In managing these patients it is best to try not to interfere with the sensory adaptations or the angle of strabismus. If there is a constant unilateral strabismus then care should be taken not to force the patient to start fixating with the strabismic eye, since this could cause fixation switch diplopia (Kushner 1995). This is only likely to happen if the practitioner prescribes a refractive correction that forces the patient either to fixate with the strabismic eye (e.g. monovision; Evans 2007b) or to look into the field of action of a paretic muscle (e.g. progressive addition lenses in a patient with a superior oblique palsy).

Occasionally, problems might also result from a refractive correction that gives a very large change in the clarity of vision in the strabismic eye (e.g. previously uncorrected anisometropia) or in the angle of deviation (e.g. corrected hyperopia for the first time in accommodative strabismus). A cautious approach in these cases would be to try the refractive correction for a few minutes in a trial frame, ideally whilst testing for any change in the sensory adaptations to the strabismus (Evans 2007a).

Adults with a recent-onset strabismus

The development of strabismus in an adult is a cause for concern because it could be a sign of ocular, orbital, or central nervous system pathology. These cases should be referred, and the speed of onset of the strabismus (and accompanying diplopia) will be a guide to the urgency of referral. An exception to this rule is if the patient is known to have a long-standing, barely compensated heterophoria, and some environmental (e.g. new job involving a change in visual activities) or systemic (e.g. febrile illness) factor has caused this to decompensate, resulting in strabismus.

In these cases, the primary care optometrist may be able to manage the condition, but careful monitoring is necessary to ensure that any management is successful and that the condition does not continue to deteriorate. If it does, then referral is required.

Children with recent-onset strabismus

It is common for parents to bring a child to an optometrist because a 'turning eye' has been noticed. If these cases are strabismus of recent onset then the prognosis is good, especially if the strabismus is intermittent. The primary care optometrist will need to determine whether there is a cause for the strabismus which can be managed in optometric practice. **Table 16.5** presents a guide to these cases.

If a refractive cause for the deviation (e.g. hyperopia in accommodative esotropia) can be found, then a pathological factor is unlikely and, as long as the binocular status does not worsen, the optometrist is in a good position to treat the problem. In another scenario, the optometrist may have been monitoring a large exophoria for some time, which then breaks down into an exotropia when the child undertakes increased near-vision activities at school. Treatment with exercises or minus lenses is entirely appropriate in optometric practice. But if a deviation develops or changes for an unknown reason, then the patient must be referred promptly so that the necessary scans and other neuro-ophthalmological tests can be carried out to determine the aetiology. For the same reason, any new or changing incomitant deviation must be referred. Finally, any case that cannot be corrected in optometric practice (see **Table 16.5**) or does not respond to optometric treatment requires referral.

An overriding factor is the need to treat strabismus of recent onset urgently. If the patient has recently had normal binocular vision, then the prospects for regaining normal binocular vision are good if treatment is timely. As the strabismus becomes more firmly established, not only does the potential for correcting the strabismus reduce, but also the risk of amblyopia increases (see below).

Children with long-standing strabismus

These cases are most commonly found in older children who have developed sensory adaptations to the strabismus (harmonious abnormal retinal correspondence and/or suppression) and therefore are probably asymptomatic. Larger deviations may need to be referred if surgery is desired for cosmetic reasons.

Microtropia has been defined in several ways (Evans 2007a), but is invariably characterized by a small-angle ($<10\Delta$) strabismus. There is typically a good cosmetic appearance and good sensory adaptations, and in some cases there is no movement on cover testing, which can make diagnosis very difficult. These cases are likely to have reduced or absent stereoacuity and suppression. Suppression can be detected with the Mallett polarized letters test (Tang & Evans 2007).

In microtropia, there is often a good argument for not attempting to treat the deviation, unless it is of recent onset and is easily managed (e.g. by correcting a refractive error). Care should be taken to ensure that any treatment aimed at correcting the strabismus does not cause intractable diplopia, which is possible if there are deep sensory adaptations. But in all children with strabismus, due attention must be paid to treating any amblyopia (see next section).

Table 16.5 Summary of the management of recent-onset paediatric strabismus in primary care optometric practice

Type of strabismus	Features	Treatment	Best setting for treatment
Incomitant strabismus	Strabismus that varies with direction of gaze and with fixating eye	Monitoring, maybe surgery	These cases require neuro-ophthalmological investigation of aetiology and often surgical management, so need referral
Fully accommodative esotropia	Esotropia that is fully corrected by refractive correction of the hyperopia	Spectacles or contact lenses	The patient will need frequent refraction, monitoring of binocular status, and checks of the spectacle or contact lens fit. Suitable for management in optometric practice
Non-accommodative basic esotropia	Esotropia at distance & near that is not significantly influenced by correction of any refractive error	Surgery	Refer to investigate aetiology & surgery The community optometrist may start treatment of amblyopia whilst referring
Partially accommodative esotropia	Esotropia whose angle is reduced by refractive correction	Spectacles & possibly surgery	Optometric practice and/or referral The optometrist can correct the full cycloplegic hyperopia, initiate amblyopia treatment, & refer
Convergence excess esotropia	Esotropia at near	Multifocals (possibly surgery)	Most cases can be corrected with multifocals and these cases can be managed in optometric practice, but should be monitored & referred if the binocular status worsens
Divergence excess exotropia	Exotropia at distance	Refractive over-minus or exercises or surgery	The presentation of the case will determine the most appropriate treatment and therefore the best setting for treatment. New or markedly changing deviations require referral
Convergence weakness exotropia	Exotropia at near	Eye exercises or refractive over-minus	Most of these cases are long-standing exophoria that has decompensated and can be treated in the primary care setting. Surgery is not usually required. Cases should be monitored & referred if the binocular status worsens.
Basic exotropia	Exotropia of similar degree at distance and near	Refractive over-minus or exercises or surgery	The presentation of the case will determine the most appropriate treatment and therefore the best setting for treatment. New or changing deviations require referral

Some children who have long-standing strabismus will have infantile esotropia syndrome: this is esotropia that occurs in the first year of life. Most of these cases do not have a refractive aetiology and require surgery, but very few ever regain normal binocular vision. These cases are often left with strabismus, no binocular vision, dissociated vertical deviation (DVD), inferior oblique overaction, and latent nystagmus. Latent nystagmus is discussed towards the end of this chapter. In the most common presentation of DVD there is the appearance of 'alternating hyperphoria': in the cover test, whichever eye is about to be covered deviates upwards.

Amblyopia

Diagnosis

Amblyopia is defined as a visual loss resulting from an impediment or disturbance to the normal development of vision (Evans 2007a). The two diagnostic criteria for amblyopia that are used most commonly are either a difference in each eye's acuity of two lines or more, or acuity in the amblyopic eye of worse than 6/9. An amblyogenic factor will also need to be present. The most common causes are anisometropia and/or strabismus.

Typically, amblyopia is detected by the primary care optometrist when a patient presents who either complains of reduced vision in one eye or is asymptomatic. Many children with amblyopia do not notice the reduced vision and are surprised when the optometrist covers the good eye during the measurement of visual acuity. When significantly reduced vision is found in one eye, then the diagnosis of amblyopia requires two stages: the exclusion of a non-amblyopic cause and the inclusion of an amblyogenic factor. The exclusion requires a careful eye examination to rule out pathology and significant refractive error. The checks for pathology can be carried out in the primary care setting and the practitioner will need to concentrate on: fundus examination, pupil reactions, and visual field testing if the patient is old enough. A careful refraction, usually with cycloplegic, is required and the best corrected visual acuities will reveal whether the reduced vision can be immediately corrected simply by a refractive correction, in which case the patient does not have amblyopia.

In addition to excluding pathology and simple refractive error, the practitioner needs to confirm the presence of amblyogenic factors. The two commonest causes of amblyopia are anisometropia and strabismus (other causes were reviewed by Evans 2007a). Anisometropia and strabismus may both be present, so each should be looked for in every case. Microtropia can be difficult to diagnose (eccentric fixation is usually present), but the diagnosis is important because the management of amblyopia is different for cases where any form of strabismus is present (**Fig. 16.7**). If an amblyogenic factor is not found, then the diagnosis of

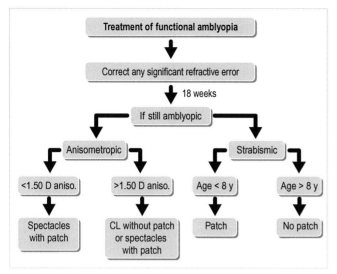

Fig. 16.7 Summary of the management of amblyopia. The second box, 'correct any significant refractive error', is known as *refractive adaptation*. CL, contact lenses. (Modified with permission from Evans 2007a Pickwell's binocular vision anomalies, Elsevier, Oxford.)

amblyopia is unsafe and the patient should be referred for more detailed investigation for ocular disease.

Management

Assuming that an amblyogenic factor is found, the first stage is to correct any significant refractive error. It has long been recognized that the treatment of amblyopia starts with correction of the refractive error (Gibson 1955), and recent research has shown that, on occasion, amblyopia can be cured by several weeks of spectacle wear, in both anisometropic and strabismic cases (Stewart et al 2004a). This research has shown that the recommended period of *refractive adaptation* is about 18 weeks, and occlusion is only indicated if the patient still meets the diagnostic criteria for amblyopia after this interval.

The mode of refractive correction is a subject that has received too little attention. All types of anisometropia experience less aniseikonia with contact lenses than with spectacles (Winn et al 1988), and contact lenses are therefore the best optical solution in anisometropia (Evans 2006a). Of course, contact lenses should only be fitted when the patient meets the usual criteria for safe contact lens wear.

If the patient is still amblyopic after the 18-week period of refractive adaptation then the approach to treatment will depend on the type of amblyopia and the patient's age (see **Fig. 16.7**). A recent review of the literature on the treatment of amblyopia reveals a distinction between the effect of age on the treatment of anisometropic and strabismic amblyopia (Evans 2007a). For this distinction, cases that have both anisometropia and strabismus (including microtropic cases) should be treated as strabismic amblyopia. In strabismic amblyopia, there is a significant effect of age, so patients under the age of about 8 years can be treated with occlusion, but patients over the age of about 8 years should not usually be treated with prolonged periods of occlusion. This cutoff at age 8 years is approximate: some authorities say 7 years, some 10 years, and some 12 years. The reasons for not treating older cases of strabismic amblyopia are that treatment is less likely to be effective and

could cause the binocular sensory adaptations to the strabismus to break down, possibly causing intractable diplopia. It is not impossible to treat strabismic amblyopia over the age of 8 years with patching (Simmers et al 1999), but such treatment should only be undertaken by experienced practitioners who can closely monitor the patient, including monitoring binocular sensory adaptations to the strabismus (Evans 2007a).

The most common form of occlusion is direct occlusion with an eye patch. The cases that are most likely to be treated in optometric practice are those aged between about 5 and 8 years. Younger children may require specialist acuity tests and more careful monitoring because of the risk of occlusion amblyopia; so these preschool cases are best managed by paediatric optometrists or other specialists. Children between 5 and 8 years of age can be managed by most community optometrists, assuming, of course, that the optometrist has the necessary expertise and is used to dealing with children. Recent studies suggest that part-time occlusion (3 hours a day) is as effective as more prolonged occlusion (PEDIG 2003a), and atropine can be of similar effectiveness to patching (PEDIG 2003b). Whatever treatment is attempted, it is likely to be enhanced if the child is encouraged to carry out detailed visual tasks. The most important factor is compliance, and poor compliance is extremely common (Awan et al 2005). Practitioners must take a realistic approach, carefully explaining the need for treatment and monitoring the patients closely. Another advantage to frequent checks is that any adverse reactions can be detected. Adverse reactions are rare, but if the patient starts to experience diplopia then patching should be stopped. When monitoring acuity improvement the test conditions should be kept similar on each occasion, the optotypes should be crowded, and the child should be prevented from memorizing the chart. Computerized test charts are particularly helpful in achieving these objectives.

For cases of non-strabismic anisometropic amblyopia, the literature indicates that treatment, including patching, can be effective at virtually any age (Evans 2007a). Although most studies have found no large effect of age on the success of treatment, it seems likely that the greater plasticity in the visual system will confer some advantage to treatment at a younger age. Therefore, anisometropic amblyopia usually should be treated when first detected in children. As noted above, contact lenses are the preferred option, from an optical point of view (Evans 2006a). The advantages of contact lenses over spectacles increase with the degree of anisometropia. Initially, contact lenses should be tried without occlusion, but if the acuity does not improve then some occlusion may also be required (see below).

Most children are able to tolerate the correction of quite high degrees of anisometropia in spectacles, but adults who have not worn spectacles to correct their anisometropia before may have difficulties tolerating them, particularly if the anisometropic correction is greater than approximately 1.50 D. Some of these cases might prefer a balance lens for the more ametropic eye, but this decision should only be made after full discussion with the patient, since some people would rather have a full correction, perhaps with contact lenses, in view of the possibility of improving the visual function in the amblyopic eye.

In paediatric cases, the full anisometropic correction (as revealed by cycloplegic) should be prescribed to bring about the best possible improvement in the amblyopic eye. If the eye does not improve with refractive correction alone, then patching is indicated. In non-strabismic anisometropic amblyopia, prolonged occlusion is contraindicated, since this could cause the binocular vision to break down; 2–3 hours a day of occlusion is usually adequate. Careful monitoring is required and the state of compensation of any heterophoria should be routinely assessed.

Cases of anisometropic amblyopia require regular refractive checks, either contact lens aftercare or regular adjustments to their spectacles and careful monitoring of visual acuities and ocular health. Anisometropic amblyopia is usually detected later than strabismic amblyopia, and most of these cases can be treated successfully in primary care optometric practice.

Any case of amblyopia that does not respond as expected to treatment should be referred in case neuroimaging is required. Current guidelines are that neuroimaging is not appropriate in cases of monocular reduced vision where an amblyogenic factor is present, but if a case does not respond to treatment and/or if the presentation is atypical in any other way, then further investigations may be necessary. It is important for practitioners who treat amblyopia to start treatment without delay and to monitor the patient closely. This means that any failure of treatment to bring about the expected improvement will be detected rapidly so that appropriate referral can take place without undue delay.

Notwithstanding the preceding comments, it must be explained as part of the informed consent to treatment that an improvement cannot be guaranteed. Some cases which do not respond to treatment may have a subtle form of optic nerve hypoplasia (Lempert 2000). There is some debate about the period of occlusion that is necessary before it can be concluded that treatment is not working (Evans 2007a). In one recent study that preceded occlusion with 18 weeks of refractive adaptation, 80% of the improvement with occlusion occurred within 6 weeks (Stewart et al 2004b).

Incomitancy

With incomitant deviations, the angle of deviation varies as the patient looks in different directions of gaze, and may also vary depending upon which eye is fixating. In this section, emphasis will be placed on the types of incomitancy that are seen most frequently in optometric practice.

Incomitant deviations can result from serious (and in some cases potentially life-threatening) pathology, and any new or changing incomitancy requires urgent referral for neuro-ophthalmological examination. When compared with long-standing incomitancies, new or changing incomitant deviations are more likely to have diplopia, an awareness of the onset, similar acuities in each eye, a markedly abnormal head posture, and past-pointing in the field of action of the affected muscle. Old photographs can be helpful to indicate long-standing deviations, and long-standing cyclovertical incomitancies typically have larger than average vertical fusional reserves opposing the deviation. It will be assumed in the rest of this section that the incomitant deviation is long-standing.

The classification of incomitant deviations is summarized in **Table 16.6**, which gives commonly encountered examples.

Diagnosis

The diagnosis of incomitant deviations may be possible from the ocular motility test alone, but in many cases it is not easy to be sure of a diagnosis from this test. It is useful to obtain a plot of the movements of each eye in different positions of

Table 16.6 Summary of classification of incomitant lesions

Classification	Description	Examples
Mechanical	Resulting from a mechanical restriction to the movement of one or more muscles	Duane's syndrome Brown's syndrome
Myogenic	Resulting from a problem affecting the muscle itself	Myasthenia gravis
Neurogenic	Caused by a problem with one of the cranial nerves that innervate the extraocular muscles	Fourth nerve palsy Sixth nerve palsy Third nerve palsy
Supranuclear or internuclear	The lesion occurs at or above the level of the nuclei in the mid-brain that control the extraocular muscles	Internuclear ophthalmoplegia

gaze when fixating with each eye in turn, i.e. a Hess screen plot. This has been made easier in the primary care setting by the development of the Thomson Software Solutions PC Hess screen (available from Thomson Software Solutions, London, www.thomson-software-solutions.com).

A careful assessment of the ocular motor status at both distance and near will also provide valuable information: for example, a lateral rectus palsy is characterized by an eso-deviation which is greater at distance than at near.

The cyclovertical incomitancies are particularly difficult to diagnose. Various algorithms are available, such as the Parks three step test, which analyse the results of a step-by-step testing method to provide a diagnosis of the underacting muscle (Evans 2007a). Although the Parks three step test is best known, an alternative approach (Lindblom's) which usually gives very clear results is described in **Table 16.7** (Lindblom et al 1997; Evans 2007a).

The incomitant deviations that are most commonly seen in optometric practice will now be described in turn. The key features relating to diagnosis will be summarized.

Duane's syndrome

Duane's syndrome is a congenital restrictive incomitancy affecting the abduction and/or adduction of one or both eyes. There are usually no symptoms, as the patient adopts a compensatory head posture and moves their head rather than their eyes when looking in the field of action of the affected muscle(s). The motility picture is characteristic: the affected eye(s) will look as if it is tethered and will not move or hardly move in abduction and/or adduction. Usually, the palpebral aperture narrows (globe retracts) in adduction. There are three types with, confusingly, two different methods of classification (Evans 2007a). It is simplest for the clinical notes to describe the appearance rather than using a classification, which may be unknown to subsequent clinicians. Previously uninvestigated cases should be referred since there are occasionally associated systemic conditions.

Fourth nerve palsy

A fourth nerve palsy affecting the action of the superior oblique muscle is often congenital or can be acquired, quite commonly from a road traffic accident or other traumatic event. In acquired cases, diplopia is usually present and is predominantly vertical

Table 16.7 Procedure for Lindblom's method of differentially diagnosing cyclovertical incomitancies

The test instructions are given on the left and the paretic muscles indicated by a given answer on the right

		Diagram representing patient's view	
If the patient has vertical diplopia then they should view, from a distance of 1 m, a 70 cm horizontal wooden rod (if a wooden rod is not available, then a 50 cm or 1 m ruler will suffice). If the patient does not have vertical diplopia, then two red Maddox rods can be used, placed in a trial frame with axes at 90°, so that when the patient views a spotlight at a distance of 1–3 m they see two horizontal red lines.			
Question 1: Move the wooden rod (or spotlight) up and down & ask: Where is the vertical diplopia (or separation of the red lines) greatest, in upgaze or downgaze?	Up gaze: RSR, RIO, LSR, LIO Downgaze: RIR, RSO, LIR, LSO	separation greatest in upgaze	separation greatest in downgaze
Question 2: In the position of maximum diplopia, are the two images parallel or torsional?	Parallel: RSR, RIR, LSR, LIR Torsional: RSO, RIO, LSO, LIO	parallel	torsional
Question 3: If parallel, does the separation increase on right or left gaze?	Right gaze: RSR, RIR Left gaze: LSR, LIR	left gaze	right gaze
Question 4: If tilted, does the illusion of tilt increase in upgaze or downgaze?	Upgaze: RIO, LIO Downgaze: RSO, LSO	tilt greatest in upgaze	tilt greatest in downgaze
Question 5: If tilted, then the two rods will resemble an arrow (< or >) or an X. If they resemble an arrow, which way does the arrow point (to the patient's right, or to the patient's left)?	The arrow will point to the side with the paretic eye. Arrow points to right: RSO, RIO Arrow points to left: LSO, LIO	arrow points to patient's left	arrow points to patient's right
Question 6: If the two rods resemble an X, does the tilt angle increase in upgaze or downgaze?	Upgaze: bilateral IO paresis (v. unlikely) Downgaze: bilateral SO paresis	tilt angle greatest in upgaze	tilt angle greatest in downgaze

Adapted with permission, from Evans 2005 Eye essentials: binocular vision. Elsevier, Oxford.

(and torsional), usually worse in downgaze. In fourth nerve palsy there is typically a head tilt and a hyperdeviation that is worse when the affected eye looks down and in, so multifocal lenses may be contraindicated.

The condition can be difficult to diagnose for several reasons. Firstly, the main action of the superior oblique muscle is intorsion, yet few practitioners test for torsional deviations. In any case of suspected cyclovertical imbalance a test of torsion is advisable. One of the best tests is a double Maddox rod test, but even the tilting arrow on the Maddox wing test will provide useful information. Secondly, the hyperdeviation of the affected eye on looking down and in can be subtle and difficult to see on motility testing because the lid and nose obscures the practitioner's view. Thirdly, secondary sequelae are often present which complicate the clinical picture. Secondary sequelae are adaptations that occur to extraocular muscle palsies over time, sometimes described as a spreading of the comitance (Evans 2007a). In a long-standing superior oblique paresis, there is often a secondary restriction of the contralateral superior rectus, which can be more apparent than the original superior oblique paresis.

Sixth nerve palsy

A sixth nerve palsy affecting the lateral rectus muscle can be congenital or acquired, for example from raised blood pressure, intracranial pressure or trauma. There is often a head turn, and predominantly horizontal diplopia which is worse when the patient looks in the distance and to the side of the affected eye. Clinically, there is likely to be an eso-deviation for distance vision which is worse when looking to the affected side. Long-standing cases can be confused with Duane's syndrome, although if globe retraction is present on adduction, this indicates Duane's syndrome.

Third nerve palsy

The third nerve is responsible for many ocular motor functions, and the clinical presentation of a third nerve palsy varies depending on which of these functions are affected. Total third nerve palsy will cause ptosis (which may prevent diplopia), a fixed dilated pupil, and an eye which is depressed and abducted. All cases of sudden onset require emergency referral.

Brown's syndrome

Brown's (superior oblique tendon sheath) syndrome is a usually congenital, restrictive (mechanical) incomitancy caused by an abnormality of the superior oblique tendon sheath which prevents this muscle from feeding out through the trochlear pulley. There is an inability to elevate the eye when abducted, which is often misdiagnosed as an inferior oblique paresis. An inferior oblique paresis is the rarest of all the extraocular muscle restrictions, and is much less likely to be present than a Brown's syndrome. In a true inferior oblique paresis there will be an overaction of the superior oblique muscle, a positive Park's three step (or Lindblom's test; **Table 16.7**); and a compensatory head posture.

Management

New or changing incomitant deviations require urgent referral for neuro-ophthalmological investigation. The urgency of the referral is indicated by the speed of onset of the symptoms. If a patient presents with an incomitant deviation that occurred suddenly that day then immediate emergency referral is indicated. If the deviation has been occurring intermittently for a year or two, but appears to be gradually increasing in frequency, then an 'early' rather than 'urgent' neuro-ophthalmological investigation would be more appropriate.

Optometrists are more likely to see long-standing stable incomitant deviations which will not require referral unless the patient is bothered by symptoms or by the cosmesis. If the incomitancy occurred in adult life there is likely to be diplopia. If the degree of diplopia is subtle, then the effect of prisms can be investigated. Although no one prism power is likely to be completely satisfactory in all positions of gaze, the prism that eliminates any diplopia or decompensated heterophoria in the primary position may be helpful by enlarging the patient's field of comfortable and single binocular vision.

Care should be taken not to prescribe an optical intervention that could cause a patient with a long-standing incomitancy to fixate with their strabismic eye, unless they already alternate. For these cases, monovision refractive correction is contraindicated. In contrast, a patient with a recent subtle incomitant deviation that is causing troublesome diplopia may find monovision to be helpful because this will encourage them to fixate with one eye at a time and to suppress central vision in the other (Evans 2006a). If this approach is used then the patient should be monitored carefully to ensure that the deviation remains stable and that, when the monovision correction is not worn, the diplopia does not worsen.

Nystagmus

Primary care optometrists only occasionally encounter nystagmus, and this will usually be long-standing. Acquired nystagmus always requires prompt referral for neuro-ophthalmological investigation of the underlying aetiology, as does early-onset nystagmus when it is first detected (usually in the first few months of life). Nystagmus that occurs early in life is nearly always either early-onset nystagmus (*synonyms*: infantile nystagmus syndrome, congenital nystagmus) or latent nystagmus. The latter condition is associated with an early interruption to binocularity, typically infantile esotropia syndrome. The differential diagnosis of the main types of nystagmus is shown in **Table 16.8**.

There is often a latent component to nystagmus: the deviation increases when one eye is covered. As the name suggests, this is particularly marked in latent nystagmus. When determining the refractive error of these cases it is better not to cover one eye, but instead to use a plus lens to blur the eye that is not being tested. The best view of the ocular fundi is often obtained with photography, where the shutter speed will usually mean that the photograph is unaffected by the eye movements.

There are no treatments for nystagmus that have been validated by randomized, controlled trials (Evans 2006b). Many

Table 16.8 Differential diagnosis of the three main types of nystagmus

Early-onset nystagmus	Latent nystagmus	Acquired nystagmus
Presents in first 6 months of life	Usually presents in first 6 months of life, and almost always in first 12 months	Onset at any age and usually associated with other symptoms (e.g. nausea, vertigo, movement or balance disorders)
Family history often present	May be family history of underlying cause (e.g. infantile esotropia syndrome)	History may include head trauma or neurological disease (e.g. multiple sclerosis)
Oscillopsia absent or rare under normal viewing conditions	Oscillopsia absent or rare under normal viewing conditions	Oscillopsia common; may also have diplopia
Usually horizontal; although small vertical and torsional movements may be present. Pure vertical or torsional presentations are rare	Always horizontal; and, on monocular occlusion, saccadic, beating away from the covered eye (so direction reverses when occluder is moved from one eye to the other)	Oscillations may be horizontal, vertical, or torsional depending on the site of the lesion
The eye movements are bilateral and conjugate to the naked eye	Oscillations are always conjugate	Oscillations may be disconjugate and in different planes
May be present with other ocular conditions: albinism, achromatopsia, aniridia, optic atrophy	Usually occurs secondary to infantile esotropia syndrome; sometimes in association with DVD	Results from pathological lesion or trauma affecting motor areas of brain or motor pathways
A head turn may be present, usually to utilize a null zone	May be a head turn in the direction of the fixating eye	There may be a gaze direction in which nystagmus is absent, and a corresponding head turn
Intensity may lessen on convergence but it is worse when fatigued or under stress	More intense when the fixating eye abducts, less on adduction	

DVD, dissociated vertical deviation.
Reproduced with permission from Evans 2005 Eye essentials: binocular vision. Elsevier, Oxford.

patients with infantile-onset nystagmus have a null zone: a position of gaze (often convergence) in which the nystagmus is lessened and in which the acuity improves. Several authors have advocated prisms or surgery to utilize the null zone, and other surgical approaches have been advocated. However, there has only been one randomized, controlled trial of a therapy for nystagmus and the result of this was negative (Evans et al 1998). Initial reports of this intervention were very positive (Mallett 1983), and the results of the subsequent randomized, controlled trial indicated that practice and placebo effects can be quite large in infantile-onset nystagmus (Evans et al 1998). It would therefore seem prudent for surgical approaches to be investigated with randomized controlled trials before they are widely advocated (Evans 2006b).

One small study that did control for the placebo effect, through an elegant experimental design, indicated that contact lenses can be helpful in early-onset nystagmus (Dell'Osso et al 1988). The mechanism appears to be via lid sensation, so rigid gas-permeable lenses will probably be most helpful. These can also correct the corneal astigmatism that often accompanies the condition.

Other conditions

Accommodative anomalies

Accommodative anomalies are characterized by inadequate amplitude or control of accommodation. Accommodation is not a binocular function, so accommodative anomalies will not be described in detail in this chapter. However, it should be noted that accommodative anomalies are often associated with binocular vision anomalies. Assessment of binocular function in pre-presbyopic patients should always be accompanied by an evaluation of accommodative status (see Ch. 15).

Visual stress/Meares–Irlen syndrome

Visual stress (Wilkins 1995), also known as Meares–Irlen syndrome (Evans 1977), is a condition characterized by symptoms of visual perceptual distortions (e.g. text moving, blurring, glare from the page; symptoms of eyestrain, headaches, and visual discomfort) when viewing text (Evans 2001). The condition is particularly common in people with dyslexia, autism, migraine, or epilepsy. Dyslexia is also sometimes associated with binocular instability, a subtle form of decompensated heterophoria, which has similar symptoms to visual stress (Evans 2001). These cases therefore require a detailed optometric assessment, including binocular vision assessment and testing for visual stress, to facilitate an appropriate differential diagnosis (Evans 2005b).

Declaration of interest

The author designed a system of eye exercises for treating convergence insufficiency and decompensated near exophoria (Evans 2000). These exercises are marketed by i.o.o. Sales, which raises funds for the Institute of Optometry, a charitable organisation. i.o.o. Sales pays a small 'award to inventors' to the author.

References

Awan M, Proudlock F A, Gottlob I 2005 A randomized controlled trial of unilateral strabismic and mixed amblyopia using occlusion dose monitors to record compliance. Investigative Ophthalmology and Visual Science 46:1435–1439

Casillas C E, Rosenfield M 2006 Comparison of subjective heterophoria testing with a phoropter and trial frame. Optometry and Vision Science 83:237–241

Convergence Insufficiency Treatment Trial Study Group 2008 Randomized clinical trial of treatments for symptomatic convergence insufficiency in children. Archives of Ophthalmology 126:1455–1456

Cooper J 1991 Stereopsis. In: Eskridge J B, Amos J F, Bartlett J D (eds) Clinical procedures in optometry. Lippincott, Philadelphia, pp 121–134

Dell'Osso L F, Traccis S, Abel L et al 1988 Contact lenses and congenital nystagmus. Clinical Vision Sciences 3:229–232

Evans B J W 1997 Coloured filters and dyslexia: what's in a name? Dyslexia Review 9:18–19

Evans B J W 2000 An open trial of the Institute Free-space Stereogram (IFS) exercises. British Journal of Optometry and Dispensing 8:5–14

Evans B J W 2001 Dyslexia and vision. Whurr, London

Evans B J W 2005a Eye essentials: binocular vision. Elsevier, Oxford

Evans B J W 2005b Case reports: the need for optometric investigation in suspected Meares-Irlen syndrome or visual stress. Ophthalmic and Physiological Optics 25:363–370

Evans B J W 2006a Orthoptic indications for contact lens wear. Contact Lens and Anterior Eye 29:175–181

Evans B J 2006b Interventions for infantile nystagmus syndrome: towards a randomized controlled trial? Seminars in Ophthalmology 21:111–116

Evans B J W 2007a Pickwell's binocular vision anomalies, 5th edn. Elsevier, Oxford

Evans B J W 2007b Monovision: a review. Ophthalmic and Physiological Optics 27:417–439

Evans B J, Evans B V, Jordahl-Moroz J et al 1998 Randomised double-masked placebo-controlled trial of a treatment for congenital nystagmus. Vision Research 38:2193–2202

Gibson H W 1955 Amblyopia. In: Textbook of orthoptics. Hatton, London, pp 170–194

Hayes G J, Cohen B E, Rouse M W et al 1998 Normative values for the nearpoint of convergence of elementary schoolchildren. Optometry and Vision Science 75:506–512

Jenkins T C A, Pickwell L D, Yekta A A 1989 Criteria for decompensation in binocular vision. Ophthalmic and Physiological Optics 9:121–125

Jenkins, T C A, Abd Manan F, Pardhan S et al 1994 Effect of fixation disparity on distance binocular visual acuity. Ophthalmic and Physiological Optics 14:129–131

Jenkins T C A, Abd-Manan F, Pardhan S 1995 Fixation disparity and near visual acuity. Ophthalmic and Physiological Optics 15:53–58

Karania R, Evans B J 2006 The Mallett fixation disparity test: influence of test instructions and relationship with symptoms. Ophthalmic and Physiological Optics 26:507–522

Kushner B J 1995 Fixation switch diplopia. Archives of Ophthalmology 113:896–899

Lempert P 2000 Optic nerve hypoplasia and small eyes in presumed amblyopia. Journal of the American Academy of Pediatric Ophthalmology and Strabismus 4:258–266

Lindblom B, Westheimer G, Hoyt W F 1997 Torsional diplopia and its perceptual consequences: a 'user-friendly' test for oblique eye muscle palsies. Neuro-Ophthalmology 18:105–110

Mallett R F J 1983 The treatment of congenital idiopathic nystagmus by intermittent photic stimulation. Ophthalmic and Physiological Optics 3:341–356

Marran L F, De Land P N, Nguyen A L 2006 Accommodative insufficiency is the primary source of symptoms in children diagnosed with convergence insufficiency. Optometry and Vision Science 83:281–289

Morgan M W 1944 Accommodation and its relationship to convergence. American Journal of Optometry and Archives of the American Academy of Optometry 21:183–195

Morris F M 1960 The influence of kinesthesis upon near heterophoria measurements. American Journal of Optometry and Archives of the American Academy of Optometry 37:327–351

North R V, Henson D B 1992 The effect of orthoptic treatment upon the vergence adaptation mechanism. Optometry and Vision Science 69:294–299

O'Leary C I, Evans B J W 2006 Double-masked randomised placebo-controlled trial of the effect of prismatic corrections on rate of reading and the relationship with symptoms. Ophthalmic and Physiological Optics 26:555–565

Payne C R, Grisham J D, Thomas K L 1974 A clinical examination of fixation disparity. American Journal Optometry and Physiological Optics 51:88–90

Pediatric Eye Disease Investigator Group (PEDIG) 2003a A randomized trial of patching regimens for treatment of moderate amblyopia in children. Archives of Ophthalmology 121:603–611

Pediatric Eye Disease Investigator Group (PEDIG) 2003b A comparison of atropine and patching treatments for moderate amblyopia by patient age, cause of amblyopia, depth of amblyopia, and other factors. Ophthalmology 110:1632–1637

Pickwell L D, Kaye N A, Jenkins T C A 1991 Distance and near readings of associated heterophoria taken on 500 patients. Ophthalmic and Physiological Optics 11:291–296

Rainey B B, Schroeder T L, Goss D A et al 1998 Inter-examiner repeatability of heterophoria tests. Optometry and Vision Science 75:719–726

Rosenfield M, Ciuffreda K J, Ong E et al 1995 Vergence adaptation and the order of clinical vergence range testing. Optometry and Vision Science 72:219–223

Scheiman M, Gallaway M, Frantz K A et al 2003 Nearpoint of convergence: test procedure, target selection, and normative data. Optometry and Vision Science 80:214–225

Simmers A J, Gray L S, McGraw P V et al 1999 Functional visual loss in amblyopia and the effect of occlusion therapy. Investigative Ophthalmology and Visual Science 40:2859–2871

Simons K, Arnoldi K, Brown M H 1994 Color dissociation artifacts in double Maddox rod cyclodeviation testing. Ophthalmology 101:1897–1901

Stewart C E, Moseley M J, Fielder A R et al and the MOTAS cooperative 2004a Refractive adaptation in amblyopia: quantification of effect and implications for practice. British Journal Ophthalmology 88:1552–1556

Stewart C E, Moseley M J, Stephens D A et al 2004b Treatment dose-response in amblyopia therapy: the Monitored Occlusion Treatment of Amblyopia Study (MOTAS). Investigative Ophthalmology and Visual Science 45:3048–3054

Tang S T W Evans B J W 2007 The near Mallett unit foveal suppression test. Ophthalmic and Physiological Optics 27:31–43

Wilkins A J 1995 Visual stress. Oxford University Press, Oxford

Winn B, Ackerley R G, Brown C A et al 1988 Reduced aniseikonia in axial anisometropia with contact lens correction. Ophthalmic and Physiological Optics 8:341–344

Yekta A A, Pickwell L D, Jenkins T C A 1989 Binocular vision, age and symptoms. Ophthalmic and Physiological Optics 9:115–120

CHAPTER 17

Examination of the anterior segment of the eye

Keith Edwards • Jerome Sherman • Joan K Portello • Mark Rosenfield

Introduction

Examination of the anterior segment of the eye includes the assessment of the external eye and adnexa, tear film, ocular surfaces, anterior chamber and crystalline lens. The choice of examination procedures is based on the structure to be examined, the level of detail required and the specific abnormality anticipated.

Evaluation is conducted either to establish baseline conditions or to evaluate specific symptoms or signs. A wide range of instrumentation can be used, ranging from the simplest, such as a hand-held slit torch (flashlight), to the more technologically complex optical coherence tomography (OCT) or ultrasound biomicroscopy (UBM). While the slit-lamp biomicroscope is the standard method for assessing the integrity of the anterior region of the eye, the need to conduct a detailed examination may also be indicated by other techniques used routinely in optometric examination.

In addition, measurement of the curvature of the anterior corneal surface is performed to quantify the power (and astigmatism) of the anterior corneal surface, the most powerful refractive element in the eye.

Corneal curvature and topography

Keratometry

The goals of keratometry are:

1. To assist with ocular refraction by estimating both the magnitude and direction of ocular astigmatism
2. To determine the site of ocular astigmatism (corneal or non-corneal)
3. To assist in the fitting of contact lenses by measuring the corneal radius of curvature
4. To gain information on corneal health from the quality of the reflected mire
5. To gain information as to whether the ocular ametropia is likely to be axial or refractive. For example, in patients having high degrees of ametropia whose keratometry findings are close to the mean value, such as a 10 D myope with corneal power around 42 D, it may be concluded that refractive error is probably axial in nature. In contrast, a 10 D myope having corneal power of approximately 52 D is likely to have refractive aetiology. Differentiating between axial and refractive ametropia is important in the treatment of anisometropia and aniseikonia (Bartlett 1987).

Optical principles

The keratometer uses the anterior corneal surface as a convex mirror. Consider **Figure 17.1**. The image (h') of an object or mire (h) contained within the

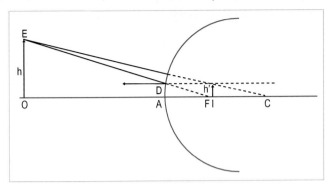

Figure 17.1 Principle of keratometry. The anterior corneal surface is considered as a convex mirror. An image (h') is formed by reflection at I from the object or mire (h) positioned at O. F and C represent the focal point and centre of curvature of the mirror, respectively.

keratometer is produced by reflection at the anterior cornea. Let C be the centre of curvature of the convex surface, F the focal point of the mirror and h and h' the height of the object and image, respectively.

Now triangles FDA and FEO are similar. Therefore FA/FO = DA/EO = h'/h.

But FA = f, where f is the focal length of the mirror.

If FO = b, then IO is approximately equal to b (since AO is large).

And h'/h = f/b.

But h'/h = m (where m is the magnification of the optical system)

Therefore, f/b = m.

Since f = −r/2 (where r = radius of curvature of the curved mirror)

Then r = −2mb.

This equation, r = −2mb, is known as the *approximate keratometer equation*, due to the approximation that IO is approximately equal to FO. Therefore, the radius of curvature of the cornea can be calculated provided b (the approximate distance from the mire to the reflected image), h (the height of the mire) and h' (the height of the reflected image) are known.

Distance from the object to the image (b)

The optics of the keratometer ensures that this distance remains constant, provided both the focusing graticule and the image are kept in focus throughout the measurement

procedure. As shown in **Figure 17.2**, the focusing graticule, objective lens and mire are all fixed within the keratometer. While the spacing between these elements is fixed and remains constant, focusing of the reflected mire is achieved by moving the whole instrument either towards or away from the patient's cornea.

The first step in keratometry is to focus the eyepiece, thereby making the observer's retina conjugate with the focusing graticule. This is achieved by turning the eyepiece fully anticlockwise, and then rotating it in a clockwise direction until the graticule just comes into focus. The instrument is then moved either towards or away from the patient's cornea until h' (the image of the mire formed by reflection) appears clear. Many keratometers use the Scheiner disc principle so that the image seen will be doubled when out of focus. At this point h' is conjugate with both the focusing graticule and the observer's retina. Since the distance between the focusing graticule and the objective is fixed, then h' will appear clear when it lies at a constant distance away from the objective lens.

Accordingly, when both the graticule and h' appear clear, the distance from h' to the objective lens is known. Additionally, the distance of the mire (h) from the objective lens is fixed and constant. Therefore, provided h' is in focus, then the distance between h' and h (i.e. b) will be constant for a particular instrument. The size of the object (h) is also fixed. To calculate r, the only unknown variable in the approximate keratometer equation is h' (the size of the reflected image). This can be measured using the principle of doubling.

Using the principle of doubling to measure the height of the image (h')

Since the cornea (the convex reflecting surface), and therefore the reflected image, is moving constantly, the height of h' cannot be assessed using a measuring graticule. Rather, the principle of doubling is used to measure the height of this image.

If a prism is introduced into the optical system, then h' will be seen diplopically, as shown in **Figure 17.3**. The magnitude of deviation (in centimetres) is equal to the product of the prism power (in prism dioptres) and the distance between the prism and the image (in metres). By varying this distance, the degree of deviation created by the prism will change. A position can be reached where the two diplopic images just touch one another. At this point

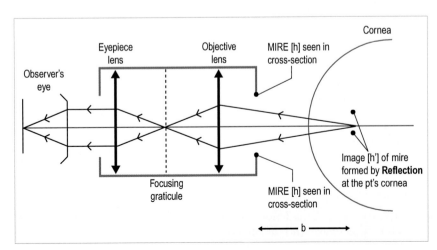

Figure 17.2 Schematic representation of the keratometer. The observer first ensures that the focusing graticule is seen in focus. A mire (h) positioned at the front of the instrument produces an image (h') by reflection at the patient's anterior corneal surface. The keratometer is moved anteroposteriorly until this reflected image appears clear when viewed through the optical system. Since the distance between the objective lens and the focusing graticule is constant, the distance between h' and the objective lens will also be constant (provided h' is seen clearly). If the distance from the object mire (h) to the objective lens is known, then b, the approximate distance between the mire and the reflected image will also be known.

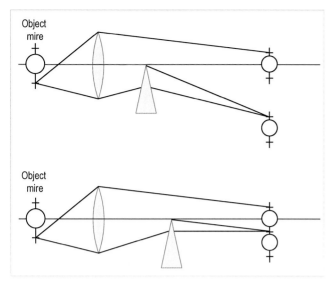

Figure 17.3 Principle of doubling. The prism produces a double image of the target (the image formed by reflection at the cornea). The position of the prism is adjusted along the optical axis until the two images just touch one another (*lower diagram*). At this point, the displacement produced by the prism (the product of the prism power and the separation of the prism from the target) is equal to the height of the reflected image. (Redrawn with permission from Goss and Eskridge 1991.)

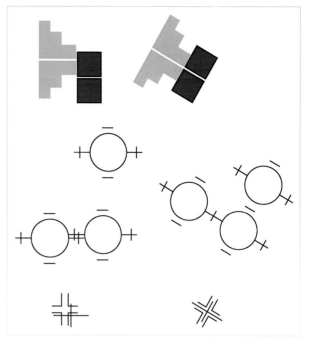

Figure 17.4 Three examples of keratometry mires. In each case, the left-hand figure shows the appearance of the mires when the instrument is not aligned along a principal meridian of the eye, and the right-hand figure illustrates the appearance of the mires when the instrument is aligned along one of the principal meridia of the eye. Mires are shown from the Javal-Schiötz/Haag-Streit (*top figures*), Bausch and Lomb (*middle figures*) and Zeiss instruments (*bottom figures*).

the amount of deviation is equal to the height of h'. For example, consider when part of the reflected image is viewed through a 4△ prism to create diplopic images. The diplopic images just touch one another when the prism lies 33 cm away from the image. Therefore, the deviation = 0.33 × 4 = 1.32 cm, and this is equal to the height of the image.

Variable and fixed doubling

In the Bausch and Lomb type keratometer, the magnitude of prismatic deviation (or doubling) is varied by altering the position of the prisms within the instrument, and therefore from h' (the image formed by reflection at the cornea). This is known as a *variable doubling* instrument. Other types of keratometers such as the Haag-Streit (or Javal Schiötz type) instrument use the principle of *fixed doubling*. Here, the degree of doubling (or prismatic deviation) remains constant since both the magnitude and position of the prisms are fixed. However, the size of the object (h) is varied until the diplopic images just touch one another. At this point, the prismatic deviation is equal to the image height. The size of the object (h) can be measured easily to calculate r.

One- and two-position keratometers

The Bausch and Lomb type of keratometer is a one-position instrument because it can measure both principal meridia without having to reposition the instrument. In contrast, the Haag-Streit (Javal Schiötz) type of instrument is termed a two-position instrument because it only measures one meridian at a time. After measuring the first principal meridian, the instrument must be rotated through 90° to determine the second meridian. One potential advantage of a two-position instrument is for patients having irregular astigmatism, i.e. where the principal meridia are not 90° apart. However, the Bausch and Lomb type of one-position instrument may still be used by aligning the lower two mires only, and treating the device as if it were a two-position

instrument. The lower two mires are aligned along one of the principal meridia, and then the instrument rotated to identify the second principal meridian, and the same two mires realigned.

Mires may be of three principal types: the circular (Bausch and Lomb) mire, the cross (Zeiss) mire and the rectangular (Javal Schiötz) mire. In all cases there are linear components to the mires which must align with each other to identify the astigmatic axes. Examples of different types of mires, and their appearance when positioned along, or away from, the principal meridia are shown in **Figure 17.4**.

Curvature or power?

Keratometers actually measure the radius of curvature of the anterior corneal surface. If this is to be expressed in terms of dioptric power, then the equation F = (n′−n)/r is applied, with n′ and n representing the refractive index of the cornea and air, respectively. Unfortunately, different manufacturers use dissimilar values of n′ in this calculation. For example, if two keratometers from different manufacturers assume a corneal refractive index of 1.332 and 1.3375, then when measuring a cornea having a radius of curvature of 8.2 mm, these two instruments would give powers of 40.49 D and 41.16 D, respectively, i.e. a difference of 0.67 D.

Procedure

The procedure described below is for the one-position, Bausch and Lomb type of keratometer. If a two-position instrument is used, then a similar procedure is adopted, except that after the first principal meridian has been identified and measured, the instrument is rotated through 90°, and the second principal meridian identified and measured.

1. Focus the eyepiece for the examiner's refractive error. This is facilitated by placing a piece of white paper in front of the instrument objective in the plane of the patient's eye, while viewing the eyepiece graticule. Alternatively, have the patient close their eyes and view the graticule against their closed eyelid. Turn the eyepiece fully anticlockwise (maximum plus) and then return it in a clockwise direction until the graticule is just seen in sharp focus.

2. Adjust the height of the instrument and/or patient's chair to be at a comfortable level for both patient and examiner. Ensure that the instrument headrest and chinrest are clean. An alcohol wipe is suitable for this purpose.

3. Explain the purpose of the test to the patient; for example, this machine will measure the shape of the front of your eye.

4. Ask the patient to place their chin on the chinrest and forehead against the headrest. Note that during the examination, patients sometimes allow their forehead to move away from the headrest. This will make obtaining accurate readings more difficult. Emphasize to the patient that they should try to keep their head and eye as still as possible during the test. Occlude the non-tested eye to ensure measurement along the visual axis.

5. The height of the instrument may be approximately aligned by raising or lowering it until the levelling markers are at the same height as the patient's outer canthus. Then turn the instrument on, and the horizontal alignment can be completed by centring the reflection of the keratometer mires on the patient's cornea. An alternative method of aligning the instrument is to place a small light source, e.g. a penlight or a transilluminator, against the eyepiece and adjust the keratometer so that the emergent light falls on the patient's cornea. The patient should now be able to see an image of their eye in the instrument and should be instructed to look at this. Complete the alignment procedure by looking into the eyepiece and making adjustments so that the graticule is centred in the lower right-hand circle.

6. Focus the instrument until the doubling mire (lower right-hand circle) is single.

7. Adjust the horizontal and vertical power wheels until the mires are in close apposition.

8. Rotate the barrel of the instrument until the horizontal markers between the two lower circles are superimposed. This aligns the instrument along a principal meridian.

9. While maintaining the exact focus of the instrument by keeping one hand on the focusing knob (it may be necessary to re-focus frequently because of movement of the patient's eye), adjust the horizontal power wheel until the horizontal plus signs are superimposed.

10. While maintaining the image in focus, adjust the vertical power wheel until the minus signs are superimposed. The correct final appearance of the mires should be as shown in **Figure 17.4**.

11. From the horizontal power wheel, record the power of the horizontal meridian.

12. From the vertical power wheel, record the power of the vertical meridian.

13. From the instrument protractor, record the location of the two principal meridia.

Recording findings

Method 1

The result may be recorded by stating the dioptric power and orientation of the two principal meridia, e.g. either:

$$42.00 \, @ \, 45/43.75 \, @ \, 135$$

or

$$42.00 \, M \, 45/43.75 \, M \, 135$$

(where M = meridian)

Method 2

The result can be quantified in terms of the radius of curvature in millimetres, e.g. either:

$$7.80 \, @ \, 25/8.05 \, @ \, 115$$

or

$$7.80 \, M \, 25/8.05 \, M \, 115$$

Method 3

The result may be recorded as the cylinder required to correct the corneal astigmatism. If minus cylinder form is preferred, then the cylinder axis corresponds with the orientation of the weaker-powered meridian. Therefore, the example shown in Method 1 above can be written as:

$$-1.75 \times 45 \, AM \, 42.00$$

(where AM indicates the power in the axis meridian, which in this case is 45°).

Extending the range of the keratometer

The normal range of the keratometer is from 36.00 to 52.00 D, but for extremely steep corneas (such as those found in keratoconus patients), the range can be extended by holding a +1.25 trial lens against the front of the instrument. Readings must be corrected by reference to a conversion table, such as that presented by Horner et al (2006). Similarly, the lower range can be extended by approximately 6 D (e.g. in a post-LASIK patient) with a −1.00 trial lens.

Javal's rule

In 1890, Javal proposed an equation to predict the ocular astigmatism from keratometric measurements, namely:

$$OA = (1.25 * CA) + k$$

where OA = ocular astigmatism

CA = corneal astigmatism

k = 0.50 D against-the-rule astigmatism.

For those patients where objective and subjective techniques to determine the refractive error of the eye (see Chs 13 and 14) are unsuccessful, this equation can be applied to the keratometry findings to estimate the magnitude and direction of ocular astigmatism.

This equation assumes that patients with a spherical cornea will have 0.50 D of against-the-rule non-corneal astigmatism; an assumption that is not born out in practice. Javal did state that the constants 1.25 and 0.50 in the equation above were not definitely established, and that a new factor as a function of age would have to be added. However, Mote and Fry (1939), Grosvenor and Ratnakaram (1990) and others have offered alternative equations. For example, Grosvenor and Ratnakaram (1990) suggested that a better equation is OA = CA + k. In addition, Portello et al (1996) reported a significant change in the relationship between ocular and corneal astigmatism with increasing age. Accordingly, while these relationships are useful for examining average data from large populations, they are of limited value when estimating the astigmatism of an individual patient.

Potential sources of error in keratometry have been reviewed elsewhere (Edwards 1997).

Topographical keratoscopy

If the cornea were a spherical surface, keratometry would be a suitable method for determining overall corneal curvature. However, on average, the corneal surface is aspheric, approximating an evolute and usually described as a flattening ellipse (Douthwaite et al 1996; Guillon et al 1986) although there is considerable variation between individuals. Additionally, the conventional keratometer measures an annulus around (but not including) the corneal apex. The precise position and area measured varies with the corneal radius of curvature, and also with the type of instrument used.

In order to gain more information about the overall shape of the cornea, it is necessary to collect data outside the central corneal cap. Corneal topography can also be assessed with off-axis keratometry. In its simplest form this can be achieved using keratometers modified with peripheral fixation targets (Wilms & Rabbetts 1977; Lam &

Douthwaite 1994). For a general review of corneal topography, see Fowler and Dave (1994).

More recently, automated keratometers have been used to assess both central and paracentral curvature and corneal asphericity (Rabbetts 1985; Port 1987). However, these may provide only limited information if only the horizontal corneal meridian is used to determine the degree of eccentricity. Small but significant differences have been observed between corneal eccentricity for the horizontal and vertical meridia (Guillon et al 1986; Douthwaite et al 1996). For a more thorough estimation of corneal shape, topographers are required that take measurements from a large number of points on the corneal surface. Two principal methods are used in topographers, based on either videokeratoscopy, which reflects concentric rings onto the corneal surface, or using scanning slits to build up elevation maps of the corneal surface.

Videokeratoscopy

By reflecting concentric rings from the anterior corneal surface, multiple data points can be analysed in each corneal meridian. The separation of the rings imaged in the cornea is compared to the known separation of the object, and corneal power can be estimated on a point-by-point basis. These analyses are used to generate colour-coded corneal power maps and show overall topographical data (**Fig. 17.5**).

While all videokeratoscopic devices are based on the same principle, the methods of image capture and analysis algorithms vary, and this can give rise to differences in output for the same cornea. Comparisons of different topographers on the same eyes have shown that their outputs cannot be used interchangeably and may not be reliable when used with young children (Cho et al 2002; Chui & Cho 2005). The reproducibility of results has also been questioned, with multiple readings being necessary to improve precision. In addition, the number of readings varies with instrument manufacturer (Hough & Edwards 1999; Cho et al 2002). There is also some doubt about the accuracy of the

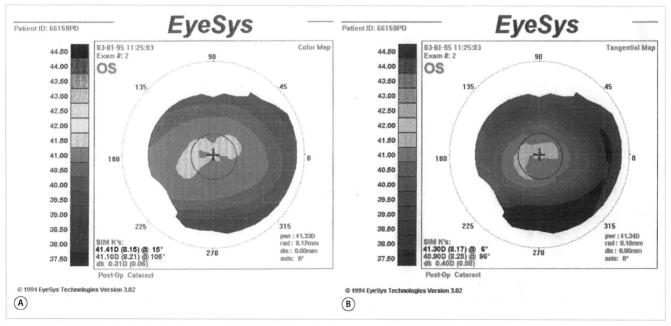

Figure 17.5 A typical print-out from a videokeratoscope; **(A)** shows the axial power map while **(B)** shows the tangential power map for the same patient.

instruments when measuring human corneas as opposed to fixed plastics surfaces (Douthwaite & Matilla 1996; Pardhan & Douthwaite 1998; Douthwaite 2003).

Different analyses can be used to measure various aspects of corneal power. Axial power can be calculated at any point by considering rays that are parallel to the axis of rotation of the cornea. A more robust optical approach is to calculate 'instantaneous' or tangential power where rays approaching normal to the surface at any given point are considered. Asymmetry in the corneal shape determined by videokeratoscopy may also be an artefact. Since the instrument is aligned around the fixation axis, which may not coincide with the axis of rotation of the cornea, some apparent tilt may become evident. As a result, further data analysis might be necessary to eliminate these artefacts (Douthwaite et al 1996; Douthwaite & Pardhan 1998; Douthwaite 2003).

More recently, experimental devices have been examined to determine their utility in assessing non-rotational, symmetric shape features of the cornea such as might arise from pathology or trauma (Sicam & Van der Heijde 2006). Preliminary results suggest that they achieve this goal without sacrificing the ability to model the normal aspects of corneal shape.

Scanning slit keratoscopy

An alternative approach to topography can be achieved by scanning the cornea with a slit object and capturing the reflected images. An elevation map can be constructed subsequently by combining the images to create a single model of the cornea being scanned. Since the output of such a reconstruction algorithm will be different from that determined by optical calculation, instruments such as the Orbscan (Bausch and Lomb Inc., Rochester, NY) also include a keratoscopic disc to allow the calculation of optical power by similar means to other videokeratoscopes. Other instruments such as the Pentacam (Oculus, Inc,. Lynnwood, WA) combine slit scanning corneal topography with a Scheimpflug camera.

Comparisons of scanning slit and videokeratoscopes have shown both to be valuable for research and clinical purposes (Gonzalez et al 2004). While the print-outs are very similar to those of videokeratoscopes, additional data can be included (**Fig. 17.6**).

A significant benefit of the scanning slit technology is that it allows imaging and therefore modelling of both the anterior and posterior cornea. As a result, corneal thickness can be calculated at any point on the cornea. Since the iris is also imaged, the anterior chamber depth can be determined. While there are differences between optical pachymetry from scanning slit devices and ultrasound pachymetry (see Ch. 24), both are capable of measuring changes in corneal thickness (Basmak et al 2006; Buehl et al 2006; Cheng et al 2006; Thomas et al 2006).

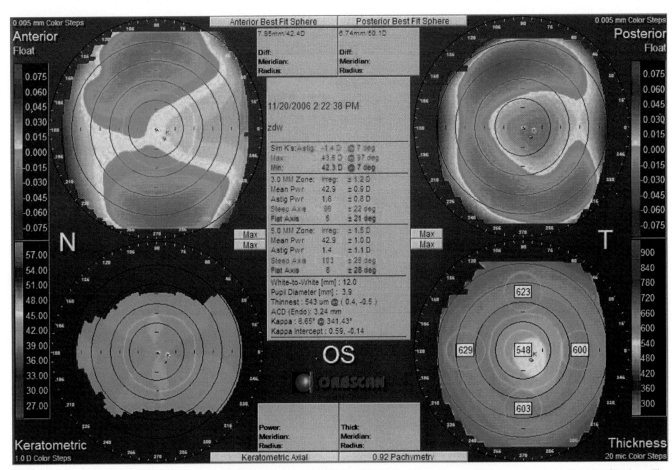

Figure 17.6 A print-out from the Orbscan scanning slit keratoscopy. The upper-left plot shows the anterior surface elevation relative to a best-fit sphere. The upper-right plot shows posterior corneal surface elevation relative to a best-fit sphere. The values of each best-fit sphere are shown between the two plots. The lower-left plot is axial power and the lower-right plot shows corneal thickness at predetermined points. Thickness at other points can be read by moving the cursor over the map. The central value is the thinnest measure and its exact location is shown.

Applications of video and scanning slit keratoscopy

There are a number of applications for corneal topographic mapping systems. Much interest has been given to the use of these systems for fitting contact lenses, especially rigid gas-permeable lenses (Arffa 1992; Szczotka et al 1994; Szczotka 1997; Jani & Szczotka 2000). This is particularly true for patients having keratoconus (Rabinowitz et al 1991; Soni et al 1991; Ucakhan et al 2006) or a corneal graft (Gomes et al 1996; Eggink & Nuijts 2001; Gruenauer-Kloevekorn et al 2005), where the corneal shape may be abnormal and where central keratometry does not show the full extent of the abnormality. In particular, both tangential power maps and the zonal corneal pachymetry associated with slit scanning systems have been shown to be useful in the detection of keratoconus (Azar et al 1996; Demirbas & Pflugfelder 1998; Auffarth et al 2000).

In addition, topographical mapping may be a prerequisite for techniques such as orthokeratology (see Ch. 23), where the impact of the lenses on the corneal shape must be evaluated fully (Edwards 2000). Further, the utility of topography in rigid lens fitting increases after refractive surgery (Choi et al 2004; Gemoules 2006; Gonzalez-Meijome et al 2006).

A more recent problem has been the calculation of intraocular lens (IOL) power for cataract patients who have had previous refractive surgery. Since IOL power is usually calculated from axial length and corneal power, any surgical changes to the corneal power will cause postoperative refractive surprises, with patients being left with significant refractive error. It has been shown that postrefractive surgery corneal topography can help improve accuracy of IOL calculation formulae (Qazi et al 2007) or can be used in conjunction with new formulae to gain the same benefit (Borasio et al 2006).

Slit-lamp biomicroscopy

When evaluating the anterior segment of the eye, the slit-lamp biomicroscope is generally the primary examination instrument. It combines an illumination system having a focusable beam with well-defined edges that may be narrowed to a slit aperture, and an observation system comprising a high-resolution microscope with variable magnification. Both systems pivot about a common centre of rotation which provides constant focus as one moves over the curved surfaces of the eye. This ensures that the structure focally illuminated by the slit beam is in focus for the observation system.

Illumination system

The slit-lamp illumination is provided by an optical system that projects an image of a mechanical aperture onto the surface being illuminated. This ensures that there is a sharp cutoff at the edges of the beam and no diffusion of light away from the area being illuminated, unless there are irregularities within the optical media being examined. The slit can be varied in both height and width and can usually be supplemented with the following filters:

- *Diffuser*: Used when general, non-focal illumination is required. This can also be used for anterior segment photography.
- *Cobalt blue*: Used in fluorescein examinations as an exciter filter for fluorescein examination.
- *Red-free*: Used to enhance contrast between blood vessels and their surroundings.

- *Neutral density*: Permitting larger slit widths to be employed without a commensurate increase in brightness as an aid to patient comfort.
- *Yellow*. Some instruments include a yellow filter for increased patient comfort during prolonged examinations.

Observation system

The observation system comprises a microscope which may have convergent or, more commonly, parallel eyepieces. This includes a turret of objective lenses to create a wide range of magnification levels. Systems with an optical zoom provide no-step progression from lowest to highest magnification. Supplementary eyepieces permit a wider range of magnification to be made available. In addition, eyepieces may be fitted with reticules for the measurement of structures or anomalies, although calibration at each magnification is necessary for absolute values to be determined.

Illumination methods

By rotating the observation and illumination systems relative to one another, the appearance of structures and anomalies within the ocular media can be altered to provide optimal visibility. Six standard illumination methods are most commonly used, as described below.

1. Diffuse illumination

A wide beam is used, typically at low magnification ($\approx 6\times$), to obtain a general overview of the eye which can then direct subsequent and more detailed investigation. The structures to be viewed with this technique include the lids, lid margins, puncta, eyelashes, bulbar and palpebral conjunctiva, cornea, pupil, and iris. An overview of the precorneal tear film is also obtained.

2. Direct focal illumination (DFI)

In this technique both the slit beam and the microscope are focused at the same point. By varying the width of the slit beam, the degree of magnification and the angle between the illumination and observation systems, one can move from a general view of the anterior segment to a three-dimensional optic section of the cornea, anterior chamber or crystalline lens.

DFI: Parallelepiped When observed with a 1–2 mm beam, a parallelepiped-shaped section is seen (**Fig. 17.7**). This method of illumination allows structures to be viewed in three dimensions. In addition, one may observe tear debris, corneal nerves, abrasions, scars, striae (subtle, thin, white vertical folds located in the posterior stroma secondary to corneal oedema which is often associated with contact lens wear), ghost and blood vessels with this illumination method. Examination of the crystalline lens, vitreous (with or without the aid of an auxiliary lens) and retina (with the aid of an auxiliary lens; see Ch. 18) can be viewed with DFI parallelepiped illumination.

DFI: Optic Section An optic section is formed with a narrow beam (approximately 0.2–0.3 mm in width) and typically a 60° angle between the observation and illumination systems (**Fig. 17.8**). After an object of regard has been located using the parallelepiped illumination, the optic section is employed to isolate the layer of tissue where the object lies. When viewing a corneal optic section, the anterior bright band is the tear film layer and epithelium, the posterior

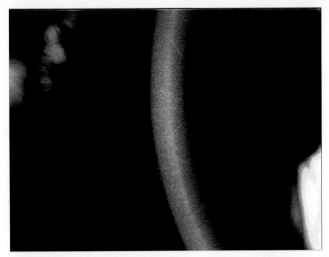

Figure 17.7 A parallelepiped section of the cornea seen under direct focal illumination (DFI) through the slit-lamp biomicroscope.

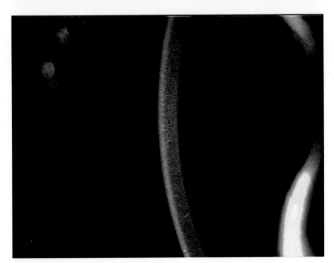

Figure 17.8 An optic section of the cornea seen under direct focal illumination (DFI) through the slit-lamp biomicroscope.

Table 17.1 Guideline for assessing cells and flare when viewing the anterior chamber

Grade	Cells	Flare
0	None	Absent
1	1–3	Mild
2	4–8	Moderate
3	9–15	Marked
4	>15	Severe

To examine the anterior chamber, a conical beam is used to produce a small patch of light having a small vertical dimension which is viewed under high magnification (25×). All ambient illumination should be extinguished when assessing the anterior chamber using this technique. To view the anterior chamber, first focus the conical section on the central cornea so that it may be observed against the dark background of the pupil. Then move the biomicroscope forward approximately 2–3 mm to bring the focus within the anterior chamber. Both the cornea and iris should now be out of focus. Observe the anterior chamber for *at least* 30 to 60 seconds to look for any floating debris. Cells and flare should be graded as shown in **Table 17.1**.

3. Sclerotic scatter

This is produced by the total internal reflection that occurs within the cornea as light is directed onto the limbus. In a clear cornea, the limbus will glow around its circumference while the central area remains dark. However, any defect within the cornea (such as oedema, haze or infiltrates) will scatter light and can be seen as an area of brightness within the cornea, and viewed against the dark background of the pupil or iris. The illumination system is generally uncoupled (out of the click stop position) from the observation system for this technique. This procedure may also be performed by the practitioner viewing the cornea directly without the microscope.

4. Indirect illumination

This occurs when the microscope is focused directly adjacent to the illuminated area. Accordingly, the illumination system must be uncoupled (out of click stop) from the observation system for this technique. This procedure is useful for observing the surface of the iris (Fleming & Semes 2006) or epithelial corneal oedema, corneal microcysts, map-dot and fingerprint dystrophy (a dystrophy of the epithelial basement membrane), pigment spots and corneal foreign bodies (Bartlett 1991).

5. Retroillumination

This is produced when areas of interest are illuminated by light reflected from a more posterior surface. For example, the cornea can be lit by light reflected from the iris. Similarly, the iris or crystalline lens can be viewed against the red reflex of light reflected from the fundus. Since the object of regard is viewed against a bright background, it will appear dark or in shadow (**Fig. 17.9**). The observation system may be coupled (direct retroillumination) or uncoupled (indirect retroillumination) from the illumination system for this technique. In direct retroillumination of the cornea, the microscope is focused on the cornea while the beam of light is reflected from the iris onto the cornea. Opacities

bright band is the endothelium, while the thicker, dim band between these two bright layers is the corneal stroma. The DFI optic section allows observation of corneal nerves located within the middle third of the stroma, changes in corneal thickness due to keratoconus, corneal scars or infiltrates, corneal abrasions or foreign bodies. When viewing an optic section of the crystalline lens, zones of discontinuity and lens opacities may be observed. This technique is also employed when estimating the depth of the anterior chamber angle by the Van Herick method (see p 269).

When examining the anterior chamber, the aqueous fluid of a healthy eye will appear optically empty when a light beam traverses it. However, in the case of an inflamed eye such as one with anterior uveitis, cells (white blood cells) and flare (excess protein) from the iris and ciliary body can be visualized within the beam of light focused on the aqueous. Red blood cells or pigment from the iris (usually due to trauma) may also be observed within the beam. Blood cells and/or pigment generally appear as floating particles whereas flare is seen as a milky haze. This phenomenon, which occurs when the scattering particles are larger than the wavelength of the radiation being scattered, is termed the Tyndall effect.

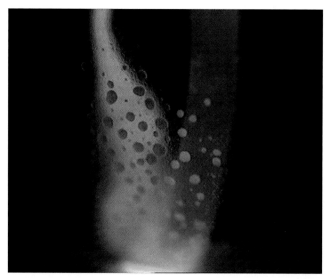

Figure 17.9 Keratic precipitates (KPs) viewed simultaneously in direct and in retroillumination. Multiple, large KPs are easily seen in this patient with recurrent iritis, secondary to sarcoid. The KPs on the right of the image are seen in direct focal illumination and appear white. The KPs on the left are viewed in retroillumination, being lit by light reflected from the iris, and therefore appear dark brown in colour.

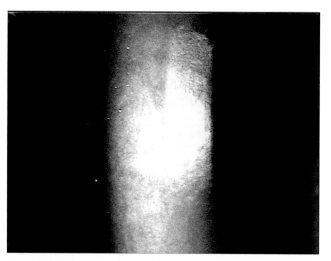

Figure 17.10 Specular reflection from the corneal endothelium. The hexagonal endothelial cells can be seen in the top right portion of the corneal section.

such as scars and blood vessels will appear dark against the bright background. Lesions which scatter light, e.g. epithelial oedema or corneal precipitates, will appear lighter.

For indirect retroillumination, the observation system is uncoupled (out of click stop) from the illumination system, and the area illuminated by light reflected from the surface of the iris will lie directly adjacent to the lesion. Light may also be reflected from the anterior crystalline lens to view the cornea or from the retina to view opacities within the cornea and/or crystalline lens. When reflecting light from the retina, the light source is positioned in the primary position and directed through the pupil. Any opacities in the crystalline lens or cornea will appear dark against the red-orange retinal reflex. One can also check for holes in the iris (transillumination) with this method.

6. Specular reflection

This can be used to image surfaces and allows assessment of surface texture. It occurs when the observation and illumination systems are set at equal angles to a line perpendicular to the structure being observed. This technique is valuable for examining the tear film, the corneal endothelium (**Fig. 17.10**) and the anterior and posterior surfaces of the crystalline lens. These surfaces are generally examined under high magnification (25–40×).

In reality, the distinctions between these methods of illumination are arbitrary since the field of view of the microscope is greater than the area illuminated by the slit beam. Therefore, several types of illumination will be evident within the field of view at the same time. For a summary of the settings for the various types of slit-lamp illumination see **Table 17.2**. In addition, during the course of a slit-lamp examination the light is moved across the eye, and the angle between illumination and observation system varied. The main methods of focal illumination will occur sequentially

Table 17.2 Summary of settings for various slit-lamp illumination settings

	Diffuse	DFI: parallelepiped	DFI: optic section	Conical section	Sclerotic scatter	Indirect	Retroillumination	Specular reflection
Beam angle	45° to 60°	45° to 60°	45° to 60°	60° to 75°	60°	45° to 60°	60° (when reflected off iris) 0° (when reflected off the retina)	Angle of illumination system = angle of observation system (usually 45°)
Beam height	Maximum	Maximum	Maximum	3–4 mm	Maximum	Maximum	Maximum	Maximum
Beam width	4 mm to wide open	1–2 mm	0.2–0.3 mm	0.5–0.6 mm	1 mm	1–2 mm	1–2 mm	1–2 mm
Magnification	Low	Start low (≈6x), and then increase	Start ≈10–12× and then increase as necessary	20–30×	Low (≈6×),	Low to high as necessary	Low to high as necessary	High (20–45×)
Illumination level	Low	Low	Moderate to high	Maximum	Moderate	Low to moderate	Moderate	Moderate

Table 17.3 Illumination and examination techniques with the slit lamp

Structure/ abnormality to be observed	Magnification	Illumination	Slit width	Filters/accessories
Lids/general view of external eye	Low–medium	Diffuse	Wide	Diffuser
Lashes	Medium	Direct focal	Narrow to medium	None
Localized oedema	Low	Sclerotic scatter	Medium	Uncoupled system
Corneal defects	Medium–high	Direct/indirect focal	Medium to narrow	None
Depth of opacity	Medium–high	Direct focal	Narrow	Observation system normal to surface and wide separation between observation and illumination system
Corneal microcysts	High	Indirect/indirect retro	Narrow	None
Corneal striae	High	Indirect	Narrow	None
Corneal vascular change/ghost vessels	Medium–high	Indirect retro	Medium to narrow	None. red-free filter may help if there is blood flow through vessel
Corneal endothelium	High	Specular reflection	Medium	None
Dystrophies	Low–medium	Direct retro/focal or sclerotic scatter	Medium	None
Fluorescein staining	Low–medium	Direct focal or diffuse	Wide	Blue exciter filter in illumination system, yellow barrier filter in observation system

for different structures within the eye. As the light passes over defects in otherwise optically clear media, areas of interest pass from one method of illumination to another and may seem, on initial observation, to become visible and then invisible with a specific method of illumination. This effect is enhanced by the sharply defined slit image, making these transitions in illumination more dramatic. Further examination can then be concentrated in that area. Specific illumination and examination techniques to enhance the visibility of various structures and/or abnormalities are shown in **Table 17.3**.

Use of the slit lamp

To ensure maximum overlap of the field of view and the area of illumination, the instrument has coincident centres of rotation for both the illumination and observation systems. This ensures that the slit image is produced in the same plane as the focus of the microscope and that the slit image is centred in the field of view. However, the microscope must be focused accurately for the observer. Before beginning the examination, it is important that the eyepieces are focused for the individual user. This is achieved either by focusing each eyepiece using the internal graticule that is normally present or by using a focusing bar that provides a suitable reference plane on which to focus. Alternatively, one can focus the instrument on the patient's closed lid or viewing the outer section of the sclera. Once a particular instrument has been focused for an individual observer, the reading on the oculars might be noted, to facilitate refocusing for that individual. If the eyepieces are not adjusted for the individual observer, then the microscope and illumination system will

not share a common focus and the slit beam will be imaged off centre within the field of view.

In normal usage, the observation system is positioned normal to the surface being examined with the illumination system to one side. The angle between observation and illumination system should be as large as possible, perhaps 70° when viewing a corneal section but much less when viewing the crystalline lens, where the view is restricted by the iris. During a comprehensive slit-lamp examination the slit width, angle between observation and illumination system and magnification are continuously varied to obtain the best view of the structures being examined.

Method of examination

The patient should be seated comfortably at the instrument with the outer canthus of the eye to be examined in line with the marker on the vertical post of the headrest. This will ensure that the instrument is at the centre of its vertical travel, thereby permitting examination of the peripheral cornea and sclera without the need to readjust the chin rest height.

For corneal examination, focal illumination is used with a moderate width slit. The microscope should be positioned normal to the surface being examined with the illumination positioned on the same side of the midline as the area being examined. Initial examination of the cornea can be completed in three sweeps as shown in **Figure 17.11**. With the patient fixating straight ahead, one sweep from temporal to nasal will examine the central area. As the patient looks down and the sweep is reversed, the superior region is examined. Finally, with the patient looking up, a third sweep examines the inferior region. At any time an area of interest

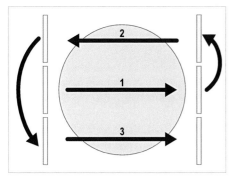

Figure 17.11 Examination of the cornea in three sweeps.

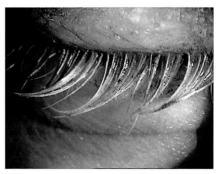

Figure 17.12 Example of white lashes. Poliosis (white lashes) as well as vitiligo (white skin patches) are observed in several rare disorders. In this case, poliosis, vitiligo and depigmented fundus lesions confirm the diagnosis of Vogt–Koyanagi–Harada (VKH) syndrome. Patients with VKH exhibit an autoimmune response to the body's own pigment. This immunological overreaction results in pigment destruction.

can be examined in detail by changing slit width, brightness and observation system magnification, as well as varying the angle between the two systems.

Structures of the anterior eye and their assessment

Ocular adnexa

A general view of the external eye, lids and lashes can be made with low magnification and a diffuse beam. Observe for abnormalities such as elevations, deposits or exudates, irregularities of the number or direction of the cilia, and/or deposits or scales on the cilia (**Fig. 17.12**). With a wide parallelepiped beam, have the patient to look up and gently pull down the lower lid. Examine the lid margin, noting the shape, tissue colour, meibomian gland openings, and look for abnormalities such as swelling, exudates, or localized growths. Examine the palpebral conjunctiva for injection, haemorrhage, swelling, wounds, discharge, concretions, follicles or papillary hypertrophy. Note if the punctum is patent, and check the caruncle for growths or unusual pigment. Subsequently, have the patient look down and gently pull up the upper lid, noting any abnormalities of the lid margin as described above. With the upper lid still raised observe the bulbar conjunctiva, noting abnormalities such as unusual pigmentation, blood vessels engorgement, growths, injection, or chemosis. Additionally, have the patient look to the right and left while observing the bulbar conjunctiva. Subsequently, evert the upper lid to examine the palpebral conjunctiva. This is achieved by pulling the upper lid downwards and away from the eye as the patient continues to look downwards. Pressure is then applied at the top of the lid with a finger or cotton bud and the lid pulled slightly outwards and upwards. The everted lid will reveal the palpebral conjunctiva and will remain in position provided it is held in place as the patient continues to look downwards.

A summary of possible findings when examining the external eye are shown in **Table 17.4**.

Examination of the lacrimal system should also include an assessment of tear layer quality or quantity. Rarely, there may be swelling of the lacrimal gland that is apparent from examination and palpation of the superior lateral region of the lid. Alternatively, there may be suspected occlusion or inflammation of the drainage system. Blockage may be assessed by examination of the nasal puncta, but is more readily tested with the introduction of fluorescein stain. Stained tears will normally drain via the puncta and be found in the nasal secretions. By shining a blue or ultraviolet light source onto the contents of the nasal passages expressed onto a tissue, the integrity of the lacrimal system can be determined. Fluorescent mucous indicates that stained tear fluid has reached the nasal passage and confirms that there is no substantial blockage. A lack of fluorescence after a suitable delay (2–3 minutes) suggests an obstruction in the nasolacrimal system.

A tender, inflamed swelling in the region of the inner canthus may suggest an inflammatory reaction in the lacrimal sac resulting in dacryocystitis. In severe cases, discharge from the puncta can be elicited by mild pressure in the region of inflammation. This may be visible to the naked eye or can be observed by the use of the slit lamp with low magnification and diffuse illumination

Tear film

An adequate pre-corneal tear film is a prerequisite for the maintenance of an intact, optically clear anterior corneal surface. The tear film comprises a superficial lipid or oily layer, an intermediate aqueous layer and an inner mucus layer. Each contributes unique properties to the tears and both the quantity and quality of the tear film will impact a patient's signs and symptoms.

Tear volume

The majority of the tear volume originates from the lacrimal gland and is contained in the aqueous layer. An inadequate volume of tears will give rise to clinically dry eye, although the aetiology may be more complex than a simple undersecretion of aqueous tears. Unfortunately, procedures to assess tear volume are prone to artefacts since anything which either comes into contact with or is added to the tear film, or requires a light bright enough to create reflex lacrimation can alter tear production. Both the Schirmer and phenyl red thread tests are used to obtain a base measure of overall tear volume.

Schirmer tear tests These comprise small strips of absorbent filter paper of pre-set dimensions. The end of the strip is bent over at a right angle and is hooked over the lower lid in contact with the bulbar and palpebral conjunctiva. Tears are absorbed onto the strip and after a predetermined time, usually 5 minutes, the strip is removed and the length of wetted strip measured. A normal eye will usually wet between 10 and 30 mm of the test strip in the 5 minute test period.

Table 17.4 Common external eye lesions

Benign lesions	Appearance	Cause
Chalazion	Painless, nearly round lump, usually affecting the upper lid	Blockage to the meibomian gland
External hordeolum	Tender, inflamed swelling at the lid margin pointing anteriorly	Infection of lash follicle and associated glands
Internal hordeolum	Tender, inflamed swelling within the tarsal plate	Infection of the meibomian gland
Cysts	Cysts are usually small, not tender and associated with sebaceous or accessory lacrimal glands	Fluid retention within the gland
Papillloma	A pedunculated or broad-based extension to the epidermis of the lids	Often associated with human papillomavirus infection
Xanthelasma	Yellow subcutaneous plaques	Deposition of cholesterol and lipid
Pigmented naevi	Flat or elevated with varying degrees of pigment and circumscription	Deposition of pigmented cells
Malignant lesions		
Basal cell carcinoma	Usually a firm, raised, indurated nodule with small, dilated surface vessels	Possible link to UV exposure
Squamous cell carcinoma	Hard nodule or roughened scaly patch developing crusting erosions	Possible link to actinic keratitis and Bowen's disease
Malignant melanoma	Pigmented spreading or nodular lesion	Some cases associated with lentigo maligna
Kaposi sarcoma	Vascular pink to red-violet or brown lesion affecting the periorbital region or conjunctiva	Associated with acquired immune deficiency syndrome

Adapted from Kanski 2007.

The main issue with the Schirmer strip is that it creates a foreign body sensation which may stimulate secretion above the normal background level. This will be exacerbated if the patient moves their eye so that the strip makes contact with the cornea. However, this effect can be minimized by placing the strips in the outer third of the palpebral aperture, and asking the patient to keep their eyes as still as possible. Some clinicians recommend the use of topical local anaesthetic prior to conducting the test as a means of avoiding the foreign body sensation. Both the volume of the drop and the initial stinging created following instillation of the anaesthetic may also increase tear production. Therefore, one should wait at least 1 minute after the anaesthetic has been instilled before introducing the strips, and, additionally, take care to wipe away any excess volume before beginning the test. Following this interval, a normal eye will moisten at least 8 mm of the test strip after a 5 minute period.

Phenyl red thread test The phenyl red thread (PRT) test was developed in the 1970s as an alternative to the Schirmer test (Tomlinson et al 2001). It consists of a thin cotton thread impregnated with phenol red dye which is hooked over the lower lid for just 15 s (Doughty et al 2007). In a review of the technique, Tomlinson et al concluded that the procedure probably measures uptake of a small amount of fluid residing in the eye while stimulating reflex tearing. They indicated that while it was more comfortable for patients than the Schirmer test, it may not offer a valid assessment of reflex tear facility. Miller et al (2004) suggested that the test provides a useful measure of tear meniscus volume, while Doughty et al (2007) noted the absence of clearly stated protocols for this procedure. To avoid misinterpretation of the results due to the rapid capillary action of the thread, it is important to measure the degree of wetting quickly as the tears advance rapidly along the thread. One advantage of the PRT test is that it can be performed while contact lenses are being worn.

Tear break-up time test

The tear break-up time (TBUT) test measures the stability of the pre-corneal film using fluorescein dye (Fleming & Semes 2006). Fluorescein solution is instilled into the lower bulbar conjunctiva using an impregnated strip. The patient should be instructed to blink several times and then asked to avoid blinking. With the cobalt filter in place, the cornea is viewed via the slit-lamp biomicroscope under low magnification ($6-10\times$) until one or more black dry spots appear (**Fig. 17.13**). A normal result is 10–15 seconds or longer (Casser et al 1997). However, Johnson and Murphy (2005) noted that TBUT values vary with the volume of fluorescein instilled, and that accurate assessment requires averaging of multiple measurements.

Rose bengal and lissamine green

To assess the integrity of the cornea and conjunctiva, either rose bengal or lissamine green stain may be employed. Rose bengal was first used by Sjögren in 1933 in patients with keratoconjunctivitis sicca (Manning et al 1995). It has an affinity for degenerated or dead cells and mucous strands. It appears to stain epithelial surfaces that have been deprived of protection from mucin or albumin. It can also be used for evaluating epithelial dendrites of herpes simplex and zoster as well as conjunctival squamous neoplasmia (Wilson 1976). The dye has significant antiviral properties,

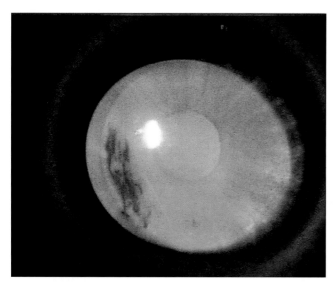

Figure 17.13 Tear break-up time (TBUT) test. Following the instillation of fluorescein and several blinks, the patient avoids blinking and the time taken for one or more black dry spots to appear is measured. A normal result is 10–15 s or longer.

and can interfere with the isolation of viruses from conjunctival or corneal cultures (Schnider 1995).

Rose bengal is supplied as both a 1% solution and an impregnated filter strip. After instillation, it can cause severe ocular irritation and stinging for up to 24 hours. Therefore, it is recommended to instil a drop of topical anaesthetic before administrating rose bengal to reduce stinging and reflex tearing. It is important to avoid getting excess dye on the eyelid, skin and clothing as it will stain these also. The volume introduced into the eye can be minimized by placing a drop onto the superior conjunctiva and allowing the dye to migrate inferiorly over the eye (Bron et al 2003). While the appearance of the stained eye can be viewed using white light (**Fig. 17.14**), coloured filters will enhance observation. For example, a red-free filter may be used to increase the contrast of the dye. Under this illumination, stained areas will appear black.

Since staining is dose dependent, the effect will be proportional to the volume of dye instilled. Therefore, if less dye is introduced to minimize stinging, this will also reduce the amount of staining observed. At the end of the examination, patients should be warned as to the possible presence of residual dye, as the red appearance may cause them to believe that blood is present in or around their eyes.

Rose bengal and lissamine green ophthalmic dyes have similar staining characteristics. Unlike rose bengal, lissamine green is not toxic to the ocular surfaces and is better tolerated by patients (Manning et al 1995). Accordingly, lissamine green is preferred, and has become more widely used than rose bengal (Kim & Foulks 1999).

Lissamine green is supplied in a 1% solution or as an impregnated filter strip. It is generally instilled without an anaesthetic because of its non-irritating properties. Staining should be evaluated 1–4 minutes after the dye has been introduced into the eye. Further, lissamine green staining is best evaluated under low illumination. Foulks (2003) suggested beginning the examination with low illumination and increasing the level until the lissamine green staining becomes most visible. However, using excess illumination will decrease the visibility of the stained regions.

Van Herick angle estimation

The Van Herick technique can be used to assess the depth of the anterior chamber (AC) angle. This is most important before any mydriatic pharmaceutical agent is instilled. With this technique the patient is directed to look straight ahead and an optic section of their cornea created on the edge of the limbus. The illumination system is positioned 60 degrees away from the microscope and the magnification set at approximately 16×. The illumination is positioned temporally when grading the temporal angle and nasally when assessing the nasal angle. The anterior chamber will appear as a black space between the cornea and the iris. With the optic section focused on the cornea, the width of the anterior chamber (i.e. the black space) is compared with the width of the corneal section.

The method of grading the angle is shown in **Table 17.5**.

Gonioscopy

While the Van Herrick technique can be used to estimate anterior chamber depth and therefore the likelihood of angle closure, detailed examination of the angle both to determine the degree to which it is open and to view the anatomical structures can only be achieved with a gonioscopy lens. Without such a lens, light reflected from the angle is totally internally reflected within the eye and is not visible externally. Gonioscopic lenses are placed in contact with the cornea, necessitating the use of topical anaesthesia and lubricating

Table 17.5 Grading of Van Herick technique to estimate the depth of the anterior chamber angle

Grade	Description	Likelihood of angle closure
1	Width of AC is less than ¼ of the width of the corneal section	Angle is extremely narrow and will probably close with full pupillary dilation
2	Width of AC is approximately ¼ of the width of the corneal section	Angle is narrow and capable of closure
3	Width of AC is ¼ to ½ of the width of the corneal section	Angle is unlikely to close
4	Width of the AC is equal or greater than the width of the optic section	This is a wide-open angle

Adapted from Casser et al 1997.

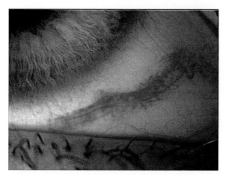

Figure 17.14 Rose bengal staining on inferior nasal conjunctiva and around limbus.

drops. Most typically, these include mirrors to obtain a clear view of the angle. For a detailed review of the history of gonioscopy, see Fisch (1993).

Gonioscopy lenses can be divided into those that require cushioning fluid to provide suction to hold the lens onto the cornea and lenses which do not use fluid to obtain suction. The most commonly used fluid lens is the Goldmann 3-mirror lens, although 1- and 2-mirror lenses are also available. The 3-mirror lens contains three mirrors and a centre lens. The centre lens (a Hruby lens) is used to view the posterior pole (see Ch. 18) while the two rectangular-shaped mirrors are utilized to view the mid-periphery and peripheral retina through a dilated pupil. The D-shaped (also termed bullet-shaped) mirror is used for assessing the anterior chamber angle through an undilated pupil. This lens has to be rotated 360° to observe all the quadrants of the angle.

The 4-mirror goniolens, which does not require cushioning solution, allows all quadrants of the angle to be viewed without the need for lens rotation. However, the field of view is smaller than with the 3-mirror lens. Although the inexperienced practitioner may initially find 4-mirror lenses more difficult to use, they are valuable for providing rapid evaluation of the angle since the overall procedure is quicker. However, the image quality may be poorer than that observed with fluid-cushioned lenses.

Method of examination

- Disinfect the lens with either 70% ethanol or isopropyl alcohol, or 3% hydrogen peroxide. Firstly, apply the disinfecting agent to a tissue, then wipe only the ocular surface of the lens. Rinse with saline or irrigating solution and wipe dry. However, Volk (Volk Optical Inc., Mentor, OH) recommend that their gonioscopy lenses be disinfected by soaking in either a 2% solution of glutaraldehyde for 20–25 min or a solution of sodium hypochlorite (household bleach) composed of 1 part bleach to 10 parts water for 10–12 min. The lens should then be rinsed thoroughly and dried.

- A lubricant drop should be used to fill the concave surface of the 3-mirror gonioscopy lens (although the 'no-flange' 3-mirror Volk lenses do not require cushioning solution). Lubricant solutions include hydroxypropyl methylcellulose (2.5%), hydroxyethylcellulose (2.5%) and carboxymethylcellulose sodium (1%). The latter is less viscous than hydroxypropyl methylcellulose, and patients seem to have less corneal reactions to this solution. Further, post-examination irrigation seems less necessary when compared with hydroxypropyl methylcellulose. However, carboxymethylcellulose may produce some degradation of image clarity.

- The patient should be seated comfortably at the slit lamp and both corneas anaesthetized with a topical anaesthetic. Since the eye without the goniolens has a tendency to dry out, in order to avoid reflex blinking (which may cause the lens to dislodge) both eyes should be anesthetized.

- Place the lens onto the eye.

  With a *cooperative patient or one with a wide palpebral aperture* the following procedure may be used. Have the patient look up, and while holding the goniolens with the thumb and index finger, gently pull the patient's lower lid down with the index finger of the free hand. Rest the edge of the goniolens onto the lower lid and release this eyelid.

At this point, hold the upper lid with the thumb of the free hand. Then, pivot the lens onto the globe (release the upper lid) and tell the patient to look straight ahead *slowly*. If they look straight ahead too quickly the lens may come off the eye. Brace the remaining fingers on the headrest band of the biomicroscope. The cushioning solution forms a partial seal between the lens and cornea, so that only a small amount of inward pressure is required once the lens is in position.

When working with an *uncooperative patient or one with a small palpebral aperture*, they should be instructed initially to look down. Hold the upper lid with the thumb of the free hand. Now tell the patient to look up. As the lens is held between the thumb and index finger, pull the lower lid down with the middle finger of the hand holding the lens. Pivot the lens onto the globe while the patient continues to look up and release the eyelids. Finally, tell the patient to look straight ahead slowly while keeping their eyes wide open. With a very uncooperative patient, have them look down. Holding the upper lid with the free hand, place the lens on the upper part of the globe as the patient continues to look as far down as they can. Then, instruct the patient to look straight ahead slowly. Release the upper lid. The appearance of the lens when centred on the eye is shown in **Figure 17.15**. If significant bubbles are trapped under the lens, it should be removed from the eye, and the insertion procedure repeated after refilling with lubricant drops. With small bubbles, it may be possible to tilt the lens towards the bubble, thereby flattening it.

- Once the goniolens is in position, set the illumination approximately 5–10° away from the centre of the biomicroscope. Start with low (approximately 6–10×) magnification and low illumination with a 3 mm-wide parallelepiped to gain orientation. If the D-shaped mirror is positioned *superiorly*, you may need to raise the microscope to focus on the mirror. Push the slit-lamp base forward until the front surface of the lens is in focus. Then move forward a further 1–2 cm to obtain a focused image of the chamber angle. The angle viewed lies 180° away from the position of the mirror. Therefore, when the mirror is superior, the inferior angle is being observed. It is customary to

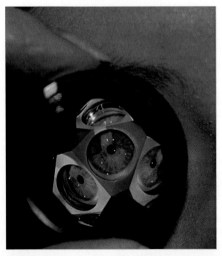

Figure 17.15 A Goldmann 3-mirror gonioscopy lens is centred on the eye. The D-shaped mirror is shown superiorly for viewing the inferior angle.

place the goniolens onto the eye first, with the D-shaped mirror superiorly. The inferior angle is typically the widest, and therefore easiest to see, whereas the superior angle is typically the narrowest. As one rotates the goniolens to evaluate the other quadrants apply slight pressure to avoid the lens popping off. When viewing both the superior and inferior angles with a vertical beam, it is important to move the illumination across the entire width of the quadrant being examined. Rotating the lens through 360° will allow the whole angle to be examined in a methodical manner.

- To remove the lens, use one of the following techniques:

  a. Instruct the patient to blink hard or squeeze their lids tightly closed. This will break the suction and the lens will release.

  b. With the index finger, push on the globe through the lid just temporal to the lens and simultaneously tell the patient to blink hard. Support the lens with the other hand to hold it when suction breaks. Occasionally, one may hear a 'popping' sound, indicating that the seal has been broken.

  c. Instruct the patient to turn their eye in and then blink hard. This utilizes the caruncle or lid margins to break the seal.

  d. If the lens does not release after performing the three procedures described above, irrigate with sterile saline solution. *Gently* rock the lens back and forth during irrigation to break the suction.

- Finally, if cushioning solution was used with the goniolens, then the eye must be irrigated after lens removal to wash out the viscous solution. Give the patient a few tissues to place on their cheek and have them tilt their head back while looking up. Pull their lower lid down and direct a stream of irrigating solution (sterile ophthalmic saline) into the lower cul-de-sac. Next, tell the patient to look down and again direct a stream of solution under the upper lid. Repeat if necessary. Do *not* spray the irrigating solution directly onto the cornea. The patient's vision will be blurry due to any residual methylcellulose, corneal punctate staining and lack of oxygen while the lens was on the eye. Reassure the patient their vision should clear in approximately 20 minutes.

Anatomy of the angle

The following structures should be visible during gonioscopic examination:

- *Iris*: This should appear flat. Any bowing (whether convex or concave) should be noted in terms of its extent and location. A concave iris configuration is more commonly seen in myopic patients.
- *Ciliary body*: Usually appears as a narrow grey or brown band beyond the iris. It tends to be wider in myopic eyes compared with emmetropic or hyperopic eyes.
- *Scleral spur*: A bright white band lying immediately anterior to the ciliary body.
- *Trabecula*: Seen as a grey band anterior to the scleral spur. It may contain more pigment on its posterior edge. Two layers may be visible, and, since the more posterior layer (the one closer to the iris) filters most of the aqueous, this is more likely to accumulate pigment or debris.

- *Canal of Schlemm*: While not normally visible, pressure on the episcleral vessels may cause it to fill with blood, in which case it will be seen as a dark band within the trabecula (**Fig. 17.16**).
- *Schwalbe's line*: Seen as a very thin white line anterior to the trabecula.
- *Iris processes*: These may be observed as thin lacy fibres or spoke-like projections that bridge the angle from the iris periphery to the uvea. They are more commonly found nasally, compared with other quadrants.

Figure 17.17 presents a diagrammatic representation of the angle, while a gonioscopic view is shown in **Figure 17.18**.

The angle is judged by the number of structures visible and by estimating the angle between the anterior surface of the iris and the posterior surface of the cornea, also known as the approach to the angle. If all structures are visible, the angle will generally be open, and the estimated angle between the iris and the cornea will be approximately 40°. If the structures between the iris and scleral spur are seen, this usually indicates a moderately open angle in

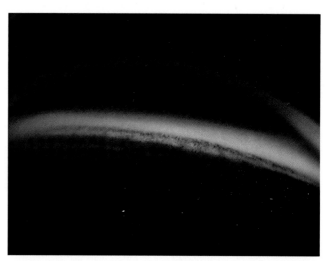

Figure 17.16 Blood in Schlemm's canal. Intentional pressure on the episcleral vessels during gonioscopy allows blood to back up into the canal of Schlemm, thereby enabling the examiner to identify the position of a lightly pigmented trabecular meshwork. Other causes of blood in Schlemm's canal include trauma and sickle cell anaemia.

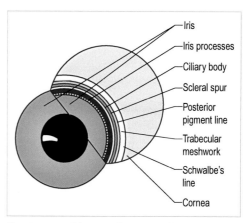

Figure 17.17 Schematic illustration of the structures of the angle seen during gonioscopy. (Reproduced with permission from Janikoun 1988.)

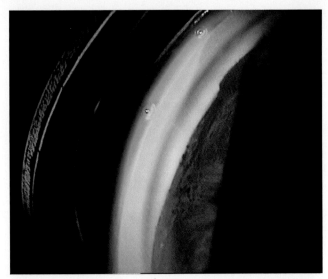

Figure 17.18 Gonioscopic view contrasting open- from closed-angle configuration. Although the trabecular meshwork is visible in most of this view, the zone at the top reveals peripheral anterior synechiae where the iris is in direct contact with the trabecular meshwork (TM), thus blocking filtration through this area. Intraocular pressure was normal, as most of the TM allowed normal aqueous filtration.

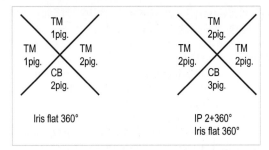

Figure 17.19 Recording gonioscopy. In each quadrant both the most posterior structure visible and the degree of pigmentation is recorded. The iris configuration, presence of iris processes (IP) and other abnormalities such as neovascularization should also be noted.

Grade 1	Anterior third of the trabecular meshwork
Grade 0	No structures seen

Additionally, pigment cells may be present in the trabecular meshwork. The amount of pigment is generally graded on a scale from 0 to 4 as follows:

Grade	*Amount of pigment*
4	Dense
3	Moderate
2	Mild
1	Minimal
0	None

The iris configuration (flat, concave, convex) and other abnormalities such as neovascularization or anomalous vessels should be noted. Furthermore, when describing the iris architecture one should observe the uniformity of the surface and note any irregularities such as a lacy or thread-like appearance.

This information is usually recorded on a cross, denoting the superior, nasal, inferior and temporal quadrants as shown in **Figure 17.19**.

Slit-lamp examination of the iris

For iris examination, focal illumination will be used and the slit should be of moderate width. The microscope should be positioned normal to the iris. In patients with a history of proliferative diabetic retinopathy or central retinal vein occlusion, it is essential to scrutinize the iris immediately adjacent to the pupil since this is often the first site to develop iris neovascularization or rubeosis. The iris examination at the pupillary border should be conducted with bright light, high magnification and good focus on the anterior region. The new blood vessels are barely perceptible and often easily missed (**Fig. 17.20**). Detection of subtle rubeosis, when present, followed by timely panretinal photocoagulation, can generally prevent the development of neovascular glaucoma.

Slit-lamp examination of the crystalline lens

A normal crystalline lens when viewed via optic section has distinct boundaries which define the various nuclei and cortex. These zones assist in the localization of lens abnormalities. The most anterior border is the interface between the aqueous humour and the anterior lens capsule. The dark zone immediately posterior includes the anterior capsule and lens epithelium. Moving further posteriorly, a second bright zone marks the anterior limit of the lens cortex. Further boundaries divide

the region of 20°. When the trabecula is not visible, the angle is closed and the angle between iris and cornea will be close to zero. However, the angle structures may also not be visible due to the iris being bowed, appositional closure or peripheral anterior synechiae (PAS).

Compression gonioscopy may be performed to differentiate between appositional and synechial closure, or in the presence of a narrow approach to the angle (i.e. the angle between the anterior surface of the iris and the posterior surface of the cornea). Use of the 4-mirror goniolens allows the cornea to be flattened due to its flatter base curve and the smaller diameter of the ocular surface. Pressure applied to the cornea pushes aqueous into the angle thereby forcing the iris away from its insertion. In the case of appositional closure, the iris will move away from the angle, thereby allowing deeper structures to become visible. However, if the iris remains attached to the wall of the angle, then synechiae are present.

In addition, it may be difficult to view the angle structures in an iris with a steep contour. This can be facilitated by using a 3-mirror goniolens and instructing the patient to look towards the D-shaped mirror. In order to determine whether an angle is at risk to closure, change the slit-lamp illumination from moderate to dim (with low ambient illumination) and note whether there is any change in the approach to the angle as the pupil dilates.

Recording

The most common method of grading the anterior angle is the Becker–Shaffer system. The most *posterior* structure visible is noted as follows:

Becker–Shaffer system	*Most posterior structure visible*
Grade 4	Ciliary body
Grade 3	Scleral spur
Grade 2	Anterior half of the trabecular meshwork

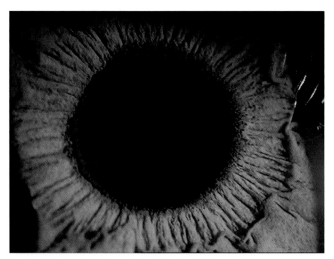

Figure 17.20 Rubeosis. Note the presence of fine blood vessels on the iris at the pupillary border from 12 to 5 o'clock. These minute vessels often appear as tiny red dots and represent early to moderate rubeosis, which in this case is due to proliferative diabetic retinopathy. Contrast this zone to the normal-appearing iris between 6 and 12 o'clock.

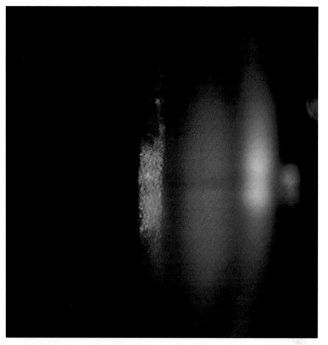

Figure 17.21 Age-related cataract. In this three-dimensional optic section of the crystalline lens, the slit beam is entering from the right side. The whole oval zone in the centre of the lens is a nuclear cataract. In addition, this view demonstrates a posterior subcapsular cataract on the left side of the image, which appears granular. Both will contribute to a reduction in vision.

the cortex from the adult nucleus, and then the adult from the fetal nucleus. On occasion, in younger subjects, a faint stripe separates the juvenile from the adult nucleus, although in most eyes the juvenile nucleus blends into the adult nucleus. The fetal nucleus surrounds the central dark area or embryonic nucleus in the very centre of the crystalline lens. A thick, bean-shaped zone defines the inner layers of the fetal nucleus. Lying posterior to the embryonic nucleus is a similar pattern of dark and light boundaries, although the posterior regions generally have steeper radii of curvature (Phelps 1992).

For slit-lamp examination of the crystalline lens, an optic section at medium magnification is most often employed since this affords the best approach to differentiate between anterior cortical, nuclear, posterior cortical and posterior sub-capsular (PSC) cataracts (**Fig. 17.21**). A dilated pupil allows improved observation of peripheral cortical spokes and PSC cataracts as well as permitting indirect retroillumination of various lens opacities. As the angle of the illumination system is decreased and nearly matches the microscope which is positioned normal to the crystalline lens, the view abruptly changes at some point and lens opacities can be seen to block the light reflected from the retina. For the inexperienced examiner, it is important to remember that an optically empty structure such as the normal anterior chamber appears black. Similarly, a normal crystalline lens appears darker than a cataract. A patient with a nuclear cataract only will reveal a milky white, yellow or brown nucleus while the remainder of the lens will appear quite dark, i.e. similar to the appearance of the normal anterior chamber. In addition, specular reflection may be used to observe any irregularities on the anterior and posterior surfaces of the crystalline lens.

Other applications

The slit lamp can be used in conjunction with accessories to provide additional examination options. These are considered below.

Pachymetry

Optical pachymetry has largely become obsolete with the introduction of ultrasound pachymeters (see Ch. 24) and slit-scanning topographical systems that can calculate corneal thickness over its whole diameter from elevation maps of the anterior and posterior surfaces (see **Fig. 17.6**). Nevertheless, optical pachymetry can still be employed through the use of special accessories. The normal thin slit section of the cornea is doubled, using a doubling eyepiece and prism introduced in front of half the image. In this way the back surface of the endothelium can be aligned with the front surface of the epithelium to provide a measure of apparent corneal thickness. A correction for corneal refractive index will permit the real corneal thickness to be determined. An automated method of optical pachymetry was developed by Holden et al (1982) to allow repetitive measures and more repeatable outcomes.

Aesthesiometry

Corneal sensitivity may be of interest in certain ocular conditions such as diabetes, dry eye and following refractive surgery or contact lens wear (Campos et al 1992; Bourcier et al 2005; Tavakoli et al 2007). This can be measured using an aesthesiometer to determine corneal sensitivity (Boberg-Ans 1955, 1956; Millodot 1977). The instrument, which is mounted on the slit lamp, includes a unit housing nylon filaments of varying lengths. Using the applicator, the filament is brought forward to touch the cornea perpendicularly and then withdrawn. The patient is asked to respond whenever they feel the stimulus. Longer filament lengths apply less pressure to the cornea than shorter filaments (Murphy et al 1998). However, Murphy et al (1996) noted that the technique could modify corneal touch sensitivity by producing slight trauma to the corneal epithelium. Other limitations of the device have also been noted, and a non-contact aesthesiometer which stimulates the cornea by directing a pulse of air of variable pressure and duration has been proposed (Murphy et al 1996, 1998).

Scheimpflug imaging

When imaging the anterior chamber, a large depth of field is required to capture the anterior segment from the cornea to the posterior capsule of the crystalline lens in a single clear image. This can be achieved with a rotating Scheimpflug camera. The Scheimpflug rule states that the image plane, the subject plane and the plane of the camera lens must converge along a single line (Drews 1964). This technique is discussed further in Chapter 19.

Most recent digital Scheimpflug cameras, such as the Oculus Pentacam (Oculus, Inc., Lynnwood, WA), allow multiple digital images of the anterior segment to be captured along different axes, thereby permitting three-dimensional reconstruction of the anterior segment (see **Figs 19.5** and **19.6**).

Specular microscopy

Routine slit-lamp examination can be used to visualize the corneal endothelium using the method of specular reflection (see **Fig. 17.10**). Indeed, routine examination of the cornea will usually provide an opportunity to see the endothelial mosaic on six occasions, once on each side of the midline in each of the three sweeps across the cornea. High magnification is required (25–45×), and even then the view obtained is only adequate to give an overall qualitative appreciation of endothelial cell structure.

Although specular reflection at very high magnification often allows the observer to view the corneal endothelial cells, the procedure requires skill, practice and perseverance. Several innovative systems, such as the Noncon Robo Pachy SP-9000 endothelial cell count (ECC) apparatus (Konan Medical Corporation, Fairlawn, NJ), provide remarkable views and photodocumentation of the corneal endothelium in less than a minute without corneal contact. Such systems allow for the quantification of the number of cells per square millimetre, the range and distribution of cell size and the percentage of cells with the normal hexagonal shape. ECC is useful prior to cataract surgery since a cell count below $1000/mm^2$ is often associated with corneal decompensation after surgery. In contrast, an ECC above $2000/mm^2$ virtually never results in postoperative corneal decompensation. ECC measurements in long-term hard or rigid gas-permeable contact lens patients may reflect damage to the endothelial cells, which could worsen with continued contact lens wear.

Other methods of examination

With developments in technology, other methods of examination for the anterior segment are more readily available. These may be used to image structures not visible to the slit-lamp biomicroscope.

Ultrasound biomicroscopy

Ultrasound has long been used to examine the eye, especially where direct visualization was prevented by media opacities, and for providing biometric information. The procedure is described in detail in Chapter 19. Ultrasound biomicroscopy (UBM) provides high-resolution imaging of the anterior segment using a frequency of approximately 50 Hz,

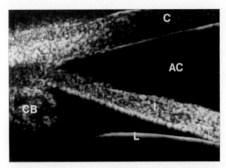

Figure 17.22 Ultrasound biomicroscope (UBM) of a normal eye. The iris (I) is flat and has a normal insertion, forming an open angle with the cornea (C). Although the ciliary body (CB) is invisible to ophthalmoscopy and slit lamp, it is clearly visible with UBM. AC, anterior chamber. Note that the iris appears to rest gently on the anterior lens capsule (L).

giving resolution of approximately 50 microns and penetration of 4–5 mm. Ultrasound provides images of structures not visible to light microscopy. **Figure 17.22** shows the normal anterior eye imaged with UBM.

To obtain good UBM images, an eyecup filled with saline is used to ensure adequate acoustic coupling between the ultrasound probe and the eye, since ultrasound energy travels much faster in a liquid medium than in air. Patient fixation can be an issue and as a result it can take some time to produce a well-aligned image of the area of interest. UBM imaging can be used to provide measurements of anterior structures such as anterior chamber depth and crystalline lens thickness as well as to identify structural anomalies or pathology. The degree to which the angle is open can also be assessed from the images. A UBM image of an iris cyst is shown in **Figure 17.23**.

Optical coherence tomography

Optical coherence tomography (OCT) is a non-invasive, interferometric technique using broadband light sources such as superluminescent diodes or femtosecond lasers. These provide interference at the short working distances required for imaging of the anterior eye and the images are created due to the different reflectivity of the structures being examined. The technique is described in detail in Chapter 18.

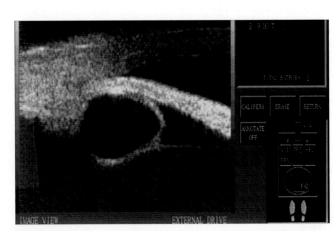

Figure 17.23 Ultrasound biomicroscope of an iris cyst. The iris is in close proximity with the corneal endothelium because of the presence of a large cyst. Note that the cyst appears sonolucent. The UBM allows differentiation between a solid lesion and a cyst.

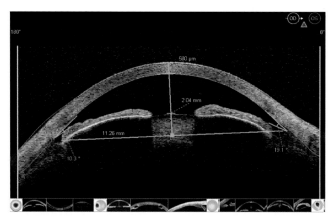

Figure 17.24 Optical coherence tomography in narrow-angle glaucoma. This anterior segment OCT demonstrates an iris that is bowed forward, forming a narrow angle. Software allows for the angle to be measured. OCT allows better resolution of anterior segment structures than UBM. However, because it utilizes light rather than sound waves, it cannot penetrate opaque tissue and therefore cannot image structures such as the ciliary body as well as UBM.

OCT is increasingly a non-contact, non-invasive technique where the accompanying software can produce cross-sectional images or build three-dimensional images. **Figure 17.24** shows an OCT image of an eye with narrow-angle glaucoma.

Unlike UBM, OCT is unable to image through the pigmented iris and so mydriasis is generally required. However, images of structures behind the peripheral iris can be obtained if a trans-scleral route is used. Resolution of detail within the structure is superior to that of UBM. Both UBM and OCT have been used to image the anterior segment either for detection of anomalies and/or disease (Radhakrishnan et al 2005) or to investigate aspects of accommodation (Ludwig et al 1999; Baikoff et al 2004). In general, both devices perform similarly but the OCT instrument, being non-contact and with an adjustable fixation target, is somewhat more user friendly (Radhakrishnan et al 2005).

Summary

Anterior segment examination is an important aspect of optometric examination. Basic hand-held instruments can provide information that suggests the need for more detailed examination. Slit-lamp examination provides the basis for many diagnoses and is supplemented by attachments that assess the anterior chamber angle, corneal sensitivity, fundus appearance or permit anterior chamber photographs.

More recent methods of imaging including UBM and OCT can provide more detailed assessment of intraocular structures and may help to diagnose abnormality.

Assessment of corneal topography and/or zonal corneal thickness may improve rigid lens fitting, diagnosis of corneal abnormalities or provide improved outcomes for refractive surgery patients and those requiring cataract extraction.

References

Arffa R C 1992 Clinical uses of corneal topography analysis. Current Opinions in Ophthalmology 3:71–77

Auffarth G U, Wang L, Volcker H E 2000 Keratoconus evaluation using the Orbscan topography system. Journal of Cataract and Refractive Surgery 26:222–228

Azar D, Salvat M, Benson A 1996 Corneal topography, ultrasound biomicroscopy, and scatterometry. Current Opinion in Ophthalmology 7:83–93

Baikoff G, Lutun E, Ferraz C et al 2004 Static and dynamic analysis of the anterior segment with optical coherence tomography. Journal of Cataract and Refractive Surgery 30:1843–1850

Bartlett J D 1987 Anisometropia and aniseikonia. In: Amos J F (ed.) Diagnosis and management in vision care. Butterworths, Boston, pp 173–202

Bartlett J D 1991 Slit lamp. In: Eskridge J B, Amos J F, Bartlett J D (eds) Clinical procedures in optometry. Lippincott, Philadelphia, pp 206–220

Basmak H, Sahin A, Yildirim N 2006 The reliability of central corneal thickness measurements by ultrasound and by Orbscan system in schoolchildren. Current Eye Research 31:569–575

Boberg-Ans J 1955 Experience in clinical examination of corneal sensitivity; corneal sensitivity and the naso-lacrimal reflex after retrobulbar anaesthesia. British Journal of Ophthalmology 39: 705–726

Boberg-Ans J 1956 On the corneal sensitivity. Acta Ophthalmologica (Copenhagen) 34:149–162

Borasio E, Stevens J, Smith G T 2006 Estimation of true corneal power after keratorefractive surgery in eyes requiring cataract surgery: BESSt formula. Journal of Cataract and Refractive Surgery 32:2004–2014

Bourcier T, Acosta M C, Borderie V et al 2005 Decreased corneal sensitivity in patients with dry eye. Investigative Ophthalmology and Visual Science 46:2341–2345

Bron A J, Evans V E, Smith J A 2003 Grading of corneal and conjunctival staining in the context of other dry eye tests. Cornea 22:640–650

Buehl W, Stojanac D, Sacu S et al 2006 Comparison of three methods of measuring corneal thickness and anterior chamber depth. American Journal of Ophthalmology 141:7–12

Campos M, Hertzog L, Garbus J J et al 1992 Corneal sensitivity after photorefractive keratectomy. American Journal of Ophthalmology 114:51–54

Casser L, Fingeret M, Woodcome H T 1997 Atlas of primary eyecare procedures, 2nd edn. Appleton & Lange, Stamford, CT

Cheng A C, Rao S K, Tang E et al 2006 Pachymetry assessment with Orbscan II in postoperative patients with myopic LASIK. Journal of Refractive Surgery 22:363–366

Cho P, Lam A K, Mountford J et al 2002 The performance of four different corneal topographers on normal human corneas and its impact on orthokeratology lens fitting. Optometry and Vision Science 79:175–183

Choi H J, Kim M K, Lee J L 2004 Optimization of contact lens fitting in keratectasia patients after laser in situ keratomileusis. Journal of Cataract and Refractive Surgery 30:1057–1066

Chui W S, Cho P 2005 A comparative study of the performance of different corneal topographers on children with respect to orthokeratology practice. Optometry and Vision Science 82:420–427

Demirbas N H, Pflugfelder S C 1998 Topographic pattern and apex location of keratoconus on elevation topography maps. Cornea 17:476–484

Doughty M J, Whyte J, Li W 2007 The phenol red thread test for lacrimal volume – does it matter if the eyes are open or closed? Ophthalmic Physiological Optics 27:482–489

Douthwaite W A 2003 The asphericity, curvature and tilt of the human cornea measured using a videokeratoscope. Ophthalmic Physiological Optics 23:141–150

Douthwaite W A, Matilla M T 1996 The TMS-1 corneal topography measurement applied to calibrated ellipsoidal convex surfaces. Cornea 15:147–153

Douthwaite W A, Pardhan S 1998 Surface tilt measured with the EyeSys videokeratoscope: influence on corneal asymmetry. Investigative Ophthalmology and Visual Science 39:1727–1735

Douthwaite W A, Pardhan S, Burek H 1996 Extent and effect of surface tilt on the data display of the EyeSys videokeratoscope. British Journal of Ophthalmology 80:986–993

Drews R C 1964 Depth of field in slit lamp photography. An optical solution using the Scheimpflug principle. Ophthalmologica 148:143–150

Edwards K H 1997 Clinical instrumentation in contact lens practice. In: Phillips A J, Speedwell L (eds) Contact lenses. Butterworth Heinemann, Oxford, pp 232–246

Edwards K H 2000 Contact lens problem solving: orthokeratology. Optician 220:20–27

Eggink F A, Nuijts R M 2001 A new technique for rigid gas permeable contact lens fitting following penetrating keratoplasty. Acta Ophthalmologica Scandinavia 79:245–250

Fisch B M 1993 Gonioscopy and the glaucomas. Butterworth Heinemann, Boston, pp 1–6

Fleming J B, Semes L P 2006 Anterior segment evaluation. In: Benjamin W J (ed.) Borish's clinical refraction, 2nd edn. Butterworth Heinemann, St Louis, pp 485–510

Foulks G N 2003 Challenges and pitfalls in clinical trials of treatments for dry eye. The Ocular Surface 1:20–30

Fowler C W, Dave T N 1994 Review of past and present techniques of measuring corneal topography. Ophthalmic Physiological Optics 14:49–57

Gemoules G 2006 Comparison of axial and tangential topographic algorithms for contact lens fitting after LASIK. Eye and Contact Lens: Science and Clinical Practice 32:158–159

Gomes J A, Rapuano C J, Cohen E J 1996 Topographic stability and safety of contact lens use after penetrating keratoplasty. CLAO Journal 22:64–69

Gonzalez P J, Cervino A, Giraldez M J et al 2004 Accuracy and precision of EyeSys and Orbscan systems on calibrated spherical test surfaces. Eye and Contact Lens 30:74–78.

Gonzalez-Meijome J M, Sanudo-Buitrago F, Lopez-Alemany A et al 2006. Correlations between central and peripheral changes in anterior corneal topography after myopic LASIK and their implications in postsurgical contact lens fitting. Eye and Contact Lens 32: 197–202

Goss D A Eskridge J B 1991 Keratometry. In: Eskridge J B, Amos J F, Bartlett J D (eds) Clinical procedures in optometry. Lippincott, Philadelphia, pp 135–154

Grosvenor T, Ratnakaram R 1990 Is the relation between keratometric astigmatism and refractive astigmatism linear? Optometry and Vision Science 67:606–609

Gruenauer-Kloevekorn C, Kloevekorn-Fischer U, Duncker G I 2005 Contact lenses and special back surface design after penetrating keratoplasty to improve contact lens fit and visual outcome. British Journal of Ophthalmology 89:1601–1608

Guillon M, Lydon D P, Wilson C 1986 Corneal topography: a clinical model. Ophthalmic Physiological Optics 6:47–56

Holden B A, Polse K A, Fonn D et al 1982 Effects of cataract surgery on corneal function. Investigative Ophthalmology and Visual Science 22:343–350

Horner D G, Salmon T O, Soni P S 2006 Corneal topography. In: Benjamin W J (ed.) Borish's clinical refraction, 2nd edn. Butterworth Heinemann, St Louis, pp 645–681

Hough T, Edwards K 1999 The reproducibility of videokeratoscope measurements as applied to the human cornea. Contact Lens and Anterior Eye 22:91–99

Jani B R, Szczotka L B 2000 Efficiency and accuracy of two computerized topography software systems for fitting rigid gas permeable contact lenses. CLAO Journal 26:91–96

Janikoun S 1988 Gonioscopy. In: Edwards K, Llewellyn R (eds) Optometry. Butterworth Heinemann, Oxford, pp 394–396

Johnson M E, Murphy P J 2005 The effect of instilled fluorescein solution volume on the values and repeatability of TBUT measurements. Cornea 24:811–817

Kanski J J 2007 Clinical ophthalmology. A systematic approach, 6th edn. Butterworth-Heinemann, Edinburgh

Kim K, Foulks G N 1999 Evaluation of the effect of lissamine green and rose Bengal on human corneal epithelial cells. Cornea 18:328–332

Lam A K, Douthwaite W A 1994 Derivation of corneal flattening factor, p-value. Ophthalmic Physiological Optics 14:423–427

Ludwig K, Wegscheider E, Hoops J P et al 1999 In vivo imaging of the human zonular apparatus with high-resolution ultrasound biomicroscopy. Graefe's Archives of Clinical and Experimental Ophthalmology 237:361–371

Manning F J, Wehrly S R, Foulks G N 1995 Patient tolerance and ocular surface staining characteristics of lissamine green versus rose Bengal. Ophthalmology 102:1953–1957

Miller W L, Doughty M J, Narayanan S et al 2004 A comparison of tear volume (by tear meniscus height and phenol red thread test) and tear fluid osmolarity measures in non-lens wearers and in contact lens wearers. Eye and Contact Lens: Science and Clinical Practice 30:132–137

Millodot M 1977 The influence of age on the sensitivity of the cornea. Investigative Ophthalmology and Visual Science 16:240–242

Mote H G, Fry G A 1939 The significance of Javal's rule. American Journal of Optometry 16:362–365

Murphy P J, Patel S, Marshall J 1996 A new non-contact corneal aesthesiometer (NCCA). Ophthalmic Physiological Optics 16:101–107

Murphy P J, Lawrenson J G, Patel S et al 1998 Reliability of the non-contact corneal aesthesiometer and its comparison with the Cochet-Bonnet aesthesiometer. Ophthalmic Physiological Optics 18:532–539

Pardhan S Douthwaite W A 1998 Comparison of videokeratoscope and autokeratometer measurements on ellipsoid surfaces and human corneas. Journal of Refractive Surgery 14:414–419

Phelps C D 1992 Examination and functional evaluation of crystalline lens. In: Tasman W, Jaeger E A (eds) Duane's clinical ophthalmology, vol 2. Lippincott, Philadelphia, Chapter 72, 1–23

Port M J A 1987 Ophthalmic instruments: keratometry and keratoscopy. Optician 193:17–24

Portello J K, Rosenfield M, O'Dwyer M et al 1996 Javal's rule and age. Optometry and Vision Science (supplement)73:214

Qazi M A, Cua I Y, Roberts C J et al 2007 Determining corneal power using Orbscan II videokeratography for intraocular lens calculation after excimer laser surgery for myopia. Journal of Cataract and Refractive Surgery 33:21–30

Rabbetts R B 1985 The Humphrey Auto Keratometer. Ophthalmic Physiological Optics 5:451–458

Rabinowitz Y S, Garbus J J, Garbus C et al 1991 Contact lens selection for keratoconus using a computer-assisted videophotokeratoscope. CLAO Journal 17:88–93

Radhakrishnan S, Goldsmith J, Huang D et al 2005 Comparison of optical coherence tomography and ultrasound biomicroscopy for detection of narrow anterior chamber angles. Archives of Ophthalmology 123:1053–1059

Schnider C M 1995 Dyes. In: Bartlett J D, Jaanus S D (eds) Clinical ocular pharmacology, 3rd edn. Butterworth Heinemann, Boston, pp 389–407

Sicam V A, Van der Heijde R G 2006 Topographer reconstruction of the nonrotation-symmetric anterior corneal surface features. Optometry and Vision Science 83:910–918

Soni P S, Gerstman D R, Horner D G et al 1991 The management of keratoconus using the corneal modeling system and a piggyback system of contact lenses. Journal of the American Optometric Association 62:593–597

Szczotka L B 1997 Clinical evaluation of a topographically based contact lens fitting software. Optometry and Vision Science 74:14–19

Szczotka L B, Capretta D M, Lass J H 1994 Clinical evaluation of a computerized topography software method for fitting rigid gas permeable contact lenses. CLAO Journal 20:231–236

Tavakoli M, Kallinikos P A, Efron N et al 2007 Corneal sensitivity is reduced and relates to the severity of neuropathy in patients with diabetes. Diabetes Care 30:1895–1897

Thomas J, Wang J, Rollins A M et al 2006 Comparison of corneal thickness measured with optical coherence tomography, ultrasonic pachymetry, and a scanning slit method. Journal of Refractive Surgery 22:671–678

Tomlinson A, Blades K J, Pearce E A 2001 What does the phenol red thread test actually measure?. Optometry and Vision Science 78:142–146

Ucakhan O O, Kanpolat A, Ozdemir O 2006 Contact lens fitting for keratoconus after Intacs placement. Eye and Contact Lens: Science and Clinical Practice 32:75-77

Wilms K, Rabbetts R B 1977 Practical concepts of corneal topography. Optician 174:7–13

Wilson F M II 1976 Rose Bengal staining of epibulbar squamous neoplasms. Ophthalmic Surgery 7:21–23

CHAPTER 18

Examination of the posterior segment of the eye

Sherry J Bass

Introduction

Although the first direct ophthalmoscope was designed by Charles Babbage, an English mathematician in 1847, the invention of the direct ophthalmoscope is often credited to Hermann von Helmholtz in 1850 (Dorion 1998). Ophthalmoscopy opened up a method to evaluate the posterior segment of the eye, thereby increasing the breadth of an eye examination. Eye care practitioners could now examine, diagnose and evaluate diseases of this part of the eye.

Since that relatively simple but extremely valuable invention, more recent developments in retinal imaging technology have expanded the ability to view the posterior segment of the eye, providing not only two-dimensional but also three-dimensional views of the retina. This 'in vivo' dissection of retinal structure allows for earlier detection and more accurate diagnosis of retinal and optic nerve disorders. In addition, these newer imaging technologies have provided a better understanding of how specific diseases affect retinal structure.

This chapter will review the current instruments available for viewing the posterior segment of the eye, the principles behind these techniques and their applicability in the detection, diagnosis and management of diseases of the posterior segment.

Standard techniques for examination of the posterior pole

Direct ophthalmoscopy

Direct ophthalmoscopy allows an examiner to view the posterior pole of the eye and obtain a 'direct' view, because the image formed is erect and real. Therefore, the retina appears in its actual orientation. For example, a lesion which appears to be superior and temporal to the macula is indeed superior and temporal to the macula. This makes direct ophthalmoscopy the easiest of the viewing techniques to learn, since the examiner does not need to reconfigure spatially the location of detected abnormalities, as is required in other forms of ophthalmoscopy. An additional advantage is the lack of light reflections seen that tend to interfere with image clarity. These reflections are a greater problem in other forms of ophthalmoscopy. Thirdly, the posterior pole may be viewed through an undilated pupil. A disadvantage of direct ophthalmoscopy is the required close working distance between examiner and patient, which can be discomforting for both individuals. Further, the view is limited primarily to the posterior pole. While more extensive views may be obtained by having a patient move their eye into various fields of gaze, the area seen is still limited, and a peripheral view of the retina cannot be accessed by this method of ophthalmoscopy, even through a widely dilated pupil. Indeed, only an area around two disc diameters can be seen in any one view (Casser et al 1997). Since the view is monocular, subtleties in depth as required for assessing cupping of the optic nerve head or abnormalities in retinal thickness are difficult to appreciate.

The posterior segment can be viewed through an undilated pupil but, for best viewing, direct ophthalmoscopy should be performed through a dilated pupil. Mydriatic (dilating) agents that are commonly used to dilate the pupil include tropicamide 1% (or 0.5% for light-coloured irides), phenylephrine 2.5% and, in children, cyclopentolate 1%, either alone or in combination with tropicamide. Darker irides, older or diabetic patients and those with small pupils may require more than one instillation of the mydriatic agent.

The technique for direct examination of the posterior pole is straightforward, but requires a logical sequence to avoid missing any structures. The examiner and patient usually remove their spectacle corrections, but contact lenses may remain in place. However, a patient with a high degree of myopia and/or astigmatism should be encouraged to wear their spectacles (if contact lenses are not available), as the high magnification obtained in uncorrected myopic patients reduces the field of view significantly. The examiner holds the direct ophthalmoscope in the right hand (for the right eye), and observes the patient's right eye with their right eye. When examining the patient's left eye, the observer holds the instrument in the left hand and views with the left eye (**Fig. 18.1**). The examiner should start out at a distance of about 1 m from the patient with a +1.00 D lens in the ophthalmoscope as the patient looks into the distance.

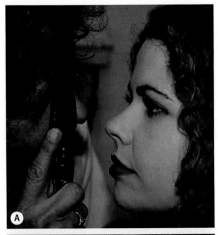

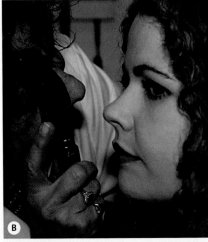

Figure 18.1 Position of examiner and patient while performing direct ophthalmoscopy of posterior pole (**A**) and retinal mid periphery (**B**)

A red reflex should be seen filling the pupil as the light is reflected from the fundus. Any media opacities should be noted. A +15.00 D lens is then introduced into the instrument, allowing examination of the anterior cornea at a viewing distance of approximately 10 cm. Next, as the examiner moves closer to the patient, the plus power is reduced to allow examination of the anterior chamber, crystalline lens and anterior vitreous. Motion parallax can be used to locate opacities observed within the media of the eye. Opacities anterior to the pupillary plane will move 'against' the motion of the ophthalmoscope, while opacities posterior to the pupillary plane will move in a 'with' motion. The power wheel in the ophthalmoscope is again turned in the minus direction until the retina appears in focus. The lens required to observe the patient's retina clearly will be approximately the sum of the patient's and observer's refractive correction, providing neither is accommodating. Therefore, if both the patient and observer are 4 D myopes, approximately a −8.00 D lens will be required. However, inexperienced young observers often find that more minus power is required to see the fundus clearly, due to the effects of proximal accommodation. To obtain the maximum field of view, the examiner should be as close to the patient as possible.

Examination of the posterior pole by direct ophthalmoscopy

Four areas of the fundus deserve special attention when performing direct ophthalmoscopy: the optic nerve head, macula, retinal vessels and the fundus background.

The optic nerve head

Examination of the optic nerve head should include an evaluation of:

- The size and shape of the nerve. The overall size of the normal optic nerve head usually ranges from 2.2 mm^2 to 2.8 mm^2 (Jonas et al 1999). The 5° spot size of a direct ophthalmoscope just about covers the normal optic disc, and can be used to estimate whether the disc is larger or smaller than normal. Large discs are usually found in high (>5.00 D) myopic patients and in certain other populations, e.g. Hispanics, Asians, and blacks. Small discs are associated with high hyperopia and optic disc hypoplasia. It should also be noted whether the disc has a normal (**Fig. 18.2A**) or oblique entrance, or whether it appears tilted (**Fig. 18.2B**)
- Disc margins. The borders of the disc should be well demarcated or distinct, since blurred, indistinct disc margins may be a sign of optic disc drusen (**Fig. 18.3A**), oedema or inflammation of the optic nerve (**Fig. 18.3B**). In addition, there may be a crescent around the optic nerve head, usually the temporal border (see **Fig. 18.2B**). These crescents may be:

  1. dark black, composed of heaped-up RPE melanocytes, termed a 'pigment crescent'
  2. dark grey, composed of choroidal pigmentation, termed a 'choroidal crescent'
  3. white, composed of sclera, and termed a 'scleral crescent'

Both choroidal crescents and scleral crescents are associated with myopic discs.

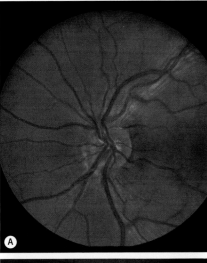

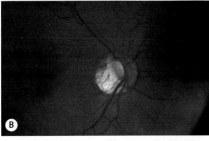

Figure 18.2 Normal optic nerve head **(A)** and a tilted optic nerve head **(B)**.

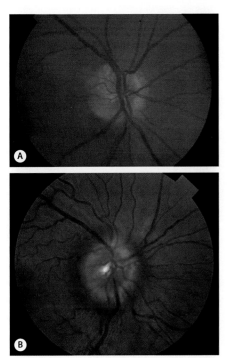

Figure 18.3 Optic disc borders can be blurred by disc drusen **(A)** and oedema or inflammation of the optic nerve head **(B)**.

- The colour of the nerve head borders. The colour of the optic nerve head rim reflects the underlying microcirculation, and the rim should be pink or reddish-orange. Any pallor (white or yellow border) may be a sign of optic atrophy. Pallor often affects the temporal rim first. Rim

pallor is not a sign of glaucoma, except in extreme end-stage glaucoma associated with severe loss of vision. Patients who have intraocular implants following cataract extraction may exhibit pallor of the temporal border of the nerve, as the intraocular lens (IOL) filters out some red wavelengths. This 'pallor' is physiological and not a sign of pathology. Disc colour that is very red or 'hyperaemic' may be an indication of inflammation. In addition to colour, the presence of any abnormalities on or around the disc surface should be noted. These include congenital anomalies of the disc, such as the 'morning glory disc' (**Fig. 18.4A**), disc tumours such as melanocytoma of the optic disc (**Fig. 18.4B**) and disc coloboma (**Fig. 18.4C**).

- Rim tissue thickness and cupping. Cupping (or the cup-to-disc ratio) represents the portion of the optic nerve head (or disc) that is occupied by the cup. The 'cup' is the central depression in the optic nerve head into which all the nerve fibres are channelled through to the optic nerve. As rim tissue decreases, a feature of glaucoma, the cup-to-disc ratio will increase. This ratio should be assessed in both the horizontal and vertical meridians, since glaucoma typically affects the vertical meridian before the horizontal meridian. The size of the cup is generally proportional to the size of the disc. Large

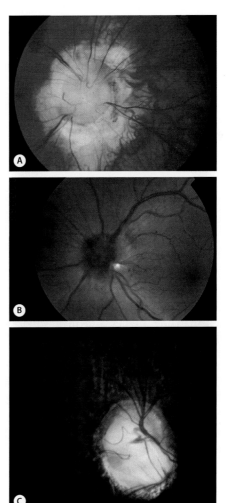

Figure 18.4 Optic disc anomalies: 'morning glory disc' **(A)**, melanocytoma **(B)** and coloboma **(C)**.

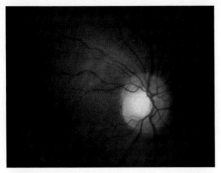

Figure 18.5 An example of a large physiological cup associated with a large disc.

discs, often seen in black, Hispanic and Asian populations, are normally associated with large cup-to-disc ratios (**Fig. 18.5**), whereas small discs normally have a small cup-to-disc ratios (=0.3) (Jonas et al 1999). A large disc with a large cup, which should be considered physiological, is often misdiagnosed as a glaucomatous optic nerve head. Likewise, a cup-to-disc ratio >0.3 in a small disc may be glaucomatous. This underlies the importance of looking at rim tissue thickness in addition to the cup-to-disc ratios. Cup depth may be assessed by noting the change in the dioptric power needed to focus from the top to the bottom of the cup. A change in power of 1 D on the direct ophthalmoscope wheel is equivalent to a change in cup depth of 0.3 mm. This is a crude but useful way of estimating cup depth; however, there are newer and better ways of doing so that are discussed in detail in later sections of this chapter. Sometimes, it is difficult to assess the cup-to-disc ratio because the borders of the cup are shallow and poorly defined. In these cases, the deviation of the blood vessels may be used to assess the ratio. However, the ratio is best assessed using stereoscopic viewing, which is not possible with the direct ophthalmoscope. Stereoscopic viewing is available with other techniques that are addressed in subsequent sections.

The retinal blood vessels

The arteries and veins of the eye (which are really smaller branches, termed arterioles and venules) are directly visible with ophthalmoscopy. The arteries are narrower than the veins (typically two-thirds the vein diameter when assessed 1–2 disc diameters from the disc), are a salmon-pink colour and reflect light (called the arterial reflex). The veins are wider and darker red than the arteries and their surfaces do not reflect light. Venous pulsation may be observed where the central retinal vein emerges. Arterioles should not pulsate. Indeed, the presence of arterial pulsation is highly abnormal. The arteriovenous crossings should also be evaluated. Narrowing of the vessels at these crossings is a potential sign of systemic disease.

The fundus background

The colour of the fundus varies depending on race and overall pigmentation. Lightly pigmented Caucasians usually have an orange fundus, with visible choroidal vessels. Darkly skinned Caucasians tend to have a tessellated or tigroid fundus due to irregularities in the choroidal pigment. The negroid fundus tends to have a dark, brownish-red appearance. In addition to the colour of the fundus

background, the presence of other abnormalities within the posterior pole should be noted, e.g. white or yellow-white lesions (drusen, exudates, cotton wool spots, fibrous scars, etc.) red lesions (haemorrhages), black lesions (retinal pigment epithelium (RPE) hypertrophy, laser burns, etc.), or grey lesions (choroidal nevi or melanomas; **Fig. 18.6**).

The macula

Examination of the macula is critical, especially in cases where a patient complains of reduced visual acuity that is not correctable with spectacles or contact lenses. To locate the macula with direct ophthalmoscopy, the observer can focus on the disc and then move about 2.5 disc diameters temporal and slightly inferior to the disc. Another way is to ask the patient to look directly into the light. Photophobic patients tend to find this particularly uncomfortable, and it seems to produce greater pupillary constriction. Therefore, the first technique described may be better. When viewing the macula through an undilated pupil, the smallest aperture and dimmest illumination level should be used to minimize pupillary constriction. A third technique is to place a circular grid or graticule into the ophthalmoscope light and ask the patient to look at the innermost circle. This grid can be used to assess the steadiness of fixation and whether the patient has central or eccentric fixation. This is useful for determining the aetiology of reduced visual acuity when the

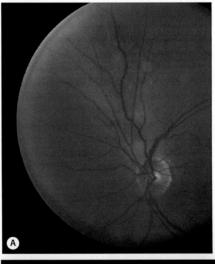

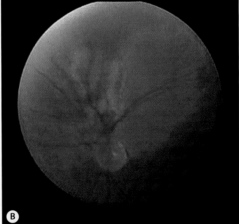

Figure 18.6 A choroidal nevus **(A)** must be monitored closely as it can transform to a malignant melanoma **(B)**.

cause is not obvious. Once the macula is located, it should appear avascular, or free of blood vessels. In addition, it should be noted whether the patient has a foveal reflex, which is a bright, pinpoint reflection. A foveal reflex is not present in all patients, and its absence is not indicative of disease. Likewise, the presence of a foveal reflex does not guarantee that the fovea is normal. Other macular abnormalities should also be noted: for example, the presence of a depression in the macula, as in a macular hole (**Fig. 18.7**), white deposits in and around the macula (drusen), yellow exudates or red haemorrhages, as can be seen in diabetic retinopathy (**Fig. 18.8**)

Apertures and filters

Apertures: Viewing with the direct ophthalmoscope can be enhanced using various aperture and filter settings. Most ophthalmoscopes have three aperture diameters. The large aperture is used for general viewing of the fundus, except for patients with small pupils. The medium aperture is useful for patients with small pupils and when determining if an optic disc is larger or smaller than normal. The smallest aperture is used to minimize the area of illuminated retina.

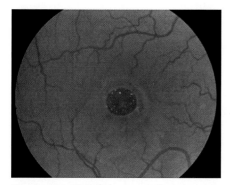

Figure 18.7 A full-thickness macular hole.

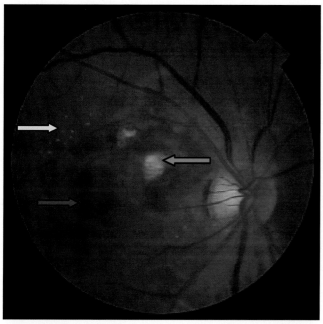

Figure 18.8 Retinal haemorrhages (*red arrow*), exudates (*yellow arrow*) and fluffy cotton wool spots (*green arrow*) in the posterior pole in diabetic retinopathy.

This is particularly useful when viewing the macula in order to reduce pupillary constriction.

Some ophthalmoscopes also have a slit aperture. This is used to identify tissue elevation or depression. It is also useful to illuminate a small portion of the retina in order to view structures in indirect illumination (the structural abnormality is viewed to the left or right of the slit beam). Certain abnormalities in the RPE are more visible in indirect illumination.

A graticule consisting of a series of concentric rings is often available. This is used to locate the fovea and to determine whether fixation is eccentric or central and steady or unsteady. This is performed by occluding the fellow eye and asking the patient to look directly into the central ring of the graticule. The fovea should be assessed for about 30 seconds under dim illumination. The graticule is also useful for estimating the size and location of a lesion. However, graticules are not standardized and may differ from one make of instrument to another.

Filters: Filters enhance the viewing of the fundus and allow for certain structures and abnormalities to be more visible than when viewing in white light. The red-free filter has a green colour and is useful for viewing haemorrhages, since the haemorrhage appears dark. This filter also increases the contrast of the vessels against the retinal background, thereby making them easier to see, although it makes differentiation between arteries and veins more difficult. This filter is also useful for viewing the nerve fibre layer, making it easier to see than in white light.

Indirect ophthalmoscopy

Examination of both the peripheral fundus and the posterior pole is possible with indirect ophthalmoscopy. This method of ophthalmoscopy should be used:

- when examining a patient for the first time
- when examining a patient with reduced best corrected visual acuity
- when examining a patient with symptoms of shadows, cobwebs, hazy vision, flashes of light, and/or floaters, which might suggest a retinal tear, detachment, or other retinal abnormality
- when following a patient for a known retinal disease or abnormality
- when following a patient who has had trauma to, or around, the eye
- when patients are taking systemic drugs with known retinal manifestations
- when following patients with systemic diseases that have retinal manifestations, such as diabetes, high blood pressure, cardiovascular disease, sickle cell disease, infectious and autoimmune diseases
- in patients with cataracts or following cataract extraction
- when a patient presents with intraocular inflammation
- for routine follow-up care (usually every 2 to 3 years)
- annually in patients with family history of retinal disease
- for older patients (>60 years) who are at greater risk for media opacities which preclude good observation without dilating, and who are at greater risk for the development of glaucoma and age-related macular degeneration.

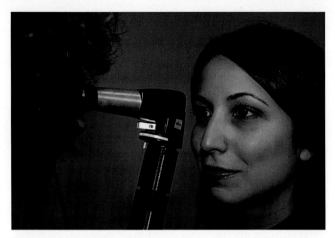

Figure 18.9 Monocular indirect ophthalmoscopy allows for increased working distance from the patient.

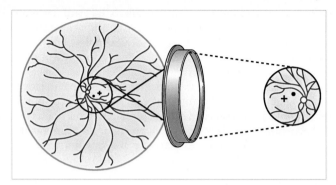

Figure 18.10 In binocular indirect ophthalmoscopy, the image is real and magnified, but inverted and reversed. (Figure redrawn with permission from Fingeret M, Casser L and Woodcome H T 1990 Atlas of primary eyecare procedures. Appleton & Lange, Norwalk, CT.)

There are two methods of indirect ophthalmoscopy.

- *Monocular indirect ophthalmoscopy*: Monocular indirect ophthalmoscopy is a hand-held technique which produces a real and erect image. The advantage over direct ophthalmoscopy is the increased field of view, albeit at lower magnification. Since the image is real and erect, the examiner also sees a direct view. An additional advantage over direct ophthalmoscopy is the increased working distance from the patient (**Fig. 18.9**). However, the examiner is still using only one eye to examine the fundus and therefore stereoscopic viewing is not possible. Accordingly, examination of elevated and excavated lesions, as well as depth of optic nerve cupping, is limited with this form of ophthalmoscopy. There are two instruments of note currently manufactured: the Welch Allyn Panoptic (Welch-Allyn, Skaneateles Falls, NY, USA) and the Keeler Wide-Angle (Keeler Instruments, Windsor, UK). The Panoptic is good with small pupils and provides a 5× greater field of view than standard ophthalmoscopy. The Keeler Wide-Angle monocular ophthalmoscope provides a 10× larger field of view and two different magnification settings.

- *Binocular indirect ophthalmoscopy*: In binocular indirect ophthalmoscopy (BIO), as its name suggests, both eyes are viewing the fundus, thereby allowing stereoscopic examination. The light from the illumination system is reflected off the retina and converged by a condensing lens held in front of the patient's eye to form an aerial image. The image is real and magnified, but inverted and reversed (**Fig. 18.10**). A greater field of view is possible compared with direct ophthalmoscopy because the lens can capture rays emanating from the peripheral fundus. Magnification varies with the power of the condensing lens. These are generally high plus, double-aspheric lenses ranging in power from +14 D to +90 D.

The general rule is that the higher the dioptric power of the condensing lens, the lower the magnification, the smaller the lens diameter and the larger the resulting field of view. The various powers of available condensing lenses, their diameter, magnification, field of view and working distances are shown in **Table 18.1**. In order to view the peripheral fundus and get an overall view of the posterior pole (at lower magnification), BIO is performed using lower-powered condensing lenses (the most commonly used is +20 D, but one can go as high as +40 D) while wearing a headset to illuminate the retina. This is referred to as headset

Table 18.1 Comparison of Volk aspheric condensing lenses used in headset binocular indirect ophthalmoscopy

Lens power	Lens size	Image magnification	Field of view (°)	Working distance (cm)
+15 D	52 mm	3.92	40	60.0
+15 D	45 mm	3.89	35	60.6
+20 D	50 mm	2.97	46	43.1
+20 D	35 mm	2.93	32	44.3
+25 D	45 mm	2.41	52	32.8
+25 D	33 mm	2.36	38	34.2
+30 D	43 mm	2.05	58	26.5
+30 D	31 mm	1.99	42	27.4
+40 D	40 mm	1.59	64	17.7
+40 D	31 mm	1.53	50	19.0
Panretinal 2.2	52 mm	2.56	56	34.1

BIO. When using condensing lenses of higher dioptric power, the magnification is so low that the fundus must be viewed via a biomicroscope to provide additional magnification. This technique, known as fundus biomicroscopy, allows a detailed view of the posterior pole, macular area, blood vessels and details of the optic nerve head. Elevation and excavation of retinal lesions within this area and cupping of the optic nerve head can be viewed under high slit-lamp magnification using higher-power condensing lenses (typically +78 D and +90 D).

Binocular indirect ophthalmoscopy requires both an illumination system and a viewing system. For headset BIO, the illumination source comes from a bulb mounted within the headset that is powered by a power supply and rheostat. Power supplies may be wall mounted or may be worn on the examiner for improved access to the patient. For fundus biomicroscopy (discussed later), the biomicroscope supplies the illumination. The viewing system for headset BIO consists of a mirror, oculars, prisms (for setting the examiner's inter-pupillary distance necessary to achieve stereopsis and optimal depth perception), the light source and various filters (**Fig. 18.11**). The oculars may also contain plus lenses (ranging from +1.75 D to +2.50 D) for presbyopic examiners in order to alleviate the need for accommodation. Myopic examiners using these oculars will need to wear their correction while doing BIO. Newer BIO models may be supplied with plano lenses for observers with active accommodation.

As in direct ophthalmoscopy, there are a variety of filters and apertures used to maximize viewing of the fundus for both headset BIO and fundus biomicroscopy. Filters consist of red-free (for viewing haemorrhages, which appear black against the background, and the retinal nerve fibre layer), cobalt blue (for better detection of fluorescence, as in optic disc drusen), yellow (for greater patient comfort) and polarized (to reduce glare from reflected light off the retina). Some systems, such as the Keeler Vantage BIO (Keeler Instruments, Windsor, UK) have a 'safety filter' designed to reduce infrared, ultraviolet and blue hazard wavelengths without compromising colour. The newer BIO models have various aperture settings to accommodate pupil size and area of detail that is being examined. For small pupils and small areas of the fundus to be viewed, a small aperture

setting is used; for diffuse views through widely dilated pupils, a larger aperture size would be used.

Procedure for binocular indirect ophthalmoscopy

Firstly, the patient's pupil must be dilated. The pupil should ideally be as widely dilated as possible to get a maximum view of the retinal periphery. Initially, instil one drop of tropicamide 0.5% for lighter-coloured irides or 1.0% tropicamide for darker irides. In patients with dark irides, or for patients who do not dilate well, one drop of phenylephrine 2.5% should be added to the tropicamide. An additional set of drops (tropicamide first, then phenylephrine if necessary) may be required for patients who typically do not dilate well, such as diabetics, patients who have had a history of uveitis with resulting iris adhesions to the lens surface (synechiae) and patients who have had cataract extraction. Cycloplegics, such as cyclopentolate 1%, may be used to dilate the pupil in children or in adults when relaxation of accommodation is desired. Since cycloplegics are longer acting than other mydriatics, this class of dilating agents is reserved only for special situations as aforementioned. After instillation of the mydriatic drops, wait at least 30 minutes before examining the retina.

Procedure for performing headset BIO

- Place the headset on the observer's head, and adjust the headband so it is snug and comfortable.
- Bring the headset as close to the observer's eyes as possible.
- Align the eyepieces to match the observer's inter-pupillary distance.
- Hold the thumb along the midline at arm's length (about 40 cm).
- Fixate on the observer's thumb with both eyes and make sure each eye can view the thumb by closing one eye at a time. If not, realign the oculars.
- Adjust the light beam and direct it to the upper third of the thumb.
- Focus the light source on the top of the thumb so that the illuminating light rays are separated from those being reflected back from the patient's retina (observation system).
- The patient can be either sitting upright or lying back in a supine position. Hold the condensing lens in the dominant hand between the thumb and index finger, making sure that the white or silver ring on the condensing lens is facing the patient, otherwise the image will be distorted. Two small circles of light or reflexes will be seen when the lens is held properly; these represent two lines of sight, one from each eye. The patient's upper lid is usually held with the examiner's thumb from the free hand, and the middle finger of the hand holding the lens is placed on the patient's lower lid. The other fingers rest on the patient's cheek or forehead (**Fig. 18.12**).
- Place the condensing lens as close to the patient's eye as possible without touching it and centre the pupil in the lens. Move the lens towards the observer until the whole lens is filled with as much of the retinal view as possible. Keep the lens perpendicular to the line of sight. The retina should be in focus: if not, the examiner must move either closer or farther away from the patient until a clear focus is seen. Media opacities, such as corneal disease, cataracts

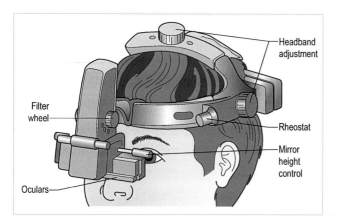

Figure 18.11 The headset BIO houses a mirror, oculars, prisms, various apertures, a light source and filters. (Figure redrawn with permission from Fingeret M, Casser L and Woodcome H T 1990 Atlas of primary eyecare procedures. Appleton & Lange, Norwalk, CT.)

Labels: Headband adjustment, Rheostat, Mirror height control, Filter wheel, Oculars

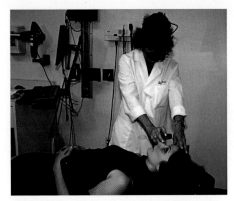

Figure 18.12 Positioning the arm and the hand for examination with headset BIO.

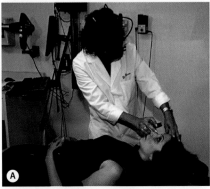

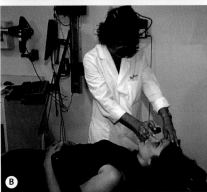

Figure 18.13 (A–B) To examine the retinal periphery, the examiner must align the light source, the lens and the line of sight when moving from side to side.

and/or vitreal haemorrhage and fibrosis will prevent the examiner from gaining a clear view of the posterior segment.

- When examining the far periphery, the pupil becomes more elongated and therefore the examiner must tilt their head in order to align both the light source and one line of sight (**Fig. 18.13**). In addition, viewing the periphery induces astigmatism, so it is important to tilt the condensing lens to compensate for this induced astigmatism. For optimal stereopsis when examining the periphery, both lines of sight must enter the pupil. This can be accomplished by adjusting the headset to the small pupil setting.

Posterior segment examination with headset BIO: procedure and sequence

Examination of the retinal periphery

Begin by viewing the peripheral retina in all directions. This is more comfortable for the patient since the light is directed to areas outside the posterior pole and light sensitivity will be less pronounced. If a patient is still photosensitive to an extent that prevents the examiner from viewing the retina, a yellow filter can be introduced in some headsets. This filter affects the resolution to a small degree but may make the patient more comfortable.

The examiner should be positioned 180° away from the quadrant to be examined and the patient directed to look in the direction of that quadrant as follows:

- Direct the patient to look up. The examiner will be below the patient's head and will be viewing the superior retina of either eye.
- Direct the patient to look up and to their right. The examiner will be situated down and to the patient's left and will be viewing the superior temporal retina of the right eye or the superior nasal retina of the left eye.
- Direct the patient to look to their right. The examiner will be situated to the left and will be viewing the temporal retina of the right eye or the nasal retina of the left eye.
- Direct the patient to look down and to their right. The examiner will be situated up and to the patient's left and will be viewing the inferior temporal retina of the right eye or the inferior nasal retina of the left eye.
- Direct the patient to look down. The examiner should be above the patient's head looking directly at the inferior retina of either eye.
- Direct the patient to look down and to their left. The examiner will be situated up and to the patient's right and will be viewing the inferior nasal quadrant of the right eye or the inferior temporal quadrant of the left eye.
- Direct the patient to look to their left. The examiner will be on the patient's right and will be viewing the nasal retina of the right eye or the temporal retina of the left eye.
- Direct the patient to look up and to their left. The examiner will be situated down and to the patient's right and will be viewing the superior nasal quadrant of the right eye or the superior temporal quadrant of the left eye.

The patient is moving their eye 360° around in an anticlockwise direction and the examiner follows the patient 180° away, also moving in an anticlockwise direction. This sequence should be followed for each patient for consistency in order to ascertain that all areas of the retinal periphery are examined.

Examination of the posterior pole

Once the periphery has been examined, the examiner directs the patient to look at the observer's right ear to examine the posterior pole of the right eye and at the observer's left ear to examine the posterior pole of the left eye. This direction will provide a view of the optic disc and macula. Since light sensitivity will be greater when viewing the posterior pole, the patient may be tempted to close their other eye. Remind the patient to keep their other eye open as this will facilitate viewing of the posterior pole.

Remember that the view in each area of the retina will be inverted and reversed. This is one of the more difficult spatial concepts for the examiner who is learning the technique. Although the examiner is examining the superior retina when the patient is looking up, for example, all of the structures seen within that view are inverted and reversed. Therefore, a larger hole that appears to be more peripheral or anterior to a smaller hole is really less peripheral, or more posterior, to the smaller hole. But both holes are in the superior retina.

Other examination points

- If the examiner wants to centre a portion of the image in the condensing lens, their body and condensing lens must pivot as a single unit.

- As for the safety of BIO, the American National Standards Institute (ANSI) recommends no more than 40 seconds of continuous viewing time when examining a specific area of the posterior segment, and the light should be set at medium intensity. However, in patients with media opacities, it may be necessary to raise the rheostat setting. However, the examiner should shorten the viewing time if using a brighter setting.

Anatomical landmarks

The peripheral fundus

- *Vortex system*: This system is made up of tributaries that look like spider's legs. The vessels vary in size and shape, are usually red and range in number from as few as 4 to as many as 15. The vortex veins are responsible for drainage of the choroid, iris and ciliary body. They empty into a dilated sac called the ampulla. These ampullae number between 4 and 10 per eye and are located at approximately 1.30, 4.30, 7.30 and 10.30 in clock hours. In a lightly coloured fundus, such as that of a fair-skinned patient, it is quite easy to view the vortex system. The vortex veins travel obliquely through the scleral canal for about 4 mm, and exit the globe posterior to the equator. The equator is not a landmark but is a description of an imaginary circle through the ampullae of the vortex veins, located about 14 mm to 15 mm from the limbus. The superior and inferior vortex veins drain into the superior and inferior ophthalmic veins, respectively.

- *Long ciliary nerves and accompanying arteries*: These nerves are easy to spot as they are elongated yellowish projections usually surrounded by pigment that appear exactly at 3 and 9 o'clock. They divide the fundus horizontally into superior and inferior halves, and run from the mid periphery out to the ora serrata. These nerves are accompanied by a long ciliary artery which lies just above the nerve; however, the arteries are more difficult to observe.

- *Short posterior ciliary nerves*: These nerves are located at the 6 and 12 o'clock positions of the fundus, and can range in number from 10 to 20 per eye. They are more difficult to identify than the long ciliary nerves. The short posterior ciliary arteries are visible in various locations in the fundus.

- *The ora serrata*: The ora serata is the most anterior portion of the fundus and is seen as a dark pigmented band. It marks the end of the sensory retina and the beginning of the ciliary body (pars plana). The ora has bays and dentate processes (teeth) that are more prominent in the nasal than the temporal retina. Viewing the ora assures the examiner that they have viewed the entire peripheral retina.

- *The vitreous base*: Just posterior to the ora, or before the ora begins, is the vitreous base. This structure runs circumferentially around the retina and is firmly attached to it. It appears as a whitish band or ridge which is wider nasally than temporally.

The examiner's ability to view all of the anatomical landmarks is dependent on the size of the dilated pupil and the absence of media opacities, especially when viewing the periphery. These landmarks help to establish the location of any abnormalities noted during the fundus examination.

Posterior pole and central 30 degrees The optic disc, macula, fovea and the quadrantic branches of the central retinal vein and artery should be viewed. This is accomplished by having the patient look at the examiner's right ear while the patient's right eye is being examined. This places the disc and macula into one view as well as most of the posterior pole. The examiner can thereby obtain a large field of view, although at low magnification. To increase magnification, the examiner can move slightly closer to the patient. To visualize the optic disc, vessels and macula in greater detail, it is necessary to perform either direct ophthalmoscopy, as described previously, or fundus biomicroscopy using a higher-powered lens, e.g. +78 D or +90 D condensing lens, described later.

Recording retinal findings

Documentation of abnormal retinal findings is an important part of good record keeping. If the retinas of both eyes are normal, one records that the retina is flat and intact 360° in both eyes (ocular uterque or OU), with no holes, tears or anomalies. If any anomalies are found, an accurate diagram of the abnormality should be drawn, paying attention to both size and location. Since the view in indirect ophthalmoscopy is inverted and reversed, it helps the novice to turn the page upside down and draw the lesion as it appears to them, rather than performing the mental exercise of inverting and reversing what was seen. Eventually, with experience, the examiner is able to do this without inverting the page. It should also be remembered that if a retinal abnormality appears to be closer to the examiner in the condensing lens, then it is actually more peripheral.

Diagrams of the eye are typically made by drawing two concentric circles, where the outer circle represents the ora serrata and the inner circle represents the equator; the optic disc is added to the drawing, placed nasally and the fovea is represented by a '+'sign. In addition to a diagram, a description of the abnormality is necessary, in which the identification, location, size and shape are denoted. For example: Right eye (OD): 1 DD (disc diameter) retinal hole at 8 o'clock surrounded by a 1/2 DD area of fluid.

The circumference of the globe is greater at the equator than at the ora. However, this concept is reversed when drawing a diagram of the retinal periphery. The circle represented by the ora is actually wider than the circle represented by the equator (**Fig. 18.14**).

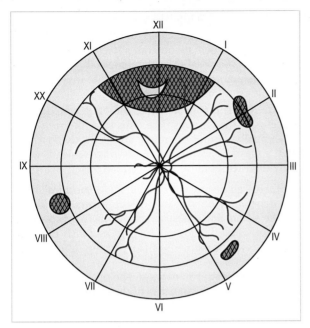

Figure 18.14 The fundus is divided into 12 sectors, like clock hours; lesions are placed within their proper location. (Figure redrawn with permission from Fingeret M, Casser L and Woodcome H T 1990 Atlas of primary eyecare procedures. Appleton & Lange, Norwalk, CT.)

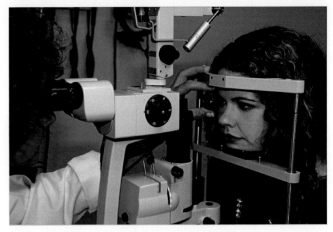

Figure 18.15 The condensing lens (usually a 78 D or 90 D lens) is held about 1 cm from the patient's eye.

Additional viewing options

Fundus biomicroscopy This procedure permits binocular viewing of the fundus while the examiner and patient are seated at a slit-lamp biomicroscope. Viewing the retina with this technique allows for higher magnification and is optimal for detailed, stereoscopic examination of the optic nerve head, retinal vasculature, and macula. The patient's pupils are dilated, as described previously and, as in BIO, a high-powered condensing lens is used to view the retina. Because an aerial image is formed from the light reflected off the retina, the resulting magnified, real image is also inverted and reversed, as in headset BIO. The most commonly used lens powers are +78 D and +90 D, although there are additional lenses that provide higher resolution, wider field of view and improved viewing through small pupils.

- The examiner and patient are seated at the slit lamp, and the patient is instructed to keep their forehead pressed against the forehead rest and their chin firmly in the chin rest. The examiner positions the patient's head so that their eyes are aligned with the positional lateral markers on the headrest supports.
- The width of the slit lamp beam is adjusted to 2–3 mm using moderate illumination and the magnification set at 6× or 10×.
- The biomicroscope is centred in front of the patient's eye with the light source in front of the biomicroscope.
- The slit lamp is moved forward until it is about 10 cm away from the eye.
- The examiner will initially see a red reflex in the pupil, which is retroillumination light from the retina. The patient should then be instructed to look at the examiner's right ear with their left eye for examination of the right eye, and at the examiner's left ear with their right eye, for examination of the left eye.

- The condensing lens is held about 1–2 cm away from the patient's eye (**Fig. 18.15**). The examiner may stabilize the lens either by using a lens holder or by resting the fingers against the patient's cheek. The examiner's middle finger and ring finger are used to raise the upper and lower lid, respectively, if necessary.
- The slit lamp is then moved back slightly until an inverted and laterally reversed image comes into focus; widen the beam of the slit lamp to a degree that is tolerable to the patient.
- Adjust the tilt of the lens to get the best focus. Examine the posterior pole as described below.
- To examine the temporal and nasal periphery, tilt the lens to the left with the patient looking in left gaze and to the right with right gaze. To examine the superior retina, tilt the inferior edge of the lens inward and closer while the patient looks up. To examine the inferior retina, tilt the lens outward and away from the eye while the patient looks downward.

Scleral indentation/depression Scleral indentation allows the examiner to view the more anterior (peripheral) aspects of the fundus. By indenting the fundus, the examiner physically moves the anterior fundus into view. In addition, a particular lesion is seen differently because it is palpated or pushed from outside the globe, or behind the lesion. A popular analogy used when describing the concept of scleral depression is that the depressor, when palpating a lesion from behind the globe, is viewed in the condensing lens as having the appearance of a 'mouse under a rug'. This is a very accurate description of this procedure when it is performed correctly.

There are various types of scleral depressors. The Schepen's thimble depressor is shaped like a sewing thimble (manufactured by Propper, Inc.; Topcon, Inc.; and Heine, Inc.). This should be held between the thumb and index finger for best stability. The articulated scleral depressor is elongated, like a pencil, and has an 's'-shaped or double-ended indentor (such as the Schocket scleral depressor) as well as a clip for insertion into a coat pocket. The more frugal practitioners can use a cotton bud, coin, or even a paper clip to indent the eye.

Applications of scleral depression include:

- The identification and localization of breaks and tears in the retina. If a break is present, it will open up in a gaping manner when indenting.
- Determining the extent of a retinal break.
- Differentiating full-thickness from partial-thickness breaks.
- Determining if fluid is present under the surrounding retinal break or hole. If fluid is present, one will see white with pressure around the hole or break.
- Differentiating a retinal haemorrhage from a retinal break. The haemorrhage remains constant in colour when indented whereas when a break is indented, the margins will blanch or appear lighter.
- Differentiating a retinoschisis from a retinal detachment. The underlying choroidal detail is visible through a retinoschisis, but not through a retinal detachment.
- Evaluating the extent of vitreal traction.

When performed properly, scleral indentation will not enlarge a retinal hole or break or cause a retinal detachment.

Three-mirror contact lens evaluation This technique permits binocular evaluation of the retina from the optic nerve all the way to the ora serrata including the vitreous and vitreoretinal interface. Once an abnormality is identified by BIO, with or without scleral depression, then this lens can be used to provide greater magnification of the area in question.

The lens consists of a 64 D central viewing lens which provides a direct view of the optic disc and macula. The three mirrors are spaced 120° apart; one mirror, inclined at approximately 59° (depending upon the specific manufacturer), is used to view the area from the ora serrata to the pars plana (and is also used in gonioscopy to view the anterior chamber angle); a second mirror, angled at approximately 67°, is used to view an area from the equator to the ora serrata; the third mirror, angled at approximately 73°, is used to view the retinal equator (**Fig. 18.16**). The mirrors are placed 180° away from the point of interest and provide an anterior–posterior inverted view. Since the lens is placed directly onto the eye, this procedure requires instillation of a topical anaesthetic in addition to mydriatic (dilating) drops.

The procedure for performing both scleral depression and three-mirror evaluation is described in detail elsewhere (Casser et al 1997) and requires a great deal of practice. Both of these procedures can be uncomfortable for the patient and should only be performed for the reasons described above. It is important to explain the purpose of these techniques to the patient before one begins the procedure.

Imaging systems for posterior segment examination

Over the past decade, eye care practitioners have witnessed the development of several devices that use scanning lasers to image the posterior segment of the eye. These technologies have expanded the practitioner's ability to examine the posterior segment and, in some cases, allow an 'in vivo' dissection of the retina. These imaging systems assess the structural integrity of the retina, retinal nerve fibre layer and optic nerve, and have many advantages over viewing the posterior segment with an ophthalmoscope. These include:

- ease of use for examiner and patient alike
- reproducibility of results
- greater field of view in some cases
- ability to image retinal layers
- ability to detect abnormalities missed by standard ophthalmoscopic viewing techniques
- quantification of size and depth, which allows better determination of progression or resolution of disease state.

These new technologies are not meant to diagnose disease. That task is still left to the clinical judgement of the examiner. The results obtained from these instruments are meant to serve as an adjunct to clinical care, providing quantifiable data that can be used to detect structural changes earlier in the course of a disease, and help practitioners provide better management through more prompt detection of abnormalities and of change over time.

Imaging devices that are currently commercially available to evaluate the structural integrity of the posterior segment include:

- Optical Coherence Tomography (OCT)
  1. Time Domain OCT
  2. Fourier Domain OCT

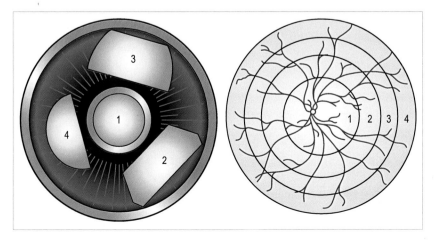

Figure 18.16 The three-mirror lens has a central lens (1), to view the posterior pole, and three peripheral mirrors 120° apart, angled at 73° (2), 67° (3) and 59° (4). These mirrors allow one to view the retinal periphery from the equator to the pars plana and anterior chamber angle. (Figure redrawn with permission from Fingeret M, Casser L and Woodcome H T 1990 Atlas of primary eyecare procedures. Appleton & Lange, Norwalk, CT.)

- Optos Panoramic 200
- GDxVCC Nerve Fibre Layer Analyzer
- Heidelberg Retinal Topography (HRT)
- Retinal Thickness Analyzer

Optical coherence tomography

Optical coherence tomography (OCT) performs cross-sectional, or tomographic high-resolution imaging of the internal microstructure of biological tissues, including the retina and optic nerve. This instrument uses low-coherence or white-light interferometry to perform B-scan ultrasonography. The original OCT devices provided high-resolution time and distance measurements, thereby determining the echo time delay and intensity of backscattered or reflected light (Hee et al 1995). Developed in the early 1990s (Huang et al 1991), OCT has evolved into a powerful imaging technology, enabling commercially available systems to offer in vivo, real-time imaging of tissues with a resolution between 3 and 15 μm. A cross-sectional image is generated by a superluminescent diode laser light (810 nm) that is scattered, reflected and absorbed by tissue. The resultant cross-sectional image is made up of hundreds of juxtaposed axial or A-scans, one-dimensional images and transverse pixels. This image is displayed using a logarithmic 'false-colour' scale, in which the log of the backscattered light intensity corresponds to a rainbow colour scale. The logarithm is used because reflected light signals from the various retinal layers vary over five orders of magnitude. The intensity of this backscattered light is dependent upon the optical properties (index of refraction) of the layers of tissue being imaged.

The principle of OCT is applicable to many tissues in the body, but has gained popularity over the last decade for imaging the eye, including the retina, optic nerve head and retinal nerve fibre layer. It may also be used for imaging the anterior chamber, including the cornea, iris, angle and lens.

In a patient with clear media and good fixation, it is possible to image up to seven or eight retinal layers with a resolution of 5–10 μm using the time-domain (TD) OCT systems. Higher-resolution Fourier-domain (FD) systems, described later, are capable of 3–5 μm of resolution. If one considers that the diameter of a red blood cell is about 7 μm, one can appreciate the exquisite resolution of OCT systems, and the opportunity to observe retinal tissue at the cellular level in some cases. The retinal layers that can be seen in TD-OCT are depicted in **Fig. 18.17**.

The procedure does not require contact with the cornea, and therefore is very comfortable for the patient. Images can be obtained by ancillary personnel and interpreted by the eye care practitioner. Pupil dilation is usually required for imaging of the posterior pole; however, imaging of the optic disc and retinal nerve fibre layer (RNFL) may be accomplished through an undilated pupil in most cases.

There are currently several commercial systems available for OCT measurements of the eye. The earlier systems were time-domain (TD-OCT) such as the widely used OCT Stratus (Carl Zeiss Meditec, Dublin, CA), which has been in clinical use for several years. More recently, a new technology in OCT has emerged, namely high-speed OCT, also known as Fourier-domain (FD), high-definition (HD) or spectral-domain (SD) OCT (Wojtkowski et al 2005).

The posterior pole may be scanned using a number of data acquisition protocols. One popular clinical scan is the 'Fast Macular Scan', in which a 6 mm area is scanned (six line scans), thereby providing a two-dimensional 360° thickness map divided into three circular macular sectors, namely 1 mm, 3 mm and 6 mm from the fovea. Quantification of retinal thickness is depicted in the parameter display of the printout and on the colour map. Thicker areas of the retina are denoted in yellows and reds; thinner retinal areas are denoted in blue. As expected, a normal fovea would be depicted in blue and is less than 200 μm thick. This particular scan provides a quick assessment of the entire macular area. One shortcoming of this scan is that should a lesion fall between the six line scans, it may be missed. In addition, information is extrapolated in areas between the six scans. **Figure 18.18** shows a patient with central serous choroidopathy, an often idiopathic condition leading to a serous detachment. An additional, higher-resolution scan can be performed, known as the 'Line Scan'. Here, only one

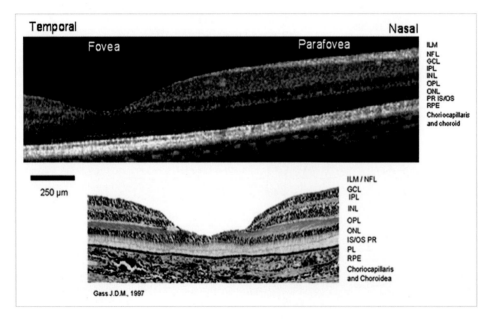

Figure 18.17 The high resolution of the newer Fourier-domain OCT systems (RTVue) allow for assessment of all the retinal layers (top) compared with a histological slide (bottom). (Reproduced with permission from Optovue, Inc.)

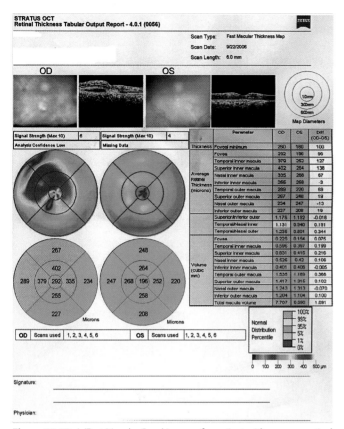

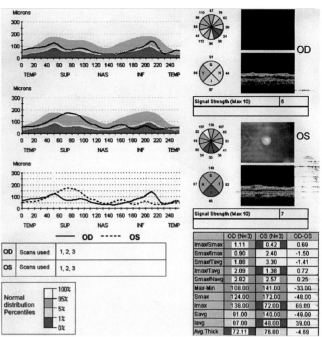

Figure 18.21 OCT technology can measure the thickness of the RNFL in an area 3.4 mm in diameter around the optic nerve head. The patient's RNFL thickness is displayed as a TSNIT curve, in black, on the left, compared with the normative database. The sectors, on the right, depict the comparison in clock hours and in quadrants. Normal sectors are depicted in green, borderline are yellow and abnormal in red. The patient in **Figure 18.20** has glaucoma in both eyes, with inferior RNFL thinning OD and greater inferior RNFL thinning OS.

Figure 18.18 A 'Fast Macular Scan' image of a patient with a serous retinal detachment secondary to central serous choroidopathy in the right eye. The thickened areas on the retinal map are depicted in yellows and reds.

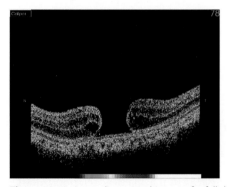

Figure 18.19 A two-dimensional image of a full-thickness macular hole.

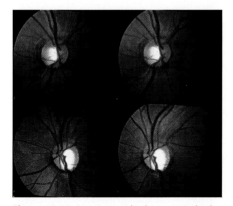

Figure 18.20 A patient with glaucoma in both eyes. Note the inferior rim thinning in both eyes, much greater in the left eye (*bottom*).

meridian is scanned at a time, but the resolution of the resulting image is greater than with the Fast Macular Scan. **Figure 18.19** shows a line scan of a patient with a full-thickness macular hole and an incomplete posterior vitreal detachment. OCT is also useful in assessing oedema resolution following treatment. This provides a more reliable indicator of treatment effectiveness than ophthalmoscopy or fundus photography, since thickness cannot be quantified using the latter techniques.

OCT is also valuable when obtaining quantitative measurements of optic disc topography and RNFL thickness. In the OCT Stratus, a series of 4 mm-long radial line scans at 12 clock hours around the disc allows for topographic measurement of disc parameters (**Figs 18.20** and **18.21**). The instrument finds the margin of the disc objectively using a signal from the end of the RPE. Disc parameters measured include cup volume, disc area, cup and rim area and cup-to-disc ratios. To determine the RNFL thickness, data are collected in a circular area 3.4 mm in diameter around the optic nerve head (when using the fast RNFL scanning protocol). A peripapillary cross-sectional image is obtained and displayed as a temporal–superior–nasal–inferior–temporal (TSNIT) curve. Using this scanning protocol, the patient's curve is displayed within a 5–95% confidence interval of normative data for that patient's age group. In addition, the RNFL thickness is quantified in 12 clock hours as well as four quadrants. The statistical significance of any abnormal areas is depicted in yellow (borderline) and red (outside normal limits). **Figure 18.21** depicts an abnormal RNFL in a patient with glaucoma. These measurements are not only important in the early detection and progression of structural damage due to glaucoma but also play a role in the detection of other optic neuropathies that affect the health of the RNFL. For additional clinical examples and more detailed explanation of TD-OCT, the reader is directed to a comprehensive text on this subject by Schuman et al (2004).

The original OCT systems were considered 'time-domain' (TD-OCT). Here, a mechanical, moving reference mirror performs the individual A-scans. The information is accumulated sequentially along the longitudinal direction of the retina, 1 pixel at a time, 1024 pixels per A-scan. In 1.28 seconds, 512 A-scans are collected and a B-scan (2-D) image is created. In FD-OCT, the reference mirror is stationary and the image is captured using a fast transfer rate CCD camera. A spectrometer analyses the signal by wavelength, and the resulting spectral interferogram is converted by Fourier transform to a typical A-scan image. In 0.04 seconds, 1024 A-scans are collected (twice the number from TD-OCT). Therefore, FD-OCT is 30 times faster than TD-OCT; this speed is faster than the velocity of eye movements, so eye movements do not affect the image as they do with TD-OCT. Since FD-OCT also collects twice the amount of data within this period of time, it results in a higher-resolution image (5 μm) than with standard TD-OCT. This allows for more precise detail and a better understanding of the histology of retinal disease at the cellular level. The data acquired by these systems also allow for 3-D imaging to be superimposed above the A-scans for better resolution and localization of pathology (**Fig. 18.22**).

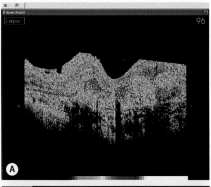

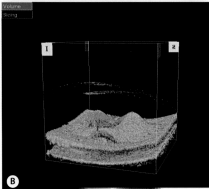

Figure 18.22 High-speed, high-resolution spectral or Fourier-domain OCT systems allow for 2-D (**A**) and 3-D (**B**) imaging, as seen in this patient with an active choroidal neovascular (CNV) membrane, in wet age-related macular degeneration.

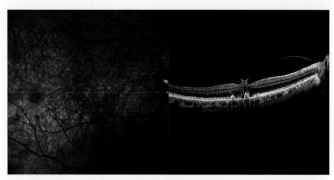

Figure 18.23 Other Fourier-domain OCT systems provide high-speed, high-resolution imaging, such as in the Spectralis™. This patient has vitreomacular traction syndrome, in which the vitreous causes traction on the macula, pulling the tissue in an upward direction. This is difficult to appreciate with an ophthalmoscope or in a fundus photograph (*left*). It can best be appreciated with high-resolution OCT (*right*). (Courtesy: Heidelberg Engineering, Inc.)

FD-OCT systems that are presently commercially available include:

- RTVue 100 (Optovue, Inc., Fremont, CA)
- Cirrus High Definition (HD) OCT (Carl Zeiss Meditec, Inc, Dublin, CA)
- Spectral OCT (SOCT) Copernicus (Reichert, Inc., Depew, NY)
- Spectral OCT/SLO (Ophthalmic Technologies, (OTI), Inc., Toronto, Canada)
- 3D OCT-1000 (Topcon, Inc., Paramus, NJ)
- Spectralis™ HRA+OCT (Heidelberg Engineering, Inc.,Vista, CA).

The Spectralis™ HRA+OCT Spectral domain (SD) OCT combines spectral- or Fourier-domain OCT technology with simultaneous HRA (Heidelberg Retinal Angiography), using either fluorescein or indocyanine green dye (the latter dye is utilized for better visualization of choroidal abnormalities). Autofluorescence, red-free imaging and infrared imaging may also be obtained. Fundus autofluorescence is a viewing technique that is gaining use in the detection and tracking of lipofuscin concentration in the macula, a potential indicator of progression of dry age-related macula degeneration (ARMD) to geographic atrophy, a later stage of dry ARMD (Holz et al 2001). Using a scan rate of 40 000 A-scans per second, the Spectralis™ HRA+OCT cross-sectional images enable visualization of nine retinal layers, with an axial resolution of 7 microns and a transverse resolution of 14 microns. **Figure 18.23** depicts a patient with vitreomacular traction. This causes a reduction in best corrected visual acuity and is difficult to appreciate with the ophthalmoscope.

Another clinical application of higher-resolution OCT systems is the visualization of the interface line between the inner segments (IS) and outer segments (OS) of the photoreceptors. This IS/OS line has recently been termed the photoreceptor integrity line (PIL). This interface is markedly affected in diseases of the outer retina, such as retinitis pigmentosa and occult outer retinopathy. The presence of this line, which is invisible with the ophthalmoscope, confirms photoreceptor integrity (see **Fig. 18.24**).

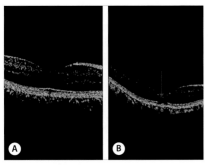

Figure 18.24 (A) The SD-OCT images the IS/OS junction line, or photoreceptor integrity line (PIL) (red arrow), as seen in a normal eye. Note the elevation of this line at the fovea. This is due to the longer outer segments of the foveal cones. **(B)** Note that the PIL in the fovea is disrupted in this patient with age-related macular degeneration (red arrow). (Reproduced with permission from Sherman et al 2008.)

There are many retinal and vitreal clinical applications for retinal imaging of the posterior pole with OCT, including:

- retinal tumours and cysts
- retinal detachment
- retinoschisis
- retinal tear; retinal hole
- multiple defects of retina without detachment
- diabetic retinopathy – all stages
- macular oedema
- macular hole
- macular pucker
- hypertensive retinopathy
- exudative retinopathy
- vascular changes
- vascular occlusive diseases
- central serous choroidopathy
- serous detachment of the RPE
- macular degeneration (dry and wet forms)
- toxic maculopathy
- vitreoretinal degenerations and dystrophies
- retinal dystrophies
- retinitis
- choroiditis
- choroidal degeneration
- pars planitis

Optos Panoramic 200

Since numerous systemic diseases have retinal and choroidal manifestations, one could argue that virtually every comprehensive medical evaluation should include a panoramic view of the fundus of the eye. Prior to the introduction of the Panoramic 200 (Optos, Inc., Marlborough, MA) the standard of care was generally considered to be a dilated fundus examination using the BIO. Clinicians experienced with the traditional procedures (headset BIO and fundus biomicroscopy), as well as the Panoramic 200, have found that the preferred method that minimizes the possibility of missing a lesion is to perform all of these procedures. However, a more efficient approach may be to obtain an 'Optomap', or fundus image, and then to decide which additional forms of ophthalmoscopy or other high-tech imaging procedures are necessary. Any lesion or an area of concern detected on the Optomap can then lead to 'targeted clinical ophthalmoscopy', where the clinician utilizes the Optomap as a roadmap to locate and then analyse the area of concern with various other technologies or procedures (e.g. BIO, fundus biomicroscopy, etc.). If, on the other hand, the Optomap is normal, the practitioner can decide based upon a number of factors whether or not to do a dilated fundus examination (DFE). For example, if a high-quality image is obtained out to 200°, and the patient is asymptomatic and free of systemic disease, the practitioner can defer a DFE until the next visit. If not, the practitioner may elect to do a DFE in addition to the Optomap.

Several attributes of this technique contribute to enhanced disease detection. The scanning device uses different frequency lasers, capable of gathering information from multiple layers of the fundus. The green laser (532 nm) captures most of its information from the neurosensory retina to the retinal pigment epithelium (RPE), whereas the red laser (633 nm) captures most of its information from the pigment epithelium posterior to the choroid. However, there is some overlap between the two.

Both the green and red separation views are obtained simultaneously and are immediately available (in addition to the composite view). Subtle findings at the level of the retina anterior to the RPE are more obvious with the green separation view, while subtle findings at the level of choroid (posterior to the RPE) are more obvious with the red separation view. This allows for differential diagnoses of most lesions within the view of the Panoramic 200. For example, retinal haemorrhages can be visualized with the high-magnification green separation view (but often not with the red), whereas a choroidal abnormality such as a naevus or inflammation can be visualized with the red separation view (but often not with the green). In addition, the ability to study the mid and far periphery under magnification allows for the identification of important findings that may be missed with conventional BIO. For example, numerous patients have been identified by Optomaps with mid- and far-peripheral haemorrhages, often associated with diabetic retinopathy, that can be missed with BIO. Retinal holes, tears, detachments and retinoschisis may be detected with BIO. **Figure 18.25** shows a

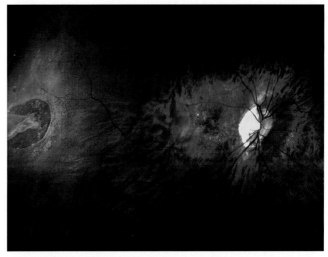

Figure 18.25 An Optomap image goes out to 200° and reveals a horseshoe-shaped retinal tear. (Courtesy of Jerome Sherman OD.)

patient who had a routine BIO examination followed by an Optos Panoramic examination. The Optomap detected a horseshoe-shaped tear in the temporal retina of the right eye. Notice how the 'U' of this tear faces the posterior retina. This is typical of these types of tears. This patient must be promptly treated with a laser to prevent retinal detachment.

Abnormal findings can be accurately identified, localized, circled, measured, and e-mailed to other clinicians for consultation using this imaging technology. Identification of incremental change is another feature of the Panoramic 200. Serial Optomaps obtained over time can be compared simultaneously to identify even subtle changes. Lesion size can be quantified. One example where this can be especially helpful is when monitoring a lesion that initially was believed to be a naevus. However, if serial images demonstrate a clear increase in size over time, then the lesion is more likely to be a melanoma. One could argue that retinal photography can monitor these changes as well. While this is true of central lesions, it is often difficult to obtain good-quality photographs in the retinal periphery.

The virtual point technology of the Optos Panoramic allows viewing of 200° of the fundus through a 2-mm pupil by bringing the green and red light to a virtual focus just posterior to the pupillary plane via an ellipsoidal mirror. In effect, the virtual scan takes place within the eye, thereby allowing an ultrawide view of the fundus anterior to the equator. The 200° panoramic view is therefore attainable, even without pupillary dilation. This is valuable in patients whose pupils do not dilate easily, cannot be dilated safely, or refuse to be dilated. The use of virtual point technology predicts vitreal opacities that are close to the scan point. They are going to appear disproportionately large because of their angular subtense.

The ultrawide field technology provided by the Optos Panoramic 200 has also been adapted for wide-field fluorescein angiography (Manivannan et al 2005). This technology introduces a way of simultaneously imaging both the central and peripheral retina while performing fluorescein angiography. This type of viewing is useful in retinal diseases such as diabetic retinopathy that affect both the central and peripheral retina.

Optos has introduced the P200 C, which provides a more natural, round look to the optic nerve head. For additional clinical cases and a more detailed description of this technology, the reader is directed to a comprehensive text of this subject (Sherman et al 2007).

GDxVCC (glaucoma diagnosis, variable corneal compensation) nerve fibre layer imaging

Most practitioners agree that the retinal nerve fibre layer (RNFL) is one of the most difficult parts of the retina to assess by ophthalmoscopy. It is often too thin, especially in older patients, to assess accurately. The thickness of this layer, which is an important parameter in the detection of glaucoma and other optic neuropathies, cannot be quantified, and perhaps only 'qualified' by standard ophthalmoscopy and red-free fundus photography.

The GDxVCC was developed specifically for assessment of RNFL thickness using technology known as scanning laser polarimetry (SLP). This specifically and objectively quantifies RNFL thickness. The RNFL is affected early in glaucoma and this is the prime reason why many clinicians will use this

technology. However, the RNFL is also affected in many other optic neuropathies. These include but are not limited to vascular, infectious, inflammatory, traumatic, toxic, autoimmune, metabolic, inherited, neoplastic, nutritional, endocrine and environmental aetiologies. Therefore, the clinician has many clinical reasons to image the RNFL on a daily basis.

As previously mentioned, RNFL thickness can be assessed by OCT technology, but assessment of RNFL by the GDxVCC involves a different methodology. RNFL measurements are comparable, meaning that an abnormal RNFL thickness detected by GDxVCC will also be abnormal when compared with findings from other technologies such as OCT. This is true even though the actual numbers, expressed in microns, are different. The reason for the absolute difference is due to variations in the methods adopted by each technique to determine RNFL thickness.

The GDxVCC relies on the principle of birefringence of the RNFL to obtain thickness measurements. The RNFL is made of highly ordered, parallel axon bundles. The axons contain microtubules, i.e. cylindrical intracellular organelles whose diameters are smaller than the wavelength of light. The highly ordered (parallel) structure of the microtubules creates birefringence within the RNFL. Birefringence is the splitting of a light wave by a polar material into two components. These two components of light travel at different velocities, thereby creating a relative phase shift between the two, termed 'retardation' (**Fig. 18.26**).

Scanning laser polarimetry takes advantage of the birefringent properties of the RNFL to measure its thickness accurately. It has been demonstrated that the amount of retardation is proportional to the thickness of the structure (Weinreb et al 1990). The cornea also has birefringent properties, but the GDxVCC employs a variable compensator to cancel out the corneal birefringence. A scanning laser polarimeter (SLP), i.e. a confocal scanning laser ophthalmoscope with an integrated ellipsometer, is used to measure retardation. The SLP directs polarized light through the eye. This light passes through the RNFL and the two components of the polarized light are phase shifted relative to each other (retarded). This light reflects off of the retina and returns to the ellipsometer, where the retardation is measured. An algorithm determines the RNFL thickness, point by point in the peripapillary region, by measuring the total retardation of light reflected from the retina.

The SLP provides both a reflected light image and a retardation map of the peripapillary retina. The magnitude of

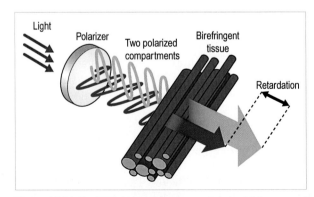

Figure 18.26 The RNFL is form-birefringent. Polarized light passes through the RNFL and splits into two rays. The ray travelling perpendicular to the RNFL undergoes a phase shift and is 'slowed down'. This is termed retardation. (Reprinted with permission from Cart Zeiss Meitec, Inc.)

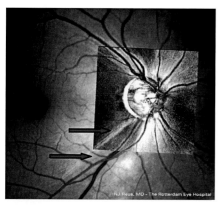

Figure 18.27 The image obtained by scanning laser polarimetry (SLP) (*inner picture*) in a glaucoma patient with an inferotemporal wedge-shaped RNFL defect (*red arrow*): the GDx overlies a red-free fundus image of the right eye, demonstrating the close correlation between the image obtained by SLP and the anatomical RNFL. (Reprinted with permission from Elsevier publishers; Reus et al 2003.)

retardation is captured by a detector, and converted into thickness. SLP measurements are taken by scanning the beam of a near-infrared laser (780 nm) in a raster pattern. This scan captures an image with a 40° horizontal by 20° vertical field, and includes both the peripapillary and macular regions. The total scan time is 0.8 seconds. The reflectance image is generated from the light reflected off the surface of the retina, and is displayed as the fundus image. The retardation image is converted into RNFL thickness based on a conversion factor of 0.67 nm/μm. Each image is made up of 256 (horizontal) × 128 (vertical) pixels, or 32 768 total pixels. The correlation between red-free photography and SLP is evident in **Figure 18.27**. Here, the GDxVCC image of a glaucoma patient with an inferior–temporal wedge defect in the right eye is superimposed on the red-free image. The wedge defect is seen better in the GDx image and this illustrates the close correlation between the image obtained by SLP and the anatomical RNFL (Reus et al 2003).

Each print-out has a wealth of information regarding the patient's RNFL. The print-out displays specific RNFL parameters (superior average, inferior average, TSNIT standard deviation, symmetry between eyes), which are highlighted when these values deviate from the normal age-matched and race-matched population. A neural network analysis is also performed to differentiate the patient's RNFL from the glaucomatous population, and this analysis is displayed as a 'Nerve Fibre Indicator', or NFI. The NFI ranges between 2 (the best possible score) and 98 (the worst possible score). The latter indicates that no more than 20 μm of RNFL remain. An RNFL with an NFI greater than 30 is considered suspicious.

The display (**Fig. 18.28**) also features the scanning laser ophthalmoscopy (SLO) fundus image, the thickness or retardation map, and the deviation map, which indicates which points of the patient's RNFL, spaced 0.7 μm apart, deviate from the age-matched normals, and the statistical significance of these deviated points. The lower display, or TSNIT curve, is a measure of the RNFL thickness within a designated circular area around the optic nerve head, termed the ellipse, and is represented by a double-peaked graph. Each peak corresponds to the superotemporal and inferotemporal thickness of the RNFL. The troughs correspond to the thinner nasal and temporal RNFL. **Figure 18.28A** shows GDxVCC findings from a patient with a normal

RNFL. Notice the rich yellow and orange colours on the thickness or retardation map that correspond to the superior–temporal and inferior–temporal RNFL, the thickest part of the RNFL. Contrast that with **Figure 18.28B**, which illustrates the findings from a glaucomatous patient. There is very little yellow or orange on this thickness map. Note also the difference in the parameters (thickness measurements) between these two patients and the amount of statistically significant deviation from normal on the deviation map (yellow and red pixels) for the glaucoma patient. Further, in **Figure 18.28** the double-peak TSNIT curve is clearly seen in the normal patient (**Fig. 18.28A**) but is reduced in the glaucoma patient (**Fig. 18.28B**). This GDx technology can also monitor RNFL change over time using serial analysis software. Any statistically significant progression is noted on the serial analysis print-out, which includes both numeric and graphic progression of the parameters over time.

Heidelberg Retinal Tomography

Previously, the optic disc rim and cup was assessed by direct observation. Initially, the direct ophthalmoscope allowed practitioners to view the colour, borders, vessels and anomalies of the optic disc. Assessment of the cup, however, with regard to contour, depth, shape, and cup-to-disc ratio, was more of a problem with this monocular technique. With the addition of indirect ophthalmoscopy using lenses of high dioptric power at the binocular slit-lamp biomicroscope, assessment of the optic cup was more accurate, given the stereoscopic viewing and high magnification. Stereophotography also afforded a better degree of accuracy regarding assessment of cupping and rim tissue loss. However, these viewing techniques were limited by examiner technique and subjective opinion. Additionally, these parameters of the optic nerve could not be quantified accurately by direct observation.

The need existed, therefore, for the development of an objective method of quantifying various parameters of the optic disc that could be followed over time. The eventual development and clinical use of imaging techniques utilizing SLO for measuring the topography of the optic disc and the quantification of optic disc parameters has proven to be valuable in the diagnosis and management of glaucoma. Heidelberg Engineering, Inc. (Vista, CA, USA) developed an imaging device using confocal scanning laser ophthalmoscopy (CSLO) which is used in the Heidelberg Retinal Tomography (HRT). The HRT uses a CSLO to produce a pseudo 3-D image of the optic nerve head, and quantifies various parameters of the optic disc surface and topography. These parameters (specified below) can be used to document change over time (Hatch et al 1997).

The HRT uses a 670 nm diode laser that can be sharply focused at various depths within the eye, scanning a series of 15° × 15° areas. It begins at the most anterior portion of the disc and scans back and forth, acquiring height measurements from 147 456 points within each plane. It then proceeds posteriorly, focusing on between 16 and 64 planes, depending on the cup depth, until it reaches the base of the cup (**Fig. 18.29**). Three sets of images are obtained to account for variability. All the data points are computed to produce a 3-D image of the optic disc in which all planes appear in focus. The quality of the image obtained is indicated by a topography standard deviation of the three sets.

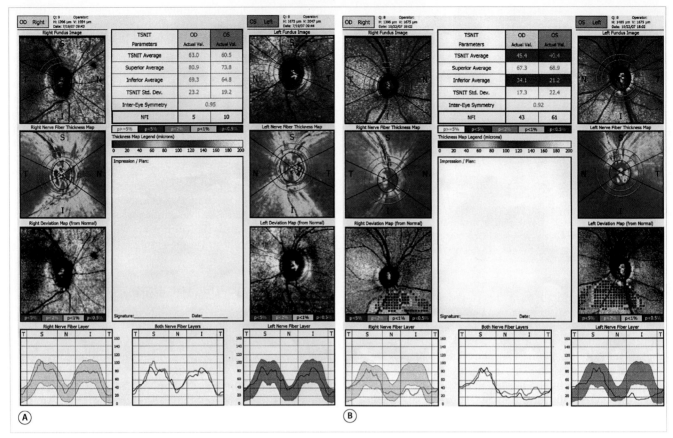

Figure 18.28 The print-out report of the GDx contains an SLO fundus image, thickness or retardation map, and a deviation map. In addition, various RNFL parameters are quantified. On the bottom of the display is the double-humped TSNIT curve, where the peaks correspond to the thickness of the superior and inferior (thickest) portion of the RNFL and the troughs correspond to the nasal and temporal (thinnest) portion of the RNFL. **(A)** A patient with normal RNFL thickness. Note the normal parameters in green, the warm yellow and red colours on the thickness map and the normal TSNIT curves. The NFIs are well below 30 in each eye. **(B)** A display from a glaucoma patient, with inferior cupping and inferior–temporal nerve fibre layer loss. Note parameters are highlighted in reds and yellows, denoting statistically significant RNFL thinning. The NFI is well above 30 in both eyes, which is abnormal. Note the red and yellow pixels on the deviation map, greater in the left eye, denoting statistically significant RNFL thinning in these areas, and the depressed TSNIT curves on the bottom.

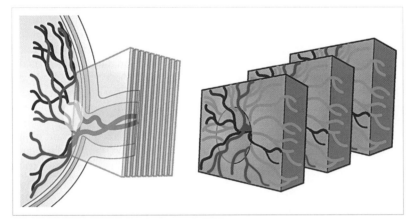

Figure 18.29 The HRT uses a 670 nm diode laser that can be sharply focused at various depths within the eye, scanning a series of 15° × 15° areas. It begins at the most anterior portion of the disc and scans back and forth, acquiring height measurements from 147 456 points within each plane. It then proceeds posteriorly, focusing on between 16 and 64 planes, depending on the cup depth, until it reaches the base of the cup; three similar images are captured and computed. (Reprinted with permission from Heidelberg Engineering, Inc.)

The generated report includes several disc parameters including disc size, linear cup-to-disc ratio, cup shape measure, rim area, rim volume and RNFL height variation contour. Mean RNFL thickness is measured at the edge of the disc using an artificial reference plane located 50 μm below the edge of the disc margin. Six sectors of the optic disc rim are analysed by the Moorfields Regression Analysis (MRA), which compares the patient's disc parameters to a normative database, and predicts the sector and global status of a patient's optic disc, generating both numeric tables and a graphic analysis. A green check mark indicates that the rim is predicted to be 'normal' for that sector; a yellow exclamation point predicts that sector to be 'borderline' and a red 'x' predicts that sector to be 'outside normal limits'. An asymmetry parameter also accounts for any difference between the two eyes. In addition to the MRA, the

HRT3, i.e. the newest software version of this technology, provides a Glaucoma Probability Score (GPS). This is a score generated by artificial intelligence known as relevance vector machine (RVM), which determines the statistical probability of an abnormal disc based on the shape of the optic disc and the RNFL compared with an ethnically matched database. Both methods classify the patient's findings as being normal, borderline or outside normal limits. This does not necessarily mean that the disc is glaucomatous, as other non-glaucomatous optic neuropathies cause damage to rim tissue and the RNFL. **Figures 18.30A and 18.30B** depict displays from the HRT3 from a normal patient and a patient with glaucoma, respectively.

HRT technology can also be used for determining the topography of the macular region in diseases that affect macular thickness, such as diabetic retinopathy. The Heidelberg Mapping Program uses the same principles for acquiring images of the optic nerve head to image the macula (Hudson et al 1998).

The primary benefit of the HRT technology in glaucoma is for monitoring changes in disc topography over time. This quantification of multiple disc parameters allows the statistical analysis of these data to determine progression. Although stereophotography and BIO can also be used to assess progression, the limitations of subjective variability are, for the most part, removed by this objective technology. In addition, objective assessment of the disc is less time consuming for both the doctor and patient. For the assessment of early glaucomatous changes, however, it has been demonstrated that confocal SLO is superior to optic disc photography (Wollstein et al 2000). However, binocular visual assessment of the optic disc as well as stereophotography are still standard-of-care techniques. Objective disc analysis is considered adjunctive and assists clinicians in following patients over time.

Retinal Thickness Analyzer

The Retinal Thickness Analyzer (RTA) (Marco, Inc., Jacksonville, FL, USA) is an ophthalmic imaging device for the mapping and quantification of retinal thickness and disc topography. It was originally designed by Talia Technology (Neve-Ilan, Israel) to detect retinal thickening at the posterior pole (Zeimer et al 1996), an application especially useful in diabetic retinopathy. However, its clinical applicability was

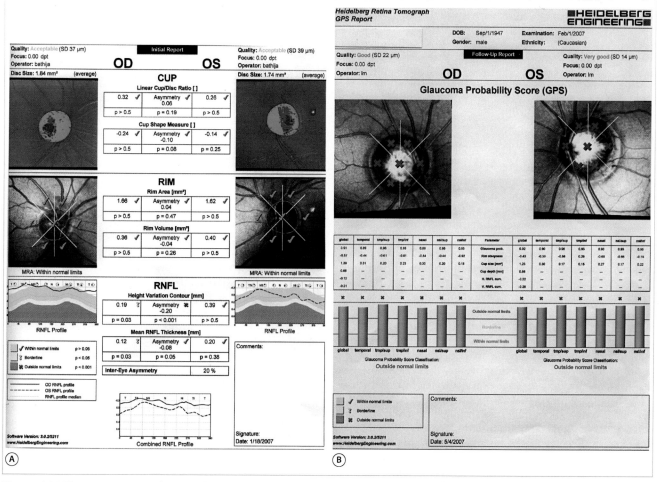

Figure 18.30 The print-out report of the HRT for disc topography displays an SLO fundus image of the optic nerve and the parameters of disc topography. There are two statistical analyses of deviation from the normative database. the Moorfields Regression Analysis (MRA), which predicts sector and global status of the disc rim, and the Glaucoma Probability Score (GPS), which determines the statistical probability of an abnormal optic disc rim and RNFL using an ethnic-specific database. **(A)** HRT print-out from a normal patient depicting normal cup, rim and RNFL topography. **(B)** HRT display from a patient with advanced glaucoma.

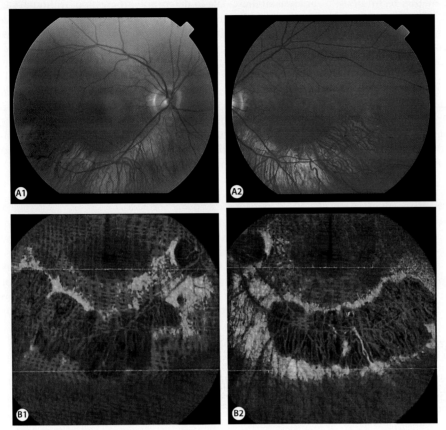

Figure 18.31 Fundus **(A1 and A2)** and fluorescein angiography **(B1 and B2)** image of a patient with a mild form of autosomal dominant retintis pigmentosa demonstrates inferior arcuate retinal and choroidal atrophy.

expanded to include optic disc topography. In addition, this technology measures thinning in the macular region secondary to loss of ganglion cells as an early sign of glaucoma.

The RTA utilizes a vertical, narrow HeNe (543 nm) laser to project an angled slit beam while a CCD camera records light backscattered from the vitreoretinal internal limiting membrane (ILM) and chorioretinal (RPE) surfaces. A 3 mm × 3 mm scan consisting of 16 optical cross-sections is obtained across the posterior pole at nine different positions. The thickness of each slit at these nine points is used to construct a three-dimensional image or retinal map. The resulting map depicts areas of retinal thickening or thinning. The eye depicted in **Figure 18.31** has a retinal dystrophy, a mild form of autosomal dominant retinitis pigmentosa. The fundus photograph shows only inferior arcuate retinal and choroidal atrophy. However, the RTA image (**Fig. 18.32**) demonstrates that the superior arcuate retina is also affected by this disease.

It should be noted that all of the imaging technologies that incorporate scanning laser ophthalmoscopy are not without limitations and do require patient cooperation. Accurate images may not be obtained in patients with dense media opacities, intraocular lens implants or poor fixation due to functional or structural abnormalities. Further, patients with peripapillary abnormalities, such as staphyloma, large scleral crescents, peripapillary atrophy, poorly defined disc borders, tilted discs with oblique entrance, etc., may also have equivocal results.

The future of posterior segment imaging

The further evolution of posterior segment examination lies in the development of even higher-resolution imaging. The principle of adaptive optics, in which higher-order wavefront aberrations of the eye are corrected, is being incorporated into eye-imaging technologies, specifically OCT (Zawadski et al 2007). The high resolution of adaptive optics, recognized in the late 1990s (Liang et al 1997), improves resolution to the cellular level, allowing the examination and even counting (Xue et al 2007) of individual cells never before possible in the examination of the retina, making histology an in vivo experience. These systems are currently used in research of hereditary retinal diseases and in glaucoma, but are not yet clinically available.

Telemedicine

The ability to digitize fundus photographs and the availability of SLO imaging has paved the way for ease and completeness of communication between eye care professionals via telemedicine. Images can be transferred immediately through the internet for on-line consultation and education between a general eye care practitioner and a specialist.

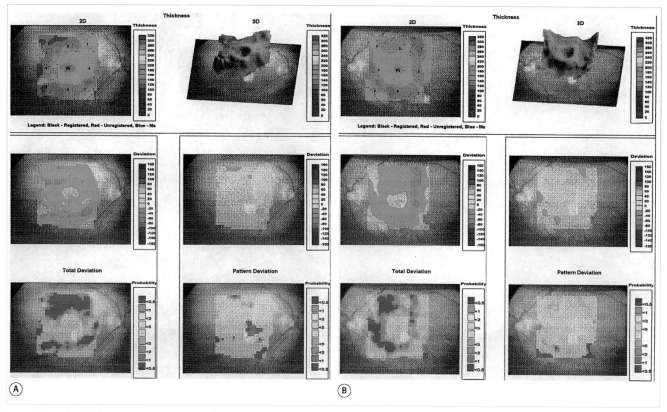

Figure 18.32 The RTA image demonstrates a circular or ring-shaped annular area of retinal thinning in both eyes (in blue). This was not evident either in the fundus image or in the fluorescein angiography image.

Access to consultation between practitioners can be performed across the street or across the world in minutes thanks to digitized imaging of the eye. The result of this is more timely diagnosis, treatment and more comprehensive follow-up of posterior segment diseases.

Summary

We have come so far in our ability to view the posterior segment of the eye. One can only wonder what Helmholtz would think if he were alive today. The quest for accurate in vivo assessment of the posterior segment continues as technologies evolve that are faster, more accurate and have higher resolution. Instead of viewing whole tissues, the higher-definition imaging technologies allow us to view individual cell layers and, in some cases, individual cells in a live patient. This chapter has reviewed the past and present standard of care, and has provided glimpses into the future. Many techniques that are currently considered 'state-of-the art' may soon be regarded as the required 'standard-of-care'. These procedures will continue to be 'adjunctive', and perhaps never replace standard ophthalmoscopy, but will provide an additional point of view in a patient. This will assist eye care practitioners to detect, manage and treat ocular diseases of the posterior segment to the highest possible standard.

References

Casser L, Fingeret M, Woodcome H T 1997 Atlas of primary eyecare procedures, 2nd edn. Appleton and Lange, Stamford, Conn

Dorion T 1998 Manual of ocular fundus examination. Butterworth-Heinemann, Hong Kong

Hatch W V, Flanagan J G, Etchells E E et al 1997 Laser scanning tomography of the optic nerve head in ocular hypertension and glaucoma. British Journal of Ophthalmology. 81:871–876

Hee M R, Izatt J A, Swanson E A et al 1995 Optical coherence tomography of the human retina. Archives of Ophthalmology 113(3):325–332

Holz F G, Bellmann C, Staudt S et al 2001 Fundus autofluorescence and development of geographic atrophy in age-related macular degeneration. Investigative Ophthalmology and Visual Science 42:1051–1056

Huang D, Swanson E A, Lin C P et al 1991 Optical coherence tomography. Science 254(5035):1178–1181

Hudson C, Flanagan J, Turner G et al 1998 Scanning laser tomography Z profile width as an objective index of macular retinal thickening. British Journal of Ophthalmology 82:121–130

Jonas J J, Budde W M, Panda-Jones S 1999 Ophthalmoscopic evaluation of the optic nerve head. Survey of Ophthalmology 43:293–320

Liang J, Williams D R, Miller D T 1997 Supernormal vision and high-resolution retinal imaging through adaptive optics. Journal of the Optical Society of America A, Optics, Image, Science, and Vision 14:2884–2892

Manivannan A, Plskova J, Farrow A et al 2005 Ultra-wide field fluorescein angiography of the ocular fundus. American Journal of Ophthalmology 140(3):525–527

Reus N J, Colen T P, Lemij H G 2003 Visualization of localized retinal nerve fiber layer defects with the GDx with individualized and with fixed compensation of anterior segment birefringence. Ophthalmology 110(8):1512–1516

Schuman J S, Puliafito C A, Fujimoto J G 2004 Optical coherence tomography of ocular diseases, 2nd edn. Slack, Inc., Thorofare, NJ

Sherman J, Karamchandani G, Jones W et al 2007 Panoramic ophthalmoscopy: Optomap image and interpretation. Slack, Inc., Thorofare, NJ

Sherman J, Yannuzzi L, Madonna R, Nath S 2008 Photoreceptor integrity line (PIL): as revealed by spectral domain OCT. Lulu.com, New York

Weinreb R N, Dreher A W, Coleman A et al 1990 Histopathologic validation of Fourier-ellipsometry measurements of retinal nerve fiber layer thickness. Archives of Ophthalmology 108:557–560

Wojtkowski M, Srinivasan V J, Fujimoto J G et al 2005 Three-dimensional retinal imaging with high-speed ultrahigh resolution optical coherence tomography. Ophthalmology 112(10):1734–1746

Wollstein G, Garway-Heath D F, Fontana L et al 2000 Identifying early glaucomatous changes: comparison between expert clinical assessment of optic disc photographs and confocal SLO. Ophthalmology 107(12):2272–2277

Xue B, Choi S S, Doble N et al 2007 Photoreceptor counting and montaging of en-face retinal images from an adaptive optics fundus camera. Journal of the Optical Society of America A, Optics, Image, Science, and Vision 24(5):1364–1372

Zawadski R J, Choi S S, Jones S M et al 2007 Adaptive optics – optical coherence tomography: optimizing visualization of microscopic retinal structures in three dimensions. Journal of the Optical Society of America A, Optics, Image, Science, and Vision 24(5):1373–1383

Zeimer R, Shahidi M, Mori M et al 1996 A new method for rapid mapping of the retinal thickness at the posterior pole. Investigative Ophthalmology and Visual Science 37:1994–2001

CHAPTER 19

Ocular biometry, colour vision testing and electrophysiology

Leon N Davies

Introduction

The scope of this chapter is quite diverse and aims to describe the clinical techniques that have not been covered hitherto. The chapter comprises three sections. Firstly, methods employed to measure and quantify ocular components are discussed (e.g. ultrasound, Scheimpflug imaging, optical coherence tomography and magnetic resonance imaging). The second section outlines the techniques utilized in colour vision assessment, while the final section covers electrophysiological techniques and their use in diagnosing patients presenting with signs and symptoms indicative of neurological or ophthalmological disease.

Ocular biometric techniques

Introduction

Clinical use of ocular biometry varies depending upon the professional setting. In ophthalmology, ocular biometry forms an integral part of the diagnosis and management process. For example, the localization and measurement of ocular tumours is facilitated by the use of ultrasound techniques, whereas more recent methods such as partial coherence interferometry (PCI) are utilized to calculate the power of intraocular lenses inserted into the eye following cataract surgery. In optometric practice, however, the use of biometric procedures is rather more limited. The advent of new, high-resolution, non-contact methods, however, may challenge that trend.

Ultrasound biomicroscopy

Ultrasound is an acoustic wave (above audible frequency) that consists of an oscillation of particles within a medium (Byrne & Green 2002). Ultrasound waves have frequencies greater than 20 KHz (i.e. 20 000 oscillations/s). Frequencies used in diagnostic ophthalmic ultrasound are in the range of 8 to 10 MHz (where 1 megahertz = 1 000 000 cycles/s). These very high frequencies produce short wavelengths (less than 0.2 mm), which enable ocular ultrasound instruments to resolve very small ocular and orbital structure. As a point of note, however, examination of larger structures (e.g. in abdominal or obstetric ultrasound) require frequencies in the range of 1 to 5 MHz. As such, the wavelengths produced by these lower frequencies enable these instruments to penetrate deeper into the body. This increase in penetration, however, is at the detriment of their resolution capability.

Ultrasound is transmitted as a longitudinal wave and, therefore, its speed is dependent upon the density of the medium it is passing through (e.g. in air, sound travels at 340 m/s, whereas in water, its speed is much faster at approximately 1480 m/s). Given this, fluid contact is essential between the transducer and the eye. To achieve this, saline is used on the open eye, or water-soluble gel is used if the reading is taken through the eyelid. Furthermore, as a longitudinal wave travels through tissue, part of the wave may be reflected back towards the probe; this reflected wave is referred to as an echo and is the basis of clinical ultrasound biomicroscopy (UBM). These echoes are produced at the junction between two media (e.g. the posterior crystalline lens and the anterior vitreous face). The greater the difference in density of these structures, the greater the echo signal becomes; this phenomenon is known as the acoustic impedance (where acoustic impedance = sound velocity × density of media). These echo signals can be further influenced by the size, shape and smoothness of the interface, and the angle of sound/probe incidence. As such, a better understanding of these potential confounding variables is imperative for the performance of reliable and repeatable ocular UBM. For a more detailed explanation of these factors, the reader is referred to the further reading section at the end of this chapter.

A-scan

Ultrasound A-scan, also known as time-amplitude ultrasonography, is produced when a static transducer is aimed along a specific line in the eye. The results of an A-scan are represented as a one-dimensional acoustic display in which echoes are represented as vertical spikes from a time baseline (**Fig. 19.1**). Echoes from structures deeper within the

eye take longer to return to the transducer for conversion back to an electrical signal, so appear further along the time baseline. The spacing between the echo spikes in the trace is dependent on the time required for the sound wave to reach a given interface and for its corresponding echo to return to the probe. The time between any two echo spikes can then be converted into a distance for biometric purposes (where distance = velocity (of wave) × time). The relative heights of the echoes along the trace give information as to the strength of the echoes and hence the nature of the intervening structures.

B-scan

In cases where a cross-sectional image of the eye is required, B-scan UBM is used. Here, a two-dimensional acoustic section of the eye is produced and displayed where each echo is represented as a spot. The strength of the echo is depicted by the brightness of the spot, the cumulative effect being a two-dimensional pictorial image (**Fig. 19.2**). To record the cross-section of tissue, an oscillating probe that emits a sound wave in the range of approximately 10 MHz is used. Again, a number of variables affect the B-scan image, including the angle of the scanning section and the speed of the probe oscillation. Indeed, the area of the eye or orbit that can be imaged at any one given time is related directly to the sector angle of the moving probe. This angle can typically vary between 45 and 60 degrees, depending on the instrument. The greyscale display is also an important factor. Instruments differ in their ability to display varying levels of grey. Intuitively, the more greyscale levels that are available, the better the instrument is at differentiating between echo intensities produced from neighbouring interfaces.

Colour Doppler imaging

A recent development in B-scan imaging incorporates the Doppler phenomenon; known as colour Doppler imaging (CDI), the technique provides information about the ocular vascular supply superimposed on a B-scan image (**Fig. 19.3**). This modality gives the approximate flow velocity of the principal vessels in the eye and the orbit, by providing a colour Doppler display for pulse Doppler examination (Lieb et al 1991; Giovagnorio et al 1993).

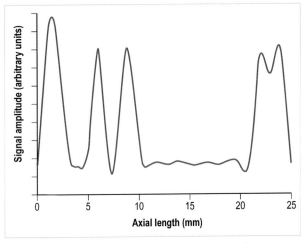

Figure 19.1 Schematic example of an A-scan ultrasound trace.

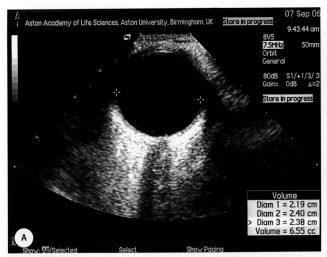 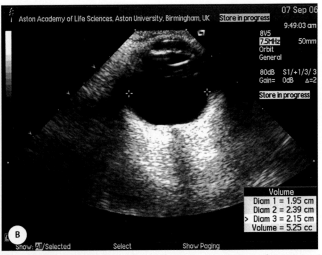

Figure 19.2 Ultrasound B-scan. (**A**) depicts the globe, optic nerve, and surrounding orbital tissues while (**B**) also highlights the position of the patient's crystalline lens.

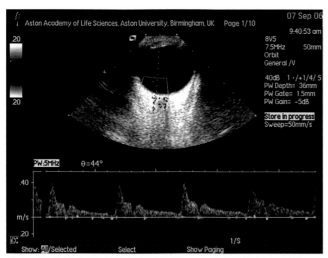

Figure 19.3 Example of a colour Doppler imaging measurement. The lower trace in the figure shows the blood flow within the optic nerve.

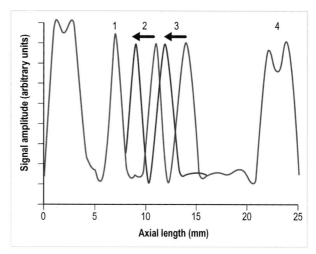

Figure 19.4 Schematic representation of an A-scan ultrasound trace with an eye cup. Here, the signal produced by the probe is separated from the peak caused by the cornea (peak 1) by approximately 5 mm. The blue trace represents the axial separations of the ocular components when the eye is in the relaxed state. Conversely, the red trace represents the axial separations of the ocular components when the eye is accommodating; hence there is an anterior shift in the crystalline lens (peaks 2 and 3), compared to the position of the peaks when the eye is relaxed.

Consequently, CDI has been proposed as a tool for diagnosis or study of vascular disorders in the eye and orbit. Several CDI studies have examined the ocular vessels, primarily via assessment of measured velocity or calculation of resistive index (RI).

CDI scans of the eye and orbit are performed with the patient lying supine with their eyes closed using an ultrasound frequency >7 MHz and a Doppler frequency >5 MHz (Tranquart et al 2003). The transducer or probe is applied to the closed upper eyelid using a thick layer of acoustic gel. Care must be taken not to exert any pressure on the globe as this might result in a decrease in blood flow velocity, thus increasing the RI with no diagnostic significance. For more detailed information on CDI the reader is directed to the further reading list at the end of this chapter.

Clinical use in biometry

A-scan ultrasonography is used principally for axial measurements of ocular components. Until recently, the A-scan was the instrument of choice; however, this has now been superseded by partial coherence interferometry (see later). It should be noted that certain crystalline lens opacities inhibit partial coherence interferometric measurements. As a consequence, many practitioners revert back to A-scan measurements in these circumstances.

The resulting echo peaks in the A-scan trace can be converted to distance to provide these ocular measurements. To facilitate the procedure, eye cups are often used. Here, the initial echo produced by the cornea is separated from the initial peak produced by the transducer. The eye cup supports a bed of saline placed on the anaesthetized cornea, meaning that the minimum transducer–cornea distance is maintained at approximately 5 mm.

Figure 19.4 shows an A-scan of an eye taken with the aid of an eye cup in both the relaxed (blue trace) and accommodated (red trace) state. Peak 1 represents the cornea (due to the resolution of the instrument, the two corneal surfaces cannot be resolved), peaks 2 and 3 represent the anterior and posterior crystalline lens surfaces, respectively, while the final peak 4 is the retina. **Figure 19.4** shows clearly the anterior shift in the crystalline lens relating to the anterior shift in peaks 2 and 3.

Scheimpflug imaging

The examination of the anterior eye segment, especially evaluation of different parameters of the anterior chamber, is important in many fields of eye care (e.g. assessing risk factors for the development of glaucoma). Anterior chamber values are also necessary when planning surgical procedures for calculation of intraocular lens (IOL) power or implantation of anterior chamber phakic IOLs.

The Scheimpflug principle images the anterior eye with a camera (often a charged couple device (CCD)) perpendicular to an optical slit beam, thus creating an optic section of the cornea and crystalline lens (**Fig. 19.5**). As with all optical and acoustic techniques, correction of the image distances needs to be made for the refractive index and the curvature of the intervening refractive surfaces (Fink 2005). The advent of the Pentacam (Oculus, Wetzlar, Germany) has increased dramatically the use of the Scheimpflug technique. The instrument

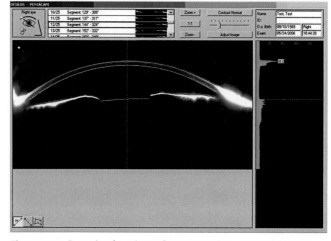

Figure 19.5 Example of a Scheimpflug image taken with the Pentacam (Oculus, Wetzlar, Germany). (Image courtesy of Dr Shehzad Naroo.)

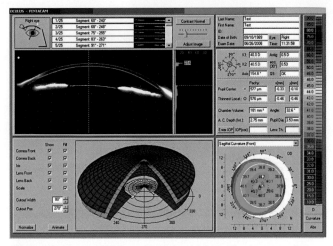

Figure 19.6 Example of three-dimensional Scheimpflug image analysis taken with the Pentacam (Oculus, Wetzlar, Germany). (Image courtesy of Dr Shehzad Naroo.)

enables evaluation of the entire anterior segment from the anterior corneal surface to the posterior lens surface using a rotating Scheimpflug camera. The non-contact measuring process takes only 2 seconds and performs 12 to 50 single captures of the anterior segment. The data can then be processed and converted to a three-dimensional model of the anterior eye segment for analysis (**Fig. 19.6**). There are five evaluation modules: Scheimpflug tomography, three-dimensional chamber analysis (depth, angle and volume), pachymetry (including adjustment of intraocular pressure (IOP)), densitometry of the crystalline lens, and corneal topography including anterior and posterior corneal surface as well as keratometry (see Ch. 17).

Partial coherence interferometry

The placement of an artificial lens within the eye after cataract surgery requires an accurate calculation of the intraocular lens power necessary for attaining the optimal postoperative refraction. Intraocular lens power is calculated using standard formulae and is dependent on the accurate measurement of the axial eye length, the corneal radius, and the anterior chamber length (Haigis et al 2000). The corneal radius is typically measured using keratometry, while the anterior chamber length is measured by slit-lamp illumination or Scheimpflug imaging. Hitherto, ultrasound biometry has been the method of choice to assess the axial length of the eye; however, partial coherence interferometry has been introduced recently as an alternative technique. This technique relies on a laser Doppler method to measure the echo delay and intensity of infrared light reflected back from intervening tissue interfaces. The technique, which is more accurate and precise than ultrasound biometry (Santodomingo-Rubido et al 2002), has now become the instrument of choice for optometrists and ophthalmologists alike. Its relatively high order of dioptric resolution for axial length (±0.03 D) is also a valuable asset in research, especially studies of myopia.

The IOLMaster (Zeiss Meditec, Jena, Germany) is a commercially available, non-contact device that performs measurement of the axial length of the eye using PCI with a spatial resolution of 0.01 mm for axial length measurements (an order of magnitude greater than A-scan ultrasound biometry). The IOLMaster uses laser interferometry instead of ultrasound to measure the axial length of the eye in approximately 0.4 seconds. It produces two beams by means of an optical delay path and reflects these beams of short coherence light from the surfaces of the cornea and then the retina. The IOLMaster compares the delay path against the optical pathway of the eye, and then evaluates that interference pattern. The instrument also enables measurement of the corneal radius using traditional keratometric principles, and measurement of anterior chamber depth by Scheimpflug imaging. The IOLMaster also includes software that uses these measurements to calculate the intraocular lens power according to standard formulas.

Optical coherence tomography

Optical coherence tomography (OCT) is a recently developed, non-invasive technique for imaging subsurface tissue structure with micrometre resolution. Depths of 1 to 2 mm can be imaged in opaque tissues such as skin or arteries, while greater depths are possible in transparent tissues such as the eye (e.g. through the cornea). Optical coherence tomography complements other imaging modalities commonly used to image subsurface tissue structure, including ultrasound B-scan and confocal microscopy; however, it has the added benefit of being non-invasive. Importantly, OCT has significant advantages over other medical imaging systems; for example, UBM, magnetic resonance imaging (MRI) and confocal microscopy are not suited to all tissue types, the former two having poor resolution, the latter lacking millimetre penetration depth.

The clinical application of OCT extends from the retina to the anterior segment. It can evaluate retinal layers to delineate preretinal, intraretinal and subretinal pathology. Furthermore, it can image disorders of the vitreoretinal interface with high resolution, and provide a quantitative analysis of macular oedema and macular holes. Optical coherence tomography can also measure retinal nerve fibre layer thickness directly to generate a two-dimensional map of the structure. Other possible applications of OCT include using the instrument to measure corneal thickness, determine the corneal ablation depth in refractive surgeries, measure the anterior chamber angle, verify anterior chamber depth and iris thickness, calculate IOL power and evaluate cataract density (Wolffsohn & Davies 2007).

In essence, OCT works via the process of low coherence interferometry. In conventional interferometry with a long coherence length (e.g. laser interferometry), interference of light occurs over a distance of metres. In OCT, this interference is shortened to a distance of micrometres by the use of a broadband light source (i.e. sources that can emit light over a broad range of frequencies). Broadband sources include superluminescent diodes, fibre amplifiers, and femtosecond pulse lasers in the wavelength range of 800 to 1550 nm.

Light in an OCT system is broken into two sections: a sample section (containing the item of interest) and a reference arm (usually a mirror). The combination of reflected light from the sample arm and reference light from the reference arm gives rise to an interference pattern, but only if light from both arms have travelled a similar optical distance (where the difference in optical distance is less than a coherence length). By scanning the mirror in the reference arm, a reflectivity profile of the sample can be obtained (this

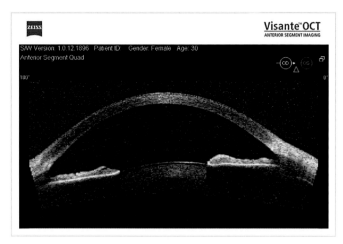

Figure 19.7 Example of an optical coherence tomography (OCT) image taken with the Visante OCT. (Zeiss Meditec, Jena, Germany.)

is time-domain OCT). Areas of the sample that reflect light back will create greater interference than areas that reflect less. Light that is outside the short coherence length will not interfere. This reflectivity profile (similar to that produced by A-scan) contains information about the spatial dimensions and location of structures within the item of interest. A cross-sectional profile (similar to that produced by B-scan) may be achieved by combining a sequence of axial depth scans (**Fig. 19.7**).

Magnetic resonance imaging

Magnetic resonance imaging (MRI) is a technique used primarily in medical settings to produce high-quality images of the internal structures of the human body. MRI is based on the principles of nuclear magnetic resonance (NMR), a spectroscopic technique used by scientists to obtain microscopic chemical and physical information about molecules. MRI began as a tomographic imaging technique, in that it produced an image of the NMR signal in a thin slice through the human body. Subsequently, however, MRI has advanced beyond a tomographic imaging method to a volume imaging technique. Medical MRI uses electromagnetic waves combined with the reception of weak radio signals to record the density or concentration of hydrogen (and other) nuclei in the human body (**Fig. 19.8**). As such, MRI frequently relies on the relaxation properties of excited hydrogen nuclei in water and fat. When the object to be imaged is placed in a

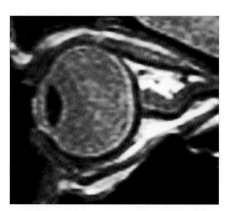

Figure 19.8 Example of a magnetic resonance image (MRI) taken with a 3-Tesla Trio (Siemens, Erlangen, Germany). (Image courtesy of Ms Liz Wilkinson.)

powerful, uniform magnetic field, the spins of the atomic nuclei with non-integer spin numbers within the tissue all align either parallel to the magnetic field or not. Common magnetic field strengths range from 0.3 to 3 teslas (the SI unit for magnetic field strength), although research instruments reach as high as 20 teslas (for comparison purposes, the Earth's magnetic field is, on average, around 50 μT).

MRI avoids health risks associated with ionizing radiation found in routine X-rays (high-energy, short-wavelength radiation which is able to pass through tissue) and computerized tomography (simultaneous X-rays from different angles) scans, but retains the ability to penetrate and image the whole human body. The clinical utility of MRI in ocular terms, however, is limited due to high cost and limited availability. Conversely, its use in ocular research is developing at a rapid pace (Strenk et al 2006; Singh et al 2006).

Clinical assessment of colour vision

Introduction

Colour sensation is derived from the interactions of various wavelengths of light energy with photosensitive pigments in the cone cells of the retina and their subsequent neural interpretation within the visual pathway. It is important to remember, therefore, that colour sensations are subjective, psychological experiences; objects and surfaces themselves do not possess colour. Moreover, the light reflected from such objects is not coloured in any way. As such, colour is a totally psychological experience produced by the effect that reflected light, from certain wavelengths of the visible spectrum, has on the nervous system. Colour does not exist even in the chain of events between the retinal receptors and the visual cortex, but only when the information is finally interpreted in the consciousness of the observer.

Normal colour vision

In the normal, healthy human eye, there are three different classes of cone photoreceptors; this leads to the term trichromacy. Each class contains a different photopigment with a maximum sensitivity in three regions of the visible electromagnetic spectrum. Consequently, all spectral hues can be matched by an additive mixture of three primary colours taken from the long-wavelength ((red) 558 nm maximum absorption), medium-wavelength ((green) 531 nm maximum absorption) and short-wavelength ((blue) 419 nm maximum absorption) regions of the spectrum. The three types of cone differ in their overall numbers and their distribution over the retina. Indeed, the short-wavelength (blue) photoreceptors are almost absent from the central fovea. As such, the phenomenon of 'small field tritanopia' often arises if colour matches are made within an area that subtends less than 0.5 degrees.

Normal colour vision can vary significantly among males and females. A large part of the diversity is due to individual differences in the optical densities of the photopigments and the relative transparency of the crystalline lens. The change in density of the crystalline lens with age is a particular problem in the elderly. Given these factors, light that reaches the photoreceptors is composed of a mixture of wavelengths and it is the dominant wavelength which determines the colour experienced.

Colour vision theories

At the level of the photoreceptors, vision is trichromatic and mediated by the three types of cones (the Young–Helmholtz trichromacy theory). The different types of cone contain one of three types of photopigment, principally but not exclusively sensitive to wavelengths that correspond to the hues of blue, green and red. Stimulation of red light produces a chromatic experience specifically due to the strong excitation of the red receptors together with a weak stimulation of the green and blue receptors; the result is a red sensation. A similar effect occurs with blue and green stimulation.

The responses from the three types of photoreceptor are transformed by the complex neural network in the retina so that at the level of the ganglion cells, colour information is coded into two opponent colour channels (red *versus* green and blue *versus* yellow), and a brightness (white *versus* black) channel (Hering's opponent-process theory). The white *versus* black channel responds when light excites any of the three types of photoreceptor. Its function is to transmit luminance rather than hue information.

The ability to match colours using a mixture of just three primaries forms the basis of an authoritative method of describing colours. In 1931 the *Committee Internationale de l'Eclairage* (CIE) devised a standard system for specifying colours based on the trichromatic colour matching characteristics of a standard observer. As it is not possible to match all wavelengths with an additive mixture of real primary colours (red, green and blue) the CIE adopted imaginary primary colours which were designated the values X, Y and Z. The relative amounts of X, Y, Z required in a colour match are represented by the lower case letters x, y, and z. Since the sum of $x+y+z$ is equal to unity, the value of z can be ascertained by subtracting $(x+y)$ from 1. All perceptible colours of a given brightness, therefore, can be represented on a graph which is known as the CIE chromaticity diagram (**Fig. 19.9**). Spectral colours are arranged along the arc of the perimeter of the diagram. White, a roughly equal mixture of the three primaries, falls in the centre of the diagram.

Defective colour vision

Trichromacy is not experienced by all. Many people are partially or completely colour deficient, confusing colours that trichromats (regardless of their individual differences in colour vision) distinguish easily. A very few, however, are completely 'colour blind', where colour discrimination is completely absent.

Inherited colour vision defects

The most common forms of colour deficiency are inherited. Congenital defects are binocular, symmetrical and do not change with time unless the individual acquires a disease that causes damage to the visual pathway. They arise from alterations in the genes encoding the opsin molecules and are characterized by abnormal colour matching and colour confusions; genes are either lost, rendered non-functional, or altered. Phenotypically, the results of the gene alterations are:

- anomalous trichromacy (where one of the three cone photopigments is altered in its spectral sensitivity, but trichromacy is not fully impaired)
- dichromacy (where one of the cone pigments is missing and colour vision is reduced to two dimensions)
- monochromacy (where two or all three of the cone pigments are missing and colour vision is reduced to one dimension).

Those inherited alterations affecting a single cone pigment are referred to by the generic names protan, deutan, and tritan, to distinguish disorders in the long/red-, medium/green-, and short/blue-wavelength photoreceptors, respectively. The term '-anomaly', when appended to the generic names, indicates a deviation or abnormality in the function of the long/red- (protanomaly), medium/green- (deuteranomaly), or short/blue-wavelength (tritanomaly) cone pigments. Similarly, '-anopia' indicates the absence of function of the long/red- (protanopia), medium/green- (deuteranopia), or short/blue-wavelength (tritanopia) cone pigments. Those inherited modifications resulting in the loss of two cone pigments are referred to as cone monochromacies. They include short/blue-cone monochromacy (affecting both the long/red-cone and medium/green-cone opsin genes), medium/green-cone monochromacy (affecting the short/blue- and long/red-cone opsin genes), and long/red-cone monochromacy (affecting the short/blue- and medium/green-cone opsin genes). Those inherited modifications resulting in the loss of function of all three cone types are referred to as rod monochromacy.

Using the CIE chromaticity diagrams, described earlier, colours which dichromats confuse lie within ellipses orientated along straight lines when plotted on a chromaticity diagram (see **Fig. 19.9**). The lines radiate from different points according to the type of defect. These lines are called isochromatic confusion loci. Dichromats will tend to confuse colours over the whole length of the confusion loci, whereas anomalous trichromats will tend to confuse colours over a more limited range.

Colour genetics

Genes that specify the red- and green-sensitive photopigments are located on the X chromosome and abnormalities are inherited as an X-linked recessive trait. Consequently,

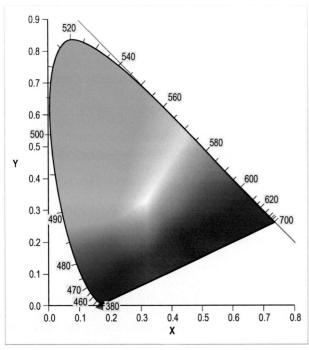

Figure 19.9 The CIE chromaticity diagram.

this results in a much higher prevalence of red–green colour deficiency in men than in women. The most usual transmission is from maternal grandfather to grandson, through the female as the carrier; this is because only one X chromosome is affected. As such, a colour vision defect will only manifest in a female when both of her X chromosomes carry similar abnormal genes; hence there is a much lower prevalence of inherited deficiency among females. Brothers of colour-deficient men have a 50% chance of being similarly affected. The different types of red–green colour deficiencies, however, do not occur with the same frequency (**Table 19.1**).

In contrast to red–green deficiencies, the gene that specifies the blue-sensitive photopigment is located on chromosome seven. Colour deficiencies derived from abnormalities of this photopigment are inherited as an autosomal dominant trait. As such, an equal number of men and women are affected. The prevalence of inherited tritanopia is equivocal, with estimates ranging from 1 in 65 000 to 1 in 1000 (Wright 1952; Kalmus 1955; Van Heel et al 1980; see **Table 19.1**). Individuals with inherited colour deficiency have normal visual acuity with the exception of monochromats, where there is a marked reduction as only one or perhaps no cone photoreceptors remain functional.

Despite the relatively high prevalence of colour vision deficiencies, the assessment of colour vision is often overlooked in optometric practice. This is usually justified on the grounds that colour vision deficiencies are not a serious handicap and even if detected there is no cure. Often, the main justification for screening for colour deficiencies, therefore, is to inform affected individuals of their problem and give appropriate advice. There are, however, a number of acquired conditions which may also lead to colour vision deficiencies, the occurrence of which add to the importance of routine screening of colour vision.

Acquired colour deficiency

Acquired colour vision deficiencies occur as a secondary feature to pathology and can arise at any time throughout life as a result of general or ocular disease, trauma, and medication, or as a result of exposure to toxic substances. Some changes in colour vision occur throughout life even in healthy individuals. As stated previously, these changes can be explained in terms of yellowing of the ocular media (Swanson & Cohen 2003) and perhaps changes in retinal sensitivity (Brown 1993; Nathan 2002). Acquired defects often fluctuate in severity, tend to be monocular and often affect blue perception. Hence, changes in colour vision can be used as a useful indicator of potentially more serious damage to the visual system.

The classification of acquired colour vision deficiencies is not as straightforward as that for congenital colour vision deficiencies. Generally, three types of colour vision defect can be distinguished:

- Type 1 (red/green): similar to a congenital protan defect
- Type 2 (red/green): similar to a congenital deutan defect
- Type 3 (blue): similar to a tritan defect.

Acquired defects, however, often show a combination of characteristics associated with more than one type; moreover, both dichromatic and anomalous trichromatic stages occur (Birch et al 1979). Clinically, acquired colour vision defects are of particular importance if they are the precursor to, or an early sign of, pathological disease. In general, however, most red–green acquired colour vision defects occur alongside ill health or a reduction in visual acuity. Conversely, type III defects can be insidious and defects can be severe before the disease manifests itself clinically. Common ocular anomalies found in clinical practice leading to colour vision defects are:

- optic neuritis: results in type 2 red–green defect; acuity may recover over time but a slight colour deficiency will remain
- glaucoma: results in type 3 colour defect
- diabetic retinopathy: early background retinopathy results in a type 3 colour defect which worsens as the disease develops
- Stargardt's disease: results in a type 1 defect
- age-related macular degeneration: results in a type 3 colour defect
- hydroxychloroquine retinal toxicity: often used to treat the autoimmune diseases systemic lupus erythematosus (SLE) and rheumatoid arthritis; can lead to a type 1 acquired colour vision defect.

Table 19.1 Types and incidences (in percentage) of inherited colour vision deficiencies in men and women

Types of colour vision	Category	Available photoreceptor types	Prevalence (%)	
			Male	Female
Trichromatism		3	92	99.5
Anomalous trichromatism	Protanomalous	3	1	0.02
	Deuteranomalous	3	5	0.40
	Tritanomalous	3	Equivocal	Equivocal
Dichromatism	Protanopic	2	1	0.02
	Deuteranopic	2	1	0.02
	Tritanopic	2	0.001	0.001
Monochromatism	Cone	1	Equivocal	Equivocal
	Rod	1	0.003	0.003

Other colour defects can also occur. Chronic exposure to industrial solvents (e.g. styrene, carbon disulphide and solvent mixtures) as well as inorganic mercury leads to type 3 defects. Moreover, patients with an inadequate diet, particularly those with vitamin A deficiencies, can present with colour vision defects. The visual acuity is often normal but rod function is affected; there is a gross constriction of the visual field and an overall reduction in hue discrimination. Improvement follows vitamin A supplementation.

Colour vision tests

Clinically available colour vision tests are used to diagnose and differentiate congenital and acquired colour deficiency. They exploit the isochromatic colour confusions and abnormal wavelength discriminations experienced by colour defectives and are designed to perform different functions.

Results of colour vision tests which use surface colours can only be considered valid if the test is administered under standardized illumination conditions, since the appearance of pigment colours changes with the spectral content of the illuminant. Tests are designed to be used with an illumination source approximating to Standard Illuminant C of the CIE, which corresponds with the blue-white appearance of overcast north sky light in the northern hemisphere (often achieved when the test is viewed with a MacBeth lamp). Usually the colour vision assessment is made at the end of a routine examination with the appropriate refractive correction in situ. For congenital defects, binocular testing is sufficient; however, it is important to remember that acquired deficiencies often present as monocular abnormalities. It is, therefore, imperative also to test colour vision in the monocular state if any acquired abnormality is suspected.

Ishihara pseudoisochromatic plates

When using a pseudoisochromatic test, observers are required to identify a figure or pattern composed of coloured dots of varying size embedded in a background of differently coloured dots. The figure and background colours are chosen so that they are confused (isochromatic) by colour defectives but are readily discernible by normal subjects. The best-known and most widely used pseudoisochromatic test is the ubiquitous Ishihara plates. Introduced in 1917, the Ishihara test is designed to give a quick, accurate and inexpensive assessment of colour vision deficiency of congenital origin. The Ishihara test has been shown to have excellent sensitivity and specificity when administered appropriately. It is designed, however, as a screening test and although some information about the severity of the test can be gleaned from the results, it is unable to differentiate reliably between anomalous trichromats and dichromats.

The full version of the test contains 38 plates, of which 25 have numerals and 13 contain 'snake-like' pathways which may be used to test young children and innumerate subjects. There is also an abbreviated 24-plate test version, and a concise test with 14 plates; however, these are considered to be an only just acceptable alternative to the 38-plate test. The test should be conducted in natural daylight or in artificial light that is as close to daylight as possible (ideally with a MacBeth lamp). Tungsten light is unsuitable (due to its bias towards long wavelengths) but daylight fluorescent light, which is available in most ophthalmic consulting rooms, is satisfactory if the illuminance is greater than 250

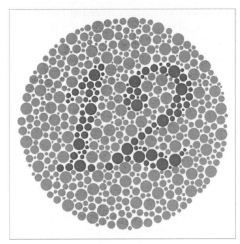

Figure 19.10 Ishihara colour vision plate used to demonstrate the test. This plate is also useful when practitioners suspect that the patient may be malingering.

lux. The plates should be held at 75 cm from the subject and tilted so that the plane of the paper is perpendicular to the line of vision. The subject should also be encouraged to answer within 3 seconds of plate presentation. Patients must be encouraged to make an immediate verbal response, as any undue hesitation on the part of the patient could suggest a slight colour deficiency.

With the 38-plate version, plate one should be seen by all subjects and be used to demonstrate the task (**Fig. 19.10**). It is also a useful test to expose subjects who are malingering. Screening plates 2 to 9 are screening transforming plates, designed so that one number is seen by the normal trichromats and another is seen by those with red–green colour deficiency (**Fig. 19.11**). Sometimes colour deficients do not see a number with these plates. Screening plates 10 to 17 are vanishing plates, and again contain numbers, which will be detected by normal trichromats but not by colour-deficient individuals. Plates 18 to 21 contain hidden digits. Here, numbers will not be detected by normal trichromats but will be detected by colour-deficient individuals. Authors have proposed that these types of plates should be omitted as they have poor sensitivity and specificity due to the fact that only 50% of colour-deficient individuals are able to see the figures (Birch 2001). The classification plates (22 to 25) are

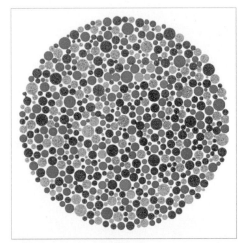

Figure 19.11 Ishihara colour vision test transforming plate.

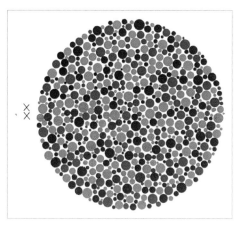

Figure 19.12 Ishihara colour vision test plate for patients who are innumerate.

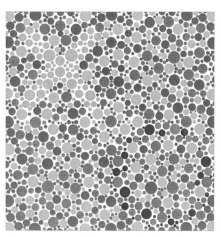

Figure 19.13 Hardy, Rand and Rittler colour vision test plate.

designed to differentiate between protan and deutan defects. Here, each plate contains two numbers printed against a background of grey dots. One number is made up of reddish-purple dots while the other consists of more bluish-purple spots. The former will be invisible (or less visible) to an individual with a protan defect while a deutan will have some difficulty resolving the later. Plates 26 to 38 can be used for those who are unable to read numerals (**Fig. 19.12**). However, as the subject is required to 'draw' over these pathways, the time taken on each plate is often too long for the test design to be effective.

Hardy, Rand and Rittler plates

In 2002, Richmond Products, a US-based ophthalmic instrument manufacturer, introduced the second edition of its version of the Hardy, Rand and Rittler (HRR) pseudoiso-chromatic test, based on the original HRR test first published by the American Optical Company in 1955 (Hardy et al 1954; Rand & Rittler 1956). Although the test is similar in appearance to the Ishihara test, importantly, the HRR is able to test for tritan colour vision defects as well as protan and deutan deficiencies. Furthermore, the HRR has additional plates to differentiate protan, deutan and tritan deficiencies and grade their severity; thus providing the clinician with more information than the Ishihara. Indeed, the HRR has been shown to be as good as the Ishihara test for detection of red/green deficiencies with the added benefit of tritan detection (Cole et al 2006a).

The HRR comprises 26 plates (plus two example plates) each displaying either one or two symbols, which can be a circle, cross, square, star or triangle (**Fig. 19.13**). As with the Ishihara test, the symbols are constructed of a series of coloured dots on a uniform grey background colour. The figure colours are such that a protan, deutan, or tritan colour defective will confuse it with the background colour. The patient is asked to describe the shape of each symbol they see and indicate its location, which can be in one of four quadrants of each plate, while the test is held at approximately 30 cm from the patient.

The 28 plates consist of:

- 2 demonstration plates, which can be seen by all observers (one of which has no symbol so that patients understand that this may occur in the main test)

- 13 screening plates: 12 for the protan–deutan defects and 1 for tritan deficiencies
- 13 diagnostic plates designed to assess the severity of the condition and to differentiate protans, deutans and tritans.

Colour deficiency is graded as mild, medium or severe, depending on whether they see or do not see the symbols on the grading plates. For example, patients who make one or more errors in the three red/green diagnostic plates with the most saturated colours are graded as severe; those who make an error in the next two most saturated plates are graded as medium. Patients who make errors only with the four least saturated plates are graded as mild deficiencies.

Arrangement tests

Arrangement tests involve the sorting of coloured samples in order of colour appearance. They classify protan, deutan and tritan defects and grade the severity of the colour deficiency. The tests demand qualitative judgements to arrange the colours in sequence and therefore are unsuitable for young children or subjects with poor communication skills. The colour samples (derived from the Munsell colour system) are spaced equidistantly around the hue circle and each colour is held within a circular cap subtending 1.5 degrees at a test distance of 50 cm to ensure that observations are made with the central rod-free retinal area. Colour confusions and the ability to discriminate fine differences in colour can be evaluated using the Farnsworth D-15 and Farnsworth–Munsell (F–M) 100-Hue tests, respectively.

Farnsworth D-15

Introduced in 1947, the Farnsworth D-15 consists of 15 Munsell colours having Munsell value 5 and chroma 4 and a reference colour as the starting point. The subject arranges the 15 mixed colour caps into a natural colour sequence corresponding to their perceived colour. Colour defectives are unable to discriminate between certain colours and will place them out of order. The order of the caps is revealed from the number on the back of each cap, which is then plotted on a circular diagram. A normal trichromat's plot would be illustrated by a complete circle with consecutive numbers of

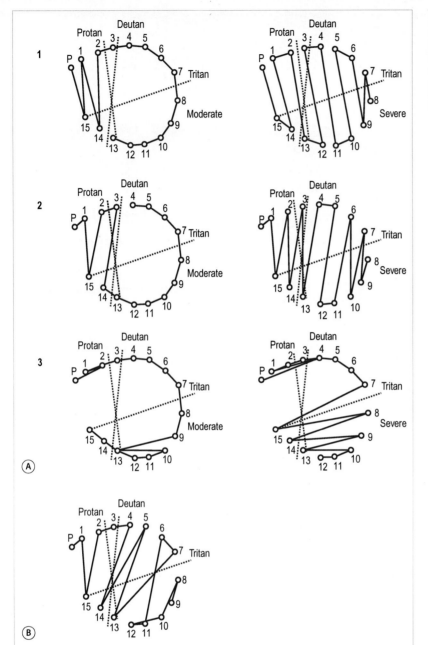

Figure 19.14 Clinical examples of D-15 colour vision test results. **(A)** Classification of moderate (left) and severe (right) colour deficiency. 1. protan defects; 2. deutan defects; 3. tritan defects. **(B)** A typical monochromat result where no overall trend is apparent in the plot. (Reproduced, with permission, from Birch 2001 Diagnosis of defective colour vision. Butterworth-Heinemann, Edinburgh, Scotland.)

1 to 15. Results from a colour deficient would show a series of lines crossing the colour circle corresponding to the axes of isochromatic colour-confusion lines (**Fig. 19.14**). A single error of two steps or more is counted as a failure. Protans show a confusion axis from red to blue-green, while deutans from green to purple and tritans from yellow to violet. The severity of the defect is indicated by the number of confusion lines that cross the diagram. The aim of the test is to divide subjects into two groups: those who have either normal colour vision or only a slight colour deficiency and those with moderate or severe deficiencies.

Farnsworth–Munsell (F–M) 100-Hue test

The F–M 100-Hue test evaluates hue discrimination ability in normal trichromats and hue discrimination losses in colour defectives and was introduced in 1943. Intuitively, the name implies that 100 hues are used; in fact, the test consists of 85 Munsell colour caps divided into four boxes. The subject arranges the colours in a linear sequence between pairs of fixed reference caps located at either end of each box. Consequently, the test can be quite time-consuming. As the test is essentially split into four sections, only confusions between hues in the same quadrant of the hue circle can be made. Isochromatic confusions cannot be demonstrated as colours from opposite sides of the hue circle are not presented simultaneously. Results are plotted on the radial line of the polar diagram representing each colour (**Fig. 19.15**). Hue-discrimination ability is calculated from the total error score, while the type of colour vision deficiency is established from the graphic representation of the results. Plots for congenital protan, deutan and tritan deficiencies demonstrate arrangement errors in two opposite positions in the polar diagram producing an axis of confusion. The magnitude of the axis of confusion and the total error score indicate the severity

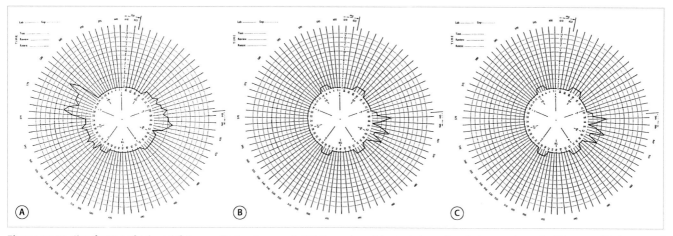

Figure 19.15 Classification of colour deficiency with the Farnsworth 100-Hue colour vision test. Axes of confusion are shown in **(A)** protan, **(B)** deutan and **(C)** tritan defects. (Reproduced, with permission, from Birch 2001 Diagnosis of defective colour vision. Butterworth-Heinemann, Edinburgh, Scotland.)

of the discrimination deficit; however, unless the subject has a dense defect along a particular colour axis, interpretation can be difficult. Indeed, the differences in axial orientation for protan and deutan plots are small and are relatively difficult to distinguish from one another. This is because the orientations of isochromatic confusion lines for protan and deutan types are very close to one another.

The key features of the 100-Hue test are that:

- The 100-Hue test is designed to provide an assessment of hue discrimination.
- The test is not reliable for colour vision screening since it is complex and can take over 20 minutes to complete.
- Only individuals with moderate or severe colour deficiencies are identified.
- The test does not reliably differentiate between dichromats and anomalous trichromats or protans and deutans.
- It has more value for occupational assessments than in diagnosis.

The City University test

The first and second editions of the City University test are derived from the Farnsworth D-15 test, in that they contain the same Munsell colours but in a book format. It was designed to overcome some of the disadvantages experienced with the D-15 test, notably soiling of the colour caps and difficulties with the concept of sequencing the colours. The second edition of the City test contains six of the original ten plates (subtending 1.5 degrees at the test distance of 35 cm; **Fig. 19.16**) and four plates (subtending 0.6 degrees at 35 cm) with desaturated colours having Munsell value 5 and chroma 2. The desaturated plates are intended to improve screening efficiency and grade the colour vision defect. However, the small size of the colour spots in the latter plates does make them vulnerable to false-positive results due to small field tritanopia. Each plate displays a central coloured circle surrounded by four other circles. Three of the comparison colours are chosen so that the centre colour and the comparison colour represent average isochromatic confusions of protanopes, deuteranopes and tritanopes. The fourth comparison colour is an adjacent colour in the D-15 sequence and, therefore, is most similar to the central colour.

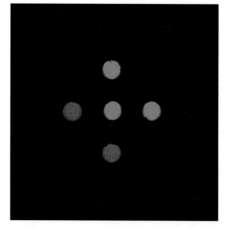

Figure 19.16 City colour vision test plate (2nd edition).

Changes were made to the coloured elements for the third edition of the test. As a part of the third edition, the task of detecting colours which differ from nearby colours was introduced. The second part of the test, however, retained the colour matching task as in previous editions. The third edition has two sections, which may be used in sequence or separately, according to clinical judgement. Section one uses four pages. It is primarily designed for screening and is the more sensitive of the two sections. Each page has four lines of coloured spots, arranged vertically in sets of three spots (**Fig. 19.17**). Subjects are required to detect differences of colour. Page 1 uses a pair of lines, which should be reported as showing no different spot, while the other two lines of spots show an obvious difference and a more subtle difference (often confused by tritans). Pages 2, 3 and 4 each carry red/green confusion colours, while two of these pages also show tritan confusions. There is, however, no obvious separation of protans from deutans; this separation is usually possible using the second part (as in the second edition of the test). Tritans are identified by the specific errors made on the bottom halves of pages 1, 2 and 4. A score giving the number of correct answers is used to indicate the number and type of confusions by each subject.

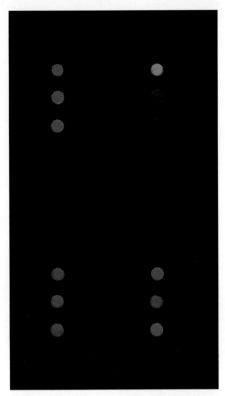

Figure 19.17 City colour vision test plate (3rd edition).

Section two of the test follows the format and requirements of earlier editions, where four spots on each of six test pages surround a central spot. Colours used follow what are considered to be 'most successful' ones from earlier editions, with some small variations. The patient is required to choose a spot most closely matching the central colour.

The test, however, is not effective for screening; moreover, classification of congenital protan and deutan defects is imprecise (due to the limited choice of confusion colours) with discrimination between dichromats and anomalous trichromats being unreliable. Thus, the test could be used as part of a battery of tests to provide additional information regarding the severity of a defect, or if other tests in the battery are unable to test for tritanopia.

Nagel anomaloscope

Introduced in 1907, the Nagel anomaloscope is the 'gold standard' reference test for red/green colour deficiencies (Squire et al 2005). The instrument consists of a Maxwellian view target where the two halves of the 3-degree circular bipartite target are illuminated by monochromatic yellow (589 nm) and a mixture of monochromatic red (670 nm) and green (546 nm) wavelengths. The subject alters the colour balance of the test half to match the yellow field. The purpose of the test is to determine the exact matching range of the subject. Normal subjects make an exact colour match within a small range of red/green mixture ratios. This instrument is widely used but is currently out of production.

Lantern tests

Lanterns are designed and used as vocational tests and employ the concept of colour naming. First introduced in the nineteenth century, the main aim of the test is to determine if signal lights can be correctly identified; however, only the Holmes-Wright lantern test contains actual signal colours. The tests usually present red, green and white lights of an angular size and point brilliance representative of maritime or aviation signal lights. The subject's task is to name the colours of the lights. If more than a defined number of errors are made naming the colours, the subject is deemed unfit for occupations in which the recognition of signal lights is critical. Lanterns used in different countries are based on different design principles. International lantern tests currently approved by the CIE are the:

- Holmes-Wright A and B lantern (UK)
- Farnsworth lantern/Optec 900 (USA)
- Beyne lantern/Tritest L3 (France).

Holmes-Wright lantern (UK)

Although no longer commercially available, the Holmes-Wright lantern is still used by the United Kingdom Armed Forces and Civil Aviation Authority (CAA). Essentially, there are two types of Holmes-Wright lantern: Type A and Type B. Type A consists of nine pairs of coloured lights separated vertically, while in Type B, colours are separated horizontally. Both systems have two reds, two greens and two whites, which are CIE-specified signal-light colours.

Farnsworth lantern/Optec 900 (USA)

Currently used by the US Armed Forces, the US Coastguard, and by the Federal Aviation Authority (FAA), the Farnsworth lantern test (or more recently the Optec 900) differs from the Holmes-Wright test. The Optec 900 (Cole et al 2006b) shows larger pairs of colours than the Holmes-Wright type A. Most notably, the colours used are not within the specifications for signal lights. Instead, the colours (red, green and yellow-white) are chosen to lie within isochromatic zones that encourage colour confusion.

Beyne lantern/Tritest L3 (France)

The Tritest L3 (previously called Beyne lantern) was developed for aviation. It shows single and paired colours derived from narrow wavelength bands in the blue, green, yellow-orange and red parts of the visible spectrum with an additional white light. The test distance is 5 m. There are six apertures for single lights, one for paired, and nine shutter speeds to vary the exposure time.

Electrophysiological techniques

Clinically, information gathered by visual electrophysiological techniques is used to diagnose patients presenting with signs and symptoms indicative of neurological or ophthalmological disease. The procedures are also of benefit to paediatric professionals when assessing young children with poor unexplained visual loss. Further clinical uses of electrophysiological techniques include the testing and diagnosis of inherited visual disorders and the monitoring of patients who are being treated with medications that have potential neuro- or retinotoxic effects.

The electroretinogram

The electroretinogram (ERG) is a technique that measures an electrical action potential recorded at, or near, the cornea when the retinal cells are activated electrically by a flash of light. The stimulus is produced by a Ganzfeldt stimulator where the light output reaches 2×10^6 cd/m^2 in order to achieve maximum amplitudes. This activation predominantly takes place within the outer and middle retinal layers (Rudduck 2006). The electrical activity produced reflects the complexity of the retinal network. The photoreceptors (rods and cones) are connected to bipolar cells (second-order neurons), ganglion cells (third-order neurons) and two types of inter-neurons called horizontal and amacrine cells. Surrounding these neurons are the structurally unique glial cells (Müller cells). The distribution of the bipolar cells and the ganglion cells is similar to that of the cone photoreceptor, in that their density peaks at the fovea centralis.

The first wave of the ERG response to a flash stimulus, the negative a-wave, is associated with the initial hyperpolarization of the photoreceptors. In the dark-adapted state, the retina is very sensitive to light, the resting potential of the photoreceptors being −40 mV compared with approximately −90 mV of other central nervous system neurons. This low resting potential is due to the fact that, in darkness, the photoreceptors are 'leaky' to positively charged ions (e.g. sodium and potassium), which flow into the cell. On exposure to light, however, the cells become more resistant to this ion flow, thus making them relatively more negative; i.e. the cell hyperpolarizes. The combined effect of numerous photoreceptors contributes to the initial a-wave in the ERG recording (**Fig. 19.18**).

The response of bipolar cells is more complex. A photon of light in the centre of the cell's receptive field hyperpolarizes one class of bipolar cells. If the surrounding region of the bipolar cell is stimulated, however, a depolarizing response will result. In other classes of bipolar cell, the converse phenomenon occurs. These depolarizing elements of the bipolar cells may contribute, in part, to the positive inflection (b-wave) seen in the ERG (see **Fig. 19.18**). Many authors now agree, however, that the Müller cells are essentially responsible for the b-wave formation.

The b-wave of the ERG is generated by current flow following the light-evoked increase in the potassium concentration in the extracellular space, causing the Müller cells to depolarize. The responses of the Müller cells, however, are caused by the balance of neuronal activity, which involves both the outer- and inner-synaptic layers. The b-wave, therefore, reflects the postsynaptic neuronal activity in the retina and is clinically the most important component of the ERG. Indeed, the ERG b-wave is selectively abolished by any agent which blocks synaptic transmission. The ascending limb of the b-wave also consists of a rhythmic superimposed feature known as oscillatory potentials, which are triggered by bright light stimulation (see **Fig. 19.18**). Amacrine cells are thought to be involved in the generation of the oscillation, although this is equivocal (La Chapelle 2006).

Analysis

a- and b-wave amplitudes

In order to compare presynaptic retinal activity (represented by the a-wave in the signal), and postsynaptic activity (represented by the b-wave in the signal), the b-wave:a-wave amplitude ratio is used. In normal healthy subjects, the b-wave should be at least twice the size of the a-wave at the highest intensity. The ratio may become reduced in cases of drug-induced visual defects or retinal vascular disease not involving the choroidal circulation. A clinical example of this would be in a case of central retinal artery occlusion, where there is a selective loss in the b-wave amplitude, the pathogenesis being that the choroidal circulation that gives nutritional supply to the photoreceptors is intact, whilst the central retinal artery that supplies the amacrine, bipolar, and ganglion cells is blocked. This results in electrical inactivity of the post-receptoral cells.

b-wave latency

The b-wave latency represents the time from the onset of the flash stimulus to the peak of the b-wave. Early changes in retinal disease often manifest as a reduction in the speed of the b-wave. The normal time for the b-wave to appear in the dark-adapted eye is approximately 40–50 msec. In early cases of pathology (e.g. retinitis pigmentosa), however, the b-wave latency is increased significantly, often presenting before any attenuation in the b-wave becomes manifest.

Common conditions and situations where the ERG is informative are:

- retinitis pigmentosa (a-wave abnormality)
- optic atrophy (b-wave abnormality)
- retinal dystrophies (b-wave abnormality)
- vascular disorders (b-wave abnormality)
- diabetes mellitus (oscillatory potentials)
- central vein occlusion (oscillatory potentials).

Pattern electroretinogram

The pattern ERG (PERG) is a retinal field potential evoked by stimulation of the retina in response to a patterned stimulus such as a chequerboard pattern. Thus, in clinical terms it provides valuable information about retinal macular function. As the subject is required to view the stimulus unhindered, the corneal recording electrodes used are fine wire or DTL electrodes (**Fig. 19.19**). Compared with the flash-evoked ERGs

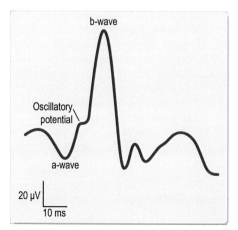

Figure 19.18 Schematic representation of a normal electroretinogram (ERG) response profile illustrating the a-wave, b-wave and oscillatory potentials.

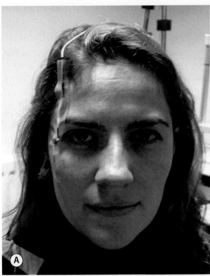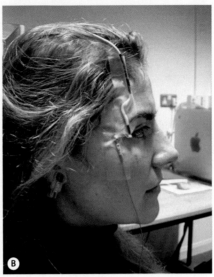

Figure 19.19 Patient set up for an electroretinogram (ERG) recording showing the positioning of the skin, corneal and reference electrodes; **(A)** front view and **(B)** side view.

described earlier, which are in the order of 100–200 μV, PERGs are in the order of 0.5–8 μV and can, therefore, only be obtained by using the technique of signal averaging.

The PERG is maximally stimulated when the chequerboard stimulus projects on to the macula and paramacular areas. The stimulus is a black-and-white chequerboard and is defined by the size (the angle subtended at the eye) of a single check. The checks change phase rapidly at a specific rate. Importantly, there is no overall change in luminance of the screen. The response to the stimulus is recorded during chequerboard pattern reversal. At low rates of reversal (e.g. 2 to 6 per second), the resultant waveform is characterized by a small initial negative component at approximately 35 ms (known as N35). This is followed by a positive inflection at 50 ms (P50), and a large negative component (N95) at the corresponding time of 95 ms post stimulation (**Fig. 19.20**).

The perception of a patterned stimulus depends upon the neuronal properties of spatial contrast discrimination rather than the detection of gross luminance changes. The neuronal ability to discriminate spatial contrast in the retina begins at the level of the bipolar cell. Importantly, there are two types of cells: those which depolarize with light and those which hyperpolarize with light. The depolarizing bipolar cells hyperpolarize when the surround is stimulated by light, whilst the hyperpolarizing bipolar cells depolarize on surround stimulation. This contrast discrimination property is established more clearly at the level of the retinal ganglion cells. Here, 'ON ganglion cells' become activated to a stimulus brighter than the background and are inhibited by a stimulus that is darker than the background. The converse occurs with 'OFF ganglion cells' (i.e. the cell fires when a light is switched off).

Consequently, when the retina is stimulated by a chequerboard pattern, the depolarizing bipolar and ON ganglion cells are excited when white squares appear at a given point in the visual field. Moreover, hyperpolarizing bipolar and OFF ganglion cells are excited when a black square appears. Whether the PERG reflects the summed activity of ON or OFF ganglion cells remains equivocal; however, there is evidence to suggest that the PERG response may be abnormal in optic nerve lesions when the conventional flash-type ERG remains normal. Authors have suggested that the N95 component in the PERG response profile may be dependent on the integrity of the ganglion cell layer, whereas the P50 component appears to receive a significant contribution from bipolar cell excitation.

Common conditions and situations where the ERG is informative are:

- optic neuropathy
- diabetic retinopathy
- early maculopathies.

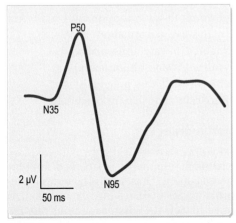

Figure 19.20 Schematic representation of a normal pattern electroretinogram (PERG) response profile showing the characteristic N35, P50 and N95 peaks.

Multifocal electroretinography

Multifocal electroretinography (mfERG) is a relatively new technique for assessing the local ERG from different regions

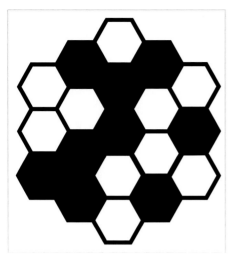

Figure 19.21 Multifocal electroretinogram (mfERG) target.

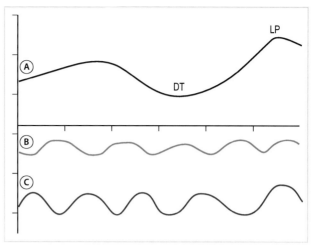

Figure 19.22 Schematic representation of an electro-oculogram recording demonstrating the dark trough (DT) and the light peak (LP) on the trace (**A**). The lower traces demonstrate amplitude differences of the ocular response measured from dark-adapted (**B**) and light-adapted (**C**) states.

of the retina (Sutter & Tran 1992). Electrical responses from the eye are recorded with a corneal electrode as in conventional ERG recordings, but the nature of the stimulus and analysis produce a topographic map of ERG responses (Marmor et al 2003). For the routine mfERG, the retina is stimulated with a computer monitor or other device that generates a pattern of elements (typically hexagons), each of which has a 50% chance of being illuminated every time the frame changes (**Fig. 19.21**). The pattern appears to flicker randomly; however, each element follows a fixed, predetermined sequence so that the overall luminance of the screen at any one given time is relatively stable. By correlating the continuous ERG signal with the on (white) or off (black) phases of each stimulus hexagon, the focal ERG signal associated with each element is calculated.

Data can be displayed in various ways such as a topographic array or a three-dimensional plot. Different stimulus patterns and flicker sequences can be used for specialized applications. Importantly, however, the tracings of the mfERG are not 'responses' in the sense of direct electrical responses from a local region of retina. Instead, the mfERG waveforms are a mathematical model of signals that correlate with a particular area of the stimulus that is illuminated at that time; thus the response from the corresponding retina is recorded. Multifocal electroretinogram signals, therefore, may be influenced by adaptation effects (from prior stimuli) and by the effects of scattered light on neighbouring retinal areas.

The electro-oculogram

The human retina consists of an electrically (negatively) charged nervous membrane. Clinical electro-oculography records the potential electrical difference between the posterior pole of the eye and the cornea. As such, the electro-oculogram (EOG) records the standing corneo-retinal potential during eye movements. A variety of ocular structures give rise to this corneo-retinal potential, but it is mainly generated at the junction between the photoreceptors and the retinal pigment epithelium (RPE). This steady DC transepithelial potential is of the order of 60 mV and is permanently present even in the absence of light. Common conditions and situations where EOGs are informative are:

- retinitis pigmentosa
- diffuse RPE disease
- Best's macular dystrophy
- Stagardt's disease
- chloroquine retinal toxicity.

EOG uses silver skin electrodes which are attached to the inner and outer canthi of each eye, while an earth (ground) electrode is placed on the patient's forehead. The patient is invited to look at two fixation lights 30 degrees apart which are successively illuminated. Following a preliminary adaptation period of 40 cd/m^2, the resting potential is recorded for 2 minutes. The patient is then placed in the dark for 12 minutes, during which time a record is made for 15 seconds each minute or until a minimum amplitude of standing potential is reached; this is known as the dark trough (DT). A light stimulus is then activated and the EOG recorded until the light peak (LP) in the EOG signal has occurred (**Fig. 19.22**).

The values corresponding to the LP and DT are recorded and a ratio of the two calculated. This light:dark ratio is usually expressed as a percentage, and is known as the Arden Index (Arden et al 1962). The Arden Index is calculated as thus:

$$(\textbf{light peak amplitude/dark peak amplitude}) \times \textbf{100}$$

Visual evoked potentials

The visual evoked potential (VEP) represents a mass response of cortical and possibly subcortical visual areas and is employed routinely in the assessment of the functional integrity of the visual pathways. Even though VEPs have been recorded and studied for over 75 years, the precise genesis of the responses remains unclear. The VEP has important applications in the identification and diagnosis of both retinal and neural pathologies.

The signals are recorded between an electrode over the visual (or occipital) cortex and a reference electrode over a non-visual part of the brain. In clinical situations, two or more recording channels may be used to sample the two halves of the visual cortex separately. Again, as with PERG, the process of signal averaging must be employed to measure the minute signals against the background of unassociated brain activity. The exact waveform generated through VEP depends upon the mode of stimulation.

The flash VEP

A series of bright flashes from a strobe evoke an averaged VEP with a series of positive and negative components, which are numbered in time sequence, occurring approximately 25 ms after the initial stimulation (**Fig. 19.23**). As the stimulus is bright and diffuse, accurate fixation by the subject is not necessary. The incidence of the early components N1, P1 and N2 in the response waveform varies with age; however, the major P2 component (at approximately 120 ms) is found in almost all subjects. Studies suggest that the flash components before 100 ms arise in the primary visual cortex, while the components after 100 ms come from higher stages of visual processing. Clinically, this method is useful for uncooperative patients and those patients whose refractive error is unknown.

The pattern VEP

In the majority of clinical cases, the pattern VEP is the most favoured method of measurement due to its low variability. A normal pattern VEP consists of a negative peak at 75 ms after stimulation (N75), a much larger positive peak (P100), and a negative peak at 135 ms (N135; **Fig. 19.24**). The amplitude of P100 is measured from N75, whereas its latency is measured from the time of the stimulus. The P100 peak is very robust in that there is very little variation between subjects, over time or between eyes of the same subject. It is, however, susceptible to changes in pattern size, contrast, luminance and pupil miosis (Rudduck 2006).

Common conditions and situations where VEPs are informative are:

- cortical blindness
- optic neuritis
- optic atrophy
- cranial inflammation or trauma.

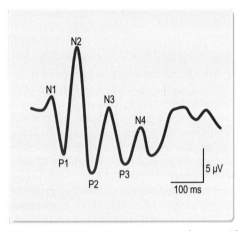

Figure 19.23 Schematic representation of a normal flash visual evoked potential (VEP). It is important to note that positive changes in the VEP signal are conventionally plotted, with positive changes shown as downward deviations.

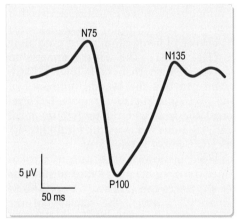

Figure 19.24 Schematic representation of a normal pattern reversal visual evoked potential (VEP).

Table 19.2 Examples of electrophysiological tests that can detect lesion in specific locations along the visual pathway

Location of lesion		Electrophysiological test
Retinal pigment epithelium (RPE)		EOG
Photoreceptor layer	Cones	Photopic ERG
		Flicker ERG
	Rods	Scotopic ERG
Müller cells		ERG (b-wave)
Amacrine cells and bipolar cells		ERG (oscillatory potentials) PERG (P50)
Ganglion cells		PERG (N95)
Optic tract		VEP
Visual cortex		VEP

Table 19.3 Examples of ERG patterns that, when considered alongside additional electrophysiological tests and clinical symptoms, are diagnostic of specific conditions

Test and results	Clinical symptoms/findings	Disease
Normal ERG Abnormal PERG	Optic disc pallor Visual field defect	Optic neuropathy
Normal ERG Abnormal EOG	Macula lesion	Best's disease
Abnormal photopic ERG Normal scotopic ERG	Macular atrophy	Cone dysfunction

Clinical application of electrodiagnosis

One of the essential features of electrodiagnosis is the ability to localize a lesion within the visual system. Through monocular stimulation and recording of the EOG and ERG from each eye and the VEP from both visual cortices, it is possible to identify whether the lesion in question occurs in the globe, optic nerve, optic chiasm or visual cortices (**Table 19.2**). Additionally, if the presenting condition is uniocular, the contralateral unaffected eye can often be used as a control. It is important to remember, however, that signals produced further along the visual system may be confounded by any lesion affecting the visual pathway more anteriorly (e.g. lesions affecting the retina, optic nerve, optic chiasm, and optic tracts).

There is a common misconception that individual electrophysiological tests are always diagnostic and can be interpreted in isolation without other tests, often without regard to the ocular signs and symptoms. Where there are certain characteristic electrophysiological tests for specific disease states, the majority of patients require a combination of tests to arrive at a satisfactory diagnosis of the presenting condition. **Table 19.3** provides examples of ERG results that, when considered with other electrophysiological tests and clinical findings, are diagnostic of specific diseases or disorders. An understanding of each test and their interrelationships, therefore, is essential to assist the diagnosis of a number of diseases relating to optometry.

References

Arden G B, Barrada A, Kelsey J H 1962 New clinical test of retinal function based upon the standing potential of eye. British Journal of Ophthalmology 46:449–467

Birch J 2001 Diagnosis of defective colour vision, 2nd edn. Butterworth-Heinemann, Edinburgh, Scotland

Birch J B, Chisholm I A, Kinnear P et al 1979 Acquired colour vision defects. In: Pokorney J, Smith V C, Verriest G et al (eds) Congenital and acquired colour vision defects. Grune and Stratton, New York, pp 243–248

Brown N A 1993 The morphology of cataract and visual performance. Eye 7(1):63–67

Byrne S F, Green R L 2002 Ultrasound of the eye and orbit, 2nd edn. Mosby, St. Louis, MO, pp 1–11

Cole B L, Lian K Y, Lakkis C 2006a The new Richmond HRR pseudoisochromatic test for colour vision is better than the Ishihara test. Clinical and Experimental Optometry 89(2):73–80

Cole B L, Lian K Y, Lakkis C 2006b Color vision assessment: fail rates of two versions of the Farnsworth lantern test. Aviation, Space, and Environmental Medicine 77(6):624–630

Fink W 2005 Refractive correction method for digital charged-coupled device-recorded Scheimpflug photographs by means of ray tracing. Journal of Biomedical Optics 10:Art No 024003

Giovagnorio F, Quaranta L, Bucci M G 1993 Color Doppler assessment of normal ocular blood flow. Journal of Ultrasound in Medicine 12 (8):473–477

Haigis W, Lege B, Miller N et al 2000 Comparison of immersion ultrasound biometry and partial coherence interferometry for intraocular lens calculation according to Haigis. Graefe's Archive for Clinical and Experimental Ophthalmology 238(9):756–773

Hardy L H, Rand G, Rittler M C 1954 HRR polychromatic plates. Journal of the Optical Society of America 44:509–523

Kalmus H 1955 The familial distribution of congenital tritanopia with some remarks on some similar conditions. Annals of Human Genetics 20:39–56

La Chapelle P 2006 The oscillatory potentials of the electroretinogram. In: Heckenlively J R, Arden G B (eds) Principles and practice of clinical electrophysiology, 2nd edn. MIT Press, Cambridge, MA pp 565–597

Lieb W E, Cohen S M, Merton D A et al 1991 Color Doppler imaging of the eye and orbit. Archives of Ophthalmology 109(4):527–531

Marmor M F, Hood D C, Keating D et al 2003 Guidelines for basic multifocal electroretinography (mfERG). Documenta Ophthalmologica 106(3):105–115

Nathan J 2002 The painter and handicapped vision. Clin Experimental Optometry 85(5):309–314

Rand G, Rittler M C 1956 An evaluation of the AO HRR pseudoisochromatic plates. Archives of Ophthalmology 56:736–742

Rudduck G 2006 The electrophysiology of vision. Optometry in Practice 7(4):131–140

Santodomingo-Rubido J, Mallen E A H, Gilmartin B et al 2002 A new non-contact optical device for ocular biometry. British Journal of Ophthalmology 86(4):458–462

Singh K D, Logan N S, Gilmartin B 2006 Three-dimensional modelling of the human eye based on magnetic resonance imaging. Investigative Ophthalmology and Visual Science 47(6):2272–2279

Squire T J, Rodriguez-Carmona M, Evans A D B et al 2005 Color vision tests for aviation: comparison of the anomaloscope and three lantern types. Aviation, Space, and Environmental Medicine 76 (5):421–429

Strenk S A, Strenk L M, Guo S 2006 Magnetic resonance imaging of aging, accommodating, phakic, and pseudophakic ciliary muscle diameters. Journal of Cataract and Refractive Surgery 32(11): 1792–1798

Sutter E E, Tran D 1992 The field topography of the ERG components in man I. The photopic luminance response. Vision Research 32 (3):433–446

Swanson W H, Cohen J M 2003 Colour vision. Ophthalmology Clinics of North America 16:179–203

Tranquart F, Berges O, Koskas P et al 2003 Color Doppler imaging of orbital vessels: personal experience and literature review. Journal of Clinical Ultrasound 31(5):258–273

Van Heel L, Went L N, Van Norren D 1980 Frequency of tritan disturbances in a population study. In: Verriest G (ed.) Colour vision deficiencies. Adam Hilger, Bristol, pp 256–260

Wolffsohn J S, Davies L N 2007 Advances in anterior segment imaging. Current Opinion in Ophthalmology 18(1):32–38

Wright W D 1952 The characteristics of tritanopia. Journal of the Optical Society of America 42:509–521

Further reading

Aminoff M 2005 Electrodiagnosis in clinical neurology, 5th edn. Churchill Livingstone, Edinburgh, Scotland

Atta H R 1996 Ophthalmic ultrasound: a practical guide. Churchill Livingstone, Edinburgh, Scotland

Birch J 2001 Diagnosis of defective colour vision, 2nd edn. Butterworth-Heinemann, Edinburgh, Scotland

Byrne S F, Green R L 2002 Ultrasound of the eye and orbit, 2nd edn. Mosby, St. Louis, MO

Elliott D B 2007 Clinical procedures in primary eye care, 3rd edn. Butterworth–Heinemann, Edinburgh, Scotland

Pavlin C J, Foster F S 1994 Ultrasound biomicroscopy of the eye. Springer-Verlag, New York, NY

CHAPTER 20

Visual field examination

John G Flanagan

Introduction

Examination of the visual field is fundamental to the measurement of visual function away from the fovea. As such, it is essential to the clinical evaluation of ocular health. The last 25 years has seen a dramatic change both in the way we examine the visual field and to the average clinician's access to the technologies and techniques used in its evaluation. This has resulted in the availability of more standardized techniques, more repeatable data, and more sophisticated and robust analysis, which might better reflect functional damage to the visual pathway. It is likely that the next decade will see further development as these functional test results are combined with the detailed structural assessment of the retina and optic nerve (see Ch. 18) to give structure–function signatures for the early diagnosis and better management of a variety of ocular diseases.

The visual field describes the visual function within an area that is defined by the limits of visual space to a steadily fixating eye. The process of measuring the visual field is called perimetry, which involves the mapping of the visual field using a perimeter. This is an instrument that enables the projection of a known visual stimulus at a fixed distance from the eye within a bowl of calibrated luminance. Automated perimeters are computer assisted, permit the standardization of testing protocols and provide statistical and interpretive analysis of the results. There are now monitor-based automated visual field instruments as an alternative to bowl-based instruments. These are not strictly perimeters and are generally restricted to the measurement of the central visual field (<30° radius from fixation), but the misnomer is commonly accepted.

A brief history of visual field assessment

Hippocrates is thought to have been the first to describe a visual field defect in 500 BC. (Lloyd 1936; http://webeye.ophth.uiowa.edu/ips/PerimetryHistory). Ptolemy later described the shape of the visual field in 150 BC. Leonardo da Vinci wrote about the temporal limits of the visual field in the early sixteenth century and a short while later, in 1668, Mariotte documented the physiologic blind spot, and surmised that it was due to the optic nerve. At the turn of the nineteenth century, Thomas Young was the first to measure the visual field, work later refined by Purkinje, who defined the limits of the visual field in 1825. Helmholtz proposed the relationship between scotomas and retinal lesions, but it was von Graefe who introduced visual field assessment into clinical practice. He plotted the field using a blackboard at a working distance of 45 cm, and a target of white chalk. In 1855, he published *Examination of the Visual Functions in Amblyopic Affections* with examples of classic defects such as ring scotomas, constrictions of the peripheral field, enlargement of the blind spot, and hemianopias.

In 1869, Aubert and Förster of Wroclaw (formally Breslau), Poland, introduced the first arc perimeter. The so-called Förster perimeter positioned the optic nerve at the centre of the visual field, an idea that remained popular for several decades. They also published novel observations on the perimetric limits of coloured targets and two-point separation in peripheral vision.

In 1873, Brudenell Carter made a simplified arc perimeter and carefully mapped the position and extent of the blind spot in degrees from foveal fixation. The term 'isopter' was first used in 1893 by Groenouw to describe the boundary of equal or isosensitivity for a given target. During these latter years of the nineteenth century it was generally considered that plotting the limits, or perimeter, of the visual field was the only information of clinical importance, and little attention was given to the central visual field. This changed in 1889 following a paper by Jannik Peterson Bjerrum of Copenhagen, who re-introduced and emphasized the detailed mapping of the central visual field. He introduced the 2 m tangent (Bjerrum) screen, and with his assistant Rønne used graduated targets of different sizes to document early, subtle glaucomatous field loss. Traquair, of Edinburgh and 'island of vision' fame (**Fig. 20.1**), used both a 2 m tangent screen and an arc perimeter, and introduced many contemporary ideas on visual field interpretation in his popular and influential book (Traquair 1938). Ferree and Rand introduced their self-illuminated combination of campimeter and arc perimeter in 1924 (Ferree & Rand 1922).

Arguably the most profound change in clinical perimetry, and the innovations that have dictated the approach of modern-day visual field assessment, were introduced by Swiss ophthalmologist Hans Goldmann of Bern in 1945. His perimeter used a hemispheric bowl, which was illuminated to control retinal adaptation, and a projection system that could control target size, brightness and colour. The unique recording system enabled unprecedented, detailed, cartographic mapping of the visual field (**Fig. 20.2**). The 'Goldmann' perimeter was manufactured by Haag-Streit and became the industry-standard kinetic perimeter, and is still available today, remaining popular in neurological practice. Of particular importance was the care given to the relationship between stimulus size and brightness, leading to the concept of coincidence.

The concept and advantages of static threshold perimetry were introduced by Sloan in 1933, but not popularized until the introduction of Aulhorn and Harms' 'Tubinger' perimeter in 1959. This perimeter was designed to enable both kinetic and static threshold assessment of the visual field and allowed for cross-sectional profiles to be plotted through the visual field. Multiple pattern, static screening techniques were introduced by Harrington and Flock in

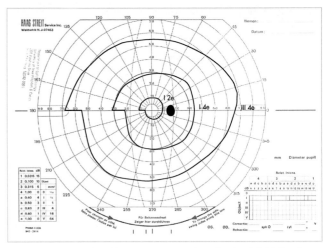

Figure 20.2 Typical Goldmann perimetry plot of a visual field showing a nasal step in the right eye of a patient with glaucoma. The plot illustrates two isopters; the inner being that found with an I4e target and the outer being a III4e. (Reproduced with permission from Alward W L M 2002 Glaucoma. The requisites in ophthalmology. Mosby, St Louis.)

1954 (Harrington 1976) and later in the Friedmann visual field analyser (Friedmann 1979) and the contemporary Henson series of perimeters (Henson & Bryson, 1986). In 1971, Armaly and Drance proposed methods for testing patients with glaucoma using both kinetic and static techniques on the Goldman perimeter (Armaly 1972). Two kinetic peripheral isopters were plotted with additional meridians around the horizontal nasal field, followed by the static assessment of the central field and blind spot using a target brightness that was just visible at 25°.

In the late 1970s, the combination of the popularity of static threshold perimetry and the advent of personal computing enabled the development of computer-assisted, or automated, static threshold perimetry. The first commercially available instrument was largely the creation of Franz Fankhauser (Fankhauser et al 1972). It was launched in 1976 and called the Octopus 201 perimeter (Interzeag AG, Switzerland). The next few years saw the launch of several computer-assisted perimeters due to pioneering work from the likes of John Lynn, Hans Bebie, Jorg Spahr, John Keltner, Chris Johnson, Erik Greve, Anders Heijl and CET Krakau. Instruments such as the Fieldmaster, Competer, Squid, Digilab, Dicon, Peritest, Perimat and Perimetron were unveiled. The following decade saw the launch of the Humphrey perimeters (Heijl & Patella 2002), which were developed as a collaboration between the Humphrey Instruments-based team led by Michael Patella and a scientific team led by Anders Heijl of Sweden. Humphrey Instruments (now Carl Zeiss Meditec, Dublin, CA) enjoyed a rapid ascendancy to international market leaders, with their perimeters and methods assuming the mantle of clinical gold standard from the Goldmann perimeter. More recent additions include the UK-based Henson range of perimeters, the Medmont from Australia (Vingrys & Helfrich 1990) and several instruments manufactured by Oculus. Other recent and more novel developments in visual field assessment involving preferential stimulation of colour mechanisms and the use of monitor-based technologies will be discussed at the end of the chapter.

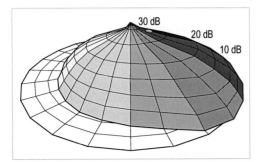

Figure 20.1 Illustration of Traquair's island of vision, typical of a left eye, from a 50-year-old measured with a Goldmann size III target. The sensitivity peaks at the fovea and declines more steeply in the nasal field than the temporal field. The optic nerve gives an absolute defect on the temporal side of fixation (for a left eye). (With permission from Heijl & Patella 2002.)

Basic concepts

There are several basic concepts that need to be clearly understood before the process of visual field assessment can be fully appreciated:

- The anatomical limits of the visual field are approximately 100° temporally, 60° nasally, 60° superiorly and 75° inferiorly.
- Visual sensitivity is greatest (lowest threshold) at the fovea and decreases towards the periphery, with the steepest slope on the nasal side. Traquair likened this topography to 'an island of vision surrounded by a sea of darkness' (see **Fig. 20.1**), not unlike Mont St Michel when viewed from the Normandy coast at high tide.
- The optic nerve head causes a physiological blind spot that is approximately 7° high and 5° wide. This can be demonstrated by closing one eye and holding a small target in the temporal field of view at approximately 15° along the horizontal meridian.
- The height and shape of the island changes with retinal adaptation, age and stimulus size. This will be discussed further in the section on instrument and physiological variables.
- Heijl and Patella (2002) define a visual field defect as 'any statistically and clinically significant departure from the normal hill (island) of vision'.
- Defects can be described in terms of general constriction or depression, shape, size and depth.
- The retinotopic projection of the visual field is reversed and inverted, such that the nasal retina projects to the temporal visual field and the inferior retina projects to the superior visual field (**Fig. 20.3**).
- Damage to the visual pathway projects to the visual field in a way that is entirely predictable when considering the anatomy of the visual system along with the retinotopic

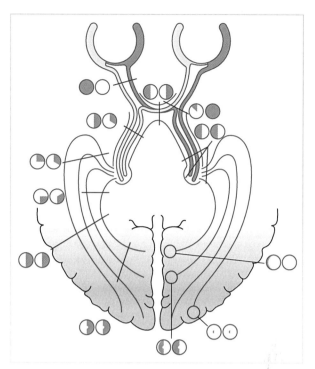

Figure 20.4 Illustration of the visual pathway showing its retinotopic organization, and the decussation at the chiasm. Classic visual field defects are shown along with their association with lesions at specific locations along the pathway. If a defect is monocular or does not respect the vertical midline then it has to originate from the retina or optic nerve. Heterogenous hemianopic defects originate from the chiasm, most commonly being bitemporal. Homonymous hemianopic defects can only originate after the chiasm, and become more congruous (similar) the further along the pathway the lesion occurs.

projection. Consideration needs to be given to the decussation at the chiasm and the hemifield-specific cortical projections (**Fig. 20.4**).

- A defect within which sensitivity is reduced from normal but not absent is called a relative defect or relative scotoma (likely from the Greek *skotos* meaning 'darkness'; or Latin meaning 'dim sight'). When there is no detectable sensitivity the defect is described as absolute, such as the physiological blind spot.
- Measuring the island of vision is a cartographic problem. As such, its topography can be mapped using contours or by defining height or sensitivity values at known locations. The former approach is called kinetic perimetry. This uses moving targets of known brightness, colour and size, to define a contour, or isopter, of equal sensitivity. The target is also used to locate and map areas of reduced sensitivity within the isopter (see **Fig. 20.2**). By measuring a series of isopters of graded sensitivity, the topography of the island of sensitivity is defined. It should be noted that the isopters are plotted by moving from non-seeing (infrathreshold) to seeing (suprathreshold) areas, or starting from within regions of reduced sensitivity. Sensitivity mapping at known locations with variable targets is known as static perimetry. At each location the stimulus is adjusted, usually with respect to its brightness, in order to determine the sensitivity. A map can be generated once sufficient locations have been measured (**Fig. 20.5**).

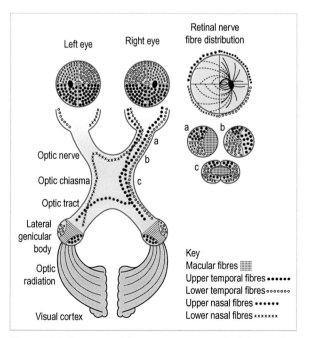

Figure 20.3 Illustration of the retinotopic mapping of the visual pathway and its relationship to the projection of the visual field.

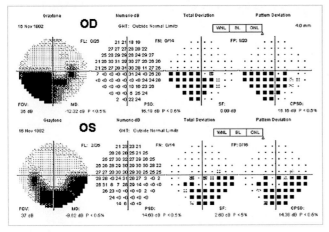

Figure 20.5 Classic inferior arcuate defects of a patient with glaucoma. The greyscale maps (left) are generated using the sensitivity data displayed immediately to their right. The darker the area the lower the sensitivity.

- Threshold perimetry, which is really sensitivity perimetry (sensitivity being the reciprocal of threshold), estimates the actual sensitivity across the visual field. Screening perimetry refers to rapid, suprathreshold testing, which attempts to find regions of obvious defect by presenting targets that would normally be seen with ease. The use of the term 'screening' is yet another misnomer associated with perimetry, as there are no visual field tests that would meet international criteria for a screening test.

Stimulus definition and units of light

Perimetric stimuli are defined with respect to their apparent size and brightness when projected against a known background for a specified amount of time (static), or at a specific speed and direction of motion (kinetic). Apparent size is defined, in degrees, by the target size and its distance from the eye, such that a 1 mm diameter circular target projected to a distance of 33.3 cm would be equivalent to a 3 mm diameter target projected to 1 m. Goldmann defined a progression of target sizes that doubled in angular subtense, and quadrupled in target area, such that size 0 was 0.055° (0.0625 mm^2), size I was 0.11° (0.25 mm^2), up to size V, which was 1.72° (64 mm^2). The standard target size used by most automated perimeters is size III (0.43°). The size V target is sometimes used in advanced field loss.

The traditional unit of light used in perimeters is the apostilb (asb), a legacy from perimetry's past. It is an old European unit of luminance popular when Goldmann was revolutionizing visual field measurement. It is equivalent to 1 lumen per square metre. The current international unit for luminance is the candela per square metre, which is related to the apostilb as a function of *pi*, hence 1 asb = 1 cdm^{-2}/3.14159 = 0.31831 cdm^{-2}. Goldmann established a maximum stimulus luminance of 1000 asb, or 318 cdm^{-2}, and a background luminance of 31.5 asb, or approximately 10 cdm^{-2}. The background luminance has remained a standard for most contemporary automated perimeters and was adopted as such by the International Council of

Ophthalmology in 1979, but the target luminance is more often 10 000 asb or 3183 cdm^{-2}.

Visual field testing is the process of measuring the differential light sensitivity, or the ability to see the contrast difference between a stimulus relative to a known background luminance. It is convention to use a logarithmic scale to measure the differential light sensitivity. As with audition, it is a more appropriate way to express sensation, as specific log units of change have the same relative magnitude across the entire measurement range; for example, 0.3 log units will always represent a doubling of stimulus intensity. Such scales are generally expressed in 0.1 log unit steps, called a decibel (dB). Unlike audition, vision scientists use a log scale of sensitivity rather than threshold, therefore 0 dB represents the brightest stimulus available, with the dimmest perceivable stimuli usually being somewhere between 40 dB and 50 dB. As an example, the Humphrey perimeter uses a 51 dB scale, with 0 dB corresponding to the brightest 10 000 asb stimulus and 51 dB being a stimulus of 0.08 asb. The dimmest target found to be observable by a young, trained observer was approximately 1 asb, or 40 dB (Heijl & Patella 2002), so the clinically useful measurement range of the perimeter is between 0 and 40 dB.

Perhaps the most difficult concept in visual field measurement is the relative scales between instruments with different measurement ranges. For example, a 3 dB change from 0 dB on the Humphrey perimeter would mean that the stimulus brightness changed from 10 000 asb to 5000 asb. However, a 3 dB change from 0 dB on the Goldmann perimeter would result in a change from 1000 asb to 500 asb. Goldmann estimated that the doubling of target area used in his target size progression would be approximately the same as a 5 dB change in target brightness (relative to a maximum stimulus brightness of 1000 asb). Comparing visual field information between instruments becomes even more complex when different background luminances are used, and different psychophysical tasks are performed, e.g. short-wavelength automated perimetry or frequency doubling perimetry.

Evaluation of the visual field

The purpose of routine visual field examination was best described by Greve (1973) as 'the early and efficient detection, the assessment and the follow-up of functional loss of the visual system'. It is considered essential for the diagnosis and management of glaucoma, is commonly used in neurological disease and aspects of retinal disease, and to evaluate vision standards and visual disability.

To understand the examination and the subsequent analysis of the results it is important to consider both the instrumental and physiological variables that can influence the examination and its outcome.

Instrument variables

It was noted that standards exist for most of the static threshold automated perimeters, that is, a background luminance of 31.5 asb and a target size of 0.43° (Goldmann size III). When considering background luminance, a notable exception is offered by the Octopus perimeters. They suggested using a more scotopic level of retinal adaptation with a background luminance of 4 asb (approximately 1 cdm^{-2}), similar to that used on earlier semi-automated static instruments such as the

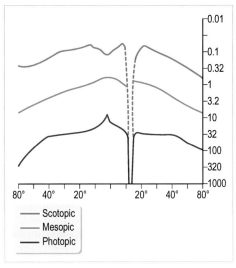

Figure 20.6 Horizontal profile of visual sensitivity (asb) through the centre of the visual field in scotopic, mesopic and photopic conditions. Note that under scotopic retinal adaptation there is a central depression. Also note the absolute defect at the blind spot.

Friedmann visual field analyser. This gave a flatter profile across the central 30° of the visual field (**Fig. 20.6**), and was argued to be more sensitive to damage in the mid-peripheral region, which is important in the detection of early glaucoma. The more recent Octopus perimeters have switched to the Goldmann standard, but their full-bowl perimeters (currently the Octopus 900) still offer the capability of using either background.

Stimulus size

Stimulus size is of less importance in contemporary perimetry as it has been largely standardized to the use of a 0.43°, Goldmann size III. However, it remains important to understand the concept by which Goldmann developed his target size progression, particularly when using the Goldmann perimeter, or the recently developed automated equivalent (Octopus Goldmann Kinetic Perimetry, available on the Octopus 900, Haag-Streit, Bern, Switzerland). Goldmann's idea was to relate change in size with a perceptually equivalent change in intensity, such that a bright, small target would be equivalent to a dimmer, larger target. The relationship between stimulus area (A) and intensity (I) is governed by spatial summation, whose properties change with retinal location and adaptation, and can be described by the equation: $A^k \times I = $ Constant. The exponent k varies with retinal location, but Goldmann used 0.8 as a compromise. With this value, a doubling of the stimulus area is equivalent to a 5 dB (0.5 log unit) increase in intensity. This also led to the concept of Goldmann equivalence whereby a I-4e (0.11°; 1000 asb) gives the same isopter as a IV-1e (0.86°; 31.6 asb) or a III-2e (0.43°; 100 asb) (equivalence being shown as the sum of the Roman and Arabic numerals). Theoretically, changing from a target size III to a V on an automated perimeter will give an increase of 10 dB for an equivalent intensity, although it tends to be less, as k was calculated for the entire visual field.

Stimulus duration

Stimulus duration is another variable that is important to understand, but is seldom adjustable on the currently available clinical instruments. Temporal summation properties ensure that there is an approximately linear relationship between threshold and stimulus duration for very rapid presentations with a doubling of threshold for every doubling of stimulus duration (Anderson & Patella, 1999). However, this relationship reaches a ceiling at approximately 500 msec. The most frequently used presentation time is 200 msec, which is considered to be relatively unaffected by temporal summation but is quick enough to prevent the tendency for re-fixation eye movements that occurs after approximately 250 msec.

Stimulus velocity

In kinetic perimetry, the speed of the moving target is an important variable, although difficult to control in manual Goldmann perimetry. It is recommended that the velocity lies between 3° and 5° per second. If too slow, it encourages the patient to lose fixation and search for the target. If too rapid, the isopters become artefactually small.

Colour

Stimulus and background colour in standard automated perimetry is white. There is little evidence of a clinical advantage over white-on-white threshold perimetry by preferentially stimulating the long- and mid-wavelength systems using red or green stimuli, projected on complementary coloured backgrounds. However, short-wavelength automated perimetry (SWAP), using a blue target on a bright yellow background, has become popular and is available on several leading projection perimeters, as discussed later. Coloured targets have long been popular in kinetic perimetry, but the simple addition of a colour target on a standard white background is unlikely to test the colour mechanism selectively. However, it does enable the measurement range of the perimeter to be extended and allows more detailed examination of central function. The concept of disproportion usually relates to a comparison between white and coloured targets that would normally give similar isopters. In certain conditions, such as optic neuritis, the coloured target, usually red, gives a smaller than expected isopter, i.e. it is of reduced sensitivity. There is no similar concept when performing automated static perimetry.

Patient variables

Perimetry is a subjective test and as such there is inherent variability within the results. Several patient-based aspects of the testing procedure have been shown to affect reliability and repeatability. These are important to understand as they can usually be distinguished from truly abnormal results.

Learning

The presence of a learning effect in perimetry is well established. It is estimated that approximately 15% of normal, first-time field takers give results that are outside normal limits (Wood et al 1987; Heijl et al 1989a; Wild et al 1989, 1991; Werner et al 1990; Heijl & Bengtsson 1996). The typical presentation is of a non-specific, mid-peripheral depression (20–30°), with a relatively normal central field (**Fig. 20.7**). Fortunately, it is difficult to produce a normal field artefactually, so if the results are within normal limits and reliable, they can generally be trusted. However, if initial results show any abnormality, it is essential that the field

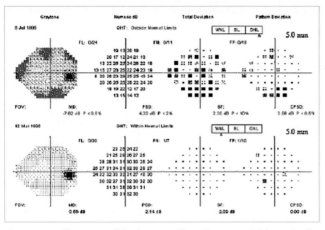

Figure 20.7 Illustration of the learning effect. The upper field was the first field performed by the patient. It shows a typical non-specific, mid-peripheral depression. The lower display shows the subsequent normal field.

be repeated. It has also been shown that the learning effect is test specific, such that experienced patients can demonstrate learning on new techniques such as SWAP or FDT (Wild & Moss 1996; Horn et al 2007; Hong et al 2007).

Fatigue

The effects of fatigue during perimetry have been recognized since the earliest days of automated perimetry (Heijl 1977; Hudson et al 1994). It has been estimated to average approximately 0.2 dB per minute of testing. In those patients who demonstrate high levels of fatigue, a similar-looking field to that produced by learning effects is often found, i.e. a mid-peripheral depression. In such cases it is best to ensure that all subsequent fields are as short in duration as possible by reducing the number of test locations (for example, 24–2 versus 30–2) and choosing the fastest available algorithm.

Pupil size

Pupils less than 2.5 mm in diameter can adversely affect visual field results by reducing the retinal illuminance, being diffraction limited, and consequently no longer falling within the limits of Weber's Law. The resulting field tends to be generally depressed. Large pupils, while creating increased aberrations, particularly spherical aberration with a myopic shift, do not affect the visual field unduly, although there can be mild reduction at the most central target locations. It is reasonable to perform perimetry while a patient's pupil is dilating, provided the test is started after the pupil diameter is 3 mm or greater, and that appropriate near vision correction is provided.

Refractive error

Uncorrected refractive error reduces visual sensitivity in standard automated perimetry by approximately 1 dB per dioptre of blur when using a Goldmann size III target (Weinreb & Perlman 1986). Smaller targets are more adversely affected. It is advisable to correct refractive error using full-aperture trial lenses. It is also important to use as few lenses as possible to minimize reflections. Astigmatism should be corrected when it exceeds 1.50 dioptres, whereas a best sphere (i.e. sphere + half cylinder power) may be used with lower amounts. Near working distance corrections should be added for presbyopic patients or those

who have been cyclopleged. When using a trial lens correction, care must be taken to align the lens system in order to avoid artefacts from the lens rim. These can usually be recognized due to their typically steep-sided, often absolute appearance in the periphery. In addition, they often do not respect the horizontal or vertical midlines. Interestingly, some of the newer vision-function-specific-perimetry techniques that generate more magnocellular system-specific stimuli are less sensitive to refractive blur, e.g. frequency doubling and flicker defined form.

Anatomy

Prominent brows, large noses, drooping lids and small palpebral apertures can all lead to artefactual abnormality of the visual field. Such features should always be documented on the field result and in the patient's record. Droopy lids can be taped, while patients can sometimes be reoriented to avoid prominent brows and noses affecting the results.

Media opacities

Cataracts and other media opacities produce veiling glare, which can depress the resulting visual field dramatically, particularly in the presence of small pupils. Most perimeters provide analytical tools that help ignore generalized depression of the field in order to expose any underlying focal defect (see Pattern deviation).

Age

Ageing reduces visual sensitivity, as might be expected. The normal databases provided on modern automated perimeters provide an age-corrected analysis (see Total deviation).

When to perform a visual field

Perimetry is essential in the diagnosis and management of many ocular and neurological diseases. This is particularly true for the glaucomas. The visual field should be evaluated in all patients with:

- Symptoms suggesting central vision loss, including non-refractive reduced vision, positive and scintillating scotoma
- Glaucoma or risk factors for glaucoma, including high intraocular pressure (IOP), family history, old age (generally regarded as over 65 years of age), thin central corneal thickness (<515 mm), abnormal appearance of the optic nerve head
- Symptoms of neurological disease, including headache, dizziness, tingling or numbness of the limbs, and for the follow-up of known neurological problems that can affect the visual system
- Symptoms or signs of retinal disease, and particularly for monitoring the effects of existing retinal disease (e.g. age-related macular degeneration) on visual function
- Repeatable, abnormal screening results from confrontation testing, Amsler grid, standard automated perimetry (SAP) or frequency doubling technology (FDT) screening, or other vision-specific perimetry tests
- A risk for developing drug-related retinopathy, such as from hydroxychloroquine or ethambutol

Threshold perimetry should be used when monitoring a known defect, other than for some neurologic defects that are absolute and stable. Typical suprathreshold screening strategies can miss the development of subtle field defects.

Test selection

Confrontation

Confrontation testing can provide information in a primary eye care setting when patients present with gross field defects, particularly when standard field testing equipment is unavailable. Elliott et al. (1997) suggested that using red targets gave the most sensitive examination of the central visual field but that any confrontation test is insensitive to all but very large, deep defects such as homonymous hemianopias, when compared to automated perimetry (Pandit et al 2001). It is recommended, whenever possible, to refer suspect patients for automated field testing rather than relying on the results of a confrontation test.

Amsler charts

The Amsler chart (grid) is a rapid, qualitative technique designed to test the central 10° of the visual field, using a standard chart with a grid of white lines on a black background (Amsler 1949). Each square of the grid is 5 mm, subtending approximately 1° at a viewing distance of 30 cm. The patient is asked whether any of the lines are missing or distorted. The Amsler chart can be used for a quick assessment of macular function and is particularly useful in cases of metamorphopsia. Standard perimetry has been shown to be more sensitive, specific and repeatable for central field defects, although Amsler charts have the advantage of being quicker, easy to apply and portable (Schuchard 1993; Achard et al 1995).

Screening fields

Central visual field screening can be considered part of a routine eye examination for asymptomatic and risk-free patients. For patients who fall into the categories outlined in the section 'When to perform a visual field' it is more appropriate to perform full-threshold testing rather than use a screening technique. Visual field screening should never be used to follow disease progression. See also Frequency doubling technology for fast screening procedures. Frequency doubling offers one of the most rapid screening tests, as well as having one of the most impressive diagnostic performances for the detection of early glaucoma.

Multiple-stimulus suprathreshold testing

The Henson perimeters continue the tradition of multiple-stimulus suprathreshold testing. The screening test uses 26 points within the central 25° visual field in eight presentations of between two and four points each. Initially, a threshold is estimated at several mid-peripheral points 10° from fixation, and the expected threshold values for the entire visual field are extrapolated. All target locations are then tested 5 dB brighter (or suprathreshold). If any point

is repeatedly missed, the programme can be extended to screen 68 or 136 points in the central field. Typical test duration is between 2 and 4 minutes. The technique will likely miss some small or shallow defects. It is by definition a procedure that is not standardized, due to the manual nature of the test.

Standard suprathreshold testing

The use of standard, single-stimulus, suprathreshold screening procedures have become largely redundant following the introduction of fast thresholding techniques. However, they are still used occasionally for full-field screening, particularly for suspected neurological defects. There are several alternate approaches that estimate a suprathreshold screening level either relative to age-matched normal values or relative to initially tested seed points (the seed point being one of four locations at 9° × 9° in each quadrant, which are tested first in a standard test; Anderson & Patella 1999). These are then tested in a two- or three-zone strategy. The three-zone strategy will test once (Octopus 2-LT) or twice (HFA three-zone, Oculus three-zone) at the screening level, and if stimuli are missed, will test again with the brightest stimulus level. If seen at the initial screening level, usually 4 dB to 6 dB brighter than the expected threshold, the location is recorded as being within normal limits. If missed at the initial screening level but seen at the maximum brightness then it is recorded as a relative defect. If missed at both screening levels the location will be designated an absolute defect. The Oculus and Humphrey perimeters offer an additional screening strategy, whereby the locations missed twice at the initial screening level are quantified using a full-threshold, staircase strategy. Suprathreshold screening is likely to miss shallow defects.

Fast threshold testing

The fast threshold estimation strategies found on most contemporary perimeters, such as SITAFast (Humphrey Field Analyser, HFA) and the Dynamic and Tendency Oriented Perimetry (Octopus perimeters), have largely replaced the need for single- or multiple-stimulus suprathreshold strategies. Although they generally provide full-range sensitivity values and can give a better idea of defect depth and area, they take approximately the same time to test the visual field as traditional screening methods (2 to 4 minutes). When compared with full-threshold techniques they are quicker but less precise, and have inferior test–retest characteristics. These strategies should be considered when defects are not suspected, but should not be used for monitoring disease unless a patient has a history of fatigue during the test. For a review of the various threshold estimation techniques see McKendrick (2005).

Peripheral field testing

Peripheral testing should be considered in some neurological disease, occasional retinal disease, for example retinitis pigmentosa, very occasionally in patients with glaucoma, when there are symptoms of poor peripheral vision and when assessing vision standards. However, the majority of visual field defects, including neurological ones, are reflected within the central 30° of a threshold visual field (**Fig. 20.8**).

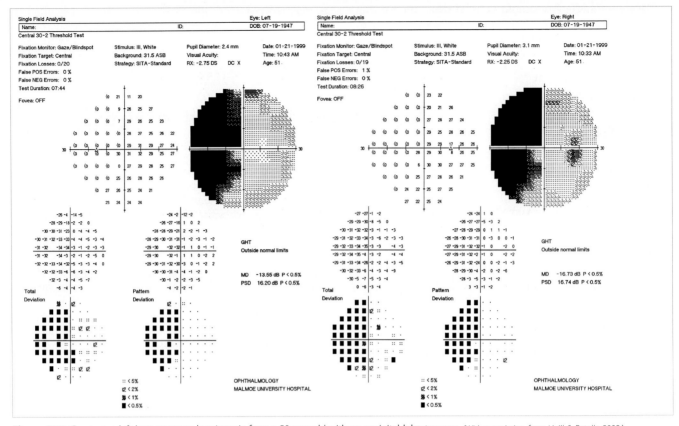

Figure 20.8 Congruous left homonymous hemianopia from a 50-year-old with an occipital lobe tumour. (With permission from Heijl & Patella 2002.)

It is recommended to use peripheral suprathreshold screening programmes that usually test between 30° and 60°, and combine them with central threshold tests. Alternatively, a full-field screening technique can be used.

Standard automated perimetry

The standard clinical application of static threshold automated perimetry entails the assessment of the central 30°, and is commonly called standard automated perimetry (SAP). The most frequently used programmes for SAP are the 30–2 and 24–2 (**Fig. 20.9**) as popularized by the Humphrey perimeters. First introduced on the original Octopus perimeter as programme 32, the 30–2 programme tests 76 locations over the central 30° in a 6° grid pattern that straddles the horizontal and vertical midlines, i.e. targets are located 3° either side of the midlines (Anderson & Patella 1999). Equivalent programmes can be found on most perimeters. The 24–2 programme examines the central 25°, with the addition of more peripheral targets in the nasal step region, and consequently testing time is reduced by approximately 20%. It was initially used in follow-up assessments and to lessen the likelihood of any fatigue effect, but increasingly it is the field of first choice. This is due to the reduced diagnostic value of many of the additional target

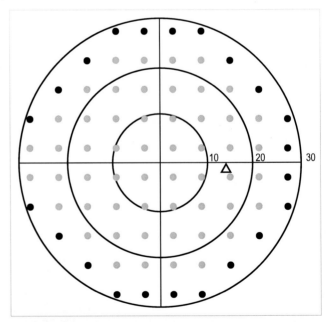

Figure 20.9 Test patterns for the 24–2 and 30–2 (Humphrey Field Analyzer). The targets are 6° apart and straddle the midlines. The dark locations in the outer peripheral ring are the additional locations used by the 30–2 pattern. (With permission from Heijl & Patella 2002.)

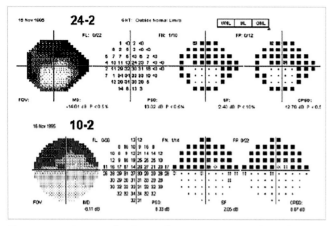

Figure 20.10 An example of using the 10–2 programme (*lower field*) to examine the macular region of the left eye of a patient with glaucoma whose defect was threatening fixation. The upper field shows the patient's regular 24–2 visual field, measured on the same day as the 10–2 field shown in the lower plot.

locations used in programme 30–2, particularly the superior locations that are adversely affected by upper lid and brow artefact.

A variety of threshold estimation algorithms are available, with the newer, faster strategies based on Baysian methods, for example the Swedish Interactive Thresholding Algorithm (SITA) strategy found on the Humphrey Field Analyzer (HFA) and the four-step, ZEST-inspired algorithm found on the Matrix (McKendrick 2005). It is important to re-test abnormal visual fields to ensure repeatability, particularly in the naive patient, as there is a clearly defined learning effect that can mimic early defects.

The macular region should be examined regularly and in more detail than that afforded by programmes 30–2 or 24–2 in patients with age-related maculopathy, when defects are threatening fixation in glaucoma, and in those taking medications that have the potential to cause maculopathy. The recommended approach to testing the macular region is to use a 10° central threshold programme with a spatial resolution of at least 2°, often referred to as a 10–2 (**Fig. 20.10**).

Interpretation

The development of standard automated perimetry has been accompanied by the sophistication of analytical techniques available to assist in the interpretation of visual field data. The most commonly used and imitated approach is that found on the Humphrey Field Analyzer (HFA; Carl Zeiss Meditic, Dublin, CA, USA). In consequence, the HFA will be used to demonstrate and illustrate the interpretation of the visual field. In order to interpret visual field results successfully, they should be scrutinized with respect to their reliability, as the result of a single visit and with respect to change over time.

Reliability indices

There are several reliability indices that are commonly used to give guidance regarding a patient's performance (Anderson & Patella 1999; Heijl & Patella 2002).

Fixation losses

The fixation loss (FL) rate provides an estimate of how steadily an eye fixates during a visual field test. The rate is estimated using the Heijl–Krakau technique, which periodically presents suprathreshold targets in the presumed location of the blind spot. If the patient responds positively to the stimulus, it is assumed that they were not fixating appropriately. If the rate is more than 20%, it is flagged, although it has been suggested that this criterion is too stringent and that 30% is a more appropriate cutoff (Katz & Sommer 1988). High fixation losses are frequently flagged when the blind spot has not been mapped accurately, and it is important to assess and document the patient's fixation subjectively during the test by observing the eye monitor. High FL rates accompanied by high false-positive rates would indicate a 'trigger-happy' patient with very low reliability.

The HFAII also employs gaze-tracking throughout the test, displayed as a bar chart on the monitor and the print-out (**Fig. 20.11**). Upward deflections indicate eye movements and downward deflections are recorded when the position of the eye cannot be determined or there was a blink. A full-scale spike indicates a 10° or greater eye movement.

False-positive catch trials

False-positive (FP) errors indicate a 'trigger-happy' patient who is responding when no stimulus is presented. It is evaluated either by monitoring for responses when one is not expected (SITA), or by going through the process of presenting a target and having the patient respond to the sound when no target is actually presented. They should be less than 15%. Intervene immediately if false-positives start to appear during the test and re-instruct the patient. If false-

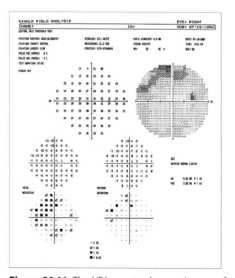

Figure 20.11 The HFA gaze-tracker monitors eye fixation throughout the visual field test, displayed as a bar chart on the monitor and the print-out (e.g. **Fig. 20.8**). The lower panel shows a magnified view of the gaze-tracker display. Upward deflections indicate eye movements and downward deflections are recorded when the position of the eye cannot be determined or there was a blink. A full-scale spike indicates a 10° or greater eye movement.

positives are greater than 33%, the result should be discarded and the field repeated. Other indicators of a trigger-happy patient include a high mean sensitivity, white areas on the greyscale print-out and larger defects on the pattern deviation plot than the total deviation plot.

False-negative catch trials

False-negative (FN) errors accumulate when a patient fails to respond to a suprathreshold target (9 dB brighter than threshold) at a given location and are associated with fatigue and/or inattention. They should also be less than 20%. If one notices FN errors accumulating, particularly toward the end of an examination, allow the patient to rest. This will often ensure that the false-negative score does not reach significance. FN rates are higher in the presence of an abnormal field, particularly in patients with glaucoma. This means that the FN error rate is of limited value when the field is outside of normal limits.

For strategies other than HFA SITA there will often be an estimate of the intra-test variance called the short-term fluctuation. This provides a score of the within-test repeatability by looking at the variances in 10 target locations where the stimulus was presented twice. The results are displayed with a probability of the score being within normal limits.

Single field analysis

The HFA single field STATPAC analysis is designed to assist in the interpretation and identification of visual field defects (see **Fig. 20.11**). Along with patient demographics and the reliability parameters, it includes the sensitivity level for each location in decibels, an interpolated greyscale display, global indices, the glaucoma hemifield test, the total deviation in decibels and probability of each point being within normal limits, and the pattern deviation in decibels and probability of each point being within normal limits. The Octopus and Oculus perimeters also include the Bebie defect curve (see later section).

The global indices

The global indices are data reduction statistics designed to describe specific characteristics of the glaucomatous visual field (Heijl et al 1987). The value of the index and the probability of it being within normal limits are stated on the print-out.

Mean deviation

Mean deviation (MD) is a measure of average sensitivity. It is useful to monitor the overall change in the visual field.

Pattern standard deviation

Pattern standard deviation (PSD) is a measure of non-uniformity in the shape of the hill of vision, i.e. it is sensitive to early scotoma that can be mapped. It has been used in several classifications of early abnormality. Note that the index gets better as the field defect advances to more severe stages, and therefore becomes more uniform once again.

Short-term fluctuation

Short-term fluctuation (SF) is a measure of the intra-test variance. It has proven to be of little clinical value. SF is not calculated when using SITA.

Total deviation

Total deviation (TD) compares the result with an age-matched normal population, and states the probability of each point being abnormal on a point-by-point basis (**Fig. 20.12**; see **Fig. 20.11**). The numeric display illustrates the deviation in decibels from the median age-matched sensitivity, such that negative and positive numbers indicate a reduction or increase from normal, respectively. It is important to understand that the normal range is greater in the periphery than centrally; consequently, a 5 dB reduction centrally can be significant with a high level of confidence that the reduction is a real abnormality, but in the periphery could be within normal limits. The accompanying total deviation probability plot illustrates graphically all sensitivity values that were found to have a 5% or lower probability of being normal. The probability values were determined empirically from a multicentre clinical trial designed to collect normal data. An abnormal classification on the TD analysis could indicate a true defect or, if the majority of values are affected, a generalized depression.

Pattern deviation

Pattern deviation (PD) compares the result with an age-matched normal population corrected for the overall level of sensitivity of the individual (see **Figs 20.11** and **20.12**). This is achieved by adjusting the TD data so that it is normalized to the seventh most sensitive non-edge value, by adding this decibel off-set to each location. The numeric display illustrates the deviation in decibels from the new zero level. The accompanying pattern deviation probability plot illustrates graphically all sensitivity values that were found to have a probability of 5% or less of being normal. This greatly enhances the ability to observe mappable defects within a generalized depression, which may be induced by small pupils or poor media. It can also be a sensitive way

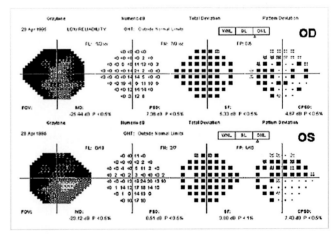

Figure 20.12 The visual fields of a patient with glaucoma showing a large difference between the total deviation analysis, comparing all points to age-matched normal data, and the pattern deviation analysis. Pattern deviation compares the result to an age-matched normal population corrected for the overall level of sensitivity for the given individual. This is achieved by adjusting the TD data such that it is normalized to the seventh most sensitive non-edge value, by adding this decibel off-set to each location. The differences in the example illustrated were principally due to cataract. The right eye (OD) illustrated in the upper panel also shows a classic cloverleaf pattern on the greyscale display, which is most frequently associated with fatigue. This is supported by the high false-negative catch trial rate.

of detecting early focal defects in a patient whose normal field is on the high side of the normal range.

The TD and PD plots provide the most useful and immediate analysis of the visual field. If there are no abnormal points on the TD and PD plots, then the patient can be considered as having a normal field. A depressed TD plot with a normal PD plot likely indicates the presence of cataract or a small pupil. A normal TD plot and an abnormal PD plot usually indicate a 'trigger-happy' patient. Clusters of two or more non-edge points together on the PD chart ($p<0.05$) should be considered suspicious. An isolated point within the central $10°$ ($p<0.05$) should also be considered suspicious. If a cluster of abnormal points exists it should be interpreted with respect to its underlying anatomical correlate and subsequent clinical significance.

Glaucoma hemifield test

The glaucoma hemifield test (GHT) analyses the relative symmetry of five predefined areas in the superior and inferior field, as well as judging the overall level of sensitivity compared with age-matched normal values (Åsman & Heijl 1992). The visual field is then classified in 'plain language' as being:

- 'Outside normal limits', when one or more zones in the superior field is significantly different from its corresponding zone in the inferior field ($p<0.01$)
- 'Borderline', when one or more zones in the superior field is classified as different from its corresponding zone in the inferior field, but does not reach the significance level required to be 'outside normal limits' (0.01 = $p<0.03$)
- 'Within normal limits', when all corresponding zones are considered to be similar ($p =0.03$)
- 'Abnormally high sensitivity', when the highest sensitivities are greater than average and the probability of being within normal limits is 0.05% or less ($p<0.05$).
- 'General reduction of sensitivity', when the highest sensitivities are lower than average and the probability of being within normal limits is 0.05% or less ($p<0.05$), provided that the hemifield asymmetry is not great

enough to classify the field as being 'outside of normal limits'.

The GHT has been accepted as one of the most reliable and successful diagnostic tools for glaucoma. However, it should be noted that the analysis is specific to glaucoma and should not be relied upon to interpret all visual field defects.

Cumulative defect curve (Bebie curve)

The cumulative defect curve, found on the Octopus and Oculus perimeters, ranks the test locations from most to least sensitive and plots relative to the 5% and 95% confidence interval for normal visual fields (Bebie et al 1989). The plot is designed for easy recognition of diffuse versus local defect, relative to age-matched normal confidence limits.

Glaucoma fields

The field defects reflect damage to the nerve fibre layer bundles as they track toward the optic nerve, although the site of damage is thought to be at the level of the lamina cribrosa within the optic nerve. Classic defects include early isolated paracentral, arcuate (**Fig. 20.13**), nasal step and occasional temporal wedge defects (**Fig. 20.14**). It is likely that generalized defects due to the diffuse loss of axons are present in many glaucomatous visual fields, but such defects have limited diagnostic value as they are difficult to distinguish from the effects of media opacities and pupil size.

Glaucoma progression analysis

It is essential to establish good-quality baseline data for both the early diagnosis and management of manifest disease. Current methods for the analysis of visual field progression include an expert inspection of the overview print-out and the glaucoma progression analysis (GPA), an updated version of the original glaucoma change probability (GCP) analysis. Caution is recommended when considering change in the visual field due to the high level of inter-test variability, particularly when a defect is present (Heijl et al 1989b). When in doubt, always repeat the test. GPA is empirically

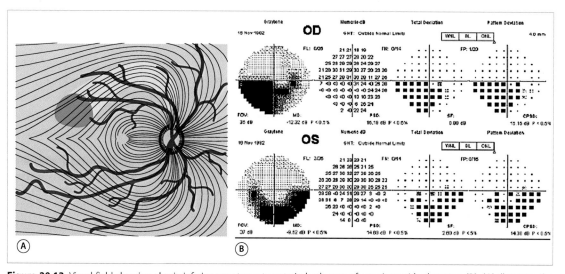

Figure 20.13 Visual field showing classic inferior arcuate scotomata in both eyes of a patient with glaucoma (**B**). (**A**) illustrates the nerve fibre layer bundle that would cause such an abnormality. (Fig. 20.13A with permission from Heijl and Patella 2002.)

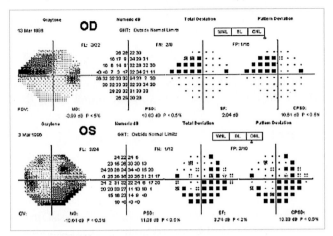

Figure 20.14 Visual field showing temporal wedge defects in both eyes. The right eye shows a superior nasal step defect and a superior temporal wedge. The left eye shows both inferior and superior defects and a superior temporal wedge.

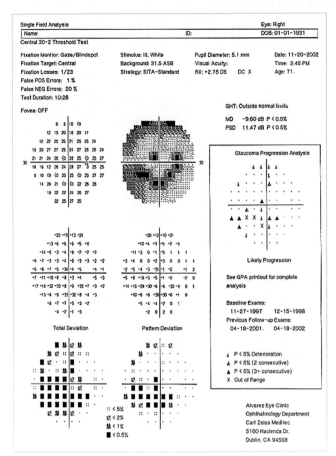

Figure 20.15 Single field analysis print-out from the Humphrey Field Analyzer (Carl Zeiss Meditec, Dublin, CA, USA) following a 30–2 field performed on the right eye of a patient with glaucoma. The result shows an inferior arcuate defect, including a nasal step, and a superior paracentral defect. Fixation is threatened both superiorly and inferiorly. The gaze tracker shows excellent fixation for the initial 25% of the test, followed by a period of excessive eye movements that eventually settle for the latter half of the test. The print-out also shows the glaucoma progression analysis comparing the pattern deviation data to two baseline fields in an event analysis based upon criteria established by the Early Manifest Glaucoma Trial (Heijl et al 2003). Note the plain English descriptor, along with a listing of the date of the previous baseline and follow-up examinations. (Reproduced with permission of Carl Zeiss Meditec.)

based, and compares a patient's pattern of change to the 'typical' change experienced by others with glaucoma. GCP was based on the total deviation of the normal database, and was criticized for being prone to error in the presence of developing cataract and changing pupil size. The GPA is based upon the analysis developed for the Early Manifest Glaucoma Treatment Trial (EMGT) (Heijl et al 2003) and uses the pattern deviation normal database allowing for an analysis that is less sensitive to the effects of cataract and reduced pupil size. GPA is available on the Humphrey Field Analyzer (HFA). The analysis uses estimates of the inherent variability of glaucomatous visual fields from data collected at 16 testing centres. This is combined with the EMGT criterion of three significantly deteriorating points repeated over three examinations. A minimum of two baseline and one follow-up examination are required. Each exam is then compared to baseline and to the two prior visual fields. Points outside the 95th percentile for stability are highlighted, as are points that progress on two or three consecutive examinations. Two additional qualifying statements alert the clinician to the likelihood of 'probable progression' (3 × 2 consecutive) and 'likely progression' (3 × 3 consecutive) (**Figs 20.15** and **20.16**). An advantage of the GPA is that it permits progression analysis across the full-threshold and SITA standard-threshold estimation strategies, thus allowing analysis of pre-SITA visual fields alongside SITA standard fields.

GPA is a good example of an event-based analysis, in which progression is quantified relative to a baseline. This is the most common type of analysis used in clinical trials and is well suited to the follow-up of patients with stable or slowly progressing disease. An alternate, but complementary approach is to use trend-based analysis whereby summary data is analysed using regression techniques. An example is the linear regression analysis of mean deviation found on the HFA (see **Fig. 20.16**). When five or more fields of the same type are plotted together using the GPA or change analysis print-out, a linear regression analysis is performed and the slope calculated. In a recent development, the progression rate is used to predict the outcome over

the next 5 years and the visual field index expresses the percentage of vision expected to be remaining (**Fig. 20.17**).

Visual-function-specific perimetry

New technologies for the testing of visual function have concentrated on selectively testing specific anatomical and/or perceptual pathways. The goal of such an approach is to detect loss of retinal ganglion cells earlier and with improved repeatability. As with most developments in perimetry, they are driven by the need to detect and monitor glaucoma better, but they are frequently useful for all types of visual field loss.

Short-wavelength automated perimetry

Short-wavelength automated perimetry (SWAP), or blue-on-yellow perimetry, uses a large Goldmann size V blue

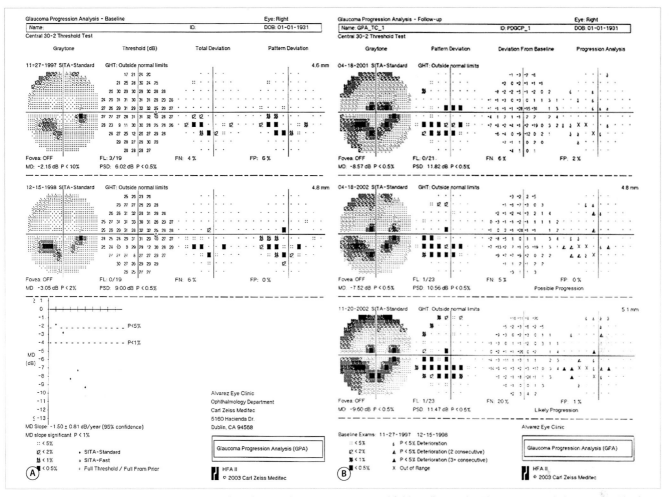

Figure 20.16 (A) and **(B)** Glaucoma progression analysis showing the same patient's visual fields as illustrated in **Figure 20.15** and **Figure 20.17**. The figure highlights the two baseline fields including greyscale and sensitivity plots (labelled Threshold) in decibels, and the total and pattern deviation probability plots. There is also a trend analysis of the mean deviation values. These are the baseline fields used to calculate the GPA presented in the single field printout shown in **Figure 20.15** and the lower part of **Figure 20.17**, and the same fields illustrated at the top of **Figure 20.17**. (Reproduced with permission of Carl Zeiss Meditec.)

stimulus (centred on 440 nm) against a bright yellow background (100 cd/m^2). The rationale is to selectively test the blue cones and their projection through the koniocellular pathway via the s-cone bipolar cells and the retinal ganglion cells, thus taking advantage of their reduced redundancy. The high luminance yellow background is necessary to saturate both the middle- and long-wavelength sensitive pathways and to suppress rod activity. It has been calculated that together this results in approximately 1.5 log units (15 dB) of isolation of the short-wavelength system. SWAP is available on several commercially available perimeters including the HFA and the Octopus.

Several longitudinal studies have found that SWAP can predict early glaucomatous SAP visual field defects, in some cases up to 5 years early (Johnson et al 1993; Sample et al 1993) (**Fig. 20.18**). SWAP is tested, analysed and displayed in an intuitively similar way to SAP. The 2002 Ophthalmic Technology Assessment on automated perimetry (Delgado et al 2002) stated that SWAP gave a sensitivity of 88% and a specificity of 92% for early glaucoma. SWAP was found to be limited by the relatively greater influence of cataracts and other media opacities, a compressed dynamic range, poor

test–retest characteristics and increased test time. The launch of SITA SWAP on the HFA has improved the test time and clinical usefulness of the technique. However, SWAP is unlikely to replace SAP and should be considered a complementary test to be used in selected situations, such as high-risk glaucoma suspects with normal SAP results. SWAP has also proven useful in cases of optic neuritis (Keltner & Johnson 1995) and for detecting the presence of diabetic macular oedema (Hudson et al 2003). Due to chromatic aberration, the optimum refractive correction for SWAP testing is approximately one dioptre more minus than that required for SAP.

Frequency doubling technology

Frequency doubling technology (FDT; Welch Allyn, NY, USA; Carl Zeiss Meditec, CA, USA) perimetry is based on the frequency doubling illusion (Kelly 1966, 1981), whereby a low spatial frequency grating (<1 cycle/degree) is flickered in counterphase at a high temporal frequency (>15 Hz). When this occurs, the spatial frequency of the grating appears to double. The technique has been applied clinically using a grating of 0.25 cycles/degree and temporal frequency of 25 Hz. It was

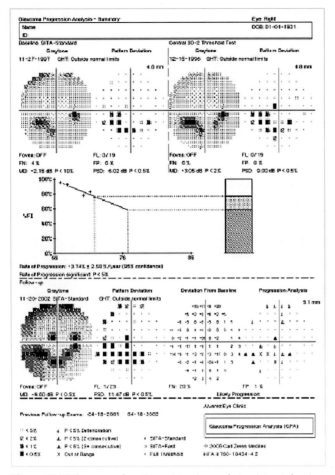

Figure 20.17 Summary glaucoma progression analysis print-out showing the two baseline visual fields and the final field (*lower*). In the centre of the print-out is a graph showing the rate of progression of mean deviation using linear regression analysis, including a forecast of the likely progression over the next 5 years. (Reproduced with permission of Carl Zeiss Meditec.)

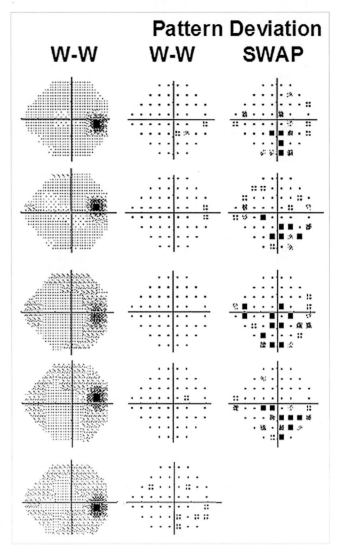

Figure 20.18 Four years of SWAP and standard automated perimetry (white-on-white, W-W) for a patient with early glaucoma. The pattern deviation probability plot for SWAP shows an inferior arcuate defect, with slight progression over the 4 years. The SAP fields show no defect.

initially proposed that the illusion was due to selective processing of the My cells, a subset of magnocellular projecting retinal ganglion cells (Maddess & Henry 1992; Anderson & Johnson 2002). However, this is now thought unlikely, as there is no evidence for such cells in primates, although the illusion is still likely to stimulate the magnocellular system preferentially. It is also likely that the stimulus, as used clinically, is a flicker contrast threshold task, and does not use the frequency doubling illusion (Quaid et al 2004a,b).

The original FDT instrument tested up to 19 10° × 10° targets in either a threshold mode or a rapid (<1 minute) screening test. During testing, the stimulus flicker and spatial frequency are held constant while the contrast is modified in a stepwise process similar to the bracketing method used in conventional perimetry. In response to concerns over the ability of such large targets to detect subtle, early defects, a second-generation machine was developed, the FDT Matrix, which uses smaller 5° targets and measures with a standard 24–2 pattern. A video camera is incorporated for fixation monitoring, and it is possible to view serial fields. A ZEST-like strategy is used to estimate the sensitivity and ensure a standardized test time, regardless of defect.

FDT has been reported to have high sensitivity and specificity for the detection of glaucoma. The 2002 Ophthalmic Technology Assessment on automated perimetry (Delgado et al

2002) indicated that FDT gave a sensitivity of 85% and a specificity of 90% for early glaucoma. Even when used in the screening mode, it may detect some defects earlier than SAP and offers good test–retest characteristics. Recent reports on the full-threshold FDT suggest that it is capable of diagnosing early disease before SAP and often prior to SWAP (Ferreras et al 2007). Patients tend to prefer FDT testing, especially when compared with SAP. FDT is relatively resistant to optical blur, small pupils and the influence of ambient illumination, which make it feasible to use in a screening environment. In a small number of patients there will be an artifactual, diffusely abnormal result in the second, generally left, eye tested. This is thought to be due to binocular rivalry. This phenomenon can be overcome by repeating the second eye examination with the first eye occluded, or by ensuring that the second eye remains light adapted during testing of the first eye.

Flicker defined form

Flicker defined form perimetry is the newest of the vision-function-specific tests and was launched commercially as the Heidelberg Edge Perimeter (HEP; Heidelberg Engineering, Heidelberg, Germany). It is based upon an illusionary stimulus called flicker defined form, in which a 5° stimulus region within a background of random dots is flickered at a high temporal frequency (15 Hz) in counterphase. This gives rise to an illusionary edge or border that is perceived as a grey circle against a mean luminance background. The stimulus targets the magnocellular projecting retinal ganglion cells and is proposed for the early detection of glaucomatous damage (Quaid & Flanagan 2005). A rapid, adaptive staircase strategy is used for threshold estimation. Targets are circular and 5° in diameter for testing standard fields such as the 24–2, and 3° for the 10–2 field. No literature yet exists to define the diagnostic performance of the HEP, but initial results indicate good test–retest characteristics and the ability to detect glaucoma earlier than SAP.

Of particular interest is the availability of the first ever combined structure–function map, in which structural data from the Heidleberg Retina Tomograph is combined with functional data from the HEP. The display combines data for specific sectors of the optic nerve upon which the visual field data is mapped, allowing for the individual-specific anatomical relationship between the optic nerve and the fovea (**Fig. 20.19**).

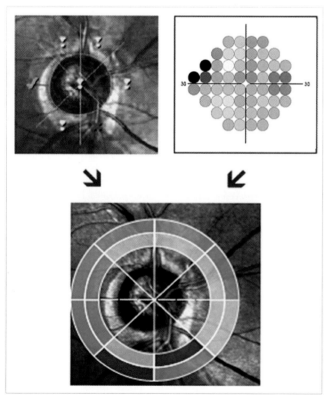

Figure 20.19 Illustration of the structure–function map from the Heidelberg Edge Perimeter (HEP). The plot combines the probability values of the Moorfields Regression Analysis (MRA) found on the Heidelberg Retina Tomograph (HRT) with the corresponding visual field data from the HEP. The inner coloured ring is the structural HRT data and uses the colour coding found on the MRA, green being 'within normal limits', yellow being 'borderline' and red indicating a high probability of being 'outside of normal limits'. The outer ring uses the same probability levels to define the visual field in each of the sectors used by the MRA. The functional field data are mapped using knowledge of the relative position of the fovea to the optic nerve, derived from the HRT map.

Pulsar perimetry

Pulsar perimetry uses a 5° diameter, circular sinusoidal stimulus that flickers at 30 Hz, and decreases in contrast from the centre to the edge (Haag Streit AG, Switzerland) (Gonzalez-Hernandez et al 2004). It is a monitor-based perimeter and the stimulus is designed to stimulate the magnocellular system preferentially.

There are other interesting and potentially useful techniques including flicker perimetry, available on the Medmont and Octopus perimeters, motion perimetry (Wall & Ketoff 1995; Verdon-Roe et al 2006), high-pass resolution perimetry (Frisén 1993) and rarebit perimetry (Frisén 2004). Also of interest but outside the scope of this chapter is the development of objective perimetry, including multifocal visual evoked potentials, electroretinograms and pupil perimetry. It is also likely that functional imaging techniques that map retinal and optic nerve metabolism, or the adaptation of high-resolution optical coherence tomography (OCT; see Ch. 18) for cellular-level optical evoked potentials will soon provide objective information about both the structure and function of the retina and optic nerve.

Summary

In 2003, the first global consensus meeting of the newly founded Association of International Glaucoma Societies (now the World Glaucoma Societies) was on the topic of 'Structure and Function in the Management of Glaucoma'. The following consensus statements were published with regard to function (Weinreb & Greve 2004):

1. A method for detecting abnormality and documenting functional status should be part of the routine clinical management of glaucoma.
2. It is unlikely that one functional test assesses the whole dynamic range.
3. Standard automated perimetry (SAP), as usually employed in clinical practice, is not optimal for early detection.
4. With an appropriate normative database, there is emerging evidence that short-wavelength automated perimetry (SWAP) and possibly also frequency doubling technology perimetry (FDT) may accurately detect glaucoma earlier than SAP.
5. There is little evidence to support the use of a particular selective visual function test over another in clinical practice because there are few studies with adequate comparisons.

- 2007 Update: The FDT N30 may provide better sensitivity than SAP–SITA or SWAP–full threshold. Evidence concerning the sensitivity of SWAP–SITA and FDT Matrix 24–2 is not yet available.

Although these consensus statements refer specifically to the evaluation of the visual field in patients with glaucoma, they summarize appropriately the development of contemporary perimetry and its clinical application. There should be little argument about the necessity for routine perimetry in our clinical armamentarium or the need to continually develop techniques capable of earlier, more precise and more repeatable measurements of visual function.

References

Achard O A, Safran A B, Duret F C et al 1995 Role of the completion phenomenon in the evaluation of Amsler grid results. American Journal of Ophthalmology 120:322

Amsler M 1949 Quantitative and qualitative vision. Transactions of the Ophthalmological Society of the United Kingdom 69:397–410

Anderson A J, Johnson C A 2002 Mechanisms isolated by frequency doubling technology perimetry. Investigative Ophthalmology and Visual Science 43:398–401

Anderson D R, Patella V M 1999 Automated static perimetry. CV Mosby, St Louis

Armaly M F 1972 Selective perimetry for glaucomatous defects in ocular hypertension. Archives of Ophthalmology 87:518–524

Åsman P, Heijl A 1992 Glaucoma hemifield test. Archives of Ophthalmology 110:812–819

Bebie H, Flammer J, Bebie T 1989 The cumulative defect curve: separation of local and diffuse components of visual field damage. Graefe's Archives of Clinical and Experimental Ophthalmology 227 (1):9–12

Delgado M F, Nguyen N T, Cox T A et al 2002 Automated perimetry: a report by the American Academy of Ophthalmology. Ophthalmology 109(12):2362–2374

Elliott D B, North I, Flanagan J 1997 Confrontation visual field tests. Ophthalmology Physiology Optometry 17(Suppl 2): S17–S24

Fankhauser F, Koch P, Roulier A 1972 On automation of perimetry. Albrecht Von Graefes Arch Klin Exp Ophthalmol 184(2):126–150

Ferreras A, Polo V, Larrosa J M et al 2007 Can frequency-doubling technology and short-wavelength automated perimetries detect visual field defects before standard automated perimetry in patients with preperimetric glaucoma? Journal of Glaucoma 16(4):372–383

Ferree C E, Rand G 1922 An illuminated perimeter with campimeter features. American Journal of Ophthalmology 5:455–465

Friedmann A I 1979 Outline of visual field analyzer Mark II. Documenta Ophthalmologica: Proceedings Series 22:65–67

Frisén L 1993 High-pass resolution perimetry. A clinical review. Documenta Ophthalmologica 83:1–25

Frisén L 2004 Vigabatrin-associated loss of vision: rarebit perimetry illuminates the dose-damage relationship. Acta Ophthalmologica Scandinavica 82:54–58

Gonzalez-Hernandez M, Garcia-Feijoo J, Mendez M S et al 2004 Combined spatial, contrast, and temporal functions perimetry in mild glaucoma and ocular hypertension. European Journal of Ophthalmology 14(6):514–522

Greve E L 1973 Single and multiple stimulus static perimetry in glaucoma: the two phases of visual investigation. Junk, The Hague

Harrington D O 1976 The visual fields. A textbook and atlas of clinical perimetry. Mosby, St Louis

Heijl A 1977 Computer test logics for automatic perimetry. Acta Ophthalmologica 55:837–853

Heijl A, Bengtsson B 1996 The effect of perimetric experience in patients with glaucoma. Archives of Ophthalmology 114(1):19–22

Heijl A, Patella V M 2002 Essential perimetry. The field analyzer primer. Carl Zeiss Meditec, Jena, Germany

Heijl A, Lindgren G, Olsson J 1987 A package for the statistical analysis of visual fields. Documenta Ophthalmologica: Proceedings Series 49:153–168

Heijl A, Lindgren G, Olsson J 1989a The effect of perimetric experience in normal subjects. Archives of Ophthalmology 107(1):81–86

Heijl A, Lindgren A, Lindgren G 1989b Test re-test variability in glaucomatous visual fields. American Journal of Ophthalmology 108:130–135

Heijl A, Leske M C, Bengtsson B et al and the Early Manifest Glaucoma Trial Group 2003 Measuring visual field progression in the Early Manifest Glaucoma Trial. Acta Ophthalmologica Scandinavica 81:286–293

Henson D B, Bryson H 1986 Clinical results with the Henson-Hamblin CFS2000. Documenta Ophthalmologica: Proceedings Series 49:233–238

Hong S, Na K, Kim C Y et al 2007 Learning effect of Humphrey Matrix perimetry. Canadian Journal of Ophthalmology 42(5):707–711

Horn F K, Link B, Mardin C Y et al 2007 Long-term reproducibility of screening for glaucoma with FDT-perimetry. Journal of Glaucoma 16 (5):448–455

Hudson C, Wild J M, O'Neill E C 1994 Fatigue effects during a single session of automated static threshold perimetry. Investigative Ophthalmology and Visual Science 35:268–280

Hudson C, Flanagan J G, Turner G S et al 2003 Correlation of a scanning laser derived oedema index and visual function following grid laser treatment for diabetic macular oedema. British Journal of Ophthalmology 87(4):455–461

Johnson C A, Adams A J, Casson E J et al 1993 Blue-on-yellow perimetry can predict the development of glaucomatous field loss. Archives of Ophthalmology 111:645–650

Katz J, Sommer A 1988 Reliability indices of automated perimetric tests. Archives of Ophthalmology 106:1252–1254

Kelly D H 1966 Frequency doubling in visual responses. Journal of the Optical Society of America 56:1628–1633

Kelly D H 1981 Non-linear visual responses to flickering sinusoidal gratings. Journal of the Optical Society of America 71:1051–1055

Keltner J L, Johnson C A 1995 Short-wavelength automated perimetry in neuro-ophthalmologic disorders. Archives of Ophthalmology 113 (4):475–481

Lloyd R I 1936 Evolution of perimetry. Archives of Ophthalmology 15:713–732

McKendrick A M 2005 Recent developments in perimetry: test stimuli and procedures. Clinical and Experimental Optometry 88(2):73–80

Maddess T, Henry G H 1992 Performance of non-linear visual units in ocular hypertension and glaucoma. Clinical and Visual Science 7:371–383

Pandit R J, Gales K, Griffiths P G 2001 Effectiveness of testing visual fields by confrontation. Lancet 358(9295):1820

Quaid P T, Flanagan J G 2005 Defining the limits of flicker defined form: effect of stimulus size, eccentricity and number of random dots. Vision Research 45(8):1075–1084

Quaid P T, Flanagan J G, Simpson T 2004a Monocular and dichoptic masking effects on the frequency doubling illusion. Vision Research 44:661–667

Quaid P T, Simpson T L, Flanagan J G 2004b Frequency doubling illusion: detection versus resolution. Optometry and Vision Science 82:36–42

Sample P A, Taylor J D N, Martinez G A et al 1993 Short-wavelength color visual fields in glaucoma suspects at risk. American Journal of Ophthalmology 115:225–233

Schuchard R A 1993 Validity and interpretation of Amsler grid reports. Archives of Ophthalmology 111:776–780

Traquair H M 1938 An introduction to clinical perimetry, 6th edn. Henry Kimpton, London

Verdon-Roe G M, Westcott M C, Viswanathan A C et al 2006 Exploration of the psychophysics of a motion displacement hyperacuity stimulus. Investigative Ophthalmology and Vision Science 47 (11):4847–4855

Vingrys A J, Helfrich K A 1990 The Opticom M-600TM: a new LED automated perimeter. Clinical and Experimental Optometry 73:3–17

Wall M, Ketoff K M 1995 Random dot motion perimetry in glaucoma patients and normal subjects. American Journal of Ophthalmology 120:587–596

Weinreb R N, Greve E L 2004 Glaucoma diagnosis: structure and function. Kugler Publications, Amsterdam

Weinreb R N, Perlman J P 1986 The effect of refractive correction on automated perimetric thresholds. American Journal of Ophthalmology 101(6):706–709

Werner E B, Krupin T, Adelson A et al 1990 Effect of patient experience on the results of automated perimetry in glaucoma suspect patients. Ophthalmology 97(1):44–48

Wild J M, Moss I D 1996 Baseline alterations in blue-on-yellow normal perimetric sensitivity. Graefe's Archives of Clinical and Experimental Ophthalmology 234(3):141–149

Wild J M, Dengler-Harles M, Searle A E et al 1989 The influence of the learning effect on automated perimetry in patients with suspected glaucoma. Acta Ophthalmologica (Copenh) 167 (5):537–545

Wild J M, Searle A E, Dengler-Harles M et al 1991 Long-term follow-up of baseline learning and fatigue effects in the automated perimetry of glaucoma and ocular hypertensive patients. Acta Ophthalmologica (Copenh) 69(2):210–216

Wood J M, Wild J M, Hussey M K et al 1987 Serial examination of the normal visual field using Octopus automated projection perimetry. Evidence for a learning effect. Acta Ophthalmologica (Copenh) 65 (3):326–333

CHAPTER 21

Contact lenses

Lyndon Jones • Kathryn Dumbleton

Introduction

Patients who attend a clinician for evaluation and correction of their refractive error deserve to be given advice on all the available options to correct their ametropia. In addition to spectacles, advice on their suitability for contact lenses and refractive surgery should also be considered.

In some cases, contact lenses would be appropriate for cosmetic reasons, whereas in certain refractive conditions (for example, keratoconus, post-corneal grafting or corneal trauma) contact lenses may be the only available option to achieve optimal vision correction.

This chapter will broadly deal with situations where contact lenses would be a suitable form of vision correction and, where this is the case, which options of lenses and solutions would be most appropriate.

General indications and contraindications for contact lenses

Patient selection is crucial for success when prescribing contact lenses. Practitioners are fortunate to have such a wide array of contact lens designs and materials available that almost every patient can be successfully fitted. However, care must still be taken to select only those patients suitable for contact lens wear and then to prescribe the most appropriate lens type for their individual optical, physiological, vocational, and environmental needs.

Patient history

A thorough history is essential, not only to assess the patient's motivation and reasons for contact lens wear, but also to evaluate their general and ocular health (see Ch. 26). Systemic disease, medications, allergies, dry eyes, and previous inflammation or infection may contraindicate certain types of contact lenses or how they are prescribed. In addition, information about the patient's occupation, work environment, and leisure pursuits is also important. For example, computer use can result in decreased blinking and patients may need supplemental lubricating drops for this situation, and regular swimming may preclude the use of extended-wear lenses.

Optical considerations

Assessment of the patient's current refractive error and binocular vision are also important when prescribing contact lenses. The majority of contact lens wearers are myopic. When these individuals are fitted with contact lenses they benefit from a relatively larger retinal image size compared with their spectacle correction, a greater field of view and a reduction in the effects of optical aberrations. These benefits are, however, attained at the expense of an increased demand for accommodation and convergence, which can be a problem for patients with higher prescriptions and emerging presbyopes. This may cause a myopic presbyope to require a reading addition with contact lenses, when their distance spectacles were adequate for comfortable near vision. While hyperopic patients also realize the benefits relating to field of view and aberrations with contact lenses, their retinal image size is decreased when compared with their spectacle correction and their visual acuity with contact lenses may be compromised. Conversely, the accommodation and convergence demands with contact lenses are reduced for hyperopic patients and such patients may avoid needing a reading addition for longer by switching to contact lenses.

The decrease in prismatic effects with a contact lens correction is also beneficial for patients with anisometropic prescriptions (see Ch. 22). This occurs as a result of the contact lenses moving with the eyes, practically removing the differential prismatic effects experienced with version movements. This is particularly helpful for vertical prism differences, allowing comfortable binocular single vision without excessive head movements. Since anisometropes often compensate for their horizontal prism differences in spectacles, they may require some time to adapt to a contact lens correction. As a result of magnification differences in the two principal meridians, astigmatic spectacle wearers have a distorted retinal image. A square, for example, will appear rectangular for with-the-rule and against-the-rule astigmats and will be tilted in cases of oblique astigmatism. These distortions are minimal with a contact lens correction, since the differences in magnification between the two meridians are reduced. Long-term spectacle wearers with high astigmatic prescriptions may require a period of adaptation to this apparent change in the retinal image and frequently report distortions when initially wearing contact lenses.

Consideration must also be made for correcting ametropia on the cornea rather than in front of the cornea. A relative decrease (myopic wearers) or increase (hyperopic wearers) in power is required when patients are corrected at the plane of the cornea compared with the spectacle plane. This difference only becomes significant for prescriptions of $> \pm4.50\,D$ in either meridian, and can be calculated from the effective power formula, or vertex distance correction tables can be consulted. In addition, when a rigid contact lens is worn on the eye, the tear film between the cornea and the back surface of the lens forms a 'liquid lens'. If the back surface of the lens is in alignment with the cornea over the optical zone, the liquid lens will have no effective power. However, if the back surface of the lens is relatively steeper than the cornea, a positive liquid lens results and must be compensated for by an increase in power for myopes and a decrease for hyperopes. The converse is true for a back surface which is relatively flatter than the cornea. Lenses which drape over the cornea or flex to conform to the corneal shape (soft lenses) result in little or no effective power from the tear layer and the contact lens power is basically the spectacle lens power, back vertexed to the corneal plane.

Baseline ocular assessments and measurements

Prior to contact lens fitting taking place, a number of measurements and baseline data are required before a suitable lens type and form can be chosen. The first of these is an up-to-date refractive error assessment. Secondly, the ocular integrity must be assessed with a thorough slit-lamp examination (Jones & Jones 2000; Bruce 2002). Factors which may affect lens choice will include evaluation of the eyelids (including lid eversion), lashes and margins, integrity of the limbal region, and a detailed examination of the conjunctiva and cornea. In addition to calculating the refractive error at the corneal plane, the corneal diameter, curvature, and topography should be carefully measured before lens fitting is commenced. Finally, pupil size and the palpebral aperture will be measured. Once these parameters are known, the potential advantages and disadvantages of various lens types for the patient should be broadly discussed with the patient.

Advantages and disadvantages of contact lenses

Contact lenses offer many benefits when compared with spectacles, including an increased field of view, an improvement in cosmetic appearance (with the eyes appearing their normal size) and practicality for sports and outdoor activities. There are three main classes of contact lenses: conventional soft lenses, silicone hydrogel soft lenses, and rigid gas-permeable (RGP) lenses, all of which are available in numerous designs. All of these lenses can be worn for daily wear or overnight wear and are replaced at intervals from 1 day (soft lenses) to 1 year or more (RGP lenses). Details of these materials, designs, and their fitting is given later, but it is important to consider these broad categories and their advantages and disadvantages when selecting the most appropriate lens for a patient.

Soft lenses

Soft lenses (conventional and silicone hydrogel) afford immediate comfort and allow more rapid adaptation than can be achieved with RGP lenses. These benefits allow flexible wearing times and may better suit the occasional wearer or patients with low refractive errors. Since these lenses are generally fitted from an inventory, they can be relatively inexpensive. The larger overall size and optical zones of soft lenses can be advantageous not only for visual performance but also to provide improved stability for sporting activities. Since soft lenses conform to the shape of the cornea, there is less likelihood of dust or foreign bodies getting under the lenses, which is particularly beneficial for patients working in dusty or windy surroundings. There are, however, a number of shortcomings of soft lenses, including variable vision as a result of fluctuations with blinking and environmental changes affecting hydration. Since these lenses tend to conform to the shape of the cornea, they offer very little correction of residual corneal astigmatism in spherical designs. Soft lenses are also more fragile and conventional materials are particularly susceptible to tearing and edge nicks. As a result of interaction with the tear film and the environment, soft lens materials are also more prone to deposition with lens age. Their surfaces can deposit with substances from the tear film (e.g. proteins, lipids, and calcium), which can lead to decreased comfort and vision. Fortunately, deposits are less of an issue now, since the majority of soft lenses are replaced before they are 1 month old. The risk of contamination of soft lenses with pathogenic microorganisms does remain a problem and can lead to possible infection if soft lenses are not properly cleaned and disinfected after wear. Historically, a major shortcoming of soft lenses was their low oxygen transmissibility. Fortunately, this is no longer an issue with the introduction of highly permeable silicone hydrogel materials.

Rigid gas-permeable lenses

The principal advantage of RGP lenses is the superior visual quality they can afford, primarily as a result of correction of any residual corneal cylinder, but also due to fewer fluctuations with environmental changes. These lenses are also more durable and easier to care for than soft lenses and many materials are available with extremely high oxygen permeability. The relatively inflexible nature of these materials also allows applications for myopia control and corneal reshaping. Nonetheless, these lenses do have some drawbacks, the foremost being the need for initial adaptation in order to achieve acceptable comfort. There is also increased potential for discomfort from foreign bodies being lodged under the lenses. The requirement for 'more parameters' at the fitting appointment results in these lenses being rarely fitted from 'stock' and they are usually more expensive than other contact lens options. In addition, increased practitioner skill is required to fit these lenses and, as a result of the drawbacks detailed above, some 90% of patients are fitted with soft lenses (Morgan et al 2008).

Corneal physiology and oxygen requirements

The cornea is avascular and derives most of its oxygen supply from the atmosphere. A sufficient oxygen supply is required to maintain corneal integrity and normal metabolism, and to provide defence against infection. Any contact lens acts as a potential barrier to oxygen transport to the anterior ocular surface, and the ability of a material to transport oxygen through the lens is a major factor in determining the clinical success of that material. The average level of oxygenation required at the anterior cornea in order to prevent oedematous complications is 10% EOP (equivalent oxygen percentage) for daily wear and 18% EOP for closed-eye conditions (Holden et al 1984; Brennan et al 1988), although individual variations are marked (Efron 1986).

To determine if contact lenses provide patients with such levels of oxygen, it is necessary to examine the ease with which oxygen is able to transfer through the lens material. To establish this, the oxygen transmissibility (Dk/t) of the lenses must be evaluated, which takes into consideration both material oxygen permeability (Dk) and lens thickness (t). The units of Dk are 10^{-11} $(cm^2/sec)(mLO_2/mL \times mmHg)$ or 'barrer' and the units of oxygen transmissibility are 10^{-9} $(cm/sec)(mLO_2/mL \times mmHg)$.

Traditional soft contact lens materials rely on water to transport the oxygen through the lens, as the oxygen dissolves into the water phase of the material and diffuses through the lens from the anterior to the posterior lens surface. This has been a severely limiting factor, since water has a Dk value of only 80 barrer (Fatt 1986). The Dk of conventional hydrogels increases logarithmically with the equilibrium water content of the material (Ng & Tighe 1976) and to determine the Dk of conventional soft lenses the non-edge-corrected Fatt formula (Dk = $2.0 \times 10^{-11}e^{0.0411WC}$) (Fatt & Chaston 1982) or boundary and edge-corrected Morgan and Efron formula (Dk = $1.67 \times 10^{-11}e^{0.0397WC}$) (Morgan & Efron 1998) can be used, in which 'WC' is the quoted water content of the material concerned. Once the Dk of the material is known, an assessment of lens thickness enables the clinician to determine the Dk/t of the contact lens in question. By contrast, rigid gas-permeable lenses transmit oxygen via the polymer phase, with no oxygen diffusion occurring through the water phase.

To establish if any given contact lens will provide sufficient oxygenation to a patient it is necessary to determine the amount of oxygen required by the individual's cornea. The most widely cited figures for the minimum acceptable Dk/t are 24×10^{-9} units for daily wear and 87×10^{-9} units for overnight or extended wear (Holden & Mertz 1984). More recently, a level of 125×10^{-9} units has been reported as a requirement to prevent stromal anoxia during closed-eye conditions (Harvitt & Bonanno 1999). However, it must be reiterated that these values are 'averages' and patients exhibit widely different corneal metabolic requirements (Larke et al 1981; Efron 1986). **Table 21.1** describes typical values of Dk/t provided by commonly fitted conventional soft lenses.

The close relationship between water content and oxygen permeability for conventional soft lenses described above has impeded hydrogel lens material development for extended wear for more than 20 years. Inspection of **Table 21.1** clearly shows that conventional hydrogel lens materials provide woefully inadequate Dk/t values for safe, oedema-free overnight wear. However, any of the new silicone hydrogel lens materials is able to supply sufficient oxygen for overnight wear. Recent work has drawn attention to the fact that while Dk/t values are adequate to describe the oxygen performance of conventional hydrogel materials, the performance of higher Dk/t materials does not follow a linear fashion and there is a progressive 'law of diminishing returns', with a doubling of the Dk/t of high-Dk materials not resulting in a doubling of the oxygen reaching the ocular surface. The work of Brennan and others has suggested that oxygen flux models may be a better predictor of oxygen performance for these highly oxygen-permeable materials (Morgan & Brennan 2004; Brennan 2005a,b).

Contact lens materials and designs

All contact lens materials are polymers, which are either 'homopolymers', which contain multiple repeat units of the same monomer, or 'copolymers', which are composed of more than one monomer type joined together. The constituent monomers that are combined to make the polymers determines the physical and chemical properties of the materials. Within this subdivision of materials are a variety of options of designs and replacement periods.

As described above, contact lenses can be broadly divided into rigid and soft (hydrogel) types.

Rigid lens materials

Perspex or polymethyl methacrylate (PMMA) lenses were first fitted in the 1940s and remained the standard for contact lens wear until the commercialization of hydrogel lenses in the early 1970s. Whilst it remains an excellent material in

Table 21.1 Common conventional hydrogel contact lens materials

Commercial name	Manufacturer	Water content	Dk (edge & boundary corrected)	CT	Central Dk/t
Frequency 38	Cooper Vision	38.0	7.5	0.070	10.8
SofLens	Bausch & Lomb	38.0	7.5	0.035	21.6
Biomedics 1 Day	Cooper Vision	52.0	13.2	0.070	18.8
Biomedics 55 Premier	Cooper Vision	55.0	14.8	0.070	21.2
Focus 1–2 Week Visitint	CIBA Vision	55.0	14.8	0.060	24.7
Focus Monthly Visitint	CIBA Vision	55.0	14.8	0.100	14.8
1-Day Acuvue	Johnson & Johnson	58.0	16.7	0.084	19.9
Acuvue 2	Johnson & Johnson	58.0	16.7	0.084	19.9
Soflens 59	Bausch & Lomb	59.0	17.4	0.140	12.4
Soflens Daily Disposable	Bausch & Lomb	59.0	17.4	0.090	19.3
Proclear 1 Day	Cooper Vision	60.0	18.1	0.090	20.1
Proclear Sphere	Cooper Vision	62.0	19.6	0.065	30.1
Focus Dailies	CIBA Vision	69.0	25.8	0.100	25.8
Precision UV	CIBA Vision	74.0	31.5	0.140	22.5

Dk, oxygen permeability; CT, centre thickness at −3.00D; Dk/t, oxygen transmissibility (for −3.00D).
Dk is edge and boundary corrected and calculated from the quoted water content using the formula derived by Morgan and Efron (Dk = $1.67 \times 10^{-11}e^{0.0397WC}$) (Morgan & Efron 1998).

terms of cost, stability, wettability and manufacturing ease, its inability to transmit oxygen obviously limits its practical use in most patients. The development of modern-day rigid gas-permeable (RGP) materials from PMMA is best understood through a full review of the patent literature in this area, which is outside the scope of this chapter but can be viewed elsewhere (Kishi & Tighe 1988; Tighe 2002a). The work of Norman Gaylord and others in the mid-1970s resulted in the development of rigid lenses which incorporated either silicon (siloxymethacrylates) or fluorine (fluorocarbon methacrylates), thereby significantly enhancing the oxygen transmissibility of rigid lenses above that of both PMMA and conventional hydrogel materials. Since the introduction of RGP lenses into clinical practice in the early to mid-1980s, manufacturers have largely adjusted the ratios of methyl methacrylate, silicon, fluorine and various wetting agents to attempt to provide the best possible balance of oxygen permeability, wettability, dimensional stability, and deposit resistance (Tighe 2002a). **Table 21.2** presents a list of several common RGP materials and their manufacturer-reported Dk values, which may be slightly higher than those reported by independent laboratories (Benjamin & Cappelli 2002). The Dk/t of the lenses is also presented for comparative purposes, at a commonly encountered centre thickness of 0.15 mm.

Rigid lens designs and replacement frequencies

The design of rigid lenses has evolved enormously over the past 50 years, as knowledge regarding the shape of the cornea has improved through the development of corneal topographers (Rabinowitz 1993; Fowler & Dave 1994; Dave 1998), and manufacturing techniques have become ever more sophisticated. The cornea can, in most cases, be approximated to a prolate elliptical shape, or one that flattens towards the periphery.

The design of most modern-day lenses can broadly be classified into those that are spherical, aspheric, and reverse-geometry in nature. Readers are referred to standard texts on RGP contact lens fitting for further information on the design of these lenses and how to fit them appropriately (Young 2002; Bennett 2004; Phillips 2006; Veys et al 2007).

- Spherical multicurve designs: Many lenses fitted today still follow the original fitting philosophies developed in the 1950s and 1960s, where lenses are fitted with the central base curve generally aligned with the central corneal curvature and then progressively flatten in the periphery, using a series of flattening spherical curves.
- Aspheric designs: As manufacturing techniques have evolved, the types of peripheral curves that may be cut onto rigid lenses have become more sophisticated. Given that the cornea can best be described as a complex asphere (Guillon et al 1986; Fowler & Dave 1994; Lindsay et al 1998), it has been suggested that aspheric peripheral designs may provide a more appropriate fit than rigid lenses that are fitted using spherical curves that attempt to mimic an aspheric surface (van der Worp et al 2002).
- Reverse geometry designs: Certain corneas have atypical shapes, where rather than flattening in the periphery they actually steepen. This can be seen in healthy eyes, in those that have undergone surgical procedures, following trauma, and also in diseases such as keratoconus. Until recently, these eyes proved difficult to fit appropriately with rigid lenses, as 'classical' rigid lenses flatten in the periphery. The development of computer-controlled lathes in the late 1980s that allowed

Table 21.2 Common rigid lens materials

Name	Material type	Manufacturer-quoted Dk	Dk/t *
Boston II	Silicone acrylate	12	8
Boston IV	Silicone acrylate	19	13
Boston EO	Fluorosilicone acrylate	58	39
Boston Equalens	Fluorosilicone acrylate	47	31
Boston XO	Fluorosilicone acrylate	100	67
Boston Equalens II	Fluorosilicone acrylate	85	57
Boston XO$_2$	Fluorosilicone acrylate	141	94
Fluoroperm 30	Fluorosilicone acrylate	30	20
Fluoroperm 60	Fluorosilicone acrylate	60	40
Fluoroperm 92	Fluorosilicone acrylate	92	61
Fluoroperm 151	Fluorosilicone acrylate	151	101
Menicon Z	Siloxanylstyrene-based fluoromethacrylate	163	125
Paragon HDS	Fluorosilicone acrylate	58	39
Paragon HDS 100	Fluorosilicone acrylate	100	67
Paraperm EW	Silicone acrylate	56	37

* Dk/t, oxygen transmissibility calculated at a 'standardized' centre thickness of 0.15 mm

peripheral curves to be cut that were steeper than the central base curve allowed the manufacture of lenses that were steeper in the mid-periphery. These so-called 'reverse-geometry' lens designs were initially developed for use in orthokeratology (OK), where the steeper peripheral curves allowed the reduction in myopia seen in OK to occur much faster and in a more predictable fashion (Dave & Ruston 1998; Mountford et al 2004; Swarbrick 2004, 2006) (see Ch. 23). **Figure 21.1** shows the fit of a reverse-geometry lens on a spherical cornea. In addition to their use in myopia reduction, reverse geometry lenses have proven extremely valuable in the management of eyes with abnormal peripheral topographies due to surgery or disease (Szczotka & Aronsky 1998; Mathur et al 1999; Lim et al 2000; Szczotka & Lindsay 2003; Lagnado et al 2004), and the use of such lenses in the management of complex cases continues to grow.

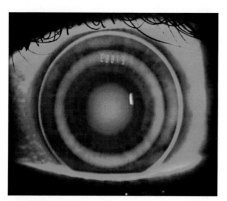

Figure 21.1 Fluorescein pattern of a reverse-geometry orthokeratology-design lens on an eye. The fit is clearly steeper in the mid-peripheral zone due to the steeper second curve. (Picture courtesy of Luigina Sorbara.)

While the acceptance of fitting soft lenses on a regular replacement basis has become standard practice, with current replacement times for the vast majority of soft lenses being anything from 1 day to 3 months, rigid lenses are typically replaced on an 'as needed' basis, with many practitioners advising that such lenses should be replaced annually to biannually. However, data do exist to suggest that frequent replacement of rigid lenses would also likely improve their clinical performance (Woods 2002) and some companies have now started to offer planned replacement schemes for rigid lenses.

Soft (hydrogel) lens materials

Hydrogels are water-absorbing, hydrophilic, polymeric materials. The first successful hydrogel (poly-2-hydroxyethyl methacrylate or polyHEMA) was developed by Otto Wichterle in the late 1960s as a general-purpose surgical material (Wichterle & Lim 1960).

Conventional hydrogel materials

Conventional hydrogel contact lens materials essentially consist of a 'backbone' material that provides, predominantly, parameter stability. The amount of water absorbed by the hydrogel is described by the term 'equilibrium water content' (EWC) and this factor strongly influences the final polymer's surface, mechanical, and transport properties. The principal backbone material used is polyHEMA, which has a water content of 38%. Various monomers are added to provide variations in wettability and oxygen transportation. Two principal strategies have historically been employed to increase the water content of hydrogels above that of polyHEMA: (1) small quantities of negatively charged groups such as methacrylic acid (MA) or (2) larger amounts of more hydrophilic, neutral groups such as polyvinyl alcohol (PVA) or N-vinyl pyrrolidone (NVP) are added

Table 21.3 FDA classification of hydrogel contact lens materials

		Water content (%)	Ionic content (mole fraction at pH=7.2, %)
Group I	Low water content, non-ionic	<50	≤1
Group II	High water content, non-ionic	>50	≤1
Group III	Low water content, ionic	<50	>1
Group IV	High water content, ionic	>50	>1

to raise the water contents to 60% or greater (White 1994; Tighe 2002b). Addition of hydrophilic monomers such as NVP or MA increases water content but reduces physical strength, whilst addition of relatively hydrophobic monomers such as methyl methacrylate (MMA) reduces water content but increases the mechanical characteristics of the materials (Tighe 2002b). The Food and Drug Administration (FDA) uses a classification system to categorize soft lens materials, based upon their water content and ionic (or negative) charge (**Table 21.3**). Materials with water contents greater than 50% are classified as being 'high water content' and those with greater than 0.2% ionic material (invariably methacrylic acid) are termed 'ionic' in nature. This classification is useful to describe the way in which materials interact with both contact lens solutions and the tear film (Jones 2002).

Silicone hydrogel materials

The relatively recent release of a new family of hydrogel materials based on silicone technology (termed 'silicone hydrogels') has introduced a new generation of lenses to the contact lens arena. These lenses were originally intended for continuous in-eye wear for up to 30 days and the term 'continuous wear' has become synonymous with their use. However, more recently, a new generation of silicone hydrogels have been made available that are intended more for the daily wear or occasional overnight ('flexi-wear') market.

In silicone hydrogel materials the 'silicone' component provides extremely high oxygen permeability, while the hydrogel component facilitates fluid transport and thus lens movement. Detailed explanations of the development and composition of silicone hydrogel materials have been described previously (Friends et al 1995; Kunzler & Ozark 1995; Kunzler 1999; Nicolson & Vogt 2001; Jones & Tighe 2004; Tighe 2004; Jones & Dumbleton 2005, 2006b; Jones et al 2006) and these reviews should be consulted for greater detail. Currently, there are seven silicone hydrogel lens types commercially available and their basic details are described in **Table 21.4**. A review of **Table 21.4** will indicate that silicone hydrogel lenses have been classified into FDA groups I and III, although the properties of these materials are not suitably described within the current FDA classification system and it may transpire that a 'fifth group' is required to adequately describe hydrogel lenses that incorporate siloxane groups.

Silicone hydrogel lenses have unique properties due to the fundamental differences between these materials and conventional hydrogels. These differences include their high oxygen transmission, rigidity, and surface wettability.

Oxygen transmissibility

Examination of **Tables 21.1** and **21.4** shows that the Dk/t of silicone hydrogel materials is vastly different from that seen with conventional materials, in which the Dk is directly related to the water content of the lens material. As a result of the increased oxygen availability, oedema levels with silicone hydrogels approved for overnight wear is similar to that seen with no lens wear, and is far lower than that measured with commercially available conventional soft lenses (Brennan & Fonn 2004; Fonn et al 2005). In addition to a reduction in acute signs of hypoxia such as corneal swelling, studies have shown that the use of silicone hydrogel lenses for overnight wear has resulted in a significant reduction in the chronic signs of hypoxia, including limbal hyperaemia, microcysts, and myopic progression (Papas et al 1997; Papas 1998; Dumbleton et al 1999, 2001; Keay et al 2000; Covey et al 2001; du Toit et al 2001; Brennan et al 2002; Morgan & Efron 2002; Sweeney et al 2004; Stapleton et al 2006).

Plasma surfacing treatments

Historically, a huge impediment to the development of silicone hydrogel lenses related to the decreased wettability, increased lipid interaction, and accentuated lens binding inherent in silicon-based materials. In order to make the surfaces of the first-generation silicone hydrogels acceptably hydrophilic, techniques incorporating plasma into the surface processing of the lens were developed (Grobe 1999; Tighe 2004; Jones & Dumbleton 2005, 2006b; Jones et al 2006). Certain silicone hydrogel materials incorporate long-chain, high-molecular-weight polymers within the lens, which aid material wettability.

The surfaces of CIBA Vision's Night & Day and O₂Optix lenses are permanently modified in a gas plasma reactive chamber to create a permanent, ultrathin (25 nm), high refractive index, continuous hydrophilic surface (Nicolson & Vogt 2001; Weikart et al 2001). Bausch & Lomb's PureVision lenses are surface treated in a gas plasma reactive chamber, which transforms the silicone components on the surface of the lenses into hydrophilic silicate compounds (Grobe 1999; Grobe et al 1999; Lopez-Alemany et al 2002; Tighe 2002b, 2004). Glassy, island-like, discontinuous silicate 'islands' result (Lopez-Alemany et al 2002), and the hydrophilicity of these areas 'bridges' over the underlying material. Johnson & Johnson's Acuvue OASYS and Acuvue Advance lenses incorporate polyvinyl pyrrolidone (PVP) into the lens matrix, which helps aid lens wettability (Steffen & Schnider 2004; Jones & Dumbleton 2006b; Jones et al 2006).

Mechanical properties and lens stiffness

Silicone-elastomeric materials are extremely elastic and tend to adhere to the cornea with a 'suction effect'. The material elasticity of the currently marketed silicone hydrogel lenses is much less, and fortunately approaches that of HEMA. This

Table 21.4 Silicone hydrogel lens materials

Proprietary name	Night & Day	O$_2$ OPTIX	PureVision	Acuvue OASYS	Acuvue Advance	Biofinity	Menicon PremiO
United States adopted name	lotrafilcon A	lotrafilcon B	balafilcon A	senofilcon A	galyfilcon A	comfilcon A	asmofilcon A
Manufacturer	CIBA Vision	CIBA Vision	Bausch & Lomb	Johnson & Johnson	Johnson & Johnson	CooperVision	Menicon
Centre thickness (@ −3.00 D) mm	0.08	0.08	0.09	0.07	0.07	0.08	0.08
Water content (%)	24	33	36	38	47	48	40
Oxygen permeability ($\times 10^{-11}$)	140	110	91	103	60	128	129
Oxygen transmissibility ($\times 10^{-9}$)	175	138	101	147	86	160	161
Surface treatment	25 nm plasma coating with high refractive index	25 nm plasma coating with high refractive index	Plasma oxidation process	No surface treatment. Internal wetting agent (PVP)	No surface treatment. Internal wetting agent (PVP)	None	Plasma oxidation
FDA group	I	I	III	I	I	I	I
Principal monomers	DMA + TRIS + siloxane macromer	DMA + TRIS + siloxane macromer	NVP + TPVC + NVA + PBVC	mPDMS + DMA + HEMA + siloxane macromer + TEGDMA + PVP	mPDMS + DMA + EGDMA + HEMA + siloxane macromer + PVP	FM0411M; HOB; IBM; M3U; NVP; TAIC; VMA	Not disclosed

DMA (*N,N*-dimethylacrylamide); EGDMA (ethyleneglycol dimethacrylate); FM0411M (α-methacryloyloxyethyl iminocarboxyethyloxypropyl-poly(dimethylsiloxy)-butyldimethylsilane); HEMA (poly-2-hydroxyethyl methacrylate); HOB (2-hydroxybutyl methacrylate); IBM (isobornyl methacrylate); mPDMS (monofunctional polydimethylsiloxane); NVP (*N*-vinyl pyrrolidone); TEGDMA (tetraethyleneglycol dimethacrylate); TPVC (tris-(trimethylsiloxysilyl) propylvinyl carbamate); TRIS (trimethylsiloxy silane); M3U (α w-Bis(methacryloyloxyethyl iminocarboxy ethyloxypropyl)-poly(dimethylsiloxane)-poly(trifluoropropylmethylsiloxane)-poly (ω−methoxy-poly(ethyleneglycol)propyl methylsiloxane)); NVA (*N*-vinyl amino acid); PBVC (poly[dimethylsiloxy] di [silylbutanol] bis[vinyl carbamate]); PVP (polyvinyl pyrrolidone); TAIC (1,3,5-triallyl-1,3,5-triazine-2,4,6(*1H,3H,5H*)-trione); VMA (N-Vinyl-N-methylacetamide).

further helps to prevent lens adhesion and promote movement and tear flow beneath the lens. Silicone hydrogel lenses are, however, 'stiffer' than their conventional hydrogel counterparts, due to the incorporation of silicon (Tighe 2004; Jones et al 2006).

Increased rigidity or stiffness has some advantages, in that the lenses handle very well and are a perfect choice for people who exhibit poor handling capabilities. The mechanical properties of these lenses may pose some problems, in that they are less able to conform easily to the shape of the eye and fitting is critical, with loose lenses exhibiting poor comfort (Dumbleton et al 2002). Additionally, the rigidity of these materials may be implicated in a variety of mechanical complications seen with silicone hydrogel lenses, including papillary conjunctivitis and superior epithelial splits (Holden et al 2001; Jalbert et al 2001; O'Hare et al 2001; Dumbleton & Jones 2002; Jones & Dumbleton 2002; Skotnitsky et al 2002). More recently released silicone hydrogels tend to not suffer from these mechanical complications to the same extent, as their oxygen permeability is lower and thus their silicone content is generally lower,

resulting in stiffness values much closer to conventional lenses (Jones et al 2006). In addition, improved back surface designs of first-generation materials have resulted in far fewer mechanical complications than originally reported.

Hydrogel lens designs and replacement frequencies

The majority of single-vision soft lenses are spherical in design. Recent interest in attempting to correct higher-order visual aberrations has resulted in the development of aspheric lenses that aim to improve visual quality, particularly at night, and of complex lenses that aim to reduce various aberrations (Jiang et al 2006; Roberts et al 2006; Sabesan et al 2007). Readers are referred to standard texts on soft contact lens fitting for further information on the design of these lenses and how to fit them appropriately (Jones & Dumbleton 2006a).

A wealth of knowledge now exists to demonstrate that clinical performance with soft lenses is improved if lenses are replaced frequently (Boswall et al 1993; Jones 1994; Brennan & Coles 2000) and evidence does support the concept that 'shorter is better', with shorter replacement periods demonstrating lower levels of deposition from the tears, fewer complications and enhanced clinical performance (Marshall et al 1992; Poggio & Abelson 1993; Hamano et al 1994; Jones et al 1996; Pritchard et al 1996; Solomon et al 1996; Donshik & Porazinski 1999; Porazinski & Donshik 1999; Suchecki et al 2000). The vast majority of soft lenses are now replaced following 1 month or less of wear, with daily disposable lenses representing a large portion of those lenses fitted, particularly in Northern Europe and Japan (Morgan et al 2008).

Presbyopic contact lens fitting

Due to the changing demographics of the age of the population, increasing numbers of current and prospective contact lens wearers require a presbyopic correction. As a result of ageing, these individuals generally exhibit reduced tear quantity and quality, reduced eyelid tonicity, and small pupils, all of which can prove to be problematic for contact lens wear. Therefore, careful prescreening, appropriate lens selection, and patient education, especially regarding expectations, must be undertaken before fitting.

Many standard texts cover the fitting of the presbyopic patient (Bennett et al 2000; Veys et al 2002; Gasson & Morris 2003; Bennett 2006). This section will cover broad principles of fitting the presbyope only, and interested readers are referred to more extensive texts for specific details regarding presbyopic lens designs and fitting procedures.

The simplest approach is to fit contact lenses with a distance correction and prescribe over spectacles with the near addition prescription for close work. Another common way of managing presbyopes, particularly early presbyopes, is by prescribing contact lenses for 'monovision', where one eye is optimally corrected for distance and the other eye for near. While this method is possible with contact lenses, the primary drawback is compromised binocular vision, which may affect performance for certain tasks, especially driving. For these patients, the prescription of distance-correcting spectacles to provide binocularity can be important for medicolegal purposes.

Recent years have seen the development of many new designs of contact lenses in both rigid and soft materials specifically for presbyopia. The two broad categories for these designs are simultaneous and alternating vision types. Simultaneous designs present a range of powers within the pupil at the same time. These designs require the wearer to suppress selectively the blurred images. Alternating (or translating) designs vary in power across the lens and rely on the lens moving to change the power presented at any one time. The vision 'alternates' between two different corrections, much like bifocal spectacles.

Simultaneous vision lenses, which are generally easier to fit than alternating designs, may be aspheric, concentric, or diffractive in design. Aspheric designs can be centre-distance or centre-near. Concentric designs can also be manufactured in each of these formats. With both of these designs there is some degree of compromise, which is largely dependent on the illumination in which they are used. In centre-distance formats, low illumination favours near vision and high illumination favours distance vision, with the reverse being true for centre-near formats. The latest designs are the 'multi-zone' bifocals, which employ alternate zones of concentric distance and near vision. Diffractive designs are used less frequently but have a central zone which focuses distance images by refraction and near images by diffraction. The diffractive and multizone bifocals have the advantage of being less dependent on pupil size.

Because alternating designs rely primarily on vertical movement on the eye, they are generally employed in RGP materials. These designs can either have a segment for the reading add or employ a concentric design. Segmented designs require prism ballasting or truncation to prevent rotation and assist translation on the eye. Although this design probably offers the best visual potential, successful fitting requires skill, time, and experience.

A further approach is to prescribe 'modified monovision', which involves either the combination of a bifocal or multifocal contact lens in one eye and a single-vision lens in the other eye, or the use of two bifocal contact lenses, with one correcting for distance and intermediate vision and the other correcting for intermediate and near vision.

There will always be some degree of compromise when fitting the presbyopic patient and additional persistence may be required on the part of the patient and the eye care practitioner to achieve success. Often, the key to successful presbyopic fitting is matching the correct design to the patient's needs and being realistic about the likely outcome.

Contact lens solutions

The development of contact lens solutions dates to the late 1940s, following the production of rigid contact lenses manufactured from polymethyl methacrylate (PMMA). These early solutions were indicated primarily for enhanced wetting and it was not until the 1970s that the 'science of contact lens solutions' was truly born. Since that time, the development and optimization of contact lens solutions has evolved rapidly to keep pace with the development of novel contact lens materials and our ever-growing appreciation of the role that contact lens care regimens play in contact lens success.

Contact lens solutions form a very important part of the overall care of contact lenses, but are just one component of many elements, which include digital rubbing, rinsing, soaking, and lens case hygiene. Over the past 30 years, solutions have gradually evolved towards simpler regimens to aid compliance and improve convenience for the patient.

Modern care regimens basically consist of a combination of antibacterial agents, surfactants or wetting agents, chelating agents, demulcents, and a number of other agents that primarily assist with control of pH and osmolality (Jones & Senchyna 2007, Jones & Christie 2008).

Rigid lens solutions

Rigid gas-permeable care regimens can be divided into three components: cleaning solutions, soaking and wetting solutions, and multifunctional solutions.

RGP cleaning solutions

The primary function of a cleaning solution is to remove loosely bound foreign matter by solubilizing contaminants such as cell debris, mucus, lipid, and protein, in addition to cosmetics and other surface contamination (Randeri et al 1995). In achieving this aim, any cleaning solution will also significantly reduce the level of microbiological burden (Shih et al 1985) prior to overnight soaking in the disinfectant.

The major component of any cleaner is the surface active agent (or surfactant). Surfactant cleaners can be either abrasive or non-abrasive. Most RGP cleaning solutions are non-abrasive surfactants because they contain detergents that, in combination with digital pressure during the cleaning process, remove lipids, mucoproteins, and other contaminants on the lens surface. As these agents are potentially toxic to the corneal tissues at the concentration at which they are present in the RGP solutions, they must be rinsed from the lens prior to lens insertion and cannot be used directly in the eye.

In addition to surfactants, other constituents include viscosity-enhancing agents, alcohols (such as isopropyl alcohol or ethanol) to assist in lipid removal, and mild abrasive particles (in the form of polymeric beads) to assist with the removal of certain strongly attached deposits. These 'abrasive' cleaners have been found to be more effective than non-abrasive cleaners for certain patients (Chou et al 1985). However, two problems have been reported with the long-term use of abrasive-containing surfactant cleaners. Small surface scratches have been observed under high magnification (Doell et al 1986) and reports exist describing the addition of minus power to RGP lenses and reduction in centre thickness (Caroline & Andre 1999), particularly where lenses are cleaned between the fingers rather than between the palm of the hand and index finger. In

situations where this is recorded, practitioners should re-educate the patient about how to clean the lenses appropriately, or switch to non-abrasive surfactants.

Some unique products of note are the two abrasive cleaners Opti-Clean II from Alcon and the original Boston/Bausch & Lomb cleaner, both of which contain small polymeric beads. In addition, the Boston Advance/Bausch & Lomb Elite cleaner also includes the principle of microscopic beads (albeit a finer 'ultra-micronized' version), incorporated with ethoxylated alkyl phenol to provide an alcohol base, which is highly effective at removing lipid deposits. Finally, Miraflow from CIBA Vision includes isopropyl alcohol, which is also very effective against lipid deposits.

RGP soaking and wetting solutions

Soaking and wetting solutions are often called 'conditioning solutions', which is, perhaps, a more accurate description of their function. Whilst a major function of the soaking solution is to disinfect the lens, an equally important function relates to the ability of the solution to 'condition' or 'wet' the lens surface. The solution should cushion the lens onto the cornea on insertion, whilst at the same time enhancing the spread of tears across the lens surface. **Table 21.5** describes the common components of many of the modern-generation soaking and wetting solutions available.

The choice of preservative can have an effect not only on the bacterial load but also upon the eye and the lens surface. One of the most effective disinfectants is benzalkonium chloride (BAK) (Penley et al 1989; Silvany et al 1991; Niszl & Markus 1998), a common cationic detergent used as a

Table 21.5 Common RGP wetting and soaking solutions

Solution	Company	Preservative and concentration	Conditioning/viscosity agents
Opti-Soak® conditioning & disinfecting solution	Alcon	Polyquad 0.001% Disodium edetate 1 mg/mL	Sodium chloride Sodium phosphates Polysorbate 80 Hydroxyethylcellulose Polyvinyl alcohol
Soaclens® soaking & wetting solution	Alcon	Polyquad 0.011 mg/mL Disodium edetate 1 mg/mL	Hypromellose (Methocel™) Boric acid Mannitol
Barnes Hind® ComfortCare®	Advanced Medical Optics	Edetate disodium Benzalkonium chloride 0.004%	Polyvinyl alcohol
Wet-N-Soak PLUS®	Advanced Medical Optics	Edetate disodium Benzalkonium chloride 0.003%	Polyvinyl alcohol
TotalCare™	Advanced Medical Optics	PHMB 0.0005% Edetate disodium 0.01%	Hydroxyethylcellulose
Original Formula Boston® Conditioning Solution	Bausch & Lomb	Edetate disodium 0.05% Chlorhexidine 0.006%	Polyvinyl alcohol Derivatized polyethylene glycol Cellulosic viscosifier Cellulose derivative polymer
Boston Advance® Comfort Formula Conditioning Solution	Bausch & Lomb	Polyaminopropyl biguanide 0.0005% Edetate disodium 0.05% Chlorhexidine 0.003%	Polyvinyl alcohol Derivatized polyethylene glycol
Delta Plus	Sauflon	Polyhexanide 0.001%	Poloxamer

preservative in ophthalmic eyedrops and contact lens solutions. However, several authors have questioned the cytotoxicity of BAK (Rosenthal et al 1986; Wong et al 1986; Begley et al 1991, 1992). BAK-containing care regimens are not used to disinfect soft lenses due to the high levels of binding of BAK to hydrogel surfaces, resulting in toxic tissue reactions. In RGP contact lens wearers, the use of a solution preserved with BAK (which may be used every day, over many months and years) can produce red, gritty eyes and reduced wearing times due to a preservative sensitivity to this low molecular weight preservative. This can be a problem with high-Dk RGP lenses (Sterling & Hecht 1988; Jones & Jones 1992), which seem to induce more preservative-based reactions when used with BAK-containing solutions than when such regimens are used with low-Dk RGP lenses.

RGP multipurpose solutions

Like the much larger soft lens market, the trend in RGP lens care is towards the use of multipurpose solutions. These one-bottle 'multipurpose' systems offer the patient convenience and combine the functions of cleaning, soaking and wetting in a single bottle (**Table 21.6**)

One interesting approach concerns Alcon's Unique pH, whose distinctive aspect is that the viscosity or 'thickness' of the solution changes as a function of pH. When the solution is exposed to human tears it changes from a thin liquid solution to a thicker solution. This theoretically provides the patient with easy lens care handling and the appropriate amount of cushioning for lens wear comfort, following insertion.

Soft lens solutions

As previously stated, soft lenses must be adequately disinfected if ocular infection is to be avoided. The development of relatively hydrophobic silicone hydrogel lenses has resulted in some unique challenges for manufacturers of soft lens solutions, as the uptake and release of preservatives from silicone hydrogels is different from that seen with conventional hydrogels, and the wettability of their surfaces also differs.

The composition of some commonly encountered soft lens solutions is described in **Table 21.7**. The primary role of the antimicrobial agent or 'biocide' is to provide a lens that is suitably disinfected such that it is 'safe' to be inserted into the eye, typically following overnight soaking. The choice of a suitable antimicrobial is technically challenging, as the choice must take into consideration three separate, yet equally important issues, namely efficacy, safety, and convenience. The agent of choice must be effective against a wide variety of pathogens, provide an effective kill against pathogens and not against ocular tissues, and be convenient and simple to use for the patient. Examples of biocides include hydrogen peroxide, polyquaternium-1 (Polyquad®), polyhexamethylene biguanide (PHMB), chlorhexidine, and benzalkonium chloride. One important difference between these agents relates to their molecular weight (mw), with small molecular weight biocides such as chlorhexidine showing much less uptake into the lens polymer than larger biocides such as polyquaternium-1, which results in much lower levels of allergic and toxicity reactions (Jones & Senchyna 2007). With the exception of the hydrogen peroxide-preserved systems, most modern regimens require no neutralization process after the lenses have been soaked overnight. The hydrogen peroxide systems all rely on 3% peroxide and most are neutralized via either a coated time-release tablet containing a catalytic enzyme (catalase) or a platinum disc system. Residual peroxide is toxic to corneal tissue when present in a sufficiently high concentration and can cause discomfort unless neutralized to a concentration of less than 100 ppm, with the subjective sensitivity threshold being 50–300 ppm (Chalmers & McNally 1988).

Surfactants are 'wetting agents' that lower the surface tension of a liquid and lower the interfacial tension between two liquids. They are usually organic compounds that are amphiphilic, meaning they contain both hydrophobic groups (their 'tails') and hydrophilic groups (their 'heads'). Examples include poloxamines sold under the trade name Tetronic® and poloxamers sold under the trade name Pluronic®. The functions of surfactants in contact lens care regimens are twofold. Firstly, they are used as 'detergents' or cleaners, removing loose debris and deposits (including microorganisms), by combining with these substances to form micelles which are more easily suspended in the

Table 21.6 Common RGP multipurpose products

Solution	Company	Preservative concentration (%)	Surfactant	Conditioning/viscosity agent (s)
Unique pH® MPS	Alcon®	POLYQUAD® (polyquaternium-1) 0.0011%; edetate disodium 0.01%	TETRONIC® 1304* *TETRONIC® is a registered trademark of BASF	Hydroxypropyl guar, polyethylene glycol, propylene glycol
Bosto® Simplus™	Bausch & Lomb	Chlorhexidine gluconate 0.003% Polyaminopropyl biguanide 0.0005% Edetate disodium 0.05%	PEO sorbitan monolaurate + Betaine surfactant	Derivatized polyethylene glycol Silicone glycol copolymer Cellulosic viscosifier
Solocare Hard	CIBA	Polyhexanide 0.0002%	Poloxamer 407 Lutrol F	Hydroxyethyl cellulose
MeniCare Plus	Menicon	Polyhexanide 0.0005%	Poloxamer	Hypromellose

Table 21.7 Principal components of common soft contact lens solutions

Manufacturer	Solution	Preservative (%)	Neutralizing agents	Other agents (e.g. surfactants, chelating agents and buffers)
Alcon®	OPTI-FREE® *Express*® MPDS	POLYQUAD® (polyquaternium-1) 0.001%; ALDOX® (MAPD) 0.0005%; edetate disodium 0.05%		Sodium citrate, sodium chloride, boric acid, sorbitol, AMP-95, TETRONIC® 1304
Alcon®	OPTI-FREE® RepleniSH® MPDS	POLYQUAD® (polyquaternium-1) 0.001%; ALDOX® (MAPD) 0.0005%		Sodium citrate, sodium chloride, sodium borate, propylene glycol, TEARGLYDE™ [TETRONIC® 1304 and nonanoyl ethylenediaminetriacetic acid (C-9 ED3A)]
Advanced Eyecare Research	Regard	0.01% hydrogen peroxide; chlorite ion (ClO_2^-)		0.15% HPMC; Pluronic® F68
Advanced Medical Optics	Complete Easy Rub	0.0001% PHMB		Phosphates; 0.02% EDTA; Poloxamer 237 (Pluronic® F87)
Advanced Medical Optics	Ultracare or OxySept 1-Step	Hydrogen peroxide (3%)	HPMC-coated catalase tablet	Phosphates, HPMC
Bausch & Lomb	ReNu MultiPlus	0.0001% PHMB		Boric acid; sodium borate; hydroxyalkylphosphonate
Bausch & Lomb	Sensitive Eyes MPS	0.00005% PHMB		Edetate disodium; poloxamine; boric acid; sodium chloride; sodium borate
CIBA Vision	AOSept	Hydrogen peroxide (3%)	Platinum disc	Phosphates
CIBA Vision	ClearCare or AOSept Plus	Hydrogen peroxide (3%)	Platinum disc	Phosphates; Pluronic® 17R4
CIBA Vision	SoloCare Aqua or Focus Aqua	0.0001% PHMB		Tromethamine; sorbitol; 0.025% EDTA; dexpanthenol (provitamin B5);
Menicon	MeniCare Soft	0.0001% PHMB		Macrogolglycerol hydroxystearate 60; glycine; glycolic acid; AMPD.
Sauflon	CyClean	0.0001% PHMB		Biopol
Sauflon	All in One Light	0.0001% PHMB		Poloxamer; sodium phosphate
Sauflon	Multi	Hydrogen peroxide (3%)	Platinum disc	Poloxamer
Sauflon	Comfort-Vue	0.00008% PHMB		Poloxamer; HPMC; sodium phosphate
Sauflon	Synergi	hydrogen peroxide; chlorite ion (ClO_2^-); 0.08% Oxipol		HPMC

MAPD, myristamidopropyl dimethylamine; PHMB, polyhexamethylene biguanide (also known as polyhexanide, Dymed®, polyhexidine and polyaminopropyl biguanide); HPMC, hydroxypropylmethylcellulose; EDTA, ethylenediaminetetraacetic acid; AMPD, 2-amino-2-methyl-1,3-propanediol.

surrounding liquid. The micelles are then removed during the rinsing procedure. The surfactants both 'soften' the deposits, preventing them from becoming irreversibly adherent to the lens surface (Phillips 1980), and also aid subsequent lens disinfection by reducing the bacterial bioburden by a factor of up to four log units (>99%) (Houlsby et al 1984; Shih et al 1985). The second function relates to their ability to enhance the wettability of hydrophobic substrates (Tonge et al 2001; Ketelson et al 2005), which is becoming of increasing importance with the development of silicone hydrogel lenses, which are generally more hydrophobic than conventional hydrogel materials (Weikart et al 1999; Bruinsma et al 2001; Cheng et al 2004). As the growth in the numbers of patients wearing silicone hydrogels

continues, the importance of surfactants for both their cleaning and enhanced wetting roles is likely to increase.

Chelating agents are added to modern care regimens either to act synergistically with other agents to improve disinfection efficacy or to aid in removal of tear film components, typically proteins. Ethylenediamine tetra-acetic acid (EDTA) is a chelating agent that binds free metals and enhances antimicrobial activity of disinfectants and is found in the majority of multipurpose products.

Sodium citrate and hydroxyalkylphosphonate (Hydranate®) are sequestering agents that aid in the passive removal of protein (Hong et al 1994; Christensen et al 1998).

Demulcents are agents that help to improve comfort through modification of the contact lens surface. Examples include hydroxypropylmethylcellulose (HPMC) (Simmons et al 2000, 2001) and propylene glycol. Issues relating to increased *Acanthamoeba* infections with a product containing these demulcents (Joslin et al 2007) saw this product being removed from the market in 2007.

Specialty applications of contact lenses

There are many specialty applications of contact lenses and only a broad overview can be given in this chapter. The interested reader is directed to many of the expansive texts giving further details of the conditions which can benefit from a contact lens correction and their individual applications (Hom & Bruce 2006; Phillips & Speedwell 2006).

Keratoconus

Keratoconus is a progressive degenerative dystrophy of the cornea, which usually results in thinning and irregularity of the cornea, resulting in visual distortion not readily corrected by spectacles lenses. The combination of the relatively inflexible surfaces of an RGP lens and the resultant tear lens can mask these irregularities and provide a regular refracting surface, resulting in superior visual performance compared with spectacles or soft lenses. Keratoconus fitting is complicated by the relative decentration of the corneal apex and atypical corneal topography. While the apex of the cornea may be extremely steep in curvature, the periphery frequently retains a relatively normal contour, particularly in the early stages of the disorder. Consequently, conventional RGP designs have been frequently fitted too 'flat', which may afford improved visual performance but may ultimately exacerbate the corneal scarring commonly observed in keratoconus patients (Edrington et al 1999; Leung 1999). Conversely, lenses can be fitted with minimal apical clearance (Korb et al 1982). Usually, this latter approach requires a small optical zone and overall diameter and very steep central radius and often results in poor visual outcomes. An alternative to these approaches has been to fit using a 'three-point-touch' method, where the weight of the lens is distributed between the cone and the mid-peripheral cornea (Leung 1999).

The optimal design to fit a cornea that exhibits keratoconus has historically used either multiple spherical curvatures or aspheric back surfaces. Unfortunately, these customized designs are frequently complicated and time consuming to work with and an optimal fit is often difficult to achieve. In an attempt to make keratoconus contact lens fitting more straightforward, a number of new designs and products specifically developed for this condition have been developed, including the Rose K lens (Rose 2005), the CLEK lens (Edrington et al 1996), and the Shepherd K lens (Ehrlich 2004; Steele 2005).

In some cases of keratoconus, and other conditions where corneal irregularity is a concern, a combination of rigid and soft lens designs may be used. This is usually referred to as a 'piggyback' correction, where a soft lens is placed on the cornea and an RGP lens is placed over the top of this soft 'carrier' lens. While historically this approach resulted in significant physiological compromise due to the very low oxygen transmissibility of the lens combination, newer silicone hydrogel and high-Dk RGP materials have made this a practical approach for many complex cases. The softer carrier lens drapes over the cornea and conjunctiva, affording comfort and stability for the RGP lens resting on it. For keratoconus patients it is often advantageous to fit a minus-powered soft carrier lens to artificially flatten the cornea and then fit the RGP lens according to the curvature of the anterior surface of this lens (Caroline & Andre 2004). This usually results in improved centration and movement of the RGP lens. Conversely, when fitting post-refractive surgery patients with very flat central corneas, a plus-powered carrier lens is fitted to artificially steepen the cornea. In both cases, the power of the RGP lens is used to correct the induced ametropia.

Another approach to improving comfort and stability when fitting keratoconic and post-refractive surgery patients is to use a hybrid lens design. The first of these, the Saturn lens, comprised a PMMA central zone and a silicone skirt. This combination was subsequently replaced by lenses with an RGP centre and a hydrogel skirt. In the same way that the original piggyback combinations provided insufficient oxygen transmission, these hybrid designs gave rise to chronic hypoxia and they became less popular over time. More recently, a hybrid design has been developed with a Paragon HDS 100 rigid centre and a hydrogel skirt (SynergEyes, Quarter Lambda Technologies, CA, USA) for post-refractive cases. While this design offers great promise, a hybrid design with a silicone hydrogel skirt would certainly be preferable and lenses of this design may become available in the near future.

Scleral lenses

An alternative method of providing a suitable fit and good visual outcome for irregular corneas is to use scleral lens designs. These lenses are considerably larger than soft or RGP designs and rest on the sclera, creating a tear-filled vault over the cornea. The first scleral lenses were fitted following impression moulding in the late 1800s. These techniques were enhanced and became more popular in the 1930s. Their popularity declined with the introduction of rigid and hydrogel lenses and currently scleral lenses are used almost exclusively in cases where an acceptable lens fit cannot be achieved with other lens designs. Interested readers are referred to supplementary texts describing this speciality area of contact lens fitting in detail (Pullum 2006). Typical cases where these lenses are beneficial include advanced keratoconus, pellucid marginal degeneration, keratoglobus, post-corneal transplant, corneal dystrophies, post trauma, and in severe dry eye conditions such as those occurring following chemical burns, ocular cicatricial pemphigoid, and Stevens–Johnson syndrome.

Therapeutic and bandage lenses

Although required by a relatively small proportion of wearers, contact lenses for therapeutic purposes are a very important indication for contact lens wear. The lenses are generally prescribed for protection and promotion of healing of the cornea and can bring about relief in a number of different ways. These include acting as a mechanical barrier, particularly in cases of eyelid dysfunction, or as a splint in cases of corneal perforation. A major use is in pain relief associated with corneal conditions, including bullous keratopathy, filamentary keratitis, and many dystrophies. In addition, pain may be relieved in conjunctival diseases and injuries where there is a risk of adhesion between the palpebral and bulbar conjunctiva. Therapeutic lenses can also aid in healing of recurrent epithelial erosions and other surface defects where the extended period of time that the lens is worn allows protection and regeneration of the epithelium (Hickson-Curran 2006).

Historically, high-water-content or thin, mid-water-content hydrogel contact lenses were used for these applications (Gasset & Kaufman 1970; Gruber 1991; Tanner & DePaolis 1992), since therapeutic lenses are generally worn for prolonged periods. Unfortunately, these lenses were not able to supply sufficient oxygen to prevent overnight corneal swelling (Holden & Mertz 1984) and the combined effects of chronic hypoxia in already compromised eyes often resulted in severe complications, including infection and inflammation (Dohlman 1974; Kent et al 1990). Silicone elastomer lenses were also used for some conditions; however, these lenses, although capable of providing sufficient oxygen to prevent overnight corneal swelling, often resulted in lens adhesion and poor wetting (Rae & Huff 1991).

The introduction of silicone hydrogel lenses has provided clinicians with a viable alternative for their therapeutic cases, since the high oxygen transmissibility of these lenses has been shown to result in little or no additional overnight corneal swelling compared to that measured following sleep with no lens in place. CIBA Vision's Night & Day, Bausch & Lomb's PureVision, and Johnson & Johnson's Acuvue OASYS lenses have received FDA and CE Mark approval for therapeutic use throughout the USA, Canada, and the European Union. Silicone hydrogel lenses are now the most widely prescribed lens type for therapeutic indications (Karlgard et al 2004) and they have proven useful in managing a number of conditions (Lim et al 2001; Kanpolat & Ucakhan 2003; Ambroziak et al 2004).

Dry eye

Contact lenses are sometimes used to maintain epithelial hydration in moderate to severe dry eye conditions, although this approach is only implemented when other therapies have been unsuccessful, as supplemental ocular lubricants are typically still required and the risk of infection is higher in severely dry-eyed patients. Scleral lenses have been useful in the management of pathological dry eye (Segal et al 2003; Dart 2005; Visser et al 2007) and silicone hydrogel lenses may also be able to offer greater success in dry-eyed patients (Ambroziak et al 2004).

Drug delivery

Soft lenses can also be used for drug delivery since they are able to provide a slow release of drugs over a prolonged period of time and this can result in greater efficacy and reduced toxicity. Common applications include the management of glaucoma and the treatment of bacterial and viral infection. Drug delivery with silicone hydrogel lenses is expected to be improved when compared with traditional hydrogel materials, as they release the drugs at a similar rate to conventional hydrogel materials but offer greater levels of oxygenation during overnight wear (Karlgard et al 2003a,b). Recent work has suggested that the delivery may be too rapid for long-term therapeutic use (Hui et al 2008) and that dedicated delivery systems would provide a better alternative.

Cosmetic and prosthetic applications

Cosmetic lenses are generally used to change eye colour, while prosthetic lenses are prescribed to improve the appearance of an unsightly eye. Prosthetic lenses are also indicated in some cases of photophobia, diplopia, aniridia and coloboma (Lazarus 2006). While both soft and RGP lenses can be manufactured for these applications, the majority of cosmetic and prosthetic lenses are soft hydrogel lenses, and it is these lenses which will be described.

Many manufacturers now offer cosmetic tinted contact lenses in a wide range of prescriptions and colours. Patients with light-coloured irides simply wishing to deepen or adjust the colour of their light-blue, grey, or blue-green irises are often fitted with enhancer tints. Lenses of this type usually have the tint across the central 11–12 mm of the lens, with no clear pupil aperture. In order to change the appearance more radically or alter the colour of an individual with dark irides, a more translucent or opaque tint is required. Newer techniques for incorporating the tints have resulted in a more natural appearance for these lenses, and pigment printing, colour variation from the pupil edge to the limbus and black limbal bands can give very convincing results. All these more complex designs do, however, require a central clear pupil aperture to reduce interference in vision. The centration of the lens and the size of this aperture are crucial for a realistic appearance. In some cases, a deliberately unnatural appearance is desired, for example by actors and entertainers or even by individuals who simply want to seek attention. Unfortunately, these lenses are often not prescribed by eye care practitioners but rather are sourced from the internet and unlicensed retailers, and issues of noncompliance with their wear and care can result (Snyder et al 1991; Leahey & Jones 1996). Tinted lenses are often used only infrequently and have been known to be exchanged between wearers, which can result in infection (Gagnon & Walter 2006).

The ideal modality for cosmetic lens wear is undoubtedly daily disposable, where the lenses are worn once and then discarded. While lenses are now available with this indication, the selection is limited and cost may be prohibitive. Consequently, the majority of cosmetic lenses are reused, requiring disinfection after each wearing period and re-disinfection at regular intervals (generally every 7 days), regardless of their frequency of use. Currently, tinted lenses are not available in silicone hydrogel materials. An issue which must be considered when prescribing tinted lenses for cosmetic reasons is the potential for a reduction in visual performance compared with a lens which is clear or tinted only lightly for handling reasons. Reductions in both contrast sensitivity and visual field have been reported (Josephson & Caffery 1987; Ozkagnici et al 2003) and patients must be counselled with respect to these alterations, particularly for activities such as driving at night.

Many different tint designs are available for prosthetic applications (Lazarus 2006) and the most appropriate generally depends on whether the pupil appears normal. Even though complex iris patterns and designs are available, often

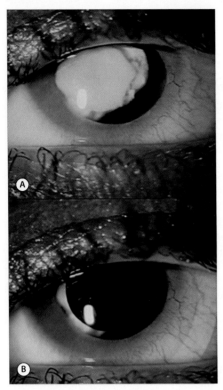

Figure 21.2 Prosthetic application of a black pupil soft lens **(B)** for a patient with a cataract formed subsequent to a retinal detachment (non-seeing eye: **A**). Note the vascularization visible in the corneal periphery resulting from long-term wear of a low oxygen transmissibility material.

employing intricate hand-painting techniques, in many cases where the pupil appears abnormal in one eye (e.g. a congenital cataract) a simple soft lens with a 4 mm black pupil can be very effective, as shown in **Figure 21.2**. Custom contact lens laboratories can be extremely helpful for practitioners in recommending an appropriate lens design. Digital photographs can be taken of the affected and contralateral eyes and sent to the laboratory to aid in selection and design.

Complications with contact lenses

A number of complications can occur with contact lens wear. These can be broadly classified into hypoxic, mechanical (including environmental), inflammatory, toxic, and infectious. Inevitably there can be some overlap between these complications. For example, a complication with a mechanical aetiology can have associated inflammation and may result in infection, but for the purpose of this overview, each type will be discussed separately. The reader is referred to supplementary expansive texts for a more comprehensive description of the prevalence, aetiology, symptoms, signs, management and prognosis for each of these conditions (Jones & Jones 2000; Efron 2004).

Hypoxic complications

Complications associated with hypoxia were historically observed frequently in contact lens wearers due to the poor oxygen supply to the cornea, particularly through thick, low-water-content soft lenses worn for extended periods of time. Fortunately, with the advance of silicone hydrogel materials and high-Dk RGP materials, these complications are now relatively rare. However, wearers of low oxygen transmissibility lenses may still experience both acute and chronic conditions, particularly when lenses are worn on an extended-wear basis. When the cornea receives insufficient oxygen, there is a propensity for corneal swelling or oedema. When oedema exceeds the normal overnight rate without lenses (approximately 3%), striae (fine vertical lines occurring at >5%) and folds (bright lines in direct illumination, dark lines in specular reflex, occurring at >10%) can be observed in the stroma (La Hood & Grant 1990). These are a transient response to acute hypoxia and resolve rapidly upon lens removal after eye opening. A more chronic response to hypoxia is the appearance of epithelial microcysts (Zantos 1984). These are small (15–50 μm) inclusions observed in the superficial epithelium, appearing after approximately 6 months of chronic hypoxia. Since they have a higher refractive index than the surrounding tissue they display 'reversed' illumination. When patients are refitted with high-Dk lenses there is frequently a transient rebound effect, where the number of microcysts is seen to increase rapidly within the first weeks of lens wear but then the numbers decrease to close to zero within a month or so of lens wear (Keay et al 2001). Other complications commonly observed with chronic anoxia include superficial punctuate keratitis, as a result of premature desquamation of stressed epithelial cells, and endothelial polymegethism, when chronic stromal acidosis results in structural damage to the endothelial cells, which may result in a loss of endothelial pump function (Schoessler 1983).

Corneal neovascularization is another frequent complication observed in wearers of low-Dk/t lenses, particularly in patients with either high myopia or those wearing toric lens designs, as a result of the thicker profile towards the edge of the lenses. In this condition, new blood vessels penetrate into the normally avascular cornea (**Fig. 21.3**). Fortunately, wearing high-Dk/t lenses prevents this complication (Dumbleton et al 2001) and when patients are refitted with high-Dk/t lenses the vessels do 'empty', leaving residual 'ghost vessels'. Limbal and bulbar hyperaemia are also frequently observed as a result of acute and chronic hypoxia (**Fig. 21.3**) and a clear correlation has been reported between oxygen transmissibility and limbal hyperaemia (Papas 1998). Other causes, including dry eye, toxic responses, and poor lens fit, have also been implicated in the development of

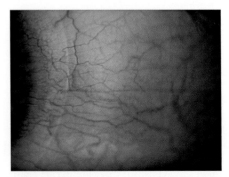

Figure 21.3 Neovascularization and hyperaemia subsequent to long-term conventional hydrogel lens wear. This appearance denoted chronic hypoxia over several years due to insufficient corneal oxygenation.

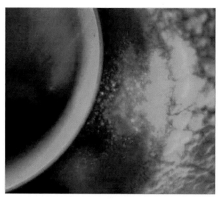

Figure 21.4 Three and nine o'clock corneal staining in a patient with poor blinking and poor-quality tear film, wearing an RGP lens with an inadequate corneal diameter and excessive edge clearance. (Picture courtesy of Desmond Fonn.)

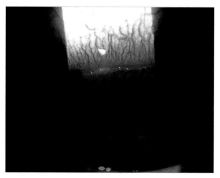

Figure 21.6 Superior epithelial arcuate lesion (SEAL) subsequent to silicone hydrogel lens wear. This is often seen in a stiffer lens with a poor fit.

neovascularization (Efron 2004). Since complications associated with hypoxia are invariably not associated with symptoms, it is particularly important for the eye care practitioner to be vigilant for these conditions.

Mechanical complications

Mechanical complications are more likely to occur with RGP lenses than conventional soft or silicone hydrogel lenses. 'Three and nine o'clock' staining occurs as a result of drying of the peripheral cornea (**Fig. 21.4**), with poor lens fit, poor wettability or incomplete blinking in RGP wearers (Businger et al 1989). Patients with this condition often report dry, irritable eyes, and a reduced wearing time. Modification to the lens fit is invariably required to rectify this condition. Extreme cases may develop into an inflamed area in the limbal region (vascularized limbal keratitis) or severe peripheral thinning (dellen).

Corneal abrasions and erosions can occur with all lens types (**Fig. 21.5**). The aetiology for these conditions is either a foreign body getting under the lens and abrading the superficial epithelial cells or the contact lens briefly becoming 'bound' to the epithelium and disturbing the cells when it regains mobility. The severity of symptoms associated with these conditions varies considerably, but in almost all cases simply removing the lens allows rapid resolution.

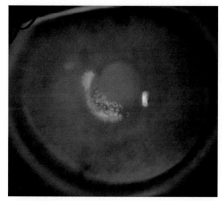

Figure 21.5 Corneal erosion secondary to transient binding of a silicone hydrogel lens. Refitting with a different silicone hydrogel lens will often eradicate this appearance.

Superior epithelial arcuate lesions (SEALs) are frequently asymptomatic, mechanically induced lesions appearing as thin white arcuate lesions in the superior cornea of soft contact lens wearing patients (Hine et al 1987). A SEAL will stain with fluorescein and the edges may be irregular, roughened, or thickened, particularly if the SEAL is associated with diffuse or focal infiltration (**Fig. 21.6**). SEALs may present unilaterally or bilaterally, but if bilateral, the appearance may be asymmetric. Patients presenting with SEALs often do not have any associated symptoms, but a mild foreign body sensation may be reported and often there is slight irritation following lens removal (Dumbleton 2003). The aetiology of SEALs is multifactorial but can mainly be attributed to mechanical trauma from an increase in mechanical pressure under the eyelid and is often associated with stiff materials, particularly silicone hydrogel lenses (Young & Mirejovsky 1993; Holden et al 2001). Management requires temporary discontinuation of lens wear for 1–2 days. Patients should be warned that their symptoms may increase initially and ocular lubricants can be dispensed to relieve discomfort. In cases of reoccurrence, refitting with a different design (e.g. change in base curve) or a lower modulus, less stiff material is indicated.

A further type of mechanical staining which has a somewhat different aetiology is inferior arcuate or 'SMILE' staining. This staining occurs commonly in soft lens wearers as a result of incomplete blinking and lens dehydration, resulting in post-lens tear film thinning and epithelial desiccation. In mild cases, blinking exercises and ocular lubricants are often sufficient, but in severe cases a change in lens material to either a lower water content material (such as a silicone hydrogel) or a thicker design may be indicated (Jones & Jones 1995).

Fluorescein staining is usually used to assess damaged epithelial cells. Since the stain also 'colours' the tear film, it will 'pool' in indentations in the epithelial surface. In the case of RGP lenses, bubbles can sometimes form under the lens as a result of poor fit, with fluorescein pools seen in the transient indentations left in the epithelium. This is referred to as 'dimple veiling'. A similar appearance can occur with stiff soft lenses, such as that seen with certain high-modulus silicone hydrogel lenses. In this case, mucin forms into small, hard spherical particles under the lenses of some individuals. When the lenses are removed, transient depressions are left in the epithelium, which pool with fluorescein. When silicone hydrogel lenses first became available, many eye care practitioners confused this appearance

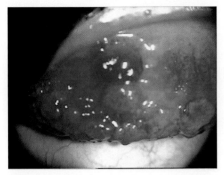

Figure 21.7 A severe case of giant papillary conjunctivitis (GPC). (Photograph courtesy of Dr Jerome Sherman OD.)

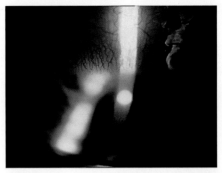

Figure 21.8 Contact lens peripheral ulcer (CLPU) in an extended-wear silicone hydrogel patient. Note the very circular nature of the infiltrate.

with true corneal staining. This presentation has since been termed 'mucin balls', and in most cases where these debris particles are seen beneath the lens no action is required, since the patient is asymptomatic and the condition has not been shown to be associated with further complications (Dumbleton et al 2000b; Tan et al 2003).

Contact lens papillary conjunctivitis (CLPC) or giant papillary conjunctivitis (GPC) presents with changes to the palpebral conjunctiva, consisting of increased hyperaemia and papillary excrescences (Allansmith et al 1977) (**Fig. 21.7**). The symptoms associated with this condition are generally rapid in onset and include foreign body sensation or discomfort, itching, and stringy or ropy mucous discharge. The aetiology of CLPC is believed to be both mechanical and immunological. CLPC had become a relatively rare finding in contact lens patients since the introduction of frequent-replacement lenses. Following the introduction of silicone hydrogel lenses, particularly for continuous wear, the prevalence of this condition initially appeared to increase, with a more localized rather than diffuse appearance (Skotnitsky et al 2002). A combination of the increased stiffness and edge designs of some of these lenses has been implicated. Newer designs and lower-modulus silicone hydrogel materials appear to have diminished the prevalence. Cases of CLPC which are mechanical in origin generally resolve very quickly, simply by ceasing lens wear and either wearing spectacles or daily disposable lenses for a period of approximately 2 weeks (Dumbleton 2003). Mast cell stabilizers may also be used to manage CLPC, particularly for immunological cases. However, the efficacy of this form of treatment is slow and the condition often resolves before these agents have started to take effect. Changes to wearing schedule, lens design and material may then be required to prevent reoccurrence.

Inflammatory complications

Several inflammatory complications may occur with contact lens wear, including contact lens peripheral ulcer (CLPU), infiltrative keratitis (IK) and contact lens acute red eye (CLARE).

A CLPU is an inflammatory response which results in lesions often termed 'sterile ulcers'. The aetiology of this condition is a hypersensitive reaction to the (usually Gram-positive) exotoxins released by pathogenic bacteria on the lids (Wu et al 2003). Signs include a single, small, circular, peripheral or mid-peripheral greyish-white lesion in the anterior stroma (**Fig. 21.8**) (Sankaridurg et al 2004). Symptoms include mild to moderate pain (foreign body

sensation), mild lacrimation and mild photophobia. Following the acute 'phase', the epithelium regenerates within a few days. Diffuse infiltration surrounding the lesion may develop. A very well-defined circular 'scar' remains, gradually fading with time, but still present several months after the event (Dumbleton 2002). Differential diagnosis from microbial keratitis (MK) is extremely important.

CLARE is a unilateral, acute inflammatory response to Gram-negative organisms which colonize the lens and release endotoxins (Holden et al 1996; Sankaridurg et al 2004). Patients with CLARE are typically woken in the early morning by a moderately painful (foreign body sensation) red eye, with associated epiphora and photophobia. Focal or diffuse subepithelial infiltrates are usually observed in the mid-periphery of the cornea close to the limbus. The infiltrates rarely stain and rapidly resolve.

IK is the term used to describe all other inflammatory events. IK can occur with both daily and extended wear and may also occur in non-lens wearers (Dumbleton 2002; Sankaridurg et al 2004). However, the incidence is higher in lens wearers, presumably as a response to toxins being concentrated against the cornea by the hydrogel lens. Many IK cases are due to the presence of Gram-positive exotoxins found on the lid margin. Symptoms vary in severity and commonly include mild to moderate irritation (often a foreign body discomfort), mild hyperaemia, lacrimation, photophobia, and occasionally mild discharge. Diffuse and/or small focal infiltrates are seen with slit-lamp examination. These infiltrates may be located anywhere in the cornea but are usually peripherally situated in the limbal area.

Most cases of inflammation in contact lens wearers are self-limiting. The first step is to discontinue lens wear temporarily until there is full resolution of signs and symptoms. In most cases, no medication is required. However, ocular lubricants may be dispensed to alleviate symptoms. Severe cases may benefit from a prophylactic topical antibiotic to reduce the chance of secondary infection. Since there appears to be a patient predisposition for inflammatory events (Dumbleton et al 2000a; Sweeney et al 2002), the introduction of lid hygiene measures (warm compresses and lid scrubs) to the daily routine for these patients is strongly recommended. Patients repeatedly experiencing inflammatory events with overnight wear should be advised to wear their lenses on a daily-wear basis only.

Contact lens wearers must also be examined for signs of inflammation of the lid margins. Blepharitis and meibomian gland dysfunction are relatively common inflammatory conditions which, although they do not occur as a

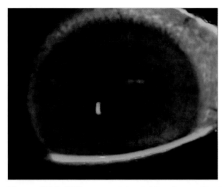

Figure 21.9 Diffuse punctate staining in a patient using a silicone hydrogel lens on a daily-wear basis with a preserved care regimen. This appearance is suggestive of a solution–lens incompatibility and requires a change of the care regimen.

result of contact lens wear, can certainly have an impact on the clinical success of lenses in contact lens wearers. These chronic conditions require regular lid hygiene with hot compresses, lid scrubs and, in some cases, systemic antibiotics. Patients with these conditions may be better suited to a daily-wear modality.

Toxic complications

Exposure to elements in contact lens care systems can result in diffuse punctate staining of the epithelium and, in some cases, bulbar hyperaemia. This was mainly a historical problem with hydrogel care systems preserved with thiomersolate and chlorhexidine, which have largely disappeared from the market. A similar appearance has recently been reported to occur when certain multipurpose care systems are used in conjunction with silicone hydrogel lenses (**Fig. 21.9**) (Jones et al 2002; Garofalo et al 2005). Patients inadvertently inserting their lenses from hydrogen peroxide systems with incomplete neutralization can also experience a toxic reaction, although this has shown to be rare when careful instructions are given (Dumbleton et al 2006).

Infectious complications

Microbial keratitis (MK) is the most serious complication associated with contact lens wear. Fortunately, the prevalence of MK within the general population is extremely low, due in part to the exceptional defence mechanisms that protect the ocular surface. The microorganisms most commonly associated with MK in contact lens wearers are the *Pseudomonas* spp (principally *aeruginosa*) but many different microorganisms have been cultured from cases of MK in contact lens patients (Willcox & Holden 2001). The major risk factors for corneal infection include overnight wear, poor compliance, epithelial trauma, smoking, and swimming in lenses (Keay et al 2006). The generally accepted figure for annualized incidence of MK in soft daily wear patients is 4 per 10 000 wearers (Poggio et al 1989; Schein et al 1989; Cheng et al 1999). Extended wear has been reported to increase this risk by approximately five times, regardless of lens material (Poggio et al 1989; Schein et al 1989, 2005; Cheng et al 1999).

Patients with MK present with marked, increasing pain, intense lacrimation, hyperaemia, and photophobia. A single paracentral or central irregular lesion may be observed with focal and often significant diffuse infiltration. The lesion is characterized by excavation of the epithelium, Bowman's layer and the stroma and usually stains. An anterior chamber reaction and lid oedema are also common. The condition is also associated with severe, progressive corneal tissue death and the formation of pus (Aasuri et al 2003).

Since most cases of MK in contact lens wearers are bacterial, treatment is with antibiotic agents unless other prognostic signs exist. Initial treatment is generally with fluoroquinolone monotherapy, and supplemental cycloplegics and analgesics are given as required. In severe cases, fortified antibiotics may also be prescribed. Prognosis for most patients is good, particularly if treatment or referral occurs early in the disease process, but it does depend upon the causative organism, and in all cases a scar will remain.

References

Aasuri M K, Venkata N, Kumar V M 2003 Differential diagnosis of microbial keratitis and contact lens-induced peripheral ulcer. Eye Contact Lens 29 (1 Suppl):S60–S62; discussion S63–S64, S192–S194

Allansmith M R, Korb D R, Greiner J V et al 1977 Giant papillary conjunctivitis in contact lens wearers. American Journal of Ophthalmology 83(5):697–708

Ambroziak A M, Szaflik J P, Szaflik J 2004 Therapeutic use of a silicone hydrogel contact lens in selected clinical cases. Eye Contact Lens 30(1):63–67

Begley C G, Waggoner P J, Hafner G S et al 1991 Effect of rigid gas permeable contact lens wetting solutions on the rabbit corneal epithelium. Optometry and Vision Science 68(3):189–197

Begley C, Weirich B, Benak J et al 1992 Effects of rigid gas permeable contact lens solutions on the human corneal epithelium. Optometry and Vision Science 69(5):347–353

Benjamin W J, Cappelli Q A 2002 Oxygen permeability (Dk) of thirty-seven rigid contact lens materials. Optometry and Vision Science 79(2):103–111

Bennett E S 2004 Lens design, fitting and evaluation. In: Bennett E S, Hom M M (eds) Manual of gas permeable contact lenses, 2nd edn. Butterworth-Heinemann, St Louis, pp 86–116

Bennett E S 2006 Bifocal and multifocal contact lenses. In: Phillips A, Speedwell L (eds) Contact lenses, 5th edn. Butterworth-Heinemann, Edinburgh, pp 311–331

Bennett E, Jurkus J M, Schwartz C 2000 Bifocal contact lenses. In: Bennett E, Henry V (eds) Clinical manual of contact lenses, 2nd edn. Lippincott, Williams & Wilkins, Philadelphia, pp 410–449

Boswall G J, Ehlers W H, Luistro A et al 1993 A comparison of conventional and disposable extended wear contact lenses. CLAO Journal 19(3):158–165

Brennan N A 2005a Beyond flux: total corneal oxygen consumption as an index of corneal oxygenation during contact lens wear. Optometry and Vision Science 82(6):467–472

Brennan N A 2005b Corneal oxygenation during contact lens wear: comparison of diffusion and EOP-based flux models. Clinical and Experimental Optometry 88(2):103–108

Brennan N A, Coles M-L C 2000 Deposits and symptomatology with soft contact lens wear. International Contact Lens Clinic 27(3):75–100

Brennan N, Fonn D 2004 Corneal hypoxia. In: Sweeney D (ed.) Silicone hydrogels: continuous wear contact lenses, 2nd edn. Butterworth-Heinemann, Oxford, pp 126–163

Brennan N, Efron N, Lg C 1988 Corneal oxygen availability during contact lens wear: a comparison of methodologies. American Journal of Optometric and Physiological Optics 65:19–24

Brennan N A, Coles M-L, Comstock T L et al 2002 A 1-year prospective clinical trial of balafilcon a (PureVision) silicone-hydrogel contact lenses used on a 30-day continuous wear schedule. Ophthalmology 109(6):1172–1177

Bruce A 2002 Preliminary examination. In: Efron N (ed.) Contact lens practice, 1st edn. Butterworth-Heinemann, Oxford, pp 367–375

Bruinsma G M, van der Mei H C, Busscher H J 2001 Bacterial adhesion to surface hydrophilic and hydrophobic contact lenses. Biomaterials 22(24):3217–3224

Businger U, Treiber A, Flury C 1989 The etiology and management of three and nine o'clock staining. International Contact Lens Clinic 16(5):136–139

Caroline P, Andre M 1999 Inadvertent patient modification of RGP lenses. Contact Lens Spectrum 14:56

Caroline P, Andre M 2004 Sometimes two lenses are better than one. Contact Lens Spectrum 19(3):56

Chalmers R, McNally J 1988 Ocular detection threshold for hydrogen peroxide: drops vs. lenses. International Contact Lens Clinic 15 (11):351–357

Cheng K H, Leung S L, Hoekman H W et al 1999 Incidence of contact-lens-associated microbial keratitis and its related morbidity. Lancet 354(9174):181–185

Cheng L, Muller S J, Radke C J 2004 Wettability of silicone-hydrogel contact lenses in the presence of tear-film components. Current Eye Research 28(2):93–108

Chou M, Rosenthal P, Salamone J 1985 Which cleaning solution works best? Contact Lens Forum 10:41–47

Christensen B, Lebow K, White E M et al 1998 Effectiveness of citrate-containing lens care regimens: a controlled clinical comparison. International Contact Lens Clinic 25(2):50–58

Covey M, Sweeney D F, Terry R et al 2001 Hypoxic effects on the anterior eye of high-Dk soft contact lens wearers are negligible. Optometry and Vision Science 78(2):95–99

Dart J 2005 Cicatricial pemphigoid and dry eye. Seminars in Ophthalmology 20(2):95–100

Dave T 1998 Current developments in measurement of corneal topography. Contact Lens Anterior Eye (Supp):s13–s30

Dave T, Ruston D 1998 Current trends in modern orthokeratology. Ophthalmic and Physiological Optics 18(2):224–233

Doell G B, Palombi D L, Egan D J et al 1986 Contact lens surface changes after exposure to surfactant and abrasive cleaning procedures. American Journal of Optometric and Physiological Optics 63(6):399–402

Dohlman C H 1974 Complications in therapeutic soft lens wear. Transactions of the American Academy of Ophthalmology and Otolaryngology 78(3):OP399–405

Donshik P C, Porazinski A D 1999 Giant papillary conjunctivitis in frequent-replacement contact lens wearers: a retrospective study. Transactions of the American Ophthalmology Society 97:205–216; discussion 216–220

Dumbleton K 2002 Adverse events with silicone hydrogel continuous wear. Cont Lens Anterior Eye 25(3):137–146

Dumbleton K 2003 Noninflammatory silicone hydrogel contact lens complications. Eye Contact Lens 29(1 Suppl):S186–S189; discussion S190–S191, S192–S194

Dumbleton K A, Jones L 2002 Silicone hydrogel lenses: Follow-up and management. Optician 223(5845):34–43

Dumbleton K A, Chalmers R L, Richter D B et al 1999 Changes in myopic refractive error with nine months' extended wear of hydrogel lenses with high and low oxygen permeability. Optometry and Vision Science 76(12):845–849

Dumbleton K, Fonn D, Jones L et al 2000a Severity and management of contact lens related complications with continuous wear of high Dk silicone hydrogel lenses. Optometry and Vision Science 77 (12s):216

Dumbleton K, Jones L, Chalmers R et al 2000b Clinical characterization of spherical post-lens debris associated with lotrafilcon high-Dk silicone lenses. CLAO Journal 26(4):186–192

Dumbleton K A, Chalmers R L, Richter D B et al 2001 Vascular response to extended wear of hydrogel lenses with high and low oxygen permeability. Optometry and Vision Science 78 (3):147–151

Dumbleton K A, Chalmers R L, McNally J et al 2002 Effect of lens base curve on subjective comfort and assessment of fit with silicone hydrogel continuous wear contact lenses. Optometry and Vision Science 79(10):633–637

Dumbleton K, Jones L, Woods C A et al 2006 Clinical performance of a hydrogen peroxide care regimen with silicone hydrogel lenses. Optometry and Vision Science 83(E-abstract 060069)

du Toit R, Simpson T L, Fonn D et al 2001 Recovery from hyperemia after overnight wear of low and high transmissibility hydrogel lenses. Current Eye Research 22(1):68–73

Edrington T B, Barr J T, Zadnik K et al 1996 Standardized rigid contact lens fitting protocol for keratoconus. Optometry and Vision Science 73(6):369–375

Edrington T B, Szczotka L B, Barr J T et al 1999 Rigid contact lens fitting relationships in keratoconus. Collaborative Longitudinal Evaluation of Keratoconus (CLEK) Study Group. Optometry and Vision Science 76(10):692–699

Efron N 1986 Intersubject variability in corneal swelling response to anoxia. Acta Ophthalmologica (Copenh) 64(3):302–305

Efron N 2004 Contact lens complications, 2nd edn. Butterworth-Heinemann, Oxford

Ehrlich D 2004 Fitting the distorted cornea. Optometry Today (Nov 19th):33–40

Fatt I 1986 Now do we need 'effective permeability'? Contax (July):6–23

Fatt I, Chaston J 1982 Measurement of oxygen transmissibility and permeability of hydrogel lenses and materials. International Contact Lens Clinic 9(2):76–88

Fonn D, Sweeney D, Holden B A et al 2005 Corneal oxygen deficiency. Eye Contact Lens 31(1):23–27

Fowler C W, Dave T N 1994 Review of past and present techniques of measuring corneal topography. Ophthalmic and Physiological Optics 14(1):49–58

Friends G, Kunzler J, Ozark R 1995 Recent advances in the design of polymers for contact lenses. Macromolecular Symposia 98:619–631

Gagnon M R, Walter K A 2006 A case of *Acanthamoeba* keratitis as a result of a cosmetic contact lens. Eye Contact Lens 32(1):37–38

Garofalo R J, Dassanayake N, Carey C et al 2005 Corneal staining and subjective symptoms with multipurpose solutions as a function of time. Eye Contact Lens 31(4):166–174

Gasset A R, Kaufman H E 1970 Therapeutic uses of hydrophilic contact lenses. American Journal of Ophthalmology 71:1185–1189

Gasson A, Morris J 2003 Lenses for presbyopia. In: Gasson A, Morris J (eds) The contact lens manual, 3rd edn. Butterworth Heinemann, Oxford, pp 298–317

Grobe G 1999 Surface engineering aspects of silicone-hydrogel lenses. Contact Lens Spectrum 14(8 (suppl)):14–17

Grobe G, Kunzler J, Seelye D et al 1999 Silicone hydrogels for contact lens applications. Polymeric Materials Science and Engineering 80:108–109

Gruber E 1991 The Acuvue disposable contact lens as a therapeutic bandage lens. Annals of Ophthalmology 23(12):446–447

Guillon M, Lydon D P, Wilson C 1986 Corneal topography: a clinical model. Ophthalmic and Physiological Optics 6(1):47–56

Hamano H, Watanabe K, Hamano T et al 1994 A study of the complications induced by conventional and disposable contact lenses. CLAO Journal 20(2):103–108

Harvitt D M, Bonanno J A 1999 Re-evaluation of the oxygen diffusion model for predicting minimum contact lens Dk/t values needed to avoid corneal anoxia. Optometry and Vision Science 76(10):712–719

Hickson-Curran S 2006 Contact lenses in other abnormal ocular conditions. In: Phillips A, Speedwell L (eds) Contact lenses, 5th edn. Butterworth-Heinemann, Edinburgh, pp 531–543

Hine N, Back A, Holden B 1987 Aetiology of arcuate epithelial lesions induced by hydrogels. Journal of the British Contact Lens Association 48:50

Holden B A, Mertz G W 1984 Critical oxygen levels to avoid corneal edema for daily and extended wear contact lenses. Investigative Ophthalmology and Visual Science 25(10):1161–1167

Holden B A, Sweeney D F, Sanderson G 1984 The minimum precorneal oxygen tension to avoid corneal edema. Investigative Ophthalmology and Visual Science 25(4):476–480

Holden B, La Hood D, Grant T et al 1996 Gram-negative bacteria can induce contact lens related acute red eye (CLARE) responses. CLAO Journal 22 (1):47–52

Holden B A, Stephenson A, Stretton S et al 2001 Superior epithelial arcuate lesions with soft contact lens wear. Optometry and Vision Science 78(1):9–12

Hom M M, Bruce A 2006 Manual of contact lens prescribing and fitting, 3rd edn. Butterworth-Heinemann, Oxford

Hong B, Bilbaut T, Chowhan M et al 1994 Cleaning capability of citrate-containing vs. non-citrate contact lens cleaning solutions: an in vitro comparative study. International Contact Lens Clinic 21(11/12):237–240

Houlsby R, Ghajar M, Chavez G 1984 Microbiological evaluation of soft contact lens disinfecting solutions. Journal of the American Optometry Association 55(3):205–211

Hui A, Boone A, Jones L 2008 Uptake and release of ciprofloxacin-HCl from conventional and silicone hydrogel contact lens materials. Eye Contact Lens 34(5):266–271

Jalbert I, Sweeney D F, Holden B A 2001 Epithelial split associated with wear of a silicone hydrogel contact lens. CLAO Journal 27(4):231–233

Jiang H, Wang D, Yang L et al 2006 A comparison of wavefront aberrations in eyes wearing different types of soft contact lenses. Optometry and Vision Science 83(10):769–774

Jones L 1994 Disposable contact lenses: a review. Journal of the British Contact Lens Association 17(2):43–49

Jones L 2002 Modern contact lens materials: a clinical performance update. Contact Lens Spectrum 17(9):24–35

Jones L, Christie C 2008 Soft contact lens solutions review: part 2 – modern generation care systems. Optometry in Practice 9:43–62

Jones L, Dumbleton K 2002 Silicone hydrogel lenses: fitting procedures and in-practice protocols for continuous wear lenses. Optician 223 (5840):37–45

Jones L, Dumbleton K 2005 Silicone hydrogels part 1: technological developments. Optometry Today Nov 18th:23–29

Jones L, Dumbleton K 2006a Soft contact lens fitting. In: Phillips A, Speedwell L (eds) Contact lenses, 5th edn. Butterworth-Heinemann, Edinburgh, pp 223–240

Jones L, Dumbleton K 2006b Soft lens extended wear and complications. In: Hom M M, Bruce A (eds) Manual of contact lens prescribing and fitting, 2nd edn. Butterworth-Heinemann, Oxford, pp 393–441

Jones L, Jones D 1992 A new high Dk elliptical lens. Optician 203 (5333):16–24

Jones L, Jones D 1995 Smile staining and dehydration. Optician 210 (5513):24–25

Jones L, Jones D 2000 Common contact lens complications. Butterworth-Heinemann, Oxford

Jones L, Senchyna M 2007 Soft contact lens solutions review: part 1 – components of modern care regimens. Optometry in Practice 8:45–56

Jones L, Tighe B 2004 Silicone hydrogel contact lens materials update – Part 1. Silicone hydrogel. Online. Available: http://www.siliconehydrogels.org/editorials/index.asp

Jones L, Franklin V, Evans K et al 1996 Spoilation and clinical performance of monthly vs three monthly group II disposable contact lenses. Optometry and Vision Science 73(1):16–21

Jones L, MacDougall N, Sorbara L G 2002 Asymptomatic corneal staining associated with the use of balafilcon silicone-hydrogel contact lenses disinfected with a polyaminopropyl biguanide-preserved care regimen. Optometry and Vision Science 79(12):753–761

Jones L, Subbaraman L N, Rogers R et al 2006 Surface treatment, wetting and modulus of silicone hydrogels. Optician 232(6067):28–34

Josephson J E, Caffery B E 1987 Visual field loss with colored hydrogel lenses. American Journal of Optometric and Physiological Optics 64 (1):38–40

Joslin C E, Tu E Y, Shoff M E et al 2007 The association of contact lens solution use and Acanthamoeba keratitis. American Journal of Ophthalmology 144(2):169–180

Kanpolat A, Ucakhan O O 2003 Therapeutic use of Focus Night & Day contact lenses. Cornea 22(8):726–734

Karlgard C C, Jones L W, Moresoli C 2003a Ciprofloxacin interaction with silicon-based and conventional hydrogel contact lenses. Eye Contact Lens 29(2):83–89

Karlgard C C, Wong N S, Jones L W et al 2003b In vitro uptake and release studies of ocular pharmaceutical agents by silicon-containing and p-HEMA hydrogel contact lens materials. International Journal of Pharmacology 257(1–2):141–151

Karlgard C C, Jones L W, Moresoli C 2004 Survey of bandage lens use in North America, October–December 2002. Eye Contact Lens 30 (1):25–30

Keay L, Sweeney D F, Jalbert I et al 2000 Microcyst response to high Dk/t silicone hydrogel contact lenses. Optometry and Vision Science 77(11):582–585

Keay L, Jalbert I, Sweeney D F et al 2001 Microcysts: clinical significance and differential diagnosis. Optometry 72(7):452–460

Keay L, Edwards K, Naduvilath T et al 2006 Factors affecting the morbidity of contact lens-related microbial keratitis: a population study. Investigative Ophthalmology and Visual Science 47(10):4302–4308

Kent H D, Cohen E J, Laibson P R et al 1990 Microbial keratitis and corneal ulceration associated with therapeutic soft contact lenses. CLAO Journal 16(1):49–52

Ketelson H A, Meadows D L, Stone R P 2005 Dynamic wettability properties of a soft contact lens hydrogel. Colloids Surfactant B Biointerfaces 40(1):1–9

Kishi M, Tighe B 1988 RGP materials: a review of the patent literature. Optician 195(5134):21–28

Korb D R, Finnemore V M, Herman J P 1982 Apical changes and scarring in keratoconus as related to contact lens fitting techniques. Journal of the American Optometry Association 53(3):199–205

Kunzler J 1999 Silicone-based hydrogels for contact lens applications. Contact Lens Spectrum 14(8 (supp)):9–11

Kunzler J, Ozark R 1995 Hydrogels based on hydrophilic side chain siloxanes. Journal of Applied Polymer Science 55:611–619

Lagnado R, Rubinstein M P, Maharajan S et al 2004 Management options for the flat corneal graft. Contact Lens Anterior Eye 27 (1):27–31

La Hood D, Grant T 1990 Striae and folds as indicators of corneal edema. Optometry and Vision Science 67(12s):196

Larke J, Parrish S, Wigham C 1981 Apparent human corneal oxygen uptake rate. American Journal of Optometric and Physiological Optics 58(10):803–805

Lazarus M 2006 Cosmetic and prosthetic contact lenses. In: Phillips A, Speedwell L (eds) Contact lenses, 5th edn. Butterworth-Heinemann, Edinburgh, pp 519–530

Leahey A B, Jones D 1996 Haemophilus influenzae central corneal ulcer associated with cosmetic lens wear. CLAO Journal 22(3):213–214

Leung K K 1999 RGP fitting philosophies for keratoconus. Clinical and Experimental Optometry 82(6):230–235

Lim L, Siow K L, Sakamoto R et al 2000 Reverse geometry contact lens wear after photorefractive keratectomy, radial keratotomy, or penetrating keratoplasty. Cornea 19(3):320–324

Lim L, Tan D T, Chan W K 2001 Therapeutic use of Bausch & Lomb PureVision contact lenses. CLAO Journal 27(4):179–185

Lindsay R, Smith G, Atchison D 1998 Descriptors of corneal shape. Optometry and Vision Science 75(2):156–158

Lopez-Alemany A, Compan V, Refojo M F 2002 Porous structure of Purevision versus Focus Night & Day and conventional hydrogel contact lenses. Journal of Biomedical Material Research (Applied Biomaterial) 63:319–325

Marshall E, Begley C, Nguyen C 1992 Frequency of complications among wearers of disposable and conventional soft contact lenses. International Contact Lens Clinic 19(3/4):55–59

Mathur A, Jones L, Sorbara L 1999 Use of reverse geometry rigid gas permeable contact lenses in the management of the postradial keratotomy patient: review and case report. International Contact Lens Clinic 26(5):121–127

Morgan P, Brennan N 2004 The decay of Dk? Optician 227(5937): 27–33

Morgan P B, Efron N 1998 The oxygen performance of contemporary hydrogel contact lenses. Contact Lens and Anterior Eye 21(1):3–6

Morgan P B, Efron N 2002 Comparative clinical performance of two silicone hydrogel contact lenses for continuous wear. Clinical and Experimental Optometry 85(3):183–192

Morgan P B, Woods C, Knajian R et al 2008 International contact lens prescribing in 2007. Contact Lens Spectrum 23(1):36–41

Mountford J, Ruston D, Dave T 2004 Orthokeratology: principles and practice. Butterworth-Heinemann, Edinburgh

Ng C, Tighe B 1976 Polymers in contact lens applications VI. The 'dissolved' oxygen permeability of hydrogel and the design of materials for use in continuous wear lenses. British Polymer Journal 8: 118–123

Nicolson P C, Vogt J 2001 Soft contact lens polymers: an evolution. Biomaterials 22(24):3273–3283

Niszl I A, Markus M B 1998 Anti-*Acanthamoeba* activity of contact lens solutions. British Journal of Ophthalmology 82(9):1033–1038

O'Hare N, Naduvilath T, Sweeney D et al 2001 A clinical comparison of limbal and paralimbal superior epithelial arcuate lesions (SEALs) in high Dk EW. Investigative Ophthalmology and Visual Science 42(4): s595

Ozkagnici A, Zengin N, Kamis O et al 2003 Do daily wear opaquely tinted hydrogel soft contact lenses affect contrast sensitivity function at one meter? Eye Contact Lens 29(1):48–49

Papas E 1998 On the relationship between soft contact lens oxygen transmissibility and induced limbal hyperaemia. Experimental Eye Research 67(2):125–131

Papas E B, Vajdic C M, Austen R et al 1997 High-oxygen-transmissibility soft contact lenses do not induce limbal hyperaemia. Current Eye Research 16 (9):942–948

Penley C A, Willis S W, Sickler S G 1989 Comparative antimicrobial efficacy of soft and rigid gas permeable contact lens solutions against *Acanthamoeba*. CLAO Journal 15(4):257–260

Phillips A 1980 The cleaning of hydrogel contact lenses. Ophthalmic Optician 20(11):375–388

Phillips A 2006 Rigid gas-permeable corneal lens fitting. In: Phillips A, Speedwell L (eds) Contact lenses, 5th edn. Butterworth-Heinemann, Edinburgh, pp 189–222

Phillips A, Speedwell L 2006 Contact lenses, 5th edn. Butterworth-Heinemann, Edinburgh

Poggio E C, Abelson M B 1993 Complications and symptoms with disposable daily wear contact lenses and conventional soft daily wear contact lenses. CLAO Journal 19(2):95–102

Poggio E C, Glynn R J, Schein O D et al 1989 The incidence of ulcerative keratitis among users of daily-wear and extended-wear soft contact lenses. New England Journal of Medicine 321(12):779–783

Porazinski A D, Donshik P C 1999 Giant papillary conjunctivitis in frequent replacement contact lens wearers: a retrospective study. CLAO Journal 25(3):142–147

Pritchard N, Fonn D, Weed K 1996 Ocular and subjective responses to frequent replacement of daily wear soft contact lenses. CLAO Journal 22(1):53–59

Pullum K W 2006 Scleral contact lenses. In: Phillips A, Speedwell L (eds) Contact lenses, 5th edn. Butterworth-Heinemann, Edinburgh, pp 333–353

Rabinowitz Y S 1993 Corneal topography. Current Opinions in Ophthalmology 4(4):68–74

Rae S T, Huff J W 1991 Studies on initiation of silicone elastomer lens adhesion in vitro: binding before the indentation ring. CLAO Journal 17(3):181–186

Randeri K, Quintana R, Masood A 1995 Contact lens cleaning. In: Kastl P (ed.) Contact lenses: the CLAO guide to basic science and clinical practice, vol ll: soft and rigid contact lenses, 2nd edn. Kendall/Hunt, Dubuque, pp 215–262

Roberts B, Athappilly G, Tinio B et al 2006 Higher order aberrations induced by soft contact lenses in normal eyes with myopia. Eye Contact Lens 32(3):138–142

Rose P 2005 Improving a keratoconus lens design. Contact Lens Spectrum 20(6):38–42

Rosenthal P, Chou M, Salamone J et al 1986 Quantitative analysis of chlorhexidine gluconate and benzalkonium chloride adsorption on silicone/acrylate polymers. CLAO Journal 12(1):43–50

Sabesan R, Jeong T M, Carvalho L et al 2007 Vision improvement by correcting higher-order aberrations with customized soft contact lenses in keratoconic eyes. Optometry Letters 32(8):1000–1002

Sankaridurg P, Holden B, Jalbert I 2004. Adverse events and infections: Which ones and how many? In: Sweeney D (ed.) Silicone hydrogels: continuous wear contact lenses, 2nd edn. Butterworth-Heinemann, Oxford, pp 217–274

Schein O D, Glynn R J, Poggio E C et al 1989 The relative risk of ulcerative keratitis among users of daily-wear and extended-wear soft contact lenses. A case-control study. Microbial Keratitis Study Group. New England Journal of Medicine 321(12):773–778

Schein O D, McNally J J, Katz J et al 2005 The incidence of microbial keratitis among wearers of a 30-day silicone hydrogel extended-wear contact lens. Ophthalmology 112(12):2172–2179

Schoessler J 1983 Corneal endothelial polymegethism associated with extended wear. International Contact Lens Clinic 10(3):148–155

Segal O, Barkana Y, Hourovitz D et al 2003 Scleral contact lenses may help where other modalities fail. Cornea 22(4):308–310

Shih K, Hu J, Sibley M 1985 The microbiological benefit of cleaning and rinsing contact lenses. International Contact Lens Clinic 12 (4):235–242

Silvany R E, Dougherty J M, McCulley J P 1991 Effect of contact lens preservatives on *Acanthamoeba*. Ophthalmology 98(6):854–857

Simmons P A, Prather W, Vehige J 2000 Improvement in wetting properties of a multipurpose contact lens solution by addition of hydroxypropyl methylcellulose (HPMC). Optometry and Vision Science 77 (12s):178

Simmons P A, Donshik P C, Kelly W F et al 2001 Conditioning of hydrogel lenses by a multipurpose solution containing an ocular lubricant. CLAO Journal 27(4):192–194

Skotnitsky C, Sankaridurg P R, Sweeney D F et al 2002 General and local contact lens induced papillary conjunctivitis (CLPC). Clinical and Experimental Optometry 85(3):193–197

Snyder R W, Brenner M B, Wiley L et al 1991 Microbial keratitis associated with plano tinted contact lenses. CLAO Journal 17(4): 252–255

Solomon O D, Freeman M I, Boshnick E L et al 1996 A 3-year prospective study of the clinical performance of daily disposable contact lenses compared with frequent replacement and conventional daily wear contact lenses. CLAO Journal 22(4):250–257

Stapleton F, Stretton S, Papas E et al 2006 Silicone hydrogel contact lenses and the ocular surface. Ocular Surfactants 4(1):24–43

Steele C 2005 Fitting the irregular cornea. Optometry Today (Oct 21st):32–39

Steffen R, Schnider C 2004 A next generation silicone hydrogel lens for daily wear. Part 1 – Material properties. Optician 227(5954):23–25

Sterling J, Hecht A 1988 BAK-induced chemical keratitis? Spectrum 3 (3):62–64

Suchecki J K, Ehlers W H, Donshik P C 2000 A comparison of contact lens-related complications in various daily wear modalities. CLAO Journal 26(4):204–213

Swarbrick H A 2004 Orthokeratology (corneal refractive therapy): what is it and how does it work? Eye Contact Lens 30(4):181–185; discussion 185–186

Swarbrick H A 2006 Orthokeratology review and update. Clinical and Experimental Optometry 89(3):124–143

Sweeney D F, Stern J, Naduvalith T et al 2002 Inflammatory adverse event rates over 3 years with silicone hydrogel lenses. Investigative Ophthalmology and Visual Science 43(4):40

Sweeney D, du Toit R, Keay L et al 2004. Clinical performance of silicone hydrogel lenses. In: Sweeney D (ed.) Silicone hydrogels: continuous wear contact lenses, 2nd edn. Butterworth-Heinemann, Oxford, pp 164–216

Szczotka L B, Aronsky M 1998 Contact lenses after LASIK. J American Optometry Association 69(12):775–784

Szczotka L B, Lindsay R G 2003 Contact lens fitting following corneal graft surgery. Clinical and Experimental Optometry 86(4):244–249

Tan J, Keay L, Jalbert I et al 2003 Mucin balls with wear of conventional and silicone hydrogel contact lenses. Optometry and Vision Science 80(4):291–297

Tanner J, DePaolis M 1992 Disposable contact lenses as alternative bandage lenses. Clinical Eye and Vision Care 4(4):159–161

Tighe B 2002a Rigid lens materials. In: Efron N (ed.) Contact lens practice, 1st edn. Butterworth-Heinemann, Oxford, pp 153–162

Tighe B 2002b Soft lens materials. In: Efron N (ed.) Contact lens practice, 1st edn. Butterworth-Heinemann, Oxford, pp 71–84

Tighe B 2004 Silicone hydrogels: structure, properties and behaviour. In: Sweeney D (ed.) Silicone hydrogels: continuous wear contact lenses, 2nd edn. Butterworth-Heinemann, Oxford, pp 1–27

Tonge S, Jones L, Goodall S et al 2001 The ex vivo wettability of soft contact lenses. Current Eye Research 23(1):51–59

van der Worp E, de Brabander J, Lubberman B et al 2002 Optimising RGP lens fitting in normal eyes using 3D topographic data. Contact Lens and Anterior Eye 25(2):95–99

Veys J, Meyler J, Davies I 2002 Managing the presbyope. In: Veys J, Meyler J, Davies I (eds) Essential contact lens practice, 1st edn. Butterworth-Heinemann, Oxford, pp 54–63

Veys J, Meyler J, Davies I 2007 Rigid contact lens fitting. Optician 234 (6113):16–27

Visser E S, Visser R, van Lier H J et al 2007 Modern scleral lenses part I: clinical features. Eye Contact Lens 33(1):13–20

Weikart C M, Miyama M, Yasuda H K 1999 Surface modification of conventional polymers by depositing plasma polymers of trimethylsilane and of trimethylsilane + O_2. II Dynamic wetting properties. Journal of Colloid Interface Science 211(1):28–38

Weikart C M, Matsuzawa Y, Winterton L et al 2001 Evaluation of plasma polymer-coated contact lenses by electrochemical impedance spectroscopy. Journal of Biomedical Matererial Research 54(4):597–607

White P 1994 A complete guide to contact lens materials. Contact Lens Spectrum (November):31–36

Wichterle O, Lim D 1960 Hydrophilic gels for biological use. Nature 185:117–118

Willcox M D, Holden B A 2001 Contact lens related corneal infections. Bioscience Rep 21(4):445–461

Wong M, Dziabo J, Kiral R 1986 Adsorption of benzalkonium chloride by RGP lenses. Contact Lens Forum 11:25–32

Woods C A 2002 Planned rigid lens replacement. In: Efron N (ed.) Contact lens practice, 1st edn. Butterworth Heinemann, Oxford, pp 237–242

Wu P, Stapleton F, Willcox M D 2003 The causes of and cures for contact lens-induced peripheral ulcer. Eye Contact Lens 29(1 Suppl): S63–S66; discussion S83–S84, S192–S194

Young G 2002 Rigid lens design and fitting. In: Efron N (ed.) Contact lens practice, 1st edn. Butterworth Heinemann, Oxford, pp 186–202

Young G, Mirejovsky D 1993 A hypothesis for the aetiology of soft contact lens-induced superior arcuate keratopathy. International Contact Lens Clinic 20(9/10):177–179

Zantos S 1984 Ocular complications – corneal infiltrates, debris, and microcysts. Journal of the American Optometry Association 55 (3):196–198

CHAPTER 22

Prescribing spectacles

Glyn Walsh

Introduction

Although many practitioners may wish it to be a science, prescribing spectacles is essentially an art. There are too many factors involved, not least the individual local variations in responsibility and requirements and the chair-side manner of the optometrist, for absolute rules about prescribing spectacles to be drafted. However, the minimum essential information to decide what lens powers (if any) to prescribe have remained unchanged since optometry evolved from simply selling spectacles. These are uncorrected monocular and binocular distance vision (also termed uncorrected visual acuity), distance refractive correction for each eye, best corrected monocular and binocular distance visual acuity and details of any binocular vision anomalies. For intermediate, near and occupational requirements, the equivalent measurements are required at the appropriate working distance, while for a presbyopic patient, the near addition (add) must be determined (Obstfeld 1988).

The practitioner must determine whether prescribing corrective lenses will be of benefit to the patient. The correction should alleviate the symptoms associated with the chief presenting complaint. This may appear obvious, but it is easy to overlook under the pressures of normal optometric practice.

When there is marked ametropia, which is clearly the cause of the patient's symptoms or could eventually lead to amblyopia, there is seldom any doubt about prescribing (Ingram et al 1990; Anker et al 2004; Holmes & Clarke 2006), although even this has been questioned in some cases (Harvey et al 2004). Myopes with visual symptoms will almost always benefit from spectacles, but for hyperopes the decision is more difficult, and there are very little data on prescribing criteria for a given refractive error (O'Leary & Evans 2003). Spectacle lenses may have a placebo effect in some circumstances (Cholerton 1955; Nathan 1957; Carter & Allen 1973; Daum et al 2004), and the success of low prescriptions either as placebos or a genuine solution may depend on both the patient's mental attitude and the practitioner's communication skills (Ball 1982). However, caution should be exercised with placebos, as they are frowned on by both regulatory and professional bodies (Blakeney 2006). It has also been indicated that some symptoms may be resolved by prescribing small amounts of vertical prism (Mallett 1974), although unwanted vertical prism in spectacles will reduce visual performance (Tunnacliffe & Williams 1985). Placebo effects have also been ascribed to prismatic correction (Kommerell & Kromeier 2002; Scheiman et al 2005). Not surprisingly, presbyopia creates symptoms only in those patients whose activities require a near addition lens (Morgan 1960).

As noted earlier, binocular function must also be considered when evaluating a patient's symptoms and, in general, it is advisable to use a binocular balancing technique to reach the final distance prescription (Amigo 1968; West & Somers 1984; Shapiro 1995). However, there is a spectrum of binocularity from the truly monocular to comfortable, clear and single binocular vision. In the case of the monocular patient, it is sufficient to correct the functional eye, but ocular dominance, suppression and retinal correspondence can become issues in binocular patients. Binocular balancing techniques (see Ch. 14) will often provide information on these factors, providing the binocular status is stable enough for the procedure to be carried out. In some instances, such as progressive pathology or a refractive change of recent onset, there may be a conflict between correcting the dominant eye and providing good acuity and stable binocular vision.

A significant number of patients will present with symptoms of headache or eyestrain (Giles 1960; Vaithilingam & Khare 1967; Graf & Flammer 1980; Hutter & Rouse 1984; Glover et al 2006). However, a relatively low proportion of headaches are solely refractive in origin (Thomas et al 2004). If an optometric solution cannot be found, then referral for a medical opinion is mandatory (Ball 1982). Often, the position is less clear (Daum 1983), with Harle & Evans (2006) indicating that migraine sufferers are more likely to be astigmatic, whilst visual stress syndrome sufferers (see Ch. 16) often benefit from other optical assistance besides the tinted spectacles commonly prescribed for this condition (Evans et al 1999; Evans 2005). A low refractive error may also cause symptoms. The management of these cases should be discussed with the patient, and if a correction is prescribed then the patient should be advised to return if their symptoms are not alleviated.

Prescribing in the very young patient

The appropriate correction for infants and many older preschool children must be obtained objectively (see Ch. 13) as subjective responses are either impossible or inadequate. Refractive error is usually determined by retinoscopy, using either conventional distance retinoscopy or by an 'estimation technique' (Mohindra 1977; Wallace et al 2006). Other retinoscopy techniques have been proposed and show variable degrees of promise (Howland 1974; Mailer 1978; Atkinson & Braddick 1983; Roorda et al 1998).

Patients having a refractive error close to emmetropia and oculomotor balance within normal limits clearly require no correction. A cycloplegic examination is necessary when there is reason to suspect significant latent hyperopia, an oculomotor imbalance produced by uncorrected ametropia or potential refractive amblyopia (see Ch. 28). Indeed, it could be argued that cycloplegia should be used on all young children, especially when cooperation issues arise, such as poor distance fixation. In some instances it is necessary to monitor the child at frequent intervals after the first examination, although for normal individuals this may be questionable in the absence of symptoms, signs of refractive error or ocular abnormality. Although spectacles may affect the emmetropization process (see Ch. 28), the effect of prescribing spectacles on a young eye remains uncertain (Troilo 1992; Saunders et al 1995; Gwiazda & Thorn 1998, 1999; Atkinson et al 2000; Ingram et al 2000).

Unfortunately, the question of 'what is a significant refractive error' does not appear to have been answered satisfactorily for any age group (O'Leary & Evans 2003). The consequences of not correcting the patient's refractive error must be considered. For example, the myopic infant without significant anisometropia is less likely to develop amblyopia when compared with hyperopes, anisometropes or astigmats, as most objects of interest for this age group are positioned at a close working distance (Ingram et al 1986; Robaei et al 2005, 2006). High degrees of hyperopia that exceed the patient's accommodative ability (absolute

hyperopia) will prevent formation of a clear image at all viewing distances and may lead to accommodative strabismus. Significant astigmatism will also produce blur at all distances and can lead to meridional amblyopia (Mitchell et al 1973). Anisometropia is generally correlated with the ultimate degree of amblyopia (Townshend et al 1993), although the magnitude of myopic anisometropia at which problems arise is much higher than for cases of astigmatic amblyopia (Tanlamai & Goss 1979).

Lyons et al (2004) observed very wide variation in prescribing practices, although surveys have shown that few ophthalmologists correct patients with hyperopia of less than 3.00 dioptres (D) (without strabismus) in children under 5 years of age (Miller & Harvey 1998; Harvey et al 2005). The College of Optometrists (2006) in the United Kingdom advises caution for prescriptions of +0.50 DS or less for any patient under 16. It has been observed that, after a short period of difficulty, infants tend to wear their spectacles without complaint, particularly if they are examined relatively frequently (perhaps 6-month intervals) and the changes in refractive correction made are small (Weale 1963; Horwood 1998).

Older children and adolescents

As the child progresses through school, the difficulty with reading material increases steadily (Maclure 1980). At the same time, there are social pressures both for (McKelvie 1997; Walline et al 2006) and against the wearing of spectacles (Terry et al 1983; Terry & Stockton 1993; Horwood et al 2005). A significant proportion of refractive errors first manifest themselves at school age, with the incidence of myopia in particular having reached epidemic proportions in some parts of the world, especially in Asia (Grosvenor 2003; Saw 2003; Woo et al 2004; Junghans & Crewther 2005). The aetiology underlying refractive development is often unclear for individual cases, although there is strong evidence for genetic factors (Jacobi et al 2005; Dirani et al 2006). Furthermore, it is uncertain whether full or partial distance correction and/or the use of bifocal or progressive addition lenses (PALs) can influence juvenile myopic progression (Goss 1994; Saw et al 2002; Gwiazda et al 2004; Adler & Millodot 2006). However, corrected hyperopia may remain relatively stable (Hirsch 1961; Sorsby & Leary 1969), particularly if a full correction is given following a cycloplegic refraction and only minimal latent hyperopia is present.

The ability to provide good subjective responses may decrease the need for cycloplegia, but further ambiguity about prescribing, such as questionable sensitivity to small changes in the refractive correction, may still exist. While the visual system is developing, amblyopia can arise if refractive errors remain uncorrected (Granet et al 2006; Cotter et al 2006). Significant degrees of myopia must be corrected for the patient to be able to resolve distant objects, and these individuals tend to use their correction without question. Higher levels of hyperopia make reading and other near activities more difficult and, whilst children have high amplitudes of accommodation, hyperopes have been shown to under-perform educationally (Wharry & Kirkpatrick 1986; Krumholtz 2000). However, particularly in lower degrees of hyperopia, the refractive correction will produce little change in visual acuity, and this may result in inconsistent lens wear. Stewart-Brown (1985) suggested that the prescribing of unnecessary spectacles to school children occurred frequently, whilst Press (1985) advised caution when prescribing small hyperopic corrections. As with younger children, the effect of prescribing spectacles on the emmetropization process remains uncertain (Gwiazda & Thorn 1998, 1999; Ong et al 1999; Ingram et al 2000).

The pre-presbyopic adult

Changes in the prescription of the pre-presbyopic adult from adolescence tend to be small (Hirsch 1961; Attebo et al 1989; Guzowski et al 2003), although sustained near work can lead to adult-onset or late-onset myopia (Adams & McBrien 1992; McBrien & Adams 1997). The potential for an increase in myopia must be reviewed if refractive surgery is being considered. With increasing age, the steady reduction in accommodation can make pre-existing hyperopia become manifest, resulting in symptoms, especially during sustained near-vision tasks.

The presbyopic patient

Conventionally, the onset of presbyopia is taken to be the age at which the near point of accommodation (see Ch. 15) lies beyond the desired near working distance (while viewing through the distance refractive correction). This commonly occurs around 40–45 years of age, and earlier in females than males (Pointer 1995a,b, 2002). The age of presbyopia onset may also depend on environmental factors such as climate and geographic location (Coates 1955; Miranda 1979; Ong 1981; Weale 1981; Jain et al 1982), although these differences, as well as those associated with variations in ethnicity, now appear to be less significant than initially claimed (Kragha 1985; Kragha & Hofstetter 1986; Hunter & Schipp 1997).

The onset of presbyopia should also be considered when advising patients about refractive surgery. The low myope may wish to be rid of their spectacles, but be unaware that eliminating their distance refractive error will necessitate the wearing of spectacles for near work.

Large changes in distance ametropia are not expected in the presbyopic individual, although there is a statistical shift of the population mean towards hyperopia between 40 and 65 years of age (Guzowski et al 2003). After 65, some patients become increasingly myopic, but this may be an early sign of ocular pathology, such as the development of lens opacities (Hirsch 1961).

The first step in determining the near correction is accurate correction of the distance refractive error. Astigmatism does not usually change significantly when switching from distance to near fixation in the presbyopic patient, although there may be measurable changes in the pre-presbyope (Nicholson & Garzia 1988; Ukai & Ichihashi 1991). The usual range of near additions (adds) is between +0.50 DS and +3.25 DS (Obstfeld 1967; Pointer 2002), although adds over +3.00 are rarely prescribed in patients with good corrected visual acuity. Equal-powered adds are usually prescribed for the two eyes except in cases of high anisometropia or unilateral pathology.

The add power is dependant on both task size and the desired viewing distance. The patient should also be questioned about task illumination, as older patients generally need more light to compensate for the loss of clarity of the ocular media (Boyce 1973), and may present with complaints of poor lighting, rather than blur, as the first symptom of presbyopia. Interestingly, near adds based purely on the patient's age have been shown to be more successful than those prescribed using other methods (Hanlon et al 1987), and the add required varies predictably with age (Blystone 1999). For a discussion of various techniques designed to determine the power of the near add lens, see Chapter 15.

A full-aperture, single-vision lens designed to correct the patient at near will blur their distance vision, and, for many emmetropes and low hyperopes who have enjoyed clear vision at all distances throughout life until this point, this change must be approached tactfully. It is wise to explain presbyopia carefully, perhaps even to the extent of indicating that not becoming presbyopic would be abnormal. Any apparent accommodation in patients over 52–54 years of age is probably due to the increase in depth of focus resulting from age-related miosis (Millodot & Millodot 1989; Ramsdale & Charman 1989).

As accommodation continues to decline, the near add should be increased concurrent with visual demands (**Fig. 22.1**). Two years is usually considered to be a reasonable interval between examinations, and changes at this rate generally permit the add to be increased without upsetting the accommodation–convergence relationship unduly, although related data have cast some doubt on the need for a slow build-up in add power (Sheedy & Saladin 1975; Wick 1985; Rosenfield et al 1995; Ciuffreda et al 1997; Baker & Gilmartin 2003). The required add power increases steadily, normally reaching its maximum around 60 years of age. If the visual performance continues to decline, higher

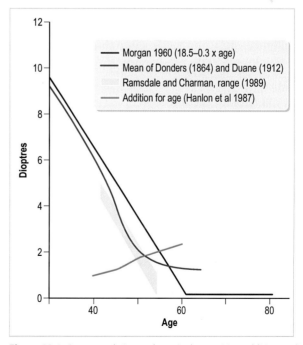

Figure 22.1 Accommodation and required near-vision addition in dioptres as a function of age in years.

adds may be needed, especially if combined with a change in near-vision habits toward a shorter working distance.

Once an add of around +1.75 has been reached, the patient may have insufficient depth of focus to see at all distances with just a distance and near correction. For these patients, correction at a third working distance may be required, and this can be achieved with a trifocal lens. In some markets, progressive addition lenses (PALs) have largely replaced bifocal and trifocal lenses even for early presbyopes, thereby eliminating this problem with intermediate distances. Further, in view of the relatively large size of even so-called 'small' print, this may be a less prevalent problem than previously suggested.

Although a detailed discussion of lens types is often not considered to be the prescriber's responsibility, he or she should at least provide general guidance on the best type of lens necessary to satisfy the patient's needs. For example, single-vision lenses are the obvious solution to a requirement for a large intermediate or near field of view.

Bifocal lenses have the advantage of two optically clear areas, but may be considered cosmetically 'ageing'. All bifocals cause objects in the field to appear to 'jump' when fixation moves across the dividing line, produced by the abrupt change in induced prism resulting from the change in lens power. Normally, the distance prescription is at the top of the lens, with the near segment at the bottom, but the lenses can be glazed upside down or with the segment at the edge of the lens should the patient's visual requirements demand. Even so-called 'no-jump' bifocals give horizontal jump at the dividing line. Bifocals need not be limited to distance and near only. For example, intermediate–near bifocals can be very successful for computer use. The near segment can vary from a 22 mm diameter circle to half the lens (E-style), with the larger near segments allowing a considerably larger field of view, when compared with PALs.

Trifocals have three distinct areas. They also have the cosmetic disadvantage of bifocals, and two lines at which jump can occur. The near area is normally smaller than bifocals, and the intermediate area is also quite shallow in most types, although it can be much wider than that found in PALs. For these reasons, the smaller segment sizes have now been largely displaced by PALs, although the larger segments still have their place.

PALs still have the distance prescription at the top of the lens and near correction at the bottom. There is no dividing line and no 'jump', although there is significant distortion over much of the lens, especially the lower part to either side of the intermediate and near areas. The intermediate zone is often very narrow, necessitating accurate horizontal centration. PALs also have a relatively small area of clear near vision, but the majority of modern designs are a good example of the tolerance of patients to blur, and cause few problems. The length of the intermediate 'corridor' in many progressive designs has reduced from the older 22 mm to as little as 12 mm in recent years, to fit contemporary fashionable shallow frames. While this results in a reduction in the area of the intermediate vision zone, most patients report surprisingly few problems with this design.

'Degressive' lenses are a variant of PALs (e.g. Essilor Computer 3V) in which the near prescription is specified and the distance is a 'negative' add. This gives a large, clear reading area, but a much reduced clear distance area. All manufacturers advise against driving in these lenses.

Spherical corrections

Although power tolerances of about ±0.12 D have been suggested (Appleton 1971; Legras et al 2004; Brown 2006) and even applied in practice (BS 2738-1, 1998), this is at variance with much of the historical literature (von Helmholtz 1924; Tassman 1932; Jackson 1932; Nathan 1957). Intra- and inter-examiner variability of 0.25–0.50 DS has been reported (Sloane et al 1954; Humphriss 1958; Jennings & Charman 1973; French & Jennings 1974; Bannon 1977; Perrigin et al 1982; Goss & Grosvenor 1996), with Rosenfield & Chiu (1995) suggesting ±0.50 DS as the minimum significant change in refractive status. However, Bullimore et al (1998) only found 0.12 DS inter-examiner variation. The depth of focus of the human eye is also quite considerable ($\approx \pm 0.40$ D), and can greatly affect both the 'accuracy' of prescribing and the tolerance to 'inaccuracy' of the finished spectacles (Campbell & Weir 1953; Morgan 1960; Wang & Ciuffreda 2006). Some practitioners round off prescriptions to the nearest half-dioptre (Aves 1926; Fletcher 1967; Obstfeld 1969), although Atchison et al (2001) observed that a refractive error of only ±0.25 D reduced visual comfort. Accordingly, the normal use of ±0.25 D steps during refraction seems justified as most patients can perceive changes of this size. However, in some cases, particularly individuals with reduced visual acuity or young hyperopes with active accommodation, larger steps may be acceptable.

Cylindrical corrections

The majority of spectacle corrections incorporate a cylindrical component, with the most frequently prescribed cylindrical power being 0.50 DC and relatively few (about 5%) being over 2.00 DC (Bennett 1965). The rounding off of cylinder powers in 0.50 D steps has also been observed (Bennett 1965; Obstfeldt 1967). A correction of 0.25 DC may be of questionable value in a distance correction and often 0.50 DC may be of little benefit in a near correction (Obsfeldt 1988). The level of repeatability of the astigmatic correction is similar to that of the spherical correction (Sloane et al 1954; Humphriss 1958; Perrigin et al 1982; Charman & Voisin 1993; Murphy et al 2002), although Johnson et al (1996) reported a repeatability of ±0.12 DC and ±5° for the cylinder axis.

Historically, the majority of practitioners used minus cylinders because of their ability to control accommodation during the subjective refraction technique (see Ch. 14). However, the widespread introduction of projector charts without a practical fan chart has brought about a shift towards the use of plus cylinders amongst some younger practitioners in the UK.

In infancy, astigmatism is unpredictable and can vary as the infant grows (Howland & Sayles 1984; Mayer et al 2001) (see Ch. 28). A majority of preschool children exhibit 'with the rule' astigmatism (i.e. the vertical meridian having the higher refractive power) rather than 'against the rule' (horizontal meridian having the higher power) or oblique astigmatism (where the orientation of the more powerful meridian does not lie within ±20° of either the horizontal or vertical meridians) (Bennett 1965; Obstfeld 1967; Hendrickson & Bleything 2001), although these observations have been questioned (Montes-Mico 2000; Huynh et al 2006a). The direction of any change in axis with age is also uncertain (Fledelius 1984; Attebo et al 1989; Gudmundsdottir et al 2000, 2005; Guzowski et al 2003). However, it is generally believed to be in the direction of more against the rule astigmatism with increasing age (Hirsch 1961).

As the magnification effects of astigmatic lenses are meridional, these corrective lenses can give rise to both binocular vision problems (Obstfeld 1982) and perceptual distortions (Langenbucher & Seitz 2003), particularly if the axes are oblique. These effects can be described to the patient on prescribing, although many patients will be entirely unaware of them, and it may not be wise to do this as a general policy (Ball 1982). They are difficult to describe in words, but rotating a trial case cylinder can provide a useful demonstration. However, the reduction of cylinder power away from that required for the best visual acuity is sometimes necessary when the glasses are dispensed, although visual standards for demanding tasks such as driving must not be overlooked. It may be possible to increase the cylinder power after a period of adaptation. The problem of meridional distortion is smaller with back surface toric lenses and minimum vertex distance (Guyton 1977). It can also be reduced on occasion by moving the axis closer to a vertical or horizontal orientation, or, for a previous spectacle wearer, towards the previously worn cylinder axis if this has been changed.

The effects of back vertex distance, lens form, bifocal/progressive near addition and ocular cyclorotation can result in a change of the astigmatic component of the correction when switching between distance and near fixation (Beau Seigneur 1946; Fletcher 1952), although these are seldom considered in practice.

Aphakia

In the developed world, the optical problems produced by aphakia have been markedly reduced since the 1980s, as a direct result of the almost universal use of intraocular lenses (IOLs) following cataract surgery. The removal of the crystalline lens without implantation of an IOL into the eye usually brings about hyperopia of 10.00 D to 13.00 D. Accommodation is also eliminated. Surgical techniques have progressed in parallel with the development of IOLs, with the result that the high degrees of astigmatism historically brought about by cataract surgery are less frequently seen, and multifocal IOLs are also available for patients in whom the loss of image quality is deemed acceptable (Avitabile & Marano 2001).

Prescribing for binocular aphakes without IOLs is very similar to other high hyperopes. There is marked magnification from the lenses, typically 20–30%. It can take some time to adapt to this, although it can compensate to some extent for reduced visual performance from other causes

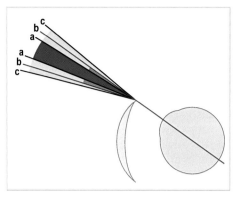

Figure 22.2 The effect of the pupil diameter on the visual field at the edge of a convex spectacle lens. The scotoma (as usually described in optical texts) when calculated for a pinhole pupil is the arc BB. However, the area of total field loss with a finite pupil size is AA, which is rather smaller. Additionally, there is a 'penumbra' (the areas between A and C) which results in the area of relative field loss being greater that the naive prediction. (After Walsh & Pearce 2006.)

(Fonda 1970). There is also a 'ring scotoma' around the edge of both full-aperture and lenticular lenses (**Fig. 22.2**), although this effect is much less than conventionally predicted (Walsh & Pearce 2006). The negative cosmesis of lenticular lenses should not be underestimated, and the success of the blended lenticular-type lenses, with their poor optical quality, may be largely attributable to the improved appearance rather than their claimed optical advantage of removing the ring scotoma.

To resolve the problem of accommodation loss, some patients slide their spectacles down their nose, thereby making use of the increased positive vergence at the eye that this brings (this will also work for high myopes). Alternatively, the same bifocal and multifocal solutions are available as for lower corrections, although the choice of lens designs and materials is very limited.

Monocular aphakia (without an IOL) can be more problematic than binocular, as the magnification effects will vary between the eyes as does the differential prism by decentration. There is no practical spectacle solution in these cases. Contact lenses are the only real option (Goar 1957), and can work well following surgery for congenital cataract (Lambert 1999), but may not be optimum even for these patients (Greenwald & Glasser 1998). Contact lenses will still give rise to magnification differences between the eyes, which may be intolerable, although they do remove the differential prismatic effect. Combined spectacle–contact lens corrections have also been suggested (Borish 1983). Asymptomatic patients wearing a full-spectacle correction have been reported, but it seems unlikely that binocular vision is present in these individuals. The usual practice is to correct the better eye, or the dominant eye if the vision is adequate, and to provide a 'balance' lens to the fellow eye.

It should also be borne in mind that removal of the crystalline lens increases the blue and ultraviolet transmission of the eye, and therefore increases the risk of damage to the retina (Kirkness & Weale 1985). Accordingly, lenses used in aphakia should not transmit these particular wavelengths.

Pseudophakia (i.e. replacement of the crystalline lens with an IOL) has replaced aphakia as the norm following cataract surgery in much of the world. Ideally, the residual refractive error in bilateral pseudophakia should be similar in both eyes, and can then be treated in a similar manner to any other presbyopic case. Unilateral pseudophakia can be more problematic, as many surgeons aim for emmetropia or low myopia in the operated eye rather than matching the pre-existing refractive error. These patients can present with marked degrees of anisometropia, but without the ability possessed by many early-onset anisometropes to suppress the poorer eye, and may require complicated optical solutions involving differential prism control at near in (usually) a bifocal lens, although a 'balance' lens is more frequently prescribed.

In pre-presbyopic patients, monocular pseudophakia will result in full accommodation in one eye with none in the treated eye. Some patients are able to adapt prescriptions with only one bifocal or progressive lens and one single-vision lens, but more frequently, they will suppress one of their eyes.

Anisometropia

Although anisometropia is a significant cause of amblyopia when present in younger patients, identical refractive corrections in the two eyes is relatively uncommon. Most interocular differences are less than 1 D (Fledelius 1984; Gupta & Gupta 2000; Mayer et al 2001; Kuo et al 2003; Hashemi et al 2004; Huynh et al 2006b; Gronlund et al 2006), and cause few problems, although the incidence of anisometropia does increase with age (Haegerstrom-Portnoy et al 2002; Weale 2002, 2003; Xu et al 2005) and may vary amongst different populations (Katz et al 1997; Wong et al 2000; Saw 2003; Quek et al 2004; Bourne et al 2004).

Anisometropic patients, when corrected with spectacles, will encounter differential prism by decentration, which (particularly in the vertical meridian) can interfere with binocular vision. Further, the eye with the more minus/less plus spectacle lens will receive a smaller retinal image, and this eye will also need to accommodate more than its fellow due to the effects of ocular accommodation (Rosenfield 1997). Aniseikonia, i.e. a difference in the size of the perceived images of the two eyes, can also be a cause of difficulty in these cases (Krzizok et al 1996). However, in view of the prismatic differences combined with the weight problems of iseikonic lenses, many practitioners do not consider the control of aniseikonia with spectacles to be a realistic option (Lebensohn 1953; Schipper 1985; Remole 1989; Achiron & Witkin 1998; Hirai et al 2004). Where differential prismatic, aniseikonic or related problems occur, contact lenses are almost always the best optical solution (Zamorini et al 1964; Winn et al 1988; Evans 2006), although isogonal (Halass 1959) or iseikonic (Nordlow 1970; Remole 1989) lenses have also been suggested. In practice, the use of a 'balance' lens (Calder-Gillie 1961) is the most frequent solution where intractable problems occur and the patient cannot wear contact lenses. Occasionally, it is necessary to occlude one eye. Masking tape, 'orthoptic'-type occluders, frosted lenses, an eye patch or just shutting or covering one eye with the hand when necessary can be useful in these situations.

A full correction is often well tolerated even by adults. Surprisingly, this can be the case not only where there is unilateral amblyopia, but where fully corrected acuity is good in each eye (Amos 1978; Krzizok et al 1996). However, results are unpredictable. If a full correction is not acceptable in adults, then the dominant eye or the eye with the better acuity should be corrected preferentially after investigating the effect on binocular performance and comfort. It is sometimes possible to increase the degree of anisometropic correction over a period of months or years until the full correction is achieved.

Anisometropic presbyopes can present a significant problem, particularly where treatment in their youth has provided good acuities and binocular function (Kozol 1996; Pouliquen de Liniere et al 1998). These patients often tend to move their head rather than the eyes, and the transition to bifocals or PALs suddenly reintroduces the prismatic problems which the patient has learned to avoid, as it becomes necessary to look through the lower part of the lens, well away from the optical centre. This problem is encountered surprisingly rarely amongst anisometropes in an optometric patient population, other than those created surgically, and suggests that the long-term results of optical and orthoptic treatment of anisometropia may be rather less successful at restoring binocular vision than believed by many of their proponents. Before supplying bifocals or PALs to an anisometropic patient who is not already a successful wearer, it is advisable to determine their likely effect. This can be done with a prism in the trial frame or by looking through the lower part of their distance spectacles if there is no significant change in the degree of anisometropia. A method of obtaining a rough estimation of the prismatic effect of sphero-cylindrical lenses is given in **Table 22.1**, which usually proves adequate for predicting potential problems, and to allow trial case prisms to be used to test the outcome before making up the spectacles.

If there is no binocular vision, and one eye is myopic and the other approximately emmetropic, then the patient may never need spectacles for distance or near. It is also possible to create a similar circumstance in patients without binocular vision, usually those with alternating strabismus where there is good acuity in both eyes. In these patients, one eye can sometimes be corrected for distance (usually the dominant eye) and the other left (or made) myopic to facilitate good near vision.

For presbyopic patients who do have binocular vision, there are solutions permitting the use of bifocal lenses, although trifocals and PALs are more problematic. However, there remain many instances in which the only satisfactory solutions are single-vision spectacles or even occluding one eye.

If the degree of anisometropia is quite low, typically less than 2–2.5 D, it is possible to set the optical centre of the lens lower than its conventional position halfway up the frame. This will have the effect of reducing the differential prism by decentration encountered during near viewing with the eyes depressed (although it will be increased for distance viewing). However, the patient's fusional reserves must be sufficient to cope with this degree of prism. This method can be applied to all types of lenses.

Another option is to 'slab off' one of the lenses. Here, the surface opposite the bifocal/progressive near addition is worked to give a base-up prism, thereby resulting in a straight line across the lens (Jalie 1980). This works well with straight-top bifocal lenses, but introduces both jump

Table 22.1 Estimation of prismatic effect in anisometropic corrections

Cylinder axis (°)	Bifocal	Progressive addition lens
180	S + C	1.5 (S + C)
30	S + 0.75C	1.5 (S + 0.75C)
45	S + 0.50C	1.5 (S + 0.50C)
60	S + 0.25C	1.5 (S + 0.25C)
90	S	1.5 S

The prism is calculated for each lens and the approximate prismatic effect is the difference between them, with base down in the more minus lens. The table assumes a reading position with a bifocal lens 10 mm (1 cm) below the distance optical centres and a progressive transition length of 15 mm (1.5 cm). The 1.5 cm value should be increased for longer and reduced for shorter transition lengths.

and a cosmetically unattractive line into PALs. An alternative 'inverse slab off' (in practice, a cast optical surface) is also available, although this is only available on 'D' segment (flat top) bifocals.

The other options listed below all leave something to be desired cosmetically, even on bifocal lenses, but may be required for some patients. Different-sized round segments can be used, with the larger segment providing more base-down prism. This is useful as a low-cost option, as only 'standard' lens types need be used. The upper limit of differential prism which can be obtained with this technique is equal to the add power (in Δ) using 25 mm and 45 mm round segments. Using a 'D' segment and a 45 mm round segment, differential prism of 1.5 times the add power can be obtained.

Franklin bifocals, constructed from separate distance and near lenses mounted in the frame, can be used to obtain almost any amount of prism. Cemented bifocals can be used similarly. Stick-on Fresnel prisms can also provide a temporary measure, and are useful for high prism powers.

Prisms

It is conventionally taught that asymptomatic patients should not be prescribed prisms, although O'Leary and Evans (2006) have questioned this statement. It is clearly untrue in cases where normal visual or educational development or safety is at risk, but it is probably valid advice when considering whether to prescribe prism for adults.

In symptomatic patients, fixation disparity (or associated heterophoria) tests (see Ch. 16) can be used to determine how much prism should be prescribed (Karania & Evans 2006), although again the validity of such methods has been questioned (Kommerell et al 2000). However, as part of the binocular vision evaluation, the prismatic effect of the lenses being worn must be considered. This is particularly true of vertical prisms, as a small difference in the vertical position of the optical centres, because of either a misaligned frame or damaged spectacles, or an error in manufacturing can bring about measurable effects. If the patient has been wearing incorrectly centred spectacles for some time, adaptation will occur (von Hofsten 1979; Henson & North 1980; North & Henson 1985), although this could still compromise stereoscopic performance (Jimenez et al 2000). In the brief period of the refractive examination

this adaptation may not have been overcome, and it may be necessary either to give a longer period of adaptation or to consider a compromise prismatic correction/centration. Conversely, it is sometimes worthwhile to decentre lenses to improve the cosmetic appearance of the spectacles, although this should be done with caution and the patient's agreement. The likely success of such a tactic can also be gauged in the examination room (Walsh 2001a).

It is common practice to determine the required prism by presenting the prism before one eye only. This is then commonly split between the two eyes in the dispensed spectacle lenses in order to improve the cosmetic appearance. This can lead to an ambiguity between writing the prescription and what is put into the lenses. Therefore, it should be indicated clearly on the final prescription whether the prism should be placed before one eye only, or as is done more commonly, split between the two eyes.

When prescribing large amounts of prism, the use of 'stick-on' Fresnel prisms should be considered. These have the advantage of being removed easily, and of being light and thin enough to wear in very high powers (up to 50Δ), which might otherwise be impossible to achieve.

Dispensing considerations for the prescriber

The optometrist should bear in mind that what is prescribed is not always what can, or will, be dispensed. One such consideration is the effect of back vertex distance (BVD) and back vertex power (BVP) of the lens combination in the trial frame or phoropter. Indeed, particular problems can arise with the latter because of the large BVD (Weiss et al 2002).

The effect of the spectacles being dispensed at a different vertex distance to that at which the refraction was carried out can be significant. British Standard BS 2738–3 (2004) states that any prescription of over ±5 D in any meridian should have a BVD included as part of the prescription. Where there is doubt about the BVP of the spectacles, such as when there are multiple lenses (including more than one relatively high-powered lens) present in the trial frame, then the trial frame should be placed in a focimeter (lensometer) and the BVP measured directly. Under such circumstances, subsequent changes in vertex distance can have an effect of 0.12 D or more. It has also been claimed (Tang

1989) that the prismatic element of the prescription may also vary with vertex distance, and aspheric lenses have been shown to be affected more by changes of BVD when compared with spherical lenses (Fontaine et al 1997).

Another BVD problem often outside the control of the prescriber is the form in which lenses are manufactured. The majority of bifocal, trifocal and PALs currently in production have the near add placed on the front surface. For minus and low plus distance corrections, this is not of great significance. However, the result of the reading area being further from the eye than the back vertex plane at which the prescription is normally measured can create a substantial error in the effective add power if compensation for the lens being produced in this way is not made at the dispensing stage (Jalie 1980). This is illustrated in **Figure 22.3**. This can easily be 0.50 D and can be as much as 1.00 D. If such an error is likely to cause the patient problems, it is perhaps as well to indicate that correction should be made by the dispenser of the final spectacles. However, care should also be taken by the prescriber, where the old prescription is being taken as a starting point, as the add in the old spectacles will have been seen as a BVP by the patient but been dispensed as a front surface add. These peculiarities come about because of the most economical method of manufacturing the majority of lenses, with the front surface being mass produced with fixed adds usually in 0.25 DS steps, and the back surface being worked later to give the astigmatic component of the correction.

Lens availability can also complicate prescribing. What one wishes to prescribe and what is available are not always the same. Ophthalmic lenses are made in fixed steps, typically 0.25 or 0.12 D. Adds for PALs are normally between +1.00 D and +3.50 D. The power range of many lens designs is also limited, and this can seriously disadvantage those with high prescriptions for whom it is not commercially viable to produce cosmetically optimal lenses. It is sometimes necessary to compromise the optimum visual performance (with the patient's agreement and understanding) in order to obtain spectacles which are both cosmetically acceptable and adequate for their purpose.

Tints

Tints are commonly prescribed for occupational and recreational use to overcome problems of safety. In some occupations, such as welding, the use of protective tints is mandatory. However, before prescribing tints it is perhaps wise to think of them as the optical equivalent of a sticking plaster or band-aid – useful only if the problem cannot be avoided. Tints can serve to reduce the visual effects of problematic lighting, to protect the eyes and to enhance visual function beyond its 'normal' level.

The most commonly prescribed tints are those to reduce excess light levels at the eye. In some instances, such as sunglasses, there must also be protection from potentially hazardous invisible radiation (infrared and ultraviolet, BS EN 1836 2005). When tints are prescribed for light reduction it should be borne in mind that the visual system does not respond linearly to lighting levels, and a tint which is dark enough to make a real difference outdoors (50 000 lux in sunshine) is likely to be unusable indoors (100 lux in typical homes) (Grundy 1988; BS EN 1836 2005), and dangerous when driving at low luminance levels. Typically, an older patient will need 50–100% more light than a younger one (Boyce 1973), and will be more vulnerable to such effects.

The majority of 'cosmetic' and 'sunglass' tints are greys and browns, which will have little effect on colour vision, and it is wise to stick with such tints for this reason, although few are truly colour-neutral. However, all tints can distort colour vision, and also can make recognition of traffic signal lights more difficult. Perhaps the most obvious candidate in this category is the yellow 'night driving spectacles', which should be avoided. Similarly, there is little or no valid evidence that tints help with sporting performance.

Polarizing tints, i.e. tints which selectively eliminate one direction of oscillation of the light waves, can cut down reflections dramatically, especially from water, ice and snow. However, there is a theoretical possibility that such tints could be hazardous in icy conditions. Commercial polarizing tints are made for reflections from horizontal surfaces, and are less efficient the further the reflecting surface lies away from the horizontal.

Tints to enhance performance can be simple contrast filters, such as using a green-tinted lens to enhance the relative

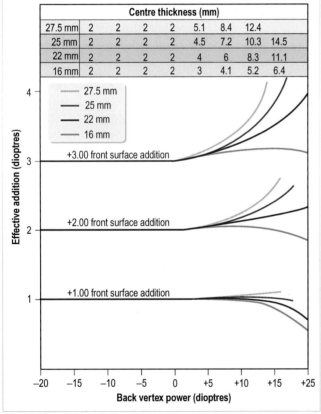

Figure 22.3 The effect of lens power on the effective near addition (D) for plano-convex and plano-concave lenses from −20 to +25. A D25 (25 mm diameter flat top) bifocal with its top set 5 mm below the distance optical centre is assumed throughout. The maximum distance from the optical centre to the lens edge is 27.5 mm (55 mm uncut lens), 25 mm (50 mm uncut), 22 mm (typical optimum full aperture for 64 mm centration distance) and 16 mm (32 mm lenticular). Other lens forms would give different errors in back vertex powers for the add, but the general trend is similar. A minimum substance of 2 mm and a refractive index of 1.5 are assumed.

luminance of green detail. Similarly, spectacle or contact lenses having different colours in the two eyes can be used to compensate for deficient colour vision, and can even be useful for normal individuals as a method to enhance colour contrast (Welsh et al 1979; Richer et al 1985). Such lenses are not adequate to replace normal colour vision, and should be used with caution. It may be possible to tint a small area of a spectacle lens to reduce the other problems created by such lenses (Walsh 2001b). Another category of tints which may be of value are the specialized tints used for the treatment of problems such as dylexia and 'visual stress' (Evans et al 1999). For most other visual disorders, it is difficult to separate placebo effects from real ones beyond the protective remit (Walsh 2001b), although many patients do benefit from the suggested lenses.

Non-tolerance

Non-tolerance is the situation in which a patient is unable to tolerate the completed spectacles after a trial period. Normally, this would be expected to be one of days or weeks, although occasionally non-tolerance becomes apparent on the initial collection of the completed spectacles. Immediate non-tolerance is usually due to a factor which could perhaps have been predicted at the time of the initial prescribing or dispensing, but which only becomes apparent on collection.

Dislike of the cosmetic appearance of the lenses or frame is not uncommon, but can often be expressed as dissatisfaction with optical performance to avoid embarrassment. Such cases can be extremely difficult to resolve, although they often involve those patients who were unable to see the spectacle frame clearly without their prescription lenses or those who have asked the opinion of a friend or partner for the first time.

Other common causes of immediate rejection include the possibility of a markedly incorrect prescription, sometimes as a result of the refractive examination, but all too frequently due to a transcription, transposition or glazing error. Such a possibility should not be discounted until the power and centration (Osuobeni & al-Zughaibi 1993) have been checked on the focimeter (lensometer). Ninety-degree transposition errors or errors in signs are easily missed, and should be consciously sought (Ball 1982). For higher-powered lenses made from low Abbe number materials, an infrared (automatic) focimeter will normally read lower than the true power because of the chromatic aberration of the lenses. Although many of these automated instruments have mechanisms for correcting these errors, they are seldom used in practice, even if the Abbe number of the lens is known.

Priest (1979) divides non-tolerance cases into prescribing and dispensing problems, and his advice to look at the dispensing aspects first remains sound, whilst Ball (1982; see **Table 22.2**) indicated that a correct refraction can also bring about a problem which did not previously exist, such as distortion, magnification or binocular difficulties. Although such problems can sometimes be predicted from the optical

Table 22.2 Possible non-pathological causes of presenting symptoms

Symptom type	Presenting symptoms	Examples of possible cause (non-pathological)
Referred or sympathetic	Headaches, giddiness, nausea, disorientation, unreality	High presbyopic additions Unintended prismatic effects (e.g. faulty centration), prismatic corrections (see also spatial distortion, below)
Ocular	Discomfort and irritation, described variously as 'drawing', 'pulling', 'straining' or 'staring' for 'clear' vision	Recent presbyopic additions
Visual		
	Micropsia	Recent myopic prescriptions Base-out prisms
	Macropsia	Recent presbyopic additions Base-in prisms
	General spatial distortions	Unaccustomed cylinders Corrected anisometropia Change of lens form
	Peripheral spatial distortions	PALs & some bifocals
	Blurred vision	Inappropriate use of prescription (e.g. blurred distance vision with near spectacles) Uncorrected residual errors Positioning of bifocal segments and interference from bifocal segment edge PAL positioning Incorrect effective power of prescription Marginally overcorrected positive powers from

Continued

Table 22.2 Possible non-pathological causes of presenting symptoms—Cont'd

Symptom type	Presenting symptoms	Examples of possible cause (non-pathological)
		maximum plus routine + finite chart distance Faulty lens centration Improperly corrected astigmatism Chromatic aberration in low Abbe number lenses (off the optical axis only)
	Diplopia	Incorrect lens centration Improperly corrected astigmatism Interference from bifocal segment edge
	Chromatopsia	Chromatic aberration in low Abbe number lenses (off the optical axis only) High addition in some fused bifocals
	Visual unease	Slight blur in dominant eye Altered muscle balance from previous prescription
	Photophobia	Contact lenses Omission of previously worn tint
	Increased contrast Unwanted clarity	Recently and fully corrected myopia
	Ghost images	Reflections from lens surfaces
Other effects		
	Lenses feel 'too strong'	Fully corrected myopia and presbyopia
	Cosmetic and allied problems	Weight and thickness of lenses, visibility of bifocal segments, weight of spectacles, poor frame choice
	Stumbling, tripping	Distorting elements of prescription (see also distortions above) Unaccustomed bifocals or PALs

Table is compiled with permission from Ball 1982.

properties of the lenses, it is harder to forecast which patients will notice them.

Apparent intolerance may also mask other factors, such as the development of pathology. For this reason intolerance should not be dismissed if it cannot be wholly resolved or explained. If the problem is not clearly one of dispensing, then a full re-examination should always be carried out.

There are few data on the causes of spectacle intolerance, but Obstfeld (1988) suggested that changes in cylindrical correction or base curve, and adds which are too high, are the most frequent causes (Hanlon et al 1987). The extensive use of computers at a longer viewing distance than that required for normal hardcopy reading has increased the frequency of the latter problem.

In the 1970s and 1980s, the weight of spectacles mounted in the large frames that were fashionable at the time could have been added to this list. More recently, the reduction in frame size has largely eliminated this problem, but replaced it with one of inadequate reading areas in bifocals and (more notably) PALs. The spatial distortions brought about by the latter (Sullivan & Fowler 1993), which increase with add power (Sullivan & Fowler 1991; Simonet & Touche 1992), are reduced with smaller frames. In the early twenty-first century, lenses have become wider, but are still very shallow and both the old thickness/weight problems and the more recent lack of reading area have recurred, although developments in lens design have offset this to some degree. However, the introduction and popularity of many low-Abbe, higher-index materials for ophthalmic lenses have also increased the relevance of transverse chromatic aberration as a cause of dissatisfaction (Tang & Charman 1992).

The 'one size fits all' approach taken by many frame manufacturers has also brought about problems in the fit of frames, particularly side lengths, although to some extent this has been offset by the massive increase in frame models available.

Occupational and recreational prescribing

The circumstances under which spectacles are to be used must be considered when prescribing. At its simplest, this is a matter of ensuring that the near add of a presbyope is correct for the range of distances over which it will be used. However, the ergonomic situation in which the patient must function should be investigated further (**Fig. 22.4**). Factors external to the visual system which must be taken into consideration include those of a purely visual nature such as lighting levels, direction and glare, contrast of the task and the resolution required. There are also non-visual considerations such as the level and nature of any concurrent and non-concurrent activities, which can influence any prescribing decisions. These may not be immediately apparent without detailed questioning or workplace investigation.

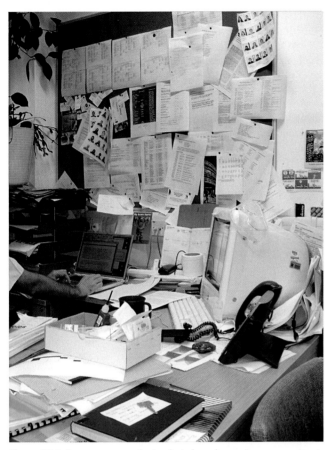

Figure 22.4 Even an apparently simple task, such as using a computer at a desk, can involve a more complex range of visual activities than it appears in the consulting room during the examination.

Occupational and recreational prescribing can have considerable overlap for any individual. What is considered an occupation for one person may be a recreation for another and vice versa. An alternative division is into hazardous and non-hazardous activities. For the appliance, this gives a natural division between formal safety standards (e.g. BS, EN, ISO, ANSI, DIN, etc.) and those for cosmetic and simple refractive eyewear. This is considered further in Chapter 29.

Occupational prescribing and disability

The UK Disability Discrimination Act (DDA) (1995) and similar legislation around the world have complicated visual task analysis and the occupational prescribing of spectacles considerably. Prior to this legislation, it was relatively easy for an employer or organization to set visual standards for any occupation. These could sometimes be justified, such as signal light recognition in maritime occupations. They could be based on a genuine but unsupported belief, such as the UK and European unaided vision standards for commercial vehicles (91/439/EEC 1991). They could even be wholly arbitrary. Requirements can be obtained from the body responsible for their enforcement, although there are also databases such as those of the Association of Optometrists in the UK (http://www.assoc-optometrists.org/services/services_visual.html).

The DDA has changed this, as it is now illegal to discriminate against anyone on the grounds of disability. Some occupational requirements are being modified on an 'evidence' basis. An example would be in police forces around the world (Sheedy et al 1983; Bachman 1994; Good et al 1998; Chisolm 2005), although even this does not take all eventualities into account (Anon 2006). A compounding factor is that required visual performance at entry into an occupation does not ensure that it will remain so throughout the potential career (Margrain et al 1996). It has been found that contact lenses may not be the obstacle they were once believed to be in some occupations (Makitie 1984; Sheedy 1986; Mittelman et al 1993), although in the case of the police, this has also been questioned (Wells et al 1997).

Although some disabilities are clearly defined, the term itself is not, and it may include non-registered individuals with any disability. 'Normal' categories such as strabismus, amblyopia and colour vision anomalies (Anon 2006), and perhaps even 'normal' refractive error and presbyopia may fall into this category. Dyslexia, with a prevalence of about 5–17% (Demonet et al 2004), has been formally accepted as a disability in the UK. Visual stress (Meares–Irlen) syndrome, with an even higher prevalence of 20–34% (Kriss & Evans 2005), is sometimes considered as such in education. Disability legislation is a legal minefield, and the optometrist should perhaps avoid involvement in the legal complexities. However, practical advice may be sought, and advice on illumination and non-standard optical aids is within the normal clinical remit.

The essential test of the UK Act is one of 'reasonable adjustment', and this should be borne in mind whenever analysis of a visual task is being done, as it has been shown that a very high proportion of occupations have what could be considered to be quite high visual demands (Parssinen et al 1987). What is considered 'reasonable adjustment', in the strict interpretation of the Act, may not be considered 'reasonable' by a school or employer, and this can cause conflict between patient, prescriber and organization. The following sections will concentrate principally on 'normal patients' and their task demands, and the reader should refer to the separate chapters on low vision, colour vision, binocular vision, etc., as appropriate.

Working distance

The working distance is one factor which must be taken into consideration when prescribing for presbyopic patients. It is essential to ask the patient about their visual requirements and not to make assumptions about the task. A typical example might be a computer user. It is common practice to assume the screen lies between 0.5 and 0.75 m away from the observer. However, this is not universal. Shorter working distances are common, particularly with laptops, while a patient with low vision could work at an extremely short distance, particularly if they are using a magnifier to view the screen. It is also widely assumed that hardcopy paperwork is carried out closer than when viewing a computer monitor, but this is a generalization best avoided (Burns et al 1993). Although 'working distance' is critical in determining the refractive correction, it should be borne in mind that for a majority of occupations, there is not just one working distance. There are no longer the great pools of copy typists and factories full of machine-tool operators that there were in the first three-quarters of the twentieth century. To this end, the prescriber must also bear in mind the availability of lens forms suitable for the overall task demands.

For a pre-presbyopic patient working within their range of accommodation, the principal effect of altering working distance is simply one of changing the angular subtense of the task detail and the accommodative demand. Reducing the working distance will clearly increase the angular subtense pro rata. An older, presbyopic patient will need an add for near work. Accommodation is usually assumed to follow the well-known decline shown by Donders (1864), Duane (1912) and others (see **Fig. 22.1**), although an effectively linear decline has also been suggested (Morgan 1960; Ramsdale & Charman 1989). The depth of focus of the eye is inversely related to pupil size (Charman 1983), which in turn is inversely related to both lighting level and age (Zinn 1972; Winn et al 1994) amongst other factors. It is therefore not surprising that many presbyopes report better visual performance from their spectacles at high illumination levels, although other factors are probably also involved.

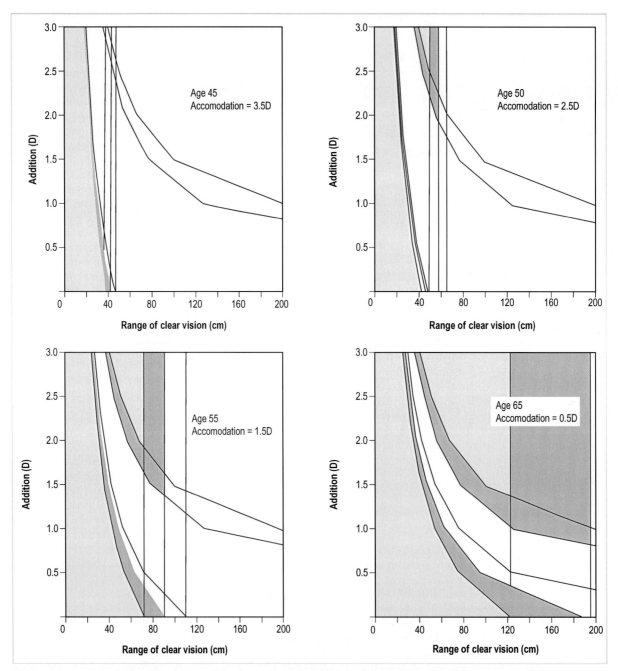

Figure 22.5 Accommodation, near addition, range of accommodation while unaided and depth of focus for nominal working distances of 33, 40, 50 and 60 cm using adds in 0.25 D steps. It is assumed that the eye can maintain 67% of its maximum accommodative effort. The addition which gives the closest near point within this distance is indicated across the bottom of each figure. The area to the top left of the diagrams represents the range of distances which are acceptably focused with only a distance correction and the patient's accommodation, assuming depths of focus of ±0.2 D and ±0.5 D. The area to the bottom right of each diagram represents the range of distances which are acceptably focused with a near correction, again assuming depths of focus of ±0.2 D and ±0.5 D. The unshaded area will be seen as out of focus with a bifocal lens for either depth of focus value, whilst the area of overlap between the two sections represents the range of distances which can be seen though either part of the bifocal lens.

The simplistic approach to accommodation, near adds and age often taken assumes zero depth of focus, even though the latter may be considerable in presbyopes. For a 3 mm pupil, the depth of focus can be as much as 1.2 D (Charman 1983). It was historically believed that the eye is able to use 67% of its accommodation for prolonged close work without discomfort (Emsley 1953; Tunnacliffe 1993), although a figure closer to 50% may be more correct (Morgan 1960; Millodot & Millodot 1989). **Figure 22.5** shows how the depth of focus affects the potential range of clear vision for the presbyopic eye exerting 67% of its accommodation, and for the eye with the lowest-powered add, in the usual 0.25 DS steps, which will allow the 'in focus' image to be just within 33 cm, 40 cm, 50 cm and 60 cm. It can be seen from **Figure 22.5** that older patients begin to get an 'intermediate distance' gap between distance and near corrections with the need for high adds/relatively short working distances at around 50–55 years of age. However, the figure for an eye nominally corrected for a longer working distance suffers less from this and the eye can often still manage to read at a 'normal' distance.

For practical purposes, working distances are often categorized into 'far' (over 2 m), intermediate (2 m to approx 66 cm), near (66–25 cm) and very near (<25 cm) (Grundy 1988). These are all rather arbitrary, although 'very near' is perhaps taken from the definition of magnification, with 25 cm being taken as 1×. With a reduced working distance, the demands on both the accommodation and convergence system increase. Thus, even a young patient may require an add for very fine tasks. It may also be necessary to prescribe prism to support the convergence system, partly because of the high demands placed upon it, but also because the use of plus power for near may compromise the established accommodation–convergence relationship (Dickinson 1998).

At extremely short working distances, binocular vision and stereopsis may no longer be viable using a simple spectacle correction (Dickinson 1998), although spectacles are readily available up to about 50 D (working distance = 2 cm), and monocular vision may have to be considered if a suitable stereomicroscope or similar device is not available.

Working position

Both the position of the observer and the location of the work must be considered. The field of view, line of sight and working distance of the principal task may be comparatively limited, as for an operator of many traditional machine tools, or much wider, such as for the controller of a modern computerized production facility overlooking both the workplace and visual display monitors.

Patients vary considerably whether they move their heads or their eyes to fixate an object at any given position, and this effect can be dependent on apparently small task variations (Proudlock et al 2003). However, when viewing for extended periods, the majority will tend to turn their eyes for objects close to the primary position and their head for greater angles. The obvious exceptions to this are bifocal and PAL users, who have to turn their eyes through quite a large angle to reach the optimum near power; typically these would be about 20° and 45°, respectively (**Fig. 22.6**). This has been reported as a source of discomfort after an extended period of computer use (Vasilieff & Dain 1986; Martin & Dain 1988; Jackson

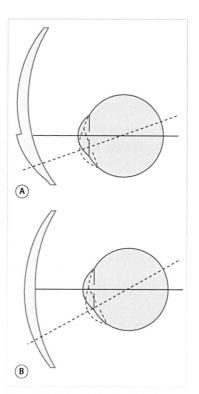

Figure 22.6 For a bifocal or PAL, the eye must turn through a considerable angle to see detail at near. For a bifocal (**A**), the top of the segment is typically 6–7 mm below the line of sight in the primary position. For a PAL (**B**), this distance can be as much as 18 mm.

et al 1997; Lyon et al 2003). Task-specific 'computer spectacles' have been shown to alleviate symptoms, although improvement of other ergonomic aspects of the workplace and lighting is also important, and it has been claimed that less than 5% of computer users need task-specific spectacles (Sheedy 1992; Bergqvist et al 1995; Thomson 1998; Balci & Aghazadeh 1998; Aaras et al 2001; Butzon et al 2002).

Symptoms are likely to arise if the observer is required to change viewing habits, such as performing a new task. Any underlying binocular vision anomalies may be exacerbated by unsuitable gaze positions, whilst the ability to converge can vary with eye position. This factor is easily overlooked in the consulting room, where convergence is conventionally tested in downgaze when a trial frame is used, but in the primary position with a phoropter. Fortunately, given a cooperative employer, it is often possible to make minor adjustments to the task, which may resolve these problems. However, there is still no simple solution for the plumber or electrician working upside down on a multiposition task in a cupboard! It should also be borne in mind that the visual performance for a static task is rather different from that of a moving one (Burg 1966), with the demands on the visual system being much higher in the dynamic situation for identical levels of task detail, particularly when the target motion is unpredictable.

Task detail and visual acuity

Figure 22.7 demonstrates that in order to resolve small details without the use of electronic or optical aids, the working distance can be reduced. However, evaluation of this, even for reading ordinary text, is seldom straightforward in

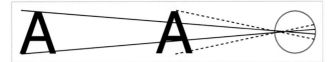

Figure 22.7 As an object is brought closer its angular subtense increases and detail becomes easier to resolve, provided it remains in focus.

a clinical setting. Apparently similar tasks such as reading a Snellen chart (composed of optotypes that are well spaced) and text are quite dissimilar, with 'crowding' serving to make the latter more difficult for some patients (Maraini et al 1963; Amos 1978). Indeed, the presence of words and a more suitable typeface can make near acuity testing easier (North & Jenkins 1951). On a purely mathematical basis, N5 upper-case 'Microsoft' Times font, which is generally considered to be good near visual acuity, subtends approximately 15′ of arc at 25 cm, which is the same overall angular subtense as a Snellen 6/18 letter. The lower case equivalent letter (N5) subtends 11.5′ of arc, which is equivalent to about 6/14.

Additionally, further difficulties arise because clinical acuity charts are far from standardized in practice. For example, contrast can vary from approximately 50% for a projector chart to 98% for a direct or rear-illuminated chart, with similar differences existing when comparing newspaper print and a high-quality textbook. Variations in font type, size and spacing must also be considered.

Task size varies not only with viewing distance but also with viewing angle. The angular subtense of detail on a plane surface decreases with the cosine of the angle through which the page has been tilted away from the normal to the line of sight. Hence, if a page is viewed at 45°, a reasonable angle for script lying flat on a desk, its vertical subtense is only 70% of that when the same script viewed normally (**Fig. 22.8**).

Grundy (1988) indicated that most people are capable of performing visual tasks requiring the perception of detail of 10′ of arc efficiently under normal lighting conditions. However, this would suggest that a person who has 6/5 acuity should be able to read N1.8 print at 25 cm. While this is possible, it is not something that many would choose to do, and certainly not for an extended period of time.

For tasks beyond the normal resolution limit of the eye, or for satisfactory visual comfort and performance with complex, demanding or prolonged tasks above that limit, magnification is required. Magnification is considered in detail under the heading of Low vision (see Ch. 30), and the situation is similar for the normally sighted individual, although the level of task detail and required working distances may differ significantly from those adopted by a low-vision patient.

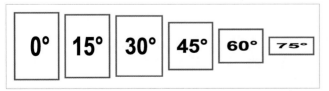

Figure 22.8 As a page is tilted from being normal to the line of sight, the angular subtense of detail decreases as the cosine of the angle through which the page has been tilted.

Conclusion

Prescribing spectacles is not a simple task. Although it is relatively easy to obtain a prescription for distance viewing, or for any given working distance, the long-term effect on visual function, the nature of the tasks being performed and the environment in which the prescription is to be used must be taken into consideration for the spectacles to function as the patient wishes.

References

91/439/EEC 1991 Second driving licence directive. European Commission, Brussels

Aaras A, Horgen G, Bjorset H H et al 2001 Musculoskeletal, visual and psychosocial stress in VDU operators before and after multidisciplinary ergonomic interventions. A 6 years prospective study-Part II. Applied Ergonomics 32:559–571

Achiron L R, Witkin N S 1998 The use of dissimilar progressives in the management of presbyopia. Survey of Ophthalmology 43:275–279

Adams D W, McBrien N A 1992 Prevalence of myopia and myopic progression in a population of clinical microscopists. Optometry and Vision Science 6:467–473

Adler D, Millodot M 2006 The possible effect of undercorrection on myopic progression in children. Clinical and Experimental Optometry 89:315–321

Amigo G 1968 Binocular balancing techniques. American Journal of Optometry and Archives of the American Academy of Optometry 45:511–522

Amos J F 1978 Refractive amblyopia: a differential diagnosis. Journal of the American Optometric Association 49:361–366

Anker S, Atkinson J, Braddick O et al 2004 Non-cycloplegic refractive screening can identify infants whose visual outcome at 4 years is improved by spectacle correction. Strabismus 12:227–245

Anon 2006 Police face legal battle over colour blindness. Glasgow Herald, 17 Oct 2006, p 4

Appleton B 1971 Ophthalmic prescription in half-diopter intervals. Patient acceptance. Archives of Ophthalmology 86:263–267

Association of Optometrists 2006 Visual Standards. Online. Available: http://www.assoc-optometrists.org/services/services_visual.html

Atchison D A, Schmid K L, Edwards K P et al 2001 The effect of under and over refractive correction on visual performance and spectacle lens acceptance. Ophthalmic and Physiological Optics 21:255–261

Atkinson J, Braddick O 1983 The use of isotropic photorefraction for vision screening in infants. Acta Ophthalmologica Supplement 1983:36–45

Atkinson J, Anker S, Bobier W et al 2000 Normal emmetropization in infants with spectacle correction for hyperopia. Investigative Ophthalmology and Visual Science 41:3726–3731

Attebo K, Ivers R Q, Mitchell P 1989 Refractive errors in an older population: the Blue Mountains Eye Study. Ophthalmology 106:1066–1072

Aves O 1926 Some notes and statistical tables on the relative distribution of refractive defects and their correction. Proceedings of the Optical Convention, 1926 (1):424–450

Avitabile T, Marano F 2001 Multifocal intra-ocular lenses. Current Opinion in Ophthalmology 12:12–16

Bachman W G 1994 Enhanced vision screening of highway patrol applicants. Optometry and Vision Science 71:286–289

Baker F J, Gilmartin B 2003 A longitudinal study of vergence adaptation in incipient presbyopia. Ophthalmic and Physiological Optics 23:507–511

Balci R, Aghazadeh F 1998 Influence of VDT monitor positions on discomfort and performance of users with or without bifocal lenses. Journal of Human Ergology Tokyo 27:62–69

Ball G V 1982 Symptoms in eye examination. Butterworth, London, pp 37–46, pp 78–85

Bannon R E 1977 A new automated subjective optometer. American Journal of Optometry and Physiological Optics 54:433–438

Bennett A G 1965 Lens usage in the Supplementary Ophthalmic Service. Optician Feb 12:131–137

Bergqvist U, Wolgast E, Nilsson B et al 1995 Musculoskeletal disorders among visual display terminal workers: individual, ergonomic, and work organizational factors. Ergonomics 38:763–776

Beau Seigneur W 1946 Changes in power and axis of cylindrical errors after convergence. American Journal of Optometry and Physiological Optics 23:111–121

Blakeney S 2006 Recent disciplinary cases and issues they raise. Optometry in Practice 7:125–130

Blystone P A 1999 Relationship between age and presbyopic addition using a sample of 3,645 examinations from a single private practice. Journal of the American Optometric Association 70:505–508

Borish I M 1983 Aphakia: perceptual and refractive problems of spectacle correction. Journal of the American Optometric Association 54:701–711

Bourne R R A, Dineen B P, Ali S M et al 2004 Prevalence of refractive error in Bangladeshi adults: results of the National Blindness and Low Vision Survey of Bangladesh. Ophthalmology 111:1150–1160

Boyce P R 1973 Age, illuminance, visual performance and preference. Lighting Research and Technology 5:125–144

Brown W L 2006 Revisions to tolerances in cylinder axis and in progressive addition lens power in ANSI Z80.1–2005. Optometry 77:343–349

BS EN 1836 2005 Personal eye protection. Sunglasses, sunglare filters for general use and filters for direct observation of the sun. British Standards Institution, London

BS 2738–1 1998 Spectacle lenses. Specification for tolerances on optical properties of mounted spectacle lenses. British Standards Institution, London

BS 2738–3 2004 Spectacle lenses. Specification for the presentation of prescriptions and prescription orders for ophthalmic lenses. British Standards Institution, London

Bullimore M A, Fusaro R E, Adams C W 1998 The repeatability of automated and clinician refraction. Optometry and Vision Science 75:617–622

Burg A 1966 Visual acuity as measured by dynamic and static tests: a comparative evaluation. Journal of Applied Psychology 50:460–466

Burns D, Obstfeld H, Saunders J 1993 Prescribing for presbyopes who use VDUs. Ophthalmic and Physiological Optics 13:409–414

Butzon S P, Sheedy J E, Nilsen E 2002 The efficacy of computer glasses in reduction of computer worker symptoms. Optometry 73:221–230

Calder-Gillie J 1961 The anisometropic presbyope. British Journal of Physiological Optics 18:174–180

Campbell F W, Weir J B 1953 The depth of focus of the human eye. Journal of Physiology 120:59P–60P

Carter D B, Allen D C 1973 Evaluation of the placebo effect in optometry. American Journal of Optometry and Archives of the American Academy of Optometry 50:94–103

Charman W N 1983 The retinal image in the human eye. Progress in retinal research. Pergammon, Oxford, pp 1–50

Charman W N, Voisin L 1993 Optical aspects of tolerances to uncorrected ocular astigmatism. Optometry and Vision Science 70:111–117

Chisolm C M 2005 New vision standards for police constable recruits. Optometry in Practice 6:131–140

Cholerton M 1955 Low refractive errors. British Journal of Physiological Optics 12:82–86

Ciuffreda K J, Rosenfield M, Chen H W 1997 The AC/A ratio, age and presbyopia. Ophthalmic and Physiological Optics 17:307–315

Coates W R 1955 Amplitudes of accommodation in South Africa. British Journal of Physiological Optics 12:76–86

College of Optometrists 2006 Section 38, Guidance for the Issuing of Small Prescriptions. College of Optometrists, London

Cotter S A, Edwards A R, Wallace D K et al 2006 Treatment of anisometropic amblyopia in children with refractive correction. Ophthalmology 113:895–903

Daum K M 1983 Accommodative dysfunction. Documenta Ophthalmologica 55:177–198

Daum K M, Clore K A, Simms S S et al 2004 Productivity associated with visual status of computer users. Optometry 75:33–47

Demonet J-F, Taylor M J, Chaix Y 2004 Developmental dyslexia. Lancet 363:1451–1460

Dickinson C M 1998 Low vision principles and practice. Butterworth-Heineman, London, pp 77–111, pp 112–120

Dirani M, Chamberlain M, Garoufalis P et al 2006 Refractive errors in twin studies. Twin Research and Human Genetics 9:566–572

Disability Discrimination Act 1995 HMSO, London

Donders F C 1864 On the anomalies of accommodation and refraction of the eye. The New Sydenham Society, London, pp 179–188

Duane A 1912 Normal values of accommodation at all ages. Journal of the American Medical Association 59:1010–1013

Emsley H H 1953 Visual optics. Butterworth, London, pp 195–223

Evans B J 2005 The need for optometric investigation in suspected Meares-Irlen syndrome or visual stress. Ophthalmic and Physiological Optics 25:363–370

Evans B J 2006 Orthoptic indications for contact lens wear. Contact Lens and Anterior Eye 29:175–181

Evans B J, Patel R, Wilkins A J et al 1999 A review of the management of 323 consecutive patients seen in a specific learning difficulties clinic. Ophthalmic and Physiological Optics 19:454–466

Fledelius H C 1984 Prevalences of astigmatism and anisometropia in adult Danes. With reference to presbyopes' possible use of supermarket standard glasses. Acta Ophthalmologica (Copenh) 62:391–400

Fletcher R J 1952 Astigmatic accommodation. British Journal of Physiological Optics 9:8–32

Fletcher T 1967 Stock keeping and the usage of various sights. FMO technical conference proceedings. Federation of Manufacturing Opticians, London

Fonda G 1970 Management of the patient with subnormal vision. CV Mosby, St Louis, pp 62–64

Fontaine N, Simonet P, Gresset J 1997 Optical performance of aspheric concave ophthalmic lenses: the effect of vertex distance. Optometry and Vision Science 74:211–221

French C N, Jennings J A M 1974 Errors in subjective refraction – an exploratory study. Ophthalmic Optician Sept 7:797–806

Giles G H 1960 The principles and practice of refraction. Hammond Hammond, London

Glover C, Greensmith S, Ranftler A et al 2006 Guidelines on the management of headaches – Part 1. Optician 231(6036):20–33

Goar E L 1957 Contact lenses in monocular aphakia. Archives of Ophthalmology 58:417–420

Good G W, Maisel S C, Kriska S D 1998 Setting an uncorrected visual acuity standard for police officer applicants. Journal of Applied Psychology 83:17–24

Goss D A 1994 Effect of spectacle correction on the progression of myopia in children – a literature review. Journal of the American Optometric Association 65:117–128

Goss D A, Grosvenor T 1996 Reliability of refraction – a literature review. Journal of the American Optometric Association 67:619–630

Graf H P, Flammer J 1980 Asthenopia in clinical practice: a comparative study of complaints, clinical findings and results of therapy in asthenopic patients. Klinische Monatsblatter fur Augenheilkunde 176:577–582

Granet D B, Christian W, Gomi C E et al 2006 Treatment options for anisohyperopia. Journal of Pediatric Ophthalmology and Strabismus 43:207–211

Greenwald M J, Glaser S R 1998 Visual outcomes after surgery for unilateral cataract in children more than two years old: posterior chamber intraocular lens implantation versus contact lens correction of aphakia. Journal of AAPOS 2:168–176

Gronlund M A, Andersson S, Aring E et al 2006 Ophthalmological findings in a sample of Swedish children aged 4–15 years. Acta Ophthalmologica Scandinavica 84:169–176

Grosvenor T 2003 Why is there an epidemic of myopia? Clinical and Experimental Optometry 86:273–275

Grundy J 1988 Ch. 33, Prescribing and patient management: occupational and recreational considerations. In: Edwards K, Llewellyn R (eds) Optometry. Butterworths, London, pp 475–485

Gudmundsdottir E, Jonasson F, Jonsson V et al 2000 'With the rule' astigmatism is not the rule in the elderly. Reykjavik Eye Study: a population based study of refraction and visual acuity in citizens of Reykjavik 50 years and older. Iceland-Japan Co-Working Study Groups. Acta Ophthalmologica Scandinavica 78:642–646

Gudmundsdottir E, Arnarsson A, Jonasson F 2005 Five-year refractive changes in an adult population: Reykjavik Eye Study. Ophthalmology 112:672–677

Gupta M, Gupta Y 2000 A survey on refractive error and strabismus among children in a school at Aligarh. Indian Journal of Public Health 44:90–93

Guyton D L 1977 Prescribing cylinders. The problem of distortion. Survey of Ophthalmology 22:177–188

Guzowski M, Wang J J, Rochtchina E et al 2003 Five-year refractive changes in an older population: the Blue Mountains Eye Study. Ophthalmology 110:1364–1370

Gwiazda J, Thorn F 1998 Development of refraction and strabismus. Current Opinion in Ophthalmology 9:3–9

Gwiazda J, Thorn F 1999 Development of refraction and strabismus. Current Opinion in Ophthalmology 10:293–299

Gwiazda J E, Hyman L, Norton T T et al 2004 Accommodation and related risk factors associated with myopia progression and their interaction with treatment in COMET children. Investigative Ophthalmology and Visual Science 45:2143–2151

Haegerstrom-Portnoy G, Schneck M E, Brabyn J A et al 2002 Development of refractive errors into old age. Optometry and Vision Science 79:643–649

Halass S 1959 Aniseikonic lenses of improved design and their application. Australian Journal of Optometry 42:387–393

Hanlon S D, Nakabayashi J, Shigezawa G 1987 A critical review of presbyopic add determination. Journal of the American Optometric Association 58:468–472

Harle D E, Evans B J 2006 The correlation between migraine headache and refractive errors. Optometry and Vision Science 83:82–87

Harvey E M, Dobson V, Miller J M et al 2004 Treatment of astigmatism-related amblyopia in 3- to 5-year-old children. Vision Research 44:1623–1634

Harvey E M, Miller J M, Dobson V et al 2005 Prescribing eyeglass correction for astigmatism in infancy and early childhood: a survey of AAPOS members. Journal of AAPOS 9:189–191

Hashemi H, Fotouhi A, Mohammad K 2004 The age- and gender-specific prevalences of refractive errors in Tehran: the Tehran Eye Study. Ophthalmic Epidemiology 11:213–225

Hendrickson K, Bleything W 2001 The visual profile of Romanian children and adults assessed through vision screenings. Optometry 72:388–396

Henson D B, North R 1980 Adaptation to prism-induced heterophoria. American Journal of Optometry and Physiological Optics 57:129–137

Hirai T, Sato M, Piao C H et al 2004 Dynamic aniseikonia measurement: prismatic effect appears on the Hess chart. Binocular Vision and Strabismus Quarterly 19:234–245

Hirsch M J 1961 Refractive changes with age. In: Hirsch M J, Wick R E (eds) Vision of the ageing patient. Hammond Hammond, London, pp 63–82

Holmes J M, Clarke M P 2006 Amblyopia. Lancet 367:1343–1351

Horwood A M 1998 Compliance with first time spectacle wear in children under eight years of age. Eye 12:173–178

Horwood J, Waylen A, Herrick D et al 2005 Common visual defects and peer victimization in children. Investigative Ophthalmology and Visual Science 46:1177–1181

Howland H C 1974 Photorefraction: a technique for study of refractive state at a distance. Journal of the Optical Society of America 64:240–249

Howland H C, Sayles N 1984 Photorefractive measurements of astigmatism in infants and young children. Investigative Ophthalmology and Visual Science 25:93–102

Humphriss D 1958 Periodic refractive fluctuations in the healthy eye. British Journal of Physiological Optics 15:30–44

Hunter H Jr, Shipp M 1997 A study of racial differences in age at onset and progression of presbyopia. Journal of the American Optometric Association 68:171–177

Hutter R F, Rouse M W 1984 Visually related headache in a preschooler. American Journal of Physiological Optics 61:711–713

Huynh S C, Kifley A, Rose K A et al 2006a Astigmatism and its components in 6-year-old children. Investigative Ophthalmology and Visual Science 47:55–64

Huynh S C, Wang X Y, Ip J et al 2006b Prevalence and associations of anisometropia and aniso-astigmatism in a population based sample of 6 year old children. British Journal of Ophthalmology 90:597–601

Ingram R M, Walker C, Wilson J M et al 1986 Prediction of amblyopia and squint by means of refraction at age 1 year. British Journal of Ophthalmology 70:12–15

Ingram R M, Arnold P E, Dally S et al 1990 Results of a randomised trial of treating abnormal hypermetropia from the age of 6 months. British Journal of Ophthalmology 74:158–159

Ingram R M, Gill L E, Lambert T W 2000 Effect of spectacles on changes of spherical hypermetropia in infants who did, and did not, have strabismus. British Journal of Ophthalmology 84:324–326

Jackson A J, Barnett E S, Stevens A B et al 1997 Vision screening, eye examination and risk assessment of display screen users in a large regional teaching hospital. Ophthalmic and Physiological Optics 17:187–195

Jackson E 1932 Norms of refraction. Journal of the American Medical Association 98:132–137

Jacobi F K, Zrenner E, Broghammer M et al 2005 A genetic perspective on myopia. Cellular and Molecular Life Sciences 62:800–808

Jain I S, Ram J, Gupta A 1982 Early onset of presbyopia. American Journal of Optometry and Physiological Optics 59:1002–1004

Jalie M 1980 The principles of ophthalmic lenses, 3rd edn. Association of Dispensing Opticians, London

Jennings J A M, Charman W N 1973 A comparison of errors in some methods of subjective refraction. Ophthalmic Optician Jan 6:6–18

Jimenez J R, Rubino M, Díaz J A et al 2000 Changes in stereoscopic depth perception caused by decentration of spectacle lenses. Optometry and Vision Science 77:421–427

Johnson B L, Edwards J S, Goss D A et al 1996 A comparison of three subjective tests for astigmatism and their interexaminer reliabilities. Journal of the American Optometric Association 67:590–598

Junghans B M, Crewther S G 2005 Little evidence for an epidemic of myopia in Australian primary school children over the last 30 years. B M C Ophthalmology 5:1

Karania R, Evans B J 2006 The Mallett Fixation Disparity Test: influence of test instructions and relationship with symptoms. Ophthalmic and Physiological Optics 26:507–522

Katz J, Tielsch J M, Sommer A 1997 Prevalence and risk factors for refractive errors in an adult inner city population. Investigative Ophthalmology and Visual Science 38:334–340

Kirkness C M, Weale R A 1985 Does light pose a hazard to the macula in aphakia? Transactions of the Ophthalmological Society of the United Kingdom 104:699–702

Kommerell G, Kromeier M 2002 Prism correction and heterophoria. Ophthalmology 99:3–9

Kommerell G, Gerling J, Ball M et al 2000 Heterophoria and fixation disparity: a review. Strabismus 8:127–134

Kozol F 1996 Compensation procedures for the anisometropic presbyope. Survey of Ophthalmology 41:171–174

Kragha I K 1985 Bifocal adds in Nigeria. American Journal of Optometry and Physiological Optics 62:781–785

Kragha I K, Hofstetter H W 1986 Bifocal adds and environmental temperature. American Journal of Optometry and Physiological Optics 63:372–376

Kriss I, Evans B J W 2005 The relationship between dyslexia and Meares-Irlen syndrome. Journal of Research in Reading 28:350–364

Krzizok T, Kaufmann H, Schwerdtfeger G 1996 Binokulare Probleme durch Aniseikonie und Anisophorie nach Katarakt-Operation. Klinische Monatsblatter fur Augenheilkunde 208:477–480

Krumholtz I 2000 Results from a pediatric vision screening and its ability to predict academic performance. Optometry 71:426–430

Kuo A, Sinatra R B, Donahue S P 2003 Distribution of refractive error in healthy infants. Journal of AAPOS 7:174–177

Lambert S R 1999 Management of monocular congenital cataracts. Eye 13:474–479

Langenbucher A, Seitz B 2003 Computerized calculation scheme for bitoric eikonic intraocular lenses. Ophthalmic and Physiological Optics 23:213–220

Lebensohn J E 1953 Anisophoria, anisometropia, and the final prescription. American Journal of Ophthalmology 36:643–649

Legras R, Chateau N, Charman W N 2004 Assessment of just-noticeable differences for refractive errors and spherical aberration using visual simulation. Optometry and Vision Science 81:718–728

Lyon J L Jr, Lillquist D R, Alder S et al 2003 An analysis of VDT monitor placement and daily hours of use for female bifocal users. Work 20:77–80

Lyons S A, Jones L A, Walline J J et al 2004 A survey of clinical prescribing philosophies for hyperopia. Optometry and Vision Science 814:233–237

McBrien N A, Adams D W 1997 A longitudinal investigation of adult-onset and adult-progression of myopia in an occupational group. Refractive and biometric findings. Investigative Ophthalmology and Visual Science 38:321–333

Maclure G M 1980 Reading type for children. British Journal of Ophthalmology 64:461–465

McKelvie S J 1997 Perception of faces with and without spectacles. Perceptual and Motor Skills 84:497–498

Mailer C M 1978 Automatic refraction and the private ophthalmologist: Dioptron II compared with subjective examination. Canadian Journal of Ophthalmology 13:252–257

Makitie J 1984 Contact lenses and the work environment. Acta Ophthalmologica Supplement 161:115–122

Mallett R F J 1974 Fixation disparity – its genesis and relation to asthenopia. Ophthalmic Optician 14:1159–1160, 1166–1168

Maraini G, Pasino L, Peralta S 1963 Visual acuity in amblyopia. II. Crowding. Ophthalmologica 145:7–12

Margrain T H, Owen C G, Woodward E G 1996 Prevalence of spectacle and contact lens wear in the UK fire service. Ophthalmic and Physiological Optics 16:11–18

Martin D K, Dain S J 1988 Postural modifications of VDU operators wearing bifocal spectacles. Applied Ergonomics 19:293–300

Mayer D L, Hansen R M, Moore B D et al 2001 Cycloplegic refractions in healthy children aged 1 through 48 months. Archives of Ophthalmology 119:1625–1628

Miller E M, Harvey J M 1998 Spectacle prescribing recommendations of the AAPOS. Journal of Paediatric Ophthalmology and Strabismus 59:983–986

Millodot M, Millodot S 1989 Presbyopia correction and the accommodation in reserve. Ophthalmic and Physiological Optics 9:126–132

Miranda M N 1979 The geographic factor in the onset of presbyopia. Transactions of the American Ophthalmological Society 77:603–621

Mitchell D E, Freeman R D, Millodot M et al 1973 Meridional amblyopia: evidence for modification of the human visual system by early visual experience. Vision Research 13:535–558

Mittelman M H, Siegel B, Still D L 1993 Contact lenses in aviation: the Marine Corps experience. Aviation Space and Environmental Medicine 64:538–540

Mohindra I 1977 A non-cycloplegic refraction technique for infants and young children. Journal of the American Optometric Association 48:518–523

Montes-Mico R 2000 Astigmatism in infancy and childhood. Journal of Pediatric Ophthalmology and Strabismus 37:349–353

Morgan M W 1960 Accommodative changes in presbyopia and their correction. In: Hirsch M J, Wick R E (eds) Vision of the ageing patient. Hammond Hammond, London, pp 83–112

Murphy P J, Beck A J, Coll E P 2002 An assessment of the orthogonal astigmatism test for the subjective measurement of astigmatism. Ophthalmic and Physiological Optics 22:194–200

Nathan J 1957 Small errors of refraction. British Journal of Physiological Optics 59:983–986

Nicholson S B, Garzia R P 1988 Astigmatism at nearpoint: adventitious, purposeful, and environmental influences. Journal of the American Optometric Association 59:936–941

Nordlow W 1970 Anisometropia, amblyopia, induced aniseikonia and estimated correction with iseikonic lenses in 4-year-olds. Acta Ophthalmologica (Copenh) 48:959–970

North A J, Jenkins L B 1951 Reading speed and comprehension as a function of typography. Journal of Applied Psychology 35:225–228

North R, Henson D B 1985 Adaptation to lens-induced heterophorias. American Journal of Optometry and Physiological Optics 62:774–780

Obstfeld H 1967 Spectacle lens prescriptions. Ophthalmic Optician 7:914–932

Obstfeld H 1969 Spectacle lens prescriptions. American Journal of Optometry and Archives of the American Academy of Optometry 46:882–885

Obstfeld H 1982 Optics in vision, 2nd edn. Butterworths, London

Obstfeld H 1988 Ch. 32, General considerations in prescribing. In: Edwards K, Llewellyn R (eds) Optometry. Butterworths, London, pp 465–474

O'Leary C I, Evans B J 2003 Criteria for prescribing optometric interventions: literature review and practitioner survey. Ophthalmic and Physiological Optics 23:429–439

O'Leary C I, Evans B J 2006 Double-masked randomised placebo-controlled trial of the effect of prismatic corrections on rate of reading and the relationship with symptoms. Ophthalmic and Physiological Optics 26:555–565

Ong J 1981 Southeastern Asian refugees' presbyopia. Perceptual and Motor Skills 53:667–670

Ong E, Grice K, Held R et al 1999 Effects of spectacle intervention on the progression of myopia in children. Optometry and Vision Science 76:363–369

Osuobeni E P, al-Zughaibi A M 1993 Induced prismatic effect in spectacle prescriptions sampled in Saudi Arabia. Optometry and Vision Science 70:160–166

Parssinen O, Saari K M, Kirjonen J 1987 Need for near vision in daily work in different occupational groups. Scandinavian Journal of Social Medicine 15:37–40

Perrigin J, Perrigin D, Grosvenor T 1982 A comparison of clinical refractive data obtained by three examiners. American Journal of Optometry and Physiological Optics 59:515–519

Pointer J S 2002 Gender-related optical aspects of the onset of presbyopia. Ophthalmic and Physiological Optics 22:126–129

Pointer J S 1995a The presbyopic add. II. Age-related trend and a gender difference. Ophthalmic and Physiological Optics 15:241–248

Pointer J S 1995b Broken down by age and sex. The optical correction of presbyopia revisited. Ophthalmic and Physiological Optics 15:439–443

Pouliquen de Liniere M, Hervault C, Meillon J P et al 1998 Anisométropie et presbytie: equipements en verres progressifs, nouvelle approche. Journal Francais d'ophtalmologie 21:321–327

Press L J 1985 Physiological effects of plus lens applications. American Journal of Optometry and Physiological Optics 62:392–397

Priest M J 1979 Non-tolerance in the NHS. Ophthalmic Optician 19:221–223

Proudlock F A, Shekhar H, Gottlob I 2003 Coordination of eye and head movements during reading. Investigative Ophthalmology and Visual Science 44:2991–2998

Quek T P L, Chua C G, Chong C S et al 2004 Prevalence of refractive errors in teenage high school students in Singapore. Ophthalmic and Physiological Optics 24:47–55

Ramsdale C, Charman W N 1989 A longitudinal study of the changes in the static accommodation response. Ophthalmic and Physiological Optics 9:255–263

Remole A 1989 Anisophoria and aniseikonia. Part I. The relation between optical anisophoria and aniseikonia. Optometry and Vision Science 66:659–670

Richer S P, Adams A J, Little A C 1985 Toward the design of an optimal filter for enhancement of dichromat monocular chromatic discrimination. American Journal of Optometry and Physiological Optics 62:105–110

Robaei D, Rose K, Ojaimi E et al 2005 Visual acuity and the causes of visual loss in a population-based sample of 6-year-old Australian children. Ophthalmology 112:1275–1282

Robaei D, Rose K A, Ojaimi E et al 2006 Causes and associations of amblyopia in a population-based sample of 6-year-old Australian children. Archives of Ophthalmology 124:878–884

Roorda A, Bobier W R, Campbell M C 1998 An infrared eccentric photo-optometer. Vision Research 38:1913–1924

Rosenfield M 1997 Accommodation. In: Zadnik K (ed.) The ocular examination. Measurement and findings. Saunders, Philadelphia, pp 87–121

Rosenfield M, Chiu N N 1995 Repeatability of subjective and objective refraction. Optometry and Vision Science 72:577–579

Rosenfield M, Ciuffreda K J, Chen H W 1995 Effect of age on the interaction between the AC/A and CA/C ratios. Ophthalmic and Physiological Optics 15:451–455

Saunders K J, Woodhouse J M, Westall C A 1995 Emmetropisation in human infancy: rate of change is related to initial refractive error. Vision Research 35:1325–1328

Saw S M 2003 A synopsis of the prevalence rates and environmental risk factors for myopia. Clinical and Experimental Optometry 86:289–294

Saw S M, Gazzard G, Au Eong K G et al 2002 Myopia: attempts to arrest progression. British Journal of Ophthalmology 86:1306–1311

Scheiman M, Cotter S, Rouse M et al 2005 Randomised clinical trial of the effectiveness of base-in prism reading glasses versus placebo reading glasses for symptomatic convergence insufficiency in children. British Journal of Ophthalmology 89:1318–1323

Schipper I 1985 Anisophoria after implantation of an intraocular lens. Journal of the American Intraocular Implant Society 11:290–291

Shapiro I J 1995 Parallel-testing infinity balance. Instrument and technique for the parallel testing of binocular vision. Optometry and Vision Science 72:916–923

Sheedy J E 1986 Contact lenses for police officers. Journal of the American Optometric Association no. 57:658–660

Sheedy J E 1992 Vision problems at video display terminals: a survey of optometrists. Journal of the American Optometric Association 63:687–692

Sheedy J E, Saladin J J 1975 Exophoria at near in presbyopia. American Journal of Physiological Optics 52:474–481

Sheedy J E, Keller J T, Pitts D et al 1983 Recommended vision standards for police officers. Journal of the American Optometric Association 54:925–928

Simonet P, Touche M 1992 Progressive addition lens channel dimension as a function of addition power. Ophthalmic and Physiological Optics 12:390–391

Sloane A E, Dunphy E B, Emmons W V et al 1954 A comparison of refraction results on the same individuals. American Journal of Ophthalmology 37:696–699

Sorsby A, Leary G A 1969 A longitudinal study of refraction and its components during growth. HMSO, London Medical Research Council, Special Report Series no. 309, pp 1–41

Stewart-Brown S 1985 Spectacle prescribing among 10-year-old children. British Journal of Ophthalmology 69:874–880

Sullivan C M, Fowler C W 1991 Reading addition analysis of progressive addition lenses. Ophthalmic and Physiological Optics 11:147–155

Sullivan C M, Fowler C M 1993 Visual detection and adaptation to optically induced curvature distortion – does curvature distortion govern progressive addition lens tolerance. Applied Optics 32:4138–4143

Tang C Y 1989 Influence of lens vertex distance changes on prismatic effect and decentration. Optometry and Vision Science 66:591–593

Tang C Y, Charman W N 1992 Effects of monochromatic and chromatic oblique aberrations on visual performance during spectacle lens wear. Ophthalmic and Physiological Optics 12:340–349

Tanlamai T, Goss D A 1979 Prevalence of monocular amblyopia among anisometropes. American Journal of Physiological Optics 56:704–715

Tassman J S 1932 Frequency of various kinds of refractive errors. American Journal of Ophthalmology 15:1044–1053

Terry R L, Stockton L A 1993 Eyeglasses and children's schemata. The Journal of Social Psychology 133:425–438

Terry R L, Berg A J, Phillips P E 1983 The effect of eyeglasses on self-esteem. Journal of the American Optometric Association 54:947–949

Thomas E, Boardman H F, Ogden H et al 2004 Advice and care for headaches: who seeks it, who gives it? Cephalalgia 24:740–752

Thomson W D 1998 Eye problems and visual display terminals – the facts and the fallacies. Ophthalmic and Physiological Optics 18:111–119

Townshend A M, Holmes J M, Evans L S 1993 Depth of anisometropic amblyopia and difference in refraction. American Journal of Ophthalmology 116:431–436

Troilo D 1992 Neonatal eye growth and emmetropisation – a literature review. Eye 6:154–160

Tunnacliffe A H 1993 Introduction to visual optics. Accommodation. ABDO, London, pp 181–233

Tunnacliffe A H, Williams A T 1985 The effect of vertical differential prism on the binocular contrast sensitivity function. Ophthalmic and Physiological Optics 5:417–424

Ukai K, Ichihashi Y 1991 Changes in ocular astigmatism over the whole range of accommodation. Optometry and Vision Science 68:813–818

Vaithilingam E, Khare B B 1967 Ocular headache and the optometrist. Journal of the American Optometric Association 38:477–479

Vasilieff A, Dain S 1986 Bifocal wearing and VDU operation: a review and graphical analysis. Applied Ergonomics 17:82–86

von Helmholtz H 1924 Treatise on physiological optics. Electronic edition 2001, University of Pennsylvania

von Hofsten C 1979 Recalibration of the convergence system. Perception 8:37–42

Wallace D K, Carlin D S, Wright J D 2006 Evaluation of the accuracy of estimation retinoscopy. Journal of AAPOS 10:232–236

Walline J J, Jones L A, Chitkara M et al 2006 The Adolescent and Child Health Initiative to Encourage Vision Empowerment (ACHIEVE) study design and baseline data. Optometry Vision Science 83:37–45

Walsh G 2001a The products we rely on: part 4. Prismatic effect on lenses. Optometry Today 41(21):36–42

Walsh G 2001b The products we rely on: part 3. Tints and coatings. Optometry Today 41(19):40–45

Walsh G, Pearce I 2006 Is the spectacle lens jack in the box phenomenon really due to the lenses. Ophthalmic Physiological Optics 26:116–119

Wang B, Ciuffreda K J 2006 Depth-of-focus of the human eye: theory and clinical implications. Survey of Ophthalmology 51:75–85

Weale R A 1963 The ageing eye. Lewis, London

Weale R A 1981 Human ocular aging and ambient temperature. British Journal of Ophthalmology 65:869–870

Weale R A 2002 On the age-related prevalence of anisometropia. Ophthalmic Research 34:389–392

Weale R A 2003 Epidemiology of refractive errors and presbyopia. Survey of Ophthalmology 48:515–543

Weiss R A, Berke W, Gottlieb L et al 2002 Clinical importance of accurate refractor vertex distance measurements prior to refractive surgery. Journal of Refractive Surgery 18:444–448

Wells G A, Brown J J, Casson E J et al 1997 To wear or not to wear: current contact lens use in the Royal Canadian Mounted Police. Canadian Journal of Ophthalmology 32:158–162

Welsh K W, Vaughan J A, Rasmussen P G 1979 Aeromedical implications of the X-Chrom lens for improving color vision deficiencies. Aviation Space and Environmental Medicine 50:249–255

West D, Somers W W 1984 Binocular balance validity: a comparison of five common subjective techniques. Ophthalmic and Physiological Optics 4:155–159

Wharry R E, Kirkpatrick S W 1986 Vision and academic performance of learning disabled children. Perception and Motor Skills 62:323–336

Wick B 1985 Clinical factors in proximal vergence. American Journal of Physiological Optics 62:1–18

Winn B, Ackerley R G, Brown C A et al 1988 Reduced aniseikonia in axial anisometropia with contact lens correction. Ophthalmic and Physiological Optics 8:341–344

Winn B, Whitaker D, Elliott D B et al 1994 Factors affecting light-adapted pupil size in normal human subjects. Investigative Ophthalmology and Visual Science 35:1132–1137

Wong T Y, Foster P J, Hee J et al 2000 Prevalence and risk factors for refractive errors in adult Chinese in Singapore. Investigative Ophthalmology and Visual Science 41:2486–2494

Woo W W, Lim K A, Yang H et al 2004 Refractive errors in medical students in Singapore. Singapore Medical Journal 45:470–474

Xu L, Li J, Cui T et al 2005 Refractive error in urban and rural adult Chinese in Beijing. Ophthalmology 112:1676–1683

Zamorini G, Merlin U, Dalfiume E 1964 Utilita delle lenti a contatto nelle anisometropie di alto grado. Annali di Ottalmologia e Clinica Oculistica 90:479–482

Zinn K M 1972 The pupil. C C Thomas, Springfield IL

CHAPTER 23

Alternative vision correction

Shehzad A Naroo

Introduction

Alternative vision correction can encompass a range of techniques, optical aids and surgery that allow the patient's refractive error to be corrected without the aid of spectacles or contact lenses. In this chapter, many methods will be discussed and these will include the latest techniques in most cases. Some of these procedures are likely to change dramatically over the next 5–10 years as new and improved techniques are developed.

History of vision correction

Optical aids for the correction of refractive error date back to ancient times. In the fourth century BC, Seneca is said to have 'read all the books in Rome' through a glass globe filled with water. Apparently, Emperor Nero watched gladiator fights through an emerald held to his eye, although no explanation of why he did this has been proposed. He either used the properties of the emerald to focus light onto his retina, suffered from photophobia or perhaps found that a red-free filter shielded an unsightly blood colour. In 1025, Abu-Ali Al-Hasan Ibn Al-Haytham (known as Alhazen in the Occident) wrote a treatise on optics, which became the blueprint on the subject for almost 500 years. In 1268, Roger Bacon mentioned a convex magnifying lens in his Opus Majus.

The identity of the inventor of spectacles is vague but is often attributed to either Salvino D'Armante or Alessandro Spina of Italy in the thirteenth century. Di Popoza, an Italian notable, wrote in 1289, 'I am so debilitated by age that without the glasses known as spectacles I would no longer be able to read or write.' The use of spectacles to correct myopia probably dates back to a similar time. Pope Leo X, painted by Raphael between 1517 and 1519, is depicted holding a concave lens, which he is famously said to have used to improve his myopia whilst hunting.

The history of contact lenses dates back to Leonardo da Vinci, who, in 1508, described several forms of rudimentary contact lenses. His suggestion of a water-filled glass to neutralize the refractive power of the cornea probably inspired Rene Descartes of France in 1632, who also suggested water to neutralize the cornea, but in this case contained in a glass tube. Later, Muller (Germany) in 1887 produced a lens designed to sit on the cornea which would allow vision and could be tolerated by the eye. There were many developments in lens designs and materials throughout the twentieth century, and in 1971 the first soft lens was commercially available, following the work of Otto Wichterle in the 1960s. The composition of rigid corneal lenses changed to gas-permeable materials in the 1970s, and gas-permeable contact lenses for overnight wear appeared in 1986. The latter sparked renewed interest in orthokeratology (also known as corneal refractive therapy), where the corneal shape can be manipulated using a contact lens to produce central flattening, thereby causing a reduction in myopia. Modern orthokeratology no longer uses this simplified approach of producing an unspecified degree of spherical myopia reduction. Instead, modern designs of orthokeratology lenses allow for the precise reduction of myopia and myopic astigmatism.

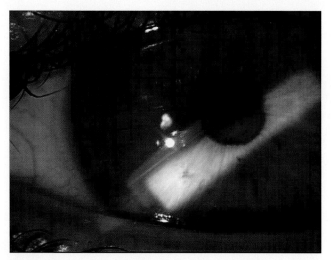

Figure 23.1 This shows an incision from successful radial keratotomy. The photograph was taken approximately 10 years after the procedure was carried out.

However, attempts to manipulate the corneal shape are not new. The ancient Chinese placed tiny bags of sand on the closed eyes of young children to flatten their corneae and thus reduce the level of myopia.

Lucciola and Lans in the 1890s showed that radial burns caused permanent changes in corneal shape. Subsequently, Sato in the 1930s and Fyodorov in the 1960s made radial incisions into the mid-peripheral cornea to produce localized flattening and thereby reduce the refractive power. This is now known as radial keratotomy (RK; **Fig. 23.1**). Some years before, Sato had actually tried placing cuts on the posterior surface of the cornea but this led to high levels of corneal decompensation.

More recently, flattening of the cornea to correct low levels of spherical myopia has been achieved using intracorneal rings (ICRs). This involves inserting circular strips of polymethyl methacrylate (PMMA) into the stroma. While this is a reversible procedure, the results were not very accurate, showed diurnal changes and the ICRs were often visible to the naked eye because of deposits within the channel. The procedure is described later in this chapter. This technique has now been largely abandoned for myopia but remains a treatment option for patients with corneal ectasia, such as keratoconus or post laser in situ keratomileusis (LASIK) ectasia, before having to resort to corneal transplantation.

Corneal treatments for refractive errors include epikeratophakia/epikeratoplasty and keratophakia. These surgeries were often used in aphakic patients to correct high levels of hyperopia by adding tissue and steepening the corneal curvature. Epikeratophakia/epikeratoplasty involve removing a corneal button from a donor cornea and reshaping it with a cryolathe. The reshaped donor button is then sutured on top of the debrided (epithelium removed) host cornea (Reidy et al 1990). The cornea will then re-epithelialize over the debrided area (which includes the donor corneal button). Keratophakia procedures involve placing a lenticule underneath a partial-thickness corneal graft (lamellar graft). The graft is sutured back onto the patient's cornea (Neumann et al 1989). The lenticule is taken from a donor cornea but recently the use of a synthetic lenticule has been advocated (Michieletto et al 2004). These two procedures may be considered for aphakic patients following intracapsular cataract extraction. It is interesting to note that Jose Barraquer conducted early versions of keratophakia, keratomileusis and intracorneal inclusion surgery in the mid-1960s and early 1970s (Barraquer 1965, 1966, 1967, 1972).

A further form of corneal surgery to reduce refractive error is keratomileusis. A corneal button is removed using a microkeratome, frozen and reshaped with a cryolathe. The net result is a flatter and therefore less powerful cornea. Indeed, the microkeratome used in this procedure is a precursor to those used in modern LASIK surgery. In fact, LASIK takes part of its name from this early surgical technique (laser in situ keratomileusis). The LASIK procedure is discussed in more detail later.

Keratectomy was used to correct myopic astigmatism. This involved excision of a piece of corneal tissue. If a crescent-shaped piece of cornea is removed and the residual cornea sutured, there will be steepening of the cornea in that particular meridian (Weber & Fagerholm 1998). Photorefractive keratectomy (PRK) takes its name from this procedure but involves the use of a laser light (hence *photo*). In PRK the laser energy is used to ablate the corneal stroma (the PRK procedure is discussed in more detail later in the chapter).

PRK and LASIK were originally refractive surgical procedures performed with an excimer laser. The term 'excimer' applies to a group of lasers where a molecule of an inert gas is forced to associate with a molecule of a halogen gas. The word 'excimer' is derived from EXCited dIMER, and is used to describe a molecule made from the two energized components. In 1982, Srinivasan in IBM's research laboratory found that the argon fluoride (ArF) excimer laser could cut organic material (Trokel et al 1983). In 1985, an ArF excimer laser was used to perform radial keratotomy (RK) on enucleated eyes (Marshall et al 1985, 1986). This process of altering the refractive power of the cornea became known as photorefractive keratectomy (PRK). In the USA, the Food & Drug Administration approved the excimer laser for PRK in October 1995, although the technique had already been widespread in the rest of the world for many years. To correct for myopia, the laser removes (ablates) tissue from the central cornea to cause a net flattening (Taylor et al 1989). If corneal tissue is removed from the mid-peripheral part of the cornea, this results in a net steepening centrally and will help to reduce hyperopia. Directional ablations can be used to correct astigmatism, and varying the created corneal shape can assist in presbyopia by creating a profile that increases depth of focus by increasing the spherical aberration.

LASIK originates from the work of Jose Barraquer, who developed keratomileusis in the 1960s, by which a thin corneal flap was removed, reshaped with a cryolathe, and then reattached onto the corneal bed (Barraquer 1967). Luis Ruiz of Columbia, in the early 1980s, took this concept further by using a manual microkeratome to excise an internal disc of corneal tissue. He later developed an automated device to create a partial-thickness slice cut into the cornea. LASIK was born from the combination of keratomileusis and PRK. LASIK was described in 1989 by Pallikaris, who used the excimer laser to treat the underlying stromal bed beneath a corneal flap, which he had created with a microkeratome (Pallikaris et al 1990). Burrato of Italy also used an excimer laser under a corneal flap but he applied the laser to the corneal cap (Buratto & Ferrari 1992; Buratto et al 1992).

The original broad-beam laser delivery systems have now been superseded by modern procedures such as scanning and flying spot, where the delivery of the laser energy is concentrated into a small spot pattern that is randomly directed across the entire desired ablation area. This is designed so that an aspheric pattern is ablated to achieve the attempted refractive outcome. The overall ablation process takes slightly longer using scanning micro-beam lasers, since they have less energy per pulse than the broad-beam lasers. Therefore, a higher pulse rate is needed. During the longer ablation periods used with micro-beam lasers, any unwanted eye movements will affect the ablation pattern. Accordingly, fixation and tracking devices were introduced that follow the direction of eye movements to prevent off-centre ablation. This is even more critical when correcting astigmatism, to ensure that the correct meridian is treated, or in hyperopic patients where a larger ablation diameter is required.

Non-corneal treatments

Changing intraocular power is an alternative to altering corneal power; this can be achieved either by replacing the crystalline lens with an appropriately powered intraocular lens (IOL) or by introducing an additional IOL without removing the crystalline lens. Lens surgery dates back to the ancients with primitive techniques of couching, where the dense cataract lens was pushed backwards into the vitreous chamber to allow light to pass through a clear entrance pupil. Surprisingly, in some African cultures this technique is still occasionally used today, and is performed by lay people. Boerhaave, in 1746, used crystalline lens removal to correct myopia and this was further popularized by Fukala in the 1890s.

Harold Ridley introduced the concept of using IOLs following cataract extraction in 1949, although the idea dates back to Tadini, an itinerant ophthalmologist in the second half of the eighteenth century. Indeed, Tadini showed Casanova a box containing artificial lenses made of glass. Tadini in all likelihood conceived the idea of the intraocular correction of aphakia. Presumably, Casanova conveyed the idea to Casaamata, an ophthalmic surgeon in Dresden. At any rate, Casaamata was the first to actually attempt the correction of aphakia by implanting an IOL.

Ridley used an IOL made of PMMA rather than glass. PMMA remains a readily available material and is used in various industries. Ridley's PMMA lens was 45 times heavier than its modern silicone acrylate equivalent. The procedure was performed without an operating microscope and also lacked the use of modern viscoelastic agents that aid current surgical techniques. At the time of his revolutionary surgery, Ridley was almost ostracized by his peers. His use of PMMA followed the experiences of World War II Royal Air Force fighter pilots, who often experienced penetrating ocular injuries resulting from their PMMA windscreens being shot out during air battles. The fragments of PMMA were found to be inert to the eye, leading to the development of PMMA IOLs and contact lenses. Modern materials have led to the introduction of phakic IOLs, i.e. IOLs that are implanted without the removal of the crystalline lens for the correction of refractive error. This is usually for patients with active accommodation.

Current techniques

An ametropic patient has many options available for correcting their refractive error. The role of the eye care professional is to offer educated and unbiased advice regarding these options. Optical aids such as spectacles and contact lenses are no longer the only choices available. A patient seeking an alternative vision correction should be carefully guided through options such as extended-wear contact lenses, orthokeratology and refractive surgery. Many patients who may be suitable for orthokeratology or contact lenses may also be suitable for surgical alternatives. Often the final choice depends on many factors including patient preference, patient motivation and the advice of their eye care professional.

Orthokeratology

Orthokeratology (Ortho-K), or corneal refractive therapy (CRT), is a reversible method of altering corneal power (**Fig. 23.2**). The fact that it can be managed in an optometry practice makes it an appealing option for optometrists to pursue for patients wishing to be freed from optical aids. It may be used by some optometrists as an alternative to refractive surgery. Many patients think of it as a treatment for their myopia rather than an option that is dependent upon an optical aid. In some ways this is correct since the orthokeratology lens is not worn to alter the refractive status but to change corneal shape, which in turn alters the refractive power of the eye. However, orthokeratology is an ongoing (but reversible) treatment as opposed to permanent refractive surgery.

The development of modern rigid gas-permeable contact lens materials and manufacturing techniques has led to

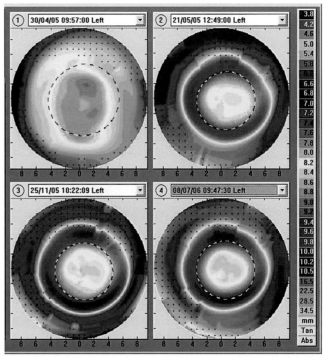

Figure 23.2 Corneal topography pictures of a 3.00 D myope who underwent successful orthokeratology. Picture 1 (*top left*) shows the pretreatment corneal shape. Picture 2 (*top right*) shows the corneal shape after 1 month. Picture 3 (*bottom left*) shows the cornea after 6 months. Picture 4 (*bottom right*) shows the cornea after more than 1 year. It is worth noting that the majority of the change in corneal shape occurred within the first month and after that the orthokeratology lenses were used to maintain this new shape. (Picture courtesy of Brian Tompkins, Tompkins, Knight and Son, Optometrists.)

contact lenses that can alter corneal curvature rapidly. Previously, orthokeratology used a flat-fitting, PMMA contact lens to reshape the cornea. The principal drawback of these earlier procedures was the lack of predictability, and the limited ability to correct even low levels of myopia. Early orthokeratology utilized the properties of the liquid lens, and used a series of progressively flat-fitting lenses over time. This often led to an unstable contact lens with even moderate levels of myopia. There are two disadvantages of fitting gradually flatter lenses: firstly, a large number of lenses are required, and secondly, controlling centration of the lens can be difficult due to superior displacement under the upper lid. This second problem often led to corneal warpage, which may cause distorted vision.

Early studies showed limited success in treating myopia, although orthokeratology was found to be safe and reversible (Winkler 1995; Ruston et al 1997). Further, a wide range of results was observed in the treatment groups, suggesting that preselection of subjects could lead to a successful outcome if a distinguishing factor were isolated. Indeed, there appears to be a relationship between the change in corneal shape and shift in refractive error. The advent of computerized video keratoscopy (more commonly referred to as corneal topography; see Ch. 17) has led to investigations into which corneal shape is best suited to manipulation by orthokeratology. The key to success was deemed to be the corneal shape, which could be described in terms of its shape factor (p), eccentricity (e) or asphericity value (Q). The relation between these terms is described in the formulae below. For example, if a patient's existing refractive correction is −3.00D and emmetropia is the desired outcome, then orthokeratology should only be attempted if the e value is at least 0.6 (note that for a spherical surface, e = 0).

The relationship between p, e and Q is given by the following formulae:

$$p = 1 - e^2$$

$$Q = -e^2$$

$$Q = p - 1$$

$$e = \sqrt{(1 - p)}$$

The cornea is a prolate shape, i.e. it is a flattening ellipse and the shape factor is determined as shown in **Figure 23.3**. Bibby (1976 a–d) and Guillon et al (1986) reported average corneal p values of 0.85 and 0.83, respectively.

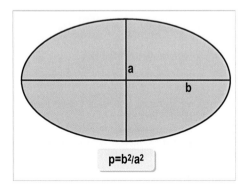

$$p = b^2/a^2$$

Fig. 23.3 The shape factor of an ellipse (p) is the ratio of the square of the major axis (b) divided by the square of the minor axis (a), i.e. b^2/a^2.

A more recent concept in orthokeratology is 'accelerated orthokeratology' (Dave & Ruston 1997; Lui et al 2000). This technique uses reverse geometry lenses, i.e. lenses where the peripheral curve is steeper than the back optic zone radius (BOZR). This shape allows lens centration to be controlled more effectively. Numerous contact lens fitting sets are available using this design and are manufactured in a range of materials. The material is selected depending on whether the patient will be using the lens for overnight use. In a reverse geometry lens design, the secondary steeper curve produces a tear reservoir in the mid-peripheral portion of the lens followed by a flatter peripheral curve. The axial edge lift can be manipulated to achieve the desired fitting pattern for the optimum result.

Additionally, further studies have shown that many factors can hinder the success of orthokeratology (Lui & Edwards 2000a,b; Tabb 2001; Joslin et al 2004; Chui & Cho 2005). Accordingly, strict patient inclusion/exclusion criteria must be observed. The list below summarizes findings which, if present, may preclude successful orthokeratology.

- where the e value and Rx do not correlate, e.g. a steep corneal shape with a high myopic prescription
- against-the-rule astigmatism, although some contact lens designs have been able to correct low levels of against-the-rule astigmatism
- with-the-rule astigmatism of up to 1.50 D may be reduced, but larger amounts of with-the-rule astigmatism may be difficult to correct
- keratoconus, corneal dystrophy or active eye disease
- deep-set eyes or loose lids
- a long-term history of rigid lens wear, as it tends to make the cornea more spherical in shape (i.e a low e value)
- a patient with a poor response to a 6-hour or overnight trial may be an unsuccessful candidate, although it is worth repeating the trial with a different type of trial lens.

Patients should first be given either a 6-hour daytime or overnight trial. After this initial trial the level of myopia will generally reduce by 0.75–1.50 D with a corresponding increase in unaided visual acuity (VA). Corneal topography should show a change in apical radius consistent with the refractive change, and a reduction in eccentricity. If no response is found, the trial should be repeated with an different contact lens design as this may give a better outcome.

An important parameter to consider when predicting success with orthokeratology is the Munnerlyn formula (Munnerlyn et al 1988). This is the basis of most modern algorithms in laser refractive surgery. It facilitates calculation of the ablation depth required to correct the level of myopia over a set diameter. The formula can be approximated to:

$$t = -(S^2 \times D)/8(n - 1)$$

where S = diameter, D = power, t = thickness (or depth in the case of orthokeratology) and n = refractive index of the anterior cornea.

According to the Munnerlyn formula, a 2.5 D reduction in myopia can be achieved if the changes from orthokeratology are purely epithelial in origin (the epithelium is typically 50–60 microns in thickness). However, since successful orthokeratology has been shown to correct up to 4.5 D of myopia, this suggests that some stromal changes must also be occurring.

Current developments in orthokeratology are directed towards better lens designs that will allow more predictable and rapid changes in corneal shape. Double reverse geometry lenses have been produced. These lenses have a second reverse curve which, although steeper than the BOZR, is flatter than the first reverse curve. The key advantage is that flatter curves can be used centrally and greater tear reservoir depths are possible without the loss of improved centration. The same pressure is applied over a smaller area of cornea, and this in turn will induce a greater level of flattening.

Refractive surgery

In a study in 1999 examining why patients chose contact lenses or refractive surgery, it was found that only around 11% of patients sought any professional guidance before attending a refractive surgery clinic, whereas a similar study by the same group in 2006 suggested this figure had risen to 30% (Naroo et al 1999; Gupta & Naroo 2006). Therefore, clinicians involved at the primary eye care level need to be fully informed on available alternative forms of vision correction. Another study by the same group in the UK suggested that the most informed clinicians, who were best placed to offer advice on refractive surgery, were optometrists, followed by ophthalmologists and finally general medical practitioners (Naroo & Ubhi 2004).

Patients opting for refractive surgery are usually from their mid-30s to about 40 years of age. Earlier studies showed approximately equal numbers of males and females, although more recent investigations have shown a slight increase in female patients. Refractive surgery patients often have more disposable income, and this is reflected by their higher socio-economic status. This may also partly explain the age groups of refractive surgery patients. **Figure 23.4** shows the occupations of these individuals. In addition, **Figure 23.5** shows the main reasons that patients opting

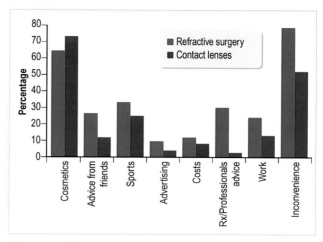

Figure 23.5 The main reasons that patients opting for refractive surgery gave as influencing their decision to cease contact lens use. The values shown on the y-axis indicate the percentage of patients offering the particular reason as an influencing factor. (From Gupta & Naroo 2006.)

for refractive surgery gave as influencing their decision to cease contact lens use.

Practitioners performing an evaluation of prospective patients for refractive surgery should first assess that the patient is suitably motivated towards undergoing the procedure. It is advisable that the patient be armed with some information before attending a consultation. The actual preoperative assessment routine may differ slightly from clinic to clinic, but the essence of the examination will be the same. The specific individual tests required are listed below, although it should be pointed out that this list is not comprehensive, and some tests may be omitted depending upon the type of refractive surgery that the patient will undergo.

The preoperative work-up of a patient for refractive surgery should include a full eye examination. The tests that need to be performed include:

- *Visual acuity* (VA): In the absence of complications, the myope will gain retinal magnification by moving the correction from the spectacle to the ocular plane, so on occasions the VA may actually improve postoperatively. However, hyperopes will lose the magnification that their spectacles provide when the correction is moved to the ocular plane and occasionally may report a postoperative decline in VA.
- *Full refraction*: Some advocate cycloplegic refraction for all patients, whereas others suggest it for hyperopes or younger patients only.
- *Slit-lamp examination* (see Ch. 17): Any anterior eye pathology that may contraindicate the procedure should be noted.
- *Dilated fundus examination* (see Ch. 18): Any pathology should be noted, especially since many patients will be high myopes who are more prone to retinal detachments.
- *Pupil diameter*: Some early excimer laser systems used small-diameter ablations, and these patients occasionally suffered with haloes around lights postoperatively. It was believed that since the pupil was wider than the treatment zone, ghost images were created similar to those

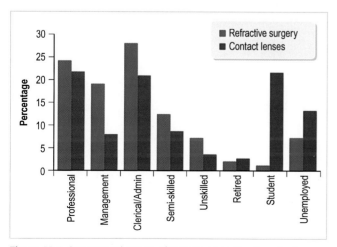

Figure 23.4 Occupational groups of patients presenting for refractive surgery compared with those presenting for contact lenses. (From Naroo et al 1999.)

observed when the optic zone of a corneal contact lens is displaced.

- *Corneal topography*: The shape of the cornea is important to assist in monitoring outcome success (see Ch. 17) as well as to help rule out any pre-existing irregularities such as keratoconus or pellucid marginal dystrophies. Furthermore, many clinicians and manufacturers now advocate excimer laser treatment profiles that try to maintain the prolate shape of the cornea, and avoid creating an oblate shape as was done by some of the earlier algorithms. This may provide better visual comfort for the patient.

- *Corneal pachymetry* (see Chs 19 and 24): Excimer lasers remove precise amounts of corneal tissue dependent upon the amount of correction attempted. The corneal thickness measurement will allow the surgeon to ensure that there is sufficient cornea for the attempted correction but, more importantly, to leave adequate corneal tissue remaining as a 'safe bed'.

- *Intraocular pressure* (IOP): Since many refractive surgery techniques involve altering the thickness of the cornea, this in turn can affect the measurement of IOP (see Ch. 24). It is worth noting that refractive surgery is unlikely to change the actual IOP but rather alters the recorded measurement. This may become an issue if the patient develops glaucoma in the future.

- *Tear tests* (see Ch. 17): Many patients complain of dry eyes following excimer laser procedures, so the quality of the tear layer should be evaluated before surgery.

- *Contrast sensitivity function* (CSF; see Ch. 12): Patients may suffer reduced CSF, especially in the healing stages or in the case of an adverse effect.

- *Oculomotor balance* (see Ch. 16): This might be considered an ancillary test, but removing the spectacle correction could affect the oculomotor balance, especially in older pre-presbyopes or presbyopes. For example, consider a 42-year-old bilateral 5 D myope who is corrected with spectacles. When reading through their glasses the patient experiences base-in prism by decentration which reduces the stimulus for convergence. When the correction is moved to the corneal plane (whether refractive surgery or contact lenses), the stimulus to convergence (as well as the stimulus to ocular accommodation) is increased.

- *Corneal sensitivity/aesthesiometry* (see Ch. 17): Again, this might be considered an ancillary test. However, corneal sensitivity may be reduced by excimer laser procedures (which may also affect tear production).

The Royal College of Ophthalmologists in the UK suggest the following criteria when considering suitability for refractive surgery:

- Suitable for treatment
  At least 21 years of age
  Stable prescription, i.e. less than 0.50 D change over the preceding 2–3 years
  Healthy eyes
  Good general health
  People with reasonable expectations

- Unsuitable for treatment
  Pregnancy/breastfeeding
  Significant keratoconus, cataract or glaucoma, herpes eye infection
  Patients on certain prescription drugs, such as oral steroids
  Excimer laser surgery may not be suitable for patients with medical conditions such as diabetes, rheumatoid arthritis or systemic lupus erythematosus.

In the author's opinion, the first decision with regard to a potential refractive surgery patient is to choose between laser and non-laser procedures. Non-laser procedures would typically be used for higher levels of ametropia with some exceptions, as detailed below.

Most refractive surgeries are excimer laser vision correction (often termed LVC). LVC can be subdivided into four main types of procedures (while the names may vary slightly between clinics, those listed below are most commonly used):

- PRK
- LASEK
- LASIK
- Epi-LASIK

PRK, LASEK and LASIK will be discussed below. Epi-LASIK is a further variation of LASIK that uses a microkeratome or a solid-state laser to make a flap cut just underneath the epithelium and includes a small amount of stroma in the flap. A fuller discussion of Epi-LASIK is beyond the scope of this chapter.

PRK (photorefractive keratectomy) and LASEK (laser-assisted epithelial keratomileusis)

Overview

Photorefractive keratectomy (PRK) involves using an excimer laser to reshape the cornea (**Fig. 23.6**). The laser energy is applied to the surface of the cornea after the epithelium has been debrided. This may be done with a blunt blade

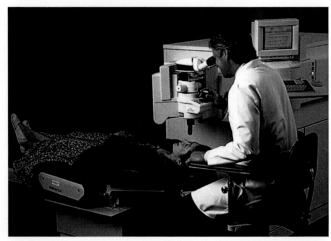

Figure 23.6 A surgeon aligning a patient's head underneath the delivery mechanism of an excimer laser in preparation for laser vision correction. (Picture courtesy of VisX Technologies.) (Reproduced with permission from Naroo & Charman 2001.)

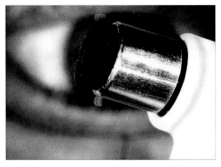

Figure 23.7 The head of the Amoil's epithelial scrubber used to debride the epithelium prior to excimer laser ablation in PRK. (Picture courtesy of Victor Spear, Innovative Excimer Solutions, Inc.) (Reproduced with permission from Naroo & Charman 2001.)

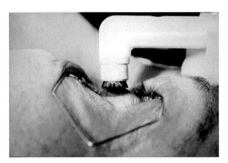

Figure 23.8 The Amoil's epithelial scrubber on a patient's cornea. (Picture courtesy of Victor Spear, Innovative Excimer Solutions, Inc.) (Reproduced with permission from Naroo & Charman 2001.)

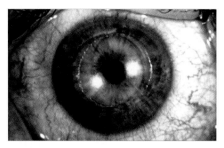

Figure 23.9 The cornea prior to excimer laser ablation in PRK after the epithelium has been removed. (Picture courtesy of Victor Spear, Innovative Excimer Solutions, Inc.) (Reproduced with permission from Naroo & Charman 2001.)

such as a beaver blade, a mechanical device such as a rotary brush (**Figs 23.7** and **23.8**) or using alcohol. LASEK is very similar but the epithelium is moved aside to allow the laser to reshape the stromal bed and then the epithelium is replaced. The most common way of moving the epithelium to the side is using alcohol as described below, although a new device called an epi-microkeratome can also be used. This is a microkeratome that separates the epithelium from the stroma and then allows the epithelium to be replaced after the laser energy has been applied to the stroma.

LASEK combines certain advantages of LASIK and PRK by being less invasive than LASIK but allowing quicker healing than PRK. This technique is safe and the epithelial healing is faster, with reduced stromal haze, quicker postoperative recovery and less postoperative pain than PRK (Verma et al 1995). In LASEK the corneal epithelium is retained in order to prevent biochemical changes in the cornea which can lead to haze formation. It is less invasive than LASIK, which may make it more attractive to some patients.

Surgical procedure

The cornea is anaesthetized by topical anaesthetics. The patient lies on a couch and is asked to focus on a flashing light. Usually, the non-operated eye is covered with an eye pad. A lid speculum is inserted in the eye to be treated. A LASEK 8.0 mm corneal trephine is used to create an epithelial incision. The circular blade is designed to perform a 270° incision with a blunt section at the 12 o'clock position for a hinge. A 9 mm corneal ring is applied, filled with 18% ethanol and left for 30 seconds. This sized corneal ring allows a 7.5 mm treatment zone to be achieved, as the

epithelium at the edges is still adhered. A flap can be raised in most eyes 20–25 seconds after application of the ethanol. The alcohol is soaked up with a mercel sponge, the cornea irrigated and a topical nonsteroidal antiinflammatory agent applied. An epithelial flap is fashioned by lifting (not debriding and not damaging the stromal bed) the edge of the loosened epithelium with a sharp beaver blade. The flap can be created either horizontally or vertically, or alternatively the epithelium is cut in the centre and a flap created in all four directions. Following the creation of the epithelial flap, the corneal stroma is exposed (**Fig. 23.9**) and laser treatment begun without delay, before the stroma dehydrates, as this might lead to overcorrection. The patient must be warned that the ablation usually produces a burning smell.

After ablation, the flap is replaced onto the cornea. A bandage contact lens is placed on the eye and left in place for 4 days. This minimizes pain and produces quicker visual recovery than standard PRK. This procedure is especially beneficial for patients with small palpebral apertures, deep-set eyes, extremely flat, steep or thin corneas or high myopia and patients who may not qualify for LASIK.

The PRK procedure is similar to LASEK as described above, but in the case of PRK the epithelium is not retained and is removed by manual, mechanical or chemical (alcohol) methods. New epithelium will subsequently grow back over the new corneal surface.

Postoperative care

Postoperative care includes topical antibiotics for 1 week. Patients are told to avoid swimming, contact sports, dust and smoke for about 1 month. They are usually reviewed after 1 week, 6 weeks and 6 months. The vision gradually improves over a few days to a few weeks (at most) depending on the size of the ablation. After LASEK, patients often wear a bandage contact lens for a few days.

Complications of PRK and LASEK

As LASEK and PRK are essentially the same procedures (with the exception of using the epithelium as a bandage in LASEK), the potential complications are similar. Haze is quite common after PRK but in the author's experience is not usually sufficient to reduce vision. More common complications are refractive. Early adverse reactions could include induced irregular astigmatism and primary under- and overcorrection. Later complications could include regression as well as under- and overcorrection. With LASEK, loss of the epithelial flap during surgery is rare, and if it occurs the procedure essentially becomes PRK. Decentred ablation, glare and haloes are possible and would affect the patient's vision. Infectious keratitis is thankfully a rare, although more serious, complication (Stephenson 2002; Abbot et al 2003).

LASIK (laser in situ keratomileusis)

Overview

LASIK is a combination of excimer laser with lamellar corneal surgery for the correction of refractive errors. LASIK is mainly carried out for the correction of myopia; however, it is also used for the correction of astigmatism and hyperopia. Most refractive surgery in the USA is now LASIK. To achieve the desired refractive power the corneal thickness and shape are altered. The excimer laser is used to ablate the corneal stromal tissue to achieve the desired refractive change.

Surgical procedure

The patient lies on a couch with the excimer laser delivery system above their head. The cornea of the eye to be operated is anaesthetized with topical anaesthetic drops. A lid speculum is inserted after instilling topical anaesthesia. The patient is asked to fixate on the laser beam and the cornea is marked with gentian violet to help realign the flap. A suction ring is applied to the limbus and the pressure increased to more than 65 mmHg to ensure a regular cut. This is confirmed using an applanation tonometer. The patient may experience transient loss of vision due to increased intraocular pressure. An automated microkeratome is activated to pass across the cornea in order to create a stromal flap. The vacuum is released and the epithelial flap reflected back to expose the stromal bed. The hinge of the flap is made either nasally or at the 12 o'clock position. Pachymetry is repeated to ensure adequate residual tissue, and excimer laser ablation is carried out on the corneal stroma. The patient is warned that they might experience a pungent smell during laser ablation. The ablation usually takes less than 90 seconds. The flap is washed with balanced salt solution and replaced. Centration is checked and the edges are smoothed down. After checking adhesion, the speculum is removed. Topical antibiotics and steroids are usually prescribed for 1 week.

Postoperative care

The patient is directed to avoid swimming, dust or smoke and any contact sport for about 1 month after the surgery. A clear eye shield should be worn for 2 weeks to avoid trauma while sleeping. The patient is normally examined 1 day, 1 week, 1 month, 3 months, 6 months and 1 year postoperatively.

Visual acuity outcomes

Clarigbold conducted a study of 222 eyes with preoperative myopia ranging from -1.25 D to -11.25 D and astigmatism up to 2.25 D. Postsurgical uncorrected visual acuity was 6/12 or better 4 days postoperatively in more than 80% of the eyes examined and 6/6 or better in 75% after 2 weeks. Additionally, the same author reported no loss of best corrected visual acuity. In a 1-year follow-up of 84 eyes, 82.0% had uncorrected visual acuity of 6/6 or better, while 100% had uncorrected visual acuity of 6/7.5 or better (Claringbold 2002). Furthermore, all eyes were within ±0.75 D of the intended correction and more than 96% of the eyes had refractive errors within ±0.5 D after 12 months (Claringbold 2002).

In a further investigation, 343 eyes with preoperative refractive errors ranging from -1.00 D to -14.00 D and astigmatism up to $+4.75$ D were followed up for 6 months. Ninety-eight per cent of these patients had postoperative unaided visual acuity of 6/12 or better (Scerrati 2001). Shahinan reported in a study of 146 eyes with myopia ranging from -1.00 D to -14.38 D that the uncorrected VA was 6/12 or better in 96% of the eyes after the 12-month follow-up (Shahinian 2002).

Visual acuity can settle quite quickly after surgery and studies have shown that 1 month postoperatively, 90% and 64% of the eyes were within $+1.00$ D and $+0.50$ D, respectively. After 12 months, 99% were within $+1.00$ D and 78% of the eyes were within $+0.50$ D. No eye lost two lines or more of best corrected VA; 92.6% and 63% had uncorrected VA of 6/12 or better and 6/6 or better, respectively. One eye lost two lines of best corrected VA while two eyes gained two or more lines (Pop & Payette 2000; Lian et al 2002).

Complications

Postoperative complications following LASIK can be divided into two broad groups, namely flap related and non-flap related.

Flap-related complications

Flap complications can include either an incomplete or completely cut flap, lost, decentred or irregular flap and flap striae (Stephenson 2002). However, in a study on 84 711 eyes, it was concluded that flap complications are low with experienced surgeons and a figure of 0.3% was quoted (Jacobs & Taravella 2002). Epithelial ingrowth (epithelium within the stromal interface) can manifest itself within a few weeks after surgery. The commonest causes of reduced VA after LASIK are often wrinkles or striae, interface infection and flap dislocations (Oliveira-Soto & Charman 2002; Stephenson 2002). It would be expected that these would not be long-term complications but could appear soon after surgery.

Non-flap-related complications

These may include under- or overcorrection, refractive regression, decentred ablation and induced irregular astigmatism due to folds or microstriae within the flap. This is often difficult to correct and produces a decrease in VA and/or the quality of vision. Small steep areas of the cornea may occur during LASIK. These are often termed central islands and are thought to be the result of an irregular scanning of the excimer laser beam (Farah et al 1998). Further excimer ablation may be required to flatten these areas if they affect the visual outcome for the patient. Haze, glare and halos are possible, and may be caused by small optic zone diameters and/or interface debris. Infectious keratitis is rare while diffuse interstitial keratitis (also known as sands of Sahara) occurs more frequently. This is an inflammatory response that takes place at the flap–bed interface. Dry eye symptoms are very common but most patients find that these subside after a few months. Night vision problems and a reduction in corneal sensitivity are also common visual complaints, but again tend to subside with time (Farah et al 1998; Oliveira-Soto & Charman 2002; Stephenson 2002). Posterior ectasia has also been reported, and is thought to be caused by insufficient corneal tissue being left as a residual 'safe bed'. However, some controversy surrounds the way that ectasia is measured, as the corneal topography devices that are able to image the ectatic posterior surface have to do so through an altered anterior surface (Joo & Tim 2000; Pallikaris et al 2001; Randleman et al 2003; Twa et al 2004). Accordingly, the prevalence of this condition may have been overestimated.

Predictability and stability

In a study of 107 LASIK-treated myopic eyes whose preoperative refractive error ranged from −1.00 D to −9.00 D, 77 of the eyes (77%) were evaluated 12 months postoperatively. Of these, 100% had postoperative uncorrected VA of 6/12 or better and 83% of the eyes achieved uncorrected visual acuity of 6/6 or better. In another study of 290 high myopic eyes (range −9.00 D to −22.00 D), the uncorrected visual acuity was 6/12 or better in 73.3% 1 month postoperatively (Pop & Payette 2000).

Further, in 131 eyes with high myopia (ranging from −9.00 D to −22.00 D) most visual performance scores were stable or improved between early and later follow-ups. For example, uncorrected VA was either stable or improved in 88% of the treated eyes after 1 month while best corrected VA was either stable or improved in 95% of the eyes after 1 month (Kawesch & Kezirian 2000).

LASIK can also be used to treat low hyperopia. In a study conducted on 376 hyperopic eyes (ranging from +1.00 D to +8.50 D), a mean postoperative refractive error of + 0.46 D was achieved after a follow-up of 8.2 months. Postoperative uncorrected VA of 6/12 or better was found in 96% of eyes with less than 4D of hyperopia and 88% of eyes with more than 4D of hyperopia (Cobo-Soriano et al 2002).

In an additional investigation of 54 hyperopic eyes (range +1.00 D to +6.00 D), it was reported that the predictability was good after 12 months, with 83% of eyes being within +1.00 D while 66% had less than 0.5 D of hyperopia (Lian et al 2002).

LASIK versus LASEK

It is difficult to state which procedure is most appropriate. Often, this is up to the individual surgeon. Most surgeons advocate LASEK for lower myopes and perhaps hyperopes and LASIK for higher myopes and hyperopes. However, other surgeons suggest LASIK for every prescription except those very high levels of refractive error that lie outside the range for the particular laser, or might benefit from lens surgery instead.

It has been suggested that LASEK is safer and more effective than LASIK since complications relating to the stromal flap are eliminated. Further, LASEK can be performed on patients where LASIK may be contraindicated, e.g. deep-set eyes or thin corneas. However, LASEK has some disadvantages over LASIK, with patients experiencing varying degrees of pain during the first 2 days after surgery and slower recovery of vision. Often, vision is somewhat blurred for the first week after LASEK. Additionally, patients may have mild recurrent epithelial erosion and require postoperative steroids for a longer period compared with LASIK (Claringbold 2002).

LASIK is preferred for high myopes because of the speed of visual recovery and predictability. There is an 'overlap' area of those between −2 D to −3 D where the advantages and disadvantages of LASIK and LASEK are about equal. LASEK is a recent modification of PRK and can be the treatment of choice in patients with lower myopia, thin or steep corneas and for patients where LASIK is contraindicated for other reasons. For example, in a patient with a history or high risk of developing an ocular vascular accident, it would be unwise to apply a suction ring (part of the microkeratome) as this will increase the intraocular pressure, possibly causing transient blockage of the central retinal artery for a few seconds with the risk of a haemorrhage (Shahinian 2002). The end results of PRK and LASIK are similar in low prescriptions (Pop & Payette 2000). One would expect comparable results between PRK and LASEK. While LASIK produces less postoperative discomfort than PRK or LASEK, these latter procedures might be considered safer as they are more superficial and do not require a microkeratome flap to be cut (Verma et al 1995; Gallar et al 2004).

In a prospective, non-randomized, comparative, paired eye trial, comprising 72 eyes of 36 patients having surgery with a Nidek EC-5000 excimer laser, eyes were divided into two groups. The first eye of each patient was treated with 20% ethanol debridement (PRK but using alcohol for the epithelial removal) and the second eye with an epithelial flap which was replaced after treatment (LASEK). After a mean follow-up of 62.6 weeks, the final mean spherical equivalent (MSE) was +0.07±0.61 D in the debridement group and −0.24±0.43 D in the epithelial flap group. There was no statistically significant difference between the two groups in the postoperative MSE. Best corrected VA was better in the epithelial flap group at all visits; this difference was statistically significant ($p<0.05$). Corneal haze was significantly less in the LASEK group ($p<0.05$) (Shah et al 2001). A further study reported better and quicker postoperative results for myopia and myopic astigmatism with LASEK compared with LASIK, as well as quicker epithelial healing and no or lesser complaints of pain (Anderson et al 2002). Accordingly, Scerrati concluded that LASEK may prove superior (Scerrati 2001). The reports of no serious or vision-threatening complications with a greater choice of patients and the elimination of stromal flap complications with LASEK may also substantiate this claim (Shahinian 2002).

Wavefront technology

More recently, ablation lasers have been linked with corneal topography units so that specific areas of the cornea can be altered to correct primary corneal irregularities. The theory of specific area ablation has now been extended to include wavefront technology.

Wavefront analysis is a method of describing the aberrations of the eye's refractive components (see Ch. 13). It includes low-order aberrations, such as refractive error (both spherical and astigmatic errors) and higher-order aberrations, such as spherical aberration and coma (which would not commonly be corrected by spectacle lenses). Spherical aberration arises from high-powered lenses and can be demonstrated as the distortions observed when viewing a grid pattern. Coma can be noted as a tail of poor image quality next to a clearer, larger image, almost like a tail on an astronomical comet. Wavefront technology is employed in astronomy where high-powered telescopes, using adaptive optics, use this wavefront information to minimize the aberrations occurring in the image. Wavefront LVC is becoming increasing popular, and is a way of customizing the surgery to the patient's individual visual blueprint.

Intracorneal ring segments (ICRs)

This procedure is based on the assumption that the refractive error can be corrected by flattening the central corneal curvature by adding tissue in the outer two-thirds of cornea. This additional tissue in the periphery will distend the outer cornea, thereby flattening the central cornea (Alio et al 2002).

This technique can be used for the correction of low myopia and astigmatism. In this procedure, half-ring segments of Perspex (Plexiglas) are inserted into channels created in the corneal stroma. The advantage of this surgical procedure is that the central cornea is not involved and the ring is positioned outside the pupillary margin. This process is easily reversible and corneal shape is intact. The levels of myopia that can be corrected by this technique are up to around 4 D. However, most surgeons feel that these levels of myopia are better treated with an excimer procedure as LVC is very predictable within this refractive range.

The ICRs operation is carried out under sterile conditions. The geometrical centre of the cornea is marked and intraoperative ultrasonic pachymetry carried out at the site of incision. The diamond blade is set at 70% of the measured corneal thickness to create a single radial incision at the steepest meridian. A stromal pocket is dissected on both sides of the incision using a modified spatula. Either a suction device is used to dissect a stromal plane to create semicircular lamellar pockets or this can be performed manually (Siganos et al 2002). After removal of the suction device, intracorneal rings are inserted into each of the semicircular channels. The rings can have different thicknesses, and selection of the appropriate ring thickness is based on the refractive error. Finally, the radial incision is closed with nylon sutures. Postoperatively, antibiotics and hydrocortisone are given to minimize the risk of keratitis.

Although the technique is rarely used nowadays for refractive surgery procedures, it remains a potential treatment option for keratoconus. The Perspex (Plexiglas) segments are inserted around the base of the cone in order to flatten the apex. The net result may be a cornea that can obtain some useful vision and/or may be refitted with a contact lens. It is often seen as a last resort treatment option for keratoconus before a corneal graft is indicated.

Thermokeratoplasty

These surgical techniques have been used for the correction of hyperopia. The application of local heat causes shrinkage of corneal collagen in the stroma, thereby causing extreme flattening at the site of treatment (Neumann et al 1990a,b). A circular treatment pattern in the mid-peripheral cornea causes a band of tightening which induces flattening of the mid-peripheral cornea and steepening of the central cornea, thus correcting low levels of hyperopia. Previous guises of this surgery have used nichrome wires and more recently Holmium YAG lasers. Spots are arranged in a circular pattern between 6 and 9 mm from the centre of the cornea and, as scar tissue forms, results

in steepening of the central cornea. Charpentier et al (1995) reported that the stability of refractive outcome is poor. This procedure was not popular when performed with heating probes, but saw a re-emergence with laser technology (Holmium lasers) and more recently in the guise of conductive keratoplasty (CK). CK uses a non-contact heating probe to alter the profile of the cornea. The technique uses thermal burns, regularly spaced in a ring around the corneal apex (outside of the visual axis), to achieve steepening of the corneal profile. A hand-held probe with a microthin disposable tip is used. The tip delivers controlled-release radio frequency radiation within the stromal layer, which acts as a natural conductor to the radio frequency, resulting in localized shrinkage. CK is now predominantly used to create 'blended vision', i.e. combination of monovision and changed corneal profile.

Phakic intraocular lenses

The word 'phakic' is derived from the Greek, *phakos*, meaning lens. Phakic intraocular lenses (PIOLs) are artificial lenses that are placed inside the eye to correct refractive error. For many years, intraocular lenses have been used following cataract removal. More recently, intraocular lenses have been designed to be placed in the eye for the correction of refractive error without removal of the natural lens. This surgical procedure is generally carried out for the treatment of high refractive errors where corneal surgery cannot be performed. Lenses made of PMMA or colorate (a soft lens composed of collagen, water and polymers) are placed inside the eye (**Fig. 23.10**). The lens is wedged between the posterior surface of the cornea and the anterior surface of the iris, clipped to the anterior surface of the iris or placed between the posterior surface of the iris and the anterior surface of the crystalline lens.

Indications for PIOL are ametropia greater than 5 D, thin corneas that cannot receive full treatment with LVC, or patients who have had previous corneal surgery (e.g. radial keratotomy) that would prevent them from having LVC.

Surgical procedure for anterior chamber lens implantation

The surgery is carried out under sterile conditions to avoid intraocular infection. The pupil is dilated, and anaesthesia

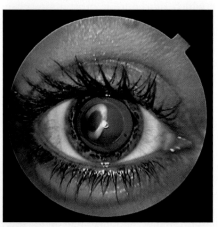

Figure 23.10 A posterior chamber phakic intraocular lens. The optic portion of the lens is clearly visible and the band haptic design can be seen. (Picture courtesy of Brian Tompkins, Tompkins, Knight and Son, Optometrists.)

administered either topically or with peribulbar injection. A temporal corneal incision of about 3 to 3.5 mm is made with a diamond blade. Sodium hyaluronate is injected into the anterior chamber to deepen it. The lens is implanted into the anterior chamber. The haptic ends are placed under the iris with a spatula and the lens centred. Peripheral iridectomy is generally performed to avoid blockage by the lens haptic. The viscoelastic material is removed by either irrigation or aspiration with balanced salt solution. Antibiotic and corticosteroid drops are usually given for 5 to 7 days postoperatively.

Surgical procedure for posterior chamber lens implantation

The pupil is dilated and the eye to be treated is anaesthetized with peribulbar injection. A temporal or nasal corneal incision of about 3 to 3.5 mm is made with a diamond blade. The silicone intraocular lens is implanted in front of the natural crystalline lens under protection of a viscoelastic substance. No sutures are necessary. A peripheral iridectomy is performed either intraoperatively or by laser after surgery. At the end of the surgical procedure antibiotics and corticosteroids are given either topically or both topically and subconjunctivally.

Advantages of PIOL include the correction of higher levels of myopia and hyperopia with preservation of accommodation. The techniques can be compatible with proven cataract and phakic IOL implantation procedures and are reversible (Baikoff et al 1998; Rosen & Gore 1998; Landesz et al 2000).

Documented complications following PIOL implantation include postsurgical astigmatism, secondary glaucoma (a major complication of an anterior chamber lens), chronic intraocular inflammation and pigment dispersion. Cataract formation can be a major complication of posterior chamber PIOLs. Glare and poor-quality vision at night with larger pupils can be associated with all types of PIOL. Endothelial cell damage has been shown in all types but is more common in anterior chamber PIOL. Infections such as uveitis and endophthalmitis are thankfully rare.

Hoyos et al reported mean best corrected VA 1 year following anterior chamber lens implantation in myopic and hyperopic eyes of 6/10.5 and 6/6.9, respectively. The study included 31 eyes (17 myopic and 14 hyperopic, with myopia ranging from −11.8 D to −26.00 D and hyperopia from +5.25 D to +11.00 D). After 1 year of follow-up, the mean spherical equivalent refractive error was −0.22 D in the myopic eyes, with 87% falling within ±1.00 D. In the hyperopic eyes the mean spherical equivalent refractive error was + 0.38 D, with 79% being within ±1.00 D (Hoyos et al 2002).

Eighteen eyes with high myopia (mean preoperative spherical equivalent −14.58±3.04 D) were evaluated by Brauweiler et al after implantation of a posterior chamber PIOL. Three eyes lost one line of best corrected VA. After 2-years' follow-up, the mean spherical equivalent refractive error was −1.33D±0.71 D (Brauweiler et al 1999).

Clear lens extraction

Indications for this procedure include high myopia or hyperopia (>6.00 D) and late presbyopia (especially in the presence of early cataractous changes). The surgical procedure is similar to cataract extraction; potential complications are similar to those of phacoemulsification cataract surgery, such as postsurgical astigmatism, chronic intraocular inflammation, endothelial cell damage and glare. Infections such as uveitis and endophthalmitis are thankfully rare. Posterior capsular opacity is not so rare and can depend on the intraocular lens design as well as other factors.

Usitalo et al, in a study on 38 eyes, reported that 71.9% gained one or more lines of best corrected VA while 40.6% gained two or more lines of corrected VA in their study of clear lens extraction on high myopic eyes (ranging from −7.75 D to −29.00 D). Of patients, 6.2% lost one line of best corrected VA after 1 year; 81.6% had a spherical equivalent refractive error within ±1.00 D while 71.1% were within ±0.5 D. In eyes with more than 18 D of myopia, 96.4% were within ±1.00 D while 85.7% were within ±0.5 D (Usitalo et al 2002).

Similarly, Pop et al examined 65 eyes with hyperopia of up to +12.25 D and reported that 1 month following clear lens extraction, the best corrected VA was 6/12 or better in 95% of eyes and 6/6 or better in 38.5% of the eyes (Pop et al 2001).

Arcuate surgery

This procedure is similar to radial keratotomy but arcuate keratotomy (AK) is only used to correct myopic astigmatism. It is sometimes used to treat corneal astigmatism alongside cataract surgery. Several nomograms are available for the incisional keratotomy to correct naturally occurring astigmatism. However, this is not the case in eyes with secondary astigmatism. Oshika et al designed a prospective, multicentre study, involving 104 pseudophakic eyes with corneal astigmatism of 1.50 D or more. All these patients were treated with arcuate keratotomy incisions. The parameter of predictability (35%) was lower than that reported for congenital astigmatism (56%) (Oshika et al 1998).

Presbyopic surgery

Surgical treatment of presbyopia is in its infancy. Surgery for presbyopia can be corneal, scleral or intraocular lens implant using either a multifocal or accommodative lens. The lens is implanted after cataract surgery on the assumption that movement of vitreous gel behind the lens will create the desired refractive error.

Corneal surgery

A multifocal cornea is developed under a LASIK flap by creating steepening of the inferior cornea or alternatively by implanting a multifocal intracorneal inlay.

Scleral surgery

Scleral surgery can be carried out using relaxing incisions and may also include expansion bands. The idea is that increasing the distance between the lens and ciliary body can reverse presbyopia, although this is not consistent with conventional theories of lens ageing. This technique has been used in various guises but without much popularity from surgeons due to variable results.

Intraocular surgery

Multifocal implants can be used in phakic IOL surgery or with clear lens extraction. The designs of these lenses are similar to multifocal contact lenses. Refractive and defractive multifocal intraocular lens are available. Again, careful patient selection is the key to success as dissatisfied patients complain of reduced contrast, haloes or glare, especially in low light levels. Use of this lens has been approved by FDA for treatment of presbyopia. A study carried out on 456 patients revealed 81% of patients treated with bilateral multifocal lens implantation could function without glasses (Hope-Ross 2002).

Accommodative IOLs are lenses with a single-power optic lens. The idea of an accommodative lens is to mimic the natural physiology of the eye whereby contraction of the ciliary muscle will change the power of the crystalline lens. These IOL designs have generated much interest by surgeons and manufacturers alike. Current designs have limited objective success but subjectively seem to be popular with patients. If the lens fails to move as intended or moves less with time then it effectively becomes a single-vision IOL. Under these circumstances, the patient may be no worse off than had a conventional IOL been used. With better designs, it is likely that this mode of presbyopic treatment will generate more success in the near future.

References

Abbot R L, Ou R J et al 2003 Medical malpractice predictors and risk factors for ophthalmologists performing LASIK and photorefractive keratcectomy surgery. Ophthalmology 110(11):137–146

Alio J L, Slem T F et al 2002 Intracorneal rings to correct corneal ectasia after laser in situ keratomileusis. Journal of Cataract and Refractive Surgery 28:1568–1574

Anderson N J, Beran R F et al 2002 Epi-LASEK for the correction of myopia and myopic astigmatism. Journal of Cataract and Refractive Surgery 28:1343–1347

Baikoff G, Arne J L et al 1998 Angle-fixated anterior chamber phakic intraocular lens for myopia of −7 to −19 diopters. Journal of Refractive Surgery 14(3):282–293

Barraquer J I 1965 [Autokeratoplasty with optical carving for the correction of myopia (Keratomileusis)] Autoqueratoplastia con talla optica para la correccion de la miopia (Queratomileusis). Anales de medicina: Especialidades 51(1):66–82

Barraquer J I 1966 Modification of refraction by means of intracorneal inclusions. International Ophthalmology Clinics 6(1):53–78

Barraquer J I 1967 Keratomileusis. International Surgery 48(2):103–117

Barraquer J I 1972 Keratophakia. Transactions of the Ophthalmological Societies of the United Kingdom 92:499–516

Bibby M M 1976a Computer assisted photo-keratoscopy and contact lens design (1). Optician 171:37–43

Bibby M M 1976b Computer assisted photo-keratoscopy and contact lens design (2). Optician 171:11–17

Bibby M M 1976c Computer assisted photo-keratoscopy and contact lens design (3). Optician 171:22–23

Bibby M M 1976d Computer assisted photo-keratoscopy and contact lens design (4). Optician 171:15–17

Brauweiler P H, Wehler T et al 1999 High incidence of cataract formation after implantation of a silicone posterior chamber lens in phakic, highly myopic eyes. Ophthalmology 106:1651–1655

Buratto L, Ferrari M 1992 Excimer laser intrastromal keratomileusis: case report. Journal of Cataract and Refractive Surgery 18:37–41

Buratto L, Ferrari M et al 1992 Excimer laser intrastromal keratomileusis. American Journal of Ophthalmology 113(3):291–295

Charpentier D Y, Nguyen-Khoa J L, Duplessix M et al 1995 Intrastromal thermokeratoplasty for correction of spherical hyperopia: a 1-year prospective study. Journal Français d'Ophtalmologie 18:200–206

Chui W S, Cho P 2005 A comparative study of the performance of different corneal topographers on children with respect to orthokeratology practice. Optometry and Vision Science 82(1):420–427

Claringbold II T V 2002 Laser assisted subepithelial keratectomy for the correction of myopia. Journal of Cataract and Refractive Surgery 28:18–22

Cobo-Soriano R, Llover F et al 2002 Factors that influence outcomes of hyperopic laser in situ keratomileusis. Journal of Cataract and Refractive Surgery 28:1530–1538

Dave T, Ruston D 1997 Current trends in modern orthokeratology. Ophthalmic and Physiological Optics 18(2):224–233

Farah S G, Azar D T et al 1998 Laser in situ keratomileusis: literature review of a developing technique. Journal of Cataract and Refractive Surgery 24:989–1006

Gallar J, Acosta M C et al 2004 Recovery of corneal sensitivity to mechanical and chemical stimulation after laser in situ keratomileusis. Journal of Refractive Surgery 20(3):229–235

Guillon M, Lydon D P M, Wilson C 1986 Corneal topography: a clinical model. Opthalmic and Physiological Optics 6:47–56

Gupta N, Naroo S A 2006 Factors affecting choice of contact lenses or refractive surgery and choice of centre. Contact Lens and Anterior Eye 29(1):17–23

Hope-Ross M 2002 Lens surgery and presbyopia. Refractive Eye News 1:11–18

Hoyos J E, Dementiev D D et al 2002 Phakic refractive lens experience in Spain. Journal of Cataract and Refractive Surgery 28:1939–1946

Jacobs J M, Taravella M J 2002 Incidence of intra-operative flap complications in laser in-situ keratomileusis. Journal of Cataract and Refractive Surgery 28:23–28

Joo C K, Tim T G 2000 Corneal ectasia detected after laser in situ keratomileusis for correction of less than −12 diopters of myopia. Journal of Cataract and Refractive Surgery 26(2):292–295

Joslin C E, Wu S M et al 2004 Higher-order wavefront aberrations in corneal refractive therapy. Optometry and Vision Science 80 (12):805–811

Kawesch G M, Kezirian G M 2000 Laser in situ keratomileusis for high myopia with VISX star laser. Ophthalmology 107:653–661

Landesz M, Worst J G et al 2000 Long-term results of correction of high myopia with an iris claw phakic intraocular lens. Journal of Refractive Surgery 16(3):310–316

Lian J, Ye W et al 2002 Laser in situ keratomileusis for correction of hyperopia and hyperopic astigmatism with the Technolas 117C. Journal of Refractive Surgery 18:435–438

Lui W-O, Edwards M H 2000a Orthokeratology in low myopia. Part 1: Efficacy and predictability. Contact Lens and Anterior Eye 23 (3):77–89

Lui W-O, Edwards M H 2000b Orthokeratology in low myopia. Part 2: Corneal topographic changes and safety over 100 days. Contact Lens and Anterior Eye 23(3):90–99

Lui W-O, Edwards M H et al 2000 Contact lenses in myopia reduction – from orthofocus to accelerated orthokeratology. Contact Lens and Anterior Eye 23(3):68–76

Marshall J, Trokel S et al 1985 An ultrasound study of corneal incisions induced by an excimer laser at 193 nm. Ophthalmology 92 (6):749–758

Marshall J, Trokel S et al 1986 A comparative study of corneal incisions induced by diamond and steel knives and two ultrasound radiations from an excimer laser. British Journal of Ophthalmology 70(7): 482–501

Michieletto P, Ligabue E et al 2004 PermaVision intracorneal lens for the correction of hyperopia. Journal of Cataract and Refractive Surgery 30(10):2152–2157

Munnerlyn C R, Coons S J et al 1988 Photorefractive keratectomy: a technique for laser refractive surgery. Journal of Cataract and Refractive Surgery 14:46–52

Naroo S A, Charman W N 2001 Refractive surgery: Review and current status. Optometry in Practice 2(1):29–46

Naroo S A, Ubhi B K 2004 Co-management in refractive surgery. Optometry in Practice 5(1):5–14

Naroo S A, Shah S et al 1999 Factors that influence patient choice of contact lens or photorefractive keratectomy. Journal of Refractive Surgery 15:132–136

Neumann A C, McCarty G et al 1989 Delayed regression of effect in myopic keratophakia versus myopia keratomileusis for high myopia. Refractive and Corneal Surgery 5(3):161–166

Neumann A C, Fyodorov S et al 1990a Radial thermoplasty for the correction of hyperopia. Refractive and Corneal Surgery 6(6): 404–412

Neumann A C, Sanders D R et al 1990b Effect of thermokeratoplasty on corneal curvature. Journal of Cataract and Refractive Surgery 16(6):727–731

Oliveira-Soto L, Charman W N 2002 Some possible longer-term ocular changes following excimer laser refractive surgery. Ophthalmic and Physiological Optics 22(4):274–288

Oshika T, Shimazaki J et al 1998 Arcuate keratotomy to treat corneal astigmatism after cataract surgery: a prospective evaluation of predictability and effectiveness. Ophthalmology 105:2012–2016

Pallikaris I G, Papatzanaki M et al 1990 Laser in situ keratomileusis. Lasers in Surgery and Medicine 10:463–468

Pallikaris I G, Kymionis G et al 2001 Corneal ectasia induced by laser in situ keratomileusis. Journal of Cataract and Refractive Surgery 27:1796–1802

Pop M, Payette Y 2000 Photorefractive keratectomy versus laser in situ keratomileusis: a control-matched study. Ophthalmology 107 (2):251–257

Pop M, Payette Y et al 2001 Clear lens extraction with intraocular lens followed by photorefractive keratectomy or laser in situ keratomileusis. Ophthalmology 108:104–111

Randleman J B, Russell B et al 2003 Risk factors and prognosis for corneal ectasia after LASIK. Ophthalmology 110(2):267–275

Reidy J J, McDonald M B et al 1990 The corneal topography of epikeratophakia. Refractive and Corneal Surgery 6(1):26–31

Rosen E, Gore C 1998 Staar Collamer posterior chamber phakic intraocular lens to correct myopia and hyperopia. Journal of Cataract and Refractive Surgery 24:596–606

Ruston D, Dave T et al 1997 An introduction to orthokeratology. British Orthokeratology Society, London

Scerrati E 2001 Laser in situ keratomileusis versus laser epithelial keratomileusis (LASIK vs. LASEK). Journal of Refractive Surgery 17: S219–S221

Shah S, Sebai Serhan A R et al 2001 The epithelial flap for photorefractive keratectomy. British Journal of Ophthalmology 85 (4):393–396

Shahinian L 2002 Laser-assisted subepithelial keratectomy for low to high myopia and astigmatism. Journal of Cataract and Refractive Surgery 28:1334–1342

Siganos D, Ferrara P et al 2002 Ferrara intrastromal corneal rings for the correction of keratoconus. Journal of Cataract and Refractive Surgery 28:1947–1951

Stephenson C 2002 Complications of PRK, LASIK and LASEK: diagnosis and treatment. Refractive Eye News 1(1):6–11

Tabb R L 2001 Surgical and non-surgical techniques to correct refractive errors. Optometry Today 41(11):34–38

Taylor D M, L'Esperance Jr F A et al 1989 Experimental corneal studies with the excimer laser. Journal of Cataract and Refractive Surgery 15(4):384–389

Trokel S L, Srinivasan R et al 1983 Excimer laser surgery of the cornea. American Journal of Ophthalmology 96(6):710–715

Twa M D, Nichols J J et al 2004 Characteristics of corneal ectasia after LASIK for myopia. Cornea 23(5):447–457

Usitalo R J, Aine E et al 2002 Implantable contact lens for high myopia. Journal of Cataract and Refractive Surgery 28:29–36

Verma S, Corbett M C et al 1995 A prospective, randomized, double-masked trial to evaluate the role of topical anaesthetics in controlling pain after photorefractive keratectomy. Ophthalmology 102(12):1918–1924

Weber B A, Fagerholm P P 1998 Plano and refractive keratectomy. Comparison of the wound healing response. Acta Ophthalmologica 76:537–540.

Winkler T D 1995 Orthokeratology. Vision Asia-Pacific March: 8

CHAPTER 24

Intraocular pressure and pachymetry

Shabbir Mohamed • Sunil Shah

Introduction

The importance of elevated intraocular pressure (IOP) has been known since ancient times, and At-Tabari in the tenth century noted a disease corresponding with firmness of the eye. Subsequently, Bannister in 1622 recognized a disease of elevated IOP encompassing long duration, loss of sight and a fixed pupil. However, it was not until the nineteenth century that the term glaucoma was clearly applied to this disease by several ophthalmologists including Demours, Guthrie and McKenzie. With a better understanding of ocular physiology and mechanics, the nineteenth century saw the development of various tonometers to measure IOP.

Adolf Weber, a student of von Graefe, designed the first applanation tonometer in 1867, but it failed to gain widespread acceptance. Schiotz, in 1910, is credited with the first clinically useful tonometer. In the mid-twentieth century, Goldmann, Schmidt and Perkins used the works of Maklakov, Imbert and Fick to design the modern instruments we commonly use to measure IOP in the clinical setting. These tonometers all measure IOP in millimetres of mercury (mmHg).

The normal range of IOP is defined from population surveys, and a cutoff value of 21 mmHg is widely used to differentiate between normal and abnormal IOP. However, these values are not strictly applicable to an individual patient (European Glaucoma Society 2003). There is increasing evidence that optic nerve damage can occur despite an IOP falling within the normal range. Furthermore, there is ample evidence from cross-sectional studies that IOP varies amongst populations (Sommer et al 1991; Mitchell et al 1996; Drance 2001; Leske et al 2001; Ekstrom 2002; Hashemi et al 2005).

The problem of measuring IOP accurately in individuals has been a central issue both in the management of patients with glaucoma and in identifying populations at risk of developing glaucoma. Accurate IOP measurement is important for several reasons, namely:

- It helps to identify individuals at higher risk of developing glaucoma.
- It helps to classify patients correctly into specific groups which have prognostic implications for the individual patient's vision.
- Initial IOP measurements guide our subsequent treatment approach and help set the desired pressure for each patient.
- Subsequent IOP measurements help us decide whether we need to be more aggressive in treating the individual's glaucoma.
- Treatment efficacy can only be monitored by measuring the IOP accurately.

In this chapter, we will discuss IOP, its measurement and the influence of ocular parameters such as central corneal thickness (CCT) on the accuracy of these values. We will try to elucidate why these parameters may influence the accuracy of IOP measurement. Subsequently, we will briefly review the currently available measuring devices and discuss their accuracy.

Measurement of CCT has also progressed from the earliest efforts. We will review the currently available measuring devices and compare them with one another. Furthermore, recent evidence indicates the importance of the biomechanical properties of the cornea in determining the true IOP. This may have a greater impact than the CCT. We will review this evidence and examine some newer methods of measuring IOP independent of CCT. Finally, we will review the clinical implications of these emerging technologies and how they can help us to manage our patient population.

Intraocular pressure and central corneal thickness

The Imbert Fick principle

Measurement of IOP using applanation tonometry is based upon the Imbert Fick principle. This states that when a flat surface with a defined area is pressed against the surface of a sphere (applanation) with a given internal pressure, equilibrium is reached when the force exerted is balanced by the internal pressure. Thus, the force required to flatten the surface of a sphere (W) is equal to the product of the pressure inside the sphere (P) and the area applanated (A), i.e. $W = P \times A$ (Gloster & Perkins 1963).

For the principle to be strictly true the sphere should be dry, thin, perfectly elastic and perfectly flexible, and the only force acting on the surface should be the pressure of the applanating surface. Furthermore, it is assumed that the displaced volume during the process of applanation from within the sphere should be small in relation to the total volume of the sphere (Goldmann 1957).

Goldmann applanation tonometry

Traditionally, the gold standard for measuring IOP has been the Goldmann applanation tonometer (GAT). This is because it is reasonably priced, fits easily into the slit-lamp examination, provides seemingly accurate IOP measurements and is based on easily understood principles.

Goldmann developed this instrument based on the Imbert Fick principle, but in addition he took into account two other forces that are of importance in relation to the eye: firstly, the surface tension (S) of the tear film attracts the tonometer prism towards the cornea, and secondly the corneal rigidity (B), which resists applanation. According to Goldmann and Schmidt (1957), these two forces were felt to cancel out one another when the area being applanated was 3.06 mm in diameter. Thus, $W + S = (P \times A) + B$.

Many of the assumptions underlying GAT do not apply strictly to the eye. This is because the cornea has a finite thickness, and the coats of the eye have significant rigidity and are not homogeneous in their elasticity. The cornea, limbus and sclera all have differing biomechanical properties (Ehlers et al 1975; Quigley et al 1991; Whitacre et al 1993; Argus 1995; Hjortdal 1996; Doughty & Zaman 2000). There is inherent resistance in the cornea to indentation, and as the corneal thickness increases, so does the force required to applanate it. Furthermore, corneal curvature can affect the degree of resistance to indentation significantly. Finally, the volume of fluid displaced by applanation produces inaccuracy in readings. Therefore, the GAT provides only a surrogate measurement of the true intraocular pressure.

Goldmann and Schmidt discussed the possible role of central corneal thickness in IOP measurements (Goldmann & Schmidt 1957). They postulated that errors can occur if the CCT value is significantly different from the mean finding, which they took as being 500 μm. However, they also suggested that variation in corneal thickness is unlikely in the absence of pathology.

Goldmann applanation tonometer procedure

Measuring IOP using GAT is a skill that is acquired with practice. The procedure requires the patient to be cooperative, able to position their head at the slit lamp, to tolerate insertion of topical anaesthesia and to keep their eye still with their eyelids open for several seconds.

At the beginning of the day, the GAT calibration is checked. This is done in position 0, 2 and 6 (corresponding to IOP values of 0, 20 and 60 mmHg). The tonometer is placed on the slit lamp with the prism in place. The feeler arm should be in free movement and should move to and fro as the dial is turned either side of the 0 mark. The calibration at position 2 and 6 is checked using the check weight supplied with the tonometer in a similar fashion.

The procedure begins with removing the prism from the disinfectant solution (usually chlorine based, but see later section on prism disinfection) and mounting it onto the tonometer with the 0° and 180° markings on the prism lined up with the white mark on the tonometer bracket. The patient's cornea is anaesthetized with topical anaesthetic drops (e.g. oxybuprocaine 0.4% or proxymetacaine) and a drop of fluorescein 1% is applied to the conjunctival sac. Excess lacrimation and drops are wiped away.

The patient is positioned at the slit lamp with the chin on the chinrest and the forehead against the bar. Once the patient is comfortable, they are instructed to stare at the examiner. The slit-lamp illumination is set on maximum with the blue filter in place and the light source is placed at approximately 60° to ensure that the tip of the tonometer is brightly illuminated. The biomicroscope magnification level is set at about 10×. The tip of the tonometer is moved forward gently until it comes into contact with the patient's cornea. It is sometimes necessary to hold the patient's eyelids open but care needs to be taken not to apply pressure onto the globe, which would induce false readings. It is best to hold the eyelids against the patient's orbital rim.

Upon contact with the cornea, one will observe two semicircles of fluorescein. At this point, the dial on the tonometer is adjusted until the *inner edges* of the two semicircles are aligned (**Fig. 24.1**). When this occurs, the diameter of the area applanated is 3.06 mm, and the IOP (in mmHg) is equal to 10 times the reading on the dial.

It is good practice to take several readings and use the average as the most accurate IOP, especially when learning to use the device. Other potential pitfalls include using too much or too little fluorescein, excessive eyelid squeezing by the patient and indenting the cornea excessively. With practice, GAT is quick and easy to perform in the majority of patients.

Accuracy of the Goldmann applanation tonometer

Since 1975, the accuracy of GAT has been disputed. Initially, Ehlers et al (1975) showed by cannulating eyes undergoing cataract surgery that GAT was most accurate when the CCT

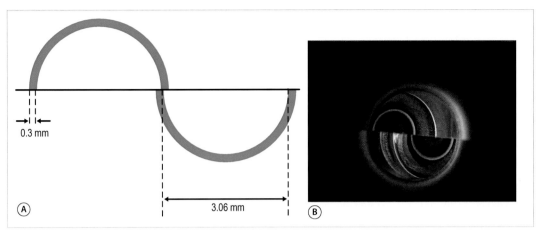

Figure 24.1 **(A)** Diagram showing the correct alignment and dimensions of the mires during Goldmann applanation tonometry. **(B)** Actual appearance of the aligned mires during Goldmann applanation tonometry.

was 520 μm. Further, true IOP varied by as much as 7 mmHg per 100 μm of CCT. Johnson et al (1978) reported a patient having a CCT of 900 μm in whom the measured IOP did not alter despite medical treatment to reduce it.

CCT has been shown to vary between populations, and evidence from work on monozygotic twins suggests that CCT is inherited (Toh et al 2005). The large Rotterdam eye study revealed a mean CCT of 537 μm (Wolf et al 1997). Other investigations have shown significant racial variations, with Afro-Caribbeans having thinner CCT values (La-Rosa et al 2001; Hahn et al 2003; Nemesure et al 2003; Shimiyo et al 2003; Herndon et al 2004).

Correction factors

As a result of these CCT findings and the previous issues relating to GAT inaccuracies, some authorities have suggested that GAT underestimates the IOP in the presence of reduced corneal thickness. Accordingly, correction factors have been proposed to compensate for changes in CCT to give a more accurate estimation of the true IOP.

The Rotterdam study (Wolf et al 1997) reported a mean CCT of 537 μm but wide variation amongst the population examined (i.e. 427–620 μm). It was suggested that for each 10 μm increase in CCT, the measured IOP increased by 0.19 mmHg. Subsequently, Bron et al (1999) and Shah et al (1999) suggested changes of 0.32 mmHg and 0.11 mmHg, respectively, for a 10 μm increase in CCT.

Doughty and Zaman (2000) performed a meta-analysis of trials of IOP and CCT. Looking at 300 data sets in the published literature between 1968 and mid-1999, they suggest that a 10% difference in CCT would result in a 3.4±0.9 mmHg change in IOP (more for diseased eyes and less for normal eyes). Using the values indicated above by Bron et al and Shah et al, we calculate a correction factor of 1.76 mmHg per 10% change in CCT, while Shah et al's correction would be 0.6 mmHg for a 10% change in CCT.

The fact that the different studies identify dissimilar correction factors indicates that this is still an unresolved issue. Furthermore, the correction factors are derived from linear trend lines that are observed within the population group as a whole. These trend lines are not necessarily accurate for an individual, and therefore doubt exists as to whether IOP measured by GAT can be corrected in such a linear fashion

to derive veridical IOP for a single patient. Additionally, the correction factor determined by Doughty and Zaman (2000) is dependent on whether the eye is normal or diseased. In the clinical situation, we are not always privileged to have this information and, in fact, the true IOP value (with appropriate correction factor) may be required to make this determination.

Additionally, the relationship of CCT to true IOP is not linear across the spectrum of IOPs. This was demonstrated in a manometric study (Whitacre et al 1993) using the Perkins applanation tonometer. They observed an underestimation in thin corneas of 4.9 mmHg and an overestimation in thicker corneas of 6.8 mmHg, giving a calculated range of correction factor of 0.18–0.49 mmHg for each 10 μm change in CCT. Further, the relationship between GAT findings and the true IOP may be influenced not only by CCT but also by corneal curvature, axial length and corneal biomechanical properties (Mark et al 2002; Mark & Mark 2003; Liu & Roberts 2005).

Central corneal thickness and ocular disease

Central corneal thickness and ocular hypertension

Numerous studies have shown that CCT is increased in patients with ocular hypertension (OHT) (Argus 1995; Herndon et al 1997; Bron et al 1999; Herman et al 2001). The Ocular Hypertension Treatment Study (OHTS) (Brandt et al 2001; Gordon et al 2002) is a major prospective, randomized, multicentre clinical trial comparing medical treatment with close observation of patients at risk of developing glaucoma due to OHT. Patients whose IOP was between 24 and 32 mmHg in one eye with both normal visual fields and optic nerve appearances were enrolled. CCT was measured 2 years after enrolment was completed. Multivariate analysis indicated that the baseline characteristic which best predicted the development of glaucoma was CCT. This landmark study also demonstrated that many patients are being misclassified solely on the basis of GAT readings. It was estimated that 30–60% of OHT and normal-tension glaucoma (NTG) patients are misclassified due to errors in measuring IOP using GAT (Argus 1995; Herndon et al 1997; Copt et al 1999; Brandt et al 2001).

Central corneal thickness and normal-tension glaucoma

It has been proposed that measurement of CCT may aid the management of glaucoma patients. In a clinic population in northwest England, Shah et al (1999) found mean CCT values of 554 μm in normal eyes, 550 μm in eyes with primary open-angle glaucoma (POAG), 514 μm in eyes with normal-tension glaucoma and 580 μm in eyes with OHT. If the IOP had been corrected on the basis of Ehler's (1975) data, 44% of the NTG patients would be reclassified as having POAG and 35% of the OHT patients would be reclassified as normal.

It is now generally accepted that NTG populations have thinner average CCT values (Morad et al 1998; Emara et al 1999). This is likely to lead to underestimation of the true IOP. However, there is also believed to be a subgroup of NTG patients who have normal CCT and true normal IOP. The pathological process in this latter group is not thought to be caused by elevated IOP, and may be related to either vascular optic atrophy or atrophy from other causes.

Central corneal thickness and open-angle glaucoma

Recent evidence suggests that thinner CCT values are correlated with more severe glaucoma at presentation and, subsequently, more aggressive glaucomatous visual field deterioration (Kim & Chen 2004; Herndon et al 2004). In addition, Medeiros et al (2003) followed 98 eyes of 98 patients with glaucoma who were diagnosed purely on optic disc assessment using stereo photographs. After 4 years, repeatable field defects were found in 46% of patients whose CCT was less than 545 μm, but only 11% of those having CCT greater than 545 μm.

However, the situation may be more complicated. Chauhan et al (2005) and Jonas et al (2005) showed that although patients with thinner corneas demonstrate more advanced field loss at presentation, if the effects of IOP are accounted for, there is no relationship between CCT and progression of visual field loss. Therefore, while CCT has implications in the progressive optic neuropathy that characterizes glaucoma, it may not be the only factor. The relationship between CCT and optic nerve damage is clearly very complex and not completely elucidated.

Possible mechanisms for the association of central corneal thickness with glaucoma damage

It is postulated that the association between reduced corneal thickness and advanced glaucoma may be due, in part, to inaccurate IOP measurements. However, CCT measurements may also be surrogate measures of posterior scleral thickness and the lamina cribrosa, through which all ganglion cell axons pass.

In experimental glaucoma, there is acquired posterior scleral thinning and increased eye wall stress, and this is thought to be due to raised IOP (Downs et al 2001).

Therefore, not only the initial scleral thickness but also the response of the peripapillary sclera to further IOP increase will affect the individual's susceptibility to develop glaucoma and also influence the aggressiveness of the glaucomatous process.

Furthermore, hydrostatic pressure around the lamina cribrosa impacts axoplasmic flow in retinal ganglion cell axons, and may lead to axonal death (Anderson & Hendrickson 1974; Minckler et al 1977; Gaasterland et al 1978; Radius & Bade 1982; Pease et al 2000). The pressure environment around the lamina cribrosa is critically affected by the thickness of the sclera at this point, and may have a significant effect on axoplasmic flow in the presence of elevated IOP (Morgan et al 1995).

It is postulated that as the coats of the eye form a continuous structure, CCT (as a surrogate measure of posterior scleral thickness) may independently affect both the risk of developing glaucoma and the rate of progression. This may account for the higher prevalence of glaucoma amongst myopic patients, as they exhibit acquired regional thinning of the sclera (Mitchell et al 1999; Jonas et al 2004). However, the relationship between CCT and scleral thickness is not established, and there is some evidence that this relationship may exist at the scleral spur but not more posteriorly (Oliveira et al 2006). It will be apparent that it remains unclear how CCT might influence glaucoma independently of the effect on IOP measurement.

Other clinically available tonometers

Several other techniques are available for measuring IOP, all of which are dependent on measurement of the physical properties of the cornea. Recently, there have been attempts to develop tonometers that are less dependent on CCT than GAT. Here, the authors will review the tonometers available and consider the influence that CCT has on their measurement accuracy.

Tono-Pen XL

The Tono-Pen XL (Reichert Inc., Depew, NY, USA) is a hand-held device based on the Mackay–Marg tonometer (Marg 1963) which provides IOP readings using microstrain gauge technology and a 1.5 mm transducer tip (**Fig. 24.2**).

Technique

The Tono-Pen XL must be calibrated when first used. The process of calibration requires the user to switch the device on and hold it pointing downwards until the LCD display shows 'UP'. At this time the user should point the tip

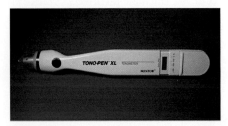

Figure 24.2 The Tono-Pen XL hand-held tonometer (Copyright Reichert).

upwards. Once calibrated, the tip of the device should be covered with a sterile disposable rubber membrane. The cornea is anaesthetized using topical anaesthetic and the instrument tip is then gently and repeatedly placed against the central corneal surface. It measures several independent readings and displays the result with a statistical coefficient. Although some practitioners have suggested that the Tono-Pen can be used without topical anaesthesia, this tends to be unpleasant for the patient and may give higher readings due to blepharospasm.

Accuracy

The Tono-Pen IOP readings are quite consistent and accurate when compared with GAT findings (**Fig. 24.3**) (Minckler et al 1987; Bhan et al 2002).

The Tono-Pen may be more 'user friendly' in the presence of corneal pathology as it applanates a smaller area of the cornea (Hines et al 1988). It has clear advantages in portability, and is less threatening when examining nervous patients such as children. However, there is evidence that Tono-Pen measurements are also affected by CCT (Li et al 2004; Sullivan-Mee & Pham 2004; Tonnu et al 2005a). In addition, it has a tendency to overestimate IOP, and therefore its measurements need to be correlated with other clinical findings.

Rebound tonometry

Rebound tonometry (RBT) is a novel way of measuring IOP. It relies on measuring the force required to decelerate a magnetized probe that is bounced off the cornea.

Technique

The Icare® tonometer (Tiolat, Finland) is a hand-held, portable instrument which utilizes the principles of RBT. A disposable probe composed of a magnetized steel wire with a rounded plastic tip is loaded onto the hand-held device. This is bounced off the corneal surface and the moving magnet induces a voltage in the enclosed solenoid of the device. The resulting impedance is detected and converted to IOP. As the contact time between the probe and the

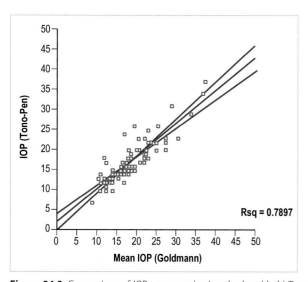

Figure 24.3 Comparison of IOPs measured using the hand-held Tono-Pen and GAT.

cornea is short, it requires no anaesthetic, reduces the risk of corneal injury and, as the probe is disposable, there is no risk of cross-infection. It is both quick and easy to use even by inexperienced operators.

Accuracy

Studies comparing GAT and RBT found that the rebound tonometer overestimates IOP by 0.6–1.8 mmHg (van der Jagt & Jansonius 2005; Martinez-de-la-Casa et al 2005; Fernandes et al 2005; Iliev et al 2006). RBT also overestimates the IOP when compared with the Perkins applanation tonometer (Garcia-Resua et al 2006). RBT measurements have also been shown to be influenced by CCT (Martinez-de-la-Casa et al 2005; Iliev et al 2006). It can be used as an alternative in cases where positioning of the head at the slit lamp is difficult, or if topical anaesthetic is contraindicated (Iliev et al 2006).

At present, RBT is still a relatively new technique and its usefulness is not clearly established, especially when compared with the older Tono-Pen XL instrument. However, its advantage of not requiring topical anaesthetic may be valuable for some groups of patients.

Non-contact tonometry

The non-contact tonometer (NCT) utilizes a puff of air to applanate the cornea. Optical detectors measure a change in the reflected light from the corneal surface. This is then correlated with an IOP reading (Regine et al 2006).

Pulsair tonometer

The Pulsair (Keeler, Windsor, UK) hand-held NCT is widely used as a screening tool for IOP in the community. It does not require corneal anaesthesia as there is no direct contact with the corneal surface to obtain a pressure reading. The examination is rapidly performed and most patients tolerate it well.

Technique

The Pulsair is an easy instrument to use. The latest generation can also be portable. The patient's cornea is aligned using an eyepiece, and the instrument gradually moved forward towards the patient. As the required distance is achieved, two green dots appear in the eyepiece, indicating that the operator is aligned correctly. At this point, the tonometer is gradually moved closer to the patient until a bow-tie pattern appears in the eye piece. The machine then automatically releases a jet of air to applanate the patient's cornea.

Accuracy

Findings from the Pulsair NCT are highly correlated with GAT within the normal range (Forbes et al 1974; Sørensen 1975; Popovich & Shields 1997; Ogbuehi 2006). CCT was found to affect IOP significantly when measured by the NCT. For each 10 μm change in mean CCT, the Pulsair NCT deviates from GAT by 0.21–0.98 mmHg (Ko et al 2005; Tonnu et al 2005a; Regine et al 2006). There is also evidence that NCT is correlated with keratometry (Yaoeda et al 2005) although keratometry values within the normal range do not significantly affect NCT findings (Paranhos et al 2000). The problem of measuring IOP during the different phases of the cardiac cycle has somewhat been addressed with the more recent NIDEK NCT-4000. This instrument measures the IOP through all phases of the cardiac cycle and can be configured to print the peak, mid and trough IOPs.

Table-mounted non-contact tonometers are also commonly available. Examples include the Reichert and American Optical non-contact tonometers and the newer Canon TX instruments. The Reichert tonometer has an icon-driven interface and the latest generation can also measure CCT through a 20 MHz ultrasound probe attached to the machine. With this instrument, the patient views a fixation target while the operator observes a red dot. This will be focused when the instrument is positioned at the correct distance from the patient's cornea. Once correctly aligned, the operator triggers the air-puff mechanism, and the reading is displayed digitally. Patients often report that they find the loud noise and sudden nature of the air puff produced by this instrument uncomfortable.

Mackie et al (1996) compared both the Keeler Pulsair and the American Optical non-contact tonometers with GAT in 45 patients (89 eyes) receiving medical treatment for primary open-angle glaucoma. Mean findings ($\pm$1SD) were 19.06$\pm$6.28 mmHg for the Pulsair, 16.27$\pm$5.93 mmHg for the American Optical instrument and 18.01$\pm$4.88 mmHg for GAT. These differences were statistically significant. In addition, the repeatability of the Pulsair was poorer than the American Optical device, while both were less repeatable than the GAT. The authors concluded that despite these limitations, both non-contact tonometers are useful for measuring IOP as part of a screening protocol for glaucoma.

The Canon TX tonometer is a fully automatic table-mounted device which has a novel eye-tracking ability that can locate the apex of the patient's cornea to improve accuracy. Tonnu et al (2005b) reported that the TX-10 significantly underestimated IOP measurements at lower IOP and overestimated those at higher IOP. Further, results from this instrument were affected by CCT significantly more than GAT (Tonnu et al 2005a).

Contact pneumotonometry: the ocular blood flow analyser

The ocular blood flow (OBF) analyser (Paradigm Medical, Salt Lake City, NV, USA) measures IOP using contact pneumotonometry, a technique first developed by Langham and McCarthy (1968). The instrument includes a 5 mm-diameter plastic tip covered by a membrane mounted on a frictionless bearing. Air at a constant pressure pushes against the membrane on one side. As the membrane comes into contact with the cornea, the membrane is deformed and air escapes from the probe. The rate of air flow that escapes is measured and converted to an IOP reading. The instrument collects 200 readings per second over 20 seconds. The results are displayed as a mean of the 4000 readings. The instrument is shown in **Figure 24.4**.

Technique

Ocular blood flow pneumotonometry is performed using the slit-lamp-mounted probe with the patient sitting upright. Each day, before measurements are taken, the air pressure generated by the instrument should be checked with a manometer and calibrated according to the

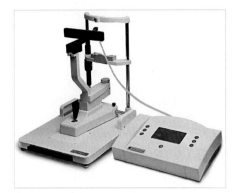

Figure 24.4 Ocular blood flow analyser. (Reproduced with permission from Paradigm Medical Instruments.)

manufacturer's instructions. Patients are instructed to look at the red fixation target within the probe. The probe tip is applied to the central cornea and, when correctly aligned, a whistling noise sounds as air escapes from the probe tip. The probe should be applied to the cornea until five pulses of equal amplitude are recorded. The mean IOP is calculated by the instrument and displayed on an LCD.

Accuracy

Studies have confirmed the accuracy of this device in the normal range when compared with GAT and manometric IOP measurement (Chidlow et al 1996; Spraul et al 1998; Yang et al 2000; Bafa et al 2001). However, the instrument has been shown to have poor intra-patient repeatability (Esgin et al 1998). When compared with GAT in patients with normal corneas, correlation coefficients of 0.77 and 0.95 have been recorded (Tuunanen et al 1996; Esgin et al 1998; Yang et al 2000). The manufacturers claim that the instrument is unaffected by CCT based on pre- and post-refractive surgery IOP measurements (Tuunanen et al 1996; Abbasoglu et al 1998). Additionally, the mathematical considerations underlying the instrument are supposed to cancel out the rigidity of the cornea (Silver & Farrell 1994). However, in a clinical setting on groups of normal (Bhan et al 2002) and pathological eyes (Browning et al 2004), it was observed that the OBF overestimates IOP when compared with GAT, and is also affected by CCT with a value of 0.26–0.28 mmHg/10 µm.

Pascal dynamic contour tonometry

The Pascal dynamic contour tonometry (DCT) is a relatively recent invention (2001). It is a slit-lamp-mounted tonometer that utilizes the principle of contour matching to measure IOP independent of CCT. The principle of contour matching is a complex one but may be summarized by noting that the cornea maintains its shape when pressure applied on the outside is equal to the pressure inside the globe. The DCT uses a pressure sensor within a concave hemisphere tip that is designed to fit on the cornea and match the corneal contour. The pressure sensor measures IOP throughout the cardiac cycle but the output is diastolic IOP (Kniestedt et al 2005). The IOP is measured through several cardiac cycles and an average reading is given with a mark for the quality of the reading (Q value).

Technique

The device is similar in shape to the GAT and fits onto the standard Goldmann tonometer mount on the slit lamp. The device has an arm, on the end of which is a concave tip having a radius of 10.5 mm. An electronic pressure sensor is integrated into the centre of the disposable contacting tip surface. After positioning the patient at the slit lamp in a fashion similar to when performing GAT, a drop of topical anaesthetic is applied to the ocular surface. The DCT tip is advanced until it makes contact with the corneal surface. Its correct positioning on the cornea is indicated by an audible signal that changes in pitch with variations in the detected pressure. When the tonometer tip contacts the cornea the tissue adopts the tip contour as if the pressure on both sides of the cornea were the same, thereby allowing the pressure sensor to measure IOP independent of corneal properties. IOP is calculated and displayed by the instrument without the examiner being able to change the result, thereby reducing possible observer bias. The readings are given a quality scale (from 1 to 4) to indicate the accuracy and reliability of the reading.

Accuracy

Investigators have found that DCT overestimates IOP, when compared with GAT, by 1.0–2.0 mmHg (Duba & Wirthlin 2004; Kamppeter & Jonas 2005; Pache et al 2005, Ku et al 2006; Schneider & Grehn 2006). DCT does seem to be less dependent on CCT, and several investigators have found only a weak association of this technique with CCT (Doyle & Lachkar 2005; Kotecha et al 2005; Ku et al 2006), while others have reported no association with CCT (Kamppeter & Jonas 2005; Pache et al 2005; Schneider & Grehn 2006). An interesting study comparing IOP readings with DCT taken before and after myopic refractive surgery correction found no significant change whereas IOP readings by GAT decreased significantly (Kaufmann et al 2003). This finding supports the argument that this instrument is not affected by changes in CCT.

The manufacturers of this instrument noted that possible sources of error could occur with extremely flat corneas, or where there may be adhesion between the cornea and the tip, leading to erroneous results. However, Scheider and Grehn (2006) found little influence of corneal curvature on IOP readings by DCT.

Another drawback of the DCT is that the sensor tip is covered with a membrane, and there may be problems with the membrane fitting poorly or wrinkling. Bubbles of air can become trapped between the tip and the eye, leading to erroneous results. Furthermore, this technique requires more cooperation from the patient as the reading can take several seconds, during which the patient is required to keep the eye still. Excessive tear film or a very dry eye can also affect the DCT reading, which means that it is not possible to get a reading in all patients.

Pressure phosphene tonometry (Proview)

The Proview (Bausch and Lomb Inc., Rochester, NY, USA) is a spring-loaded device which is pressed against the closed nasal eyelid until the patient visualizes a phenomenon described as a phosphene. It consists of a probe with a flat applicator of 3.06 mm diameter (the same size as the GAT). A phosphene spot is a self-perceptible visual phenomenon composed of a bright light. The technique has clear advantages in that it does not require topical anaesthesia, is portable and can be performed by a suitably trained patient at home to derive tonometry readings over a long period of the day when it is impractical to check IOP in the clinical setting. However, the influence of the eyelid and scleral rigidity would lead to inaccuracies. A further limitation of this technique is that not all patients can recognize phosphenes.

Technique

The Proview device is recommended to be applied to a closed eyelid without topical anaesthetic with the patient abducting and depressing the eye. The device is then placed on the superior nasal portion of the eyelid. Increasing force is gently applied. A phosphene can be induced initially with greater force than needed in order to familiarize the patient with the sensation. Subsequently, the patient is instructed to apply just enough force to induce a phosphene. The IOP level can then be read off a graticule. Several readings can be taken in this manner and the average calculated. It is important to pause between readings to allow the eye to recover from the previous deformation.

Accuracy

Fresco (1998) first described the use of phosphene phenomena, and utilized the pressure phosphene tonometer (PPT) to determine IOP. He found that this method obtained valid results when compared with GAT, although the mean finding with the PPT was 0.3 mmHg lower than the GAT value when measured in 192 eyes of 100 patients. However, only 74.9% of values were within ±2 mmHg of the GAT finding and the correlation coefficient between GAT and PPT was 0.71. Later, Naruse et al (2005) reported poor correlation between PPT and GAT, but suggested that PPT was not affected by CCT. Other studies have reported that the PPT measures higher (Chew et al 2005; Herse et al 2005), lower (Li et al 2004; Chew et al 2005; Rietveld et al 2005) or more variable pressure readings (Lam et al 2004; Brigatti & Maguluri 2005; Naruse et al 2005) when compared with GAT.

The Reichert ocular response analyser

The Reichert ocular response analyser (ORA) is a recent device (2004) that is claimed to measure IOP independent of CCT. However, before discussing this instrument, the concepts behind its development will be described.

Corneal biomechanics: recent understanding

So far, we have concentrated on how corneal thickness can affect IOP measurements obtained using different instrumentation. However, CCT is only one corneal dimension, and our more recent understanding of its biomechanical properties has cast doubt on the value of measuring CCT and trying to adjust the measured IOP based on this single parameter. There is increasing evidence of the role of corneal biomechanics in influencing IOP measurements (Liu & Roberts 2005; Pallikaris et al 2005; Bauer et al 2005).

To understand this concept better, consider the following example. If pressure is applied to a wooden bar of finite thickness, less force is required to break the wooden bar when compared with a steel bar of the same thickness. This difference is due to the mechanical ability of the two materials to withstand stress. As the corneal structure differs between individuals, the resistance to externally applied forces will vary, and this can significantly impact one's ability to measure IOP using the devices discussed in this chapter.

Further, if two individuals have the same corneal thickness, it does not necessarily mean that the resistance of these corneas will be the same. For instance, an oedematous cornea having a thickness of, say, 640 μm would be thick but easy to indent. This would lead to an underestimation of the IOP as measured by GAT. However, a healthy, clear cornea having the same 640 μm thickness would be harder to indent, thereby leading to an overestimation of IOP. The oedematous cornea can be thought of as having poor resistance to stress (like wood) compared with the healthy but thick cornea, which can be thought of as being made of steel and therefore harder to applanate. In the same way, there is inter-individual variation in the 'rigidity' of even a normal-thickness cornea, leading to IOP inaccuracies with applanating devices. The ability of the cornea to withstand external stresses varies between individuals, and since all IOP measurements relate to this 'resistance', significant inter-subject variation may exist for a given measurement procedure.

To overcome these limitations, newer devices are being developed that measure other biomechanical properties of the cornea, thereby increasing the accuracy of IOP measurement.

Stress, strain, elasticity and viscosity

It is important to define these terms in order to understand the newer concepts emerging in the measurement of IOP.

Stress is defined as the force applied to a material over its cross-sectional area. *Strain* is the amount of deformation (change in shape due to applied stress) that occurs within the material. A perfectly *elastic* substance is one that deforms under stress but which returns to its original shape when the stress is removed by following the same path that led to the original deformation. *Viscosity* is a substance's resistance to flow, and can be thought of as a measure of friction within a fluid. For example, honey has a higher viscosity than water. Further, solids are structures with a higher viscosity than liquids.

The cornea has both viscous and elastic properties and can therefore be thought of as a viscoelastic material. It undergoes deformation under stress, but returns to its original configuration by a slightly different path than the one that leads to the deformation.

Liu and Roberts (2005) derived a corneal biomechanical model to show how CCT, corneal curvature and corneal biomechanics affect IOP readings. They have shown that tonometry readings using GAT are not always reliable, and that corneal biomechanics have a much greater influence on IOP measurements than either CCT or corneal curvature.

In order to overcome the potential problem of corneal biomechanics, Reichert Inc. (Buffalo, NY, USA) developed the ocular response analyser (ORA). This is a non-contact device to measure IOP that uses the principle of bi-directional applanation. A pulse of air initially deforms the cornea, and an optical detector identifies the peak of reflected light from the corneal surface as it is flattened.

A second reflected optical peak occurs as the cornea overcomes the deformation and returns to its original shape. These two peaks of light are converted to IOP readings and the mean of the two measurements is the Goldmann-correlated IOP.

The difference between the two measured IOP peaks is termed 'corneal hysteresis' (CH). The device also derives a corneal resistance factor (CRF), which is calculated using proprietary algorithms. The manufacturers claim that the CH is a measure of the biomechanical properties of the individual cornea and further information to enable a better understanding of the individual corneal mechanical properties can be gained from this parameter. It may be possible to use this information to derive a corrected IOP which is tailored to the individual. Shah et al (2006) have found that CH, CCT and CRF are significantly, but only moderately, correlated with one another. This suggests that CH and CRF are additional measurements of corneal rigidity. These variables may be useful when trying to correct IOP measurements for altered ocular rigidity.

Other investigators have also found that CH is weakly related to CCT (Luce 2005; Shah et al 2006). CH is low in patients with keratoconus, Fuchs' corneal dystrophy and following LASIK surgery (Luce 2005). Congdon at al (2006) reported that in a population of mainly primary open-angle glaucoma patients, CH correlated better with progressive visual field than CCT, but this association was not significant when axial length was included in the regression model.

Clinical application of the understanding of the relationship between intraocular pressure and central corneal thickness

Intraocular pressure measurements in the post-refractive surgery patient

Currently, there is an increasing population of patients who have undergone refractive surgery (see Ch. 23). It is not always easy to know who has had refractive surgery upon examination alone, and therefore it is important to ask the patient specifically whether they have undergone such a procedure. Even then, some patients may not volunteer the information.

There is evidence that ablative corneal refractive surgery can result in erroneous postoperative IOP readings (Faucher et al 1997; Chatterjee et al 1997; Fournier et al 1998; Argento et al 1998; Recep et al 2000; Montes-Mico & Charman 2001; Munger et al 2001; Duch et al 2001; Rashad & Bahnassy 2001). Falsely low IOP readings may be achieved after myopic correction using laser refractive surgery (Siganos et al 2004). This might be due to a reduction in corneal thickness or curvature, or a change in the corneal biomechanics. The scarring process associated with corneal remodelling after refractive surgery may complicate matters by changing the corneal biomechanics over time.

To date, the effects of LASIK surgery on the visual field are unclear. There is anecdotal evidence of contrast sensitivity loss in some patients, and there is some evidence that LASIK can even cause visual field loss (Bushley et al 2000; Weiss et al 2001). Proposed mechanisms include LASIK-associated barotraumas and compression of the ganglion cells at the optic nerve head, LASIK-induced ischaemic optic neuropathy, primary open-angle glaucoma, steroid-induced glaucoma or anterior ischaemic optic neuropathy.

There is no straightforward solution for measuring IOP accurately following refractive surgery. Therefore, it is important to classify the patient's risk of developing glaucoma according to known risk factors, such as age, race, family history, central corneal thickness, etc. If there is suspicion that the patient has an above-average chance of developing glaucoma, perform preoperative visual field tests, obtain optic disc images or photos and take several preoperative IOP measurements, as these will all help to set a baseline from which it is possible to follow the patient longitudinally.

Postoperatively, it is advisable to perform visual field testing and obtain disc images and IOP readings on several occasions both while the patient is using steroids and afterwards. If the patient does not have a pre-LASIK IOP assessment, it is possible to make a rough estimate as to the level of IOP by examining the quantity of tissue removed and using previously documented findings. Longitudinal follow-up of these patients' optic disc appearance and visual fields is essential. One should consider using more than one device to measure IOP in these patients, and bear in mind that the IOP measurements may be still be totally inaccurate.

Tonometer sterilization techniques

Reusable tonometer prisms can be a source of potential cross-infection, and several epidemics of adenoviral keratoconjunctivitis may have arisen from cross-contamination. Other viruses, corneal epithelial cells and proteinaceous materials have also been retained on the tonometer prism tip following decontamination by standard regimens. Further, patients using glaucoma medications tend to leave a significantly higher number of epithelial cells on the tonometry prism than those not using any topical medication. In addition, this material is a potential source for the transmission of Creutzfeldt–Jakob disease (CJD), since the infectious agent is a prion protein. However, there are no documented cases of transmission of CJD through IOP measurement using GAT. Only one probable and two possible cases of CJD transmission have been reported following penetrating keratoplasty (Duffy et al 1974; Heckmann et al 1997; Hammersmith et al 2004).

The cleaning regimens recommended by the United States Centers for Disease Control and Prevention (CDC) and the American College of Ophthalmology (AAO) state that, after use, the tonometer prism should be wiped with a dry cloth or tissue and then immersed in a 0.5% solution of sodium hypochlorite (5000 ppm of available chlorine) for a minimum of 5 minutes. Alternatively, a 3% hydrogen peroxide or 70% isopropyl alcohol solution is recommended. The tonoprisms should then be rinsed under running water and wiped dry. They also recommend that two prisms should be made available for each practitioner to ensure adequate soak time between patients. The hypochlorite solution should be changed daily and the hydrogen peroxide solution twice daily.

The Royal Australian and New Zealand College of Ophthalmologists (RANZCO) have adopted similar guidelines but with the alternative of 70% isopropyl alcohol wipe or immersion in 2% glutaraldehyde solution. The Spongiform Encephalopathy Advisory Committee (SEAC), the UK College of Optometrists and the Association of British Dispensing Opticians advise a 1-hour soak time in 2% hypochlorite solution containing 20 000 ppm of available chlorine. They suggest this regimen is effective at inactivating prion proteins, and should be used for all ophthalmic devices touching the eye.

A recent survey (Hillier & Kumar 2007) of all ophthalmic units with training recognition in the UK found that 23% use only disposable tonometer prisms (see below). Of the remaining 77%, most use reusable tonometer heads, whilst some use a combination of reusable and disposable tonometry tips. For the reusable heads, 67% used hypochlorite-based immersion sterilization techniques, with the remaining using a variety of other methods. Of particular concern were the findings that only 6% of units used chlorine concentrations of 20 000 ppm, the concentration of chlorine in the soak was below 5000 ppm in many units, and none of the units used a 1-hour soak time.

Disposable prisms in tonometry

With the recent appreciation of the potential for cross-infection within ophthalmic departments, and since GAT is performed routinely on most patients, there is significant risk for transmission of microorganisms and in particular a variant of Creutzfeldt–Jakob disease (vCJD). Studies have shown persistent protein and epithelial cell remnants despite cleaning (Amin et al 2003; Lim et al 2003). As a result, disposable tonometers have been suggested as a means to reduce the risk of such infection (Amin et al 2003). There are three adaptations to the Goldmann tonometer that are currently available.

The Tonoshield (Oasis Medical, Glendora, CA, USA) is a silicone cap that fits over the standard Goldmann prism. The Tonosafe (Clement Clarke, UK) is a two-piece, acrylic biprism that fits on the end of the standard Goldmann tonometer. The Tonojet (Luneau, France) is a one-piece acrylic biprism similar to the Goldmann prism.

Studies looking at the performance of these disposable prisms and cover have shown that the Tonosafe and Tonojet show the closest agreement to Goldmann readings. However, the Tonoshield seems to elevate the reading by about 2 mmHg (Maldonado et al 1996; Bhatnagar & Gupta 2005; Maino et al 2006).

Although disposable prisms reduce the risk of cross-infection, they do not eliminate it, due to the technique employed by the person measuring IOP. For instance, operators may inadvertently touch the tip with a previously contaminated finger or surface or may not have thoroughly disinfected their hands. Rajak et al (2006) concluded that while disposable prisms may reduce the risk of transmission of prion disease, they are not aseptic and still carry a risk of infection for the patient.

Pachymetry

Pachymetry determines corneal thickness. This procedure is essential prior to refractive surgery in order to ascertain whether the proposed treatment is feasible. It is also important for monitoring corneal conditions such as Fuchs' corneal endothelial dystrophy, keratoconus or post-surgical corneal oedema. In addition, as detailed above, corneal thickness directly influences IOP readings when using most tonometers.

There are several methods available for this procedure including ultrasound pachymetry, ultrasound biomicroscopy, optical pachymetry (including orbscan pachymetry), pachymetry combined with specular microscopy, optical coherence tomography (OCT), optical low coherence reflectometry and Scheimpflug imaging.

Ultrasound pachymetry

Thornton (1984) noted that ultrasound (US) pachymetry was a reliable method of measuring CCT with little interobserver variability and low levels of bias. The technique is easy to perform, can be incorporated into the standard ophthalmic examination, is well tolerated, the instruments are relatively inexpensive and easily available and it can be performed quickly on most patients in the clinical setting. The Ocular Hypertension Treatment Study (OHTS) (Brandt et al 2001) utilized US pachymetry to assess the risk of progression of this condition. This technique has become accepted as the gold-standard method of performing pachymetry in the clinical setting.

US pachymetry takes a series of axial scans of the eye using a US probe of varying frequency (20 MHz being the current standard). The US probe is placed on the corneal surface after application of topical anaesthetic. The probe is held perpendicular to and centrally aligned on the cornea. The probe is composed of an emitter and a transducer. The emitter sends out a US wave and the transducer picks up the reflected wave from the endothelial surface of the cornea. Using the known speed of sound through the cornea (1640 m/s), the corneal thickness can be calculated (see Ch. 19).

Several readings should be taken for improved accuracy. The resolution of US pachymetry is about 100 μm and is limited by the wavelength used. Several different instruments are available and the resolution may differ by up to 75 μm (Reader & Salz 1987). However, modern devices have accuracies of ±5 μm.

Some manufacturers claim that the sampling rate of the reflected wave affects the accuracy of the data, with higher sampling rates improving the accuracy of the readings. Placing a soft contact lens on the eye is said to reduce any error associated with identifying the initial peak on the patient's cornea. Further errors can be introduced by measuring away from the centre of the cornea and by overdepressing the cornea during measurement. If pachymetry is performed after lubricating cream has been applied to the ocular surface during the clinical examination, an erroneous reading may be obtained. Commercially available clinical ultrasound pachymeters include the SP 3000 (Tomey, Phoenix, AZ), PalmScan AP 2000 (MicroMedical Devices, Calabasas, CA) and the DGH 500 (DGH Technology, Exton, PA).

Ultrasound biomicroscopy

As noted above, the limit of resolution of ultrasound pachymetry is dependent upon the wavelength used, and as all ultrasound pachymeters use sound waves, their resolution is limited. Higher-frequency probes are now generally available with frequencies of 50 MHz. Probes emitting frequencies of 75 MHz are in development with a claimed resolution of 30 μm (Silverman et al 2006).

This technique is called ultrasound biomicroscopy, and requires an immersion or coupling fluid to be used on the surface of the cornea, thereby limiting its use. However, it has a higher resolution than ultrasound pachymetry with the 20 MHz probe, and pathology in the corneal layers is more easily discernable (see **Figs 17.22** and **17.23**). It is not used routinely as it is more invasive than standard-frequency ultrasound and immersion of the anterior eye is not always well tolerated by patients. Further, the quality of the obtained images is dependent upon the skill of the operator.

Optical pachymetry

Haag-Streit slit-lamp-mounted optical pachymeter

Optical pachymetry avoids the need for corneal contact and therefore anaesthesia. The Haag-Streit pachymeter is a slit-lamp-mounted device fitted on a swing arm. The slit-lamp illumination system is set at minimal width (0.05–0.1 mm) and at an angle of 40° to the observation system. The right eyepiece of the biomicroscope is replaced with a split-image objective. This incorporates a prism which divides the image of the cornea into two. The two images are aligned using a graticule on the pachymeter so that the anterior corneal epithelium is aligned with the posterior surface of the endothelium. A measurement of the corneal thickness can be read off the device at this point. The device can measure in the range of 0–1.2 mm in steps of 0.02 mm.

As can be appreciated, the technique is quite difficult to master and is time consuming. There are few pachymeters of this type available and, from personal experience, interobserver error is considerable. With the advent of newer devices, this technique is becoming obsolete.

Orbscan optical pachymeter

The Orbscan (Bausch & Lomb, Rochester, NY, USA) is a scanning slit corneal topographer that also measures corneal thickness. It projects 40 optical slits of light at 45° to the corneal surface and records the reflected images. It also measures anterior and posterior corneal elevation relative to a best-fit sphere as well as the corneal surface curvature. The instrument software analyses over 9000 data points in about 1.5 seconds to calculate the curvature of the anterior and posterior corneal surface (see Chs 17 and 19).

Pachymetry is calculated indirectly by the difference in elevation between the anterior and posterior corneal surfaces (see **Fig. 17.6**). The central corneal thickness is displayed as the average value in the central 2 mm, and eight further corneal thickness readings are provided for the periphery of the cornea. The output identifies the thinnest point on the cornea and displays the measurement in the appropriate quadrant (Liu et al 1999; Liu & Pflugfelder 1999).

The Orbscan has been shown to give reliable and repeatable readings, although these tend to be higher than ultrasound pachymetry (Marsich & Bullimore 2000). A proposed correction factor of 0.92 has been suggested by some investigators, and this has been incorporated into the instrument. Despite this correction, the measurements tend to be inaccurate at extremes of corneal thicknesses, leading some authorities to suggest that the over-reading is due to the pre-corneal tear–mucus film. Accordingly, a subtraction correction of 42.65 μm has been suggested (Cheng et al 2006).

Disadvantages of Orbscan pachymetry include the instruments being expensive and requiring a lot more space than the ultrasound pachymeter. Additionally, considerable training is needed to obtain good-quality images, a significant amount of cooperation from the patient is required and readings may be unobtainable due to poor tear film, a small palpebral fissure, unsteady fixation or extreme pathology such as advanced keratoconus (Wong et al 2002). It is also unreliable in the presence of anterior surface pathology or following refractive surgery.

Specular microscopy

Automated specular microscopes with pachymeters are commercially available. One such instrument is the Topcon SP2000P (Tokyo, Japan), which has the advantage of being non-contact and utilizes light to image the posterior cornea and endothelium together with measuring corneal thickness. The readings are lower than those obtained with US pachymetry in both normal (Bovelle et al 1999; Suzuki et al 2003) and post-LASIK eyes (Kawana et al 2004). The instrument is easy to use, well tolerated and has low inter-observer error due to the high degree of automation (see Ch. 17).

Optical coherence tomography

Optical coherence tomography (OCT) is a noninvasive technique used to measure the anterior segment, and was described in detail in Chapter 18. Although initially developed to image the retina and the macula region, recent modifications have produced a system which images the anterior segment of the eye in detail.

In the Visante system (Carl Zeiss Meditec, Dublin, CA), a 1310 nm superluminescent diode (SLD) light source beam is split into two. One beam acts as a reference while the other beam is reflected off the ocular structures. Multiple scans are taken and the resultant beams analysed to create an image based on the difference in phase of the two beams (Hirano et al 2001). The resolution of the image is very high (18 μm) with developments underway to allow ultrahigh resolution of 1.4 μm (Linnola et al 2005). Not only is the OCT system capable of measuring CCT, it can also give detailed qualitative images of the whole anterior segment (see **Figs 17.24** and **19.7**)

Drawbacks are that the system is quite expensive and requires a significant amount of training to get good-quality images. Studies show that the OCT pachymetry measurements are higher (by 23 μm) compared with US pachymetry (Leung et al 2006) but they are highly correlated with one another (Bechmann et al 2001). Thus, a simple correction factor might be sufficient to adjust the readings to US values (Wong et al 2002; Leung et al 2006; Thomas et al 2006). Further, OCT readings are highly reproducible (Fishman et al 2005). Other recent developments include the use of OCT imaging during LASIK so that information can be gathered on the ablation as it is occurring (Wirbelauer & Pham 2004). Recently, OCT has been used to examine trabeculectomy bleb morphology (Leung et al 2006).

The technology of OCT is emerging and will continue to evolve. While pachymetry is most commonly performed at present using ultrasound techniques, the non-contact OCT procedure which allows imaging of the anterior segment in great detail may hold significant advantages. Instruments incorporating OCT technology are getting better and more user friendly. However, they are still more time consuming and expensive for CCT measurement when compared with ultrasound pachymetry using a 20 MHz probe.

Optical low coherence reflectometry

This device was initially developed to determine the axial length of the eye, but has been adapted to measure CCT. It is marketed by Haag-Streit (Konitz, Switzerland). The instrument fits onto the slit-lamp biomicroscope and uses a similar principle to the OCT by using an SLD and measuring the coherence of diffracted waves of light with a claimed resolution of 1–20 μm (Schmid et al 2001; Sobottka Ventura et al 2001). Measurements are comparable but lower than US pachymetry (Gillis & Zeyen 2004; Much & Haigis 2006) and are also comparable with those from the Pentacam Scheimpflug system (see below) (Barkana et al 2005).

Scheimpflug imaging

The Scheimpflug principle of imaging (see Chs 17 and 19) uses multiple images of the anterior segment taken with a camera that is aligned perpendicular to a slit beam of light, thereby creating an optical section of that part of the anterior segment. When these multiple images are combined, a composite image can be created. The Pentacam (Oculus Systems, Wetzlar, Germany) is an example of a system that uses the Scheimpflug technique. In addition to pachymetry, the Pentacam also provides information relating to corneal topography, anterior chamber structures, cataract analysis, keratometry and tomography, and the findings may be utilized for ocular biometry (see **Figs 19.5** and **19.6**).

Pentacam measurements take about 2 seconds to complete, and the device incorporates software to correct for minor eye movements during the examination. The output of the system is quite detailed, but a simpler version of the Pentacam (the Pachycam) is also available.

Comparison between the Pentacam, US pachymetry and the Orbscan optical instrument have shown good correlation and reproducibility (Lackner et al 2005). However, the readings with the Pentacam are lower than those obtained using US (Lackner et al 2005; O'Donnell & Maldonado-Codina 2005). The readings of Pentacam are also well correlated with the optical low coherence reflectometer (OLCR) but doubt exists as to the validity of using these measurements interchangeably (Barkana et al 2005).

Advantages of the Scheimpflug system include the non-contact nature of the procedure and repeatability of the measurements. However, the instrument is more expensive than a standard US pachymeter, is more time consuming and requires more practitioner training. It may have a greater role in refractive surgery practice where more of the data generated will be utilized.

Conclusion

The authors hope this chapter has highlighted the importance of accurate IOP measurements and the way in which CCT can affect the accuracy of its measurement. They have also discussed some of the more recent technologies that are attempting to measure IOP independently of CCT.

Understanding of corneal biomechanics is developing and the authors have discussed potentially significant alternatives to measure IOP with the benefit of improved knowledge. They have also tried to show how IOP may have different levels of importance in the development and course of the disease in any individual patient.

Infection risk with IOP measurement is becoming more important and the authors have addressed the available disposable prisms to measure IOP and have looked at their accuracy. They have also covered the available devices to measure intraocular pressure and discussed how each can be affected by changes in CCT.

It is important to consider that individual patients do not always fit into our perceived understanding of the underlying knowledge base. It may be that more than one device is needed to estimate the true IOP. Furthermore, if the clinical situation changes, we need to be prepared to question our assumptions regarding the patient's condition, and to consider what further information is required to assist in making the most appropriate decisions for clinical care.

References

Abbasoglu O E, Bowman W, Cavanagh D et al 1998 Reliability of intraocular pressure measurements after myopic excimer photorefractive keratectomy. Ophthalmology 105:2193–2196

Amin S Z, Smith L, Luthbert P J et al 2003 Minimising the risk of prion transmission by contact tonometry. British Journal of Ophthalmology 87:1360–1362

Anderson D R, Hendrickson A 1974 Effect of intraocular pressure on rapid axoplasmic transport in monkey optic nerve. Investigative Ophthalmology 13:771–783

Argento C, Cosentino M J, Moussalli M A 1998 Intraocular pressure measurement following hyperopic LASIK [letter]. Journal of Cataract and Refractive Surgery 24:145

Argus W A 1995 Ocular hypertension and central corneal thickness. Ophthalmology 102:1810–1812

Bafa M, Lambrinakis I, Dayan M et al 2001 Clinical comparison of the measurement of the IOP with the ocular blood flow tonometer, the Tonopen XL and the Goldmann applanation tonometer. Acta Ophthalmologica Scandinavica 79:15–18

Barkana Y, Gerber Y, Elbaz U et al 2005 Central corneal thickness measurement with the Pentacam Scheimpflug system, optical low-coherence reflectometry pachymeter, and ultrasound pachymeter. Journal of Cataract and Refractive Surgery 31(9):1729–1735

Bauer S, Lyubimov G, Tovstik P 2005 Mathematical modeling of Maklakoff's method for measuring the intraocular pressure. Fluid Dynamics 40:20–33

Bechmann M, Thiel M J, Neubauer A S et al 2001 Central corneal thickness measurement with a retinal optical coherence tomography device versus standard ultrasonic pachymetry. Cornea 20(1):50–54

Bhan A, Browning A C, Shah S et al 2002 Effects of corneal thickness on intraocular pressure measurements with the Pneumatonometer, Goldmann Applanation Tonometer, and Tono-Pen. Investigative Ophthalmology and Visual Science 43:1389–1392

Bhatnagar A, Gupta A K 2005 Disposable devices for measuring intraocular pressure: a clinical study to assess their accuracy. Eye 19:752–754

Bovelle R, Stephen K C, Kaufman S C et al 1999 Corneal thickness measurements with the Topcon SP-2000P Specular Microscope and an Ultrasound Pachymeter. Archives of Ophthalmology 117:868–870

Brandt J D, Beiser J A, Kass M A et al 2001 Central corneal thickness in the ocular hypertension treatment study (OHTS). Ophthalmology 108:1779–1788

Brigatti L, Maguluri S 2005 Reproducibility of self-measured intraocular pressure with the phosphene tonometer in patients with ocular hypertension and early to advanced glaucoma. Journal of Glaucoma 14:36–39

Bron A M, Creuzot-Garcher C, Goudeau-Boutillon S et al 1999 Falsely elevated intraocular pressure due to increased corneal thickness. Graefe's Archives of Clinical and Experimental Ophthalmology 237:220–224

Browning A C, Bhan A, Rotchford A P et al 2004 The effect of corneal thickness on intraocular pressure measurement in patients with corneal pathology. British Journal of Ophthalmology 88 (11):1395–1399

Bushley D M, Parmley V C, Paglen P 2000 Visual field defect associated with laser in situ keratomileusis. American Journal of Ophthalmology 129(5):668–671

Chatterjee A, Shah S, Bessant D A et al 1997 Reduction in intraocular pressure after excimer laser photorefractive keratectomy; correlation with pretreatment myopia. Ophthalmology 104:355–359

Chauhan B C, Hutchison D M, LeBlanc R P et al 2005 Central corneal thickness and progression of the visual field and optic disc in glaucoma. British Journal of Ophthalmology 89: 1008–1012

Cheng A C, Tang E, Mohamed S et al 2006 Correction factor in Orbscan II in the assessment of corneal pachymetry. Cornea 25 (10):1158–1161

Chew G S, Sanderson G F, Molteno A C 2005 The pressure phosphene tonometer: a clinical evaluation. Eye 19:683–685

Chidlow G, Nash M S, Crowhurst C et al 1996 The ocular blood flow tonograph: a new instrument for the measurement of intraocular pressure in rabbits. Experimental Eye Research 63:463–469

Congdon N G, Broman A T, Bandeen-Roche K et al 2006 Central corneal thickness and corneal hysteresis associated with glaucoma damage. American Journal of Ophthalmology 141(5):868–875

Copt R P, Thomas R, Mermoud A 1999 Corneal thickness in ocular hypertension, primary open-angle glaucoma, and normal tension glaucoma. Archives of Ophthalmology 117:14–16

Doughty M J, Zaman M L 2000 Human corneal thickness and its impact on intraocular pressure measures: a review and meta-analysis approach. Survey of Ophthalmology 44:367–408

Downs J C, Ensor M E, Bellezza A J et al 2001 Posterior scleral thickness in perfusion-fixed normal and early-glaucoma monkey eyes. Investigative Ophthalmology and Visual Science 42: 3202–3208

Doyle A, Lachkar Y 2005 Comparison of dynamic contour tonometry with Goldman applanation tonometry over a wide range of central corneal thickness. Journal of Glaucoma 14:288–292

Drance S 2001 Chronic open angle glaucoma: risk factors in addition to intraocular pressure. Acta Ophthalmologica Scandinavica 79:545

Duba I, Wirthlin A C 2004 Dynamic contour tonometry for post-LASIK intraocular pressure measurements. Klinische Monatsblätter für Augenheilkd 221:347–350

Duch S, Serra A, Castanera J et al 2001 Tonometry after laser in situ keratomileusis treatment. Journal of Glaucoma 10:261–265

Duffy P, Wolf J, Collins G et al 1974 Possible person to person transmission of Creutzfeldt-Jakob disease. New England Journal of Medicine 290:692–693

Ehlers N, Bramsen T, Sperling S 1975 Applanation tonometry and central corneal thickness. Acta Ophthalmologica (Copenh) 53:34–43

Ekstrom C 2002 Incidence studies on open-angle glaucoma. Archives of Ophthalmology 120:522

Emara B Y, Tingey D P, Probst L E et al 1999 Central corneal thickness in low-tension glaucoma. Canadian Journal of Ophthalmology 34:319–324

Esgin H, Alimgil M L, Erda S 1998 Clinical comparison of the ocular blood flow tonograph and the Goldmann applanation tonometer. European Journal of Ophthalmology 8:162–166

European Glaucoma Society 2003 Terminology and Guidelines for Glaucoma, European Glaucoma Society, 2nd edn, vol 1.1. Dogma, Savona, pp 1–3

Faucher A, Gregoire J, Blondeau P 1997 Accuracy of Goldmann tonometry after refractive surgery. Journal of Cataract and Refractive Surgery 23:832–838

Fernandes P, Diaz-Rey J A, Queiros A et al 2005 Comparison of the ICare rebound tonometer with the Goldmann tonometer in a normal population. Ophthalmic and Physiological Optics 25:436–440

Fishman G R, Pons M E, Seedor J A et al 2005 Assessment of central corneal thickness using optical coherence tomography. Journal of Cataract and Refractive Surgery 31(4):707–711

Forbes M, Pico G, Grolman B 1974 A noncontact applanation tonometer. Archives of Ophthalmology 91:134–140

Fournier A V, Podtetenev M, Lemire J et al 1998 Intraocular pressure change measured by Goldmann tonometry after laser in situ keratomileusis. Journal of Cataract and Refractive Surgery 24:905–910

Fresco B B 1998 A new tonometer – the pressure phosphene tonometer: clinical comparison with Goldmann tonometry. Ophthalmology 105:2123–2126

Gaasterland D, Tanishima T, Kuwabara T 1978 Axoplasmic flow during chronic experimental glaucoma. 1. Light and electron microscopic studies of the monkey optic nervehead during development of glaucomatous cupping. Investigative Ophthalmology and Visual Science 17:838–846

Garcia-Resua C, Gonzalez-Meijome J M, Gilino J et al 2006 Accuracy of the new ICare rebound tonometer vs other portable tonometers in healthy eyes. Optometry and Vision Science 83:102–107

Gillis A, Zeyen T 2004 Comparison of optical coherence reflectometry and ultrasound central corneal pachymetry. Bulletin de la Société Belge d'ophtalmologie (292):71–75

Gloster J, Perkins E S 1963 The validity of the Imbert-Fick law as applies to applanation tonometry. Experimental Eye Research 2:274–283

Goldmann H 1957 Applanation tonometry. In: Newell W (ed.) Glaucoma. Transactions of the Second Conference 167–220 Josiah Macy, Jr Foundation New York, NY

Goldmann H, Schmidt T 1957 Über applanationstonometrie. Ophthalmologica 134: 221–242

Gordon M O, Beiser J A, Brandt J D et al 2002 The Ocular Hypertension Treatment Study: baseline factors that predict the onset of primary open-angle glaucoma. Archives of Ophthalmology 120:714–720

Hahn S, Azen S, Ying-Lai M et al 2003 Central corneal thickness in Latinos. Investigative Ophthalmology and Visual Science 44:1508–1512

Hammermith K M, Cohen E J, Rapuano C J et al 2004 Creutzfeldt-Jakob disease following corneal transplantation. Cornea 23(4):406–408

Hashemi H, Kashi A H, Fotouhi A et al 2005 Distribution of intraocular pressure in healthy Iranian individuals: the Tehran Eye Study. British Journal of Ophthalmology 89(6):652–657

Heckmann J G, Lang C J, Petruch F et al 1997 Transmission of Creutzfeldt-Jakob disease via a corneal transplant. Journal of Neurology Neurosurgery and Psychiatry 63:388–390

Herman D C, Hodge D O, Bourne W M 2001 Increased corneal thickness in patients with ocular hypertension. Archives of Ophthalmology 119(3):334–336

Herndon L W, Choudhri S A, Cox T et al 1997 Central corneal thickness in normal, glaucomatous and ocular hypertensive eyes. Archives of Ophthalmology 115:1137–1141

Herndon L W, Weizer J S, Stinnett S S 2004 Central corneal thickness as a risk factor for advanced glaucoma damage. Archives of Ophthalmology 122:17–21

Herse P, Hans A, Hall J et al 2005 The Proview Eye Pressure Monitor: influence of clinical factors on accuracy and agreement with the Goldmann tonometer. Ophthalmic and Physiological Optics 25:416–420

Hillier R J, Kumar N 2007 Tonometer disinfection practice in the United Kingdom: a national survey. Eye Apr 20; [Epub ahead of print]

Hines M W, Jost B F, Fogleman K L 1988 Oculab Tono-Pen, Goldmann Applanation Tonometry, and Pneumatic Tonometry for intraocular pressure assessment in gas-filled eyes. American Journal of Ophthalmology 106:174–179

Hirano K, Ito Y, Suzuki T et al 2001 Optical coherence tomography for the noninvasive evaluation of the cornea. Cornea 20:281–289

Hjortdal J O 1996 Regional elastic performance of the human cornea. Journal of Biomechanics 29:931–942

Iliev M E, Goldblum D, Katsoulis K et al 2006 Comparison of rebound tonometry with Goldmann applanation tonometry and correlation

with central corneal thickness. British Journal Ophthalmology 90(7):833–835

Johnson M, Kass M A, Moses R A et al 1978 Increased corneal thickness simulating elevated intraocular pressure. Archives of Ophthalmology 96:664–665

Jonas J B, Berenshtein E, Holbach L 2004 Lamina cribrosa thickness and spatial relationships between intraocular space and cerebrospinal fluid space in highly myopic eyes. Investigative Ophthalmology and Visual Science 45:2660–2665

Jonas J B, Stroux A, Velten I et al 2005 Central corneal thickness correlated with glaucoma damage and rate of progression. Investigative Ophthalmology and Visual Science 46:1269–1274

Kamppeter B A, Jonas J B 2005 Dynamic contour tonometry for intraocular pressure measurement. American Journal of Ophthalmology 140:318–320

Kaufmann C, Bachmann L M, Thiel M A 2003 Intraocular pressure measurements using dynamic contour tonometry after laser in situ keratomileusis. Investigative Ophthalmology and Visual Science 44(9):3790–3794

Kawana K, Tokunaga T, Miyata K et al 2004 Comparison of corneal thickness measurements using Orbscan II, non-contact specular microscopy, and ultrasonic pachymetry in eyes after laser in situ keratomileusis. British Journal of Ophthalmology 88:466–468

Kim W J, Chen P P 2004 Central corneal pachymetry and visual field progression in patients with open-angle glaucoma. Ophthalmology 111:2126–2132

Kniestedt C, Lin S, Choe J et al 2005 Clinical comparison of contour and applanation tonometry and their relationship to pachymetry. Archives of Ophthalmology 123:1532–1537

Ko Y C, Liu C J, Hsu W M 2005 Varying effects of corneal thickness on intraocular pressure measurements with different tonometers. Eye 19:327–332

Kotecha A, White E T, Shewry J M et al 2005 The relative effects of corneal thickness and age on Goldmann applanation tonometry and dynamic contour tonometry. British Journal of Ophthalmology 89:1572–1575

Ku J Y, Danesh-Meyer H V, Craig J P et al 2006 Comparison of intraocular pressure measured by Pascal dynamic contour tonometry and Goldmann applanation tonometry. Eye 20:191–198

Lackner B, Schmidinger G, Pieh S et al 2005 Repeatability and reproducibility of central corneal thickness measurement with Pentacam, Orbscan, and ultrasound. Optometry and Vision Science 82(10):892–899

Lam D S, Leung D Y, Chiu T Y et al 2004 Pressure phosphene self-tonometry: a comparison with Goldmann tonometry in glaucoma patients. Investigative Ophthalmology and Visual Science 45:3131–3136

Langham M E, McCarthy E 1968 A rapid pneumatic applanation tonometer. Comparative findings and evaluation. Archives of Ophthalmology 79:389–399

La-Rosa F A, Gross R L, Orengo-Nania S 2001 Central corneal thickness of Caucasians and African Americans in glaucomatous and nonglaucomatous populations. Archives of Ophthalmology 119:23–27

Leske M C, Connell A M, Wu S Y et al 2001 Incidence of open-angle glaucoma: the Barbados Eye Studies. The Barbados Eye Studies Group. Archives of Ophthalmology 119:89–95

Leung D Y, Lam D K, Yeung B Y et al 2006 Comparison between central corneal thickness measurements by ultrasound pachymetry and optical coherence tomography. Clinical and Experiment Ophthalmology 34(8):751–754

Li J, Herndon L W, Asrani S G et al 2004 Clinical comparison of the Proview eye pressure monitor with the Goldmann applanation tonometer and the Tonopen. Archives of Ophthalmology 122:1117–1121

Lim R, Dhillon B, Kurian K M et al 2003 Retention of corneal epithelial cells following Goldmann tonometry: implications for CJD. British Journal of Ophthalmology 87:583–586

Linnola R J, Findl O, Hermann B et al 2005 Intraocular lens-capsular bag imaging with ultrahigh-resolution optical coherence tomography: pseudophakic human autopsy eyes. Journal of Cataract and Refractive Surgery 31:818–823

Liu J, Roberts C J 2005 Influence of corneal biomechanical properties on intraocular pressure measurement: quantitative analysis. Journal of Cataract and Refractive Surgery 31:146–155

Liu Z, Pflugfelder S C 1999 Corneal thickness in dry eye. Cornea 18:403–407

Liu Z, Huang A J, Pflugfelder S C 1999 Evaluation of corneal thickness and topography in normal eyes using the Orbscan corneal topography system. British Journal of Ophthalmology 83:774–778

Luce D A 2005 Determining in vivo biomechanical properties of the cornea with an ocular response analyzer. Journal of Cataract and Refractive Surgery 31(1):156–162

Mackie S W, Jay J L, Ackerley R et al 1996 Clinical comparison of the Keeler Pulsair 2000, American Optical MkII and Goldmann applanation tonometers. Ophthalmic and Physiological Optics 16:171–177

Maino A P, Uddin H J, Tullo A B 2006 A comparison of clinical performance between disposable and Goldmann tonometers. Eye 20 (5):574–578

Maldonado M J, Rodriguez-Galietero A, Cano-Parra J et al 1996 Goldmann applanation tonometry using sterile disposable silicone tonometer shields. Ophthalmology 103(5):815–821

Marg E 1963 A report on Mackay-Marg tonometry in optometry. Journal of the American Optometric Association 34:961–965

Mark H H, Mark T L 2003 Corneal astigmatism in applanation tonometry. Eye 17:617–618

Mark H, Robbins K P, Mark T L 2002 Axial length in applanation tonometry. Journal of Cataract and Refractive Surgery 28:504–506

Marsich M W, Bullimore M A 2000 The repeatability of corneal thickness measures. Cornea 19(6):792–795

Martinez-de-la-Casa J M, Garcia-Feijoo J, Castillo A et al 2005 Reproducibility and clinical evaluation of rebound tonometry. Investigative Ophthalmology and Visual Science 46:4578–4580

Medeiros F A, Sample P A, Zangwill L M et al 2003 Corneal thickness as a risk factor for visual field loss in patients with preperimetric glaucomatous optic neuropathy. American Journal of Ophthalmology 136:805–813

Minckler D S, Bunt A H, Johanson G W 1977 Orthograde and retrograde axoplasmic transport during acute ocular hypertension in the monkey. Investigative Ophthalmology and Visual Science 16:426–441

Minckler D S, Baerveldt G, Heuer D K et al 1987 Clinical evaluation of the Oculab Tono-Pen. American Journal of Ophthalmology 104:168–173

Mitchell P, Smith W, Attebo K et al 1996 Prevalence of open-angle glaucoma in Australia. The Blue Mountains Eye Study. Ophthalmology 103:1661–1669

Mitchell P, Hourihan F, Sandbach J et al 1999 The relationship between glaucoma and myopia: the Blue Mountains Eye Study. Ophthalmology 106:2010–2015

Montes-Mico R, Charman W N 2001 Intraocular pressure after excimer laser myopic refractive surgery. Ophthalmic and Physiological Optics 21:228–235

Morad Y, Sharon E, Hefetz L et al 1998 Corneal thickness and curvature in normal tension glaucoma. American Journal of Ophthalmology 125:164–168

Morgan W H, Yu D Y, Cooper R L et al 1995 The influence of cerebrospinal fluid pressure on the lamina cribrosa tissue pressure gradient. Investigative Ophthalmology and Visual Science 36: 1163–1172

Much M M, Haigis W 2006 Ultrasound and partial coherence interferometry with measurement of central corneal thickness. Journal of Refractive Surgery 22(7):665–670

Munger R, Dohadwala A A, Hodge W G et al 2001 Changes in measured intraocular pressure after hyperopic photorefractive keratectomy. Journal of Cataract and Refractive Surgery 27:1254–1262

Naruse S, Mori K, Kinoshita S 2005 Evaluation of the pressure phosphene tonometer as a self-tonometer. Ophthalmic and Physiological Optics 25:421–428

Nemesure B, Wu S Y, Hennis A et al 2003 Corneal thickness and intraocular pressure in the Barbados eye studies. Archives of Ophthalmology 121:240–244

O'Donnell C, Maldonado-Codina C 2005 Agreement and repeatability of central thickness measurement in normal corneas using ultrasound pachymetry and the OCULUS Pentacam. Cornea 24 (8):920–924

Ogbuehi K C 2006 Assessment of the accuracy and reliability of the Topcon CT80 non-contact tonometer. Clinical and Experimental Optometry 89(5):310–314

Oliveira C, Tello C, Liebmann J et al 2006 Central corneal thickness is not related to anterior scleral thickness or axial length. Journal of Glaucoma 15(3):190–194

Pache M, Wilmsmeyer S, Lautebach S et al 2005 Dynamic contour tonometry versus Goldmann applanation tonometry: a comparative study. Graefe's Archives of Clinical and Experimental Ophthalmology 243:763–767

Pallikaris I G, Kymionis G D, Ginis H S et al 2005 Ocular rigidity in living human eyes. Investigative Ophthalmology and Visual Science 46:409–414

Paranhos A Jr, Paranhos F R, Prata J A Jr et al 2000 Influence of keratometric readings on comparative intraocular pressure measurements with Goldmann, Tono-Pen, and noncontact tonometers. Journal of Glaucoma 9:219–223

Pease M E, McKinnon S J, Quigley H A et al 2000 Obstructed axonal transport of BDNF and its receptor TrkB in experimental glaucoma. Investigative Ophthalmology and Visual Science 41:764–774

Popovich K S, Shields M B 1997 A comparison of intraocular pressure measurements with the XPERT noncontact tonometer and Goldmann applanation tonometry. Journal of Glaucoma 6:44–46

Quigley H A, Dorman-Pease M E, Brown A E 1991 Quantitative study of collagen and elastin of the optic nerve head and sclera in human and experimental monkey glaucoma. Current Eye Research 10:877–888

Radius R L, Bade B 1982 Axonal transport interruption and anatomy at the lamina cribrosa. Archives of Ophthalmology 100:1661–1664

Rajak S N, Paul J, Sharma V et al 2006 Contamination of disposable tonometer prisms during tonometry. Eye 20(3):358–361

Rashad K M, Bahnassy A A 2001 Changes in intraocular pressure after laser in situ keratomileusis. Journal of Refractive Surgery 17: 420–427

Reader A L, Salz J J 1987 Differences among ultrasonic pachymeters in measuring corneal thickness. Journal of Refractive Surgery 3:7–11

Recep O F, Cagil N, Hasiripi H 2000 Correlation between intraocular pressure and corneal stromal thickness after laser in situ keratomileusis. Journal of Cataract and Refractive Surgery 26: 1480–1483

Regine F, Scuderi G L, Cesareo M et al 2006 Validity and limitations of the Nidek NT-4000 noncontact tonometer: a clinical study. Ophthalmic and Physiological Optics 26:33–39

Rietveld E, van den Bremer D A, Volker-Dieben H J 2005 Clinical evaluation of the pressure phosphene tonometer in patients with glaucoma. British Journal of Ophthalmology 89:537–539

Schmid G F, Petrig B L, Riva C E et al 2001 Measurement of eye length and eye shape by optical low coherence reflectometry. International Ophthalmology 23(4–6):317–320

Schneider E, Grehn F 2006 Intraocular pressure measurement: comparison of dynamic contour tonometry and Goldmann applanation tonometry. Journal of Glaucoma 15:2–6

Shah S, Chattejee A, Mahai M et al 1999 Relationship between corneal thickness and measured intraocular pressure in a general ophthalmology clinic. Ophthalmology 106:2154–2160

Shah S, Laiquzzaman M, Cunliffe I et al 2006 The use of the Reichert ocular response analyzer to establish the relationship between ocular hysteresis, corneal resistance factor and central corneal thickness in normal eyes. Contact Lens and Anterior Eye 29(5):257–262

Shimiyo M, Ross A J, Moy A et al 2003 Intraocular pressure, Goldmann applanation tension, corneal thickness, and corneal curvature in Caucasians, Asians, Hispanics, and African Americans. American Journal of Ophthalmology 136:603–613

Siganos D S, Papastergiou G I, Moedas C 2004 Assessment of the Pascal dynamic contour tonometer in monitoring intraocular pressure in unoperated eyes and eyes after LASIK. Journal of Cataract and Refractive Surgery 30:746–751

Silver D M, Farrell R A 1994 Validity of pulsatile ocular blood flow measurements. Survey of Ophthalmology 38(suppl):S72–S80

Silverman R H, Cannata J, Shung K K et al 2006 75 MHz ultrasound biomicroscopy of anterior segment of eye. Ultrasonic Imaging 28 (3):179–188

Sobottka Ventura A C, Böhnke M et al 2001 Central corneal thickness measurements in patients with normal tension glaucoma, primary open angle glaucoma, pseudoexfoliation glaucoma, or ocular hypertension. British Journal Ophthalmology 85:792–795

Sommer A, Tielsch J M, Katz J et al 1991 Relationship between intraocular pressure and primary open angle glaucoma among white and black Americans. The Baltimore Eye Survey. Archives of Ophthalmology 109:1090–1095

Sørensen P N 1975 The noncontact tonometer. Clinical evaluation on normal and diseased eyes. Acta Ophthalmologica 53:513–521

Spraul C W, Lang G E, Ronzani M et al 1998 Reproducibility of measurements with a new slit lamp-mounted ocular blood flow tonograph. Graefe's Archives of Clinical and Experimental Ophthalmology 236:274–279

Sullivan-Mee M, Pham F 2004 Correspondence of Tono-Pen intraocular pressure measurements performed at the central cornea and mid-peripheral cornea. Optometry 75:26–32

Suzuki S, Oshika T, Oki K et al 2003 Corneal thickness measurements using scanning-slit corneal topography and noncontact specular microscopy versus ultrasonic pachymetry. Journal of Cataract and Refractive Surgery 29:1313–1318

Thomas J, Wang J, Rollins A M et al 2006 Comparison of corneal thickness measured with optical coherence tomography, ultrasonic pachymetry, and a scanning slit method. Journal of Refractive Surgery 22(7):671–678

Thornton S P 1984 A guide to pachymeters. Ophthalmic Surgery 15 (12):993–995

Toh T, Liew S H M, MacKinnon J R et al 2005 Central corneal thickness is highly heritable: the twin eye studies. Investigative Ophthalmology and Visual Science 46(10):3718–3722

Tonnu P A, Ho T, Newson T et al 2005a The influence of central corneal thickness and age on intraocular pressure measured by pneumotonometry, noncontact tonometry, the Tono-Pen XL, and Goldmann applanation tonometry. British Journal of Ophthalmology 89:851–854

Tonnu P A, Ho T, Sharma K et al 2005b A comparison of four methods of tonometry: method agreement and interobserver variability. British Journal of Ophthalmology 89:847–850

Tuunanen T H, Hamalainen P, Mali M et al 1996 Effect of photorefractive keratectomy on the accuracy of pneumatonometer readings in rabbits. Investigative Ophthalmology and Visual Science 37:1810–1814

Van der Jagt L H, Jansonius N M 2005 Three portable tonometers, the TGDc-01, the ICARE and the Tonopen XL, compared with each other and with Goldmann applanation tonometry. Ophthalmic and Physiological Optics 25:429–435

Weiss H S, Rubinfeld R S, Anderschat J F 2001 Case reports and small case series: LASIK-associated visual field loss in a glaucoma suspect. Archives of Ophthalmology 119(5):774–775

Whitacre M M, Stein R A, Hassanein K 1993 The effect of corneal thickness on applanation tonometry. American Journal of Ophthalmology 115:592–596

Wirbelauer C, Pham D T 2004 Continuous monitoring of corneal thickness changes during LASIK with online optical coherence pachymetry. Journal of Cataract and Refractive Surgery 30 (12):2559–2568

Wolf R C W, Klaver C C W, Vingerling J R et al 1997 Distribution of corneal thickness and its association with intraocular pressure. The Rotterdam Study. American Journal of Ophthalmology 123:767–772

Wong A C, Wong C C, Yuen N S et al 2002 Correlational study of central corneal thickness measurements on Hong Kong Chinese using optical coherence tomography, Orbscan and ultrasound pachymetry. Eye 16(6):715–721

Yang Y C, Illango B, Cook A et al 2000 Intraocular pressure and pulse rate measurement by the OBF tonograph – comparison to reference instruments. Ophthalmic and Physiological Optics 20:401–407

Yaoeda K, Shirakashi M, Fukushima A et al 2005 Measurement of intraocular pressure using the NT-4000: a new noncontact tonometer equipped with pulse synchronous measurement function. Journal of Glaucoma 14:201–205

CHAPTER 25

Objectives of the eye and vision examination

Kent M Daum

Introduction

Objectives are the aims of an examination. 'He who aims at nothing, always hits his mark' is an ancient Chinese proverb and a true one at that. Unsurprisingly, good clinicians know what they are trying to accomplish during a vision examination and achieve their aims. Since it directs the entire examination sequence, recognizing one's objectives in completing a vision examination is one of the most important and fundamental aspects of any effective assessment. Failing to achieve the aims of an evaluation may have significant consequences for the patient, possibly leading to the loss of sight. This is more likely if the examination objectives are not established and clear. Not achieving one's aims also increases the risk of liability and carries with it the potential for poor healthcare, as well as financial and other penalties.

The aim of this chapter is to examine several important features about the objectives of a vision examination. The chapter considers factors involved in defining objectives, and also discusses many different aspects of objectives with particular emphasis on how they may change with different types of patients and vision examinations. Other subtle factors can also modulate objectives and these issues will also be discussed. In terms of the funding of healthcare, the examples given relate to the contemporary medical system in the United States. Additionally, the possible imposition of specific testing requirements by a third-party payer also describes the current situation in the USA. However, political and economic developments may result in significant changes in this system in the future. Of course, the funding of optometric and other eye care services, as well as legislative requirements, will vary from country to country. Indeed, within the USA, they can even vary between states.

The dictionary defines an objective as 'something aimed at or striven for' (Neufeld & Guralnik 1991). In the case at hand, the activity is the appropriate examination of a patient's eyes and visual system. Simply, the objective of the examination describes what the clinician is trying to accomplish. A clinician should be able to state explicitly the objective for their examination. Beginning an examination without a clear understanding of its objectives and goal(s) is a common mistake of a novice clinician. Often, this premature beginning is associated with anxiety and/or impatience and, in these cases, the clinician may complete testing that may not be appropriate and, therefore, may not serve the patient's needs. The result is inefficient, costly and wasteful and could be avoided if the objectives were properly set and followed.

Objectives are typically rather general. The more specific activities designed to achieve certain aspects of the objectives are known as goals. For example, for an objective of a comprehensive vision examination, the goals would be the examination of the principal aspects of the patient's vision, such as refractive status, binocular vision and eye and systemic health.

Sources of objectives

There are several different sources of objectives for a vision examination. The elements of a comprehensive vision examination have been explicitly defined by statute in the United States (Cooper 2006) and world-wide (http://www.worldop tometry.org/). In North America, insurance contracts have also defined specifically the elements of most, if not all, types of vision examinations (National Center for Health Statistics 2006). Perhaps the best source of objectives for comprehensive vision examinations for US optometrists are the Clinical Practice Guidelines of the American Optometric Association (AOA) (Scheiman et al 2002; Casser et al 2005) and the Preferred Practice Patterns of the American Academy of Ophthalmology (AAO) (Bateman et al 2002a,b,c; Mandelbaum et al 2005). These documents represent the best collective thinking of their organizations, comprising thousands of optometrists and ophthalmologists in each group. In the UK, the College of Optometrists publishes guidelines on professional conduct, which includes objectives for a routine eye examination (www.college-optometrists.org). The College develops its guidance via its Guidance Review Group, which includes observers from the Association of Optometrists, the Association of British Dispensing Opticians, the Federation of Dispensing Opticians and the General Optical Council (see Ch. 27 for further details of these bodies). As the process used in adopting these documents is elaborate, they are accurate and complete statements of current thinking about the desirable elements of various types of examinations.

In practice, clinicians rarely use written guides regarding which elements they should include in their examination. That is, a clinician does not refer to a chart to determine the objectives and goals of the examinations they provide. There may, of course, be exceptions for some situations where the clinician may not be familiar with the care that is appropriate or for optometry students in training. Most examinations include testing selected by the clinician to address the needs of the patient directly. For a substantial portion of the time, the clinician is performing a comprehensive examination of the patient. In these cases, there are clear expectations derived from several different sources with regard to the testing involved and the areas being tested. Other types of examinations do not involve comprehensive care, such as when a patient presents with a specific problem such as a red eye or for a contact lens check. It is inappropriate to complete testing unrelated to the issue concerning the patient and, therefore, other objectives for the examination must be formulated and followed. Since there are many different patient presentations, the formation of objectives is a major and ongoing task for the clinician performing eye and vision examinations. Interestingly, although the significance of the formulation is high, the time devoted to the formulation is often minimal and may not even be apparent to anyone observing the clinician during the examination.

The objectives for an examination primarily depend on the type of examination and to some extent on the clinician performing the examination. For example, consider the objectives and specific goals for a comprehensive vision examination of a 1-year-old infant versus those for a comprehensive examination of a 55-year-old college professor. Since both are comprehensive examinations, they have the same general objectives. These would include an assessment of the patient history as well as their refractive, binocular and ocular and systemic health status. Although the objectives would be similar for both patients, the specific goals, as well as the specific testing, would differ considerably.

Even though both of these patients would receive comprehensive examinations, the amount, type and nature of the testing would differ considerably. Therefore the art of assessment is not simply to be able to make general statements about the objectives of an examination but rather to include the derivation of goals to achieve the objectives and, in so doing, to fit these appropriately to each patient. Accordingly, a clinician whose concept of setting objectives is 'a comprehensive examination' does not have an optimal depth of understanding regarding the diversity of patients and the best methods necessary to address their widely varying needs. Since there are many different types of patients with widely varying needs, there are a large number of objectives and associated goals.

Fortunately, the overwhelming majority of vision examinations can be classified into relatively few types of examinations. Frequently, each of these has elements in common with other examinations. A good clinician establishes both objectives and goals for the examinations of all patients. The objectives are more general and should always be explicit, while the goals are more specific and free flowing and can be developed or modified as testing proceeds.

Significance of objectives

The formulation of an objective for an examination is an essential part of the provision of good vision care. Particularly for less experienced clinicians, an awareness of the objectives of the examination may greatly support a favourable and efficient outcome.

Inexperienced clinicians tend to treat all patients similarly. Since patients and their needs differ greatly, this may extend the time necessary for an examination and/or result in needless expenditure of effort or money for services, equipment or tests that were not required.

Objectives and goals for comprehensive adult eye and vision examinations

Consider a simple and common objective for vision care for an adult patient: a comprehensive examination. The goals of the comprehensive adult eye and vision examination as developed by the American Optometric Association (AOA; Casser et al 2005) are to:

- evaluate the functional status of the eyes and vision system, taking into account special vision demands and needs
- assess ocular health and related systemic health conditions
- establish a diagnosis and formulate a treatment plan
- counsel and educate the patient regarding their visual, ocular, and related systemic healthcare status, including recommendations for treatment, management, and future care.

Similarly, the objectives of a comprehensive adult eye and vision examination as developed by the American Academy of Ophthalmology (AAO; Mandelbaum et al 2005) are to detect and diagnose vision-, health- or life-threatening disease, and to initiate a plan of treatment as necessary. The goals of the comprehensive adult eye and vision examination are to:

- detect and diagnose ocular abnormalities and diseases
- identify risk factors for ocular disease
- identify risk factors for systemic disease based on ocular findings
- establish the presence or absence of ocular signs or symptoms of systemic disease
- determine the refractive and health status of the eye, visual system, and related structures
- discuss the results and implications of the examination with the patient
- initiate an appropriate management plan (e.g. determine the frequency of future visits, further diagnostic tests, referral, or treatment as indicated).

The objectives of a comprehensive adult vision examination as provided by these organizations of vision care providers demonstrate a significant degree of similarity. Both address the assessment, detection and diagnosis of conditions that may affect the vision and systemic health of the patient. Both suggest an assessment of fundamental areas of vision, visual acuity and refractive status, binocular and oculomotor status and eye and systemic health. Both note the significance of arriving at a diagnosis and plan for the management of the patient's health. And, finally, both note that the communication of findings to the patient should include explanations of diagnoses and alternatives available for management as well as the provision of advice regarding future care, including a discussion of risk factors for conditions likely to affect the patient.

The testing associated with the goals of a comprehensive examination usually includes a patient history (with defined elements; Haine 2006) as well as testing with regard to refractive (Borish & Benjamin 2006), binocular (Saladin 2006), ocular (Fleming & Semes 2006; Semes & Amos 2006) and systemic health status (Casser et al 2005; Mandelbaum et al 2005). The identification of risk factors, an assessment of the patient's status in each basic area and the formulation, presentation and explanation of a plan to manage the patient's condition are other important aspects of the examination.

Although the examination has required elements for each of the basic areas, a clinician has substantial latitude in choosing the precise testing procedures. In accomplishing the examination, the clinician generally has specific goals tailored for each patient. The effect of these specific goals may require somewhat different methodology in completing the evaluation of the basic areas. The effect is that although the examination differs from patient to patient, it still meets the requirements for the comprehensive examination.

A comprehensive examination of the college professor noted above should include a direct and extensive case history with the patient (see Ch. 26) (Casser et al 2005). In addition, the clinician should conduct complete and extensive testing in each of the basic areas of the vision examination and include both objective and subjective testing. The examination of the college professor should include an

evaluation of refractive error (Goss et al 2001; Moore et al 2001; Mandelbaum et al 2002) and presbyopia (Mancil et al 2001; Mandelbaum et al 2005) and discuss an appropriate spectacle lens design for daily use. It may also include recommendations of lens designs for more specific uses such as the computer or conducting a hobby (see Ch. 22). An assessment of binocular vision and other oculomotor aspects of the eye is important. Eye and systemic health of the patient may be evaluated using a variety of instrumentation such as biomicroscopy and direct and indirect ophthalmoscopy. The examination also may include a discussion of contact lens options (Weissman et al 2000) such as bifocal, monovision or distance-only alternatives with their respective strengths and weaknesses. After diagnosis and the formulation of a plan for management of the patient's eye and visual welfare, the case presentation may include a discussion of ageing changes (Mandelbaum et al 2005; Masket et al 2006) potentially affecting the eye such as cataract (Murrill et al 1999; Masket et al 2006), macular degeneration (Cavallerano et al 2004; Chew et al 2006) or dry eye syndrome (Matoba et al 2003; Semes et al 2003). Finally, the presentation may include a discussion of risk for conditions such as glaucoma (Jackson et al 2001; Lewis et al 2002; Gaasterland et al 2005a,b,c), diabetic retinopathy (Cavallerano et al 2002; Chew et al 2003) or systemic factors, e.g. diabetes mellitus (Cavallerano et al 2002), that may affect vision.

In performing the testing during the comprehensive examination of this professor, the precise elements may have been defined both by legal statute and perhaps also by a relevant insurance contract. The elements required in a case history have been set out previously (Haine 2006) (see Ch. 26). Specific portions of the eye and visual system as well as precise testing methods also have been defined by the same sources. A typical list of testing in a comprehensive examination, laid out in the subjective, objective, assessment and plan (SOAP) format, is provided in **Table 25.1**.

Objectives for comprehensive paediatric eye and vision examinations

The objectives of a comprehensive paediatric eye and vision examination as developed by the AOA (Scheiman et al 2002) are to:

- evaluate the functional status of the eyes and visual system, taking into account each child's level of development
- assess ocular health and related systemic health conditions
- establish a diagnosis and formulate a treatment plan
- counsel and educate parents/caregivers regarding their child's visual, ocular, and related healthcare status, including recommendations for treatment, management, and preventive care.

The purpose of the comprehensive paediatric eye and vision examination as developed by the AAO (Bateman et al 2002a) is: 'A comprehensive medical eye evaluation is performed to evaluate abnormalities detected on screening, to identify risk factors for and to detect and diagnose sight- and health-threatening disease, and to initiate a plan of treatment as necessary.' The specific goals of this process are to:

Table 25.1 Typical elements of a comprehensive eye and vision examination

Area	Testing element	Area examined
Subjective	Case history (specific areas required)	All
Objective	Visual acuity	All
	Pupil testing	Oculomotor status
	Eye movements	Oculomotor status
	Visual field screening and/or evaluation	All
	Objective and subjective refraction	Refractive status
	Evaluation of near addition	Refractive status
	Biomicroscopy	Ocular and systemic health status
	Tonometry	Ocular and systemic health status
	Ophthalmoscopy	Ocular and systemic health status
Assessment	Assessment of oculomotor, refractive and ocular and systemic health status and discussion with the patient	All
Plan	Plan for management of oculomotor, refractive and ocular and systemic health status and discussion with the patient	All

- identify risk factors for ocular disease
- identify risk factors for systemic disease based on ocular findings
- identify factors that may predispose to visual loss early in a child's life
- determine the health status of the eye, visual system and related structures, and assess refractive errors
- discuss the nature of the findings of the examination and their implications with the parent/caregiver, primary care physician (with report) and, when appropriate, the patient
- plan and initiate an appropriate response (e.g. treatment, counselling, further diagnostic tests, referral, follow-up, early intervention services).

As developed by both organizations, a comprehensive examination of a paediatric patient has the overall objective of providing an assessment of the major areas related to vision for each patient. In this sense, the comprehensive examination of a paediatric patient is similar to that described for adult patients. A careful review of the paediatric examination reveals a somewhat greater emphasis on an assessment of the functional status of the visual systems in conjunction with an evaluation of areas that have the potential to impact sight, such as refractive, binocular, eye or systemic health conditions.

A comprehensive paediatric vision examination usually includes a patient history (with defined elements) as well as testing with regard to refractive, binocular and ocular and systemic health status (Scheiman et al 2002; Bateman et al 2002a). Although the examination has required elements for each of these areas, a clinician has substantial latitude in choosing the precise testing procedure. In accomplishing these general objectives, the clinician should have specific aims or goals tailored for each patient. The effect of these specific aims is to provide a methodology appropriate for completing the evaluation of the basic areas of a comprehensive examination for a paediatric patient. Although the examination may differ from patient to

patient, it still meets the requirements of a comprehensive examination.

The specific testing for the examination of the 1-year-old should include a comprehensive case history with the parent. The refractive and binocular vision portion of the examination will only include objective testing (Scheiman et al 2002; Bateman et al 2002a). It should also include an evaluation of visual acuity (see Ch. 28). Other objective testing appropriate to binocular vision would include an assessment of pupil reactions, version eye movements and assessment of binocular status using the cover test, Krimsky or Hirschberg tests (Choi & Kushner 1998; Rutstein & Daum 1998). Refractive evaluation will be limited to an evaluation with retinoscopy, probably under cycloplegia (Choong et al 2006). The health portion of the examination includes external examination (Threlkeld et al 1999), which should comprise elements of a biomicroscopic examination. Ophthalmoscopy, typically using binocular indirect with a condensing lens of somewhat higher power than normally used in adults, will extend the field of view (Semes & Amos 2006). Together, these tests cover the basic areas of a comprehensive vision examination for the infant. The clinician is responsible for the determination of relevant diagnoses and plans for management of any observed conditions. The case presentation is made to the parent or guardian and should include a discussion of the clinician's assessment and plan including any recommendations for refractive correction or follow-up care to assess risk factors for amblyopia (Rouse et al 1998; Bateman et al 2002b), strabismus (Rutstein & Daum 1998; Bateman et al 2002c), learning-related developmental and visual anomalies (Garzia et al 2001) or any other elements potentially significant to the patient.

Types of vision examinations

There are, of course, several different types (or levels) of examinations besides the comprehensive examination. The various types of examinations can be considered in two

Table 25.2 Objectives of examinations as defined by CPT codes

Type of vision examination	Description	Possible objectives
Screening	Brief examination with limited elements of testing	Assess risk factors and determine presence or absence of potential risk factors. Recommend appropriate treatment pathway and timing.
Vision plan	Comprehensive	Medical diagnosis unnecessary, often routine care. Examine all basic areas of vision including refractive, oculomotor and eye and systemic health.
Medical	Problem focused	Patient reports with medically related diagnosis. Assess the significance of problem reported at patient presentation including diagnosis and plan.
	Intermediate	Patient reports with medically related diagnosis. Survey all basic areas of vision including refractive, oculomotor and eye and systemic health with emphasis on one area.
	Comprehensive	Patient reports with medically related diagnosis. Examine all basic areas of vision including refractive, oculomotor and eye and systemic health.
	Complex	Patient reports with medically related diagnosis. Examine all basic areas of vision including refractive, oculomotor and eye and systemic health with particular emphasis on diagnoses critical to sight and life.
Refraction (only or re-check)	Brief examination devoted only to refractive status	Medical diagnosis unnecessary, often routine care. Examine only refractive status, new or re-evaluate.
Contact lens	Basic or complex evaluation and fitting	Medical diagnosis unnecessary, often routine care for fitting, re-fitting or other assessment of contact lens status. Examine refractive and eye and systemic health status as applied to contact lens wear, new or re-evaluate.
	Check	Medical diagnosis unnecessary, often routine care to check contact lens status. Examine refractive and eye and systemic health status as applied to contact lens wear, new or re-evaluate.

ways (**Tables 25.2** and **25.3**). Firstly, they can be classified according to the Current Procedural Terminology (CPT) code maintained by the American Medical Association (Gordy et al 2005). These codes are used in the USA to provide a technical description of the elements contained within an examination, and are also used for filing insurance-related claims. While the CPT code is exact and serves a useful purpose in describing an examination, there are other more understandable descriptions of the objectives of an examination. Therefore, a second, more general way of describing the examination is simply in terms of the procedure(s) that need to be completed. Using task-related descriptions can also be a useful way of considering objectives (see **Table 25.3**). Although this dimension may not provide the most technical description of an examination, clinicians frequently use these terms to communicate their objectives. For a full description of an examination, it may be wise to consider both formats.

Formulating objectives for a particular examination can range from a simple decision, e.g. a routine comprehensive examination or refraction check, to more complex objectives that may encompass many aspects of the patient's vision, health and social context. The best clinicians match the objectives of their examination with the needs of the patient. Sometimes the patient may not recognize some (or any) of their needs, and in such cases it is incumbent upon the clinician to explain the necessity of additional testing and secure the patient's consent before proceeding.

Parties to the objectives of an examination

Conceptually, there can be many parties involved in an eye examination. In other words, multiple individuals and organizations may care about the outcome of the testing, albeit with individual interests. Therefore, the objectives of an examination require clinicians to be aware of the many different perspectives that affect the milieu of vision care. Some of these interested parties are listed in **Table 25.4**.

Patients and their family are interested in objectives that provide a thorough, accurate and competent examination of their eye and visual health. Although efficiency is a significant desire, the overriding concern is usually sufficient testing to ensure that the exam is complete and accurate. Since additional or redundant testing is likely to add cost and/or time, the patient views the objectives with their associated goals as those sufficient to be complete but not excessive. Similarly, the participating clinician's perspective is also aimed at objectives that allow an accurate and complete examination. Since the clinician has an economic stake in being efficient, i.e. providing proper care to the maximum number of patients, they should set objectives to ensure a complete and accurate examination with optimum efficiency and minimum redundancy.

Insurers are stakeholders in an overwhelming percentage of vision examinations provided in the United States. The number of people in the USA with health insurance coverage

Table 25.3 Objectives as a function of the task

Type of vision examination	Description	Possible goals, testing
Refractive assessment and management	Refractive error Presbyopia Anisometropia Aniseikonia	Case history Visual acuity Keratometry Retinoscopy Subjective refraction
Oculomotor/binocular vision assessment and management	Accommodation Binocular vision Strabismus Oculomotor effects of refractive correction	Case history Visual acuity Accommodative amplitude, facility Cover test, Modified Thorington, von Graefe, Maddox rod phorometry, Krimsky and Hirschberg tests Versions and ductions Stereopsis
Disease assessment and management	Ocular adnexa Anterior segment Crystalline lens Vitreous Posterior eye including retina, optic nerve, choroids Optic pathway, eye to cortex	Case history Visual acuity External examination Biomicroscopy Fundus biomicroscopy Ophthalmoscopy, direct or binocular indirect Pachymetry Visual fields Photography, digital imaging Electronic assessment of eye and visual system (e.g. GDX, HRT, OCT)
Systemic conditions assessment and management	Diabetes Hypertension Other	Case history Visual acuity Blood pressure Disease assessment and management testing (above)
Visual function, standard evaluation	Employment Colour vision Visual acuity Binocular vision Ergonomic	Case history Visual acuity Other specific testing as described in protocol

in 2005 was 247.3 million (84.1% of the population; DeNavas-Walt et al 2006). Unfortunately and correspondingly, 46.6 million (15.9%) of persons in the USA were without health insurance coverage (DeNavas-Walt et al 2006). The insurance companies have a great interest in the economics of the examination, and, at the same time, they also desire to provide a service to assist in the healthcare of their clients. In achieving these somewhat competing objectives, insurance companies have often mandated the frequency of examinations and also determine whether periodic, routine examinations are covered or not. Obviously, the more frequent the examination, the greater the likely costs to the company. However, more frequent examinations by consumers would allow the early detection of problems and the best, most efficient management of those conditions. In many cases, studies into the outcome of different approaches have not been undertaken, and are unlikely to be completed due to the large expenses involved. Unfortunately, consumers are often ill-informed about the true differences between competing insurance plans and have difficulty making choices. Consumers are often unaware of poor management that plagues some plans, which allows them to continue despite poor service and relationships with healthcare providers.

Under the current system in the USA whereby health insurance is frequently covered through one's occupation, employers certainly have a stake in the determination of healthcare objectives for their employees. At the heart of it, employers wish to retain healthy, and therefore productive, employees. In the business world, with competition fiercer than ever, these companies also have a vested interest in obtaining healthcare for their employees at the lowest possible cost. This may drive the employer to seek minimalist coverage for vision and healthcare and, in some cases, may actually work against their main objective of retaining healthy, productive employees. Decisions about what and how much healthcare to make available have been especially difficult with rapidly rising costs in the healthcare sector in the United States.

The role that educators and research scientists (particularly clinical researchers) have in setting the objectives of a vision examination may not be obvious but can actually play a significant role due to a number of different factors. As science advances, the expectations for the standard of care changes. For example, a dilated fundus examination (DFE) in most cases is now the standard of care for a routine vision examination (Classe 1989). Previously, a direct ophthalmoscope used to view the fundus through an undilated pupil represented the standard for care for most optometrists. As educators recognized the greater efficacy for a DFE with a binocular indirect ophthalmoscope and taught

Table 25.4 Parties with interest in the outcome of a vision examination

Party	Interest
Patient	Self interest
Patient's family	Family interest
Provider clinician	Provision of good care Fulfilling legal and ethical responsibility
Insurers	Corporate interest in achieving company goals Economic and legal interest in completion of contracted services
Employers	Good workers with good vision enhance profitability Good visual health works to reduce absenteeism and absences
Educator or clinic supervisors	Business is training and educating good clinicians Reputation affected by products, i.e. examinations of their clinicians
Optometric/vision care community	Vision care by each practitioner affects the perception of all patients toward the overall community
Healthcare community	Collective interest in efficient, effective healthcare
Society at large Government Economists Educators Employers	The burden of healthcare expenses is shared by the entire society Visual health affects the outcome of numerous tasks such as education

this procedure in their educational institutions, the standard has gradually changed as new practitioners have taken their place alongside their older colleagues. This evolving standard now often includes automated visual fields, and photography and digital imaging of various structures of the eye. It may also be moving toward the inclusion of objective measurement of retinal thickness and other parameters with the HRT, GDx and OCT devices (Coops et al 2006; Brusini et al 2006) (see Ch. 18).

The vision care community, both optometric and ophthalmologic, also plays an important role in setting objectives for eye and vision examinations (Soroka et al 2006). They design testing procedures that mandate the skills and knowledge to be possessed by new practitioners. And, sometimes indirectly, they negotiate with insurers and employers to reach a balance point for appropriate care for their patients at an acceptable cost with payoffs for individual and collective clinicians. Likewise, the larger healthcare community has a great stake in the inclusion of healthcare in society with eye and vision care as an appropriate part of that care. Finally, society at large has a substantial stake in ensuring that adequate eye and vision care is provided for its members.

Informed consent for objectives of the examination

Informed consent is a fundamental aspect of eye and vision examinations. In some cases, e.g. contact lens fittings or minor surgical procedures, a patient could be provided with a written explanation of the procedures including any associated risks and potential benefits and charges. This methodology has been designed to provide adequate information for the patient in managing their healthcare and also documents the appropriate provision of informed consent to the patient by the professional.

In many routine cases, such as a patient returning to have their refraction checked after receiving spectacles, the objectives of the examination may be obvious. However, even in these cases, a clinician should verbally describe the procedures to be undertaken, answer any questions the patient may have, and obtain their consent before proceeding with the examination. Often, the consent may be non-verbal and takes the form of the clinician in conjunction with the patient establishing an understanding that informed consent has been completed. Any time the clinician is not sure that informed consent has been completed, the clinician should take the time to deal with the patient directly and document the consent in the chart. If the clinician suspects that the patient does not understand all aspects of the examination or the associated fees, the best policy is to address the matter directly and document its resolution in the patient's record.

Objectives in special situations

Optometrists are required to set objectives in a variety of special situations (Soroka et al 2006; **Table 25.5**). Some of these occur quite commonly and routinely such as contact lens examinations or when patients return with problems concerning their glasses. Other situations may arise only for a subset of clinicians who provide specialized care such as screenings in schools or in the community, low-vision examinations, examinations for computer/ergonomic problems or binocular or developmental vision examinations for children.

Table 25.5 Special situations requiring objectives

Situation	Objectives required
Problem solving	Refractive problems (issues with glasses or contact lenses)
	Computer/ergonomic examination
	Other
Survey and evaluation	Screening
Standard evaluation	Contact lenses
	Driver's or pilot's licence exam
	Pre- or postoperative exam
	Insurance evaluation
	Employment evaluation, e.g. FBI
	Low vision, binocular vision or developmental vision exams
	Monitoring actual or potential disease states
	Athletic vision assessment evaluation
	Clinical research examinations

Some relatively infrequent special situations occur for practitioners when certifying patients for drivers' or pilots' licences or aspects of vision for military service. Most clinicians encounter situations where it is necessary to monitor actual or potential disease states, e.g. cataracts, dry eye, pterygium, glaucoma or glaucoma suspects, Plaquenil (hydroxychloroquine) therapy, corneal dystrophies, diabetic or hypertensive retinopathy or pre- or post-surgical evaluations.

In these special situations, the clinician must establish objectives and goals for the examination in advance. Extra consideration should be given to link the care provided in the past and with what might potentially come in the future. Communication of these objectives with the patient is, of course, necessary and appropriate.

A patient having issues with glasses or contact lenses is a relatively common occurrence. Most of the time, the patient states their objective for the examination, e.g. to determine if the glasses or contact lenses (or uncorrected state) are the correct (i.e. optimal) prescription. The clinician typically addresses the examination by restating the objective and follows through with questions designed to illuminate the problem and testing necessary to solve it. In these cases, the role of the clinician may be to provide assent to the stated objective of the patient. Alternatively, if the objective was not stated by the patient, one should formulate an objective by careful questioning, and confirm this objective with the patient before beginning testing.

On occasions, a clinician may be performing an examination to provide the best refractive correction for the patient's workplace. Most frequently, this option is agreed upon before initiating the examination. Sometimes the patient requests this type of examination, while on other occasions it will be suggested by the clinician. The statement of objectives by the practitioner is important in outlining the scope of the examination and to clarify the patient's expectations toward the testing involved, the precise outcome of the examination, perhaps a tentative spectacle design, and with regard to the costs (in both time and money) involved.

Clinicians may be involved in examinations that are designed to be a screening test. Often, these occur in settings where the expectations of the patient are clarified from the outset. A good example is glaucoma screening. Patients participating in this type of event generally recognize that the screening is designed to provide an estimate of the likelihood of glaucoma for an individual. In many cases, the setting itself is a plain statement of the objective of the examination and it is not necessary for the clinician to make any additional statements about the objective unless the patient asks. If the advanced publicity or announcement does not explain the purpose of the screening adequately, then the clinician or their assistant must provide this information to each participant. Clinicians should take care to point out to participants that the screening is not a complete vision examination and to present the significance of regular eye and vision care.

On occasion, clinicians may enter a setting where the objective varies. In nursing homes, for example, both screenings and comprehensive examinations may be provided. Before beginning, all participants must be informed about the type of examination to be provided, and this explanation should include the likely outcomes and any costs involved. Since some patients in a nursing home may be compromised in some manner, the objectives should be provided to an appropriate person who could assist in allowing the patient to make a decision about participation or who is authorized to speak for the patient.

Clinicians and patients participate in a variety of examinations designed to evaluate the patient's suitability for driving, flying or acceptance into an insurance policy. In most cases, the objective of the examination is requested by the patient, and acknowledgement by the clinician is all that is necessary to proceed. Sometimes, one of the two parties to the examination, either the practitioner or the patient, may be unsure of the scope, potential outcome or some other aspect of the examination. In these cases, a brief discussion with the patient goes a long way to ensuring that the examination is able to proceed without incident or question. In particular, the clinician should verify for the patient whether the examination is considered a part of the standard comprehensive examination and if an additional fee (and/or extra time) is necessary.

Contact lens examinations merit special attention to clarify their objectives for the patient. Even before initiating the comprehensive examination, most clinicians, or their staff, ask patients whether or not they are interested in contact lenses. If the patient is a current or potential contact lens wearer, the clinician should pay special attention to educating the patient about the lenses. Many clinicians provide a detailed written description of the various types of contact lens examinations with their associated costs and ask the patient to examine the information sheet, ask any questions and sign or initial it before the examination begins. The contact lens sheet generally contains information about the types of contact lens examinations including progress check, basic fitting, complex fitting, bifocal fitting, complex bifocal fitting, insertion and removal training and perhaps a keratoconus fitting. The explanation of the objectives of the examination should include a statement of the costs involved, the number of visits covered (and whether any additional visits are required as well as their costs). Material costs should be described. Finally, the way that contact lens patients are charged for their yearly comprehensive examinations should be made clear. In addition, the policy toward contact lens prescription release should be clearly stated. Many patients may not recognize that a contact lens fit requires a period of successful wear with an evaluation before being finalized. In this regard, a statement on the contact lens information sheet may be of great help and a comment by the clinician would clarify it.

Special evaluations for employment or recreation purposes (e.g. fitness to participate in a specific sport or leisure activity) are relatively unusual for most clinicians. In these cases, the examination may resemble a comprehensive examination, perhaps with the addition of a summary letter to a third party. In other cases, the examination may require unusual testing, e.g. special colour or stereopsis testing or oculomotor examination. Additionally, testing may be similar to a driving fitness evaluation (e.g. visual acuity, visual fields, colour vision) and be quite short. Since the testing is variable, and the individual or agency paying for the examination may also depend on the circumstances, special testing requires care to establish with the proper individual(s) the objectives of the examination including details such as the type of testing, time requirements, fees and payments required, and an understanding of the nature of the feedback expected. Although not always required directly, a detailed informed consent process is critical to allow matching of the varying objectives of the patient, clinician and the authority responsible for the examination.

Monitoring actual or potential disease states (e.g. cataract, glaucoma or glaucoma suspects, diabetic or hypertensive retinopathy, dry eye, pterygium, Plaquenil therapy, corneal dystrophies) is a common reason for a vision examination. In most of these cases, once the initial diagnosis has been made, the optometrist's objective is to determine whether any change has occurred that warrants further treatment or alternative management. For each patient, the examination may change depending upon the patient's previous status. Many of these examinations will be completed under medical insurance plans. Therefore, specific portions of the case history and additional testing may be required. Commonly, the examination is billed as a 'detailed' or 'intermediate' examination.

On occasions, clinicians undertake examinations with specific objectives. These might be for a low-vision patient or one with a binocular or developmental abnormality such as dyslexia. In some of these examinations, the objectives of the examination are directed toward making a complete and accurate diagnosis. The objective may stem from the complexity of the situation or the need for additional testing not readily incorporated into a comprehensive examination. In either case, appropriate management of the patient depends on the diagnosis. However, in other situations, the diagnosis is already available, and the primary objective of the examination is directed toward management. Thus, the clinician must have a practical understanding of how certain treatments might affect the patient. An example is the selection of the best type of magnifier for a low-vision patient. Stand, hand-held or even electronic magnifiers all have strengths and weaknesses. The examination should be aimed at educating the patient about these choices, and offering them first-hand experience. In binocular vision examinations, working with a patient in the selection of prism, lenses or orthoptic exercises/vision therapy can offer similar challenges. Developmental vision examinations may require education on the use of several different therapeutic approaches. The chosen treatment plan may be selected as a result of the clinician's observations in conjunction with the patient's input.

Clinical research projects often involve examinations with more than one objective. Of course, whenever patient care is undertaken, the welfare of the patient must be foremost. When clinical research is involved, the welfare of the patient is combined with another objective specified by the research project. The latter has the potential to affect any part of the examination, assessment, diagnosis or management. Ethical treatment of the patient requires informed consent before the initiation of any aspect of the examination. When a research protocol is undertaken, the design must be appropriate to provide clinical care as well as to achieve the objective of the research. Obviously, this requires careful thought and planning as well as approval by an ethics committee and adherence to the tenets of the declaration of Helsinki.

Modulation of objectives

Clinicians often modulate the objectives of their examination depending on a wide variety of factors. These could include the information already at hand, time consideration, the expertise of the clinician, degree of compensation and the equipment available.

Setting the objectives of an examination depends on the clinician understanding the clinical situation. This will vary based upon the amount of information available. On occasion, a patient may present with only a rudimentary understanding of their visual problem. The clinician may formulate a preliminary objective for exploring the visual concerns of the patient and when these are clarified, proceed to an appropriate assessment. When patients are referred, the clinician receiving the referral depends on the referring practitioner to describe the patient's problem(s). If the referring clinician does not communicate fully or accurately, the objectives of the subsequent examination may be inappropriate or incomplete. Communication, either between clinicians, or from patient to practitioner (or vice versa) is important when formulating examination objectives.

Although clinicians would often deny that time is a factor when setting the objectives for an examination, in a practical sense the time available to complete testing will affect the objectives being considered. Time constraints, whether from the patient or the practitioner, will inevitably lead to limitations. Particularly for routine care, such limitations may lead to the rescheduling of the patient for the completion of the examination. Most clinicians have sufficient flexibility in their schedules to accommodate the needs of their patients. On occasion, however, due to findings during the course of the examination, the clinician may have difficulties completing the objectives and the patient is scheduled for additional time for their completion at a later date. An important exception to the potential effect of time on the objectives of an examination is when the suspicion or discovery of an emergency condition such as diabetic retinopathy or retinal detachment occurs. Then the patient must be given priority and other activities set aside.

A clinician's expertise with regard to a patient's condition may affect the objectives of the examination. Clinicians with more experience and expertise are likely to set objectives aimed at a complete and accurate diagnosis of the patient's anomaly. For example, a clinician expert in corneal anomalies is more likely to aim toward a complete diagnosis, e.g. granular dystrophy, whereas a less knowledgeable clinician may simply settle for a determination of corneal anomaly with the aim of referring the patient to a specialist. Obviously, students often have limited examination objectives due to their inexperience and incomplete knowledge.

As with time constraints, most clinicians would strongly deny that financial considerations have any effect on the objectives that are set for a patient. If the clinic is sparsely equipped because of a relative lack of finance, then the objectives set may be more modest and less complete than if the examination were conducted in a lavishly equipped clinic. Although it is difficult to admit, patient resources may also play a role in the objectives set by a clinician for the examination. Unfortunately, in the absence of universal health coverage, indigent patients are sometimes given less testing and overall care than the well-off, even though the same level of care should be provided for all patients. Unfortunately, lack of insurance coverage (or the ability to pay for the examination themselves) may play a role in reduced objectives for diagnosis and treatment of those patients. However, the code of ethics for optometrists demands equal care for all in every case.

In this age of technology, the clinical equipment available will influence the objectives that can be set by the clinician. Perhaps this is most obvious in the area of glaucoma. Expensive technology such as fundus imaging, pachymetry, and objective assessment of the optic disc with devices such as the HRT, GDx and OCT (see Ch. 18) now allow exquisite diagnosis and allow changes to be measured more accurately. Clinicians with access to such equipment have the luxury of setting a much higher level of diagnosis and management. Similarly, clinicians performing examinations in settings such as screenings or remote clinics may have to adjust their objectives to account for the more limited diagnostic equipment available.

Objectives for students

It is appropriate for students and optometrists in training to have varying objectives for their examinations as a function of their training and experience as well as the setting of the examination. Often, novice clinicians have objectives for the complete and accurate performance of certain procedures. With additional experience and training, objectives are extended to the performance of all testing appropriate to the patient. The cognitive aspects of the examination including diagnostic acumen are usually the last objectives to be accomplished as they require understanding and perspective about the various aspects of the patient's condition.

Objectives related to specific symptoms and signs

When carrying out an examination, there may be one or more critical symptoms and signs that, when present, must be addressed when setting objectives. Examples of these are shown in **Table 25.6**. Often, these are the reasons that the patient is seeking care and so their inclusion in the objectives set by the patient is obvious. On occasion, however, one or more of these critical factors may present in an examination that has other objectives. When this occurs, the objectives of the examination must be altered immediately to determine the aetiology of the critical sign or symptom. An example is a routine examination for glasses on a

Table 25.6 Examples of key symptoms and signs that must be included in setting objectives whenever they are present

Key symptoms	Key signs
Sudden loss of vision	Papilloedema
Diplopia	Recent onset, incomitant strabismus
Severe headache	Anisocoria
Photophobia	Discharge, especially purulent
Foreign body sensation	Proliferative diabetic retinopathy (e.g. preretinal haemorrhage)
Soreness in the temple	Clinically significant macular oedema

diabetic patient. Many critical aspects of potential vision loss may be present, such as proliferative diabetic retinopathy or clinically significant macular oedema. The clinician must recognize the importance of an overall assessment of ocular health given the significance of the medical condition.

Monitoring versus exhaustive testing issues in setting objectives

The objectives of a vision examination may not facilitate a specific diagnosis for each anomalous finding. For example, consider an individual with a small haemorrhage near the macula of the right eye with no other significant ocular findings, a non-contributory case history, and an absence of suspect systemic conditions such as diabetes or hypertension.

In accomplishing the objectives such as a comprehensive examination for this patient, a clinical judgement must be made. In the absence of supporting data to enable a diagnosis, one option is to simply note the finding, and to monitor it on subsequent visits (in this case, perhaps a month later) at a problem-focused examination of the macula and posterior pole of each eye. Another option is to continue testing in an attempt to determine the aetiology of the haemorrhage. This approach may include fundus imaging, extended ophthalmoscopy of both eyes and perhaps visual fields or systemic testing with referral to a physician.

Either choice may be valid under certain circumstances. There is often more than one appropriate way to manage a particular patient. The decision may depend upon the clinician's competence as well as their confidence and the patient's tolerance for risk. Those with more diagnostic acumen may press for a definitive diagnosis while others may elect to assess the condition periodically or refer for a second opinion.

Subtle but real objectives

Practitioners may, on occasion, undertake certain unstated objectives. Clinical decisions may affect the patient in many ways over time. The clinician may elect to provide emotional support for a patient experiencing challenging situations such as the effects of macular degeneration or diabetic retinopathy. At their best, clinicians aim to reassure patients of their competence and that medical science can be an important source to preserve their vision. At their worst, clinicians have the potential to scare or undermine the confidence of their patients. Recognizing the potential for these effects will be useful to optometrists as they interact with patients having many different problems and needs.

Minimal required objectives

The Code of Ethics of the American Optometric Association (http://www.aoa.org/x4878.xml) states: 'It shall be the ideal, the resolve, and the duty of the members of the American Optometric Association:

- TO KEEP the visual welfare of the patient uppermost at all times;

- TO PROMOTE in every possible way, in collaboration with this Association, better care of the visual needs of humankind;
- TO ENHANCE continuously their educational and technical proficiency to the end that their patients shall receive the benefits of all acknowledged improvements in visual care;
- TO STRIVE TO SEE THAT no person shall lack for visual care;
- TO ADVISE the patient whenever consultation with an optometric colleague or reference for other professional care seems advisable;
- TO HOLD in professional confidence all information concerning a patient and to use such data only for the benefit of the patient;
- TO CONDUCT themselves as exemplary citizens;
- TO MAINTAIN their offices and their practices in keeping with professional standards;
- TO PROMOTE and maintain cordial and unselfish relationships with members of their own profession and of other professions for the exchange of information to the advantage of humankind.'

The objectives set by each optometrist for each patient encounter must be consistent with the spirit of this code of ethics.

References

Bateman J B, Christmann L M, Dankner S R et al 2002a American Academy of Ophthalmology. Pediatric eye evaluations, preferred practice pattern. San Francisco: American Academy of Ophthalmology. Online. Available: www.aao.org/ppp

Bateman J B, Christmann L M, Dankner S R et al 2002b American Academy of Ophthalmology. Amblyopia, preferred practice pattern. San Francisco: American Academy of Ophthalmology. Online. Available: www.aao.org/ppp.

Bateman J B, Christmann L M, Dankner S R et al 2002c American Academy of Ophthalmology. Esotropia and exotropia, preferred practice pattern. San Francisco: American Academy of Ophthalmology. Online. Available: www.aao.org/ppp

Borish I M, Benjamin W J 2006 Monocular and binocular subjective evaluation. In: Benjamin W J (ed.) Borish's clinical refraction, 2nd edn. Butterworth Heinemann Elsevier, St Louis, pp 790–898

Brusini P, Salvetat M L, Zeppieri M et al 2006 Comparison between GDx VCC scanning laser polarimetry and Stratus OCT optical coherence tomography in the diagnosis of chronic glaucoma. Acta Ophthalmology Scandinavia 84(5):650–655

Casser L, Goss D A, Keller J T et al 2005 Optometric Clinical Practice Guideline, Comprehensive Adult Eye and Vision Examination, Second Edition, Reference Guide for Clinicians, Prepared by the American Optometric Association Consensus Panel on Comprehensive Adult Eye and Vision Examination, American Optometric Association, St. Louis. Online. Available: http://71.153.51.135/x4813.xml

Cavallerano J, Cooppan R, Alexander L et al 2002 Optometric Clinical Practice Guideline, Care Of The Patient With Diabetes Mellitus, Reference Guide for Clinicians, Third Revision, Prepared by the American Optometric Association Consensus Panel on Diabetes, American Optometric Association, St. Louis. Online. Available: http://71.153.51.135/documents/CPG-3.pdf

Cavallerano A A, Cummings J P, Freeman P B et al 2004 Optometric Clinical Practice Guideline, Care Of The Patient With Age-Related, Macular Degeneration, Reference Guide for Clinicians, Prepared by the American Optometric Association Consensus Panel on Care of the Patient with Age-Related Macular Degeneration, American

Optometric Association, St. Louis. Online. Available: http://71.153.51.135/documents/CPG-6.pdf

Chew E Y, Benson W E, Boldt H C et al 2003 American Academy of Ophthalmology. Diabetic Retinopathy, Preferred Practice Pattern. San Francisco: American Academy of Ophthalmology. Online. Available: www.aao.org/ppp

Chew E Y, Benson W E, Boldt H C et al 2006 American Academy of Ophthalmology. Age-Related Macular Degeneration, Limited Revision, Preferred Practice Pattern. San Francisco: American Academy of Ophthalmology. Online. Available: www.aao.org/ppp

Choi R Y, Kushner B J 1998 The accuracy of experienced strabismologists using the Hirschberg and Krimsky tests. Ophthalmology 705:1301–1306

Choong Y F, Chen A H, Goh P P 2006 A comparison of autorefraction and subjective refraction with and without cycloplegia in primary school children. American Journal Ophthalmology 142:68–74

Classe J G 1989 Legal aspects of optometry. Butterworths, Boston, p 739

Cooper S L 2006 State statute and board rule reference to the definition of practice of optometry. American Optometric Association, Revised 3 November 2006

Coops A, Henson D B, Kwartz A J et al 2006 Automated analysis of Heidelberg retina tomograph optic disc images by glaucoma probability score. Investigative Ophthalmology and Vision Science 47(12):5348–5355

DeNavas-Walt C, Proctor B D, Lee C H 2006 U.S. Census Bureau, Current Population Reports, Income, Poverty, and Health Insurance Coverage in the United States: 2005. US Government Printing Office, Washington, DC, pp 60–231

Fleming J B, Semes L P 2006 Anterior segment evaluation. In: Benjamin W J (ed.) Borish's clinical refraction, 2nd edn. Butterworth Heinemann Elsevier, St Louis, pp 485–510

Gaasterland D E, Allingham R R, Gross R L et al 2005a American Academy of Ophthalmology. Primary Angle Closure, Preferred Practice Pattern. San Francisco: American Academy of Ophthalmology. Online. Available: www.aao.org/ppp

Gaasterland D E, Allingham R R, Gross R L et al 2005b American Academy of Ophthalmology. Primary Open-Angle Glaucoma, Preferred Practice Pattern. San Francisco: American Academy of Ophthalmology. Online. Available: www.aao.org/ppp

Gaasterland D E, Allingham R R, Gross R L et al 2005c American Academy of Ophthalmology. Primary Open-Angle Glaucoma Suspect, Preferred Practice Pattern. San Francisco: American Academy of Ophthalmology. Online. Available: www.aao.org/ppp

Garzia R P, Borsting E J, Nicholson S B et al 2001 Care of the Patient with Learning Related Vision Problems, Reference Guide for Clinicians, Prepared by the American Optometric Association Consensus Panel on Care of the Patient with Learning Related Vision Problems: American Optometric Association, St Louis. Online. Available: http://71.153.51.135/documents/CPG-20.pdf

Gordy T R et al 2005 Current procedural terminology CPT 2005, standard edition. AMA Press, Chicago

Goss D A, Grosvenor T P, Keller J T et al 2001 Optometric Clinical Practice Guideline, Care Of The Patient With Myopia, Reference Guide for Clinicians, Prepared by the American Optometric Association Consensus Panel on Care of the Patient with Myopia, American Optometric Association, St Louis. Online. Available: http://71.153.51.135/documents/CPG-15.pdf

Haine C L 2006 The ophthalmic case historian. In: Benjamin W J (ed.) Borish's clinical refraction, 2nd edn. Butterworth Heinemann Elsevier, St Louis, pp 195–216

Jackson J, Carr L W III, Fisch B M et al 2001 Optometric Clinical Practice Guideline, Care Of The Patient With Primary Angle Closure Glaucoma, Reference Guide for Clinicians, Prepared by the American Optometric Association Consensus Panel on Care of the Patient with Primary Angle Closure Glaucoma, American Optometric Association, St Louis. Online. Available: http://71.153.51.135/documents/CPG-5.pdf

Lewis T L, Barnebey H S, Bartlett J D et al 2002 Optometric Clinical Practice Guideline, Care Of The Patient With Open Angle Glaucoma, Second Edition, Reference Guide for Clinicians, Prepared by the American Optometric Association Consensus Panel on Care of the Patient with Open Angle Glaucoma, American Optometric

Association, St Louis. Online. Available: http://71.153.51.135/documents/CPG-9.pdf

Mancil G L, Bailey I L, Brookman K E et al 2001 Optometric Clinical Practice Guideline, Care Of The Patient With Presbyopia, Reference Guide for Clinicians, Prepared by the American Optometric Association Consensus Panel on Care of the Patient with Presbyopia, American Optometric Association, St Louis. Online. Available: http://71.153.51.135/documents/CPG-17.pdf

Mandelbaum S, de Luise V P, Driebe W Jr et al 2002 American Academy of Ophthalmology. Refractive Errors, Preferred Practice Pattern. San Francisco: American Academy of Ophthalmology. Online. Available: www.aao.org/ppp

Mandelbaum S, Chew E Y, Christmann L M et al 2005 American Academy of Ophthalmology. Comprehensive Adult Medical Eye Evaluation, Preferred Practice Pattern. San Francisco: American Academy of Ophthalmology. Online. Available: www.aao.org/ppp

Masket S, Chang D F, Lane S S et al 2006 American Academy of Ophthalmology. Cataract in the Adult Eye, Preferred Practice Pattern. San Francisco: American Academy of Ophthalmology. Online. Available: www.aao.org/ppp

Matoba A Y, Harris D J Jr, Meisler D M et al 2003 American Academy of Ophthalmology. Dry Eye Syndrome, Preferred Practice Pattern. San Francisco: American Academy of Ophthalmology. Online. Available: www.aao.org/ppp

Moore B D, Augsburger A A, Ciner E B et al 2001 Optometric Clinical Practice Guideline, Care Of The Patient With Hyperopia, Reference Guide for Clinicians, Prepared by the American Optometric Association Consensus Panel on Care of the Patient with Hyperopia, American Optometric Association, St Louis. Online. Available: http://71.153.51.135/documents/CPG-16.pdf

Murrill C A, Stanfield D L, VanBrocklin M D et al 1999 Optometric Clinical Practice Guideline, Care Of The Adult Patient With Cataract, Reference Guide for Clinicians, Prepared by the American Optometric Association Consensus Panel on Care of the Adult Patient with Cataract, American Optometric Association, St Louis. Online. Available: http://71.153.51.135/documents/CPG-8.pdf

National Center for Health Statistics 2006 Health, United States, 2006 with Chartbook on Trends in the Health of Americans, Hyattsville, MD. Online. Available: http://www.cdc.gov/nchs/hus.htm

Neufeld E V, Guralnik D B 1991 Webster's new world dictionary of American English, Third College Edition. Prentice Hall, New York, p 934

Rouse M W, Cooper J S, Cotter S A et al 1998 Optometric Clinical Practice Guideline, Care Of The Patient With Amblyopia, Reference Guide for Clinicians, Prepared by the American Optometric Association Consensus Panel on Care of the Patient with Amblyopia, American Optometric Association, St Louis. Online. Available: http://71.153.51.135/documents/CPG-4.pdf

Rutstein R P, Daum K M 1998 Anomalies of binocular vision. Mosby Yearbook, Chicago

Rutstein R P, Cogen M S, Cotter S A et al 2004 Optometric Clinical Practice Guideline Care of the Patient with Strabismus: Esotropia and Exotropia, Reference Guide for Clinicians, Prepared by the American Optometric Association Consensus Panel on Care of the Patient with Strabismus: American Optometric Association, St Louis. Online. Available: http://71.153.51.135/documents/CPG-12.pdf

Saladin J J 2006 Phorometry and stereopsis. In: Benjamin W J (ed.) Borish's clinical refraction, 2nd ed. Butterworth Heinemann Elsevier, St Louis, pp 485–510

Scheiman M M, Amos C S, Ciner E B et al 2002 Pediatric Eye And Vision Examination, Reference Guide For Clinicians, Second Edition. Reviewed by the American Optometric Association Consensus Panel on Pediatric Eye and Vision Examination, American Optometric Association, St Louis. Online. Available: www.aoa.org/documents/CPG-2.pdf

Semes L P, Amos J F 2006 Posterior segment evaluation. In: Benjamin W J (ed.) Borish's clinical refraction, 2nd ed. Butterworth Heinemann Elsevier, St Louis, pp 511–543

Semes L P, Bright D C, Pensyl C D et al 2003 Optometric Clinical Practice Guideline, Care Of The Patient With Ocular Surface Disorders, Reference Guide for Clinicians, Second Edition, Prepared by the American Optometric Association Consensus Panel on Care of the Patient with Ocular Surface Disease, American Optometric Association, St Louis. Online. Available: http://71.153.51.135/documents/CPG-10.pdf

Soroka M, Krumholz D, Bennett A 2006 The practice of optometry: National Board of Examiners in Optometry survey of optometric practitioners. Optometry 77:427–437

Threlkeld A B, Fahd T, Camp M et al 1999 Telemedical evaluation of ocular adnexa and anterior segment. American Journal Ophthalmology 127(4): 464–466

Weissman B A, Barr J T, Harris M G et al 2000 Optometric Clinical Practice Guideline, Care Of The Contact Lens Patient, Reference Guide for Clinicians, Prepared by the American Optometric Association Consensus Panel on Care of the Contact Lens Patient, American Optometric Association, St Louis. Online. Available: http://71.153.51.135/documents/CPG-19.pdf

CHAPTER 26

Communication skills in optometry – case history and case disposition

Catherine Pace Watson

The doctor may also learn more about the complaint from the way the patient tells the story than from the story itself.

James B Herrick 1861–1954

Introduction

Good communication skills play a crucial role in the delivery of high-quality optometric care. These skills allow for practitioner–patient interaction that facilitates a good relationship for the remainder of the encounter as well as for subsequent visits. During the case history, the clinician will learn a great deal about their patient. Some of that information may be of an extremely personal nature. Some questions may uncover areas over which the patient has experienced variable levels of anxiety. Some issues may require intervention on the part of the optometrist, while others may fall within the realm of other medical disciplines. Experience will teach the young clinician when to solicit the help of other professionals. Thus, the optometrist may have to play other roles such as counsellor, educator, philosopher, and social worker.

There are many myths associated with communication. Some of these are:

1. *Myth*: We communicate only when we consciously and deliberately choose to communicate.

   Reality: We are communicating both verbally and non-verbally (e.g. by our facial expressions or body posture) with patients whether we are consciously aware of it or not.

2. *Myth*: Words mean the same thing to the listener as they do to the speaker.

   Reality: Words alone do not provide meaning; it is the interpretation of the words that influences how others receive communication.

3. *Myth*: We communicate primarily with words.

   Reality: The majority of our messages are communicated through non-verbal symbols.

Good communication skills are not taught by experience alone. These skills must be practised and reviewed many times in order to be improved.

In some ways, the case history is the most important part of the entire examination. This is when the patient gains their initial impression of the optometrist, while the optometrist is both listening to and observing the patient for the first time. The first few comments or questions should be more of a general 'meet and greet', rather than jumping in to clinical questions. Simple, friendly comments about general matters such as the weather, what type of transportation the patient used to reach the practice or upcoming holidays can help the patient to relax and feel more at ease with the practitioner. If it is a returning patient, then asking about something that was discussed at a previous visit, such as a new child or grandchild, a previous vacation or other major event will often be greatly appreciated by the patient. Throughout the interview, the clinician should both listen to and observe the patient carefully, since a tentative diagnosis can often be suggested by the case history alone. Today, many clinical settings use written questionnaires to complete some or all of the case history. While this is an efficient way of working, since the questionnaire can be completed before the patient arrives at the practice, it does limit the scope for practitioner–patient interaction. A disadvantage of such questionnaires is that, on occasion, patients will answer a question even when they do not understand it. Unless the optometrist reviews every question on the form, thereby eliminating the advantage of using the written form, then these errors could potentially be missed.

Types of questions

There are many ways of collecting the data necessary for an optometric examination. Two of the most commonly employed are questionnaires completed by the patient and the direct verbal interview. During the interview, the clinician will use different types of questions to gain the knowledge necessary for a thorough examination.

Open-ended questions are those which provide a simple frame of reference yet give the patient maximum freedom for expression and reply. These questions ask the patient for general information. One use of an open-ended question is to identify the chief complaint or reason for the examination. This is typically the first formal question asked during a case history. An example of an open-ended question is 'Are you having any problems with your eyes?'

Direct questions are structured to gain information about a specific thing. These are generally used after an open-ended question to add detail to the information already obtained. An example is 'When do your eyes tear?' A focused direct question can be used to explore areas of the patient history that have not yet been covered by the information already provided.

Some question types should be avoided. These are ambiguous yes–no types of questions that leave the clinician unsure of what the response means, for example, 'Have you been using your eye drops?' If the patient responds 'yes', the clinician can infer that the patient has been using the drops, but there is still uncertainty as to whether the proper dosing instructions are being followed. A better way to phrase that question is 'How often do you use your drops?'

Questions that ask about more than one issue should be avoided. For example, a question like 'Does anyone in your family have glaucoma, cataracts or macular degeneration?' can be confusing to the patient and they may respond incorrectly. Each disease should be a question unto itself. The clinician should ask 'Does anyone in your family have glaucoma?' and then wait for the patient's response before inquiring about another disease.

Leading questions are to be avoided during a case history. This type of question suggests to the patient what the proper response should be, and therefore may influence the answer that the patient ultimately gives. An example of a leading question is 'You have been using your eye drops, haven't you?' In the desire to please the clinician, the obvious answer is 'yes' even though it may not be the case.

Questions should be concise and understandable. Medical terms or jargon should not be used as most patients will not understand them. Patients may become alarmed if they are asked to respond to a question they do not understand.

Facilitative responses

During the history, the clinician should verbally communicate interest in what the patient is saying by the use of facilitative responses. For example, phrases like 'go on' and 'please explain' encourage the patient to expand upon what they have just said. The clinician should allow the patient to continue without interruption. Other means to facilitate a patient response can be to repeat or paraphrase the statement the patient has just made.

Jargon

When discussing a case with other clinicians while the patient is present, the use of jargon or medical terms may cause the patient to become anxious. The terms used in these conversations may be descriptive of a completely benign phenomenon, but because the patient does not comprehend what is being said, the whole conversation can be very disconcerting. If a discussion with colleagues must take place in the examination room, assurance must be given to the patient that the discussion will be repeated to them in lay terms. However, it is better either to conduct the discussion outside the patient's range or hearing or to use terminology that can be understood by the patient, and to allow them to contribute to the conversation.

Emotional terms

Early in any clinical career, a new clinician is bound to be exposed to ocular or medical phenomena that have not been previously experienced. As exciting as this may be for the new practitioner, care must be taken to avoid emotional terms ('Holy Cow!', 'I've never seen this before', 'What is that?' or 'Oh my goodness') when examining a patient.

Similarly, quantifying a condition early in one's career as the worst case one has ever seen may cause the patient unnecessary anxiety. Lack of experience can make what is a clinically mild presentation to the seasoned clinician seem to be a more severe presentation to a new observer. Terms that quantify some of the more subjective components of a disease should be kept to a minimum.

Non-verbal communication skills

Much of the communication that occurs in a case history is non-verbal. There are many different means to facilitate positive, non-verbal communication. These include eye contact, posture, movement and facial expression

During a case history, the clinician should sit at an appropriate distance from the patient. Distances greater than

1.5 m are impersonal, while sitting less than 0.8 m from the patient invades the patient's 'personal space'. Therefore, the clinician should sit at a distance of approximately 1.2 m from the patient

Eye contact is an important means to communicate interest, so the clinician should sit at about eye level with the patient. There should be no barriers in the examination room that prevent eye contact between the clinician and the patient.

Body posture and positioning also communicate interest. Body language can give insight as to how information is being given and received. Interpretation of body language is a two-way process. Just as the patient observes the clinician, the clinician can observe the patient. There are many interpretations of behaviour and body language, which can vary significantly across cultures. People use these interpretations daily as they assess the full meaning of a conversation between individuals. For example, shaking of the legs or wetting the lips frequently can be indicative of stress, while a head tilt can indicate interest. Other behaviours and their interpretations are listed in **Table 26.1**.

The clinician should sit and maintain an open posture. This will be interpreted as relaxed and honest. The arms should not be folded across the chest as this can project an attitude of authority or dominance over the patient. Placing the patient in a situation where they are made to feel inferior to the clinician may interfere with the overall progress of the history.

Facial expressions such as smiling and frowning are a well-used means of non-verbal communication. Nodding the head in agreement with a patient's statement will show understanding. Similarly, shaking the head in a negative fashion can acknowledge the patient's negative feelings when they reveal a situation that was difficult for them to handle.

Distractions from external sources will disrupt the progress of the case history. Closing the door to the examination room will keep distractions to a minimum, as well as maintaining privacy. Mobile (cell) phones and pagers should at least be placed on silent mode if they cannot be turned off.

Table 26.1 Summary of body gestures or non-verbal behaviours and their common interpretation

Body gesture/non-verbal behaviour	Interpretation
Tilted head	Interest
Looking down, face turned away	Disbelief
Biting nails	Insecurity, nervousness
Stroking chin	Trying to make a decision
Pinching bridge of nose, eye closed	Negative evaluation
Sitting with hands clasped behind head, legs crossed	Confidence, superiority
Touching face or scratching the nose, shifting in the seat, fidgeting with the hands	Lying
Tapping or drumming the fingers	Impatience
Crossed or folded arms, leaning back	Rejection

Verbal communication skills

The tone and level of the clinician's voice should be that used for any personal conversation. Raising the voice seems angry or authoritative, while whispering may interfere with the patient being able to hear the entire question.

One exception is the patient who is hearing impaired. Experience will help the young clinician handle this situation. While raising the volume would seem to be the obvious solution, it becomes difficult to maintain the required level of privacy. The clinician should sit directly in front of the patient if they lip-read. Ask the patient if it is necessary for the clinician to speak louder. If necessary, the questions can be written down so the patient can read them and respond in the most appropriate fashion.

Another circumstance that can be upsetting to a young clinician is when the patient is dysphasic. These patients have limited ability to speak. This most common occurs following a stroke or a cerebral lesion. Even though the patient may appear unresponsive, they can be completely aware of the conversation taking place around them. In cases like this, the questions should be structured to keep the length of response necessary to a minimum. Yes–no questions are best in this situation. If the patient is still unable to respond to the question verbally, the clinician can ask the patient questions and have them respond either in writing or by nodding yes or no.

As simple as it may sound, a very effective way to communicate is to listen to the patient. Do not attend to other matters while the patient is speaking. Sensitive listening is being present, not just physically but mentally and emotionally as well. Do not anticipate what the patient might say. Ask for clarification only when necessary.

Developing a rapport

Developing a rapport with the patient is a critical element of the examination. This will help the patient feel understood and supported by the clinician. It can also reduce any potential conflict between the clinician and the patient. Good rapport creates an environment that improves the efficiency of information gathering, explanation of findings, and planning for the remediation of the patient's visual complaints.

Developing good rapport begins with how the clinician is perceived by the patient. The clinician must exude confidence from the first moment they greet the patient. This can be especially hard for a new student or inexperienced clinician. Nothing will get a clinician–patient relationship off on the wrong foot faster than a practitioner who appears timid or insecure. The new clinician must greet their patient with the self-assurance and poise of a 10-year veteran. Of course, this only applies when one is meeting a new patient for the first time. If the patient has been seen on multiple occasions over an extended period, then a rapport will have already been established (presumably successfully, since the patient has chosen to return). The practitioner's appearance is also significant in getting the examination off to a good beginning. Depending on the specific culture, patient's have certain expectations of how their healthcare professionals should look. While one could make a valid argument that the important issue is the competence of the optometrist rather than their clothing, hairstyle or grooming, an unconventional appearance may make some patients feel less confident about divulging personal information to the practitioner.

The history is the time when the practitioner is getting to know the patient (as well as the patient getting to know the practitioner). A great deal of information will be exchanged. All information related by the patient to the clinician should be accepted in a non-judgemental manner. The patient's personal views and feelings should always be accepted as legitimate even when they are different from the clinician's. For example, there are times when a patient will relate information that causes them great concern, even though the clinician knows that the issue is insignificant. It is important to accept the patient's concerns as legitimate, and to retain one's composure until the patient can be educated about the issue. There are also situations when a patient may reveal information about themselves or their lifestyle that the clinician finds objectionable, such as drug use, or certain sexual practices. The clinician must accept the information in a non-judgemental manner, in order to understand the patient's history and solve the problem.

Expressing concern and support for the patient communicates empathy on the part of the clinician. Acknowledging appropriate self-care and coping efforts made by the patient convey a sense of understanding. This will foster the patient's sense that the clinician's purpose is to help solve the problem.

Often, the questions in the history will touch on issues that are embarrassing or disturbing to the patient. Delicate handling of these areas on the part of the clinician will help maintain the patient's level of trust and comfort as they answer the questions posed.

The patient's perspective

The clinician may find it helpful to incorporate the patient's perspective on their visual problem. This will help to determine the patient's ideas or concerns regarding the cause of the problem. To gain the patient's perspective, the clinician can ask questions that help determine the effect the problem has had on the patient's life. Questions should also be posed as to the patient's expectations regarding the solution to the problem.

Social and cultural issues

The world has become a blend of many diverse cultures, races, religions and ethnicities. Patients are increasingly asking their healthcare practitioners to incorporate solutions that address personal beliefs as well as evidence-based solutions for their visual problems. Patients who feel that their problem has not been listened to or understood are far more likely to be non-complaint with any proposed treatment or recommendations. Clinicians must listen to, and learn from, their patients in order to increase patient satisfaction and improve the effectiveness of treatment rendered.

Social and cultural practices also vary from group to group. Manner of dress varies and can be culturally significant. A simple gesture such as a handshake is a basic ritual

for some cultures but is not practised universally and may be inappropriate in some groups. Clinicians must be aware of the major cultural practices of different groups that use their healthcare facility.

The patient

Most optometrists find that a great deal of the satisfaction with their profession comes from talking to their patients. No two patients are alike. Each presents a special challenge and learning experience. One must strive to ensure that all patients are treated courteously and with respect at all times.

The talkative patient

The talkative patient presents a challenge to all clinicians, but especially those with less experience. These patients have long answers to even yes–no questions and will completely dominate the examination if allowed. Open-ended questions should be avoided. Verbal facilitations and open-ended questions serve to encourage the patient to continue talking. Many clinicians are afraid that it would be rude to interrupt the patient. Gentle, polite interruptions followed by direct questions will help to keep the history on track without insulting the patient.

The questioning patient

Questioning patients have a seemingly insatiable desire for information. They often feel that despite adequate explanations, their questions have not been answered. These patients must be handled in a firm, yet non-condescending manner. Information can be reiterated to ensure understanding or a direct question about the area that the patient still has concern about can be posed. The patient can be given printed material if this is available. A definite closing statement to end the session should be used. If necessary, the patient can be given an additional appointment for further evaluation and discussion, or referred to another provider for continuing care.

The demanding patient

The demanding patient makes unreasonable demands of everyone involved in their healthcare experience, including the clinician and other support staff. The patient may use intimidation and guilt to force others to care for them. Despite good care, the patient still views themselves as neglected. The patient may have outbursts of anger directed towards the clinician and others involved in their care because of their feelings of neglect. Reasoning with this type of patient is usually futile. Referral to another provider may be the best course of action, as an alternative practitioner may establish a more productive relationship with the patient.

The elderly patient

With increasing life expectancies (see Ch. 31), optometric practices are seeing a significant increase in elderly patients. Advancing age brings many new issues. The changes in the eyes and vision are a small but significant part of the overall picture. Many older individuals maintain busy and productive lives even though changes in self-image and bodily functions can provide a new source of stress for the patient.

The clinician should never assume that a patient's complaints are just 'normal for their age'. Signs and symptoms may be the indications of a disease process, not simply ageing. These patients should be approached like all others in a friendly, respectful manner. A patronizing or condescending tone should never be used.

Some elderly patients are unable to care for themselves. A family member or other attendant usually accompanies these patients to the examination. The clinician should use these individuals as additional sources of information regarding the patient's visual problems and other health issues.

Unfortunately, advancing age brings loss of a spouse or other loved one. Loss of significant persons in one's life may cause the patient to suffer from loneliness or depression. The clinician should be sensitive to situations where the patient may not be caring for themselves adequately. Although the optometrist is not qualified to handle a situation like this alone, help can be sought from a social worker or other medical practitioner.

The 'SOAP' format and the problem-oriented examination

The 'SOAP' format, standing for subjective, objective, assessment and plan, is a method of patient examination, record keeping and case analysis that was originally designed to streamline the patient encounter by making it more problem oriented (Barresi 1984). The purpose is to identify the patient's problem and find the means to satisfy it in as efficient a manner as possible. Without the problem-oriented approach, the optometric examination would comprise the same tests irrespective of the presenting complaint. However, in many cases this results in an excessive amount of information, much of which is not useful or necessary for solving the patient's problem.

The problem-oriented approach is not a means to cut corners. Although efficiency is important, the examination must be extended to identify problems of which the patient may be unaware. This is important with all patients but especially for those who are at high risk of ocular disease based on existing systemic conditions, family history, environment or exposure.

The subjective (S) component consists of the case history including the chief complaint, other ocular signs and symptoms, previous ocular history, personal and family medical history and visual history. This information is given to the clinician by the patient or their representative (e.g. parent, family member or guardian.). The information gathered can be used by the clinician to formulate a list of differential diagnoses for the patient's complaints. Diagnoses should be organized with the more likely or most common cause at the top of the list, with less prevalent conditions lower down the list.

The objective (O) component consists of all examination findings, observation of the patient by the clinician, and test results that may relate to history, that identify high-risk situations or are required by an institution (or licensing authority) for baseline data collection. Testing should be structured to eliminate differential diagnoses from the most to the least common. Basic testing will either confirm or eliminate common diagnoses as a cause. The more uncommon diagnoses often require more specific tests to identify or eliminate them as a cause.

The assessment (A) and plan (P) are linked together. The assessment brings all the subjective and objective information together into diagnoses and the plan spells out the recommended treatment for each item. The assessment is broken up further into three main subcategories, namely refractive error, binocular (including oculomotor) status, and ocular health. In a comprehensive examination, the clinician should document information in all three categories. When writing an assessment and plan for a follow-up visit, the clinician need only document information for the particular subcategory that the diagnoses apply to.

The plan outlines the recommended treatment, patient education and follow-up schedule. Like the assessment, the plan is also broken up into three subcategories: refractive error, binocular status and ocular health. Each item in the assessment should have a corresponding item in the plan that dictates what action is to be taken.

The first three areas build from one to the next. The case history (S) should help to drive what testing (O) will give the most information about items identified by the patient in the case history as areas of concern. The assessment and plan (A and P) should explain all of the concerns expressed by the patient in the case history as well as any other significant findings noted during the examination. When used properly, this method directs the clinician to the most informative testing, and therefore minimizes the steps required to reach an accurate final diagnosis.

Documentation using the SOAP format

When writing a patient's medical record using the SOAP method, the assessment and plan require additional consideration. The three subcategories used in the assessment and plan, i.e. refractive error, binocularity and ocular health, should be prioritized based on their importance to the overall understanding of the case and documented in that order. In most cases, the patient's chief complaint is addressed first and the subcategory in which it falls is given priority. For example, if the chief complaint is 'blurred vision at distance' and a small change in the patient's distance refractive correction is found, then when documenting the assessment and plan, the refractive error subcategory should be listed first. However, if during the same examination the clinician discovers that the patient has a sight-threatening condition such as glaucoma, then the ocular health category should be listed first, even if the patient is unaware of any symptoms from the condition.

The comprehensive case history

Many clinicians consider the case history to be the most important 'test' in the entire examination. One mark of a good clinician is the ability to take a good case history within an appropriate period of time. Questions should be structured to extract relevant clinical information. This will help to establish the differential diagnoses, or probable causes, for the patient's complaint. With experience, the young clinician will be able to differentiate between important aspects of the case history versus incidental areas.

The case history, in many instances, will set the tone for the examination. Each clinician will develop their own technique that is reflective of their personality. It is important that one makes a polite, professional first impression. When first greeting a patient, address them by their correct title, e.g. Mr, Mrs, Ms or Dr as appropriate. If the patient prefers to be addressed in another manner, they will indicate that and the clinician should oblige. Introduce yourself and any other persons who may be present during parts of the examination (e.g. observing students or ancillary staff). Consent must be obtained from the patient for these other individuals to observe the examination. Their role should be explained fully, and the patient should be informed that it is their right that these ancillary personnel be removed.

In the examination room, be sure that the patient can sit comfortably with the chair at a comfortable height and position for them. Find a place for the patient to deposit safely any materials (bags, coats, etc.) that they have brought with them. To ensure privacy while taking the case history, the examination room door should be closed.

In most cases, the case history will use the same basic format. The clinician will work from a standard group of questions, but some may be excluded while others will be expanded upon, depending on the patient's problem. It takes experience to be able to select the questions that will give the most information. Four parts should be included in every case history. They are the chief complaint, history of this presenting complaint, review of systems, and family and social history. These areas are common to the case histories taken in most medical disciplines.

Observation

Long before the first question of the formal case history, the experienced clinician will have already observed many things about the patient. A patient who walks to the examination room feeling along the wall may have a visual field defect. A constant head tilt may be indicative of a problem with the ocular muscles. The clinician at some point in the history should then explore other facial features noted by direct observation such as lid droop, eye turn, or redness in one or both eyes. If the patient is brought into the examination room by an assistant, and the clinician does not see the patient until they are already seated in the chair, they may miss the opportunity to observe this information.

Chief complaint

The chief complaint is a concise statement describing the symptoms, problem, condition, diagnosis or other factor that is the reason for the encounter. In other words, the chief complaint is the primary purpose of the visit.

To elicit the patient's chief complaint the clinician will generally use an open-ended question such as 'Are you having a problem with your eyes?' or 'What brings you in for an examination today?' Using open-ended questions allows the patient to express their concerns fully. The clinician should listen attentively without interrupting. Ask for clarification if the meaning of the patient's statement is not clear.

The chief complaint is usually documented using the patient's own words, and may be noted as a phrase or sentence. For example, the chief complaint may simply be noted as 'My right eye is red'. Tentative diagnoses or treatment plans that are based on the patient's chief complaint should not be included at this stage. For example, if the

patient complains of 'blurred distance vision', the chief complaint should be recorded using these terms rather than as myopia. Additional details are gathered in the history of presenting complaint (see below).

The patient may use a medical term or diagnosis in their statement of the chief complaint. The clinician should ask the patient to explain the term, as they understand it. Often the patient will use a term incorrectly. Understanding what the patient is trying to communicate may prevent any subsequent misunderstandings based on the patient's misuse of a medical term.

Other information that should be obtained and documented is the age, gender and race of the patient. This information is important to the case because many diagnoses are more prevalent within certain age ranges, genders, or racial backgrounds. This information can be obtained directly from meeting and speaking with the patient, or can be obtained from information provided by the patient before the beginning of the examination.

In a more racially blended world, racial background has become more difficult to obtain without making a specific inquiry to the patient. Some clinicians ask the patient what race they consider themselves or ask the background of their parents. As this can be a sensitive topic, questions must be asked carefully. The topic of collecting racial and ethnic information is controversial, and differing opinions have been expressed regarding its validity (e.g. Werner 1997; Bhopal & Donaldson 1998; Leroi 2005).

History of the presenting complaint

History of the presenting complaint (HPC) is a chronological description of the development of the patient's present condition from the first sign and/or symptom, or from the previous encounter to the current visit. The HPC seeks to discover the what, where, when and maybe even the why of the chief complaint. The questioning becomes more direct to gather specific information. It may include the following elements:

- location
- quality
- severity
- duration
- onset
- frequency
- provocative factors
- modifying factors
- associated signs and symptoms.

Location, quality and severity deal with the more geographic and tangible portion of the patient's chief complaint. Location may be as simple as right or left eye. A lesion may be ocular, orbital, cranial, or facial. For refractive complaints such as blurred vision, note whether it is present at distance, near or both. In other situations, when the problem arises from systemic- or disease-based causes, larger areas of the face, head or body may be involved. Specific information about the location of other areas that are affected should be recorded in the patient's record.

Quality seeks to understand the patient's experience. This is best assessed by asking them to describe the problem in their own words. For example, if the patient complains of a headache, the clinician should ask about the type of pain experienced. Words such as dull, achy, stabbing or throbbing can be used to describe the headache. In refractive cases, 'can't read the fine print' or 'can't see the street signs' may be the appropriate response.

Severity looks for the patient to describe the intensity of the event. The patient may also describe severity in terms of the degree of interference with visual tasks or even its effect on activities of daily living. One of the most common ways to accomplish this is by the use of a scale. For example, if the patient complains of pain, use a scale from 1 to 10, with 1 being mild and 10 being the worst pain ever felt. The same scale can be applied to other conditions, such as a complaint of ocular redness.

Duration, onset, and frequency are based on the timing and recurrences of the event. The clinician asks questions to determine when the problem started (onset) and how long it lasts (duration). The patient may describe the onset of the problem as sudden, gradual, or intermittent. Temporal terms such as daily, hourly, or constant can be used to describe the duration. The clinician may also use descriptions such as acute, chronic or recurrent. Frequency indicates how often the event occurs. The patient might report having headaches daily for the past 2 weeks. In addition, the frequency may be associated with work, exercise, body rhythms, cycles, or seasons. In some cases, patterns will emerge, such as a patient who suffers headaches at the end of the work day. This frequency pattern may identify the underlying cause of the condition.

The purpose of questions about provocative and modifying factors as well as associated signs and symptoms is to determine whether any other issues are associated with the event. Provocative factors are potential triggers that might cause the event. A provocative factor may be associated with an activity such as computer use, or a sustained near-vision task. It may also be related to the patient's diet. For example, diabetics with poorly controlled blood glucose levels may experience fluctuations in the clarity of their vision. Modifying factors may cause the patient's symptoms to increase or decrease. The patient who experiences eyestrain after sustained near work may say that if they take a break every 30 minutes they can avoid the eyestrain.

When asking about the HPC, one must also question the patient regarding the progression of the condition. Does the patient feel that the problem is getting worse, better, or remaining the same? For a chronic problem, ask if the patient has sought professional advice previously. In these cases, questions about any previous treatments (and the level of success achieved) are valuable.

Visual history

The optometric history should also be expanded to encompass questions about other aspects of the patient's visual system. This will improve the clinician's overall understanding of the patient's vision and any special visual needs. Some of these areas may have been evaluated in the chief complaint and therefore do not have to be repeated. Any areas that evoke a positive response should be evaluated using the same type of questions adopted in the history of presenting complaint (i.e. location, severity, frequency, etc.). While these issues might not have been the primary reason for the visit, they should still be evaluated and treated appropriately.

The most obvious area for an optometrist to explore is the clarity of vision. The clinician should inquire about clarity at different distances, and the patient's use of their current correction (if any). More than one inexperienced clinician has spent time asking about the patient's blurry vision only to find out later that they only experience blur when they are not wearing their glasses!

If the patient wears contact lenses, the clinician should inquire about the wearing schedule and disinfecting methods used as well as the date of the last aftercare visit. The wearing schedule includes not only the number of hours that the lenses are worn per day but also the replacement regimen in the case of disposable lenses. Is the patient replacing the lenses as directed? Any identifying information about the brand and parameters of the contact lenses such as base curve, power and diameter should be confirmed either from the prescription or by collecting the information from the supply of lenses that the patient already has in their possession.

Headaches, eyestrain, and asthenopia are common occurrences often associated with prolonged computer use or other sustained near visual tasks. They are so common that many patients feel that these symptoms are just part of daily living, and therefore they do not report them until prompted by a clinician's inquiry.

Flashes and floaters are other frequently reported visual phenomena. Since they can be either benign or a sign of a serious ocular condition, several follow-up questions should be asked. Questions that elicit the onset, timing, location and frequency of the flashes and floaters should be raised. If the patient experiences both flashes and floaters, the chronologic development of the symptoms can be especially important.

The patient should always be questioned about the presence of diplopia or double vision. When asking about diplopia the clinician should use the lay term – double vision – rather than the clinical term. It is useful to clarify whether the patient is actually seeing two separate and distinct images of the same thing or if they are seeing one blurry image. The patient may report that the double vision goes away when one eye is covered. This indicates that the diplopia is the result of a binocular problem. In rarer cases, the patient may report that the diplopia is present even when only one eye is open. Here, the clinician will look to refractive or ocular media issues as the cause. It may also be useful to ascertain whether the double vision occurs with or without the proper refractive correction in place. On occasion, use of a properly centred, accurate refractive correction will eliminate the diplopia.

If the patient reports true diplopia, additional questions should be asked to clarify all aspects. These should include where it occurs (distance, near or both) and whether it is horizontal, vertical or oblique. The clinician should also ask the patient if they have found a way to relieve the problem. Sometimes, patients will report that closing one eye, altering their head position, avoiding looking in a particular direction of gaze or stopping the particular task being performed will relieve the problem.

Tearing, burning, itching, and redness are general symptoms that can occur in a variety of conditions. The presence of any or all of the symptoms should be thoroughly explored, especially noting the onset, duration and frequency. Associated signs and symptoms will help to determine the underlying cause. For example, red, itchy, watery eyes are common when the patient is experiencing an ocular allergic reaction to an environmental allergen such as pollen or ragweed.

Ocular history: patient and family

The patient's ocular history should also be explored during the initial visit. After the first recording of this information in the patient's record, simple follow-up questions can be asked at subsequent visits to determine whether significant changes have occurred.

The patient should be asked about a history of ocular trauma. This should include trauma to or around the eye and adnexa. For each reported incident, the clinician should inquire about any treatment or visual sequelae resulting from the trauma.

The history of strabismus or amblyopia should be documented both for the patient and their immediate family. Patients often use different terms for these two visual problems. Strabismus is more commonly called an eye turn, crossed eye or squint (while the latter term is used to refer to both strabismus and partial closing of the eyelids in the United Kingdom, in the United States its meaning is generally restricted to partial eyelid closing), while amblyopia is more commonly referred to as a lazy eye. Some patients may even use these terms interchangeably. There is also a tendency for patients who have poorer uncorrected vision in one eye compared with the fellow eye to describe the eye with the poorer vision as a lazy eye. Follow-up questions should be asked to ensure that what the patient means is clearly understood by the clinician.

Any personal or family history of eye disease such as glaucoma or macular pathology must be noted. Frequently, patients are unaware of the actual cause of a family member's vision impairment, so including a general question about any family members who are blind or visually impaired may give some useful information.

General visual demands

Visual demands for each patient should be explored. Inquiry should be made as to both vocational and avocational vision requirements. Some occupations have specific visual requirements, and therefore may need a customized ophthalmic correction. For example, police officers, train drivers or military personnel may have very specific regulations regarding the type and form of correction required. The optometrist should be sure to determine the specific requirements in the area where the patient works. Other occupations may also require individualized refractive corrections, such as a lathe operator or an individual who spends the greater part of the day viewing a computer monitor. Many patients have hobbies or other interests outside of their employment that require specific visual requirements (e.g. playing a musical instrument, sewing, DIY activities).

Patients who play racquetball, squash or other contact sports must be advised of the need for protective eyewear (see Ch. 29).

Medical history/review of systems

The review of systems (ROS) is an inventory of the body systems obtained through a series of questions that identify medical problems that the patient may be experiencing currently or has experienced in the past. Obtaining this information is important because many systemic diseases have ocular manifestations (see Ch. 10). Additionally, some medications used in the treatment of systemic disease can have side effects that involve the visual system (see Ch. 9). A thorough ROS should be obtained during the patient's first visit. This can be accomplished verbally or through use of a questionnaire. On subsequent visits, the clinician can use the initial ROS as a guide, and question the patient as to any changes that have occurred since the last visit.

A full ROS is usually conducted from the head down. The following systems are recognized:

- constitutional symptoms (see below)
- eyes
- ear, nose and throat
- cardiovascular
- respiratory
- gastrointestinal
- genitourinary
- musculoskeletal
- integument (including the skin and breast)
- neurological
- psychiatric
- endocrine
- haematological/lymphatic
- allergic/immunologic

The ROS as part of the case history in an optometric examination differs from that conducted by a general physician. The optometrist is concerned about any diagnosed disease or problem in one of the systems, but not with specific symptoms that the patient may experience. The relevance of the ROS in the optometric examination is to develop a 'big picture' of the patient's general health. No ROS would be complete without asking the patient the date of their last medical examination. This can recorded as the month and year of the examination, as the actual date is not usually critical. This also provides an indication as to how regularly the patient receives medical care. In cases where a significant amount of time has elapsed since the last medical examination, the optometrist may want to make that one of the recommendations to the patient at the end of the examination.

Constitutional symptoms concern how the patient is feeling overall. Questions may include general well-being, any recent fever or significant changes in weight. Since these questions are more relevant for a visit to a general physician, most optometrists do not routinely ask questions in this area. A general inquiry may be made as a matter of polite conversation at the beginning of the history. For example, once the patient has entered the examination room the clinician may ask, 'How are you today, Mr Jones? Are you feeling well?' or more specifically, 'How is your general health'. As the patient's response is considered, the clinician should be aware that if the patient is truly unwell and their ocular problem is not urgent, it might be better to reschedule the eye examination for a later date.

The eye/visual system is one of the elements of a full ROS. As one might surmise, optometrists will take a very thorough eye history, and therefore this item can be skipped from this section.

Many systemic diseases can have side effects on the visual system. Two of the most common systemic diseases with ocular side effects are hypertension and diabetes. Both can cause changes within the retina that may affect the patient's vision. Ear, nose and throat history should be a general inquiry. Patients who have sinus problems may have accompanying ocular symptoms such as pain or pressure around the eyes. There should be a basic inquiry as to the presence of any systemic issues relating to the remaining systems.

Allergies

Allergies require careful documentation. The patient should be questioned specifically about allergies to medications, as well as to foods and environmental factors. Thorough documentation should include the types of reactions (e.g. rashes, itching and anaphylaxis) that the patient suffers if they are exposed to a specific allergen.

Medications

The patient should be asked what medications they are taking. In some instances, a patient may report taking a medication but not state that they actually have a disease. This usually occurs when the patient suffers from a chronic condition. Patients sometimes feel that taking the medication eradicates the disease. For example, a patient taking antihypertensive medication may report that they have normal blood pressure.

The dosage of the medication is less important than the fact that the patient takes the drug. Any medications that the patient takes, for any reason, may contraindicate the use of other therapy as part of the treatment plan determined later in the examination.

Personal, family and social history

The personal, family and social history consists of a review of these three areas. A review of the patient's personal history should include questions about their occupational history and previous environmental experiences. The purpose here is to discover any exposure to disease-producing substances or environmental conditions.

Family history provides information about the general health of the patient's immediate family members, whether living and dead. Questions should relate to inherited conditions, such as glaucoma, hypertension or diabetes.

Social history is an age-appropriate review of past and current activities. In the case of a child, questions may include schooling, normal development and immunizations. For an adult, questions may include an educational history, use of alcohol, tobacco products or so-called recreational or 'street' drugs. Care must be taken to ask these questions in a non-judgemental fashion. A sexual history may be included when appropriate. Questions might include exposure of the patient to a partner with a sexually transmitted disease as many of these diseases have ocular manifestations.

Follow-up visits

If the patient has returned for follow-up of a previously diagnosed condition, the questioning process need not be as involved as for the initial visit. The questions should be structured around any changes in symptoms, compliance with recommended treatment, and any new developments since the last visit. If the disease is chronic in nature, questions should focus on the progression or stability of the disease.

Emergency visits

If a patient's initial visit is an emergency, the case history should be altered to focus on the immediate problem. A complete history of the presenting complaint should be documented as well as a full ROS. This information is necessary in the event that medication is required for treatment of the patient's problem. Other questions can be eliminated as the clinician sees fit in order to obtain the details of the acute problem rapidly. The remainder of the history can be obtained from the patient on subsequent visits.

Paediatric case history

While the actual eye examination for a child is somewhat different from that of the adult, the case history follows the adult format. There is one important difference, however. Since a child is generally unable to answer many of the questions, the clinician will refer to the parent or guardian for input. The clinician should include the child in as many questions as possible, especially regarding the chief complaint. Of course, the language used must be appropriate for the age of the child. The paediatric case history is discussed further in Chapter 28.

A final tip

Any positive responses should be explored thoroughly. Pertinent positive responses are those which have an impact on the differential diagnosis. A pertinent negative response is the lack of a symptom or finding that also has an impact on the differential diagnoses or overall assessment of the case. Therefore, the lack of a symptom for a particular differential diagnosis may require further explanation. When recording a history, one must document any positive responses as well pertinent negative responses. From a medicolegal standpoint, one might argue that all negative responses should also be recorded. It is generally accepted that the absence of any recording in a record implies that the question was not asked.

Summarizing the case history

At the end of the case history, the clinician usually summarizes what has been learned from the patient, thereby communicating their understanding of what the patient has said. This gives the clinician a chance to develop differential diagnoses. It also helps to structure the examination by allowing the clinician to select tests that will be most effective in identifying the underlying cause of the patient's problem.

The patient also benefits from a summary of the case history. They are then sure that the practitioner heard what they said. It also gives them an opportunity to correct any errors. The patient can also raise any additional concerns or issues that have not yet been discussed. Perhaps the greatest benefit is that a collaborative relationship is being built between the patient and clinician as they begin to solve the patient's problem.

Beginning a case summary is quite simple. Some phrases to use are 'Let's recap . . .' or 'Let me make sure that I understand this . . .'. Then the clinician should rephrase the chief complaint and the pertinent positive and negative responses of the case history. Make the patient aware that they can interrupt at any time to make any corrections they feel are necessary. The practitioner can also chose to read back a list of the important details of the history, checking with the patient as they go by including statements such as 'Is that right?' or 'Have I got that right?'.

In summary

Although the material described above may seem to be a scripted task, it is important for the clinician to realize that every history is dynamic and must be tailored to the individual case. There is no limit to the questions that can be asked. Experienced clinicians are aware that although the formal case history may be over, certain groups of findings or statements made by the patient may require additional history questions to be asked, even as the examination continues. Experience teaches that a case history never ends until the patient leaves the examination room. In fact, patients have been known to reveal pertinent information only after they have stood up to leave the room at the end of the examination, thereby necessitating additional discussion and testing!

Case disposition

While the case history is primarily for the optometrist, the case disposition is primarily for the patient. This is the time that the clinician will give the patient information and explain the results of the examination. It is also the time when potential treatments are discussed. This should be an interactive session, not one dominated by the clinician.

The clinician should consider many things as they are presenting the case to the patient. The amount and type of information given to the patient can be difficult to gauge. Lay terms should generally be used. If a medical term is introduced, it should always be followed by a thorough explanation.

The patient's prior knowledge should be assessed early in the case disposition. This sets the starting point for the clinician and can help to establish the quantity of information that the patient wishes to receive. The clinician can elect to ask the patient directly how much information they would like. Some patients prefer an overview while others want a full explanation of the cause of their problem. A good case disposition should neither restrict nor overload the patient with information.

The information should be delivered in parts or discrete sections, not all at once. The sections should be presented in a logical sequence. The clinician should repeat and summarize the information presented to the patient in order to reinforce it. After the delivery of discrete pieces of information, the clinician should stop and ask the patient if they understand the details presented up to that point. The clinician should review all of the items in the history that were of concern to the patient, and be prepared to discuss each one. Models, diagrams and written materials can be used, if available, to aid in understanding.

The discussion should include pertinent positive and negative test results. Any relationship between findings should also be covered. The information should be presented in a general form. For example, if the patient complained of blurred distance vision, the finding should not be reported to the patient as 6/18 unless it is followed by an explanation of what that means, for example, 'Mrs Jones, you stated earlier that your felt your distance vision was blurry. We found today that your distance vision is 6/18, which means that you see at 6 metres what a person with normal vision would be able to see at 18 metres.'

Treatment options should be presented to the patient. A discussion of the risks and benefits associated with each type of treatment is advisable. The clinician and patient should decide together what course of action is best for the individual case. A discussion of the patient's role in the treatment should take place. This should include how and when to use any glasses prescribed as well the dosage of any prescribed medications.

The patient should be aware of what is to be expected from the treatment. This discussion can be wide ranging. The most common topic of discussion is the adaptation to new glasses. Side effects and potential adverse reactions should be covered if the treatment plan includes medications.

In the case disposition, the optometrist must explain the diagnosis to the patient, relate it to the patient's symptoms (or lack of symptoms), and discuss treatment plans and prognosis. All of these must be clearly understood by the patient. If glasses are to be prescribed, the patient must know when they are to be worn (e.g. all day or only for specific tasks), their role, limitations and potential prescription changes. The young myope should understand that the myopia might increase as the patient matures. The presbyope should know that the need for stronger prescriptions is influenced not by the new glasses but rather a physiological change over time, as well as of the potential difficulties when receiving progressive or bifocal lenses for the first time.

Occasionally, a patient may elect to decline treatment. It can be as simple as declining a change in prescription or electing not to take medications. Refusal of care is within the patient's rights. They must, however, be counselled as to the outcome of the condition if it goes untreated. It must also be clear that they understand what they have been told. These situations require detailed documentation including a synopsis of the information that was given to the patient. Be careful to document that the patient verbally acknowledged that this information was understood, or perhaps have the patient sign a written statement indicating that they chose to decline the recommended therapy.

In the case disposition, the optometrist must be careful not to promise more than can be delivered. Symptoms that may be the result of multiple causative factors do not usually disappear if only one potential cause is eliminated. As a final check at the end of the case disposition, the patient should be asked if they have any questions and if all their concerns were addressed.

No case disposition is complete without a discussion of when the patient should return for re-examination. A good practice management technique is to have the patient make the follow-up appointment before they leave the practice. Alternatively, a reminder card can be written out, to be posted nearer the time of the appointment. The clinician should also address what the patient should do if a problem arises before the next scheduled appointment, and how they can be contacted.

Patient involvement in the care process

With the explosion of information available through the internet and other media outlets, many patients today are well informed regarding the treatments available to them. Allowing the patient to be involved in the decision-making process will increase their commitment to the final treatment plan.

Patients are not limited to being involved only in the decision-making process. Before this stage is reached, the clinician should involve the patient in the examination in several ways. Explaining the rationale for those parts of the examination that might seem to be unrelated to the primary reason for the visit will make the patient feel that they are receiving a personal and careful evaluation.

Another way of involving the patient in the decision-making process is for practitioners to share their thoughts as decisions about the treatment plan or course of action are made, and even the dilemmas as plans are formulated. Choices should be offered in the treatment plan whenever possible. The clinician should present these as suggestions rather than directives. Each proposal should be accompanied by enough education so that the patient can make an informed choice. With this method, the final plan for a case is made through discussion.

Breaking bad news

At some point, most clinicians will diagnose a patient with a disease that will cause them to lose some or all of their sight. They will face the difficult task of breaking this bad news to the patient. Good communication and rapport are vital parts of this task. External distractions should be controlled as much as possible. The practitioner should be sitting down for this discussion, thereby putting the patient in a less defensive position. There should be enough time set aside so that the clinician and patient will be undisturbed. The clinician should organize his or her thoughts, and prepare what will be said ahead of time, anticipating the questions the patient may ask, and being prepared to answer them. During the discussion, the clinician should find out what the patient knows about the disease and try to estimate how much they want to know at that time. The clinician should continue to assess the patient's understanding of the information being presented to them.

Communication with other professionals

Clinicians, who are skilled at presenting a case in lay terms to a patient, must be equally skilled at presenting a case to another optometrist or healthcare professional. One must also consider that there are privacy laws to protect the healthcare information of an individual, so no information may be released without express permission from the patient. This applies whether the communication is verbal or in written form.

Optometrists may also receive referrals from other healthcare providers for patients who have either poor vision or a systemic disease with known ocular manifestations such as diabetes. When the visit is complete, the optometrist should send a letter back to the referring physician listing the pertinent examination findings, diagnosis, and treatment plan where appropriate.

When a systemic disease evaluation is necessary or a more specialized evaluation of an ocular or systemic condition is required, optometrists refer the patient to another healthcare professional. In any of these situations, a letter should accompany the patient indicating the reason for the referral, pertinent findings and possible diagnoses.

Conclusion

Effective communication with a patient is a crucial requirement for success in optometric care. Good communication skills are a building block in a good optometrist–patient relationship and will improve the patient's compliance with the recommended advice or treatment plan. It may require significant effort on the part of the clinician. Although each patient is a new and challenging experience, gaining practice over time will help a new practitioner to develop this critical skill.

References

Barresi B J 1984 Problem orientation. In: Barresi B J (ed.) Ocular Assessment. The manual of diagnosis for office practice. Butterworths, Boston, pp 3–10

Bhopal R, Donaldson L 1998 White, European, Western, Caucasian or what? Inappropriate labelling in research on race, ethnicity and health. American Journal of Public Health 88:1303–1307

Leroi A M 2005 A family tree in every gene. New York Times op-ed article. 14 March

Werner D L 1997 'A 43-year-old black male...': conventional wisdom, racism or noise? Journal of the American Optometric Association 68:681–684

Bibliography

Argyle M 1990 Bodily communication, 2nd edn. International Universities Press, Madison, CT.

Ball G V 1982 Symptoms in eye examination. Butterworths, London

Elliott D B 1997 The problem-oriented examination's case history. In: Zadnik K (ed.) The ocular examination. Measurements and findings. W B Saunders, Philadelphia, pp 2–18

Fletcher S W 1996 Clinical decision making: approach to the patient. In: Claude Bennett J, Plum F (eds) Cecil textbook of medicine, 20th edn. W B Saunders, Philadelphia, pp 72–75

Grosvenor T 2002 Primary care optometry. Butterworth Heinemann, Boston, pp 115–130

Ledford J K 1999 The Complete Guide to Ocular History Taking. Slack, Thorofare, NJ

Michaels D D 1985 Visual optics and refraction: a clinical approach, 3rd edn. C V Mosby, St. Louis

Swartz M H 2002. Textbook of physical diagnosis: history and examination, 4th edn. W B Saunders, Philadelphia, pp 3–78

CHAPTER 27

Legal aspects of optometry in the United Kingdom

Susan Blakeney

Introduction

This chapter describes legal aspects of optometry as practised in the United Kingdom. It covers the principles of professional service delivery, including the legal framework governing optometry in the UK, complaints procedures, and an outline of the 'Fitness to Practise' procedures of the General Optical Council (GOC).

There are several bodies in UK optometry and optics: the GOC regulates the professions of optometry and dispensing optics; the College of Optometrists is the professional body for optometry; the Association of Optometrists (AOP) is the representative body for optometrists; the Association of British Dispensing Opticians (ABDO) is the professional and representative body for dispensing opticians; and the Federation of Ophthalmic and Dispensing Opticians (FODO) represents the larger optical companies. The AOP, ABDO and FODO provide professional indemnity cover for their members.

The GOC (www.optical.org) produces Codes of Conduct for business and individual registrants (www.optical.org/en/our_work/Standards/Standards_in_conduct. cfm). The College of Optometrists and the ABDO produce guidance for their members which includes how to interpret this Code of Conduct in various situations. If an optometrist (or dispensing optician) appears before a fitness to practise hearing, often part of the evidence that would be considered would be the guidance of the appropriate professional body.

The principles of ethics in this chapter will be largely drawn from guidance issued by the College of Optometrists.

The College of Optometrists

The College is the professional, scientific, and examining body for optometry in the UK and was established in 1980 as the successor body to the British Optical Association and the Scottish Association of Opticians. The College also incorporates the examining function of the Worshipful Company of Spectacle Makers (SMC) for optometrists. Although the SMC (www.spectaclemakers.com) exists today, it no longer examines optometrists or dispensing opticians. The College is a registered charity and was granted a Royal Charter in 1995. It has four objectives. These are: the improvement and conservation of human vision; the advancement for the public benefit of the study of and research into optometry and related subjects and the publication of the results thereof; the promotion and improvement for the public benefit of the science and practice of optometry; and the maintenance for the public benefit of the highest possible standards of professional competence and conduct. Further detail about the history of the College can be found on the College's website (www.college-optometrists.org/index. aspx/pcms/site.college.history.history_home/).

The College of Optometrists publishes a Code of Ethics and Guidelines for Professional Conduct. This is freely available on the public section of the website (www.college-optometrists.org/index.aspx/pcms/site.publication.Ethics_Guidelines. Ethics_Guidelines_home/) and sets the standards of good practice by which members agree to abide. The Guidelines are regularly reviewed and updated to reflect the changing nature of optometric practice in the UK.

All members agree to abide by the Code of Ethics and Guidelines for Professional Conduct ('The Guidance') that is issued by the College. The Code of Ethics gives members guidance on, inter alia, professional integrity, inter- and intra-professional relationships, the patient–practitioner relationship and patient–practitioner communication.

Association of Optometrists

Formerly the Association of Optical Practitioners and founded in 1946, the Association of Optometrists (AOP), as the representative body for optometrists, provides advice to its members. The AOP advice is not direct guidance on professional conduct, but includes topics such as employment issues and vocational matters, e.g. the visual standards required for various occupations. The AOP also offers advice on areas that are covered by the College guidance, such as record keeping. Although it may seem duplicatory, both bodies provide recommendations on record keeping, as it both directly affects patient care and may have legal implications for the optometrist if done improperly. Further information can be found at www.aop.org.uk

Federation of Ophthalmic and Dispensing Opticians

The Federation of Ophthalmic and Dispensing Opticians (FODO) is the representative body for the corporate bodies in optics. Its members include the larger companies providing optical services. FODO offers information and guidance to its members including a (voluntary) Code of Practice for Domiciliary Eyecare. Further information can be found at www.fodo.com

General Optical Council

The General Optical Council (GOC) regulates optometrists and dispensing opticians. The function of the Council is to promote high standards of professional education, conduct, and performance amongst registrants. The GOC has seven main committees, which are listed in part 1 of the Opticians Act 1989.

The GOC maintains the registers of optometrists, dispensing opticians, and bodies corporate, as defined by the 1989 Act. Extensive amendments were made to the Opticians Act in 2005 (see later) and since these amendments the GOC also regulates student optometrists and student dispensing opticians. Further information can be found at www.optical.org.

Principles of professional service delivery

Difference between a profession and a trade

The first guideline from the Code of Ethics published by the College is that 'The optometrist has a duty to place the welfare of his/her patients before all other considerations, to apply to each patient the full extent of his/her knowledge and skill, and to maintain and develop his/her professional competence throughout his/her professional life.' This differentiates between a profession and a trade. A tradesman may be very skilled and act with the greatest integrity, but he /she does not necessarily put his/her clients before all other considerations.

The fact that optometrists put their patients first does not, of course, preclude them from charging for their services, but it means that the optometrist should direct the patient to appropriate care if the patient is unable or unwilling to pay for the optometrist's services. Optometrists in the UK are not funded as an emergency service and as such do not tend to provide out-of-hours care, although the long opening hours of some practices – for example those sited in shopping centres – may mean that they are often the first port of call for patients suffering from acute eye problems.

Status of College Guidelines

One question that often arises at the College is whether the Guidance can be more specific to account for individual circumstances in practice. College Guidance is meant as a framework to help optometrists exercise their professional judgement, and is not a set of 'rules' or 'tick boxes'. The Guidance indicates the factors that the optometrist should (or, if there is a legal requirement, must) consider. The optometrist can then decide how to apply these principles to the particular case being considered. As mentioned above, the GOC will often consider College Guidelines as evidence of the benchmark of reasonable practice, should this be questioned.

College Guidance is regularly reviewed to ensure it is as up to date as possible and the most recent version is always available on the College website.

Commercial pressures

Intra-professional referrals

Most optometrists spend at least part of their working week in commercial community settings. These are often in a high street or commercial location. National Health Service (NHS) sight tests are provided under the General Ophthalmic Services (GOS). Over time, the GOS sight test fee has failed to keep pace with inflation (although Scotland now has a different fee structure from the rest of the UK, with higher fees being paid for the eye examination). This, coupled with the increasing (and expensive) technology that is available to optometrists for use during the eye examination, has lead to the GOS sight test being subsidized significantly by the sale of optical appliances, although this is less so in Scotland. Even with the privatization of the sight test in the late 1980s, competition kept private eye examination fees low, and the cross-subsidy of the clinical/eye examination by the retail side of the optometrist/dispensing optician's work continued. This has several knock-on effects, one of which is the professional reluctance for one optometrist to refer a patient to another, particularly one working in a similar commercial environment because they fear 'losing' the patient – particularly the more lucrative dispensing – to their colleague. Unlike General Medical Practitioners' (GMP) patients, optometric patients in the UK do not register with optometric practices in order to have an eye examination or GOS sight test – they simply present themselves at the practice of their choice. The fear therefore is that if an optometrist refers a patient to a colleague – even though the colleague may be more expert in the particular area required – they will 'lose' the patient's business to them. The originating optometrist may prefer that the patient is seen by a general medical practitioner, rather than another optometrist.

This may be exacerbated by local NHS co-management schemes in which patients who are referred (often via their GMP) may be redirected by the NHS, via a referral centre or other mechanism, to an optometrist with a special interest (OPwSI). The OPwSI will have undergone some additional training to enable them to triage referrals from their colleagues and deal with patients who can be appropriately managed within primary care. The advantage to the NHS of these schemes is that it may be more cost-effective, and is often more convenient for the patient, if they can be seen in a practice setting rather than having to travel to hospital. The disadvantage is that local optometrists may resent colleagues seeing 'their' patients, thereby leading to distrust and poor support for such a scheme. Any such scheme should ensure that the recruitment of the OPwSIs is transparent and open to all, and has a clear-cut protocol for the OPwSIs seeing the patients who are referred to them. This should include guidance so that the OPwSI directs the patient back to the originating optometrist for their ongoing routine care.

Similar considerations apply for optometrists providing co-managed services, such as screening for sight-threatening diabetic retinopathy. The College has guidance on these issues in College guidance paragraph 04.05 which states that:

'It is recognised that there are circumstances when a patient is directed to a named optometrist for a specific aspect of their eye care, for example in co-management schemes or when second opinions are arranged within the profession. In all cases practitioners participating in such schemes or accepting referrals from colleagues should make it clear to these patients that they should return to their usual eye care practice for routine eye examination and/or dispensing of optical appliances unless the patient expresses a wish not to do so.'

Such concerns about patients being tempted to go elsewhere can be allayed by having the OPwSI service provided in a location other than a commercial practice. The location could be a physician's surgery, community hospital, etcetera. However, one disadvantage of this arrangement is that the location must be equipped adequately. Another disadvantage over an optometric practice is that the OPwSI may be attending the clinic location only at specific times, whereas if the patients are seen in their own practice, they will be able to fit the OPwSI patients into the practice timetable. For these reasons it may not be practicable to run a part-time OPwSI service in a location other than community optometric practice.

Repeat clinical tests

If, during the eye examination, the optometrist finds an anomaly, there are two options: the optometrist may refer the patient, or they may decide to manage the patient within the practice by asking the patient to return for additional, or repeat diagnostic tests, such as visual field tests. Some areas have NHS schemes to enable optometrists to be paid for repeating diagnostic tests such as visual fields and/or intraocular pressure measurements, but at the time of writing these are far from universal. The exception is in Scotland where, since 2006, there is NHS funding for a supplementary examination when required. Without such schemes, the optometrist must decide whether to repeat these tests at no charge to the patient, or to ask the patient to pay for the tests being repeated. The underfunding of the clinical aspect of the service means that the optometrist may feel pressured into referring patients rather than managing them within the practice. Further, if the optometrist does refer, the patient may be seen by an OPwSI colleague who is funded by the NHS to perform the repeat or additional tests. For the reasons discussed above, the referring optometrist may feel uncomfortable referring the patient to be seen by a colleague in another optometric practice and can be faced with a difficult choice.

Separation of prescribing and supply of spectacles

An additional side effect of the cross-subsidy that can lead to ethical considerations occurs when patients decide to have the eye examination and dispensing of spectacles carried out in separate locations. If both activities were funded equitably, this would not be a problem, but because dispensing is considerably more profitable than the eye examination, the optometrist whose patient decides to purchase their spectacles elsewhere is in a difficult position. College guidance states that optometrists are responsible for a prescription that they issue. If the patient returns to the prescriber after spectacles have been dispensed elsewhere, the prescriber should first ask the patient whether they have returned to the dispenser to ensure the spectacles were made up as prescribed. If the spectacles were correctly made up, the prescribing optometrist then has to decide whether to re-examine the patient to see if there is a prescription error, or whether the patient is simply failing to tolerate the type of lens dispensed.

The prescriber also has a responsibility to make a recommendation to the patient as to the most suitable form of optical appliance for their needs. The author has designed her prescription forms to include a 'tick box' list of types of lenses (single-vision distance, single-vision intermediate, single-vision near, bifocals or progressive addition lenses) that are being recommended. The list is concluded with a statement stating that should the patient decide to have a different type of lens, they are strongly advised to contact the prescriber before doing so. Patients often do not realize that a single type of lens may be particularly suitable for them. The prescriber may have a very good reason for suggesting that the patient is most suited for a particular form of lens (such as single-vision reading spectacles rather than progressive addition lenses). If the dispensing is performed at the practice where the patient had their eyes examined, a dialogue can occur between the prescriber and the dispensing optician as to the most suitable type of lens for that patient. The prescriber may modify their original recommendation in the light of this discussion. However, if the patient decides to have their spectacles dispensed elsewhere this may not be possible. By specifying the type of optical appliance, one can prevent instances such as the first-time presbyopic emmetropic patient, for whom single-vision reading spectacles have been prescribed, receiving progressive addition lenses which are not tolerated because they are not suitable for their needs.

Alternatively, if a patient brings in an outside prescription to an optometrist ('the dispenser') to have made up and subsequently develops difficulties, the dispenser should first ensure that the spectacles are made up as prescribed. If they are made up correctly, the dispenser should resist the temptation to examine the patient's eyes themselves, but rather contact the prescriber to agree a course of action (College guidance 04.04). The reasoning here is that only the prescriber knows why a particular prescription was issued. For example, the patient may have been deliberately over- or undercorrected for a clinical reason that will not be apparent to the dispenser.

The College advises that, although it is the patient's right to have their spectacles made up wherever they choose, '*it is often more difficult to resolve any problems you may have with your spectacles when prescribing and supply are separated*' (www.college-optometrists.org).

Working for lay employers

Optometrists are bound by their legal and professional obligations regardless of their employment status. Lay employers are not bound by the same codes of conduct, and this may cause tension if the optometrist feels unable to fulfil their obligations to the patient. The principle that the optometrist should put their patients first may mean them having no alternative but to seek alternative employment, even though that may be a difficult decision to make.

General Ophthalmic Services

New General Ophthalmic Services (GOS) regulations came into force in England on 1 August 2008 (Statutory Instrument (SI) 1185 of 2008). It should be noted that the GOS in Scotland is now markedly different from that in England, and is much more geared towards the clinical aspects of the eye examination.[1] A detailed discussion of the differences between the English and Scottish schemes is beyond the scope of this chapter, but suffice to say that the difficulties posed by patients who would benefit from repeat or additional tests do not occur in the Scottish GOS system. This is because the Scottish system enables the optometrist to claim a supplementary examination fee for further investigation or refinement of their clinical findings. At the time of writing (September 2008), it is anticipated that both the Welsh and Northern Irish GOS will be reviewed shortly, but the outcome is unclear. The discussion below therefore only relates to the 2008 English contract.

Whilst much of what happens in the examination room is unchanged when compared with the previous GOS regulations, the contract imposes specific obligations upon the contractor which were not as explicit under the old arrangements. They also prohibit the contractor from refusing to see 'uneconomic' patients (see point 3 below). Examining the detail of the GOS regulations is beyond the scope of this chapter, but some points that relate to ethical considerations are discussed below:

1. The GOS regulations (para 16(2)) specifically prohibit contractors from accepting or demanding any fee or remuneration from a patient or someone who has

requested services under the GOS contract for themselves or a family member. This ensures that the GOS sight test is free at point of service for the patient.

2. The contractor must disregard their own financial interests when deciding what services to recommend or provide to a patient who is seeking a GOS sight test or when deciding to refer them (para 16(4)).

3. Contractors are prohibited from refusing to provide services for eligible patients on grounds that relate to their race, gender, social class, age, religion, sexual orientation, appearance, disability, or medical or ophthalmic condition. In addition they cannot refuse to provide services to a person in relation to the person's decision or intended decision to accept or refuse private services in respect of himself or a family member (Sch 1, para 1(5)(b)).

Unlike the situation where optometrists see private patients, this prohibits GOS contractors from refusing to see patients if they purchase their spectacles elsewhere. The College provides guidance as to when optometrists can refuse to see patients. The relevant para is 01.15 which states:

While practitioners have a right to exercise a professional freedom in deciding whom they will or will not accept as patients, this right should never be abused. The decision whether or not to accept a patient should not be made on the basis or race, gender, belief, disability or lifestyle. If the practitioner considers it appropriate to refuse, it is good practice to explain the reason to the patient and record the reason.

Legal framework

Opticians Act 1989

The main piece of legislation that governs the professions of optometry and dispensing optics in the UK is the Opticians Act. This was first enacted in 1958 and its most recent revision was by SI 848 of 2005. The Act set up the GOC and regulates various functions, namely the testing of sight, fitting and supply of contact lenses, and supply of optical appliances to various classes of people.

Under s.24 of the Opticians Act it is a summary offence to test the sight of another person without being a registered medical practitioner or a registered optometrist (or someone training as a medical student or optometry student). The Act also specifies certain duties to be performed when a person's sight is being tested (section 26). If a registered optometrist (or medical practitioner) conducts a sight test and does not fulfil the duties required by section 26, and regulations made under that section – the Sight Testing (Examination and Prescription (No2) Regulations 1989) – it is not a criminal offence. However, it may lead to fitness to practise proceedings (see later) being taken by the GOC.

The sale and supply of optical appliances is governed by s.27 of the Act. This section underwent major revisions in 2005 and now covers the supply of all contact lenses, including 'zero-powered contact lenses', which are specifically mentioned as a separate category of contact lenses. A detailed analysis of the complexities of this section is beyond the scope of this chapter, but readers are referred to the College of Optometrists' Guidelines for Professional

---

[1]See Scottish Statutory Instrument no 135 of 2006.

Conduct, particularly Chapters 28–30 inclusive, for an interpretation of the duties and responsibilities of optometrists when they are fitting and/or supplying contact lenses (available on www.college-optometrists.org/index.aspx/pcms/site.publication.Ethics_Guidelines.Ethics_Guidelines_home/). The GOC made a statement (30 October 2006) on the issue of patient health and safety regarding the sale and supply of optical appliances and has confirmed its position in relation to the three main categories of appliance, namely spectacles, zero-powered contact lenses, and sight-correcting contact lenses. The GOC statement is available on www.optical.org/en/news_publications/news_item.cfm?id=16C87627–8069–458A–A315EF85F774E825. Failure to comply with this section of the Act could lead to criminal proceedings and/or fitness to practise procedures (see below).

Under sections 27(1), (3), and (10) of the Act, it is a summary offence for a person who is not a registered optometrist, dispensing optician, or medical practitioner to sell or supply a contact lens unless certain conditions apply. One of these conditions is that the sale is done under the supervision or general direction of a registered optometrist, dispensing optician, or medical practitioner. The GOC may prosecute contact lens sellers if they do not comply with the Act. In 2008, the internet retailer Vision Direct pleaded guilty at Hendon Magistrate's Court to selling contact lenses without a valid specification and without the supervision of a registered doctor or optician.[2]

The view of the GOC mentioned above is that plano contact lenses, being specifically mentioned in s.27(1)(b), can only be sold by or under the supervision of a registered optometrist, dispensing optician or medical practitioner, and not under their general direction as for other contact lenses. This is echoed in College Guidance para 29.05.

Since 1984, an unregistered individual can supply spectacles to patients over the age of 16 with a prescription that is less than 2 years old, providing that patient is not registered as sight impaired or severely sight impaired, and the other conditions imposed by the 1984 Sale of Optical Appliances Order are met.

Difference between criminal offences and fitness to practise

As mentioned above, the Opticians Act prohibits a person from performing certain activities (such as sight testing and fitting contact lenses) unless they are on one of the appropriate registers. It is a criminal offence for these restricted functions to be carried out by an unregistered person, and that person is subject to summary proceedings and a fine if found guilty. If the activity is done (legally) by a registered optometrist, the clinical competence of the service may, however, be questioned by the fitness to practise procedures (see below). Non-registrants are not regulated by the GOC and therefore cannot be bound by the fitness to practise procedures.

Delegation

Optometrists may choose to delegate part of their activities, but the protected functions of sight testing and contact lens fitting cannot be delegated (College guidance section 05.07).

The College of Optometrists has a chapter (Chapter 5) providing guidance on delegation. This states that the optometrist has a duty to ensure that the person performing the delegated task is competent and suitable to do so. This may be particularly difficult for a locum optometrist who is unaware of the competence of individual members of staff. Advice in these instances suggests that if the optometrist is in doubt about the reliability of the test performed by a colleague, they should repeat the test themselves, as the optometrist '… *at all times retains responsibility for the patient, for the work of the person to whom functions are delegated, and for the outcome of the examination findings*' (College of Optometrists Guidance 05.02).

All optometrists must ensure that the results of any tests that they delegate to a colleague are shown to them so that they can make an appropriate patient management decisions. College guidance states that '*Non-optometrists to whom functions are delegated should not be expected or asked to interpret the findings obtained by them*' (College of Optometrists Guidance 05.03).

Medicines Act 1968

This legislation governs subjects including the manufacturing, supply, and administration of drugs and has been extensively amended over the years by various pieces of delegated legislation. The most pertinent aspects relating to optometrists are those contained in the statutory instruments (SI) including SI 1923 of 1980 (The Medicines (Sale or Supply) (Miscellaneous Provisions) Regulations); SI 1924 of 1980 (The Medicines (Pharmacy and General Sale – Exemption) Order); SI 1830 of 1997 (The Prescription Only Medicines (Human Use) Order) and SIs 1507 and 1520 of 2005.

By virtue of the legislation, optometrists are able to acquire, write a signed order for, and/or supply various eyedrops in certain circumstances. The 2005 drug legislation amendments complemented the 2005 changes to the Opticians Act which created an additional category of optometrist – the Additional Supply optometrist. Additional Supply optometrists have access to a wider range of ophthalmic drugs than do non-additional supply colleagues. The 2005 changes in legislation also enabled optometrists to qualify as supplementary prescribers, and in 2008 legislation was passed (SI of 2008) enabling optometrists to be registered as independent prescribers.

A detailed review of the drug legislation is outside the scope of this chapter, but a brief discussion is included here because the wider use of ophthalmic drugs by optometrists does bring considerations of professional conduct. These relate to the issues of self-prescribing and treatment, and interprofessional relationships.

Chapter 40 of the College Guidelines deals with the Use and Supply of Drugs or Medicines in Optometric Practice. The Guidelines mirror those of the General Medical Council and state that '*Optometrists should avoid self-prescribing or treatment wherever possible*'(40.16). There are exceptions for minor ailments, but the aim is that the optometrist should not subject themselves to a lower standard of treatment than they would expect for a patient. The College also advises that optometrists should not prescribe or prepare written orders for prescription-only medicines for members of their close family.

Until April 2005, optometrists could only supply pharmacy medicines (such as artificial tears) to their patients in an emergency. Although the word 'emergency' was not defined, it may

---

[2]www.optical.org/en/news_publications/news_item.cfm?id=F4198519–4BD9–43C1–BC607E4726A02D58 (accessed 19 September 2008).

well have been difficult to argue that a dry eye fell within this category of urgency. If it was not considered an emergency, optometrists were effectively prohibited from selling artificial tear drops, which were classed as pharmacy medicines (as opposed to contact lens solutions, which were classed as medical devices). Their only alternative was to direct their patients to a pharmacy for supply. In April 2005 the emergency requirement was lifted and optometrists are now able to supply pharmacy medicines provided it is in the course of their professional practice. This again brings professional conduct considerations into play, and the College Guidance (40.11) states that 'In order to separate prescribing and supply, it is good practice for the supply of therapeutic agents to be made by pharmacists wherever possible. Optometrists should not supply therapeutic drugs to patients unless it is in the patient's best interest for them to do so.' The separation of prescribing and supply not only enables a double check on the suitability of the drug for the patient, but also discourages overprescribing for commercial reasons.

An interesting comparison can be drawn between the prescribing and supply of spectacles and the prescribing and supply of ocular drugs. For drugs, the separation of prescribing and supply is encouraged. For spectacles, however, experience has shown that if patients separate prescribing and supply, should they have problems it can be more difficult to sort out, even though – as discussed above – the underfunding of the eye examination leads to commercial pressures on optometrists because they rely so heavily on the dispensing revenue.

Further details on the drugs legislation can be found at www.mhra.gov.uk/home/idcplg?IdcService=SS_GET_PAGE&nodeId=152 (accessed 19 September 2008)

Patient complaint procedures

1. NHS complaints procedure

It is a requirement of the General Ophthalmic Services Contract (s.22) that those providing GOS have a complaints procedure and take reasonable steps to ensure patients are aware of the procedure. The NHS sets out timescales for responding and replying to complaints (GOS regulations Sch 1 para 25). The first stage of the complaint is for the patient to raise the issue with the practice, and aims for what is termed 'local resolution'. If this fails, the patient can complain to the relevant NHS organization, which would normally be the local primary care organization. If the patient is still unhappy with how the complaint has been handled the patient can complain to the Healthcare Commission, which carries out independent reviews of NHS complaints.

Further details of the NHS complaints system can be found at www.dh.gov.uk/PolicyAndGuidance/Organisation Policy/ComplaintsPolicy/NHSComplaintsProcedure/NHS ComplaintsProcedureArticle/fs/en?CONTENT_ID=4086786 &chk=HQcXVD and www.healthcarecommission.org.uk/contactus/complaints.cfm

2. Complaints about professional conduct

If a patient has a complaint about an eye examination conducted under the GOS, they can complain using the NHS complaints system (see above). In addition, regardless of whether the eye examination or consultation was conducted under the NHS or privately, the patient may complain to the

GOC (see below). Complaints can also be brought to the GOC by other parties (such as NHS organizations). The GOC will consider whether the complaint raises an issue of the optometrist's (or dispensing optician's) fitness to practise. The fitness to practise scheme is described in more detail below.

3. Optical consumer complaints service

If the patient has a complaint about a contractual matter, such as the quality or supply of their spectacles or contact lenses, they can complain to the Optical Consumer Complaints Service (OCCS). The OCCS is an independent body that is funded by all registered optometrists and dispensing opticians via their annual retention fee which they pay in order to remain on the Opticians Register. Further information can be found at www.opticalcomplaints.co.uk.

4. Law

Patients may also, of course, decide to seek redress in the courts. Detailed discussion of negligence is outside the scope of this chapter.

Fitness to practise

The extensive revisions to the Opticians Act that were enacted in 2005 (SI 848 of 2005) included a fundamental review of the disciplinary procedures.

Serious professional misconduct

Until the amendments to the Opticians Act that came into force on 30 June 2005, the only complaint that came before the GOC's Disciplinary Committee was that the optometrist or dispensing optician was guilty of serious professional misconduct. The Disciplinary Committee hearings were formal and usually held in public. Verbatim transcripts of the hearings are publicly available on the GOC's website. Reading of these documents reveals that there was quite a range of misdemeanours that were considered by the GOC to be serious professional misconduct. Examples include being found guilty of a criminal offence (commonly fraud), failing to refer a patient with pathology, and inadequate record keeping.

It should be noted that conviction for a criminal offence often led to the registrant being found guilty by the GOC of serious professional misconduct. This could result in the optometrist/dispensing optician not only losing their liberty via the criminal courts but also their livelihood via the GOC disciplinary process. This possibility remains under the 2005 amendments, and it should be remembered that accepting a police caution involves an acceptance of guilt and as such could lead to the optometrist/dispensing optician being subject to fitness to practise proceedings without having gone to a criminal trial.

The fitness to practise procedure

The 2005 amendments to the Opticians Act led to a considerable change in the disciplinary processes at the GOC. The Disciplinary Committee was abolished and in its place stands a fitness to practise (FTP) panel which is independent of the GOC. Members of the FTP panel are drawn from the two professions that are regulated by the GOC, together with lay members. The composition of the FTP Committee is publicly available on the GOC website. Since their inception, the FTP Committee have heard a wide variety of cases and outcomes are not necessarily the same as under the Disciplinary Committee. This may be partly because the FTP panel has a wider range of sanctions and orders available to it (see later section).

One of the criticisms of the old procedures was that the GOC were unable to investigate an allegation of misconduct adequately. The procedure was that a complaint was received in writing by the GOC. This allegation was then sent to the optometrist/dispensing optician, who was given the right to reply. The optometrist/dispensing optician's reply was then sent to the complainant to correct any factual inaccuracies in the optometrist/dispensing optician's statement. The Investigating Committee of the GOC then decided whether the evidence in front of them prima facie could lead to a charge of serious professional misconduct. If so, the case was sent for a hearing.

The new procedure is different in several respects. Firstly, rather than relying purely on written submissions, the GOC can now interview the complainant. They also have access to the original patient records, rather than copies. The Investigation Committee (the successor to the old Investigating Committee) can also, if it wishes, ask for an assessment of the practitioner to be carried out in their practice. If this is requested, the assessment is conducted by one or two assessors who are independent of both the GOC and the FTP panel. The assessor(s) will be peers of the practitioner who is the subject of the complaint. The assessor(s) visit the practitioner in their practice; they will watch them at work with patients and may question the practitioner. If desired, the practitioner can ask for their legal adviser to be present during this questioning. The assessor(s) draft a report to be considered by the Investigation Committee. This committee will then decide whether further action is required. Possible actions include sending the practitioner for an FTP hearing, to issue a warning to the practitioner, or to send them for informal training.

The Investigation Committee can investigate allegations about fitness to practise where there is evidence of:

- misconduct
- deficient professional performance
- a caution or conviction in relation to a criminal offence
- adverse physical or mental health
- a finding of impaired fitness by another regulatory body in the United Kingdom
- an absolute discharge or a specified statutory penalty (Scotland only).

If the practitioner is found to have impaired fitness to practise, the powers of the FTP Committee are considerably wider than those of the old Disciplinary Committee. The Committee may:

- impose a financial penalty order of up to UK£50 000 (although in some cases this is limited to UK£1600)
- impose an order for conditional registration of up to 3 years (this restricts the way in which a person can practise).

- suspend registration for up to 12 months (or in some cases indefinitely)
- erase registration

If the practitioner is found not to have impaired fitness to practise, the Committee can issue a warning.

Comparison of the old (disciplinary) and new (fitness to practise) procedures

The FTP process has many advantages over the disciplinary system. Firstly, the performance assessment that can now be ordered by the GOC enables a more rounded view of whether the complaint was the result of one single lapse of judgement, or whether it is symptomatic of something more fundamental in the practitioner's practice. Secondly, the range of orders imposable by the Committee is far wider and can be tailored to meet the practitioner's need. Thirdly, the range of situations in which the FTP Committee can hear a case is far greater than simply being 'serious professional misconduct' as it was under the old Disciplinary Committee. One of the constraints of the old system was that for any sanction to be imposed the conduct had to fall within the remit of being 'serious professional misconduct'. Therefore, if the optometrist or dispensing optician was guilty of misconduct but this was not deemed to be *serious professional* misconduct, this lay outside of the jurisdiction of the GOC. The practitioner could therefore practise unimpeded. Similarly, if the practitioner's fitness to practise was impaired by an issue such as a health problem, the GOC was unable to restrict their registration in any way as this was, understandably, not considered to be serious professional misconduct. This no longer applies, and the FTP Committee can hear cases that fit each of these examples.

Another difference between the pre- and post-2005 systems is that the old Disciplinary Committee's remit was (as suggested by its name) disciplinary, and so the orders available to them were purely punitive. There was an 'all or nothing' approach in that the registrant could be erased, suspended, or fined. There was no mechanism by which the registrant could be allowed to practise subject to conditions. Conditional registration is now an option open to the FTP Committee and cases in which this has been used include a dispensing optician who had a conviction for class A drug use and an optometrist who was found by the FTP Committee to have poor record keeping. In the latter case, the conditions included provisions regarding to further training and supervision with respect to record keeping. This is in contrast to the pre-2005 disciplinary system, where poor record keeping had been held to be serious professional misconduct.

Students and pre-registration trainees

Until the 2005 changes, students were unregulated in that anyone (providing they met the university's entrance requirements) could become a student and study optometry or dispensing optics. The 2005 changes to the Opticians Act now enable the GOC to hold a register of student optometrists and dispensing opticians (s.8A). In order to be included on such a register the student must satisfy the Council that they are fit to undertake training as an optometrist or a dispensing optician (s.8A(3) Opticians Act).

After graduation in optometry, trainee optometrists practise under supervision for 1 year whilst undergoing regular assessments. The year is overseen by the College of Optometrists. They then take the College's final assessment. Until the 2005 changes to the Opticians Act, these trainees were not registered until they had successfully completed the Professional Qualifying Examination of the College (which preceded the Scheme for Registration). Now they, like undergraduate students, have to be registered with the GOC under section 8A and need to satisfy the GOC that they are fit to undertake training as an optometrist.

Fitness to undertake training proceedings cannot be brought against students (including pre-registration trainees) on the grounds of deficient professional performance, but they can be brought on the grounds of misconduct, the student having a conviction or caution, or the student having adverse physical or mental health (s.13D(2)). Examples are a student optometrist who was denied registration because of a conviction for theft, and a student dispensing optician who was suspended from the register for 3 months after admitting theft of spectacle frames. The FTP Committee may also consider imposing an interim order on student registrants and as an example a student optometrist had an interim order for suspension which was initially granted in March 2008 reviewed and renewed in September 2008 for unprofessional behaviour.

Details of these, and other hearings, can be found on the website of the GOC www.optical.org/en/our_work/Hearings/index.cfm (accessed 19 September 2008).

Conclusion

The practice of optometry has unique issues: as healthcare professions, optometrists strive to do their best for their patients, but the situation in which they practise and the funding of the GOS bring their own pressures to bear. The expansion of the range of services available in optometric practice and the advances in diagnostic techniques that have occurred in recent years have, in many ways, only added to these pressures. The granting of independent prescriber status to optometrists heralds great promise with regard to optometrists' clinical abilities to deliver a full range of services to their patients, but the GOS contract of 2008 does not capitalize on these additional clinical opportunities as much as many had hoped. Policies for utilizing the services of optometry in primary care are largely left to local arrangements rather than a national contract. This has the advantage of flexibility in both protocol and fees paid, but the disadvantage that there is no guarantee that these services will be commissioned, and protocols may differ between locations, which might lead to problems for practices which see patients from more than one area.

Many primary care organizations are engaging with their local practitioners in ways that were undreamt of a few years ago, and this is a time of considerable change in optometry. Like all periods of change, there is the chance that greater opportunities will become available, but also a natural wariness of what is round the corner.

Acknowledgement

The author would like to thank Caroline Withall for her very helpful comments on an earlier draft of this chapter, and David Parkins for his comments on the final version. Any errors and opinions expressed are those of the author.

Paediatric assessment

Susan J Leat

Introduction

The assessment of children's vision has 'grown up' in recent years. Since the 1970s, two new techniques have improved our clinical assessment of infants and children, and our knowledge of visual development in the early years. These two developments were forced-choice preferential looking and photo (or video) refraction. The former was conceived by Davida Teller, first published at ARVO in 1974, and based on the already known fact that infants and young children will preferentially fixate a patterned stimulus compared with a plain field. What was new was the making of this technique into a two-alternative forced-choice procedure such that an observer was forced to make a decision based on the infant's looking responses or other behaviour (Dobson et al 1978). It was assumed that when the child could no longer resolve or detect the stimulus, there would be no reliable means by which the observer could judge the position of the stimulus above a chance level. This method is called forced-choice preferential looking and has been used to study the development of visual acuity (VA), contrast sensitivity, stereopsis and many other visual functions in infants in the laboratory setting. It has enabled us to add vastly to our knowledge compared with what was known previously. The technique has also been developed into the acuity card technique (McDonald et al 1985), which is faster and is now used clinically to measure VA (the most frequent application) and stereopsis.

The second technique, photorefraction, was first described by Howland and Howland (1974) and was further developed in the laboratory of Atkinson and Braddick (Atkinson & Braddick 1983a, Howland et al 1983), leading others to the videorefraction technique that is available today. Because of its quick and less invasive nature, it enabled the rapid measurement of refractive error, and thus the study of refractive error development in large cohorts of infants. It is also useful in visual screening programmes (Atkinson & Braddick 1983b). This technique, although less often used as a clinical measure, has been of enormous benefit for the management of infants and children by giving reliable data of the natural history of refractive development, upon which clinical decisions may be based.

Children are not just small adults and for their clinical examination a very different approach is required. Infants and young children do not have the ability to attend for long periods of testing, as do most adults, nor are they able to answer questions (or at least answer reliably). Because of their reduced attention span, it is more important that the examination of an infant or child be problem specific, and that the tests chosen will provide the best, most accurate and relevant information to determine a diagnosis and management. At the same time, it is necessary to cover the bases of a complete eye examination, which normally must include a case history and an assessment of sensory, oculomotor, refractive and ocular health status.

The author tends to think in terms of either a standard or routine eye examination when there are no symptoms or concerns, or a case-specific examination when there is a specific sign or symptom which is the reason for presentation. However, some testing in a routine examination may uncover a finding that will make the clinician change into 'specific eye examination' mode. For example, reduced monocular VA may be detected during a routine eye examination, in which case the optometrist must determine the underlying cause, which may require a cycloplegic refraction, which would not normally be part of a routine eye examination.

The order of testing and the tests that are included in a routine paediatric eye examination should be based on: (1) the child's developmental age, (2) the invasiveness and level of threat and proximity imposed by each test, and (3) whether the tests are binocular or monocular, as we do not want to break down a tenuous binocularity before assessing it. Thus, we often undertake binocular testing such as cover test or stereopsis before attempting occlusion for monocular acuities, as most young children find occlusion disturbing and because it is usually better to measure binocularity before prolonged occlusion in case of an intermittent strabismus. Tests of ocular health, intraocular pressure or cycloplegic refraction can be left until later, once some rapport and level of trust has been developed with the child. These same considerations are important in a case-specific examination, but the clinician must also consider what is the key information that must be collected. A classic example is the case where a parent's chief concern is the appearance of a white pupillary reflex. Here, the ocular health examination is crucial, and would be moved up earlier in the examination so as to ensure that it is completed satisfactorily before the child's attention and cooperation wanes.

Case history

Of course, the case history will be taken from the parent or guardian for young children, although some questions may be addressed to children of 4 years and upward. However, until the age of about 8–12 years, the responses from a child may not be reliable. Children are especially susceptible to being 'led' with questioning. Therefore, open-ended questions are important. If the parent is concerned with possible poor vision and the optometrist asks the child 'Is your vision blurry?' the child may well answer 'Yes' as they see the optometrist as an authority figure with whom they should agree. If, however, they are asked 'When is your vision blurry?' the child may be able to give more accurate information. Giving examples (is it blurred when watching TV, looking at books or both) and allowing a 'don't know' option can also help.

It is important to remember that children listen to the conversation of adults from a very young age, even though they may not understand everything. Therefore, it may be wise to take the case history while the child plays nearby, if the waiting room can be set up this way. This may allow a more frank discussion between the parent and optometrist. However, it is important with children to include them later in discussions, as appropriate for their age. The use of a written case history questionnaire is also useful, but it is still important to explore verbally the details of the chief complaint with the parent, together with other information deemed particularly important.

The case history should use the usual scanning and probing technique for signs and symptoms: scanning the areas of vision, pain, headache, double vision, presence of eye turn and 'probing' for each sign or symptom that is present. **Table 28.1** gives an outline for taking the case history of a child. Parents' observations and concerns should be taken

Table 28.1 Paediatric case history outline

Case history outline
1. Open the consultation and determine chief complaint/concern, e.g. for a first visit 'So what brings you along with Sarah today?' For a subsequent visit 'So how has Sarah been doing since she was last here?' If treatment has been on-going 'How is Sarah getting on with the glasses/patching/exercises?'
2. Investigate chief complaint/concern Use the FOLDAR format F = frequency of symptoms (every day, once a week, once a month) O = onset (how long ago did it start?) L = location (for example, for a headache or eye pain) D = duration (when it occurs, how long does it last?) A = association (what factors are associated with it, tend to bring it on? Is it worse at any time of day?) R = relief (is there anything that brings relief, e.g. stopping reading?)
3. Scan for other signs/symptoms. Ask specifically about presence of eye pain, headache, blurred vision, double vision, eye turn if not already mentioned in chief concern. For any sign or symptom that is positive, use the FOLDAR technique to probe for more information.
4. Background information; The child's ocular history, general health history, medications, allergies, family ocular and general health history should be covered. The presence of risk factors should be checked, e.g. mother's pregnancy, pre- or post-maturity, birth complications, birth weight, Apgar score.
5. End with a general open-ended question. For example, 'Is there anything else that we haven't covered, or that you think I should know about Sarah?'

seriously as parents are often a good judge that something 'is not right'. They see the child every day and in more varied situations than the clinical examination room.

It is useful to observe the child before starting the formal examination. This can occur during the case history. Sometimes, an intermittent strabismus or a motility abnormality will be seen which may not be elicited during testing. Also, observe the general responsiveness of the child, e.g. making of eye contact, visually guided reach. Does the child appear to have reached the normal developmental milestones for its age? Is there a large interpupillary distance or prominent epicanthus, which might give the appearance of an exotropia or esotropia, respectively?

General tips on the examination of children

It is generally a good idea to give the child choices during the examination (as long as either choice is acceptable to the examiner). This allows the child to feel less vulnerable and that they have some measure of control. For example, it is better to say to a child 'Would you like to sit in the big chair by yourself or on Mum's lap?' rather than to say 'Would you like to jump up into the chair?' In the former case, most children will make a choice, and it usually does not matter for the start of the examination whether they are seated alone or on Mum. In the latter case, if the child says 'No' the examiner is in the unenviable situation of having either to overrule the child or to test the child in another chair. Giving the child a choice when the outcome does not matter leads to more cooperation when there is no choice.

Motivation can be improved by the use of rewards (as opposed to bribes). Small sweets or treats such as cereal, raisins or small candies may be used, but always check with the parent that they are in agreement with this beforehand. An alternative is to use non-food rewards, such as stickers or stars. It is a good idea to ask the parent to bring their choice of treat to the examination, so that the parent is happy with what is being given out (and to be sure that any dietary restrictions, whether medical, religious or ethical, are not being compromised). However, the optometrist should be the one who controls when they are given to the child. They should be used to reward cooperative behaviour, and this has to start near the beginning of the examination to be effective in extending cooperation. Otherwise, once cooperation is lost, they may end up being used as bribes, such as 'If you do this for the doctor, you can have a sweet', which seldom works.

The format for this chapter is that tests for various functions will be described in the order that they are usually done. **Table 28.2** shows tests that can be included in the examination according to age. The emphasis is on testing which is available to clinicians in general practice. For example, there is no discussion of electrodiagnostic testing, although this is often completed by optometrists in a hospital or clinic setting. There is also an emphasis on the examination of the infant and toddler, as school-aged children can cooperate with more standard forms of testing.

Fixing and following/motility

The examination of a young child usually begins with tests of fixing and following (and ocular motility), alignment, and stereopsis. The examiner uses a small toy target to observe if the child can fix and follow. Motility is checked at the same time (**Fig. 28.1A**). A 4-month-old should be able to fixate a penlight or toy. The examiner should look for steady fixation, smooth eye movements, the absence of nystagmus, and for commitancy. A variety of toys are needed as an infant will tire of observing one toy after a short time. If a penlight is used, the Hirschberg test (see Ch. 16) can be done concurrently. Some infants are more interested in a person's face and sometimes the author has used her own face as the target, i.e. moved around physically herself. Often it is necessary to gently hold the child's head, otherwise the child will follow with head rather than eye movements. For a child less than 4 months of age, it is necessary to rotate the child rather than move the target in order to check for these movements.

Tests of alignment (including stereopsis)

The unilateral cover test is the procedure of choice for the detection of strabismus. The cover test at near can be attempted even with young infants. It is performed as for adults (see Ch. 16) but with modifications according to the child's age. Obviously, a suitable target must be chosen,

usually a small toy (or better still, several interchangeable toys to keep the child's attention). This toy should be small and have sufficient detail to stimulate accommodation. This is most important in cases of accommodative esotropia. In these patients, the esotropia may be manifest only when accommodation is active, and may be missed if a non-accommodative stimulus is used. Generally, the smallest toy that will keep the child's attention is preferred. Other options, for slightly older children, are a range of small stickers on lollipop sticks or tongue depressors. These can even be stuck on the examiner's nose if one wishes to amuse the child and have both hands free, e.g. when using prism bars. Be sure to keep talking to the child and, depending on age, asking questions or making up a story about the toy. The other main modification for infants is to use your thumb (or your hand) as an occluder. The fingers of the hand are rested on the top of the head or forehead and the thumb can be brought down (**Fig. 28.1B**) These modifications work well for the unilateral cover test and even for the alternate cover test, with practice. By about 1 year of age a distance cover test can be performed, best done with a parent or helper holding a toy at about 3 m. The helper should be the person who talks to gain the child's attention, e.g. asking questions about the toy. At this age an alternating cover test (see Ch. 16) can also be attempted.

For newborns and less cooperative children, when the cover test may not be successful, the next usual test of choice is the Hirschberg test. This is not as sensitive as the cover test, as it only detects deviations of 11° or more. However, most heterotropias in younger children tend to be large. A modification of the Hirschberg test is to hold an interesting toy underneath the light or, alternatively, a translucent finger puppet slipped over the penlight with a small hole for the light to pass through, to attract the child's attention and to stimulate accommodation. Sometimes it can be seen that there is a deviation, but it is not so easy to judge which eye is deviated. This tends to occur in children whose fixation is poor or brief. Covering each eye in turn can help to determine which is the deviated eye. A modification of the Hirschberg test, which allows a more quantitative assessment of the angle of deviation, is the Krimsky test (Rosenbloom & Morgan 1990). Here, prisms are added in front of the dominant eye until the reflex in the strabismic eye is symmetric with that of the dominant eye.

The Bruckner test (Rosenbloom & Morgan 1990) may also be useful at times. Light from a direct ophthalmoscope or binocular or monocular indirect ophthalmoscope is directed so as to illuminate both eyes. An eye which is strabismic will have a brighter, whiter reflex and sometimes the appearance of a larger pupil than the fellow eye (Tongue and Cibis 1981).

An additional test is the 10, 15 or 20Δ base-out test. This is a test of fusion, which has its mean onset around 10 weeks of age (Aslin 1977; Riddell et al 1999). A 10 to 20Δ loose base-out prism is introduced before one eye, and the examiner looks for the expected fusional vergence movement, which should be present if the infant has developed fusion. By 4 and 6 months of age, 13% and 72% of children, respectively, will show a positive response to 10Δ base-out (Aslin 1977), although the use of a larger prism, e.g. 20Δ, may allow the response to be elicited at an earlier

Table 28.2 Suitable tests according to age for a normally developing child

Unless otherwise stated, the tests suitable at a younger age can also be used at older ages, i.e. the tests can be added to those for younger ages.

Newborn	VOR OKN Hirschberg Motility: Turn head to examine commitancy VA: Teller or Keeler cards for acuity or occlusion preference test Retinoscopy: Mohindra with hand-held lenses or lens bars Cycloplegic retinoscopy (but use 0.5% cyclopentolate only – max. dose = 2 drops) Pupils with transilluminator Anterior chamber with transilluminator External eye by direct observation or loupe or Burton lamp Hand-held slit lamp Ophthalmoscopy; Direct, MIO or PanOptic/Wide Angle
3–4 months	NPC Fixing and following Unilateral CT at near with thumb, Krimsky or Bruckner tests Saccades Fixation preference test Can use 1% cyclopentolate 'Flying baby' for major slit-lamp exam Tonopen or Pulsair tonometry Dynamic retinoscopy
6 months	MOKN rather than binocular OKN VOR probably difficult for this age onwards – depends on physical strength of examiner 10, 15 or 20Δ base-out test Stereopsis (with Lang or Stereo Smile tests)
1 year	Possibly alternating cover test at near Possibly distance cover test Cardiff cards for VA Distance fixation retinoscopy (with fogging glasses and hand-held lenses or lens bars) BIO
2 years	Other tests of stereopsis: Frisby, Randot Pre-school test, Titmus Fly Confrontation fields
2.5 years	Matching tests for VA with simple symbols, e.g. LEA test
3 years	Fusional reserves with prism bars (in some children) Worth 4 Dot (in some children, but counting may not be reliable until age 5–6 years) Most tests of stereopsis; TNO, Randot 4Δ base-out test for suppression Matching tests for VA with letters (Cambridge crowding cards but may have difficulty with crowded versions) LEA symbols for contrast sensitivity Goldmann fields using eye movements for response
4 years	Crowded versions of VA matching charts Near acuity: HOTV, LEA symbols or MassVAT charts Colour vision using anomaloscope or City test Major slit lamp
5 years	VA: Some may be able to do Snellen acuity, but clinician should point to letters. May be better to use matching test for reliability. Retinoscopy: May be able to use child's trial frame Goldmann fields using response buzzer Colour vision using D-15
6 years	Snellen VA Some may be able to do a simple, shortened subjective refraction Near VA with Lighthouse Chart for Children or McClure near reading chart Pelli–Robson low contrast chart Tonometry with table non-contact tonometer Slit-lamp fundus biomicroscopy
8 years	Refraction using phoropter Subjective refraction Accommodation facility testing Subjective amplitude of accommodation Ishihara test

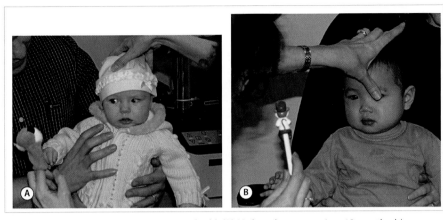

Figure 28.1 (A) Motility testing in a 4-month-old. **(B)** Unilateral cover test in a 12-month-old.

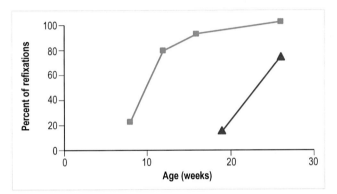

Figure 28.2 Percentage of refixation movements with the introduction of a base-out prism before one eye. (After Aslin R N 1977 Development of binocular fixation in human infants. Journal of Experimental Child Psychology 23(1):133–150 with permission from Elsevier for a 10Δ base-out prism (*triangles*) and after Riddell P M, Horwood A M, Houston S M et al 1999 The response to prism deviations in human infants. Current Biology 9(18):1050–1052 with permission from Elsevier for a 20Δ base-out prism (*solid square*.))

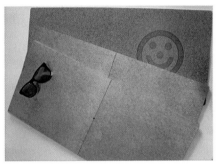

Figure 28.3 Stereo Smile test, showing the demonstration card at the back and the two test cards in front.

age (Riddell et al 1999) (**Fig. 28.2**). Therefore, this test can be useful clinically from about 6 months onwards, or from 4 months of age with a larger prism. It is assumed that, if fusion is present, there is no obstacle to binocular development, such as misalignment.

Stereopsis is also an indirect test of alignment, as well as a direct assessment of the development of sensory binocular vision. Development of fine stereopsis requires good visual acuity in each eye and binocular alignment (at the time of the test), and therefore obtaining a measurement of good stereopsis on a child helps to eliminate the possibility of poor VA or misalignment. This may be very useful information when a child refuses occlusion for measurement of monocular VA. There are many tests of stereopsis, and the ones that will be described here are those that have been specifically developed for infants and young children. Preferential looking tests and visual evoked potential (VEP) studies have shown that the onset of stereopsis occurs between 3 and 5 months of age (Birch 1993; Birch & Petrig 1996). Therefore, stereopsis is typically measured clinically from the age of 6 months onwards. There are two commercially available tests which are suitable for this young age group: the Stereo Smile test (Stereo Optical Inc) and the Lang Stereotest®. The Stereo Smile test (**Fig. 28.3**; Ciner et al 1996) is based on a preferential looking format and uses polarized dissociation and polarized filters. There are two testing cards with a random-dot stereo image of a smiley face to the left or right of the card and also on both sides of the card, so that the card can be flipped and the image will be shown on the opposite side. The cards are the same total size as the Teller acuity cards and therefore the same surround screen can be used. There is also one demonstration card with a binocularly visible face. The test is calibrated for a 0.55 or 1.1 m testing distance so that a total of four different disparity levels can be achieved, namely; 480, 240, 120 and 60 seconds of arc. Age-related normative data are provided for ages 6–17 months (Ciner et al 1996). Leat et al (2001), using a slightly different procedure, showed that 73% of 0.5–2 year olds could cooperate with this test, but found a modal threshold of 480", which is a poorer level of stereopsis than found by Ciner et al, who reported a mean of 300" for both 6–11-month-olds and 12–17-month-olds. The Stereo Smile test works well, its main disadvantages being that the child must be persuaded to wear the polarized glasses and that observing eye movements behind these filters can be difficult. A light angled onto the child's eyes from above can help.

The Lang test may also be used in a similar manner, i.e. as a preferential looking test, although it is much smaller so the resulting fixation movements are harder to observe. The Lang stereotest is a random-dot stereogram. It makes use of small cylinders over parts of the image. Under some areas, the random dots are divided into black and white areas which are refracted by the cylinders at different angles, so that the right eye's image is shifted compared with the left eye. This creates areas of disparity in shapes such as a car or a cat. A significant advantage is that the child does not need to wear filters. There are two versions of the card. The Lang I has three shapes with disparity of 1200, 600 or 550". The Lang II has shapes with 600, 400 and 200" disparity plus one image that can be seen monocularly. The purpose of the monocular image is to allow any child to perform at least part of the test, thus not leaving children with the feeling that they have failed. With younger children, the Lang is used by holding the card while observing if the child fixates the areas of disparity. Older children can be asked to point to the targets. Broadbent and Westall (1990) showed that 50% of 6-month-olds and 75% of 1-year olds can perform the Lang I test. While administering this test, it is important not to jiggle the plate as the position of the targets can be identified by an apparent movement, thus not measuring stereopsis. It is also important to keep the test perpendicular to the line of the sight, otherwise the targets are not visible. However, the levels and areas of disparity are large and some children with microtropia can pass the test (Broadbent & Westall 1990). Therefore, this test should be considered as a screening test; it does not measure a true stereothreshold. Unfortunately, the targets on the Lang II can be seen monocularly by most people and therefore it is not a true measure of stereopsis. Accordingly, it is difficult to recommend the Lang II despite its finer disparity stimuli.

For children of 2 years of age and upwards there are other stereopsis tests available. The Frisby test (Haag Streit, UK) does not require filters as it relies on real depth brought about by printing the random-dot patterns on either side of a plastic plate. There are three plates of varying thickness, and the disparity can also be varied by changing the viewing distance. At 40 cm the disparities for the different plates correspond to 340, 170 and 55". The pattern is made up of four squares, one of which includes the disparate circle. The child's task is to point to the circle or 'ball' seen in depth. The plate can be rotated to present the target any number of times. Most children of 2 years and upwards can perform this test (Saunders et al 1996; Leat et al 2001). The Randot Pre-school Stereoacuity test (Stereo Optical Inc.), which requires the child to match shapes but also requires them to wear filters, and the TNO test (Lameris Ootech BV, Nieuwegein, Netherlands), which also requires filters, can also be used from 2 years and upwards (Broadbent & Westall 1990, Birch et al 1997). After 3 years of age, the Randot or Titmus Wirt circles can be used. As with any test, it is important to compare a given patient's performance with age-related data, and these values are provided for some commonly available stereotests in **Table 28.3**.

Visual acuity

Before describing individual tests of visual acuity (VA), here are a few general tips. For matching and naming tests, a 3 m testing distance is generally more effective than 6 m. This is because it is hard to maintain a preschooler's attention at the further distance of 6 m. It is worthwhile doing a few trials at a very short distance, e.g. 0.5 m, to check that the child understands the procedure and to make sure that the examiner understands the child's responses. Speed is of the essence. In order to obtain an acuity result on both eyes, it

is vital not to spend too much time at suprathreshold levels. The Cambridge Crowding Cards, the Cardiff cards and the Teller cards use a specific protocol of starting above threshold and presenting one letter or card at each (or every other) acuity level until an error or a hesitation is made. Then the examiner jumps back one level and presents more at that and the subsequent levels to determine the end point. This is generally a good procedure to use with any of the quantitative acuity tests. The principle is to determine the approximate acuity level quickly, and then to refine the exact threshold according to the criterion for the test. For tests that have published age-related data, it is important to adopt the same protocol that was used in obtaining the age norms. Otherwise, a true comparison cannot be made.

Occlusion can be tricky; often children from around 6 months to 2.5 years do not accept this well. The author has found that younger children, e.g. those for whom preferential looking is appropriate, are less disturbed when occlusion is performed only during the presentation of the card. The parent is asked to cover the child's eye with the palm of the hand just before the card is presented until the looking response is determined (**Fig. 28.4B**). The hand can be removed while the examiner changes to another card. This brief occlusion seems to disturb the child less than occluding for the whole period of testing. The Cambridge Crowding Cards come with two pairs of brightly coloured occluding glasses and the child can be given the choice of which to wear. For the optometrist who does not have this test, similar glasses could be made up from discontinued frames. A range of stickers should be available to occlude a child who already wears glasses. Alternatively, a tissue can be placed behind the glasses.

Children are very clever. It is very easy to give clues to the child by your responses, e.g. hesitating when a wrong choice is made, in which case the child may make another guess. Or, with matching tests, the child may let its hand wander over the response card, waiting for the examiner to give a clue when the hand is over the correct response. Therefore, accept the first answer or response that the child makes (unless the child has obviously lost attention) and respond in the same way whether the answer is correct or incorrect, i.e. keep encouraging the child whether the answer is right or wrong, e.g. saying 'well done'. Also, discourage parents from being too involved, as they may also give clues to the child, wanting the child to perform well.

Preferential looking tests

For children under 2 years of age, preferential looking tests are the only method which will give a quantitative assessment of resolution (as opposed to detection) visual acuity (see Ch. 12) for the optometrist in practice. Presently, there are three main tests on the market. For children under the age of 1 year the Teller and Keeler acuity cards are available (**Fig. 28.4A**). These are based on the work of McDonald, Teller and Dobson (McDonald et al 1985) and are made up of square-wave gratings printed on one side of a card with no grating on the other. There are several cards containing gratings of varying spatial frequencies. They differ in that the Keeler cards have a circle on both sides of the card (only one being filled with a grating), which avoids the problems of edge artefacts and exact matching of the mean luminance of the gratings with the grey surround. The spatial frequency

Table 28.3 Testing success rates and age-related normal data for stereotests

Lang I: 50% of 6-month-olds can perform the test and 75% of children over 1 year (Broadbent & Westall 1990)

Stereo Smile test: 60% of 0.5–2-year-olds could perform this test (Leat et al 2001)

(Ciner et al 1996)	6–11 months old	Mean = 301″ Upper limit of 95% range = 373″
	12–17 months	Mean = 300″ Upper limit of 95% range = 336
(Leat et al 2001)	0.5–2-year-olds	Mode = 480″ Upper limit = 480″

Frisby test: With small modifications to train a child and give rewards, 96% of 18 month upwards can perform this test (Saunders et al 1996) and all children over 2 years (Leat et al 2001)

(Simons 1981)	3–5-year-olds	75 percentile = 250″
(Leat et al 2001)	2–5-year-olds	Mean = 46″ Upper limit of 95% range = 150″
(Leat et al 2001)	5–9-year-olds	Mode = 20″ 95 percentile = 40″
(Simons 1981)	Adults	75 percentile = 250″

TNO test: Only suitable for children over 2 years (Broadbent & Westall 1990)

| (Simons 1981) | 3–5-year-olds
Adults | 75% achieved 120″
75% achieved 30″ |
| (Walraven & Janzen 1993) | 4–18-year-olds | 93% achieved 240″ |

Randot circles; 93% of 2–5-year-olds (Leat et al 2001) and 97% of 3–5-year-olds could perform the Randot circles (Simons 1981)

(Simons 1981)	3–5-year-olds Adults	75 percentile = 70″ 75 percentile = 20″
(Lam et al 1996)	4.5–5.5-year-olds	98.7% achieved at least 70″
(Leat et al 2001)	2–5-year-olds 5–9-year-olds	Upper limit of 95% range = 170″ Upper limit of 95% range = 50″

Titmus circles: 60% of 3–4s and 100% of 4+ could do the Titmus circles (Cooper et al 1979)

| (Tatsumi & Tahira 1972) | 3-year-olds
4–5-year-olds | 200″ (75 percentile)
100″ |

Randot Preschool Stereoacuity Test: 70% of 2-year-olds, 90% of 3-year-olds and 100% of 4+ could perform test (Birch et al 1997)

| (Birch et al 1997) | 2-year-olds
3–4-year-olds
5-year-olds | Mean = 100″
Mean = 50″
Mean = 40″ |

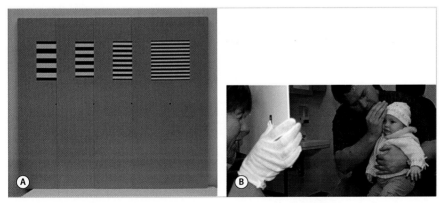

Figure 28.4 (A) Teller cards. **(B)** Teller cards being used with a 4-month-old.

increases in steps of 0.5 octaves (an octave is a doubling or a halving). Clinically, the acuity card procedure is used. Although there are slight differences in routine (McDonald et al 1985; Mayer et al 1995), the essential component is that the clinician judges the highest spatial frequency to which the infant makes a clear looking response. A flow diagram of this is seen in **Figure 28.5**. An older child can respond by pointing. The Teller cards are calibrated for distances of 38, 55 or

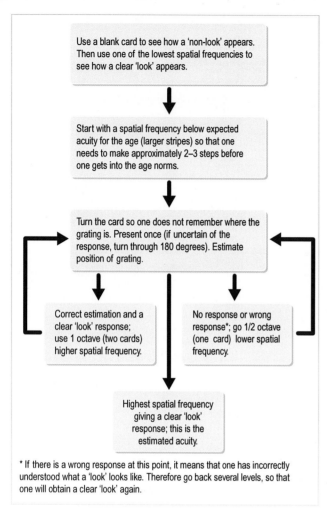

Use a blank card to see how a 'non-look' appears. Then use one of the lowest spatial frequencies to see how a clear 'look' appears.

↓

Start with a spatial frequency below expected acuity for the age (larger stripes) so that one needs to make approximately 2–3 steps before one gets into the age norms.

↓

Turn the card so one does not remember where the grating is. Present once (if uncertain of the response, turn through 180 degrees). Estimate position of grating.

Correct estimation and a clear 'look' response; use 1 octave (two cards) higher spatial frequency.

No response or wrong response*; go 1/2 octave (one card) lower spatial frequency.

↓

Highest spatial frequency giving a clear 'look' response; this is the estimated acuity.

* If there is a wrong response at this point, it means that one has incorrectly understood what a 'look' looks like. Therefore go back several levels, so that one will obtain a clear 'look' again.

Figure 28.5 Flow diagram for an acuity card procedure.

80 cm, with the most commonly used distance being 55 cm. The child is usually positioned on the parent's lap or held over the shoulder. A grey screen (although this is not currently commercially available) prevents distractions and allows the test to be made into a peep show. For children up to 1 year of age, using the perimeter screen does not affect the acuity results (Clifford-Donaldson et al 2006) but it does appear to help reduce distractions for children 17 months old. The new Teller cards (TACII), available from Stereo Optical Inc., Chicago, give a 0.5 octave lower threshold (poorer acuity) than the older cards on which the age-related data was collected (Clifford et al 2005). The cards indicate the equivalent Snellen acuity such that 30 cycles per degree = 6/6 (20/20). Recently, sets of preferential looking 'paddles' have become available, the Patti Pics (Precision Vision, La Salle, IL) and LEA (Good-Lite Co., Elgin, IL) paddles. These are much less costly than the Teller or Keeler cards, but there are no known data on reliability or validity or published norms as yet, and therefore they may be considered as giving an estimate of visual acuity at this point in time.

The Cardiff cards (Keeler, UK; Adoh et al 1992; **Fig. 28.6**) were produced for children between 1 and 2.5 years of age. These children soon tire of looking at stripes, but most are too young to undertake matching tests. The Cardiff cards use the vanishing optotype principle to produce pictures. The outline of each picture is composed of a white line surrounded by black lines having half the thickness of the white line. At threshold for resolving the thickness of the white line, the line dissolves into the background grey. Thus, the detection threshold equals the resolution threshold. The cards are designed to give rise to a vertical, rather than a horizontal looking response. This design feature was used with nystagmus in mind, which is usually horizontal in direction, and would therefore make horizontal looking responses more difficult to see. There are three cards at each acuity level in 0.1 log (one-third octave) steps, which results in an acuity range of 6/60 to 6/6 at 1 m and 6/120 to 6/12 at 0.5 m. The picture is at either the top or bottom. The child looks or points to the 'hidden picture' and is told what picture to look for. When well above the acuity threshold, they will be able to name the picture, but not at the acuity threshold. Thus, if the child names the picture before being told, the examiner knows that they are well above

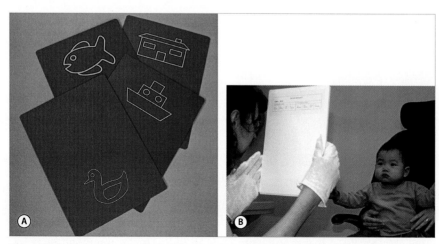

Figure 28.6 (A) Cardiff cards. **(B)** Cardiff cards being used with a 1-year-old.

threshold and can make a large jump towards a better acuity. The general procedure is similar to **Figure 28.5**. When a clear response is obtained (looking or pointing) only one card need be presented and the examiner may jump several cards to a higher acuity. Once close to threshold (responses are less clear or incorrect), present four cards (which means presenting one twice), as the threshold is taken when three out of four presentations are correct (Saunders 1999). Note that the acuity limit is taken as when the child can identify *where* the picture is, not *what* it is.

Teller, Keeler and Cardiff cards measure resolution acuity. Several studies have shown that resolution acuity does not always relate directly to recognition acuity, such as Snellen acuity (Mayer et al 1984; Kushner et al 1995). In the presence of amblyopia or visual impairment due to a variety of conditions such as foveal abnormalities, optic disc hypoplasia or cataract, grating acuity may exceed optotype acuity. Accordingly, the clinician should be aware of these differences, and that these methods of measuring resolution acuity may not always detect mild amblyopia (Geer & Westall 1996). However, in the younger age groups they are the best clinical acuity procedures currently available. Age-related norms for these and other recommended acuity tests are given in **Tables 28.4 and 28.5**.

Unfortunately, these acuity tests are quite expensive. The ideal situation, for a practice which has a paediatric emphasis, would be to have either the Teller or the Keeler cards (for ages 0–1 year) and the Cardiff cards (for ages 1 year until the child can do a matching test). The Teller cards are available in a half or full screening set, which includes spatial frequencies in octave steps. If only one set of cards is possible,

Table 28.4A Norms for preferential looking visual acuity: Teller Acuity Cards

Teller Acuity Cards

Acuity (cycles per degree)

Age (months)	Binocular upper and lower 90% limits (modified from Sebris et al 1987)	Monocular upper and lower 95% limits (modified from Mayer et al 1995)
Newborn	0.5–1.5	
1	0.5–2.0	0.5–1.7
2.5		1.2–3.9
4	2.0–6.2	1.4–5.1
6	2.6–12.0	2.95–10.8
9		3.75–12.3
12	2.6–12.0	4.3–9.6
18	5.0–18.0	5.15–14.3
24	6.6–26.3 (Courage & Adams 1990)	6.6–13.9
30	12.0–32.0	5.94–22.36
36	9.3–37.1 (Courage & Adams 1990)	13.26–35.9
48		16.17–38.07

Table 28.4B Norms for preferential looking visual acuity: Cardiff Acuity Cards

Cardiff Acuity Cards

Upper and lower 95% limit of normal (modified from Adoh & Woodhouse 1994)

Age	Binocular	Monocular
12–<18	6/12–6/50	6/14–6/39
18–<24	6/8–6/27	6/8–6/34
24–<30	6/6–6/18	6/6.8–6/21
30–36	6/5.5–6/12	6/6.4–6/13.5

Table 28.5 Norms for matching tests of visual acuity

Lea symbols uncrowded (after Becker et al 2002)	Mean of the better eye (3 out of 4 correct threshold)	10% quantiles for the better eye
21–30 months	6/9.5	6/18
31–36 months	6/4.7	6/9.5
37–48 months	6/4.7	6/6
49–60 months	6/4.2	6/7.5
60–93 months	6/3.8	6/6

Lea symbols (logMAR chart) (after Cyert et al 2003) for 3–3.5 years		62% obtained 6/15 or better
CCC (interaction free) (Oladeji 1999)		
3–<3.5 years	96% 6/9 or better	
3.5–<4 years	97% 6/9 or better	
4–<4.5 years	97.5% 6/9 or better	
4.5–<5 years	99% 6/9 or better	
5–<5.5 years	97% 6/9 or better	

then the best choice would be either the Teller or the Keeler cards, as they can cover the whole age range from 0 to 2 or 2.5 years. If none of these tests is available, other methods can infer the presence of amblyopia or unequal vision between the two eyes.

Tests to infer the presence of amblyopia

The fixation preference test makes use of the length of time that each eye maintains fixation, and the fact that an amblyopic eye or an eye with reduced VA due to other causes is unlikely to maintain fixation for as long as the dominant eye. A 10Δ base-up prism is introduced before one eye, and fixation is observed while the child is encouraged to view a toy of interest. This test is reliable for detecting differences of two or more lines of VA (Wright et al 1981; Whittaker et al 2000). The outcomes and inferences from this test are shown in **Table 28.6**.

Table 28.6 10Δ Fixation Preference test for use with and without an obvious deviation (Wright et al 1981)

Observation	Implication	Response type
Spontaneous alternation of fixation	Equal VAs or half a line of acuity difference between the eyes	Normal response
If fixation does not alternate, occlude the fixing eye to force fixation of the non-dominant eye. Then uncover. If the non-dominant eye holds fixation for 5 seconds or through a pursuit or blink or freely alternates, i.e. 'holds well'	Equal VAs or one line of acuity difference	
Non-dominant eye holds for 1–3 sec, but not through a blink or pursuit, i.e. 'holds briefly'	1–2 lines of acuity difference	Abnormal response
Fixation promptly reverts to dominant eye	2 or more lines of acuity difference	

If binocular vision is developing normally, monocular optokinetic nystagmus (MOKN) is asymmetric until the age of 6 months. Eye movements for temporalward OKN (i.e. OKN for a stimulus moving from the nasal to the temporal visual field) have lower velocity and frequency than for the nasalward direction. By the age of 5–6 months, MOKN is roughly symmetric, although not completely adult-like (Lewis & Maurer 2005). However, any obstacle to binocular development, such as strabismus or amblyopia, will interrupt this development and MOKN remains asymmetric. The percentage of children showing asymmetric MOKN decreases as the age of onset of strabismus increases up to about 5 years. Those with earlier onset tend to show the asymmetric pattern in both eyes, while those with later onset may demonstrate it in only the deviating eye (Steeves et al 1999). Thus, an observation that MOKN is still asymmetric after the age of 6 months infers the presence of amblyopia. An OKN drum can be used, or a large area such as a striped scarf moved in the patient's field of view (Leat et al 1999b). OKN can also be used to test for the presence of gross form vision, although again temporalward MOKN should be employed, since there is evidence that nasalward OKN can be driven by subcortical pathways (Steeves et al 1999) and will dominate during binocular OKN testing.

For infants who show no evidence of form vision by MOKN or PL, the vestibulo-ocular reflex may be tested. The examiner holds the baby so as to observe the eyes and spins with the baby for a few rotations and then stops. The after-nystagmus which occurs when spinning ceases is observed. In a child with normal vision, there would be one or two beats of after-nystagmus, but a child with severe visual impairment from an early age or with cerebellar disease will show more beats, indicating that visual damping from the VOR is absent (Leat et al 1999b).

Detection tests

There are tests that measure detection acuity (see Ch. 12), rather than resolution or recognition acuity, which a child under 2 years may be able to perform. These include the Stycar test and the Catford drum. For example, the child is offered a raisin either in one of two hands or placed on a white table in front of the child. The testing distance and the size of the object (parts of a raisin or hundreds and thousands (sprinkles)) can be varied until the child no longer makes a choice. Alternatively, the Catford drum makes use of a tracking eye movement response to an oscillating dot of varying size. This results in a more quantitative measure of acuity than the raisin test, but it might be criticized for measuring detection acuity. Detection acuity is an order of magnitude higher than resolution or recognition acuity, typically around 0.5 seconds of arc, rather than 0.5–1 minute (Saunders 1999), and therefore cannot be related directly to Snellen acuity measurements. These tests should only be used in the absence of a preferential looking test, which is the current test of choice for children under 2 years.

Matching tests using symbols and pictures

Once a normally developing child reaches 2.5 to 3 years of age, there are numerous matching tests that may be used. These include picture, symbol and letter tests. Some of these give rise to a slightly higher measurement of visual acuity than others (Graf et al 2000; Cyert et al 2003; Dobson et al 2003). It is important, therefore, to know the age-related norms for the test (and its specific version) being used and its repeatability (**Tables 28.5** and **28.7**). Unfortunately, many tests do not have published age-related normal data. Since it is outside the scope of this work to describe all of these tests, the chapter will concentrate on those that most closely meet the criteria of a good test of VA for children and which are readily available to the clinician. These criteria are: (1) logMAR design (as for adults (Lovie-Kitchin 1988)); (2) using a true M notation, i.e. the given size is

Table 28.7 Repeatability of visual acuity tests

Teller acuity cards (McDonald et al 1986; Mayer et al 1995)	Intraocular clinically significant difference = 1 octave = 2 levels
Cardiff acuity test (Adoh & Woodhouse 1994)	Intra-ocular clinically significant difference = 2 levels Significant improvement from one visit to next = 4 levels Significant decrease from one visit to next = 3 levels
LEA symbols (singles) for children 12–93 months (after Becker et al 2002)	Intra-ocular differences >1 line in 20% of children
Cambridge Crowding cards (Saunders 1999)	Intra-ocular clinically significant difference = 2 cards
Glasgow Acuity Cards (McGraw et al 2000) using by-letter scoring	Test–retest repeatability = 0.1 log units Intra-ocular clinically significant difference = 0.075 log units, i.e. 3 letters

based on the Snellen size at 6m so that distances can easily be changed; (3) design based on the Snellen principle of angular subtense; (4) pictures or shapes that are not strongly culturally dependent or out of date; (5) tests should include contour interaction (Richman 1990) although a version without crowding is also useful; (6) symbols that have equal recognizability at threshold; and (7) there should be published age-related normal data. A commonly used test, the Allen symbols, does not meet any of these criteria. The pictures are now out of date or strongly culturally dependent (e.g. the telephone and jeep). They were not developed based on the Snellen principle, but were 'calibrated' against Snellen acuity with adult subjects whose vision was degraded with optical blur (Saunders 1999). Additionally, they do not follow a logMAR progression, and do not control for contour interaction. For similar reasons, the Lighthouse test, which uses three shapes, umbrella, apple and house, also does not meet these criteria. At threshold, the umbrella is easier to recognize than the other shapes, so recognition is not dependent on the widths of the lines or gaps (as for Snellen acuity) but on the overall shape of the symbol. Therefore, these tests are not optimal and there are many better tests available now.

Firstly, tests using shapes or pictures will be described. The LEA symbols (Good-Lite Co., Elgin, IL) use four shapes; a square, circle, house (or arrow) and heart (or apple) (**Fig. 28.7A**). The Patti Pics symbols (Precision Vision, La Salle, IL) are very similar (**Fig. 28.7B**) and have just included a fifth shape, a star. They are available with a matching card, so that the child may name the symbols or match them. They are based on the Snellen principle, and at threshold all of the shapes tend to look like circles. They are available in many formats, including flip cards with single or crowded symbols and a full logMAR chart format or with a surrounding box for crowding. In the flip card the crowding is achieved with bars around the central symbols, which is cognitively easier than being surrounded by other symbols. They are also reasonably priced, so that an optometrist may easily obtain both a crowded and uncrowded version for distance and near. They can be used with most 30-months-olds or even some 21-month-olds (Hered et al 1997; Becker et al 2000, 2002).

Most studies show that the LEA symbols overestimate acuity compared with letter tests or Landolt Cs (Graf & Becker 1999; Dobson et al 2003) but this is probably format dependent (Cyert et al 2003). The only disadvantage of this test is that, when in the flip chart format, it is not easy to quickly flip from one acuity level to the next.

The Kay picture test (Kay Pictures, Tring, UK; **Fig. 28.7C**) uses a logMAR and crowded format. It comprises eight pictures (five pictures at each acuity level) and therefore may be more fun for a child than the LEA symbols, but on the other hand it may be more cognitively demanding. It does have a matching card, although it is intended for the child to name the pictures. However, the pictures are not equally recognizable at threshold, with the duck being more easily resolvable from its outline. It can be used with children of 3 years and above (Jones et al 2003) and has been shown to agree well with a logMAR letter chart when scored using by-picture scoring.

The Landolt C test is based directly on the Snellen principle (see Ch. 12). The child is required to identify the orientation of the C or the position of the gap. One caution of the Landolt C is that young children tend to confuse left and right, which may result in a lower acuity than the true one. The examiner should be aware of this, and only use the verticals and one horizontal orientation or ignore laterality errors (Simons 1983). Landolt Cs are available in logMAR chart format. Tumbling Es are also available in logMAR chart format. The same problem with laterality exists with these optotypes.

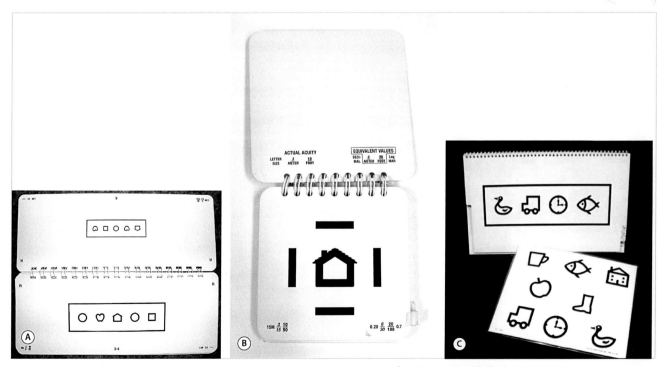

Figure 28.7 (**A**) Lea symbols in the MassVAT version. (**B**) Patti Pics showing the crowded flip chart version. (**C**) The Kay picture test.

Matching tests using letters

The Cambridge Crowding Cards (CCC, Haag Streit UK; **Fig. 28.8A**; Atkinson et al 1988) was one of the earliest letter matching tests based on the criteria specified above. They were developed by the Atkinson group for their large-scale study of refractive error. These come in flip charts, one set with single letters and the other with crowded letters, the crowding being achieved with different letters surrounding the target central letter. They are calibrated for the normal 3 m viewing distance used with children, and both the acuity level and correct letter are printed on the back of the flip card, so it is easy to see this before it is flipped over and presented to the child. There is a standard protocol for the CCC, with which the normal data were established (Atkinson et al 1988; Oladeji 1999). The protocol is as follows. Allow the child to choose which colour of glasses (and therefore which eye will be occluded) they will wear first (this increases compliance), unless you have a particular reason for testing one eye before the other. Familiarize the child with the test and with the expected response by presenting either the large uncrowded or crowded letters at near (whichever you have decided to use). Generally, slightly younger children can respond to the uncrowded letters, as they are cognitively easier. If the examiner starts with the crowded letters, and the child seems unable to respond to the test, move to the uncrowded chart. When satisfied that the child understands the test and can respond accurately, the examiner moves back to 3 m. The examiner starts above the expected acuity and presents one letter at each acuity level until the child makes an error or hesitates for a long time. This first phase is to determine the approximate acuity. When the first mistake or hesitation is made, the examiner goes back one step in VA. All three letters are presented at each VA level, once only. If they are correct for two out of three letters, this is recorded as their acuity. If they are 100% correct, the examiner goes to the next acuity level and shows the remaining letters. The

final acuity is where the patient identifies at least two out of three correctly. Thus, this final phase establishes the acuity threshold. If, during this process, the examiner suspects that poor responses are due to lost attention, the examiner presents one card at a much larger acuity and then returns to threshold testing. The disadvantages of the CCC are that they are not based on a logarithmic scale, and that letters are used to provide crowding, which makes the crowded task cognitively more complex.

The logMAR Crowded Test, previously called the Glasgow Acuity Cards (Keeler Ltd, UK; **Fig. 28.8B**; McGraw & Winn 1993), is a letter matching test, with a logMAR scale and contour interaction provided by boxes which surround the target letter, making them cognitively easier than the crowded letters of the CCC. The bars are placed at 0.5 letter-width distance, which means that the amount of contour interaction produced is greater than for other tests such as the Bailey-Lovie, CCC or LEA symbols (Flom 1991; Leat et al 1999a). It uses letters of approximately equal recognizability which are symmetric around the vertical meridian. There are screening plates with one letter at each level and threshold plates with four at each level. There are three versions, with letters in different orders, so that a child will not learn the order if frequent testing is required. It can be used with children of 3 years and above, but fewer younger children will be able to perform this than a picture or symbol test, such as the Kay (Jones et al 2003) or the LEA symbols.

The HOTV is a letter matching test which is available with a contour interaction surround box, similar to the Glasgow test, a crowded flip book format or full logMAR chart.

Near acuity

With infants and young children, if their distance acuity is good, stereopsis within normal limits and the visual system developing normally, then it is generally assumed that accommodation is normal and near acuity is good.

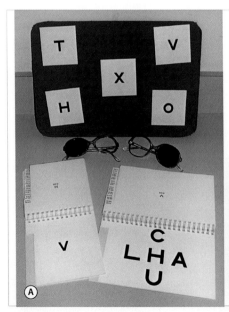
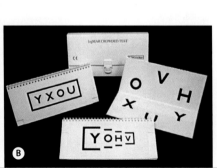

Figure 28.8 (A) The Cambridge Crowding Cards. **(B)** The logMAR Crowded Test (Glasgow Acuity cards).

Measuring near acuity in addition to distance acuity does not add a lot of information in the examination of a child, when attention span is limited. Similarly, accommodation is not measured routinely (although it could be, using dynamic retinoscopy). Of course, preferential looking tests actually measure acuity at an intermediate distance, so when these are used, measuring near acuity would be neither possible nor useful. Near acuity should be included routinely once a child is of school age, and particularly for children who may be having reading or learning difficulties at school. There are specific clinical situations when it becomes important to include a measure of near acuity, such as children with low vision or special needs. Near acuity is very relevant to the everyday near-world tasks of these children, and may also provide more readily understandable information for parents, care workers and teachers (see Ch. 32).

The criteria for a good test of near acuity are similar to those for distance testing. The LEA symbols and the HOTV test are available in a logMAR chart or 'MassVAT' (i.e. Massachusetts Visual Acuity Test) format. Tumbling Es and Landolt Cs are also available in logMAR format.

For older children who are just starting to read, the McClure plates (Haag Streit, Harlow, UK) include grade-appropriate texts (in both font style and reading level) in a range of N notation sizes, and the Lighthouse Chart for Children (Lighthouse International, NY) is a logMAR reading chart with simple text.

Refraction

General comments

It is more accurate, and there is less chance of error, to use trial lenses (using a combination of sphere and cylinder) rather than lens bars. Therefore, this is the method of choice if the child will tolerate a paediatric trial frame, or trial lenses can be hand-held over one eye.

As with other tests, speed is of the essence when refracting young children. The child may only fixate for a short period of time. It is important to obtain information on both eyes quickly. Once an approximate finding is reached on one eye (especially if the result appears in the normal range for their age), switch to the other eye. One can always return to the first eye and refine the result later.

Optometrists will have their own preference for using either a spot or streak retinoscope (see Ch. 13), and either can give accurate results with children. However, the spot retinoscope does have one advantage. Both meridians of an eye can be observed at one time, particularly at the neutral point, and this means that there is no fear of accommodation changing while the streak is rotated to view the other meridian. Therefore, the spot retinoscope has an edge over the streak model for work with infants and patients with limited cooperation.

The clinical test of choice for determining refractive error in children is retinoscopy, and for all younger patients, a high reliance will be placed on these findings. Opinions differ as to whether a cycloplegic refraction should be undertaken on all children and, in some jurisdictions, this may be required. Alternatively, the optometrist may undertake non-cycloplegic retinoscopy first, followed by a cycloplegic refraction when indicated.

Objective refraction: Mohindra retinoscopy

For infants and other children, Mohindra or near retinoscopy (Mohindra 1977) is used. The author prefers the term Mohindra retinoscopy, so as not to be confused with dynamic retinoscopy (see Ch. 15), which also uses a near fixation target. The Mohindra retinoscopy technique was developed for young infants and babies, who cannot fixate a distant target, and can also be used on patients with multiple challenges who have the same difficulty. The method is as follows. All the room lights are extinguished (slowly and with warning, so as not to surprise the child or others in the examination room) and the child encouraged to fixate the retinoscope light by calling their name and talking reassuringly. Babies will instinctively fixate the light. Allowing the child to be bottle fed during this procedure works well. Accommodation will relax, and the child will usually fixate on the light. Retinoscopy is performed monocularly at a working distance of 50 cm. Hand-held trial lenses, a trial frame or lens bars can be used, as appropriate for the child. Wesson et al (1990) showed that occluding one eye made little difference to the result, but this may depend on the model of retinoscope being used. The author has observed that some retinoscopes give reflections from the housing, which may act as a stimulus for accommodation. If using a streak retinoscope, once neutral has been determined, it is wise to check that the astigmatism is fully corrected by rotating the retinoscope streak quickly between the meridians. This will ensure that accommodation has not changed between finding neutral for each meridian.

Originally, Mohindra recommended a working distance correction of 1.25 D be subtracted for all patients, which allows for accommodation tonus of +0.75 D and the working distance (−2D). Thus, instead of subtracting the normal 2 D (assuming a working distance of 50 cm), 1.25 D is subtracted from the gross retinoscopy result to obtain the net finding. Mohindra retinoscopy makes two assumptions: (1) that the retinoscope light is not a stimulus to accommodation and that the eye therefore assumes its tonic accommodative level, and (2) that tonic accommodation (with a possible contribution from proximal accommodation) is 0.75 D. The first assumption has been shown to be correct (Owens et al 1980), but tonic accommodation varies significantly between individuals, ranging between 0 and 4 D. Tonic accommodation may also be refractive-error dependent, as hyperopes tend to have higher mean tonic accommodation than myopes (Maddock et al 1981). For these patients the degree of hyperopia would be underestimated. Additionally, tonic accommodation is greater in children than in adults (Zadnik et al 1999), and this is reflected in the study by Saunders and Westall (1992), which suggested the following correction factors:

- children under 2 years: 0.75 D
- children over 2 years: 1 D
- adults: 1.25 D

Other inaccuracies are introduced when the child has poor cooperation, poor fixation or variable pupil size. Therefore, the results from Mohindra retinoscopy must be interpreted with caution, and when high refractive errors are found (particularly high spherical errors) or when there is poor fixation, poor cooperation or variable pupil, a cycloplegic refraction is indicated.

Despite the uncertainty of determining the spherical error, the Mohindra technique can give a good estimation of astigmatism and the spherical balance between the eyes. It can also be used in combination with distance retinoscopy in the so-called Barratt method (Harvey & Franklin 2005). This is useful if one can only obtain a result with distance fixation in just one meridian of one eye, which can be used as a 'baseline measure'. The Mohindra method can then be performed on both eyes, and the distance fixation value used to adjust the spherical results accordingly.

Objective refraction: static retinoscopy

Distance fixation retinoscopy can be used for children from about 2 years upwards, depending on the child and what target is used to gain the child's attention. The best target is a small television with video or DVD player so that films can be shown. The parents may be asked to bring the child's favourite film, which can be used to gain attention during retinoscopy. The TV set can be positioned at a viewing distance of about 3–4 m, which would lead to a potentially small error of focus of only 0.25–0.3 D due to accommodation if the child were not fully fogged. Other possible fixation targets include toys with lights and music held by the parent or other helper. For children around 7+ years, the author asks the child's preference, i.e. either looking at the TV or the red–green stimulus habitually used for adults.

Fogging is critical to relax accommodation (see Ch. 14). The easiest way of achieving this for a child who does not wear glasses is to use a series of (maybe discontinued) children's frames that have been filled with +2 D, +4 D, +6 D or +8 D spheres in each eye. The child is asked to put on the +2 D 'TV' glasses before retinoscopy starts, and the retinoscopist can use hand-held trial lenses or lens bars over these. If hyperopia more than +2 D is detected, then change to higher-power fogging glasses, so that the power of the lens held over the glasses is not more than about +1 D. This will ensure some level of fogging. If a significant prescription is found, which the optometrist would consider prescribing, then it is recommended to change to a trial frame for the final check if possible, as the trial frame will allow a more accurate estimate of the cylinder axis. For older children, a trial frame can be used from the outset.

For a child who already wears spectacles, it is often useful to undertake retinoscopy over the glasses, but it is still important to fog, which means holding a plus lens over the eye not being tested. With practice, this is possible while the spherical portion of the prescription is being measured or, alternatively, Halberg (Janelli) clips can be used.

Cycloplegic retinoscopy

Cycloplegic refraction should be considered in the following situations:

- any refractive error which is outside the normal range for which the optometrist is considering prescribing glasses, including anisometropia
- the presence of strabismus
- an uncooperative child (although if the child is so uncooperative that the optometrist can barely get a glimpse of the retinoscopy reflex, or the child will not allow the optometrist anywhere near, then cycloplegic refraction will not help!)
- a child with reading or learning difficulties
- fluctuating pupils or constricted pupils during dry retinoscopy or Mohindra retinoscopy.

Typically, either 0.5 or 1% cyclopentolate is used. Two drops of 0.5% separated by 5 minutes gives good cycloplegia in most cases. There are few complications or contraindications to using this drug at low concentrations. Edwards (1991) undertook a longitudinal study of 158 Hong Kong infants in which two drops of 1% cyclopentolate were instilled at each visit. She noted a facial flush lasting up to 2.5 hours in none of the infants following the first instillation, 2.5% after the second, 7.6% after the third and 16% after the fourth instillation. Note that they did not repeat the instillation on any child who showed a reaction. However, none of these children exhibited behavioural changes or other side effects. In the author's own experience, drowsiness is the most common reaction. With 0.5% cyclopentolate there are no serious adverse reactions mentioned in the literature (Cramp 1976). Side effects start to be documented when a 1% concentration is utilized, and usually only when several drops are instilled, or when a 2% concentration is used.

Cycloplegia (or mydriasis) is contraindicated in children with abnormally formed anterior chambers, e.g. microphthalmos, microcornea, glaucoma, aniridia or Peter's anomaly. Cyclopentolate is contraindicated in cases when there was a previous adverse reaction, and 1% cyclopentolate should not be used in children under the age of 3 months (Moore 1990). There is little evidence that cyclopentolate is specifically contraindicated in children with developmental delays. There are a few anecdotal cases of seizures occurring after cyclopentolate instillation in children who may be prone to seizures (one case of a child with cerebral palsy and another with a history of seizures) (Fitzgerald et al 1990; Mwanza 1999). There is also some evidence that children with Down's syndrome may have more sensitivity to the dilation effects of atropine (Doughty & Lyle 1992), but there is little mention in the literature of increased sensitivity following instillation of cyclopentolate (see Nandakumar and Leat 2009 for a discussion). Similarly, children with albinism may demonstrate a different duration of action of the drug compared with normals (Doughty & Lyle 1992).

There are various methods for instillation. Some authors have recommended the use of a spray, as it causes less stinging. Another possibility is the use of anaesthetic prior to instillation of cyclopentolate. This reduces stinging but makes little difference to the effectiveness and only a slight lengthening of the time course of the drug (Lovasik 1986; Mordi et al 1986). However, cooperation may be exhausted during the instillation of the anaesthetic, i.e. the child may be less cooperative for the instillation of the actual cyclopentolate. Therefore, the author finds that simply instilling the cycloplegic drops as quickly as possible is most effective. The child soon calms down and can be sent out to play in the waiting room while the drops take effect. A younger child should be seated on a parent's lap and the head tilted back. If the child will not open its eyes, the drops may be placed on the eyelid margin with the head tilted back. When the child opens the eyes, the drug comes into contact with the cornea. The author finds it is better not to give the child a tissue, as it will be used to wipe away tears in the eyes and some of the drug will be lost. Instead, the examiner should use a tissue to wipe drops that have run down the cheeks (so as to minimize any dermatological reaction) and should also occlude the puncta to minimize systemic absorption. Allowing the child to close (but not rub) its eyes after instillation will also reduce systemic absorption.

Twenty minutes after instillation of the cycloplegic agent, the child can be recalled into the examination room for a dilated fundus examination. By the time this is completed, generally a further 10 minutes will have elapsed and the cycloplegic refraction can be performed. Refraction should be undertaken between 30 and 60 minutes after instillation.

Cyclopentolate does not eliminate all accommodation. Typically, up to 1.75 D of accommodation remains (Ehrlich 1953; Lovasik 1986). Therefore, it is still optimal to use distance fixation during retinoscopy. When this is not possible, e.g. with a younger child, then allow the child to fixate the retinoscope in a similar way to Mohindra, but subtract the full working distance, i.e. assuming there is little or no tonic accommodation left.

For older children who will fixate a distant target during retinoscopy, tropicamide may be used. Egashira et al (1993) found that two drops of 1% tropicamide was as effective as two drops of 1% cyclopentolate. Both gave similar cycloplegic retinoscopy and subjective results in 6–12-year-old children. Tropicamide is a very safe drug and therefore the drug of choice in older cooperative children. For children of African ancestry with darkly pigmented irides, it has been suggested that, rather than two or more drops of 1% cyclopentolate (with potential adverse effects), one drop of 1% tropicamide followed by one drop of 1% cyclopentolate could be used. Kleinstein et al (1999) found similar reductions in accommodation in African-American children over 6 years of age with this combination compared with two drops of cyclopentolate or two drops of tropicamide in children with light irides. The additional advantage of the combination of tropicamide with cyclopentolate is the stronger mydriatic effect of tropicamide for concurrent dilated fundus examination.

Objective refraction: other methods

Autorefraction demands that the child maintain fixation and relax accommodation for several seconds. Due to proximal accommodation, an underestimation of hyperopia is likely to occur, unless cycloplegia is used. Additionally, a table-mounted autorefractor is likely to intimidate a young child and generally cannot be used with infants. Newer hand-held autorefractors, such as the Retinomax K (RightMedical Products, Virginia Beach, VA) and the Welch Allyn SureSight (Welch Allyn Inc., Skaneateles Falls, NY) can be used on children from 3 years of age, but the former underestimates hyperopia when used without cycloplegia, and the latter tends to overestimate hyperopia (Suryakumar & Bobier 2003). They may have been developed for vision screenings, and can be useful with uncooperative children. Standard autorefraction may be considered in 8–10-year-olds, although by this age an accurate distance retinoscopy can usually be obtained.

Photorefraction has largely been developed either as a screening tool or for large-scale population studies (Suryakumar & Bobier 2003). Again, cycloplegia is required for accurate results. Cycloplegic retinoscopy is still the gold standard against which these instruments are compared, and is relied upon for prescribing. In the Pediatric and Special Needs Clinic at the School of Optometry, University of Waterloo, hand-held autorefractors or photorefractors are only used in a very small percentage of infants or children on whom a retinoscopy result cannot be obtained. These tend to be special needs patients or children with behavioural difficulties. In other words, the clinician in private practice should still rely on skilful retinoscopy for the vast majority of child patients.

Subjective refraction

Subjective refraction, in a shortened form, can be performed on some children of 6 years and upwards. This is *very* dependent on the cognitive abilities of the child. With some children, a 'shortened refraction' may be possible, e.g. checking the sphere, but they may not have sufficient attention span for a full refraction or may become confused with too many questions. Additionally, the examiner may have to slow down the procedure. It is better to ask just a few questions and get reliable answers than ask too many questions, which confuses the child. Using slightly larger lens changes (e.g. 0.5 D rather than 0.25 D) may give more reliable responses.

It is important to remember that all children are easily led with questions, i.e. they are *very* attuned to what they think that an adult wants them to say. Therefore, always give two alternatives, e.g. 'Is it clearer with this lens or just the same?', not 'Is it clearer with this lens' as they will invariably say 'Yes'. Also check the subjective answers by VA. For example, if a child has accepted an additional −0.50 D, the clinician would expect there to be an improvement in VA if that minus is genuinely required. If there is no improvement in VA, suspect that the child is accommodating. Similarly, if there is a significant change in the cylinder, use VA to determine whether the change is genuine. During crossed-cylinder routine (and during sphere checking) the examiner can check the child's consistency by reversing the options, i.e. 'changing' lens 1 into 2 and lens 2 into 1. Binocular balancing may be inconclusive, and the final prescription is often a combination of the objective and subjective findings.

Ocular health

External ocular heath

Many assessments of ocular health can be undertaken in a similar fashion and with similar instrumentation to adults, e.g. pupil responses, visible iris diameter and proptosis measurements. Direct observation of the anterior eye with magnification as provided by a Burton lamp is useful, and can be used with ultraviolet illumination after instillation of fluorescein to examine the integrity of the cornea. A transilluminator (or penlight) and 10–20 D loupe can also be used. The anterior angle may be assessed using a transilluminator or penlight shone parallel to the iris plane from the temporal limbus. The percentage of the nasal iris that is seen in shadow is assessed (**Fig. 28.9; Table 28.8**). Hand-held slit lamps are available from several suppliers, although these do not give high magnification. Examinaion at the major slit lamp can be undertaken for almost any age group. For

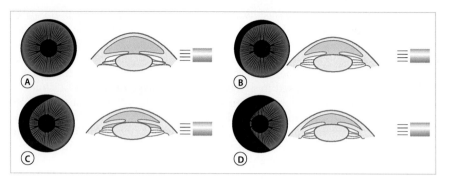

Figure 28.9 Penlight anterior chamber angle estimation. **(A)** Grade IV, **(B)** Grade III **(C)** Grade II, **(D)** grade I. (From Elliott D B 2003 Clinical procedures in primary eye care. Butterworth-Heinemann, Edinburgh, p 247.)

Table 28.8 Penlight grading of angle

Penlight grade	% nasal iris in shadow	Probability of angle closure
Grade 0	100	100%
Grade I	75	Very likely
Grade II	50	Possible
Grade III	25	Unlikely
Grade IV	0	Impossible

From: Elliott D B 2003 Clinical procedures in primary eye care, p 247, with permission from Elsevier.

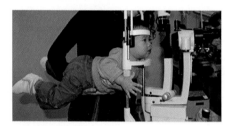

Figure 28.10 'Flying baby' for examining an infant at the major slit lamp.

infants, the 'flying baby' technique can be used, whereby a helper holds the child (**Fig. 28.10**). Children of 3 years and upwards can be positioned at the slit lamp sitting on a parent's lap, kneeling on the examination chair or standing on the foot rest. Interesting fixation targets are required for the child to maintain fixation, such as an assistant holding a finger puppet by the examiner's ear. Even the TV with video player, used for retinoscopy, can be positioned for use during slit-lamp examination.

Internal ocular health

Children older than 6 months have fairly large pupils compared with adults, and therefore a good view of the fundus can often be obtained without dilation. As with cycloplegic refraction, opinions differ whether dilation should be undertaken for all first examinations, and again some jurisdictions may require it. Dilation in babies will require 0.5% cyclopentolate, but for toddlers and older children 0.5% or 1% tropicamide is sufficient, provided cycloplegia is not also desired.

What makes fundus examination difficult in young children is their tendency to stare at the ophthalmoscope and/ or constantly move their eyes. One of the best instruments for internal examination of an infant is the old American Optical (AO) monocular indirect ophthalmoscope (see **Fig. 18.9**) or the more recent Welch Allyn PanOptic or Keeler Wide Angle ophthalmoscopes, and these are useful even when the pupil is undilated. They allow a good field of view and a not-too-close examining distance, which is less threatening and allows the child to maintain fixation better than with the direct ophthalmoscope. For viewing the posterior pole, a TV can again be used to maintain the child's fixation. To obtain a view of the peripheral fundus, an assistant or the parent can hold toys in different directions of gaze. If the child is dilated, there is no reason why the binocular indirect ophthalmoscope cannot be used. The direct ophthalmoscope is useful for a more magnified view of the posterior pole, including optic disc and macula. Children of about 6 years upwards may be able to cooperate for slit-lamp fundus biomicroscopy (see Ch. 18).

If a thorough fundus examination is indicated and the child is uncooperative, the optometrist may have to reschedule the child for another day, or resort to referring for examination under sedation or general anaesthetic.

Intraocular pressure

Although not measured routinely in children, there are occasions when intraocular pressure (IOP) measurement is indicated. For young children there are three current instruments which are suitable for a child who is not sedated or anaesthetized: the Perkins, Pulsair and Tono-Pen® tonometers. Advantages and disadvantages of these instruments are reviewed in Chapter 24. The latter two instruments are most likely to result in a successful reading on a young child. The Pulsair (Keeler Instruments, Windsor, UK) is a hand-held, non-contact tonometer, but requires frequent recalibration by the manufacturer. The Tono-Pen® (Mentor O & O Inc, Santa Barbara, CA) is an indentation tonometer which takes a measurement in less than 1 second, but has been shown to read low for pressures over 20 mmHg (Kao et al 1987). The Perkins tonometer (Haag-Streit USA, Inc.) is closest to the standard Goldman technique, but may not always give a reading on a child. Sihota et al (2006) obtained measurements on 50–65% of non-sedated, supine 1 to 3-year-olds. Most published normative data of IOP in young children were obtained under general anaesthetic or sedation (which can change the readings) and therefore is not relevant to most optometric practices. The limited data obtained without general anaesthetic are shown in **Table 28.9**. It can be

Table 28.9 Intraocular pressure according to age (not under general anaesthetic)

	Newborn	1 mo–1yr	1–2 years	2–3 years	3–4 years	4–5 years	5–6 years	6–8 years	8–11 years	11–12 years
Perkins (Goethals and Missotten 1983)	11.4±2.4	8.4±0.06								
Pulsair (Pensiero et al 1992)	9.56±2.3	10.61±3.1	12.03±3.1	12.58±1.4	13.73±2	13.56±2				
Pulsair (Kohl et al 1989)			7.5			13.0				
Perkins (Sihota et al 2006)		8.0±2.3	8.68±2.8	10.3±2.3	10.57±3.64	11.6±2.5	12.41±3.3	12.96	14.39	14.88±2.7

seen that IOP increases with age, with adult values being reached by about 8–12 years of age.

Other assessments

Contrast sensitivity

Contrast sensitivity (CS) (see Ch. 12) is not generally useful for screening or diagnostic purposes (Leat et al 1999b), but can be valuable as part of a functional assessment of a child already diagnosed with visual impairment or special needs. For children who cannot yet recognize letters and perform the Pelli–Robson test, the LEA symbols are available in a CS format (symbols of constant size but decreasing contrast). This test has been validated against the Pelli–Robson test (Leat & Wegmann 2004). Another test that is commercially available for children is the Hiding Heidi (Precision Vision, La Salle, IL), but this does not correlate well with the Pelli–Robson and has a more significant floor effect (Leat & Wegmann 2004). Of these two tests, the LEA symbols would give the most useful information of CS in young children. Recently, a contrast sensitivity version of the Cardiff cards has become available (Keeler Ltd, UK), but there do not appear to be any published validation studies yet.

Visual fields

Visual fields can be estimated in young children with a simple confrontation test. This requires an assistant. The assistant stands behind the child in a room with dimmed lights while the examiner observes the child and gets its attention (**Fig. 28.11**). A penlight covered with a finger makes a good target, as it is not too bright or large. The assistant brings this from behind the child in an arc centred on the child's head. The examiner notes when the child makes an eye or head movement towards the target, and estimates the extent of the visual field. This is repeated for all of the major meridians and can be undertaken either monocularly or binocularly, as desired. For children of 3 years and upwards, it may be possible to undertake Goldmann fields by removing the telescope, presenting the stimulus statically and relying on the child's eye movements for a response (Cummings et al 1988).

Colour vision

Unfortunately, there is no current, commercially available test of colour vision (see Ch. 19) which is suitable for infants or young children. Perhaps surprisingly, anomaloscopes can give reliable results on children 4 years and upwards, but pseudoisochromatic plate tests are not reliable until 8–12 years of age (Leat et al 1999b). This means that a pass on the Ishihara test before this age indicates that colour vision is normal, but a failure (even on the paediatric plates) is not reliable. The City University test (Keeler Ltd, UK) may be used with children from 4 years onwards, but is less sensitive. The Farnsworth D-15 test (Richmond Products Inc., Albuquerque, NM) can be used from the age of about 5–6 years, although children may become careless and make mistakes towards the end of the test. Recent developments for younger children are the Minimalist test and the Farnsworth F-2 plate, but neither of these is in production at the time of writing. Hovis and Leat (Hovis et al 2002) developed the Waterloo 4-dot test, based on a preferential looking format and the concept of the Minimalist test, i.e. the child has to determine the coloured circle from a number of grey ones. This test can be used on children as young as 2.5 years, with modified pass criteria. This test is not available commercially but could be constructed by the keen optometrist.

Accommodation testing

There are occasions when it is important to assess accommodative function. These include when a child has a suspected learning disability, cases of esophoria at near and in the special needs and low-vision populations (Woodhouse et al 1993; Leat 1996; Evans 1998; Leat et al 1999b; Cregg et al 2001) (see Chapter 32). Parameters that can be measured include the amplitude of accommodation, accommodative facility and the accuracy of the accommodative response (see Ch. 15). Amplitudes can be determined using the standard

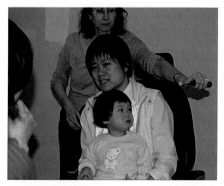

Figure 28.11 Confrontation visual field examination in a 2.5-year-old.

push-up or push-up/push-down methods (Elliott 2003) from about 8–10 years onwards. Accommodation facility also is unreliable before the age of 8 years. Scheiman et al (1988) found that many visually normal 6–7-year-old children had a facility of zero cycles per minute. Since it is an objective technique, dynamic retinoscopy may be used to assess both the accuracy of the accommodative response and the amplitude of accommodation (Leat et al 1999b) in younger children and those with development delays or other communication difficulties. Although there are few data at present, measurement of accommodative lag may turn out to be important in deciding whether to prescribe glasses for young hyperopes (Mutti 2007).

Saccades

Saccadic eye movements may be examined from the age of 3–4 months onwards. This testing could be undertaken on children with reading or learning disabilities, suspected ocular motor dyspraxia or conditions such as cerebral palsy which may influence eye movements. Two small toys (the ideal are collapsible puppets or internally illuminated finger puppets that can be lit successively) may be used as stimuli. The child's attention is directed from one to the other and the accuracy of fixation is judged. If refixations are obvious or the eye movements are slow (taking over a second to complete), then saccades are classed as inaccurate (Leat et al 1999b).

Management of refractive error in children

This section will concentrate on the management of refractive error. Management of binocular vision and ocular health disorders are reviewed in Chapters 16 and 10, respectively. When considering whether to prescribe glasses for young children (0–6 years), one must consider the following points.

1. It has been suggested that wearing either a full or partial prescription may interfere with the normal process of emmetropization. The evidence for this statement, however, is equivocal and there are few randomized, control studies in humans. Atkinson et al (2000) reported no significant difference in the reduction of hyperopia between 3-year-olds who were fitted with a partial correction and a control group who received no glasses. Ingram et al (1991) also did not find a significant overall difference in the final refraction between hyperopes with and without a partial spectacle prescription. Only when they re-analysed their intervention group according to the amount of spectacle lens wear did they find a difference. The children who wore their spectacles showed less emmetropization. However, the latter analysis violates the advantage of randomization, i.e. other factors may be influencing the difference. Interestingly, a study of adult monovision contact lens wearers found that a refractive difference subsequently developed between the two eyes (Wick & Westin 1999). If the refractive state of adults can be influenced by the degree of correction, then one might anticipate that this would also occur in children. Animal studies clearly indicate that the degree of refractive

correction influences refractive error development (Wallman & Winawer 2004; Wildsoet 1997). Therefore, based on the current information, it behoves the clinician to be conservative. We should assume that prescribing glasses may influence refractive development.

2. The normal range of refractive error as a function of age should also be considered (see Ch. 11). There is some evidence that children with very high refractive errors are less likely to emmetropize. This is suggested by animal studies (Smith & Hung 1999) and some human data (Ehrlich et al 1997). Ehrlich et al observed that hyperopes greater than 6 D did not emmetropize.

   With regard to anisometropia, occurrences before 3.5 years of age may be transient (Abrahamsson et al 1990b). Unfortunately, there is currently no way of telling whether a child's anisometropia is temporary or will remain into adulthood (with the risk of amblyopia). However, if the anisometropia is greater than 3 D, the risk of it remaining and resulting in amblyopia is high (Abrahamsson & Sjostrand 1996). It is important to monitor the child over a period of 4–6 months and to consider the level of VA. If amblyopia is already present, it should be treated, and this might also suggest that the anisometropia has been present for some time. Amblyopia would not be expected to develop with anisometropia of recent onset.

   Additionally, Gwiazda et al (1993) showed that hyperopes emmetropized differently depending on whether they had with-the-rule (WTR) or against-the-rule (ATR) astigmatism. Although the magnitude of astigmatism reduced subsequently in both groups, the hyperopes with ATR astigmatism at 6 months of age maintained their hyperopia. However, this was not confirmed by Ehrlich et al (1997), who found that the type of astigmatism did not influence the rate of change of spherical ametropia. Finally, children with low vision are less likely to emmetropize fully (Du et al 2005), although recent data from the author's laboratory shows that even these children show some degree of emmetropization.

3. The presence of uncorrected refractive error may interrupt normal visual development. High refractive errors (especially hyperopia, astigmatism and anisometropia) are risk factors for amblyopia. Based on the findings of Abrahamsson et al (1990a) and Ingram et al (1990), there is an increased chance of monocular or binocular amblyopia in: (1) 1-year-olds with at least 3.5 D of hyperopia in one meridian; (2) 4-years-olds when the most hyperopic meridian is at least 2 D, particularly when there is WTR or oblique astigmatism; (3) children between 1 and 4 years of age with increasing or unchanged ametropia; and (4) persistent anisometropia. Atkinson et al (1996, 2007) showed that the partial correction of hyperopia >3.5 D reduced the incidence of esotropia and may improve VA, although the second, similar study did not find a significant difference in esotropia. Aurell and Norrsell (1990) observed that infants who maintained >4 D hyperopia were more likely to develop esotropia. Gwiazda et al (1989) reported that the most sensitive period for astigmatism to cause meridional amblyopia was between 15 and 24 months. There is some evidence that uncorrected hyperopes (>2.5 D) under 4 years of age are more likely to have deficits in

either visual perception or the acquisition of literacy skills (Rosner & Rosner 1986; Shankar et al 2007). Visual perception problems may cause reading or learning difficulties in this group of children. Although visual perceptual difficulties have not been shown to account for learning disabilities in general, they may be one cause of reading or learning difficulties in a group of children who are usually excluded from studies of children with learning disabilities.

4. The clinician should also consider the optimization of current visual function.

With these criteria in mind, the author has developed the following guidelines for when spectacle prescription would be *considered*:

- *Hyperopia*
  ≥3.5 D at 1 year of age
  >2 D at 4 years
  give a partial prescription (unless aphakic or strabismic), i.e. leave 1–2 D of hyperopia undercorrected
- *Persisting or high astigmatism*
  astigmatism >2 D after 1.5 years of age (give partial correction, i.e. decrease cylinder by 1 D)
  >1.5 D after 3 years of age (give partial Rx up to 3 to 4 years, by which time emmetropization is largely completed) (Atkinson et al 1980; Gwiazda et al 1984, 1993)
- *Anisometropia*
  persisting after 4–6 months of monitoring or anisometropia in the presence of amblyopia
  >2 D after 1 year of age
  >1.5 D after 3 years of age
  if amblyopia is present, give the full balance correction, but correct hyperopia according to age (above); if amblyopia is not present, a partial correction of the balance between the eyes and cylinder may be considered
- *Myopia*
  correct for function, but usually a reduced prescription is given until school age
  >2 D myopia from 1 year or when child is walking – give a reduced correction
- *Reduced VA which appears refractive in origin*
- *Aphakia* – definitely prescribe
  overcorrect by 3 D (since a child's world is close) during the first months, reducing to 1 to 1.5 D overcorrection by 1 year
  distance correction with bifocals from 3–4 years onwards
  consider contact lenses
- *Near esophoria*. Consider correction of hyperopia or a near add

In cases of anisometropia with amblyopia, full refractive correction usually results in some improvement of visual acuity, most of which occurs in the first 4 months (Cotter et al 2006). However, some improvement may continue to occur up to 1 year. If the VA is still reduced after this time, a short period of occlusion (1 to 2 hours per day) is usually effective (Wallace et al 2006). Longer durations (6 hours per day or more) may result in the onset of strabismus in some

cases (Repka et al 2005). Thus, refractive correction is usually the initial management option. Occlusion therapy may not be necessary in all cases, and for those who do require occlusion, the improved VA after a period of spectacle wear makes for better compliance.

During the school years, there are slightly different considerations. Emmetropization is complete by 6 years of age (Gwiazda et al 1993), and the critical period is mostly over (although various aspects of vision may not be adult-like until 8 years and older, and there may be different types of critical period) (Gwiazda et al 1997; Gordon & McCulloch 1999; Madrid & Crognale 2000; Lewis & Maurer 2005). During these school years, hyperopia tends to remain unchanged (Pointer 2001; Jones et al 2005) although early-onset myopia may commence. Thus, during these years, correction is more for function, with a consideration of symptoms and school performance. The following guidelines are given:

- *Myopia*: Correct for function with full correction. There is no evidence that a partial correction reduces the progress of myopia (Adler & Millodot 2006). The current best evidence regarding bifocal correction to slow myopia progression comes from the COMET study. This found a small (≈0.20 D), statistically significant mean difference between the myopes fitted with progressive addition lenses (PALs) and those with single-vision lenses, but this difference was not considered clinically significant (Gwiazda et al 2003). However, a sub-analysis showed that myopes with near esophoria or a larger lag of accommodation (which can be measured with dynamic retinoscopy) did benefit from PALs (Gwiazda et al 2004).
- *Hyperopes, anisometropes or astigmats*: Consider correcting if asthenopia, suspected learning difficulties, headaches or reduced uncorrected VA are present. Provide full Rx for part-time or full-time wear.

Conclusion

Paediatric eye care is a rewarding area of optometry, and by acquiring a few of the more recently developed tests, an optometrist can undertake a full examination in most children. For routine examination, the optimum time to examine a young child is within the first year (this is when infantile esotropia and amblyogenic factors such as high refractive errors can be detected) and before the 'terrible twos' when testing is more challenging. This is in agreement with the Canadian Association of Optometrists, which recommends a first eye examination by the age of 6 months, and the American Optometric Association, which similarly recommends a first examination 'at about 6 months'. The next routine examination should be at 2.5–3 years of age, which is the time when accommodative esotropia often becomes manifest (note: the American Public Health Association recommends examinations at 6 months, 2 years and 4 years). Despite these recommendations, only a minority of children receive their first routine eye examination before the age of 2 years (Ng et al 2005). It is hoped that as we move into the future, optometrists will become more active participants in the healthcare of children.

References

Abrahamsson M, Sjostrand J 1996 Natural history of infantile aniso-metropia. The British Journal of Ophthalmology 80(10): 860–863

Abrahamsson M, Fabian G, Andersson A K et al 1990a A longitudinal study of a population based sample of astigmatic children. I. Refraction and amblyopia. Acta Ophthalmologica 68(4):428–434

Abrahamsson M, Fabian G, Sjostrand J 1990b A longitudinal study of a population based sample of astigmatic children. II. The changeability of anisometropia. Acta Ophthalmologica 68(4):435–440

Adler D, Millodot M 2006 The possible effect of undercorrection on myopic progression in children. Clinical and Experimental Optometry 89(5):315–321

Adoh T O, Woodhouse J M 1994 The Cardiff acuity test used for measuring visual acuity development in toddlers. Vision Research 34(4):555–560

Adoh T O, Woodhouse J M, Oduwaiye K A 1992 The Cardiff Test: a new visual acuity test for toddlers and children with intellectual impairment. A preliminary report. Optometry and Vision Science 69(6):427–432

American Optometric Association. Infant's Vision. Online. Available: http://www.aoa.org/x738.xml 18 Jan 2007

American Public Health Association 2001 Improving early childhood eyecare. Policy Statement No. 20011. APHA, Washington DC

Aslin R N 1977 Development of binocular fixation in human infants. Journal of Experimental Child Psychology 23(1):133–150

Atkinson J, Braddick O 1983a The use of isotropic photorefraction for vision screening in infants. Acta Ophthalmologica. Supplementum 15736–15745

Atkinson J, Braddick O 1983b Vision screening and photorefraction – the relation of refractive errors to strabismus and amblyopia. Behavioural Brain Research 10(1):71–80

Atkinson J, Braddick O, French J 1980 Infant astigmatism: its disappearance with age. Vision Research 20(11):891–893

Atkinson J, Anker S, Evans C et al 1988 Visual acuity testing of young children with the Cambridge Crowding Cards at 3 and 6 m. Acta Ophthalmologica 66(5):505–508

Atkinson J, Braddick O, Robier B et al 1996 Two infant vision screening programmes: prediction and prevention of strabismus and amblyopia from photo- and videorefractive screening. Eye (London, England) 10(Pt 2)(Pt 2):189–198

Atkinson J, Anker S, Bobier W et al 2000 Normal emmetropization in infants with spectacle correction for hyperopia. Investigative Ophthalmology and Visual Science 41(12):3726–3731

Atkinson J, Braddick O, Nardini M, Anker S 2007 Infant hyperopia: detection, distribution, changes and correlates – outcomes from the Cambridge Infant Screening Programs. Optometry and Vision Science 84:84–96

Aurell E, Norrsell K 1990 A longitudinal study of children with a family history of strabismus: factors determining the incidence of strabismus. The British Journal of Ophthalmology 74(10):589–594

Becker R H, Hubsch S H, Graf M H et al 2000 Preliminary report: examination of young children with Lea symbols. Strabismus 8 (3):209–213

Becker R, Hubsch S, Graf M H et al 2002 Examination of young children with Lea symbols. The British Journal of Ophthalmology 86(5):513–516

Birch E E 1993 Stereopsis in infants and its developmental relation to visual acuity. In: Simons K (ed.) Early visual development: normal and abnormal. Oxford University Press, New York, pp 224–236

Birch E, Petrig B 1996 FPL and VEP measures of fusion, stereopsis and stereoacuity in normal infants. Vision Research 36(9):1321–1327

Birch E, Williams C, Hunter J et al 1997 Random dot stereoacuity of preschool children. ALSPAC 'Children in Focus' Study Team. Journal of Pediatric Ophthalmology and Strabismus 34(4):217–222; quiz 247–248

Broadbent H, Westall C 1990 An evaluation of techniques for measuring stereopsis in infants and young children. Ophthalmic and Physiological Optics 10(1):3–7

Canadian Association of Optometrists. Online. Available: http://www.opto.ca/en/public/04_eye_info/04_01_exam_frequency.asp 7 Feb 2007

Ciner E B, Schanel-Klitsch E, Herzberg C 1996 Stereoacuity development: 6 months to 5 years. A new tool for testing and screening. Optometry and Vision Science 73(1):43–48

Clifford C E, Haynes B M, Dobson V 2005 Are norms based on the original Teller Acuity Cards appropriate for use with the new Teller Acuity Cards II? Journal of AAPOS 9(5):475–479

Clifford-Donaldson C E, Haynes B M, Dobson V 2006 Teller Acuity Card norms with and without use of a testing stage. Journal of AAPOS 10(6):547–551

Cooper J, Feldman J, Medlin D 1979 Comparing stereoscopic performance of children using the Titmus, TNO, and Randot stereo tests. Journal of the American Optometric Association 50(7):821–825

Cotter S A, Pediatric Eye Disease Investigator Group, Edwards A R 2006 Treatment of anisometropic amblyopia in children with refractive correction. Ophthalmology 113(6):895–903

Courage M L, Adams R J 1990 Visual acuity assessment from birth to three years using the acuity card procedure: cross-sectional and longitudinal samples. Optometry and Vision Science 67(9):713–718

Cramp J 1976 Reported cases of reactions and side effects of the drugs which optometrists use. Australian Journal of Optometry 59:13–25

Cregg M, Woodhouse J M, Pakeman V H et al 2001 Accommodation and refractive error in children with Down syndrome: cross-sectional and longitudinal studies. Investigative Ophthalmology and Visual Science 42(1):55–63

Cummings M F, van Hof-van Duin J, Mayer D L et al 1988 Visual fields of young children. Behavioural Brain Research 29(1–2):7–16

Cyert L, Schmidt P, Maguire M et al 2003 Threshold visual acuity testing of preschool children using the crowded HOTV and Lea Symbols acuity tests. Journal of AAPOS 7(6):396–399

Dobson V, Teller D Y, Lee C P et al 1978 A behavioral method for efficient screening of visual acuity in young infants. I. Preliminary laboratory development. Investigative Ophthalmology and Visual Science 17(12):1142–1150

Dobson V, Maguire M, Orel-Bixler D et al 2003 Visual acuity results in school-aged children and adults: Lea Symbols chart versus Bailey-Lovie chart. Optometry and Vision Science 80(9):650–654

Doughty M J, Lyle W M 1992 Ocular pharmacogenetics. In: Fatt H V, Griffin J R, Lyle W M (eds) Genetics for primary eye care practitioners. Butterworth-Heinemann, Boston, pp 179–193

Du J W, Schmid K L, Bevan J D et al 2005 Retrospective analysis of refractive errors in children with vision impairment. Optometry and Vision Science 82(9):807–816

Edwards M 1991 The refractive status of Hong Kong Chinese infants. Ophthalmic and Physiological Optics 11(4):297–303

Egashira S M, Kish L L, Twelker J D et al 1993 Comparison of cyclopentolate versus tropicamide cycloplegia in children. Optometry and Vision Science 70(12):1019–1026

Ehrlich D L, Braddick O J, Atkinson J et al 1997 Infant emmetropization: longitudinal changes in refraction components from nine to twenty months of age. Optometry and Vision Science 74(10):822–843

Ehrlich L H 1953 Evaluation of a new cycloplegic. New York State Journal of Medicine 53(24):3015–3017

Elliott D B 2003 Clinical procedures in primary eye care. Butterworth-Heinemann, Edinburgh, p 138, 247

Evans B J W 1998 The underachieving child. Ophthalmic and Physiological Optics 18(2):153–159

Fitzgerald D A, Hanson R M, West C et al 1990 Seizures associated with 1% cyclopentolate eyedrops. Journal of Paediatrics and Child Health 26(2):106–107

Flom M C 1991 Contour interaction and the crowding effect. Problems in Optometry 3:237–257

Geer I, Westall C A 1996 A comparison of tests to determine acuity deficits in children with amblyopia. Ophthalmic and Physiological Optics 16(5):367–374

Goethals M, Missotten L 1983 Intraocular pressure in children up to five years of age. Journal of Pediatric Ophthalmology and Strabismus 20 (2):49–51

Good-Lite Company. Online. Available: http://www.good-lite.com 8 Sept 2008

Gordon G E, McCulloch D L 1999 A VEP investigation of parallel visual pathway development in primary school age children. Documenta Ophthalmologica. Advances in Ophthalmology 99(1):1–10

Graf M, Becker R 1999 Determining visual acuity with LH symbols and Landolt rings. Klinische Monatsblatter Fur Augenheilkunde 215 (2):86–90

Graf M H, Becker, R, Kaufmann H 2000 Lea symbols: visual acuity assessment and detection of amblyopia. Graefe's Archive for Clinical and Experimental Ophthalmology 238(1):53–58

Gwiazda J, Scheiman M, Mohindra I et al 1984 Astigmatism in children: changes in axis and amount from birth to six years. Investigative Ophthalmology and Visual Science 25(1):88–92

Gwiazda J, Bauer J, Held R 1989 From visual acuity to hyperacuity: a 10-year update. Canadian Journal of Psychology 43(2):109–120

Gwiazda J, Thorn F, Bauer J et al 1993 Emmetropization and the progression of manifest refraction in children followed from infancy to puberty. Clinical Vision Sciences 8(4):337–344

Gwiazda J, Bauer J, Thorn F et al 1997 Development of spatial contrast sensitivity from infancy to adulthood: psychophysical data. Optometry and Vision Science 74(10):785–789

Gwiazda J, Hyman L, Hussein M et al 2003 A randomized clinical trial of progressive addition lenses versus single vision lenses on the progression of myopia in children. Investigative Ophthalmology and Visual Science 44(4):1492–1500

Gwiazda J E, Hyman L, Norton T T et al 2004 Accommodation and related risk factors associated with myopia progression and their interaction with treatment in COMET children. Investigative Ophthalmology and Visual Science 45(7):2143–2151

Harvey W, Franklin A 2005 Eye essentials: routine eye examination. Elsevier Butterworth-Heineman, London, p 89

Hered R W, Murphy S, Clancy M 1997 Comparison of the HOTV and Lea Symbols charts for preschool vision screening. Journal of Pediatric Ophthalmology and Strabismus 34(1):24–28

Hovis J K, Leat S J, Heffernan S et al 2002 The validity of the University of Waterloo Colored Dot Test for Color Vision Testing in adults and preschool children. Optometry and Vision Science 79(4):241–253

Howland H C, Howland B 1974 Photorefraction: a technique for study of refractive state at a distance. Journal of the Optical Society of America 64(2):240–249

Howland H C, Braddick O, Atkinson J et al 1983 Optics of photorefraction: orthogonal and isotropic methods. Journal of the Optical Society of America 73(12):1701–1708

Ingram R M, Arnold P E, Dally S et al 1990 Results of a randomised trial of treating abnormal hypermetropia from the age of 6 months. The British Journal of Ophthalmology 74(3):158–159

Ingram R M, Arnold P E, Dally S et al 1991 Emmetropisation, squint, and reduced visual acuity after treatment. The British Journal of Ophthalmology 75(7):414–416

Jones D, Westall C, Averbeck K et al 2003 Visual acuity assessment: a comparison of two tests for measuring children's vision. Ophthalmic and Physiological Optics 23(6):541–546

Jones L A, Mitchell G L, Mutti D O et al 2005 Comparison of ocular component growth curves among refractive error groups in children. Investigative Ophthalmology and Visual Science 46(7):2317–2327

Kao S F, Lichter P R, Bergstrom T J et al 1987 Clinical comparison of the Oculab Tono-Pen to the Goldmann applanation tonometer. Ophthalmology 94(12):1541–1544

Kleinstein R N, Mutti D O, Manny R E et al 1999 Cycloplegia in African-American children. Optometry and Vision Science 76 (2):102–107

Kohl P, Samek B M, Sabre M 1989 Intraocular pressure measurements in children birth–5 years of age using the Keeler Pulsair non-contact tonometer. Investigative Ophthalmology and Vision Science 30 (Suppl):241

Kushner B J, Lucchese N J, Morton G V 1995 Grating visual acuity with Teller cards compared with Snellen visual acuity in literate patients. Archives of Ophthalmology 113(4):485–493

Lam S R, LaRoche G R, De Becker I et al 1996 The range and variability of ophthalmological parameters in normal children aged 4 1/2 to 5 1/2 years. Journal of Pediatric Ophthalmology and Strabismus 33 (5):251–256

Leat S J 1996 Reduced accommodation in children with cerebral palsy. Ophthalmic and Physiological Optics 16(5):385–390

Leat S J, Wegmann D 2004 Clinical testing of contrast sensitivity in children: age-related norms and validity. Optometry and Vision Science 81(4):245–254

Leat S J, Li W, Epp K 1999a Crowding in central and eccentric vision: the effects of contour interaction and attention. Investigative Ophthalmology and Visual Science 40(2):504–512

Leat S J, Shute R H, Westall C A 1999b Assessing children's vision: a handbook. Butterworth-Heinemann Oxford, Boston, pp 151–154, 199, 276–279, 302–303

Leat S J, Pierre J S, Hassan-Abadi S et al 2001 The moving Dynamic Random Dot Stereosize test: development, age norms, and comparison with the Frisby, Randot, and Stereo Smile tests. Journal of Pediatric Ophthalmology and Strabismus 38(5):284–294

Lewis T L, Maurer D 2005 Multiple sensitive periods in human visual development: evidence from visually deprived children. Developmental Psychobiology 46(3):163–183

Lovasik J V 1986 Pharmacokinetics of topically applied cyclopentolate HCl and tropicamide. American Journal of Optometry and Physiological Optics 63(10):787–803

Lovie-Kitchin J E 1988 Validity and reliability of visual acuity measurements. Ophthalmic and Physiological Optics 8(4):363–370

McDonald M A, Dobson V, Sebris S L et al 1985 The acuity card procedure: a rapid test of infant acuity. Investigative Ophthalmology and Visual Science 26(8):1158–1162

McDonald M, Ankrum C, Preston K et al 1986 Monocular and binocular acuity estimation in 18- to 36-month-olds: acuity card results. American Journal of Optometry and Physiological Optics 63(3):181–186

McGraw P V, Winn B 1993 Glasgow Acuity Cards: a new test for the measurement of letter acuity in children. Ophthalmic and Physiological Optics: 13(4):400–404

McGraw P V, Winn B, Gray L S et al 2000 Improving the reliability of visual acuity measures in young children. Ophthalmic and Physiological Optics: 20(3):173–184

Maddock R J, Millodot M, Leat S et al 1981 Accommodation responses and refractive error. Investigative Ophthalmology and Visual Science 20(3):387–391

Madrid M, Crognale M A 2000 Long-term maturation of visual pathways. Visual Neuroscience 17(6):831–837

Mayer D L, Fulton A B, Rodier D 1984 Grating and recognition acuities of pediatric patients. Ophthalmology 91(8):947–953

Mayer D L, Beiser A S, Warner A F et al 1995 Monocular acuity norms for the Teller Acuity Cards between ages one month and four years. Investigative Ophthalmology and Visual Science 36(3):671–685

Mohindra I 1977 Comparison of 'near retinoscopy' and subjective refraction in adults. American Journal of Optometry and Physiological Optics 54(5):319–322

Moore A 1990 Refraction of infants and young children. In: Taylor D, Avetisov E S (eds) Pediatric ophthalmology. Blackwell Scientific, Boston, pp 65–70

Mordi J A, Lyle W M, Mousa G Y 1986 Does prior instillation of a topical anesthetic enhance the effect of tropicamide? American Journal of Optometry and Physiological Optics 63(4):290–293

Mutti D 2007 To emmetropize or not to emmetropize? The question for hyperopic development. Optometry and Vision Science 84: 97–102

Mwanza J C 1999 Cyclopentolate and grand mal seizure. Bulletin De La Societe Belge d'Ophtalmologie 27:317–318

Nandakumar K, Leat S J 2009 Bifocals in Down syndrome study (BiDS) – study design and baseline results of visual function. Optometry and Vision Science, Feb. In Press

Ng L, Leat S J, Jones D 2005 Parents' awareness of vision care issues in children aged four to six. Canadian Journal of Optometry 68: 21–30

Oladeji M M 1999 Visual acuity of preschool children in the oxford county study. Masters thesis, University of Waterloo, Ontario, Canada, 1999. University of Waterloo, Ontario, Canada, p 38

Owens D A, Mohindra I, Held R 1980 The effectiveness of a retinoscope beam as an accommodative stimulus. Investigative Ophthalmology and Visual Science 19(8):942–949

Pensiero S, Da Pozzo S, Perissutti P et al 1992 Normal intraocular pressure in children. Journal of Pediatric Ophthalmology and Strabismus 29(2):79–84

Pointer J S 2001 A 6-year longitudinal optometric study of the refractive trend in school-aged children. Ophthalmic and Physiological Optics 21(5):361–367

Precision Vision. Online. Available: http://www.precision-vision.com/index.cfm 8 Aug 2007

Repka M X, Holmes J M, Melia B M et al 2005 The effect of amblyopia therapy on ocular alignment. Journal of AAPOS 9(6):542–545

Richman J E 1990 Assessment of visual acuity in preschool children. In: Scheiman M (ed.) Problems in optometry – Pediatric optometry. JB Lippincott, Philadelphia, p 330

Riddell P M, Horwood A M, Houston S M et al 1999 The response to prism deviations in human infants. Current Biology 9(18): 1050–1052

Rosenbloom A A, Morgan M W 1990 Principles and practice of pediatric optometry. Lippincott, Philadelphia, pp 173–174

Rosner J, Rosner J 1986 Some observations of the relationship between the visual perceptual skills development of young hyperopes and age of first lens correction. Clinical and Experimental Optometry 69(5):166–168

Saunders K J 1999 Visual acuity. In: Leat S J, Shute R H, Westall C A (eds) Assessing children's vision: a handbook. Butterworth-Heinemann, Oxford, pp 171–193

Saunders K J, Westall C A 1992 Comparison between near retinoscopy and cycloplegic retinoscopy in the refraction of infants and children. Optometry and Vision Science 69(8):615–622

Saunders K J, Woodhouse J M, Westall C A 1996 The modified Frisby stereotest. Journal of Pediatric Ophthalmology and Strabismus 33(6):323–327

Scheiman M, Herzberg H, Frantz K et al 1988 Normative study of accommodative facility in elementary schoolchildren. American Journal of Optometry and Physiological Optics 65(2):127–134

Sebris S L, Dobson V, McDonals M et al 1987 Acuity cards for visual acuity assessment of infants and children in clinical settings. Clinical and Vision Sciences 2(1):45–58

Shankar S, Evans M A, Bobier W R 2007 Hyperopia and emergent literacy of young children: pilot study. Optometry and Vision Science 84:1031–1038

Sihota R, Tuli D, Dada T et al 2006 Distribution and determinants of intraocular pressure in a normal pediatric population. Journal of Pediatric Ophthalmology and Strabismus 43(1):14–18

Simons K 1981 Stereoacuity norms in young children. Archives of Ophthalmology 99(3):439–445

Simons K 1983 Visual acuity norms in young children. Survey of Ophthalmology 28(2):84–92

Smith E L 3rd, Hung L F 1999 The role of optical defocus in regulating refractive development in infant monkeys. Vision Research 39(8):1415–1435

Steeves J K, Reed M J, Steinbach M J et al 1999 Monocular horizontal OKN in observers with early- and late-onset strabismus. Behavioural Brain Research 103(2):135–143

Stereo Optical Company Inc. Online. Available: http://www.stereooptical.com/MainPages/TellerCards.htm 8 Aug 2007

Suryakumar R, Bobier W R 2003 The manifestation of noncycloplegic refractive state in pre-school children is dependent on autorefractor design. Optometry and Vision Science 80(8):578–586

Tatsumi S, Tahira K 1972 Study on the stereotest (Titmus). Folia Ophthalmologica Japan 23:620–632

Tongue A C, Cibis G W 1981 Bruckner test. Ophthalmology 88 (10):1041–1044

Wallace D K, Paediatric Eye Disease Investigator Group, Edwards A R et al 2006 A randomized trial to evaluate 2 hours of daily patching for strabismic and anisometropic amblyopia in children. Ophthalmology 113(6):904–912

Wallman J, Winawer J 2004 Homeostasis of eye growth and the question of myopia. Neuron 43(4):447–468

Walraven J, Janzen P 1993 TNO stereopsis test as an aid to the prevention of amblyopia. Ophthalmic and Physiological Optics 13(4):350–356

Wesson M D, Mann K R, Bray N W 1990 A comparison of cycloplegic refraction to the near retinoscopy technique for refractive error determination. Journal of the American Optometric Association 61(9):680–684

Whittaker K W, O'Flynn E, Manners R M 2000 Diagnosis of amblyopia using the 10-diopter fixation test: a proposed modification for patients with unilateral ptosis. Journal of Pediatric Ophthalmology and Strabismus 37(1):21–23

Wick B, Westin E 1999 Change in refractive anisometropia in presbyopic adults wearing monovision contact lens correction. Optometry and Vision Science 76(1):33–39

Wildsoet C F 1997 Active emmetropization – evidence for its existence and ramifications for clinical practice. Ophthalmic and Physiological Optics 17(4):279–290

Woodhouse J M, Meades J S, Leat S J et al 1993 Reduced accommodation in children with Down syndrome. Investigative Ophthalmology and Visual Science 34(7):2382–2387

Wright K W, Walonker F, Edelman P 1981 10-diopter fixation test for amblyopia. Archives of Ophthalmology 99(7):1242–1246

Zadnik K, Mutti D O, Kim H S et al 1999 Tonic accommodation, age, and refractive error in children. Investigative Ophthalmology and Visual Science 40(6):1050–1060

Further reading

Atkinson J 1993 Infant vision screening: prediction and prevention of strabismus and amblyopia from refractive screening in the Cambridge Photorefraction Program. In: Simons K (ed.) Early visual development, normal and abnormal. Oxford University Press, New York, pp 335–348

Biswas S, Lloyd C 2004 Paediatric eye disorders: cataract, retinopathy and visual dysfunction. In: Harvey W, Gilmartin B (eds) Paediatric optometry. Butterworth-Heineman/Optician, Edinburgh, pp 61–66

Biswas S, Lloyd C 2004 Paediatric eye disorders: congenital and neuromuscular conditions. In: Harvey W, Gilmartin B (eds) Paediatric optometry. Butterworth-Heineman/Optician, Edinburgh, pp 67–74

Evans B 1996 The optometric investigation of children with dyslexia. In: Barnard S, Edgar D (eds) Paediatric eye care. Blackwell Science, Oxford, pp 191–209

Leat S J, Shute R H, Westall C A 1999 Assessing children's vision: a handbook. Butterworth-Heinemann, Oxford

Logan N 2004 Myopia: prevalence, progression and management. In: Harvey W, Gilmartin B (eds) Paediatric optometry. Butterworth-Heineman/Optician, Edinburgh, pp 27–34

CHAPTER 29

Eye protection

Christine Purslow • Rachel North

Introduction

Ocular trauma has been described as a 'neglected disorder' (Parver 1986). At best, it is uncomfortable and alarming; at worst, it can cause permanent visual loss. There is a conservative estimate of approximately 23 million people worldwide with significant visual loss due to ocular injuries (Negrel & Thylefors 1998). Indeed, in the developing world, corneal trauma is a significant cause of unilateral blindness (Whitcher & Srinivasan 1997; Whitcher et al 2001). Prevention of ocular trauma is not always possible, but many injuries can be avoided if suitable eye protection is worn, and visual loss can often be reduced with prompt treatment. The toll of ocular injury across the world, in terms of suffering, disability, and the resulting economic impact, can only be imagined.

How many eye injuries occur each year?

It is estimated that 55 million people throughout the world each year will suffer an eye injury that will limit their activity by at least one day (Negrel & Thylefors 1998). In the UK it is estimated that 120 000 people (4–5 per 1000 population) report an eye injury each year (Department for Trade & Industry 2002), and that 8.14 per 100 000 will require hospitalization as a result (Desai et al 1996b). The USA reports a similar incidence rate for casualty-reported injuries of 3.54 per 1000 population (McGwin & Owsley 2005a). The Beaver Dam study reported a cumulative lifetime prevalence of almost 20% amongst adults (Wong et al 2000). Ocular trauma accounts for almost half the patients presenting at UK eye casualty departments (Vernon 1983; Chiapella & Rosenthal 1985).

Who is most at risk of eye injury?

Whilst no age group escapes the risk of eye injury, it is children and younger adults who appear to suffer most (Schein et al 1988). The majority of adults presenting with eye injuries are males below their mid-30s (Canavan et al 1980; Chiapella & Rosenthal 1985; Wykes 1988; MacEwen 1989; Desai et al 1996a; Mela et al 2005). The risk of having an eye injury requiring hospital admission is over nine times higher for men than for women between the ages of 15 and 64 years (Desai et al 1996b). Most injuries in adults do not threaten sight, but children appear more likely to suffer visual loss of some degree; eye injuries in children account for a disproportionate number of the cases that require hospital admission (Canavan et al 1980; Niiranen & Raivio 1981; Schein et al 1988; MacEwen et al 1999). Trauma is a significant cause of monocular visual loss in children, particularly for school-aged boys (Niiranen & Raivio 1981). However, the number of children being admitted with serious eye trauma appears to be improving: in a study based on subjects admitted to a Northern Ireland hospital with ocular trauma, 33.8% were children (Canavan et al 1980), whereas in a later study based in Scotland, only 18% were identified as children (MacEwen 1989).

Where do most eye injuries occur?

Over 70% of ocular injuries in adults occur whilst at work (MacEwen 1989). During 2005–2006, a total of 1764 employees required more than 3 days off work due to ocular trauma, of which 820 had a major injury, and 95 people actually lost the sight in one eye through an accident at work (data from Health and Safety Executive, 2006).

Interestingly though, the people who need hospitalization following severe ocular trauma are more likely to have injured themselves at home rather than at work: 30–40% of such severe cases have actually happened either at home or during sporting activities (MacEwen 1989; Desai et al 1996b). This highlights the areas where eye protection is not being worn. Similarly, if we look at children aged 14 and under with eye injuries, more than 50% of hospital admissions within this group also arise from accidents in the home (MacEwen et al 1999). This appears to be an increasing phenomenon when compared with previous studies (Canavan et al 1980; Niiranen & Raivio 1981), and one possible reason for this may be the relative amount of time spent in the home by the current generation of children.

What are the typical causes of ocular trauma?

Causes of ocular trauma vary according to the age of the patient and the social demographics of the region in which people live. In very young children, toys and tools are a common cause, but in children aged 5–14, sporting activities and assault appear to be the most common causes (MacEwen et al 1999).

For a total of 5671 patients (of all ages) seen at busy eye casualty units in Scotland during one year (MacEwen 1989), the various causes of injury are shown in **Figure 29.1**. Nearly a quarter of all serious ocular injuries in 1 year in Scotland occurred as a result of using tools or machinery at home or work (Desai et al 1996a). Occupations involving press and machine tools, or buffing/grinding seem to be most at risk (Chiapella & Rosenthal 1985; MacEwen 1989).

Road traffic accidents are less responsible for penetrating eye injuries since the introduction of compulsory seatbelt wearing in the UK in 1983, prior to which windscreen glass caused serious injury (Canavan et al 1980). However, although significant decreases in penetrating injuries have been recorded since then (Johnson & Armstrong 1986; Cole et al 1987), safety airbags in vehicles are recognized as an increasing cause of blunt ocular trauma and contusion following motor vehicle collisions (Pearlman et al 2001; McGwin & Owsley 2005b).

Sports-related eye injuries have shown a steady increase over the past few decades (Barr et al 2000). The typical sports causing ocular trauma, presented as part of a 1-year

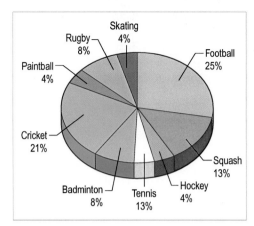

Figure 29.2 Causes of sports-related eye injuries. (After Pardhan et al 1995.)

survey at Bradford Royal Infirmary, UK, are shown in **Figure 29.2** (Pardhan et al 1995).

In the USA, the greatest number of eye injuries result from baseball, ice hockey and racket sports (Napier et al 1996). From 1976 on, the amateur hockey associations in the USA mandated that all players under the age of 20 wear a full face mask. In 1978, the Canadian Standards Association established standards for facial protection in junior hockey, and in the 1977–78 season, the NCAA (National Collegiate Athletic Association) mandated full face masks. The International Ice Hockey Federation (IIHF) requires women and minors to wear full face masks, and visors are a minimum requirement for everyone else born after 1974 (http://www.iihf.com//education/rulebook.htm; accessed July 2007). However, even when mandatory face masks are used in ice hockey, sticks can still travel up under the face visor to assault the orbit/eye (Morris 2006). In the UK and most other European countries, racket sports and football account for the majority of sports eye injuries (Jones 1988; Pardhan et al 1995; Barr et al 2000; Capao Filipe et al 2003). Interestingly, sports-related injuries account for less than 5% of casualty attendances, but for at least a quarter of severe ocular trauma that warrants hospital admission (MacEwen 1987, 1989; Jones 1988; Schein et al 1988; Fong 1995). The 1-year survey at Bradford revealed that, in the case of squash and tennis injuries, follow-up treatment and/or admission to hospital was required in 100% of cases (Pardhan et al 1995). In a study by Barr et al, it was trauma due to squash and football that was most frequently responsible for hospital admission (**Fig. 29.3**).

The speed and size of the ball in racket sports frequently determine the nature and severity of the eye injury. A squash ball may reach speeds of 224 km/h (140 mph), a racket ball and tennis ball 192 km/h (120 mph), and a shuttlecock 232 km/h (145 mph). There is also the risk of being hit by a racket itself. Despite the ocular hazards of racket sports, particularly squash, there is prevailing ignorance of the need for protective eyewear among players (Finch & Vear 1998).

Modern sports such as paintball are an alarming cause of serious eye injury (Farr & Fekrat 1998; Capao Filipe et al 2003). Even fishing and golf have recorded incidences of severe ocular trauma where no eye protection has been worn (Weitgasser et al 2004; Alfaro et al 2005).

There are numerous potentially hazardous products and activities in every home, and eye injuries can occur from

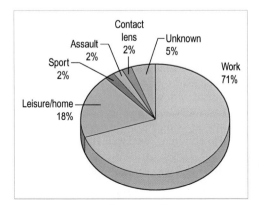

Figure 29.1 Causes of ocular injuries amongst 5671 patients in Scotland. (Modified from MacEwen 1989.)

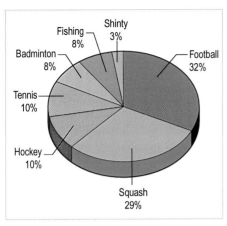

Figure 29.3 Percentage of patients suffering sports-related ocular trauma sufficiently severe to warrant hospital admission. (After Barr et al 2000.)

the most unlikely causes. For example, there have been reports of ocular injuries resulting from ostriches, thrown eggs and exploding eggs from microwave ovens (Goyal et al 2004; Chaudhry et al 2005; Stewart et al 2006).

What kind of ocular injury is most typical?

Ocular hazards can be divided into mechanical and non-mechanical. Mechanical hazards include particles, dust, compression and hot solids. Non-mechanical hazards include chemical, thermal, electrical and those due to radiation.

Contusion of the eye can cause exterior damages such as: subcutaneous haemorrhage (black eye), ptosis, ectropion, and fractures of the orbit. Damage to the anterior segment may result in corneal abrasions, hyphaema and associated damage to the ciliary body, iris or lens. In the posterior segment, contusion can cause retinal oedema (commotio retinae), haemorrhage, retinal detachment, and an interruption of the nervous supply to the extraocular muscles. For non-mechanical hazards, the most urgent condition is that of a chemical burn, which requires immediate action; the eye should be irrigated as soon as possible.

The most common type of ocular trauma is foreign bodies (FBs), causing superficial abrasions or actual penetration of the globe. In a sample of 3184 American patients, severe injuries totalled 5.1% (ruptured globe, intraocular foreign body, hyphaema, orbital/facial fracture) and 94.9% were superficial injuries and contusions (Schein et al 1988). The possible presence of an intraocular foreign body (IOFB) should always be investigated, as retained objects can frequently lead to a loss of vision, especially when containing vegetable matter, iron or copper. On average, only 2–3% of all eye injuries presenting at casualty departments require patients to be admitted to hospital (Chiapella & Rosenthal 1985; MacEwen 1989).

Preventing ocular injury

Role of the optometrist

Many patients are unaware of the ocular hazards they face, particularly at home or playing sport, and therefore it is an important role for the optometrist to inform them and to discuss the eye protection available. A thorough history of patients should be taken and a detailed analysis of the visual requirements made. For example:

- What are their hobbies?
- Do they play sports?
- Do they enjoy gardening?
- Do they carry out home improvement work?
- What is their occupation, and does this involve potential ocular hazards?

From this information, potential ocular hazards can be discussed, along with the need for eye protection where necessary. This can be particularly important for the monocular or amblyopic patient. To effectively change health-related behaviour, there is a four-level model that we can follow when in discussion with our patients (Good et al 2006):

- perceived susceptibility: belief that eye injury can happen to them (testimonials)
- perceived severity: belief that the consequences can be severe (pictures)
- perceived benefit: belief that eye protection is effective (demonstrate)
- perceived barriers: cosmesis, comfort, disruptive (demonstration) (after Good et al 2006).

Eye protection programmes in the workplace

There is widespread wearer resistance to using eye protectors in industrial situations. MacEwen (1989) found that in 85% of injuries that occurred at work, eye protection was not being worn when it should have been.

Most developed countries have now adopted strategies to protect the employee in the workplace. In the European Union, member states have legislation and enforcement routes to ensure that the basic legal requirements relating to occupational safety and health at work are met. An employer in the UK is primarily responsible for the safety of the employees as a direct result of The Health and Safety at Work Act 1974 and related Acts and Regulations (see last section in this chapter). Increasingly in the UK, the regulatory trend is turning away from prescriptive rules, and towards risk assessment. The main aim of an *Eye Protection Programme* (EPP) is to identify potential ocular hazards, and then eliminate or control them. This will not only fulfil legal obligations but also have economic advantages such as a reduction in insurance and medical expenses, minimizing lost production and less re-training and compensation costs incurred for those injured.

An eye protection programme usually consists of the following parts:

- plant environment survey
- vision screening
- implementation of the programme
- maintenance of the programme.

The strategy for eliminating injury starts with elimination of the hazard and ends with personal protective equipment. Once a hazard has been identified, it should be controlled or eliminated: the wearing of eye protectors should really be the last option. If eye protectors *are* required, then the areas where they should be worn must be clearly marked. An active safety committee plus continuing education and training in the need for, and use of, eye protectors will be an essential part of any programme.

In the USA, different states take varying approaches to legislation, regulation, and enforcement. In the USA, the Occupational Safety and Health Act of 1970 created both the National Institute for Occupational Safety and Health (NIOSH) and the Occupational Safety and Health Administration (OSHA). OSHA is responsible for developing and enforcing workplace safety and health regulations. NIOSH is focused on research, information, education, and training in occupational safety and health.

In Canada, workers are covered by provincial or federal labour codes depending on the sector in which they work. Workers covered by federal legislation (including those in mining, transportation, and federal employment) are covered by the Canada Labour Code; all other workers are covered by the health and safety legislation of the province in which they work.

In Malaysia, the Department of Occupational Safety and Health (DOSH) is responsible for ensuring that the safety, health and welfare of workers in both the public and private sector are upheld. DOSH is responsible for enforcing the Factory and Machinery Act 1969 and the Occupational Safety and Health Act 1994.

Forms of safety eyewear

Types of eye protectors

If the potential ocular hazards cannot be eliminated or controlled at source, the appropriate type of eye protection must be provided and worn. Eye protectors can be used in conjunction with screens or fixed shields to further guard against potential hazards. Eye protectors should not only be provided to fulfil legal obligations at work, but also be considered for the many other leisure activities, such as DIY, skiing and squash. Eye protectors come in various forms: spectacles, goggles, screens, visors or helmets.

Safety spectacles

Frames can be manufactured in both metal and plastic form, with nickel alloys most commonly used for metal frames, and polyamide, polycarbonate and cellulose acetate the most common plastic materials (**Fig. 29.4**). Styling is somewhat limited by functionality, and although metal frames may be more cosmetically acceptable to the wearer than plastic, plastic frames are often safer. Metal frames tend to cause more injury when a blow forces the frame against the face, due to the frame itself and the toggle pads (Clarke et al 2002). Glass lenses (even when toughened) within metal frames are prone to chipping, particularly if glazed too tightly, and screws can work loose. It has been recommended that rim screws in metal safety frames should be

secured by a lock nut, peening, or adhesives that bond the thread (Grundy 1982).

Side shields on safety spectacle frames must be transparent so as not to hinder the wearer's peripheral vision, and not discolour with age. Injection-moulded side shields made from polycarbonate are best, as their shape does not alter (unlike those made from a flat sheet, which tend to warp). Any warping of the side shield will produce gaps between the shield and the front, allowing particles direct access to the eye. Side shields may also be made from wire gauze or perforated plastics, to allow a better air flow and so prevent condensation.

Safety spectacles can be made to fit well, and different sizes are usually readily available. However, according to BS EN 166 (European Standard 166; more about standards in the final section) they are unsuitable for protection against such hazards as medium- or high-energy impact, dusts, gases, molten metal, hot solids, liquid droplets or splashes. For particular situations, part-frames can be supplied to insert within goggles and respirators.

Afocal one-piece eye protector

This is the moulded, wrap-around type that is suitable for emmetropes (**Fig. 29.5**). They are often just one size and may not be adjustable, especially when directly supplied by the employer. If not fitted correctly, eye protectors will not provide the necessary protection and eye injury may still occur. As it is often people who don't normally wear spectacles using these, they tend to have characteristic complaints about this type of eye protector:

- restricted field of view, due to the frame
- small magnification effects caused by the shape of the lenses (base curve)
- reflections from the lens surfaces giving rise to unwanted ghost images
- discomfort around ears and across bridge of nose.

Safety goggles

In many working environments it is possible to simply provide over-goggles, particularly to spectacle wearers, but these should not be seen as a long-term solution as physical and visual comfort will be limited. Safety goggles are most useful to protect from splashes and/or provide high-impact resistance. In such instances, inserts can be supplied that provide refractive correction.

There are two main types of goggle: cup and box, each with different uses, advantages, and disadvantages (Rousell 1979; Grundy 1982).

Cup-type goggles

The elastic headband provides a tight fit to the face and can provide protection against molten metal, flying particles,

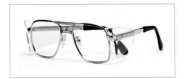

Figure 29.4 Safety spectacles. (By kind permission of UVEX and The Norville Group Ltd.)

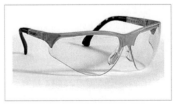

Figure 29.5 Afocal eye protector. (By kind permission of UVEX.)

dust, etc. The housing is generally made of polyvinyl chloride (PVC). They sometimes have adjustable nasal fitting and, if the rims have screws, the lenses can be replaced or exchanged for another type of lens, e.g. tinted or impact resistant. Some cup-type goggles also have large bridge aprons to protect the nose. However, they have some disadvantages: they cannot be worn over prescription spectacles, and ventilation is often poor, which causes the lenses to mistup. If present, the ventilation holes must be screened to prevent penetration and blocking by dust or chemicals, etc. They are sometimes uncomfortable, as the cup is hard, and the frequently wide separation of the lenses with obscure sides can obstruct central and peripheral vision (**Fig. 29.6**).

Box-type goggles

These have a one-piece lens made of cellulose acetate, polycarbonate, or possibly toughened glass, and the housing is made of PVC, which gives a good fit around the brows and cheeks. They are often lightweight with good ventilation with no obstruction of vision. It is possible to wear prescription spectacles underneath but comfort can vary. However, there is no adjustment possible across the bridge (**Fig. 29.7**).

Face shields

These are headband-supported visors that cover the face and neck, and are used to provide protection from flying particles, molten metal, and chemical splashes (**Fig. 29.8**). One major advantage is that they can easily be worn over prescription spectacles or other types of eye protection, if required. They also provide an excellent field of view. The face shield is generally made from either polycarbonate or cellulose acetate. They can also be made so that they can be hand-held, e.g. the arc welding screens, which have a filter as the ocular (i.e. a tinted window). Face shields are also used to provide protection in occupations such as motorcycling, cricket, and the security industry.

Helmets

Helmets are commonly worn during welding. They provide protection of the entire face and neck from the intense radiation and spatter. An ocular containing a filter prevents harmful radiation from reaching the eyes. The filter may be designed so that it can be flipped up to expose a clear, impact-resistant lens, which can be used for grinding and chipping operations. Superior versions are becoming more commonplace, where the window is fitted with a polarizing cell, which darkens to welding density as soon as the arc is struck (**Fig. 29.9**). There can be a tendency for helmets to mist over, but this can be counteracted by the inclusion of respiratory equipment, a feature essential where the gases from welding rods are toxic.

Table 29.1 summarizes the suitability of different types of eye protection for specific ocular hazards according to BS EN 166.

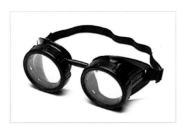

Figure 29.6 Cup-type goggles.

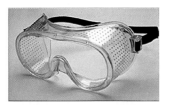

Figure 29.7 Box-type goggles.

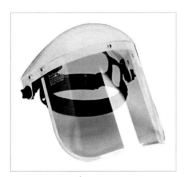

Figure 29.8 Face shield.

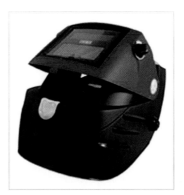

Figure 29.9 Welding helmet with flip front and auto-darkening filter.

Table 29.1 Type of eye protectors available for ocular hazards according to BS EN 166

	Spectacles	Goggles	Face shields
Mechanical strength standard:			
Increased robustness	✔	✔	✔
Low-energy impact	✔	✔	✔
Medium-energy impact		✔	✔
High-energy impact			✔
Liquid droplets/splashes		✔	✔
Large dust particles		✔	
Gas, fine dust particles		✔	
Short-circuit electric arc			✔
Molten metals/hot solids		✔	✔

Obtaining safety eyewear

Afocal eye protectors can be purchased together with other protective equipment from specialist suppliers, but if a spectacle prescription needs to be incorporated, the wearer must obtain this from an optical prescription manufacturer, such as Norville, Bolle or Uvex (UK suppliers), amongst others, with professional input from an optician. In the case of employees, the employer frequently has a contract with the supplier for this work, and the usual procedure is for the employer to send employees requiring protective spectacles to a local optician. The optometrist or optician will receive direction about which type of lenses and frames are required from the employer (safety or occupational health department), and then dispense the spectacles, charging a variable professional fee for this service to the supplier.

Note: It is not a legal requirement in the UK for employers to provide an eye examination prior to the selection of spectacles, but it is in everyone's interest if the prescription is as up to date as possible.

Lenses for eye protectors

In protective eyewear the lenses are generally thicker: the impact resistance of general-purpose spectacle lenses will be lower than in protective safety eyewear made of the same material, usually due to a toughening process or increased thickness.

Glass lenses for eye protectors

These may be:

- heat toughened
- chemically toughened
- laminated.

It must be remembered that toughened does not mean unbreakable. Glass is clearly unsuitable for an eye protector unless it is heat toughened or, less commonly, chemically toughened.

Heat-toughened glass

Crown glass lenses are toughened to a standard or industrial specification, by the application of heat almost to melting point, followed by rapid cooling, which strengthens the structure of the glass by compressing the molecules into a closer mass at the lens surface, creating a compression–tension coat (compression envelope). The heating time depends on the weight, size, and average thickness of the lens. As glass is stronger in compression than tension, the compression envelope improves the impact resistance. Heat toughening is a comparatively quick and cheap process that does not require skilled labour. However, there are some disadvantages:

- High plus lenses (>+5.00 D) tend to be unsuitable for this process, as the bulk of glass requires prolonged heating, which in turn can cause warping and degrade the optical qualities.
- A heat-toughened lens will always be thicker than a non-toughened lens of equivalent power, typically 2.4 mm centre substance and 1.8 mm edge thickness.
- Impact resistance is markedly reduced by scratches and other surface abrasions, so lenses will not retain the

same level of impact resistance throughout life. As the lens surface will naturally become scratched with use, lenses should be inspected regularly, and replaced when distinct scratches are present.

- The heat-toughening process has an adverse effect on the salts present in photochromic lenses. It reduces the range of activity and can only be partially restored by a secondary annealing process.
- When heat-toughened glass lenses are viewed through a polariscope or strain tester, a shadow or strain pattern can be seen; the 'Maltese cross' shape is typical. This pattern is induced during the heat-toughening process when the lens is cooled.

Chemically toughened glass

As with heat toughening, the impact resistance is formed by the creation of a compression–tension coat, but this time by a chemical process. The lenses are first preheated and then immersed in a tank of potassium nitrate solution. The compression coat is produced by the larger potassium ions present in the solution exchanging with the smaller sodium ions present in the glass. As this treatment occurs on the surface of the glass only, it produces a very thin, but very tough, compression coat (100 microns thick). This process does not generally affect the activity of photochromic lenses.

Advantages:
- Although chemically toughened lenses are thinner than heat-toughened lenses, they have been shown to possess a greater impact resistance.
- The toughening process takes the same time for all types of lenses.
- The temperature required for chemical toughening is lower than that used in the heat treatment of lenses. Warping is therefore not a problem, and no stress pattern will be observed.

Disadvantages:
- Chemical toughening is an expensive process, as it requires equipment that must withstand the chemicals and the temperatures involved.
- It is not ideally suited for crown glass; a more expensive type of glass is needed for the best results.
- Scratches on the lens surface reduce the impact resistance significantly because of damage to the very thin compression coat (Woodward & Melling 1977). Scratching reduces impact resistance by 20% for heat-toughened lenses and by more than 30% for chemically toughened lenses (Woodward & Melling 1977).
- It is difficult to determine whether the lens has been toughened by visual inspection.
- When chemically or heat-toughened glass lenses fracture they usually show a radial fracture pattern, although concentric cracks can also occur. Therefore, only a few splinters of glass are produced and the fragments tend to stay in the spectacle frame.

Laminated glass

Laminated glass lenses are made by the adhesion of two layers of crown glass to an inner layer of plastics material. This type of lens has an impact resistance only slightly higher than crown glass. If it shatters, the glass is supposed to stick to the plastics interlayer. However, large, low-velocity missiles may result in slivers of glass from the back glass surface injuring the eye. This method of toughening glass is more frequently found in the automotive and construction industry.

Plastic lenses for eye protectors

Thermoplastic materials (polycarbonate and Trivex) have the greatest impact resistance of all standard lens materials. If impact resistance is a priority, due to a patient's hobbies, or perhaps for dispensing to a child, then these materials should be used. Considering other lens materials, plastic lenses are more impact resistant than equivalent glass lenses and mostly retain this property even when scratched (Fowler & Petre Latham 2001). They are also lighter, and when broken the fragments tend to be larger and relatively blunt. A plastic lens can be thinner than a toughened glass lens of equivalent power, as it may not be necessary to thicken the lens as much to maintain the impact resistance. Plastics also generally withstand molten metal splashes and hot sparks better than glass, as the metal does not fuse with the lens surface. Condensation is also less of a problem due to the lower thermal conductivity (Jalie 1999). However, the softness of plastic can be a problem, and the addition of hard coatings can decrease impact resistance (Chou & Hovis 2003). Chromatic aberration can also increase in the plastics with relatively low refractive indices.

The types of plastics used in eye protectors are:

- polymethyl methacrylate (PMMA)
- allyl diglycol carbonate (CR39)
- polycarbonate
- Trivex®
- cellulose acetate.

Polymethyl methacrylate and Columbia Resin 39

Polymethyl methacrylate (Perspex, ICI) was the first plastics material used in the UK for prescription lenses (Igard/Igard Z). These lenses have, to a large extent, been replaced by the thermosetting plastics Columbia Resin 39 (CR39) (allyl diglycol carbonate). CR39 offers a greater impact resistance than PMMA but, when the lens breaks, it produces sharper fragments. However, both of these materials are suitable for certain grades of eye protectors. Lenses can be made up as a combination of PMMA and CR39. Prescription lenses for eye protectors are commonly made from CR39, which can easily be tinted if required, using a dying technique. This method of tinting cannot be applied to PMMA lenses, as it causes deformation of the lens.

Polycarbonate

Polycarbonate is a thermoplastic material which, when polymerized, forms long polymer chains independent of one another. This allows the material to be reformed and gives greater impact resistance. Polycarbonate lenses are made by injection moulding under high pressure (Fowler & Petre Latham 2001). This has the highest impact resistance of all lens materials (**Fig. 29.10**) and the lightest lens material available (specific gravity 1.2). When made for industrial purposes, polycarbonate lenses will be thicker than standard versions. For example, safety spectacles

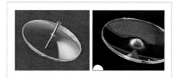

Figure 29.10 Impressive examples of impact resistance of polycarbonate lenses. The image on the left shows a nail driven though a polycarbonate lens. The polycarbonate lens on the right demonstrates its ability to withstand an 8 mm steel ball travelling at over 90 mph. (Reproduced by kind permission of The Norville Group Ltd.)

with polycarbonate lenses that fulfil the regulations for low-energy impact (grade F) are often made with a minimum centre thickness of 3 mm. A general-purpose polycarbonate spectacle lens, however, will have a centre thickness of around 1.5 mm (Fowler & Petre Latham 2001). Unfortunately, polycarbonate lenses have a very soft surface, which is easily abraded, and hard coatings are often used. However, scratch-resistant coatings decrease the impact resistance of polycarbonate lenses substantially (Chou & Hovis 2006), but even a coated polycarbonate lens is several times more impact resistant than a thermosetting plastic lens.

Polycarbonate is commonly used for plano eye protectors where the lenses and front are made in one piece by injection moulding.

Advantages

- Polycarbonate has a much greater impact resistance than heat-toughened glass. If the lens does fracture upon impact, it cracks; it does not break into particles.
- There is no age-related warping, chipping, or discoloration.
- Polycarbonate has a fairly high refractive index (1.586).
- The material absorbs UV radiation.

Disadvantages

- Compared with glass or CR39, the surface quality of polycarbonate is poor.
- Polycarbonate lenses can be tinted only by a vacuum coating process.
- The V-value (measure of dispersive power) is poor (30) and causes colour fringes. This is most marked when viewing through the periphery of the lens, especially with high-power prescriptions.
- Multiple antireflection and abrasion-resistant coatings can significantly decrease the impact resistance (Chou et al 2005).
- It is very susceptible to attacks from liquids in the hydrocarbons and ketones family, so often unsuitable for chemical hazards. If acetone is used inadvertently to clean polycarbonate lenses, they will discolour and become opaque immediately.

Trivex®

Trivex® is a plastic lens monomer developed by PPG Industries. It is a strong, light and thin material with a very high impact resistance equivalent to polycarbonate. Trivex® is distributed by Hoya as PNX and by Younger Optics as Trilogy®. Trivex material is both thermosetting (like CR39) and thermoplastic (like polycarbonate) and, as a result,

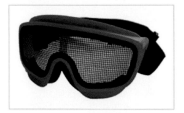

Figure 29.11 Goggles with gauze protection.

combines properties of both. It is more resistant to chemicals than polycarbonate, and can be easily tinted (Norville 2005).

Cellulose acetate

This is only used for basic eye protectors due to its relatively poor impact resistance compared with polycarbonate. However, it does have good resistance to chemical splashes and is more often used for chemical visors and box goggles.

Wire gauze goggles

Goggles made from wire gauze (**Fig. 29.11**) have a very good impact resistance but are rarely used because they impair vision and give no protection against splashes of molten metal, etc. Wire gauze is sometimes found as part of a face shield into which lenses are fitted.

Performance of protective lenses

The lenses used in eye protectors must be tested to establish whether they are suitable for the specific hazard for which they were designed. The following factors may be assessed:

- impact resistance
- surface hardness
- chemical resistance
- thermostability
- flammability
- resistance to hot particles
- radiosensitivity.

Impact resistance

The impact resistance of a lens will be influenced by its thickness and material, as well as the size and speed of the missile/particle. Scratches or abrasions on all types of lenses will reduce the impact resistance. Failure to resist impact takes two forms, which partly depend upon the size of the missile. Large particles (>16 mm) hitting a lens cause it to bend and so the failure is initiated on the back surface. Therefore, any scratches that occur on the front surface due to wear and tear will not have a significant effect on the impact resistance. Smaller particles do not cause the lens to bend upon impact, so the fracture is generally initiated on the front surface. As a result, the impact resistance to smaller particles will be reduced for all types of lenses when the front surface has been abraded (Welsh et al 1974).

In general, as the missile size decreases, the impact resistance of the lens (described as the fracture velocity) increases. When a 3 mm heat-toughened glass lens is hit by a large missile (19.1–28.6 mm) it demonstrates more impact resistance than a CR39 lens of similar thickness. However, when the missile is small (3.2–6.3 mm) the CR39 lens performs best (Chou et al 2005). It has also been shown that for small missiles (<6.4 mm), chemically toughened lenses are not as resistant as heat-toughened lenses, whereas for larger missiles (>6.4 mm) they have a slightly superior performance (Woodward & Melling 1977).

As the lens thickness increases, the impact resistance also increases; impact resistance also increases slightly as the lens is curved. The strength increases with increasing base curve (6.00–10.00 D) with both heat-toughened and CR39 lenses (Wigglesworth 1971).

The type of material used for an eye protector gives an indication of the mean fracture velocity that can be tolerated. Uncoated polycarbonate offers the greatest fracture resistance of all lens materials (Welsh et al 1974).

Hardness

There have been many efforts to study the problems associated with surface abrasion, not all of which represent natural wear and tear. There are distinct advantages in coating plastics lenses, particularly polycarbonate, which is a soft thermoplastic. A thinly coated (5 μm) polycarbonate lens is superior to an uncoated CR39 lens.

Chemical resistance

Glass lenses are resistant to most chemicals. Plastics, however, may show crazing and surface clouding with some strong chemical solutions. CR39 has quite good chemical resistance and is frequently used for chemical visors and box goggle windows.

Thermostability

Polycarbonate and polymethyl methacrylate are prone to distortion more readily than glass under extremes of temperature.

Flammability

All plastic materials are flammable. However, as their ignition temperatures are high, they are still considered safe for use.

Resistance to hot particles

Eye protectors must be able to withstand hot particles impinging upon them, as can occur in such processes as grinding or welding. A glass surface is very easily pitted by these particles, as they fuse with the surface. Plastics, on the other hand, do not pit easily. This is possibly due to the elasticity of the surface when heated by the particle.

Radiosensitivity

This is a feature of the lens material which can become important in the case of lens fracture and intraocular penetration of lens fragments. A series of X-rays taken from different angles may locate the particle(s). Glass fragments greater than 0.5 mm can be observed by X-ray techniques, but plastics particles are very difficult to find. **Table 29.2** compares lens material types for performance against these features.

Table 29.2 A comparison of the properties of glazing materials for eye protectors

Material	Impact resistance		Hardness	Chemical resistance	Thermostability	Fracture pattern	Resistance to hot particles	Weight
	Large missile	Small missile						
Glass								
Heat-toughened	Good	Good	Good	Very good	Very good	Fair	Poor	Heaviest
Chemically toughened	Good	Poor	Good	Very good	Very good	Fair	Poor	Heavy
Plastics								
PMMA	Fair	Fair	Poor	Good	Fair	Good	Very good	Light
CR39	Good	Good	Fair	Good	Good	Fair	Good	Light
Polycarbonate	Very good	Very good	Poor	Fair	Good	Very good	Good	Light

Modified from Grundy 1987, courtesy of J Grundy and Optometry Today.

Eye protectors for sports

As mentioned in the introduction to this chapter, an increasing number of serious eye injuries are resulting from sports. In the USA, it is estimated that these eye injuries account for clinical care in excess of US$175 million per year. Regular spectacles offer very little protection from flying objects; indeed, ocular trauma from the spectacles themselves, with the current trend for smaller frames, may complicate matters (Clarke et al 2002). In the UK, flying and motor sports have regulations for participants, and eye protection is mandatory in ice hockey, horse racing, for bobsleigh drivers, fencing, squash juniors (<19 years of age) and doubles. For further information refer to current texts (Loran & MacEwen 1995) and UK practitioners should refer to the Members Handbook and website provided by the Association of Optometrists (http://www.aop.org.uk/services/services_visual.html).

The following recommendations have been made regarding eye protectors for sports:

- Guidelines for frames
  - lightweight frame but resistant to strong impact
  - fitted with curl sides
  - fitted with an elasticated sports band
  - metal frames should be fitted with a padded bridge.
- Guidelines for lenses
  - made of impact-resistant plastics, preferably polycarbonate
  - glass lenses should be avoided
  - for indoor use, lenses should not be tinted and should have an antireflection coat
  - for outdoor use, it is recommended that ultraviolet protection in spectacle and contact lenses should be integral
  - where contact lenses are worn, eye protection should be used over them to prevent loss, dryness, or complications through ocular trauma.

Squash in particular is recognized as a significant cause of severe ocular trauma, and the 'British Standard for Eye protectors for Racket Sports – Part 1 Squash', BS7930–1 was published in 1998. Since that date, numerous manufacturers have submitted their eye protectors for testing. The standard applies to safety eyewear with polycarbonate oculars (including prescription lenses, but not over existing spectacles): the test procedure is that the appliance has to withstand a yellow dot squash ball at 40 m/s. It has been recommended that open eye guards should not be used for racket sports as the ball changes its shape in motion and flattens, so that it makes contact with the eye through the guard. In addition, frames with flexible hinges are not sufficiently rigid to prevent the frame hitting the eye if a racket or ball strikes it (Napier et al 1996).

Cricketers are required to wear head and face protection during batting (BS 7298: 1998; Specification for head protection for cricketers), which in turn provides essential protection from blow-out fractures and globe contusion injuries.

Current UK legal requirements and safety standards

Optometrists should be aware of current legislation in the particular state or country where they practise, and there is a need to keep up to date with such rules and regulations. In the USA, the OSHA is responsible for development and enforcement of standards (www.osha.gov), but this section outlines the current standards surrounding eye protection in the UK.

The two regulations of particular relevance to eye protection in the UK are the Management of Health and Safety at Work Regulations 1992, and the Personal Protective Equipment at Work Regulations 1992, which both were introduced via statutory instruments (SIs) under the Health and Safety at Work Act 1974.

The Management of Health and Safety at Work Regulations 1992

This legislation requires employers to identify and assess the risks to health and safety present in the workplace. Then the most appropriate method of reducing the risks to an acceptable level can be decided. The regulations clearly state that the provision of *personal protective equipment* (PPE) should be viewed as a last resort, and that risks should be controlled by other means wherever possible. For example, a fixed shield placed in front of a grinding wheel could provide more efficient protection against flying particles than eye protectors.

Personal Protective Equipment at Work Regulations

The Personal Protective Equipment at Work Regulations 1992 were amended and consolidated in 2002 (SI 1144, 2002). The regulations cover protective clothing, e.g. fluorescent vests, gloves and footwear, and protective equipment, e.g. life jackets and eye protectors. The PPE regulations are divided into 2 parts: Part 1 includes 13 regulations about PPE and Part 2 aims to assist employers with their responsibilities for selection, use and maintenance of PPE, as shown in **Table 29.3**.

Table 29.3 Personal Protective Equipment Regulations 1992

Part 1	
Regulation 1	Citation & commencement – 1st January 1993
Regulation 2	Interpretation
Regulation 3	Disapplication of these regulations
Regulation 4	Provision of personal protective equipment
Regulation 5	Compatibility of personal protective equipment
Regulation 6	Assessment of personal protective equipment
Regulation 7	Maintenance & replacement of personal protective equipment
Regulation 8	Accommodation for personal protective equipment
Regulation 9	Information, instruction and training
Regulation 10	Use of personal protective equipment
Regulation 11	Reporting loss or defect
Regulation 12	Exemption certificates
Regulation 13	Extension outside Great Britain
Part 2: Selection, use and maintenance of personal protective equipment	
	Head protection
	Eye protection
	Foot protection
	Hand & arm protection
	Protective clothing for the body
Appendices	

PPEs: Part 1

It is the responsibility of employers to make sure that any PPE supplied to their employees is appropriate for the risks concerned.

The employer must

- Identify the hazard/s present, such as chemicals, flying particles or radiation sources.
- Assess the degree of risk, for example the probable size and velocity of any flying particles.
- Select a suitable type of PPE from the range of 'CE' marked equipment (indicating that the equipment has a certificate of conformity from the 'European Community').
- Ensure that PPE should fit correctly, after adjustment if necessary.
- Ensure that where more than one type of PPE is necessary, they are compatible and remain effective against the risks.

Maintenance of PPE

The PPE should be maintained so that it continues to provide the protection required. This may include cleaning, examination, replacement, repair and testing. A stock of spare parts, when appropriate, should be made available to the wearers.

Use of PPE

The regulations also require employers to provide suitable information, instruction and training, so that effective use of PPE will be made by the employees. They must be trained in the correct use of the equipment and how to correctly fit, wear and store it. Employees also have a responsibility to wear PPE provided and to report any loss or defect to the employer as soon as possible.

PPEs: Part 2

Part 2 of the regulations (the actual selection, use and maintenance of PPE) lists the various types of ocular hazard as:

- impact
- splashes from chemicals or molten metal
- liquid droplets
- dusts
- gases
- welding arcs
- non-ionizing radiation
- laser.

The types of eye protection listed include:

- safety spectacles
- eye shields (one piece)
- safety goggles
- face shields.

Actual maintenance of PPE

Advice regarding the maintenance of PPE includes wet and dry cleaning. Dry cleaning involves the removal of grit with a brush and use of a silicone-treated, non-woven cloth to wipe the lenses (note: polycarbonate and other plastics lenses should not be dry cleaned). Anti-static and anti-fog lens solutions may be required; scratched or pitted lenses should be replaced, and suitable storage cases should be used for eye protectors.

The UK Health and Safety Executive (HSE) has published guidance on the PPE regulations (PPE Regulations Guidance L25, 2005). It states each regulation and then a section on guidance is given, which can be very helpful to optometrists (employers should consult the actual regulations).

EN and BS standards

The regulations relating to eye protection in the workplace are now taken as the European Normals, more commonly known as the BS EN standard, of which EN 166 Personal Eye Protection (PEP) is one of the most relevant to optometrists. Other standards, particularly those for sport, remain under the guidance of the British Standards Institute (adopting the BS prefix).

Guidance about British and European standards is available from British Standards (www.bsi.org.uk).

Relevant standards include:

- BS EN 165 PEP – Vocabulary
- *BS EN 166 Personal eye protection – Specifications*
- BS EN 167 PEP – Optical test methods
- BS EN 168 PEP – Non-optical test methods
- BS EN 169 PEP – Filters for welding
- BS EN 170 PEP – Ultraviolet filters
- BS EN 171 PEP – Infrared filters
- BS EN 172 – Sun glare filters for industrial use
- BS EN 174 PEP – Ski goggles for downhill skiing
- BS EN 175 PEP – Equipment for eye and face protection during welding and allied processes
- BS EN 207 – Filters and eye protectors against laser radiation
- BS EN 208 – Eye protectors for adjustment work on lasers
- BS EN 379 – Welding filters with transmittance variable by time and zone
- BS EN 13178 PEP – Eye protectors for snowmobile users
- BS 7930 (1998) Eye protectors for racket sports Part 1 – Squash
- BS 4110 (1979) Eye protectors for vehicle users
- BS 7298 (1998) Specification for head protection for cricketers
- BS 7028 (1999) Eye protection for industrial and other uses. Guidance on selection, use and maintenance
- BS EN 1836 – Sunglasses and sunglare filters for general use

Markings and symbols on personal eye protectors

Protective spectacles are looked upon as a complete unit, and therefore both frames and lenses must be marked with the relevant standard, class of protection and manufacturing mark to ensure they are traceable. Any PPE supplied in the workplace must comply with current UK legislation incorporating the relevant EC directives concerning design and manufacture (listed in Schedule 1 of the Regulations). Most PPE must be certified (CE marked; certificate of conformity) to demonstrate that an independent inspection body has ensured the PPE meets the basic safety requirements. It is illegal for suppliers to sell PPE without the 'CE' mark. The CE mark should appear somewhere on the product. Even where sunglasses are supplied for general use, a CE mark must appear to guarantee required standards of protection. In the case of personal protective equipment (PPE), the numbers after the CE marking refer to a Notified Body which has been involved in the examination of the product according to the PPE Directive 89/686/EEC. The presence of numbers indicates that the product is a complex design intended for protection against hazards which present a risk of mortal danger or irreversible harm.

A distinctive KITEMARK symbol on protective spectacles in the UK indicates that the manufacturer is licensed and assessed on a regular basis by an independent test authority (i.e. the British Standards Institute), who audit the manufacturing system to confirm compliance with the relevant British/EU standard (Norville 2005).

The following standards specify the markings or symbols that should be found on PEP appropriate to the hazard and the protection they give. Ideally, when presented with an item of PEP, an optometrist should be able to recognize the intended level of protection.

Markings on the ocular (lens or 'window')

These should occur in a particular order, shown in **Table 29.4**.

Filters

The first number refers to the type of *filter* that may be present in the eye protector, and these numbers are specified in the relevant standards (BS EN 169, 170, 171 and 172). Filters for welding just have a shade number, but filters for ultraviolet (UV) and infrared (IR) have two numbers: a code and a shade number. A code number of 2 or 3 is relevant to UV protection, whereas codes of 4, 5 or 6 pertain to infrared protection (**Table 29.5**).

Ultraviolet and infrared radiation

BS EN 170 and BS EN 171 deal with filters for protection against ultraviolet and infrared radiation, respectively. The selection of filters for protection against infrared radiation is made according to the mean temperature of the source.

Table 29.4 Order of markings or symbols on the ocular

Order of ocular marking	Symbol
Filter scale number (where appropriate)	Combination of *code* (2 to 6) & *shade* number (1.1 to 16)
Manufacturer's identification mark	
Optical class	1, 2, or 3
Symbol for mechanical strength	S, F, B, or A
Symbol for non-adherence of hot metal/hot solid	9
Symbol for resistance to surface damage by fine particles	K
Symbol for resistance to fogging	N

Table 29.5 Filter codes used on safety lenses

Filter code number	Filter property
(no code number)	Welding filters
2	UV filters where colour recognition may be affected
3	UV filters with good colour recognition
4	IR filter
5	Sunglare filter without IR specification
6	Sunglare filter with IR specification

When the level of radiation is very high, filters with reflective surface treatment are recommended for IR protection because the reflection permits a smaller rise in filter temperature. **Table 29.6** shows the filter codes pertaining to the application level of infrared radiation. Filter codes and their specificity will be found within the documents BS EN 170 and 171.

Sunglare
Filters for protection against industrial sunglare listed in EN 172 have code number 5 and 6 for without and with infrared specification, respectively, and the shade numbers range from 1.1 to 4.1.

Table 29.6 BS EN 171 – filters for protection against infrared radiation

BS EN 171: code & scale number	Typical application in terms of mean temperature sources, °C
4 – 1.2	Up to 1050
4 – 1.4	1070
4 – 1.7	1090
4 – 2	1110
4 – 2.5	1140
4 – 3	1210
4 – 4	1290
4 – 5	1390
4 – 6	1500
4 – 7	1650
4 – 8	1800
4 – 9	2000
4 – 10	2150

Welding
BS EN169 specifies a range of permanent filter shades of gradually increasing optical density which limit exposure to radiation emitted by different welding processes at different currents. The filters need to provide protection against ultraviolet, intense visible and infrared radiation. BS EN 379 defines requirements for the photosensitive variable-density lenses that are now available. Generally speaking, the higher the current applied, the higher the shade number required. Readers are advised to obtain copies of the relevant standards for their own reference. It should be remembered that anyone working regularly within 2 m of a welding arc needs to be protected against skin and eye exposure in the same way as the welder. Tinted anti-flash safety spectacles (scale number 1.2–4 for example) can be obtained from specialist suppliers for this purpose.

Optical class of ocular

The *optical class* of the ocular falls into one of three categories according to optical tolerance (**Table 29.7**). For appliances incorporating an optical correction, Class 3 would not be permitted.

Mechanical strength of ocular

Table 29.8 shows how the symbol indicates the type of protection afforded by the ocular. 'Increased robustness' is defined by the ability of the oculars to withstand the impact of a 22 mm diameter steel ball weighing 43 g travelling at 5.1 m/s.

Newer symbols on oculars (BS EN 2002)

- **R** Enhanced resistance to IR (reflects 60% IR 700–2000 nm)
- **0** Original lens
- ▼ Replacement lens
- **T** Placed after impact resistance code letter means protection against extreme temperature (55°C to −5°C).

Examples of symbols on oculars

- **12** ® **1** denotes a welding filter and optical class 1
- **3–1.7** ® **1** denotes an ultra violet filter and optical class 1
- ® **3 B N** denotes optical class 3, medium-energy impact and non-fogging properties
- ® **S K** denotes increased robustness and resistance top damage by fine particles

(® represents the manufacturer's mark).

Table 29.7 Optical class of ocular tolerances

Optical class	Spherical refractive power $(D_1+D_2)/2m^{-1}$	Astigmatic refractive power $|D_1-D_2|m^{-1}$	Difference in prismatic refractive power cm/m		
			Horizontal		Vertical
			Base-out	Base-in	
1	±0.06	0.06	0.75	0.25	0.25
2	±0.12	0.12	1.00	0.25	0.25
3	±0.12−0.25	0.25	1.00	0.25	0.25

Note: D_1 and D_2 are the refractive powers in the two principal meridians. For optical class 3, the axes of the principal meridians shall be the parallel within ±10°.

Table 29.8 Mechanical strength grading of oculars in personal eye protectors

Symbol	Mechanical strength grading
S	Increased robustness
F	Low-energy impact
B	Medium-energy impact
A	High-energy impact
9	Non-adherence of molten metal & resistance to penetration of hot solids
K	Resistance to damage by fine particles
N	Non-fogging properties

Symbols on the lens housing

The housing must also be marked as well as the oculars to indicate the protection that it provides. The markings must be given in the order:

- identification of manufacturer
- the standard number (EN166)
- the field of intended use (3, 4, 5, 8, 9)
- symbol of resistance to high-speed particles (-F, -B, -A)
- fit small head (H)
- two scale numbers: range which housing can be used
- use underwater (W)
- resistant to radiant heat (G)

Field of intended use

Table 29.9 indicates the coding used on the frame to denote suitability.

Mechanical strength of housing

A minimum standard of 'increased robustness' for the lens housing means that the 'unmounted' eye protector must withstand the impact of a 22 mm diameter steel ball weighing 43 g travelling at 5.1 m/s. Resistance to particles at greater speed is shown in **Table 29.10** (6 mm diameter steel ball, 0.86 g).

Examples of frame/housing markings:

- ® BS EN 166 3 9 -B denotes protection against liquids (droplets or splashes), molten metals and hot solids, medium-energy impacts

Table 29.9 BS EN 166 – symbols to indicate field of use

Symbol	Designation	Field of use
No symbol	Basic use	
3	Liquids	Liquid droplets or splashes
4	Large dust particles	>5 µm
5	Gas & fine dust particles	Gases, vapours, sprays, smoke & dust particles <5 µm
8	Short-circuit electric arc	Electric arc due to short circuit in electrical equipment
9	Molten metals & hot solids	Splashes of molten metals & penetration of hot solids

Table 29.10 BS EN 166 – grades of impact resistance on lens housing

Resistance to high-speed particles

Symbol	Level of impact resistance	Types of eye protector
-F	Low energy 45 m/s	All types
-B	Medium energy 120 m/s	Goggles & face shields
-A	High energy 190 m/s	Face shields

- ® BS EN 166 4 denotes protection against large dust particles
- ® BS EN 166 -F denotes protection against low-energy-impact particles

(® represents the manufacturers mark).

A summary of the markings found on PEP is given in **Table 29.11**.

Table 29.11 Summary of the markings found on the main types of eye protectors

	BS EN 166		Type of eye protector			
	Housing	Oculars	Spectacles	Goggles	Face shields	
Optical class						
		1	Yes	Yes	Yes	
		2	Yes	Yes	Yes	
		3	Yes	Yes		
Mechanical strength						
Increased robustness		S	Yes	Yes	Yes	
Low-energy impact	-F	F	Yes	Yes	Yes	
Medium-energy impact	-B	B		Yes	Yes	
High-energy impact	-A	A			Yes	
Field of use						
Liquid droplets/ splashes	3			Yes	Yes	
Large dust particles	4			Yes		
Gas, fine dust particles	5			Yes		
Short-circuit electric arc	8				Yes	
Molten metals/ hot solids	9	9		Yes	Yes	
Resistance to fogging		N	Yes	Yes	Yes	
Resistance to surface damage		K	Yes	Yes	Yes	

Conclusion

To summarize, this chapter has outlined the causes of eye injuries and the various types of eye protectors available. It is important to note that whilst various regulations and standards relating to eye protection have been presented here, the relevant documentation should always be consulted for full, up-to-date information.

References

Alfaro D V 3rd, Jablon E P, Rodriguez Fontal M et al 2005 Fishing-related ocular trauma. American Journal of Ophthalmology 13: 488–492

Barr A, Baines P S, Desai P et al 2000 Ocular sports injuries: the current picture. British Journal of Sports Medicine 34:456–458

Canavan Y M, O'Flaherty M J, Archer D B et al 1980 A 10-year survey of eye injuries in Northern Ireland, 1967–76. British Journal of Ophthalmology 64:618–625

Capao Filipe J A, Rocha-Sousa A, Falcao-Reis F et al 2003 Modern sports eye injuries. British Journal of Ophthalmology 87:1336–1339

Chaudhry I A, Al-Sharif A M, Hamdi M 2005 Severe ocular trauma caused by an ostrich. British Journal of Ophthalmology 89:250–251

Chiapella A P, Rosenthal A R 1985 One year in an eye casualty clinic. British Journal of Ophthalmology 69:865–870

Chou B R, Hovis J K 2003 Durability of coated CR-39 industrial lenses. Optometry and Vision Science 80:703–707

Chou B R, Hovis J K 2006 Effect of multiple antireflection coatings on impact resistance of Hoya Phoenix spectacle lenses. Clinical and Experimental Optometry 89:86–89

Chou B R, Gupta A, Hovis J K 2005 The effect of multiple antireflective coatings and center thickness on resistance of polycarbonate spectacle lenses to penetration by pointed missiles. Optometry and Vision Science 82:964–969

Clarke J, Newsom R, Canning C 2002 Ocular trauma with small framed spectacles. British Journal of Ophthalmology 86:484

Cole M D, Clearkin L, Dabbs T et al 1987 The seat belt law and after. British Journal of Ophthalmology 71:436–440

Department of Trade and Industry 2002 (Ed, database, Home and Leisure Accident Surveillance System) Royal Society for the Prevention of Accidents

Desai P, MacEwen C J, Baines P et al 1996a Epidemiology and implications of ocular trauma admitted to hospital in Scotland. Journal of Epidemiology and Community Health 50:436–441

Desai P, MacEwen C J, Baines P et al 1996b Incidence of cases of ocular trauma admitted to hospital and incidence of blinding outcome. British Journal of Ophthalmology 80:592–596

Farr A K, Fekrat S 1998 Eye injuries associated with paintball guns. International Ophthalmology 22:169–173

Finch C, Vear P 1998 What do adults squash players think about protective eyewear? British Journal of Sports Medicine 32:155–161

Fong L P 1995 Eye injuries in Victoria, Australia. Medical Journal of Australia 162:64–68

Fowler C W, Petre Latham K 2001 Spectacle lenses: theory and practice. Butterworth-Heinemann, Oxford

Good G W, Weaver J L, Hitzeman S A et al 2006 Eye safety – You can make the difference. Optometry – Journal of the American Optometric Association 77:201–204

Goyal S, Choong Y F, Aclimandos W A et al 2004 Penetrating ocular trauma from an exploding microwaved egg. British Medical Journal 328:1075

Grundy J W 1982 Eye protectors constructed with metal spectacle frames. Ophthalmic Optician: July 550–552

Grundy J W 1987 A diagrammatic approach to occupational optometry and illumination; Part 3: Industrial hazards and eye protection. Optometry Today 12:562–564

Jalie M 1999 Ophthalmic lenses and dispensing. Butterworth-Heinemann, Oxford

Johnson P B, Armstrong M F J 1986 Eye injuries in Northern Ireland two years after seat belt legislation. British Journal of Ophthalmology 70:460–462

Jones N P 1988 One year of severe eye injuries in sport. Eye 2(Pt 5):484–487

Loran D, MacEwen C J 1995 Sports vision. Butterworth-Heinemann, Oxford

MacEwen C J 1987 Sport associated eye injury: a casualty department survey. British Journal of Ophthalmology 71:701–705

MacEwen C J 1989 Eye injuries: a prospective survey of 5671 cases. British Journal of Ophthalmology 73:888–894

MacEwen C J, Baines P S, Desai P 1999 Eye injuries in children: the current picture. British Journal of Ophthalmology 83:933–936

McGwin G Jr, Owsley C 2005a Incidence of emergency department-treated eye injury in the United States. Archives of Ophthalmology 123:662–666

McGwin G Jr, Owsley C 2005b Risk factors for motor vehicle collision-related eye injuries. Archives of Ophthalmology 123:89–95

Mela E K, Dvorak G J, Mantzouranis G A et al 2005 Ocular trauma in a Greek population: review of 899 cases resulting in hospitalization. Ophthalmic Epidemiology 12:185–190

Morris D S 2006 Ocular blunt trauma: loss of sight from an ice hockey injury. British Journal of Sports Medicine 40:5

Napier S M, Baker R S, Sanford D G et al 1996 Eye injuries in athletics and recreation. Survey of Ophthalmology 41:229–244

Negrel A D, Thylefors B 1998 The global impact of eye injuries. Ophthalmic Epidemiology 5:143–169

Niiranen M, Raivio I 1981 Eye injuries in children. British Journal of Ophthalmology 65:436–438

Norville Prescription Companion 2005 Online. Available: http://www.norville.co.uk//pdfs/Companion05.pdf January 2006

Pardhan S, Shacklock P, Weatherill J 1995 Sport-related eye trauma: a survey of the presentation of eye injuries to a casualty clinic and the use of protective eye-wear. Eye 9(Pt 6 Suppl):50–53

Parver L M 1986 Eye trauma. The neglected disorder. Archives of Ophthalmology 104:1452–1453

Pearlman J A, Au Eong K G, Kuhn F et al 2001 Airbags and eye injuries: epidemiology, spectrum of injury, and analysis of risk factors. Survey of Ophthalmology 46:234–242

Rousell D 1979 Eye protection. Publication No. 1S126, obtainable from: the Royal Society for the Prevention of Accidents, Cannon House, The Priory, Queensway, Birmingham

Schein O D, Hibberd P L, Shingleton B J et al 1988 The spectrum and burden of ocular injury. Ophthalmology 95:300–305

Stewart R M K, Durnian J M, Briggs M C 2006 'Here's egg in your eye': a prospective study of blunt ocular trauma resulting from thrown eggs. Emergency Medicine Journal 23:756–758

Vernon S A 1983 Analysis of all new cases seen in a busy regional centre ophthalmic casualty department during 24-week period. Journal of the Royal Society of Medicine 76:279–282

Weitgasser U, Wackernagel W, Oetsch K 2004 Visual outcome and ocular survival after sports related ocular trauma in playing golf. Journal of Trauma 56:648–650

Welsh K W, Miller J W, Kislin B et al 1974 Ballistic impact testing of scratched and unscratched ophthalmic lenses. American Journal of Optometry and Physiological Optics 51:304–311

Whitcher J P, Srinivasan M 1997 Corneal ulceration in the developing world – a silent epidemic. British Journal of Ophthalmology 81:622–623

Whitcher J P, Srinivasan M, Upadhyay M P 2001 Corneal blindness: a global perspective. Bulletin of the World Health Organization 79:214–221

Wigglesworth E C 1971 The impact resistance of eye-protector lens materials. American Journal of Optometry Archives of the American Academy of Optometry 48:245–261

Wong T Y, Klein B E, Klein R 2000 The prevalence and 5-year incidence of ocular trauma. Ophthalmology 107:2196–2202

Woodward A, Melling R 1977 Glass, the basic material. Ophthalmic Optician March:231–233

Wykes W N 1988 A 10-year survey of penetrating eye injuries in Gwent, 1976–85. British Journal of Ophthalmology 72:607–611

CHAPTER 30

Low vision

Jan Lovie-Kitchin

Introduction

The care of low-vision patients is termed vision rehabilitation, and optometrists have an essential role to play in the provision of vision rehabilitation services. Ideally, if patients stay with one optometrist or practice, their low-vision care becomes part of a continuum of eye care, from the time when they had normal vision. If progressive vision loss occurs, the role of the optometrist changes from primary eye care only to one of monitoring vision loss and gradually introducing low-vision care, especially magnification and advice on lighting and contrast, in conjunction with other vision rehabilitation professionals.

Defining the low-vision population

As the world population increases and there is a growing predominance of the older age groups, the number of people at risk of visual impairment continues to increase (World Health Organization 2004). In addition, the prevalence of chronic, age-related eye diseases, particularly age-related macular degeneration, appears to be increasing at a rate greater than the ageing population would suggest (Evans & Wormald 1996; Congdon et al 2004). Thus, in coming years more services for people with low vision will be needed.

What is low vision?

In the 2006–2011 Action Plan for Vision 2000, Global Initiative for the Elimination of Blindness, the World Health Organization (2007), together with the International Agency for the Prevention of Blindness, defined a person who could benefit from low-vision services as follows:

> A person with low vision is someone who, after medical, surgical and/or optical intervention, has a corrected visual acuity in the better eye of <6/18, down to and including light perception, or a central visual field of <20 degrees, but who uses or has the potential to use vision for the planning and/or execution of a task.

This definition is termed 'functional low vision', to distinguish it from a definition based on visual acuity alone. The important aspect for optometrists is that anyone with measurable vision is potentially able to be assisted through optometric low-vision care. Even those with visual acuity better than 6/18 (20/60) might need some low-vision care, and those with no measurable vision can be assisted through referral to other rehabilitation services.

The recommendation contained in the International Classification of Functioning and Disability (ICIDH-2), based on the tenth revision of the International Classification of Diseases (ICD-10) (World Health Organization 2001), formalized the relationship between body functions and structure, activity and participation (**Table 30.1**). It is useful to consider low vision and the different dimensions of vision functioning in these terms. This then indicates the impacts of vision loss and different optometric or rehabilitation services required at different points of the vision functioning spectrum.

Table 30.1 Relationships between disorder, impairment, activity limitation and participation restriction

DIMENSION	Description	Level of functioning
DISORDER (Disease, Injury, Anomaly) ↓	A deviation from normal structure	
IMPAIRMENT (of Body Function or Structure) ↓	Organ function, e.g. visual acuity or visual field	Body (vision)
ACTIVITY LIMITATION (formerly Disability) ↓	To perform a certain task, e.g. read, write, orientation & mobility	Individual (person's daily activities)
PARTICIPATION RESTRICTION (formerly Handicap)	Manner or extent of involvement in life situations; this is related to individual and society responses	Society (life situations)

It should be noted that, in 2009, the term 'low vision' will be deleted from the tenth revision of the ICD (ICD-10), leaving the terms 'moderate visual impairment (presenting visual acuity of <6/18 to 6/60)' and 'severe visual impairment (<6/60 to 3/60)' (World Health Organization 2007).

Patients with low vision present because of limitations with everyday activities (describing their vision disability). All optometrists are expert at assessing the ocular disease and the visual functions (disorder and impairment). When working with a person with low vision, the optometrist needs to expand on these experiences to assist the person to continue functioning independently.

Classification of vision performance

Leat et al (1999) reviewed the common measures of visual functions, visual acuity, visual fields and contrast sensitivity, in an attempt to define the levels of vision loss which constitute vision impairment (or low vision) and vision disability. As they and others (e.g. Colenbrander 1994; Rubin et al 1994) have observed, there are few studies which provide normative data for the common visual functions and even fewer which indicate the level of vision impairment likely to cause disabilities in common tasks. However, based on previous studies and the author's own clinical and research experience, **Table 30.2** provides a basis for classifying vision performance in terms of impairment, disability and handicap. The assessment of each of these visual functions is discussed below.

Distribution of low vision

The distribution of low vision varies considerably with age, gender and geographical region, but the majority of vision-impaired people are aged 50 years and over (World Health Organization 2004). Various studies have consistently shown that vision impairment is more prevalent in females than males (Attebo et al 1996; Elliott et al 1997; Taylor et al 1997). The main causes of vision loss in developed countries are cataract, age-related macular degeneration (AMD), glaucoma and diabetic retinopathy, with AMD being the most common cause of permanent vision loss (Taylor et al 2005).

In developed countries, the prevalence of blindness and low vision among children is low, but the length of time they live with low vision is considerably longer and therefore the cost to society is higher than for adults with low vision. Children aged 0–15 years constitute between about 3% and 7% of the world's total low-vision population (Resnikoff et al 2004).

Low-vision assessment

The purpose of any vision assessment depends on the patients and their current vision status. The purpose may be:

- to detect vision loss
- to diagnose the cause of a vision loss
- to monitor progressive vision loss, and/or
- to predict functional impairment and inform vision rehabilitation (Lovie-Kitchin & Feigl 2005).

Assessment for vision rehabilitation differs fundamentally from assessment for diagnosis and management of the ocular disorder. The objective of diagnostic assessment is to identify and characterize the cause of a vision loss, so that, if possible, the disorder may be corrected or treated so that further deterioration is prevented. Vision rehabilitation cannot take such a mechanistic approach because functional performance, which is the object of a rehabilitation programme, varies within and across individuals (Whittaker & Lovie-Kitchin 1993).

The assessment procedures outlined below apply to most visually impaired patients irrespective of age or vocational status. In the case of a low-vision child, if possible involve the parent and teacher or special education advisor. Ask the parent or teacher for advice on the best ways of approaching and managing a young child or intellectually handicapped young person. To identify the specific needs of school students or working adults, ask them to bring examples of their work to the consultation. If the adult patient has a spouse, partner or carer, it may be useful to obtain information from that person also, but if possible, allow any patient a private consultation so he or she can speak freely.

First and most importantly, the optometrist must talk with the patient.

Case history

In the management of any patient, careful history-taking and effective communication are the keys to success (see Ch. 26), but this is particularly so for low-vision patients. From listening to the patient the optometrist must:

- understand the patient's wants and needs, i.e. define the patient's goals. There is a need to understand the patient's underlying motivations, e.g. does he/she, in fact, want help or prefer to remain dependent on others?
- gain his/her confidence; be eager to listen and sensitive to his/her difficulties.
- ask open-ended questions, encourage the patient to elaborate.

Table 30.2 Classification of vision performance

(NEAR-) NORMAL		LOW VISION		BLINDNESS		
Normal	Near-normal	Moderate	Severe	Moderate	Severe	Total

VISION IMPAIRMENT

Visual acuity

None	Slight	Moderate	Severe	Profound	Near-total	Total
6/3.8–6/7.5	6/9–6/19	6/24–6/48	6/60–6/120 (3/60)	6/150–6/300 (3/75) (3/150)	LP (<6/300)	NLP
logMAR −0.2–0.1	0.2–0.5	0.6–0.9	1.0–1.3	1.4–1.7	≥1.8	NLP

Visual field (diameter of horizontal field)

None	Slight	Moderate	Severe	Profound	Near-total	Total
≥120°	119–60°	59–25°	24–10°	9–4°	3–1.5°	<1.5° (NLP)

Contrast sensitivity (Pelli–Robson score, log CS)

None	Slight	Moderate	Severe	Profound	Near-total	Total
>1.60	1.60–1.30	1.25–0.95	0.90–0.60	0.55–0.25	0.20–0.05	0(NLP)

ACTIVITY LEVEL (VISION DISABILITY)

(NEAR-) NORMAL		LOW VISION		BLINDNESS		
Normal	Near-normal	Moderate	Severe	Moderate	Severe	Total
Can perform all visual tasks		Needs devices for detailed visual tasks		Needs devices/other senses for gross visual tasks		
		Near-normal with devices	Limited with devices	Devices as adjunct	Vision as adjunct	No vision

PARTICIPATION (VISION HANDICAP)

(NEAR-) NORMAL		LOW VISION		BLINDNESS		
Normal	Near-normal	Moderate	Severe	Moderate	Severe	Total
Can meet own or society expectations visually				Cannot meet own or society expectations visually		
Meets all		Meets most	Meets many	Fails many visually	Fails most visually	Fails all visually

Adapted from Colenbrander 1977, 1994; Johnston 1991; Rubin et al 1994; Leat et al 1999.

- continue history-taking throughout the examination.
- summarize his/her conclusions out loud to the patient to demonstrate an accurate grasp of the problems.

The case history of the low-vision patient needs to cover each of the dimensions listed in **Table 30.1**.

Ocular disorder and vision impairment

Information about the patient's medical, ocular and family history and previous treatments, including low-vision devices, will guide the optometrist in forming a diagnosis and developing a treatment programme. This reveals whether the patient understands the nature of the eye condition and has come to terms with having a serious ocular disorder. These matters should be taken into account when the clinician gives advice at the end of the examination. Determine which eye the patient believes has the better vision (which may be based on either their visual acuity or the extent of the visual field).

Activity limitations

The limitations to daily activities are what the patient presents as their chief complaint(s). Endeavour to keep the patient positive and goal oriented. Try to emphasize what the patient can still do while determining what specific tasks the patient is seeking assistance with.

Define the patient's goals

Prioritize the difficulties the patient presents as primary, secondary and other goals. Define these specific goals in objective, behavioural terms (Whittaker & Lovie-Kitchin 1993). The goals should not imply specific means or modality, e.g. 'read the paper like I used to' [visually], as this necessarily constrains the optional paths to the goal. The goal should be defined in terms of both the specific task, e.g. reading, and the performance level required, e.g. reading rate. Objective goal definition also enables the practitioner to determine when a vision rehabilitation programme has been completed and if the outcome is successful. Unfortunately, patients often present without well-defined goals. In this case, the first goal of the vision rehabilitation programme would be to help the patient define specific goals. Some of their goals may require input from other health or rehabilitation professionals.

Look at all interests of the patient, not only work or school, but hobbies, social and other recreational activities, when considering their goals. To help the patient set specific goals or to determine specific functional disabilities with which the optometrist can assist, the optometrist should question the patient on his/her vision performance on a range of visual tasks and illumination difficulties and needs.

- *Distance tasks*: driving; mobility-related tasks such as reading street signs, pedestrian crossings; cinema; sports.
- *Intermediate tasks*: daily activity tasks such as cooking, shopping, watching TV.
- *Near tasks*: 'survival' reading such as medicine and food labels, invoices and personal mail, as well as school, work and recreational reading such as computer screens, textbooks, newspapers, magazines, novels, TV guide.
- *Illumination needs*: under what lighting conditions can the patient see best? Do they have indoor and outdoor glare difficulties? Under what circumstances do they find light and dark adaptation slow or difficult?

Social participation

If the optometrist is going to accept responsibility for advising low-vision patients on all things that have become difficult due to the reduction of vision, then there is a need to ask a wide range of questions about the patient's daily living activities and general lifestyle. This means touching on topics not normally explored in general optometric practice, such as living environment, social support, travelling abilities, social activities, familiarity with rehabilitation services, etc. Many questionnaires have been developed to examine the impact of vision loss on daily functioning and quality of life of people with low vision (Margolis et al 2002; de Boer et al 2004). For example, two recently developed, relatively short questionnaires are the 25-item Low Vision Quality-of-Life questionnaire (Wolffsohn & Cochrane 2000) and the (recently revised) 28-item Impact of Vision Impairment questionnaire (Lamoureux et al 2006). Such questionnaires could be used by the optometrist to examine social participation and quality of life and to indicate when referral to other health, rehabilitation or community services may be needed. Use of a validated questionnaire before and after low-vision care also provides a measure of the outcome of vision rehabilitation.

Ocular health

Knowledge of the cause of vision loss assists in the assessment and management of low vision. For the purpose of this chapter it is assumed that all necessary ocular health testing, including anterior and posterior segment examinations, tonometry, keratometry, etc., has been carried out to determine the underlying cause of the vision loss (see Chs 17 to 19). If medical or surgical treatment is indicated, referral for such treatment should be initiated before proceeding further with vision rehabilitation. Make it clear to the patient that if medical treatment cannot help, other assistance is available so they understand that they must return to the optometrist for on-going care.

Distance visual acuity

An accurate measure of visual acuity (VA) is very important for the optometric management of low-vision patients. The traditional Snellen chart adapts poorly to low-visual-acuity measurement because it is not accurate at the reduced test distances often required (see Ch. 12). In the past, this led eye care practitioners to use tests with no scientific basis for low-visual acuities (unfortunately some still do!). Eleanor Faye in 1976 stated:

> The commonly-used term 'finger-counting' is a vague, negative, inaccurate and careless vision test. A numerical designation for everything except light projection and light perception is more accurate and psychologically more positive for practitioner and patient (Faye 1976).

Charts using uniform letter-spacing and a logarithmic progression of letter sizes such as the Bailey–Lovie charts (Bailey & Lovie 1976) or ETDRS charts (Ferris et al 1982) give accurate and positive measures (**Fig. 30.1**). Portable, externally illuminated charts are preferable to projector charts to allow for easy changes in test distance (it is easier to move the chart than the patient).

For young children who cannot read letters, there is a range of charts available (see Ch. 28). The LH symbol charts follow the Bailey–Lovie principles and can give accurate VA measures for young children (Harper 2004; Hyvarinen 2005).

To create a sense of achievement and give encouragement to the low-vision patient, start with the chart at a close test distance (preferably less than 3 metres). Use test distances that follow the same progression as the letter sizes on the chart, i.e. 6, 4.8, 3.8, 3.0, 2.4 metres (20, 16, 12, 10, 8 feet) etc. If a very close test distance is needed, a plus addition is not necessary as the small amount of blur induced will not significantly affect the low-visual acuity measured.

To ensure obtaining a threshold measure, encourage the patient to guess as they approach their limit of resolution. Give 'permission' to use whatever head and eye positions give best VA (many patients will feel they are 'cheating'). Measure VA for each eye and binocularly, with and without

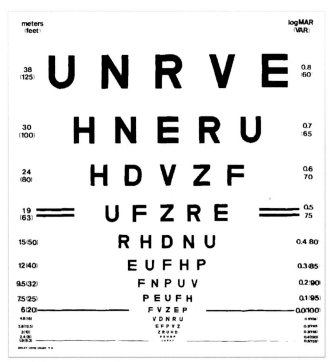

Figure 30.1 The Bailey–Lovie (or ETDRS) distance letter chart is preferred for measuring low visual acuities. These charts are available from the National Vision Research Institute of Australia or the University of California, Berkeley, School of Optometry.

the current spectacles and before and after distance refraction for an accurate assessment of whether the current or new spectacle prescription helps. Note the position of missed letters and the head/eye movements used. These give an indication of the presence and the position of scotomas and the use of eccentric viewing by the patient with a central scotoma. Some coaching on the use of eccentric viewing to see smaller letters can take place during VA testing, e.g. by instructing the patient to look above the letters they are trying to read.

If patients report that they cannot see the largest letters on a chart, always check whether or not they can see smaller letters. Some visual field losses (including hemianopia with macular sparing) may leave small islands of vision which enable small letters to be resolved but not larger ones.

To score VA, record all letters read correctly; letter-by-letter scoring doubles the sensitivity of the VA test to detect changes in vision compared with scoring row-by-row (Bailey et al 1991). It is easiest to score VA using the logMAR notation, with a correction for the reduced viewing distance (**Table 30.3**). However, always convert to the 6 m (20 ft) equivalent Snellen notation and record this for use in all communications with other eye care and health professionals as it is the most widely understood visual acuity notation. **Table 30.3** gives examples of the use of Bailey–Lovie-style charts for measurements of low visual acuities. Work through these examples with a chart (see **Fig. 30.1**) so that the line labels can be used. Useful facts to remember are that a three-step change represents a factor of two times and 10 steps a factor of 10 times.

Distance refraction

If the patient has been under regular eye care, the spectacle prescription may be up to date and correct, but low-vision refraction requires a little more patience and some modifications to routine procedures (see Ch.14). The aim is to ensure the patient has the best vision possible, so he/she will often need to use head and eye movements, which should be observed by the examiner. This can only be done using a trial frame or lens clips for over-refraction (preferred), rather than a phoropter (**Fig. 30.2**).

Retinoscopy (see Ch. 13), particularly over the current spectacles, is invaluable for refraction of low-vision patients as some patients with quite low acuity will have poor discrimination for subjective refraction. If media opacities make it difficult to obtain a satisfactory reflex, try to get some result by moving closer or off-axis ('radical retinoscopy'; Borish 1975).

For subjective refraction, use the distance letter chart as the test target at a close test distance, i.e. 3 m or less, and letters which the patient can see. Do not use the duochrome test. For spherical refraction, start with very large steps, e.g. ±4 D or ±6 D, which enables the patient to notice differences. Then use bracketing, i.e. excess plus and excess minus, systematically changing the midpoint of the range being bracketed and reducing the size of the bracketing range (Bailey 1991a).

For the astigmatic refraction, use a ±0.50 D hand-held Jackson crossed-cylinder, although higher powers such as ±0.75 D or ±1.00 D might be required for some patients. Again, work in large steps of axis and power. Use the distance chart as the test target, and ask, 'With which view can you read further down the chart?' (Borish 1975).

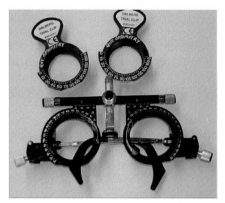

Figure 30.2 Lens clips or a trial frame is recommended for low-vision subjective refraction.

Table 30.3 Examples of the use of charts with logarithmic (geometric) progression of letter sizes for measuring low visual acuities

	CASE A	CASE B	CASE C	CASE D
Viewing distance				
Metres	4.8	3.0	2.4	1.5
Feet	16	10	8	5
Log steps closer than standard 6 m (20 ft) test distance (correction factor)	1 (0.1 log unit)	3 (0.3 log unit) – half the distance	4 (0.4 log unit)	6 (0.6 log unit)
Threshold size the patient reads	0.3 logMAR (labelled 6/12 or 20/40)	0.6 logMAR (labelled 6/24 or 20/80)	0.8 logMAR (labelled 6/38 or 20/125)	0.9 logMAR (labelled 6/48 or 20/160)
Corrected VA (logMAR)	0.3 + 0.1 = 0.4	0.6 + 0.3 = 0.9	0.8 + 0.4 = 1.2	0.9 + 0.6 = 1.5
Equivalent Snellen	6/15 (20/50) (1 line larger than line read)	6/48 (20/160) (double the size read)	6/95 (20/320) (10 times worse than 0.2 logMAR, 6/9.5 or 20/32)	6/150 (20/500) (10 times worse than 0.5 logMAR, 6/15 or 20/50)

Bailey & Lovie 1976.

If one is confident that retinoscopy does not indicate a significant change in prescription (within ±0.50 D), do not waste time on a subjective refraction, as this can become tiring and disheartening for the patient. During subjective refraction, slow down everything one does, to allow the patient time to make judgements. While sometimes slow, patients may be able to discriminate small changes in prescription. Bailey (1991a) recommended making coarse estimates of each component of the prescription (sphere, axis and cylinder power) and then refining one or more times as needed. Significant changes in spectacle correction may be detected through careful retinoscopy and/or subjective refraction if time is taken, where other practitioners in the past may not have done so.

Near vision assessment

Assistance with reading tasks is the most common request from low-vision patients. Thus, assessment of near vision is probably the most important part of the low-vision examination. For low-vision patients, both near VA and reading rate should be assessed.

Near VA

To measure near VA, record both print size, using either M units (Sloan 1959) or point size (see Ch. 12), and viewing distance. Especially for a low-vision patient, print size without the reading distance is not helpful. For example, 1.5M (12 point) print read at 20 cm subtends twice the visual angle (two times worse VA) when compared with the same print size read at 40 cm. Snellen notations should not be used for near, as they can be ambiguous (Bailey 1991b).

Use a reading acuity chart with words or text (**Fig. 30.3**), not letters, with print small enough to determine threshold size. MNRead charts (Ahn et al 1995) or Bailey–Lovie text charts (Cheong et al 2002) with short sentences at uniformly

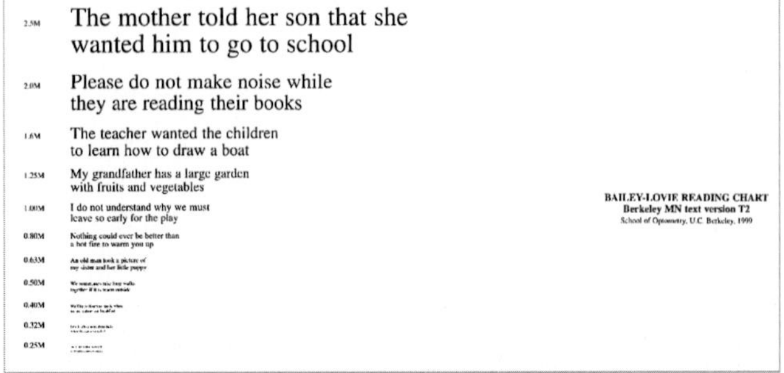

Figure 30.3 Bailey–Lovie text charts for assessing near visual acuity. These charts use sentences from the MNRead corpus (http://vision.psych.umn.edu/~gellab/MNREAD/) and are available from the University of California, Berkeley, School of Optometry Alumni association http://optometry.berkeley.edu/opt_txtpp/alumni/alumni_materials.html

decreasing print sizes are recommended. Note that many commonly used near charts do not have sufficiently small print to measure threshold near resolution for patients with normal vision or low-vision patients using magnification devices. As for distance VA, encourage the patient to read to their limit of resolution. To assess the effects of changes in illumination, test with usual room lighting and then increase and decrease the illumination level (see below).

For children, the McClure Reading Test (Harper 2004) provides reading material of varying difficulty appropriate for various ages, but the smallest print is 5 point (0.6M), which may not be small enough to determine threshold print size for many children with normal or low vision (see Ch. 28).

A useful check for presbyopic patients is to compare the dioptric equivalent of the clearest viewing distance with the current near addition. If they are not approximately equal, this could be indicative of a change in refractive error (especially if the viewing distance is longer than expected, indicating excess minus) or the patient may simply be holding the print closer to enlarge the retinal image (relative distance magnification) and tolerating some blur.

For most patients, text reading acuity is poorer than distance letter acuity because words give a crowding effect (Lovie-Kitchin & Brown 2000). If near VA seems a lot worse than distance VA, a hemianopia or paracentral scotoma is probably impeding reading vision (Lovie-Kitchin et al 2001).

When measuring near VA it is useful to have in mind the print sizes used for common reading tasks for comparison with the patient's threshold print size (**Table 30.4**). For example, reading newsprint is a common task for which patients seek help; the text of most newspapers is 1M or 8 point print (but see Ch. 12), although the contrast is usually lower than most near charts.

As for distance VA, patients with constricted visual fields or with islands of remaining vision within a central scotoma may read small letters or words on a chart but not larger ones. If the patient reads letter by letter rather than whole words, it is likely that a visual field loss is impeding reading.

Reading rate

While reduced reading rate may reflect early cognitive changes in some older people, it may also be one of the first symptoms of vision impairment, before there is noticeable vision loss (Lovie-Kitchin & Feigl 2005). Assessing reading rate may be worthwhile as a possible means of detecting early vision loss in older patients.

In practical terms, it is easiest to assess reading rate (fluency) by simply listening to the patient read print of decreasing sizes (Lovie-Kitchin & Whittaker 2000). At larger print sizes, well above threshold (plenty of acuity in reserve), the patient will read quickly. As he/she approaches threshold print size, reading rate will slow down. The print size one line above the size at which the first noticeable decrease in reading rate is heard (the smallest giving maximum reading rate) is termed the critical print size (Legge et al 1992). The difference between critical print size and threshold print size is the 'acuity reserve' and on average is three lines above threshold, although this varies for patients of different ages and with different causes of low vision

Table 30.4 Print sizes in different notations and their common uses

Points[a](N)	M units[b]	LogMAR at 25 cm	Uses
2.0	0.25	0.0	(Normal near VA at 25 cm)
2.5	0.32	0.1	
3	0.4	0.2	(Normal near VA at 40 cm)
4	0.5	0.3	
5	0.63	0.4	Small ads, bibles
6	0.8	0.5	Telephone book
8	1.0	0.6	Newspaper
10	1.25	0.7	Magazines, books
12	1.6	0.8	Books, type
16	2.0	0.9	Children's books
20	2.5	1.0	Large print books
25	3.2	1.1	
32	4.0	1.2	
40	5.0	1.3	Sub-headlines
48	6.0	1.4	
64	8.0	1.5	
80	10	1.6	
100	12.5	1.7	Headlines

Lovie-Kitchin & Whittaker 1999.
Note: Shaded rows (every 3 lines) indicate multiples of 2× or 0.3 log units.
[a] Point is a printer's measure specifying the distance from the top of the ascending letters to the bottom of the descending letters. One point equals 1/72 inches or 0.0353 mm. The height of a lower-case letter (x height) is usually half the overall point size.
[b] The M unit is the distance in metres at which lower-case letters subtend 5 minutes of arc. The x height of 1M print subtends 5 minutes arc at a distance of 1 metre (Sloan 1959).

(Whittaker & Lovie-Kitchin 1993; Lovie-Kitchin & Whittaker 2000). The acuity reserve and near VA (threshold print size and viewing distance) are most important for calculating the required magnification for reading.

Visual fields

For vision rehabilitation, the visual field assessment is not for diagnostic purposes, but to determine or explain functional abilities. Information on the patient's visual field loss is most important for reading and mobility tasks. Essentially, two questions need to be answered. Is the visual field reduced to the point where mobility might be impaired? Is there a central scotoma which is likely to impede reading? The type of field loss present is largely predictable from the cause of low vision, and this helps direct the type of visual field assessment.

As mobility is a binocular task, logically, visual fields should be assessed binocularly for this purpose. This can be done with a simple confrontation test, but some quantification of the visual field extent is useful, especially when the patient has a condition known to affect the peripheral

visual field such as glaucoma or retinitis pigmentosa (RP). This information may be important in determining the patient's eligibility for welfare payments due to vision impairment, although in this case monocular visual field results are usually required.

When the binocular visual field is constricted to within about 40° of fixation (80° diameter) mobility will first become impaired (Lovie-Kitchin et al 1990, 2002). When the field loss is greater than this, especially if the inferior field is affected, mobility may be significantly impaired and the patient should be referred for an orientation and mobility assessment. Thus, being pragmatic, a central visual field assessment to determine if the field loss is within 30° of fixation (60° diameter) will identify the patient at risk of mobility impairment; peripheral testing is not necessary. If the patient can maintain stable, central fixation, an automated visual field assessment such as the Humphrey Field Analyzer 30–2 programme (see Ch. 20) can be performed binocularly. Turn off the blind spot monitor and monitor fixation by direct observation. If fixation is not stable, this suggests some macular involvement.

Many recent studies have used scanning laser ophthalmoscopy to plot the central field loss accurately in patients with AMD (Fletcher & Schuchard 1997; Schuchard et al 1999; Watson et al 2006) but this is not a clinically available instrument and the detail it provides is more than is needed for vision rehabilitation. The modified tangent screen technique described below is both easier for the patient and less time-consuming.

Information is commonly needed about the quality of the central 15° or 20° (diameter) field as this is most important for reading (Whittaker & Lovie-Kitchin 1993; Lovie-Kitchin & Whittaker 1998a). Visual field assessment for reading purposes should be done monocularly as the close reading distance of low-vision devices often forces monocular reading, while the nature of any central scotoma can provide an indication as to which eye the patient should use for reading.

The use of Amsler charts is not recommended as there are too many false-negative results; i.e. if the patient says everything appears intact, it cannot be assumed there are no central scotomas or disturbances as patients shift fixation and/or cortically interpolate within the field to 'fill in the gaps'.

To quantify the size and position of any 'central' scotomas and to identify the areas of intact field, *a modified tangent screen technique* is recommended (Lovie-Kitchin & Whittaker 1998a). This provides sufficient information on the nature of the visual field loss to make vision rehabilitation decisions. If the patient has macular degeneration, he/she is likely to have established or be starting to use one (or more) parafoveal positions for fixation (preferred retinal locus, PRL (Timberlake et al 1986; Whittaker et al 1988)). The position, size and stability of this eccentric viewing position have a significant effect on reading (Raasch 2004).

Use a 1 m tangent screen with a large central fixation target having detail that the patient can resolve, e.g. a black letter on a white background (**Fig. 30.4**). (If a tangent screen is not available, use a 1 m square area of white wall and reverse the contrast of the fixation and test targets.) Instruct the patient to fixate *so that the target is seen clearly*. This will enable most patients with central vision loss to maintain stable *eccentric* fixation. This is how the patient is likely to read and it is easier

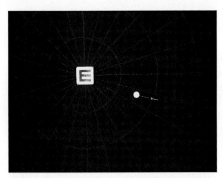

Figure 30.4 Modified tangent screen technique using a large central fixation target which the patient can see (using eccentric viewing) and a large stimulus to assess the position and size of any scotoma and the largest area of intact visual field.

for the patient to maintain stable fixation on a target he/she can see rather than using paracentral cues and expecting the patient to interpolate a central target that cannot be seen, as has been recommended in the past (Lovie-Kitchin & Bowman 1985; Nowakowski 1994). Accurate threshold assessment of the central field is not needed, so use a large test target, e.g. a 10 mm or 20 mm white stimulus. If possible, plot the blind spot. This will indicate the size and direction of the eccentric fixation, but it may not be possible if there is a large scotoma encompassing the blind spot. Plot the position and size of the central scotoma and the largest area of intact field, which is the area that should be used for reading (Lovie-Kitchin & Whittaker 1998a).

If the scotoma is positioned to the left and/or above fixation, i.e. the right and inferior visual fields are open, then reading (in English) should not be impeded severely by the scotoma. If the right field is not open, eccentric viewing training may be needed for reading, but most patients independently learn to position their scotoma appropriately for the task. In some cases, the right (reading) field will be open in one eye but not the other. Even if this eye has slightly worse visual acuity, this is the eye that should be recommended for reading, so it is important to assess the central field of each eye.

This visual field assessment technique can be used to assess the binocular field size as well. For mobility, it is desirable that fixation is below any binocular scotoma so that the inferior field is open (Lovie-Kitchin et al 1990; Hassan et al 2002). Patients often adopt different eccentric fixation positions for different tasks or for different lighting conditions (Lei & Schuchard 1997).

Contrast sensitivity

While contrast sensitivity is known to reduce with progression of vision loss and to be related to performance of everyday activities (Leat & Woodhouse 1993; Hawkins et al 2003; Monés & Rubin 2005) (see Ch. 12), in the author's clinical experience, assessment of contrast sensitivity does not greatly assist the vision rehabilitation of the majority of low-vision patients.

Contrast sensitivity can be assessed using a number of chart-based tests (Woods & Wood 1995) but they are not commonly available in clinical practice and their reliability has been questioned (Rubin 1988). None of the chart-based contrast sensitivity tests available today give an accurate and comprehensive measure of the contrast sensitivity function. However, the Pelli–Robson chart (**Fig. 12.12**) (Pelli et al 1988), because it uses letters, is the easiest test to determine a patient's contrast threshold. The test was not designed for low-vision application, but it can be used with modifications to its administration, to measure patients' letter contrast sensitivity (Whittaker & Lovie-Kitchin 1994). Use the chart at a 1 m test distance, possibly with different illuminances also, although this will alter contrast slightly. As the patient approaches threshold contrast, encourage him/her to guess and allow time (at least 20–30 seconds) for the patient to achieve best contrast sensitivity. If further reductions in test distance or increased illuminance improve contrast sensitivity, this indicates that appropriate magnification and/or lighting for reading may enhance performance, but this information can be easily determined from other assessments such as distance and near visual acuities and examining the effects of varying illumination (see below).

When contrast sensitivity is reduced, there are limited strategies to improve performance. Optimum lighting, minimizing glare, reversing or increasing print contrast, and using electronic devices such as closed-circuit TVs are the only interventions for enhancing contrast. If contrast sensitivity is severely impaired, non-visual techniques (e.g. books on CD) may be required.

Effects of varying illumination

Adaptation is abnormal in many ocular diseases, such as retinitis pigmentosa, age-related macular degeneration, albinism, etc. Accordingly, the optometrist should advise patients on appropriate lighting conditions, sunglasses and other means of illumination control, for safety and maximum vision performance.

From the case history and other assessments, it is important to determine the low-vision patient's illumination preferences, glare difficulties and any light and dark adaptation difficulties. In addition, the effects of different levels of illumination on visual acuity and reading rate can be assessed. Assessment of glare recovery (Bailey & Bullimore 1991) can be used to demonstrate the need to avoid sources of glare, the time they need to allow for adaptation when they have been subject to glare or large changes in illumination and/or the need for sunglasses.

For many low-vision patients, especially those with AMD, vision and reading performance improve at high illumination levels (Lovie-Kitchin & Bowman 1985; Eldred 1992; Bowers et al 2001). Conversely, some patients show marked reductions in VA and reading rate at moderate and high illuminances (Sloan 1969; Sloan et al 1973; Lovie-Kitchin & Bowman 1985; Bowers et al 2001). Each patient's response to varying illumination needs to be assessed. Dimmer controls on room lights and internally illuminated charts, and adjustable reading lamps are very useful for this purpose.

Bowers et al (2001) recommended that near VA and reading rate be assessed using dim room lighting (5–20 lux), normal room lighting (100–300 lux) and with a reading lamp 20 cm or less from the reading material (2000–5000 lux). Using the results of these assessments, optometrists can advise on appropriate, adjustable lighting for reading and writing, positioned to the side away from the writing hand, to avoid glare and shadows. Advice on the use of sunglasses, caps, umbrellas, etc. to manage changes in illumination is based largely on the patient's own reports.

Binocular vision

For low-vision patients, binocular vision is often absent because of a large difference in VA between the two eyes. As a general guide, if the right and left visual acuities differ by three lines (0.3 log units) or more, the patient probably functions monocularly. However, depending on their spectacle prescription, they may be using monovision, i.e. one eye for distance and the other for near.

For vision rehabilitation purposes a simple cover test at distance and near to determine if binocular vision is present or absent is usually sufficient. If the patient is binocular, convergence should be assessed as this may influence the type of near low-vision device prescribed; if convergence is poor, binocular devices are contraindicated.

Colour vision

Colour vision is not assessed routinely, but again it may be assessed (see Ch. 19) for functional, non-diagnostic purposes, to illustrate to the patient the colour confusions they might make. The Farnsworth Panel D15 is the test of choice when VA is 6/12 or less. Large chip versions of this test (PV-16) are available (Hovis et al 2003; Harper 2004).

Discussion with the patient

Following the low-vision assessment, it is important to discuss the findings with the patient.

- Explain the condition causing the low vision.
- Discuss the prognosis. In general, the more information the patient and family have, the more accepting they will be in the long term and more likely to respond to vision rehabilitation.
- Reassure patients that their functional difficulties are commensurate with the vision impairment.
- Explain the difference between reduced vision due to refractive errors and due to their ocular disease. Explain that their spectacle prescription may improve vision slightly by providing best focus but that because of their cloudy media or retinal degeneration (or whatever the underlying cause of the low vision might be) the image seen is still degraded (and will be even with magnification).
- Explain that optometric low-vision management (magnification in particular) is aimed at assisting the patient with specific tasks but will not return vision to 'normal'.
- Advise the patient that while magnification will assist reading tasks, reading rate probably will not return to their pre-vision-loss rate.
- For many patients, the optometrist will have to discuss whether the patient's vision meets the legal requirements for driving and whether or not driving with bioptic telescopes is permitted where they live. If the patient wants to drive, referral to a vision rehabilitation service is indicated for fitting and extensive training with bioptic telescopes (see below).

Optometric low-vision management

Optometric care is aimed at reducing the vision loss if possible (by refraction or referral for treatment) but vision rehabilitation is aimed at alleviating the vision disability due to the vision impairment. Management of the low-vision patient can involve any or all of the following:

- distance prescription
- magnification, to improve performance on specific tasks
- non-optical devices to improve task performance, especially lighting.
- referral to other rehabilitation services.

Distance prescription

A change in spectacle or contact lens prescription may give some general improvement in vision performance to reduce the vision loss. The decision to prescribe a change in prescription is a clinical judgement made in consultation with the patient, taking into account their visual tasks, as it is with any patient. Note, however, that a change in VA from 6/60 to 6/30 (an improvement of three lines or halving the minimum angle of resolution) is equivalent to a change in VA from 6/12 to 6/6 and may give substantial functional assistance to the patient. If in doubt, have the patient wear the new distance prescription (in a trial frame or lens clips over the current spectacles) while walking around the office or viewing outside to allow him/her to judge if the change gives noticeable improvement.

Occasionally, a general purpose monovision correction may be prescribed, particularly if the patient is not binocular, where one eye is used for distance and the other has a moderate near addition (up to +4 D) for reading.

As many low-vision patients are troubled by glare, it is important to discuss the prescription of sunglasses or tinted lenses to fit over their clear lenses, and when these should be used.

Prescribing magnification

The prescription of magnification devices is quite task specific. Rarely can one magnification device assist a patient with a range of tasks. More than one device is often required to meet the patient's goals. Those tasks that can be helped best with magnification are those in which both the patient and the task are stationary and which require resolution of detail over a small field of view. This encompasses most tasks that involve reading print, at near or distance, and these are the tasks that low-vision patients commonly request assistance with.

Tasks that involve movement are more difficult to assist with magnification devices. For example, recognizing the faces of people moving towards them or driving tasks are difficult or perhaps impossible to perform using magnification. Some activities of daily living may be assisted with magnification but may be more efficiently assisted by modifying the task, for example, commonly used telephone numbers can be programmed into the telephone or listed in large print rather than having to be read from the telephone book with a magnifier.

Magnification, when defined in simple terms, is an enlargement of the retinal image size. This can be done equally well (Lovie-Kitchin & Whittaker 1998b) by either relative size magnification or relative distance magnification, or a combination of the two, for distance, intermediate or near tasks.

- *Relative size magnification* (RSM): the size of the object (the task) is increased, e.g. large print books for children. This is not practical for many 'real world' tasks, but may be necessary or easiest for some activities of daily living or recreational tasks, especially if a wide field of view is important, e.g. large-print copy to read sheet music, or when other people are involved in the task, e.g. large-print playing cards (**Fig. 30.5**).
- *Relative distance magnification* (RDM) (sometimes called proximal magnification): the object is brought closer to the eye, e.g. moving closer to see the television (**Fig. 30.6**), such that the retinal image is enlarged. Children with low vision use accommodation to achieve RDM at near, by holding reading material at close distances. For adults, plus lenses supplement accommodation, either partially or fully, enabling reading tasks to be in focus. It is the reduced viewing distance which magnifies the retinal image, the lenses simply provide focus. In fact, patients may hold material closer than their near point, despite blur, to achieve additional magnification.

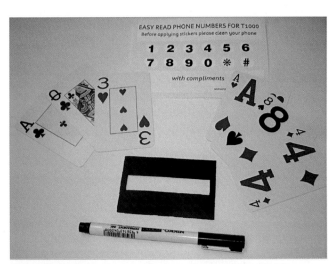

Figure 30.5 Relative size magnification – the size of the object is physically enlarged, e.g. large-print playing cards and telephone numbers. Also shown are other non-optical devices, a typoscope or signature guide and a thick, felt-tip pen.

The magnification provided by different devices, including telescopes and electronic devices, is essentially a variation on one or both of these methods.

Determining required distance magnification

Common distance tasks that patients may request help with are viewing TV, recognizing faces, reading the board in the classroom, reading street signs and viewing sporting and entertainment events.

A closer viewing distance is the first (and sometimes only) recommendation for assisting the patient with these distance tasks, provided it is practical and safe to do so, e.g. TV, reading street signs, reading the board in school, etc.

Distance VA is the starting point for determining the required viewing distance (or optical magnification) for such tasks, remembering that the linear size of detail that can be resolved is proportional to the viewing distance. For example, a person who reads the 60M line at 6 m (20 feet) on the VA chart can be expected to resolve detail equivalent to 30M from 3 m (10 feet), 15M from 1.5 m (5 feet) and so on. From this, a 1.5 m or 1 m viewing distance might be recommended for television viewing for a patient with a distance VA of 6/60 (20/200) (**Fig. 30.6**). Many older patients do not like to move to such close distances for fear of 'ruining their eyes'. The optometrist needs to reassure such a patient that it is safe to move closer and recommend the patient sits to the side of the worse eye so their better eye is aligned. If this interferes with the viewing of other family members, there are low-powered ($\approx 2\times$) telescopic spectacles available, such as the Eschenbach MaxTV spectacles (**Fig. 30.7**).

As well as enlarging the retinal image, a decreased viewing distance also reduces the central visual field or the linear extent of any central scotoma (Lovie-Kitchin & Bowman 1985). Thus, a closer viewing distance for TV and other tasks helps the patients with AMD in particular, but not the patients with RP or advanced glaucoma who have small remaining fields.

If a closer viewing distance is not practical, telescopic or electronic devices are used to reduce the distance optically. Some estimate of the required VA to carry out the task is needed, although for most distance tasks a VA of about 6/12 should suffice. The required distance magnification is calculated from the current VA and the estimated VA required for the task. Two examples of this calculation are shown in **Table 30.5**.

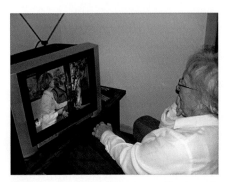

Figure 30.6 Relative distance magnification – the viewing distance to the object is reduced to enlarge the image, e.g. to view the television.

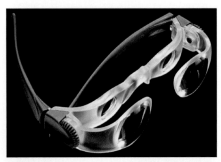

Figure 30.7 MaxTV spectacles (Eschenbach 16241) – 2× Galilean telescopes with ±3 D focus adjustment for use at a 2–3 m viewing distance. (Photograph provided by Eschenbach through European Eyewear Australia.)

Table 30.5 Determining required distance magnification

Procedure	Example 1 (20-year-old college student with albinism)	Example 2 (45-year-old lawyer with Stargardt's disease)
1. Measure distance VA	6/60 (20/200)	6/38 (20/120)
2. Identify required task	Reading the slides in lectures	Reading street signs
3. Estimate required acuity	6/12 (20/40)	6/9 (20/30)
4. M = VA required/VA habitual	(6/12) / (6/60) = 60/12 = 5× (20/40) / (20/200) = 200/40 = 5×	(6/9) / (6/38) = 38/9 ≈ 4× (20/30) / (20/125) = 125/30 = 4×
5. Test performance with this magnification	6/12 (20/40) with 5.5 × 25 Beecher Mirage spectacle-mounted binoculars	6/12 (20/40) with 4 × 12 hand-held telescope
6. Modify if expected performance not realized		6/7.5 (20/25) with 6 x 16 hand-held telescope [NOTE – 5× hand-held telescope not made]
7. Loan distance telescope for trial		

Distance magnification devices

As a consequence of the restricted field of view through most distance telescopes, it is strongly recommended that those patients needing a magnification device for extended distance tasks, especially where the person and/or the task may be moving, should be referred to a specialist low-vision practitioner or vision rehabilitation service. For example, if a person needs a telescope as an aid to independent mobility, driving or in school or university classrooms, the range of optical and electronic devices available and the specialized training required is beyond the scope of primary care optometrists.

A few simple devices may be useful to have available to demonstrate to those who need assistance with TV, theatre or viewing sports, tasks where the patient is stationary. A useful reminder for some patients is that any regular binoculars or opera glasses, which many people have at home, could be useful for sporting events, concerts, etc. As indicated above, low-powered, spectacle-mounted telescopic spectacles may be useful for TV or theatre viewing. These are preferable to a hand-held device for ease of use. These should be loaned to the patient for trial before final prescription.

The selection of a distance telescope is dependent on the needs of the patient. The type of telescope, e.g. monocular or binocular, is often determined by the availability in the magnification required. The decision between a spectacle- or head-mounted telescope, such as Beecher Mirage binoculars or a Designs for Vision bioptic telescope, or a hand-held telescope (**Fig. 30.8**) will be largely made on the basis of the

duration of the tasks for which it is to be used, cost to the patient and dexterity of hand and head movements. The Beecher Mirage head-mounted binoculars (4× to 10×) were originally designed for birdwatchers and use mirrors rather than prisms, so they are considerably lighter than most other telescopes of the same powers.

As indicated above, referral to a vision rehabilitation service is recommended for prescription of and training with distance telescopes. For more details on the optical principles and dispensing of telescopic devices, see low-vision texts (e.g. Nowakowski 1994; Dickinson 1998; Brilliant 1999).

Determining required near magnification

Reading is crucial for everyday education, work and daily living activities, and therefore is the most common task for which low-vision patients request help. Tasks with which patients may have difficulties range from simple 'survival'-type reading, such as labels on medications, bills, letters, etc., to demanding educational, vocational and recreational reading. A common presenting request from older adults with low vision is to be able to read the newspaper, perhaps because it is the task with which they first notice difficulty with reducing vision.

Relative size magnification (RSM) is commonly used to assist young children with low vision through the use of large-print books, but this is not practical for older children or adults. As indicated above, there may be some tasks for which RSM is more practical than using magnification devices, such as large-print clocks or watches, large-print labels on filing cabinets, etc.

However, for most near tasks, a closer viewing distance is needed to provide magnification. Children with low vision adopt quite close reading distances without any instruction or training, commonly between 10 cm and 20 cm. Obviously, adults do not have the accommodation to focus at such close distances, so need an appropriate optical correction, in the form of simple plus lens spectacles or magnifiers, to focus at the near viewing distance required for magnification.

As it is the viewing distance which determines the retinal image size, it is logical to record near VA in terms of print size and viewing distance, and to express the magnification

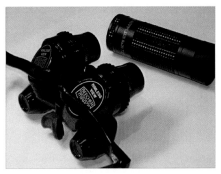

Figure 30.8 Examples of distance telescopes – 4× Beecher Mirage head-mounted binoculars and an 8× Gerber hand-held telescope.

of any system in terms of the equivalent viewing distance it provides. The author strongly advocates that the magnification of any device should be specified in terms of the equivalent viewing distance (or equivalent dioptric power). This avoids the confusion of different manufacturers or practitioners using different formulae for magnification of plus lenses.

Lovie-Kitchin and Whittaker (1999) proposed a step-by-step approach to determine the equivalent viewing distance and select an appropriate optical device for reading, as follows.

Establish the patient's reading goal

As the required magnification depends on the print size and required reading rate of the task, the patient's reading goal or goals should be specified in these terms. Some patients will present simply requesting help with reading. The first task of the optometrist is to discuss with the patient the types of reading tasks he/she wishes to do. For example, the patient might want to be able to read technical magazines or to read personal bills or emails from friends. As indicated above, reading the newspaper is a common reading goal.

For children or adults with early vision impairment, their reading task may be achievable but with difficulty. For children in particular, the goal may be to make it easier to read their school books, i.e. relieve the accommodative demand. Obtain information from the child, parent or teacher on the child's visual tasks and samples of the child's school books.

Define goal print size and reading rate

Besides the task requirements, the required print size and reading rate must also be defined. The required print size can be determined from examples of the patient's reading materials if they have them (or see **Table 30.4**). Reading rate needs to be estimated, at least qualitatively, as described on p 481.

For short-term reading tasks, such as reading an address label, the reading rate required is minimal. Whittaker & Lovie-Kitchin (1993) called this 'spot' reading, which is about 40 words per minute (wpm). For tasks such as reading the newspaper or magazines, fluency is required in order to understand the meaning; this needs to be about 100 wpm or more. For educational or business materials, much faster reading rates may be required. For a given print size, the acuity reserve (and magnification) requirements are different for each of these reading rates (**Table 30.6**).

For example, the reading goal for a patient who wants to read the newspaper would be defined as reading 1M (8 point) print fluently.

Determine required threshold print size for required reading rate

As indicated above, reading rate depends on acuity reserve, i.e. the print size being read relative to threshold print size. Lovie-Kitchin & Whittaker (1999) proposed acuity reserve requirements for different reading rates. A slightly modified version is given in **Table 30.6** with examples for reading 1M (8 point) print at different reading rates. These are generalized from different studies but subsequent research (Cheong et al 2002) and clinical experience suggest that they apply to most patients.

Thus, the patient who wishes to read 1M (8 point) print fluently requires sufficient magnification to achieve a threshold print size of 0.5M (4 point) print (i.e. three lines of acuity in reserve when reading 1M print).

Measure current near visual acuity at normal and high illuminations

The assessments of near VA and the effect of varying illumination are described above. Note that the near addition being used is not important; it is the viewing distance which determines current retinal image size, so threshold print size and viewing distance are the important parameters for determining the new (equivalent) viewing distance.

As a working example, the patient can just read 2M (N16) at 30 cm and 1.5M (N12) at 30 cm with increased illumination.

Calculate required equivalent viewing distance for the goal task

The calculation of the new equivalent viewing distance (EVD) can be done by ratios, as follows:

$$\text{Required EVD} = (\text{required print size}/\text{current print size}) \times \text{current EVD}$$

In the example given:

$$\text{Required EVD} = (0.5/1.5) \times 30$$

or

$$\text{Required EVD} = (4/12) \times 30$$

Therefore:

$$\text{Required EVD} = 10 \text{ cm}$$

The next steps are to select one or more optical devices that can provide this required EVD and test the reading performance with these devices. Low-vision children will always use some accommodation, so the equivalent power of the device selected needs to allow for this.

Table 30.7 summarizes this assessment for reading and the calculation of the required EVD with two different examples.

Table 30.6 Acuity reserve requirements for different reading rates

Reading performance	Approximate reading rate	Minimum acuity reserve	Required TPS[a] to read 1M (N8)
Spot	40 wpm	1.3:1 (1 line, 0.1 log unit)	0.8 m (N6)
Fluent	100 wpm	2:1 (3 lines, 0.3 log units)	0.5 m (N4)
Maximum or near-maximum	250 wpm	3:1 (5 lines, 0.5 log units)	0.3 m (N2.5)

[a] TPS, threshold print size.

Table 30.7 Calculating required equivalent viewing distance

Procedure	Example 1 (15-year-old student with congenital nystagmus)	Example 2 (75-year-old person with AMD)
1. Establish reading goal	Read maths text book more easily	To read telephone book
2. Define goal print size and reading rate	N10 (1.25M) rapidly	N6 (0.8M) slowly
3. Determine acuity reserve and required threshold print size for required reading rate	5 lines acuity reserve for max. reading of N10 (1.25M) give N3 (0.4M) required threshold print size	1 line acuity reserve for 'spot' reading of N6 (0.8M) give N5 (0.6M) required threshold print size
4. Measure current threshold print size and viewing distance at normal and high illuminations	N6 (0.8M) @ 10 cm with DRx (accommodation only) No change with high illumination	N20 (2.5M) @ 25 cm[a] with +3 D add No change with high illumination
5. Calculate required EVD	$(3/6) \times 10 = 5$ cm $(0.4/0.8) \times 10 = 5$ cm	$(5/20) \times 25 \approx 6$ cm $(0.6/2.5) \times 25 = 6$ cm
6. Test reading performance with a magnification system giving required EVD	N10 (1.25M) rapidly at 5 cm with +12 D near add & 8 D accommodation	N6 (0.8M) with difficulty at 6 cm with 16 D hand-held mag
7. Decrease EVD by repeating this procedure if expected performance not achieved, or assess visual fields		N5 (0.6M) just, N6 (0.8M) slowly at 5 cm with 20 D hand-held mag

[a] This is satisfactory, although not ideal focus. Decreased viewing distance increases retinal image size (with slight blur). If viewing distance is *longer* or substantially shorter than focal length of current near add, the distance prescription needs to be checked.

Near magnification devices

There is a wide range of near optical devices as well as closed-circuit TVs (CCTVs) and other electronic devices which can be used for reading with low vision, as follows:

- spectacle lenses
- hand-held magnifiers
- stand magnifiers
- head-mounted loupes
- near vision telescopes
- electronic devices.

Well-controlled research is needed to compare the efficacy of different types of optical devices for reading (Virgili & Acosta 2006) but in most cases, the requirements of the task and viewing distance preferences of the patient determine the type of low-vision device prescribed.

The features, advantages and disadvantages of each type of near magnification device are briefly discussed below. For more details on these devices see low-vision texts (e.g. Nowakowski 1994; Dickinson 1998; Brilliant 1999).

Spectacle lenses

Characteristics of spectacle lenses:

- available up to +50 D
- hands free
- close working distance
- widest field of view.

They are available as:

- single-vision high-plus lenses (sometimes called microscopic lenses); use CR39 aspheric lenticular lenses for ≥+10 D (diameter decreases with higher powers)
- diffraction glass lens (Noves mono) of 4 mm thickness from Eschenbach +12 D to +24 D in spectacles with balance lens (considerably more expensive than conventional lenses)
- prism half-eye spectacles (**Fig. 30.9**) for binocularity, +4 D to +12 D with base-in prism 2^Δ greater than dioptric power, available in conventional aspheric CR39 from various suppliers or as diffraction glass lenses (Noves bino) from Eschenbach (considerably more expensive); stock spectacles do not allow for distance correction, so effective near addition will alter with distance prescription
- bifocals; most conventional types available to +4.00 D add; >+4 D, Younger CR-39 round segment bifocal
- some stand magnifiers such as the Peak Lupe can be spectacle-mounted, such that it is effectively a high-plus lens with a spacer (cannot incorporate refractive correction).

High near add (microscopic) spectacles should be the first choice for patients with central visual field loss as the close viewing distance not only provides magnification but also reduces the linear extent of the scotoma. However, they are not suitable for patients with poor hand control or those who cannot adapt to a close viewing distance. For low-vision children, bifocal or near spectacles are commonly prescribed to relieve the accommodative demand.

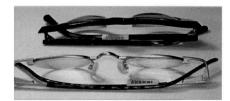

Figure 30.9 Prism half-eye spectacles +12 D R and L with 14^Δ base-in prism (*top*) and +12 D Noves mono diffractive R lens with frosted balance L lens (*bottom*).

As most adult patients have one eye better than the other, monocular near additions are most commonly prescribed, although prism half-eye spectacles may be an inexpensive alternative provided the image from the poorer eye does not interfere with the image from the better eye. If this is the case, the patient can be advised simply to patch the poorer eye.

Some older patients with low vision resist the use of a close viewing distance, in which case other devices need to be offered. Even if a patient has opted for a hand-held or stand magnifier, as they become experienced with it, they may adjust to a closer viewing distance and become amenable to high near addition spectacles at a follow-up consultation.

Binocularity with high near adds If the patient has binocular vision, it is not too difficult to achieve binocularity with additions of +8.00 D or less. To ensure that the patient looks through the optical centres of the lenses, proper decentration is required. Higher additions are difficult, and require base-in prism as in the stock half-eye prism spectacles described above.

An accurate formula for calculating the required near PD for binocular near adds is:

Near PD = Distance PD × (working distance[mm]/ working distance + 27)

where 27 mm = 12 mm vertex distance + 15 mm from cornea to centre of rotation.

Alternatively, a practical 'rule of thumb' to avoid unwanted BO prism is that total decentration should be 1.5 times the dioptric power of the addition. For example, a presbyopic patient with a +10 D add has a distance PD of 65 mm. The required decentration is 1.5 × 10 = 15, so the near PD must be 65 − 15 = 50 mm.

Hand-held magnifiers

The characteristics of hand-held magnifiers:

- available to +50 D, but most +8 D to +24 D
- one hand required for use
- flexible eye–lens distance but field of view greatest when eye is close to the lens
- use with distance Rx if eye–lens distance is > focal length of magnifier

- use with near add if eye–lens distance is ≤ focal length of magnifier.

They are available in:

- wide range between +4 D and +10 D, but many of low quality; +8 D to +20 D range of hand-held magnifiers are most useful
- some illuminated hand-held magnifiers available.

Hand-held magnifiers (**Fig. 30.10**) are particularly useful for 'spot' reading such as checking prices in the supermarket or reading an address label, as they are small and portable. As with any optical device, the closer the eye–lens distance, the wider is the field of view. For higher powers, the illuminated magnifiers overcome the lack of illumination due to the short magnifier-to-page distances and are useful for patients whose reading performance improves with increased illumination.

Stand magnifiers

The characteristics of stand magnifiers:

- up to 22× (labelled)
- posture and lighting can cause problems
- most fixed lens-to-object magnifiers have divergent light emerging from them, i.e. the image is not at infinity. This affects the equivalent power and EVD of the magnifier (Bailey et al 1994), as is discussed further below.

They are available as:

- fixed-focus stand magnifiers, +12 D to +24 D most useful
- a few focusable stand magnifiers available from COIL (Hi-power series)
- stand magnifiers with in-built illumination very useful
- paperweight magnifiers.

Stand magnifiers, like hand-held magnifiers, are useful for spot reading tasks but they can also be used for extended reading. The illuminated magnifiers (**Fig. 30.11**) are very useful for patients whose reading performance improves with increased illumination and where a close reading distance reduces other illumination.

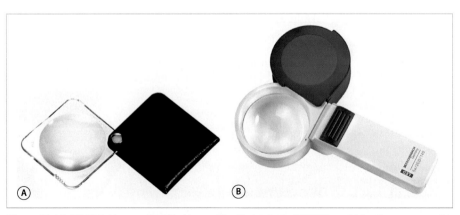

Figure 30.10 (A) 10 D biconvex hand-held magnifier (Eschenbach 1752150) useful for short-term reading tasks. **(B)** 20 D aspheric illuminated hand-held (pocket) magnifier (Eschenbach 151054). (Photographs provided by Eschenbach through European Eyewear Australia.)

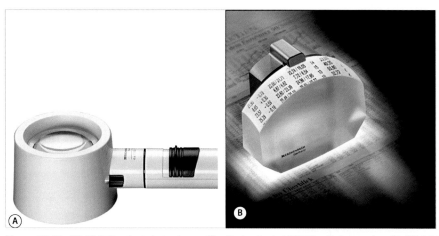

Figure 30.11 (A) 16 D illuminated stand magnifier (Eschenbach 155491) with battery handle. **(B)** A 2.2× segment bright field paperweight stand magnifier (Eschenbach 1436) comes with (shown here) or without LED illumination. (Photographs provided by Eschenbach through European Eyewear Australia.)

The solid paperweight stand magnifiers (often generically referred to as Visolettes) are popular with children with low vision who need some assistance to reduce their accommodative demand. The paperweight magnifiers can be left in place when doing schoolwork, are robust for children's use and (especially the 'Bright field' range from Eschenbach) provide good image brightness. The eye–image distances are short but children can accommodate to these distances, but they are not often used by presbyopic low-vision patients because of the need for high near additions in conjunction with the magnifiers.

Stand magnifiers provide easier hand control than hand-held magnifiers because the magnifier is designed to sit on the page. If the patient lifts the magnifier off the page to read, they are increasing the eye–image distance to bring the image into focus. In this case, the near spectacle prescription needs to be increased to allow the patient to sit the magnifier on the page or select a different magnifier.

For stand magnifiers, *both* magnification and field of view decrease as the eye–lens distance increases. The patient therefore needs to be encouraged to use stand magnifiers (and hand-held magnifiers) as close to the eye as possible but, as indicated above, the near spectacle prescription may need modifying (discussed further below).

Head-mounted loupes

The characteristics of head-mounted loupes:

- available to +30 D
- like spectacles, but with lenses mounted in front of the spectacle plane, allowing a slightly longer working distance
- may be useful for manipulative tasks.

They are available as:

- binocular loupes on headband
- lens clipped over spectacle frame.

These head- or spectacle-mounted loupes are not commonly prescribed for patients with moderate or severe low vision as the field of view is generally small. However, for those with mild low vision, if the goal task requires both hands free and a longer working distance than provided by the equivalent near add, these devices or near telescopes may be suitable. In general, though, the author would suggest referral to a low-vision clinic for patients with these goals, as a full range of optical and electronic devices and/or advice on other ways of doing the tasks are available.

Near vision telescopes (telemicroscopes)

The characteristics of near vision telescopes:

- available up to 20× magnification and higher
- frees both hands
- small field of view
- reading distance fixed but is approximately double that of equivalent spectacle lens
- can be used binocularly to 5×.

They are available as:

- stock spectacle-mounted telescopes
- distance telescopes with near caps.

Many distance telescopes can be focused to relatively short distances (e.g. a 4 × 12 telescope will focus to 20 cm), but as they are hand-held they are not useful for extended reading.

Near telescopes are not as commonly used as simple plus lens magnifiers but, as described above, for some patients' tasks they may be the best option. Referral to a multidisciplinary low-vision clinic for such devices is recommended.

Other optical devices

Various other optical devices are available for providing magnification or managing visual field restriction but they are used infrequently. These devices include: contact lens telescopes, implantable miniature telescopes, reverse telescopes or concave lenses for expanding the visual field (with loss of acuity) and mirrors or prisms for shifting images within the visual field. If these devices are indicated, specialist management and training would be required from a vision rehabilitation service. For more details on these devices, see low-vision texts.

Electronic devices

Many patients can benefit from electronic video magnifiers **(Fig. 30.12)**, which include closed-circuit television systems (CCTVs) as well as computer hardware and software to provide enlarged near, intermediate and distant images. They are particularly suited to students and adults doing paid, volunteer or recreational tasks with extensive near visual

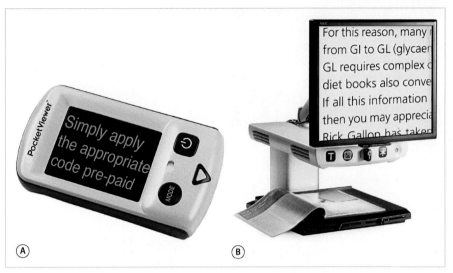

Figure 30.12 (A) Portable hand-held (Pocketviewer, up to 8× enlargement) electronic video magnifier. **(B)** Fixed camera and monitor (Smartview) electronic video magnifier. (Photographs provided by HumanWare.)

demands or requiring links to home or work computer systems. However, most patients who use electronic devices will usually use optical and non-optical devices as well in different situations.

Electronic devices have a number of advantages compared with optical devices, but a few disadvantages too. The cost is often a significant disadvantage and some patients experience nausea from the motion of print across the screen.

One important thing to remember is to ensure that any patient using a screen-based device has an intermediate or near correction appropriate for their viewing distance.

Electronic video magnifiers The characteristics:

- up to 60× linear magnification
- magnification can be varied to suit task
- positive and negative contrast and colour options
- field of view larger than optical devices (other than spectacles) for equivalent magnification
- flexible viewing distance, therefore ergonomic advantages over optical devices
- can be used for many near tasks, including writing
- some can be used for distance tasks also
- contrast enhancement
- can be interfaced with computers
- may require one hand to move $x–y$ platform or hand-held camera
- some are less portable than optical devices
- expensive to purchase, repair or update.

They are available as:

- hand-held cameras with TV or computer link
- portable hand-held CCTVs with small monitors, battery operated, limited magnification, near tasks only
- portable CCTVs with larger screens, distance and writing options; some link to TVs
- fixed cameras with own monitor, some with automatic scanning
- fixed cameras with TV or computer link

- head-mounted or spectacle-mounted cameras with computer link.

One readily available version of a hand-held camera that can be used for both reading and distance viewing is a portable video camera ('camcorder') (**Fig. 30.13**). The device provides high magnification, can focus over a range of distances, and the image is viewed on the screen. For reading, a near addition is needed to allow the person to see the screen at a close viewing distance.

Large-print or speech-output computer displays The options are:

- large monitors
- colour, contrast and font variations in display options (e.g. accessibility options on PCs)
- text enlargement software
- text-to-speech systems; screen reading software
- scanners with print and/or speech output.

As technology develops, these devices are changing regularly. If an optometrist is interested in providing information on electronic devices to low-vision patients, contact

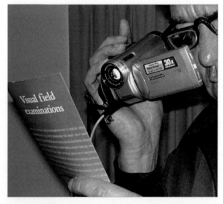

Figure 30.13 A portable video camera used to provide high magnification for reading – note that high near addition spectacles are needed to focus on the screen.

local suppliers for up-to-date catalogues or consult their websites.

Given the wide range of video magnifiers, computer and web-based systems which can display enlarged images on TV monitors or computer screens or can provide speech output, the author strongly recommends referral for specialized assessment, training and supply of these devices. As with all individual computer systems (or optical devices for that matter!) the most appropriate for any individual depends on the task requirements, ergonomics and compatibility with other systems.

Selecting a near magnification device for trial

As discussed above, before suggesting the patient try near low-vision devices, it is important to explain to him/her that conventional spectacles cannot provide the magnification required to perform their goal tasks. The patient should be advised of the requirement to use a closer-than-normal viewing distance, and that there are different magnifying devices that can assist with this.

Depending on the EVD required, any of the near devices described above might meet the patient's needs. For example, the following systems all give an EVD of approximately 10 cm (and there are many other choices too):

- +10 D spectacle addition
- +5 D addition with +5 D accommodation
- +10 D hand-held magnifier used at the focal length
- COIL 5214 4× (12 D) stand magnifier (used at an eye–lens distance of about 10 cm)
- Schweizer 14500 Okulux 8 D illuminated magnifier (used at an eye–lens distance of about 2.5 cm)
- CCTV viewed at 40 cm with print enlarged 4×.

Unfortunately, manufacturers of magnifiers do not specify the power or magnification of the devices in terms of equivalent power or equivalent viewing distance. More usually, if a dioptric power is given, it is a vertex power and, since the equivalent power is lower, the actual power or magnification of devices is almost always less than that indicated by the manufacturers' labels.

Bailey et al (1994) described the optical parameters of many magnifiers available at the time, including the EVDs for different eye–lens distances. Bailey and colleagues have updated these parameters for many magnifiers from most manufacturers and provided them in tables (known as his 'Yellow Pages') among his low-vision spreadsheet collections at the University of California, Berkeley website (Bailey 2006). The author encourages every optometrist to use these tables to assist in the selection of magnifiers of the required EVD, which can then be tried out by the patient. **Table 30.8** lists a few examples from these tables as recommended devices for optometrists to have in stock.

If the required EVD is equal to or greater than 10 cm (i.e. the equivalent power is ≤ 10 D), as a general rule in deciding which magnifier is best for the patient, the author recommends a trial with a high near addition first. If the patient has used only conventional +2.50 D or +3.00 D near adds previously, it would be wise to gradually increase the near add in a few steps in order to coach the patient on the need for a close reading distance. For example, if an EVD of 10 cm is required, work up to the indicated +10 D add in two or three steps, e.g. +5 D, +8 D and then +10 D. If the goal reading performance is achieved, discuss the options available in spectacle magnifiers (as described above) and select one for home trial.

If the required EVD is less than 10 cm (equivalent power >10 D), or the patient resists the close viewing distance demanded of the high near addition, try stand or hand-held magnifiers.

If a stand magnifier is the device of choice, determine the eye–lens distance the patient will comfortably use. A 10 cm eye–lens distance may be the closest that patients will accept at first, but the closer the better. Knowing the

Table 30.8A Some optical low-vision devices for private practice

Manufacturer & ID #	Manufacturer's description		
TELESCOPES			
Eschenbach16421	MaxTV spectacles (2×)		
Various	4 × 12 and/or 6 × 16 monocular (if likely to see low-vision children who are in regular schools)		
PRISM HALF-EYE SPECS			
Eschenbach 16801(6–10) or local optical supplier	Half-eye specs (6 D–10 D) with BI prism 2Δ more than D power		
HAND-HELD MAGNIFIERS			

Manufacturer & ID #	Manufacturer's description	Measured Fe (D)	EVD (cm)
Eschenbach 2655–150	7.6D/3×, aspheric, 100 × 50 mm	7.5	13.4
Eschenbach 2655–750	10D/3.5×, aspheric, 75 × 50 mm	9.1	11.0
Eschenbach 1740(x)60 pocket series	10D/3.5×, biconvex round folding 60 mm (x = different colours)	9.5	10.5
Eschenbach 151044	16D/4× aspheric LED illum magnifier, 60 mm	15.0	6.7
Eschenbach 2655–60	20D/5×, aspheric, 58 mm	18.8	5.3
Eschenbach 2655–50	23D/6×, aspheric, 50 mm	22.1	4.5

Bailey et al 1994; Bailey 2006.

eye–lens distance to be used, select a stand magnifier from the tables that gives the required EVD at this distance. In the Bailey tables (Bailey 2006), the eye–image distances for each magnifier for two different eye–lens distances are also given. The eye–image distance determines the near spectacle prescription needed to be used in conjunction with the magnifier. If there is a choice of stand magnifiers giving the required EVD, select one that has an eye–image distance between 25 cm and 40 cm so that the patient can use their own spectacles (near add between +2.50 D and +4 D), thereby minimizing the financial outlay.

For example, in **Table 30.8B**, both the Schweizer 190 illuminated stand magnifier and the COIL 4206 stand magnifier give an EVD of 5.8 cm (equivalent power of +17 D) when used at an eye–lens distance of 10 cm. The Schweizer 190 has an eye–image distance of 21.4 cm, necessitating a near addition of about +4.50 D to be used in conjunction with the magnifier. The COIL 4206 stand magnifier has an eye–image distance of 59.1 cm, requiring an intermediate

addition of about +1.75 D to keep the print in focus with the magnifier sitting on the page.

With the selected device(s), assess near visual acuity and reading rate (as described above). The patient should be able to read their goal print size at a similar rate to large print (critical print size and larger) with their conventional near add at the initial assessment. Have the patient try out the device on samples of the reading materials for which they requested assistance, such as newspapers, magazines, invoices, etc. If the goal reading performance is achieved (reading rate at goal print size and threshold print size as required), discuss the options available (as listed above) and select a magnifier for home trial.

If VA and reading rate are less than expected, calculate a new (shorter) EVD (higher equivalent power) from the results of the assessment with the trial device, as described in **Table 30.7**. In example 2 (**Table 30.7**), performance was one line (0.1 log unit) less than predicted, so the EVD needed to be decreased by 0.1 log unit, from 6 cm to 5 cm

Table 30.8B Some stand magnifiers for private practice

z = eye–lens distance

Manufacturer & ID #	Manufacturer's description	Measured Fe (D)	z = 2.5 cm EVD (cm)	z = 2.5 cm eye–im (cm)	z = 10 cm EVD (cm)	z = 10 cm eye–im (cm)	z = 25 cm[a] EVD (cm)	z = 25 cm[a] eye–im (cm)
ILLUMINATED								
Eschenbach 158063	7.6D/3× aspheric 100 × 50mm tilt with 4D yellow line guide	7.2	8.7	19.1	12.1	26.6	19.0	41.6
Schweizer 193	12D/4× aspheric 70 mm	11.5	6.3	16.6	9.2	24.1	15.0	39.1
Eschenbach 155493	16D/4× aspheric 70 mm with line guide	14.9	5.6	21.4	7.6	28.9	11.5	43.9
Eschenbach 155393	20D/5× aspheric 60 mm with line guide	17.8	5.0	24.6	6.5	32.1	9.6	47.1
Eschenbach 155273	24D/6× aspheric 50 mm	21.8	4.3	31.0	5.3	38.5	7.4	53.5
Schweizer 190	28D/8× aspheric 35 mm	23.9	3.7	13.9	5.8	21.4	9.8	36.4
	HANDLES							
Eschenbach 15593	Mains plug-in	Also available in battery form						
Schweizer 182	Mains plug-in							
Eschenbach 159940	2 battery LED							
NON-ILLUMINATED								
Eschenbach 1436	2.2X Bright field aspheric paperweight 70 mm	10.2	6.3	13.1	9.9	20.6	17.1	35.6
Schweizer 320/65	16D/4× Visolette paper weight 65 mm	15.6	4.2	7.6	8.4	15.1	16.8	30.1
COIL 4206	20D/6× Hi-power aspheric	18.7	5.1	51.6	5.8	59.1	7.3	74.1

Bailey et al 1994; Bailey 2006.
[a] For most of the higher-powered devices (e.g. EVD < 6 cm), an eye–lens distance of 25 cm is not practical because the field of view is too small.
The dioptric equivalent of the eye–image (eye–im) distance determines the accommodation or spectacle prescription to be used in conjunction with the stand magnifier. Note that Schweizer magnifiers have short eye–image distances, so higher accommodation or near additions are required in conjunction with these magnifiers.

(equivalent power increased by 0.1 log unit, from 16 D to 20 D). If the patient's near VA was improved with increased illumination, select an illuminated magnifier or increase illumination by using a reading lamp close to the task.

If the goal reading performance is still not achieved with increased magnification and/or illumination, this indicates that vision impairments other than visual acuity loss are limiting reading performance, most probably due to a visual field loss. Assess (or reassess) the central visual field of each eye using the modified tangent screen method described previously. If a scotoma is positioned in the right field of each eye, fluent reading is unlikely to be achieved. Spot reading may be possible with the high magnification and wide field of view provided by a CCTV.

Often, there is little choice in the type of near device selected for trial once the required EVD, eye–image distance and immediate preferences of the patient are known, but if alternative devices are possible, show these to the patient. The choice of the near magnification device(s) from the range described above will depend on a number of additional factors, such as hand steadiness and dexterity, if the task entails a fixed or variable viewing distance, whether one or both hands are required for the task, and the types of device, such as portability, cost, etc.

Instruction and training

Once a low-vision device is selected, instruction on its use is required and short-term loan of the device (perhaps with part payment) is strongly recommended. Particularly for elderly patients, if they have multiple goals and more than one device is to be used, it may be prudent to loan them one at a time. An instruction sheet for each device is an effective way for the patient and others to become familiar with the appropriate use and care of the low-vision device. Such information sheets are available in low-vision texts (e.g. Lovie-Kitchin & Bowman 1985; Nowakowski 1994; Freeman & Jose 1997).

Distance devices

If the patient is going to use a distance telescopic device in a seated position for a relatively static task, such as viewing TV or a concert, little training will be required. The optometrist can instruct the patient on how far from the TV to sit, how to focus the device for this distance and, if it is a hand-held device, how to support the arm holding the device (Grosvenor 2007). It is advisable to loan the device for trial at home to ensure it meets the patient's requirements before finalizing the prescription.

However, if the telescope is hand-held and/or the task involves movement such as walking, driving, sporting events, etc., training in a systematic approach for locating and tracking the task is needed because of the limited field of view. This training is best given by optometrists and orientation and mobility instructors with particular experience with these tasks and devices, so referral to a comprehensive vision rehabilitation service is recommended.

Near devices

Training in the use of near optical devices and coaching to adapt to a close viewing distance begins during the low-vision assessment as the devices are tried out. Once a device is selected, in-office instruction and practice followed by short-term loan of the device is recommended. For experienced users,

reading rate with the magnifier is equivalent to their reading rate for large print (critical print size and above) (Lovie-Kitchin et al 2000). For new users, reading rate initially reduces, but with practice it increases (Cheong et al 2005).

As discussed above, it is important to ensure that patients do not leave the office with unrealistic expectations. Advise that their reading rate is unlikely to return to what it was prior to vision loss, especially for patients with AMD. Depending on the size and position of their scotoma, maximum reading rate achievable with magnification (whether using large print, optical devices or closed-circuit TV systems) is usually between 30 and 100 words per minute for people with AMD; patients with other causes of low vision will read faster (Legge et al 1985; Whittaker & Lovie-Kitchin 1993). Despite the relatively slow reading rate achievable with central vision loss, many patients are satisfied with this 'spot' rate for short-term, daily reading tasks. Other electronic devices can be used for accessing information more quickly for work or recreational tasks if necessary (Whittaker & Cummings 1999; Hensil & Whittaker 2000).

Some authors have suggested extensive training programmes for use of optical and electronic devices (Nilsson & Nilsson 1994; Goodrich et al 2000) but well-controlled studies are needed to prove their efficacy. Recently, it has been found that provided sufficient magnification is prescribed, patients with AMD using illuminated stand magnifiers did not need extensive training to achieve their maximum, albeit slow, reading rate (Cheong et al 2005). A few short sessions of in-office instruction and practice with the device over 2 weeks enabled most patients to read close to their maximum reading rate (equivalent to large-print reading rate) with the magnifier.

Instruction on the use of near low-vision devices also involves advice on:

- spectacles to use in conjunction with magnifiers
- adequate posture, perhaps recommending a bookstand or bookrest
- appropriate lighting with an adjustable reading lamp
- how to change the batteries of illuminated hand-held and stand magnifiers and how to turn them off and on
- reading for only short duration at first.

Advise the patient to first practise reading on slightly larger print than their goal task. If they have difficulties with this, ensure they are using sufficient illumination. In the case of stand magnifiers, stress the required eye–lens distance. Some patients using hand-held or stand magnifiers may prefer to hold the magnifier steady and move the reading material under it (steady-eye strategy, Dickinson 1998). Most place the reading material on a table or reading stand and move the magnifier. Recommend that they raise the height of the reading material so they are not bending their neck or back excessively. The most common difficulty patients have using hand-held and stand magnifiers is finding the start of the next line but such page navigation errors are not well predicted by vision measures or magnifier parameters (Bowers et al 2007). A finger or ruler beside the start of the line can act as a guide in locating the next line.

For the patient with good hand control using a high near addition, adaptation to and control of the reduced reading distance will require regular reinforcement during in-office practice. It may be easiest to first hold the material too close (against their nose) and gradually move the print out until it is in focus and then maintain that distance.

Review the patient's performance after 2 weeks' home trial with the device before finalizing its prescription. Regular follow-up is needed thereafter (see below).

Care of low-vision devices

The lenses of most optical devices can scratch easily. Instruct patients to keep their devices in the case or box provided and to ensure that these do not become dusty. Most optical devices should not be immersed in water. To clean lenses, use a soft cloth moistened with white spirit. If dust or grit builds up around the magnifier casing, a small soft brush can be used to clean this out or, alternatively, advise the patient to return to the prescribing optometrist to have the device cleaned.

Eccentric viewing training

In the past, extensive eccentric viewing training programmes have been recommended to assist the patient with a central scotoma for reading and other daily activities (Nilsson & Nilsson 1994; Freeman & Jose 1997). However, the necessity and effectiveness of these programmes is not proven (Stelmack et al 2004). In the author's clinical experience, most patients who read left to right will learn without training to develop a relatively stable preferred retinal locus (PRL) below the scotoma, i.e. shift the scotoma up to open the inferior and right fields, whereas those who read from right to left will shift fixation to open the left field (Rohrschneider 2007).

As described above, some idea of the direction of eccentric viewing can be determined during VA testing and, if it is inappropriate, the patient can be coached during both VA testing and central visual field assessment. If a scotoma is elongated vertically, fixating below the scotoma will not be possible. In this case, fixating to the right of the scotoma (shifting the scotoma to the left) may assist with reading. The author has found the training exercises provided by Freeman and Jose (1997) to be useful for those few patients who have required eccentric viewing training.

It is important to note that most patients with AMD first develop a paracentral scotoma (Swann & Lovie-Kitchin 1991). If this becomes a partial or complete annulus affecting the right field, a small central island will remain, giving relatively good distance letter VA but poor near VA and reading rate. In this case, reading rehabilitation including eccentric viewing training is unlikely to be successful. The visual field assessment is extremely important in these cases. The spurious situation arises that low-vision care is more likely to be successful when the AMD has progressed and vision is worse because the central island of relatively good vision has gone. Under these conditions, an eccentric PRL will develop and reading is likely to be possible with higher-magnification low-vision devices.

Optical low-vision devices for the optometric practice

It is important for optometrists to know one or more local suppliers from whom a range of optical and electronic devices can be ordered. The companies will usually provide printed catalogues and price lists, and often these can be downloaded from their websites.

Most optometrists in general practice cannot stock a wide range of low-vision devices. However, a small range of commonly used equipment is needed for in-office assessment and trials by the low-vision patients. If the device required for prescription is not in the optometrist's stock, it can be ordered (often 'on-approval') from the supplier.

Tables 30.8A & 30.8B list a few optical devices which it is recommended that optometrists hold in stock. Most of the recommended instrumentation is manufactured by Eschenbach, simply because they are the most familiar to the author, but other manufacturers produce similar devices (see Bailey's tables for comparison (Bailey 2006)).

Higher-powered devices are not commonly used in private practice, as patients requiring these will usually need referral for a full range of vision rehabilitation services.

Non-optical low-vision devices

For other activities of daily living, including mobility, non-optical devices and/or training can provide assistance, in addition to or sometimes instead of optical or electronic low-vision equipment. As well as a small stock of optical devices and information on electronic equipment, the optometrist should either have the following equipment available for demonstration, or at least know where they are available for purchase. Some of these devices may be accessed only through vision rehabilitation services or agencies for visually impaired individuals.

- *Filters*: i.e. tints and fit-over sunglasses; recommend sunshields, umbrellas, hats, caps, etc. to manage changes in illumination.
- *Reading lamps*: adjustable fluorescent tube with a 'warm' colour temperature, but cool lamp temperature (**Fig. 30.14**) is preferred as the lamp can be comfortably placed close to near tasks. Demonstrate the use of the lamp, positioned to the opposite side to the writing hand, to avoid glare and shadows.
- *Portable flashlight*: recommended for safer mobility at night. For more extensive advice on lighting in the home, referral to an occupational therapist or rehabilitation teacher may be necessary
- *Large-print books and books on CD*: available from most public libraries and/or book stores.
- *Reading stand*: book rest, music stand or typing stand, especially one that will hold heavy books such as large-print books.

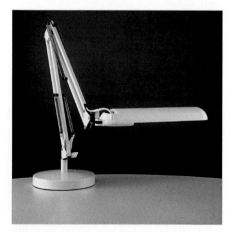

Figure 30.14 Adjustable, portable fluorescent reading lamp. (Photograph provided by Daylight Company Pty Ltd.)

- *Typoscope/signature guide*: a locator or frame of reference made of stiff black cardboard or plastic in which a small window is cut of a length and width appropriate to the size of print normally read or with sufficient space for the patient's signature (**Fig. 30.5**). The typoscope helps the reader to keep to the line while reading or signing their name, and reduces glare from the surrounding page. Often, family members will make these for the patient.
- *Felt-tipped pens*: thick black pens for labels or writing letters. Family members and others who write letters to the person with low vision should be encouraged to use these also.

Sometimes, a combination of optical and non-optical devices may be required. For example, a musician needing a wide field of view for reading music might use an increased spectacle addition together with a music stand or typing stand at a decreased viewing distance. If this is not sufficient, a photocopy enlargement of the music may be needed.

Many other non-optical devices are available for activities of daily living such as: communication, e.g. writing, telephoning; telling the time; money identification; home management, e.g. cooking, laundering, sewing; self-care, e.g. eating, hygiene and safety; community skills, e.g. shopping and recreational pursuits. These are available, and often need some training in their use by occupational therapists or rehabilitation teachers, through low-vision clinics or other agencies for visually impaired people.

Referral to other rehabilitation services

The needs of low-vision patients vary greatly depending on the cause of low vision, the level of vision, the visual tasks, the patients' motivation, the degree of family and social support, etc. There are many low-vision patients for whom optometric care alone will be sufficient to meet their goals and enable them to continue to function independently.

Patients in other circumstances, with different goals or with severe vision impairment, will require additional assistance from vision rehabilitation services and/or community resources to assist them to function as independently as possible. There are many public and private agencies that offer their resources to the optometrist, the patient and the patient's family. Optometrists should be aware of what resources exist, who offers these services and where to locate them in their community. Local government sources or branches of national agencies for visually impaired people can often provide this information.

The optometrist may choose to continue to provide both the primary eye care and optometric low-vision care to the patient and coordinate the other rehabilitation services through local resources. Alternatively, other optometrists prefer to refer patients with moderate to severe vision impairment to multidisciplinary low-vision clinics where specialist optometrists can provide the low-vision care in conjunction with the other rehabilitation professionals.

Remember, low-vision clinics often do not provide primary eye care, so the referring optometrist needs to stress to the patient that this is still required regularly through the optometrist's practice.

The rehabilitation professionals and services that might be required include: social workers, occupational therapists, orientation and mobility instructors, rehabilitation teachers, psychologists, vocational counsellors, special education teachers and other generic community groups for in-home assistance, social activities, etc. In the case of working adults, for example, work place visits by an occupational therapist or a rehabilitation or vocational counsellor may be necessary to identify the best solutions for the individual with low vision and his/her co-workers and employers. For detailed information on the roles of these rehabilitation professionals, see low-vision texts (e.g. Corn & Koenig 1996; Fletcher 1999; Scheiman et al 2007).

Such services may be particularly required by a person who has had a recent, sudden and severe vision loss. Both they and their family or carers will need a range of assistance, information and counselling to accept and learn to cope with the vision loss. Until such a person accepts that the vision loss is permanent, they are unlikely to accept optometric low-vision care.

In the provision of many of these rehabilitation services, the patient's family members and/or carers need to be involved. In the case of a severely visually impaired person it is important that sighted guide training is provided to those who live or work closely with the person with low vision.

Review

A telephone follow-up to the patient a week after low-vision devices have been loaned for home, school or work trial to reinforce instructions on their use will be appreciated by most patients and/or carers. Then an in-office review a further 1 to 3 weeks later (2 to 4 weeks after the loan) of the patient's performance with the trial low-vision device is recommended. Reassess the patient's distance and near VA at this visit and have the patient demonstrate his/her use of the low-vision device. If the patient's goal is met with the device and they are using it appropriately it can be prescribed with instructions on its care (see above).

If further goals need to be addressed, undertake the appropriate assessments as described above and prescribe devices or refer for further services as indicated.

Regular on-going review of low-vision patients' vision and their needs is required. If the patient has a progressive ocular disease, this might need to be quite frequent (e.g. every month or two). If they have stable vision, the first review after the delivery of services might occur 3 or 6 months later and then annual review is recommended if the patient is managing well. Advise the patient to return immediately there is any change in their circumstances as below.

Regular review, e.g. 6-monthly or annually, is necessary because:

- vision may change
- instruction on use of devices may need clarification/reinforcement
- the patient's goals/needs may change, e.g. with change in employment, education and/or hobbies, etc.
- other factors may arise which affect their use of devices, e.g. poor general health, stroke, etc.

Vision rehabilitation is a valuable and rewarding service that optometrists can provide to the ever-increasing numbers of people with low vision. In 1975, Mehr and Freid stated, 'it is the technique of the low-vision examination rather than the use of unusual lenses, which in the majority of these cases is responsible for the favourable results' (Mehr & Freid 1975). This remains true today. By following the systematic approach outlined here, the optometric practitioner can assist many visually impaired people to maintain independent functioning.

References

Ahn S J, Legge G E, Luebker A 1995 Printed cards for measuring low-vision reading speed. Vision Research 35(13):1939–1944

Attebo A K, Mitchell P, Smith W 1996 Visual acuity and the causes of visual loss in Australia. The Blue Mountains eye study. Ophthalmology 10:357–364

Bailey I L 1991a Low vision refraction. In: Eskridge J B, Amos J F, Bartlett J D (eds) Clinical procedures in optometry. JB Lippincott, Philadelphia, pp 762–768

Bailey I L 1991b Low vision visual acuity. In: Eskridge J B, Amos J F, Bartlett J D (eds) Clinical procedures in optometry. JB Lippincott, Philadelphia, pp 745–761

Bailey I L 2006 Low vision yellow pages: YP2Technical_data.xls. Online. Available: http://optometry.berkeley.edu/class/, University of California, Berkeley. Accessed 17 Dec 2008

Bailey I L, Bullimore M A 1991 A new test for the evaluation of disability glare. Optometry and Vision Science 68(12):911–917

Bailey I L, Lovie J E 1976 New design principles for visual acuity letter charts. American Journal of Optometry and Physiological Optics 53: 740–745

Bailey I L, Bullimore M A, Raasch T W et al 1991 Clinical grading and the effects of scaling. Investigative Ophthalmology and Vision Science 32(2):422–432

Bailey I L, Bullimore M A, Greer R X 1994 Low vision magnifiers – their optical parameters and methods for prescribing. Optometry and Vision Science 71:689–698

Borish I M 1975 Clinical refraction. Professional Press, Chicago

Bowers A R, Meek C, Stewart N 2001 Illumination and reading performance in age-related macular degeneration. Clinical and Experimental Optometry 84(3):139–147

Bowers A R, Cheong A M Y, Lovie-Kitchin J E 2007 Reading with optical magnifiers: Page navigation strategies and difficulties. Optometry and Vision Science 84:9–20

Brilliant R L 1999 Essentials of low vision practice. Butterworth-Heinemann, Boston

Cheong A M, Lovie-Kitchin J E, Bowers A R 2002 Fixed versus individualised acuity reserve methods for determining magnification for low vision reading. Clinical and Experimental Optometry 85:229–237

Cheong A M, Lovie-Kitchin J E, Bowers A R et al 2005 Short-term reading practice improves reading performance with stand magnifiers for people with AMD. Optometry and Vision Science 82:114–127

Colenbrander A 1977 Dimensions of visual performance. Transactions of the American Academy of Ophthalmology and Otolaryngology 83:332–337

Colenbrander A 1994 The functional vision score. In: Kooijman A C, Looijestijn P L, Welling J A et al (eds) Low vision – research and new developments in rehabilitation. IOS Press, Amsterdam, pp 552–561

Congdon N, O'Colmain B, Klaver C C W et al 2004 Causes and prevalence of visual impairment among adults in the United States. Archives of Ophthalmology 122(4):477–485

Corn A L, Koenig A J 1996 Foundations of low vision: clinical and functional perspectives. AFB Press, New York

de Boer M R, Moll A C, de Vet H C W et al 2004 Psychometric properties of vision-related quality of life questionnaires: A systematic review. Ophthalmic and Physiological Optics 24(4):257–273

Dickinson C 1998 Low vision: principles and practice. Butterworth-Heinemann, Boston

Eldred K B 1992 Optimal illumination for reading in patients with age-related maculopathy. Optometry and Vision Science 69(1):46–50

Elliott D B, Trukolo-Ilic M, Strong J G et al 1997 Demographic characteristics of the vision-disabled elderly. Investigative Ophthalmology and Visual Science 38(12):2566–2575

Evans J, Wormald R 1996 Is the incidence of registrable age-related macular degeneration increasing? British Journal of Ophthalmology 80:9–14

Faye 1976 Clinical low vision. Little, Brown, Boston

Ferris F L, Kassoff A, Bresnick G H et al 1982 New visual acuity charts for clinical research. American Journal of Ophthalmology 94:91–96

Fletcher D C 1999 Low vision rehabilitation: caring for the whole person. American Academy of Ophthalmology, San Francisco

Fletcher D C, Schuchard R A 1997 Preferred retinal loci relationship to macular scotomas in a low-vision population. Ophthalmology 104 (4):632–638

Freeman P B, Jose R T 1997 The art and practice of low vision. Butterworth-Heinemann, Boston

Goodrich G L, Kirby J, Keswick C et al 2000 Training the patient with low vision to read: Does it significantly improve function? In: Stuen C, Arditi A, Horowitz A et al (eds) Vision rehabilitation. Swets & Zeitlinger, New York, pp 230–236

Grosvenor T P 2007 Primary care optometry, Chapter 19. MO Butterworth-Heinemann/Elsevier, St Louis, MO

Harper R A 2004 Low vision assessment and management. In: Harvey D, Gilmartin B (eds) Paediatric optometry. Churchill Livingstone, Edinburgh, pp 91–97

Hassan S, Lovie-Kitchin J, Woods R 2002 Vision and mobility performance of subjects with age-related macular degeneration. Optometry and Vision Science 79:697–707

Hawkins A S, Szlyk J P, Ardickas Z et al 2003 Comparison of contrast sensitivity, visual acuity, and Humphrey visual field testing in patients with glaucoma. Journal of Glaucoma 12(2):134–138

Hensil J, Whittaker S G 2000 Visual reading versus auditory reading by sighted persons and persons with low vision. Journal of Visual Impairment and Blindness 94:762–771

Hovis J K, Leat S J, Epp K 2003 The UWCdot colour vision test and low vision. Ophthalmic and Physiological Optics 23(2):125–131

Hyvarinen L 2005 Visual assessment of the infant and child: Assessment of vision in infants and children with vision loss. In: Hartnett M E (ed.) Pediatric retina. Lippincott Williams & Wilkins, Philadelphia, pp 29–44

Johnston A W 1991 Making sense of the M, N, and logMar systems of specifying visual acuity. In: Rosenthal B P, Cole R G (eds) Problems in optometry: a structured approach to low vision care. J B Lippincott, Philadelphia, pp 394–407

Lamoureux E L, Pallant J F, Pesudovs K et al 2006 The Impact of Vision Impairment questionnaire: an evaluation of its measurement properties using Rasch analysis. Investigative Ophthalmology and Visual Science 47(11):4732–4741

Leat S J, Woodhouse J M 1993 Reading performance with low vision aids: relationship with contrast sensitivity. Ophthalmic and Physiological Optics 13:9–16

Leat S J, Legge G E, Bullimore M A 1999 What is low vision? A re-evaluation of definitions. Optometry and Vision Science 76(4):198–211

Legge G E, Rubin G S, Pelli D G et al 1985 Psychophysics of reading – ii. Low vision. Vision Research 25(2):253–266

Legge G E, Ross J A, Isenberg L M et al 1992 Psychophysics of reading: clinical predictors of low vision reading speed. Investigative Ophthalmology and Visual Science 33(3):677–687

Lei H, Schuchard R A 1997 Using two preferred retinal loci for different lighting conditions in patients with central scotomas. Investigative Ophthalmology and Visual Science 38(9):1812–1818

Lovie-Kitchin J E, Bowman K J 1985 Senile macular degeneration – management and rehabilitation. Butterworths, Boston

Lovie-Kitchin J E, Brown B 2000 Repeatability and intercorrelations of standard vision tests as a function of age. Optometry and Vision Science 77(8):412–420

Lovie-Kitchin J E, Feigl B 2005 Assessment of age-related maculopathy using subjective vision tests. Clinical and Experimental Optometry 88:292–303

Lovie-Kitchin J E, Whittaker S G 1998a Low vision assessment for reading rehabilitation: Indications for visual field assessment. In: Vision '96, Proceedings of the International Conference on Low Vision 1996. Madrid, Organizacion Nacional de Ciegos Espanoles. Book I: 268–275

Lovie-Kitchin J E, Whittaker S G 1998b Relative-size magnification versus relative-distance magnification: effect on the reading performance of adults with normal and low vision. Journal of Vision Impairment and Blindness 92:433–446

Lovie-Kitchin J E, Whittaker S G 1999 Prescribing near magnification for low vision patients. Clinical and Experimental Optometry 82 (6):214–224

Lovie-Kitchin J E, Whittaker S G 2000 Prescribing magnification for reading with low vision: What are the criteria? In: Stuen C, Arditi A, Horowitz A et al (eds) Vision rehabilitation – assessment, intervention and outcomes. Swets & Zeitlinger, Lisse, pp 314–318

Lovie-Kitchin J E, Mainstone J, Robinson J et al 1990 What areas of the visual field are important for mobility in low vision patients? Clinical and Vision Sciences 4:249–263

Lovie-Kitchin J E, Bowers A R, Woods R L 2000 Oral and silent reading performance with macular degeneration. Ophthalmic and Physiological Optics 20(5):360–370

Lovie-Kitchin J, Devereaux J, Wells S et al 2001 Multi-disciplinary low vision care. Clinical and Experimental Optometry 84:165–170

Lovie-Kitchin J E, Woods R L, Hassan S E et al 2002 Critical visual field size for mobility of low vision adults. (Vision 2002 abstract a6:30) Online. Available: http://www.islrr.org/vision02/160.html International Society for Low Vision Research and Rehabilitation

Margolis M K, Coyne K, Kennedy-Martin T et al 2002 Vision-specific instruments for the assessment of health-related quality of life and visual functioning: A literature review. Pharmacoeconomics 20 (12):791–812

Mehr E B, Freid A N 1975 Low vision care. Professional Press Incorporated, Chicago

Monés J, Rubin G S 2005 Contrast sensitivity as an outcome measure in patients with subfoveal choroidal neovascularisation due to age-related macular degeneration. Eye 19(11):1142–1150

Nilsson U L, Nilsson S E G 1994 Educational training in the use of aids and residual vision is essential in rehabilitation of patients with severe age-related macular degeneration. II. Results of a prospective study. In: Kooijman A C, Looijestijn P L, Welling J A et al (eds) Low vision – research and new developments in rehabilitation. IOS Press, Amsterdam, pp 151–154

Nowakowski R W 1994 Primary low vision care. Appleton & Lange, Connecticut

Pelli D G, Robson J G, Wilkins A J 1988 The design of a new letter chart for measuring contrast sensitivity. Clinical and Vision Sciences 2 (3):187–199

Raasch T W 2004 What we don't know about eccentric viewing. British Journal of Ophthalmology 88(4):443

Resnikoff S, Pascolini D, Etyaale D et al 2004 Global data on visual impairment in the year 2002. Bulletin of the World Health Organization 82:844–851

Rohrschneider K 2007 Low vision: the morphofunctional approach. In: Midena E (ed.) Perimetry and the fundus: an introduction to microperimetry. Slack Inc., Thorofare, NJ, pp 215–224

Rubin G S 1988 Reliability and sensitivity of clinical contrast sensitivity tests. Clinical and Vision Sciences 2(3):169–177

Rubin G S, Roche K B, Prasada-Rao P et al 1994 Visual impairment and disability in older adults. Optometry and Vision Science 71 (12):750–760

Scheiman M, Scheiman M, Whittaker S 2007 Low vision rehabilitation: a practical guide for occupational therapists. Slack Inc, Thorofare, NJ

Schuchard R A, Naseer S, de Castro K 1999 Characteristics of AMD patients with low vision receiving visual rehabilitation. Journal of Rehabilitation Research and Development 36(4):294–302

Sloan L L 1959 New test charts for the measurement of visual acuity at far and near distances. American Journal of Ophthalmology 48:807–813

Sloan L L 1969 Variation of acuity with luminance in ocular diseases and anomalies. Documenta Ophthalmologica. Advances in Ophthalmology 26:384–393

Sloan L L, Habel A, Feiock K 1973 High illuminations as an auxiliary reading aid in diseases of the macula. American Journal of Ophthalmology 76(5):745–757

Stelmack J A, Massof R W, Stelmack T R 2004 Is there a standard of care for eccentric viewing training? Journal of Rehabilitation Research and Development 41(5):729–738

Swann P G, Lovie-Kitchin J E 1991 Age-related maculopathy: II. The nature of the central visual field loss. Ophthalmic and Physiological Optics 11:59–70

Taylor H R, Livingston P M, Stanislavsky Y L et al 1997 Visual impairment in Australia: distance visual acuity, near vision, and visual field findings of the Melbourne visual impairment project. American Journal of Ophthalmology 123(3):328–337

Taylor H R, Keeffe J E, Vu H T V et al 2005 Vision loss in Australia. Medical Journal of Australia 182(11):565–568

Timberlake G T, Mainster M A, Peli E et al 1986 Reading with a macular scotoma: I. Retinal location of scotoma and fixation area. Investigative Ophthalmology and Visual Science 27(7):1137–1147

Virgili G, Acosta R 2006 Reading aids for adults with low vision. Cochrane Database of Systematic Reviews Issue 4. (Art No.: CD003303): DOI: 10.1002/14651858.CD14003303.pub14651852

Watson G R, Schuchard R A, De L'aune W R et al 2006 Effects of preferred retinal locus placement on text navigation and development of advantageous trained retinal locus. Journal of Rehabilitation Research and Development 43(6):761–770

Whittaker S G, Cummings R W 1999 New approaches for vision rehabilitation. In: Berger J, Fine S, Maguire M (eds) Age-related macular degeneration. Mosby, St Louis, pp 443–450

Whittaker S G, Lovie-Kitchin J E 1993 Visual requirements for reading. Optometry and Visual Science 70(1):54–65

Whittaker S G, Lovie-Kitchin J E 1994 The assessment of contrast sensitivity and contrast reserve for reading rehabilitation. In: Kooijman A C, Looijestijn P L, Welling J A et al (eds) Low vision – research and new development in rehabilitation. IOS Press, Amsterdam, pp 88–92

Whittaker S G, Budd J M, Cummings R W 1988 Eccentric fixation with macular scotoma. Investigative Ophthalmology and Visual Science 29(2):268–278

Wolffsohn J S, Cochrane A L 2000 Design of the low vision quality-of-life questionnaire (LVQOL) and measuring the outcome of low-vision rehabilitation. American Journal of Ophthalmology 130(6):793–802

Woods R L, Wood J M 1995 The role of contrast sensitivity charts and contrast letter charts in clinical practice. Clinical and Experimental Optometry 78:43-57

World Health Organization 2001 International classification of functioning, disability and health. World Health Organization, Geneva

World Health Organization 2004 Magnitude and causes of visual impairment. Fact sheet no. 282, World Health Organization. Online. Available: http://www.who.int/mediacentre/factsheets/fs282/en/print/html. Accessed 17 December 2008

World Health Organization 2007 VISION 2000 THE RIGHT TO SIGHT. Global initiative for the elimination of avoidable blindness: Action Plan 2006–2011. WHO Press, World Health Organization, Geneva. Online. Available at http://www.who.int/blindness/en/index.html. Accessed 17 December 2008

CHAPTER 31

Ageing populations

Bruce P Rosenthal

Epidemiology

The world's population clock continues to tick furiously, standing at over 6.5 billion people, while the population of the United States is now over 300 million. The past century has witnessed an even more dramatic growth in the cohort of 65+ and 85+ year-olds in the USA. The 65+-year-old age group comprised only 4% of the US population in l900, but grew to 12% by the year 2000. During the same period, the 85+ cohort went from less than 1% of the population in 1900 to 2% by the year 2000. Projecting these statistics out to 2050 and beyond reveals a huge increase of over 20% in those over 65, and an increase of 5% of those over 85 (**Fig. 31.1**). The actual numbers of these individuals, which stood at 3.1 million in the 65+ group, will soar to over 71 million by the year 2030. This represents almost a 25-fold increase, as illustrated in **Figure 31.2**.

Future issues on health costs to society

According to Saaddine et al (2005), blindness and visual impairment are among the 10 most common causes of disability in the USA, and are associated with a shorter life expectancy as well as a lower quality of life (**Table. 31.1**). Vision 2010, a programme of the National Eye Institute (NEI), has advocated addressing this problem of the twenty-first century through prevention; specifically with early detection, treatment, and rehabilitation. Additionally, *Healthy People 2010* set forth two goals, namely the elimination of health disparities and an increase in both the quality and duration of healthy living. A memorandum of understanding has been developed between the American Optometric Association (AOA) and the US Department of Health and Human Services regarding activities related to *Healthy People 2010*.

The vision objectives listed in *Healthy People 2010* state that the national goal is to 'improve the visual health of the nation through prevention, early detection, treatment, and rehabilitation'. This chapter will address visual impairment due to conditions such as diabetic retinopathy, age-related macular degeneration (AMD), glaucoma, cataract, and refractive error, since 'visual impairment is associated with loss of personal independence, decreased quality of life, and difficulty maintaining employment. For older adults, visual problems have a pronounced negative impact on their quality of life, equivalent to those of life-threatening conditions such as heart disease and cancer.'

With the increasing numbers of older individuals in the twenty-first century, vision care must be addressed with innovative, inexpensive, and accessible screening and preventative measures. Screening for genetic predispositions that lead to age-related vision conditions will probably become commonplace in the future. In fact, disease-causing genetic mutations are associated with many ocular diseases, such as glaucoma, cataract, corneal dystrophies and a number of retinal abnormalities including AMD and retinitis pigmentosa.

Ojha and Thertulien (2005) refer to four distinct issues of universal importance to healthcare policy and society that have been spawned by the genetic revolution: genetic privacy, regulation and standardization of genetic tests, gene patenting

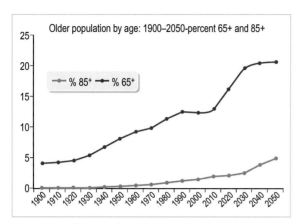

Figure 31.1 Older population by age: 1900–2050. (From: http://www.aoa.gov/prof/Statistics/online_stat_data/AgePop2050Chart-pct.asp.)

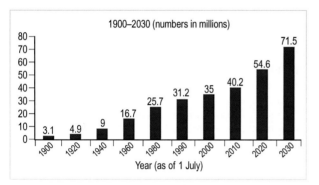

Figure 31.2 Number of persons 65+, 1900–2030 (number in millions). (Source: Projections of the population by age are taken from the January 2004 Census Internet Release. Historical data from: 65+ in the United States, Current Population Reports, Special Studies, pp 23–190. Data for 2000 from: The 2000 Census. 2002 data from: The Census estimates for 2002.)

and education. But continuing ethical concerns and political controversy are sure to accompany and surround any radical changes and concepts that are intended to decrease the burgeoning health costs to society.

Crews and Campbell (2004) stated that older adults with vision loss may experience a higher rate of falls, hip fractures, depression and family stress. Indeed, a higher risk of depression in individuals with vision loss was also observed by Branch et al (1989), Campbell et al (1999), and Caraballese et al (1993).

Horowitz and Reinhardt (2000) reported that depression is common in visually impaired older adults, and stated that it may have a significant impact on both functional ability and the quality of life. Rizzo and Kellison (2004) noted that visual disability may also impact other areas such as driving, where drivers may not only cause injuries to themselves but to their passengers and other road users.

Rein et al (2006) reported that the estimated cost to the USA of major vision problems in people over 40, such as visual impairment, blindness, refractive error, AMD, cataracts, diabetic retinopathy, and primary open-angle glaucoma, was US $35.4 billion. This can be broken down to direct medical costs of US$6.8 billion for cataracts, US$5.5 billion for refractive error, US$2.9 billion for glaucoma, US$575 million for AMD and US$493 million for diabetic retinopathy. Since many of the conditions are treatable, early detection with routine eye examinations will not only translate into huge healthcare economic savings, but will also result in significantly improved quality of life. Well-planned health programmes will reduce substantially the costs for future generations as well.

The rising economic cost to society from an increasing elderly population, as well as the specific cost to the healthcare system, is becoming apparent around the world. This may be visualized by the projected population pyramids for 2025 and 2050. The population pyramids for the USA are shown in **Figures 31.3–31.5**. However, the population pyramids for Italy (**Figs 31.6–31.8**) and Japan (**Figs 31.9–31.11**) are more dramatic illustrations of two other developed nations where the birth rate has fallen substantially, while the number of older individuals continues to grow. This demonstrates the increasing healthcare burden that will be borne in the future. The dramatic increase in the older population is not only seen in the more developed nations but also in less developed countries. This is shown in **Table 31.2**.

Resources and impact on health

The rapidly approaching 'golden era' of older persons will bring many questions and issues that have to be addressed. These include access to 'affordable' healthcare and prescriptive medications, as well as liability issues (Gingrich & Gill 2006). An increased number of trained medical and ancillary personnel will be needed. Additional concerns include appropriate living arrangements for these older individuals,

Table 31.1 Prevalence of blindness and low vision among adults 40 years and older in the USA.

Age, years	Blindness**		Low vision**		All vision impaired	
	Persons	(%)	Persons	(%)	Persons	(%)
40–49	51 000	0.1%	80 000	0.2%	131 000	0.3%
50–59	45 000	0.1%	102 000	0.3%	147 000	0.4%
60–69	59 000	0.3%	176 000	0.9%	235 000	1.2%
70–79	134 000	0.8%	471 000	3.0%	605 000	3.8%
>80	648 000	7.0%	1 532 000	16.7%	2 180 000	23.7%
Total	937 000	0.8%	2 361 000	2.0%	3 298 000	2.7%

From: http://www.nei.nih.gov/eyedata/pbd_tables.asp
**Blindness, as defined in the USA, is the best-corrected visual acuity of 6/60 (20/200) or worse in the better-seeing eye; low vision is defined as best-corrected visual acuity less than 6/12 (20/40) in the better-seeing eye (excluding those categorized as being blind).

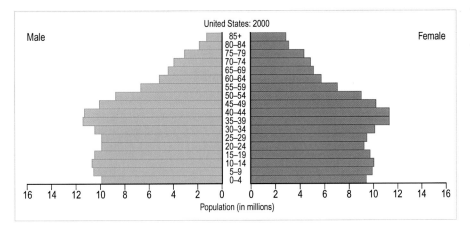

Figure 31.3 United States population (in millions) in 2000. (Data from: http://www.census.gov/ipc/www/idbpyr.html 24 Aug 2006.)

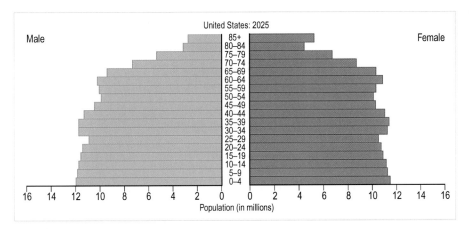

Figure 31.4 Projected United States population (in millions) in 2025. (Data from: http://www.census.gov/ipc/www/idbpyr.html (24 Aug 2006.)

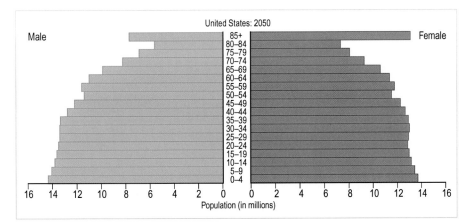

Figure 31.5 Projected United States population in millions in 2050. (Data from: http://www.census.gov/ipc/www/idbpyr.html 24 Aug 2006.)

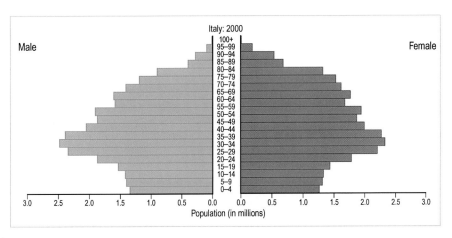

Figure 31.6 Italian population (in millions) in 2000. (Data from: http://www.census.gov/ipc/www/idbpyr.html 24 Aug 2006.)

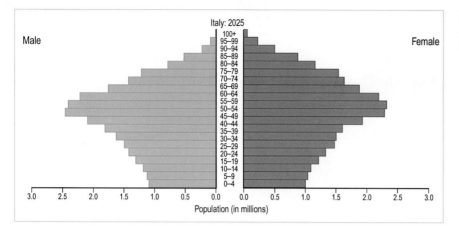

Figure 31.7 Projected Italian population (in millions) in 2025. (Data from: http://www.census.gov/ipc/www/idbpyr.html 24 Aug 2006.)

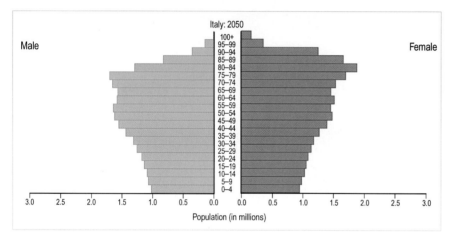

Figure 31.8 Projected Italian population (in millions) in 2050. (Data from: http://www.census.gov/cgi-bin/ipc/idbpyrs.pl?cty=IT&out=s&ymax=200)

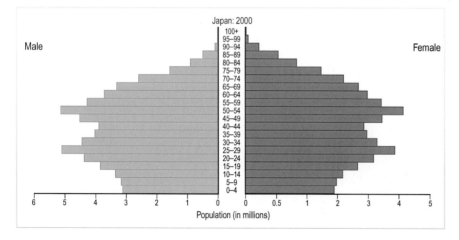

Figure 31.9 Japanese population (in millions) in 2000. (Data from: http://www.census.gov/ipc/www/idbpyr.html 24 Aug 2006.)

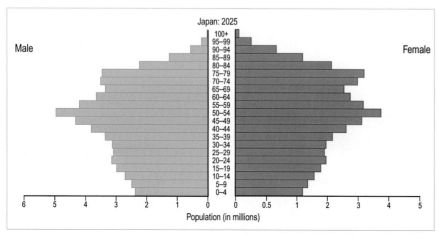

Figure 31.10 Projected Japanese population (in millions) in 2025. (Data from: http://www.census.gov/ipc/www/idbpyr.html 24 Aug 2006.)

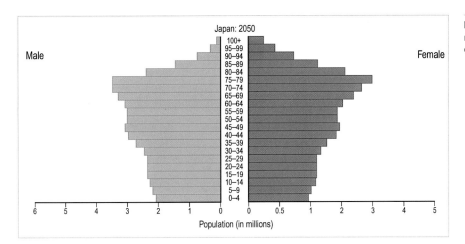

Figure 31.11 Projected Japanese population (in millions) in 2050. (Data from: http://www.census.gov/cgi-bin/ipc/idbpyrs.pl?cty=JA&out=s&ymax=200)

Table 31.2 Older population in both more and less developed countries in 2002 and projected numbers for 2025

Region and country or area	Total population by age group, region, and country: 2002	
	65–79 years	80 years and over
WORLD	363 177	77 138
Less developed countries	226 944	36 998
More developed countries	136 234	40 140

Region and country or area	Total population by age group, region, and country: 2025	
	65–79 years	80 years and over
WORLD	668 912	164 400
Less developed countries	476 869	95 131
More developed countries	192 043	69 269

Midyear population in thousands. Figures may not add to totals because of rounding.
Data from: http://www.census.gov/ipc/prod/wp02/tabA-07b.xls

adequate mental health and socio-economic status, and special adaptive equipment. Preventative measures must be given high priority on the healthcare agenda.

The National Eye Health Education Program (NEHEP) has prioritized goals to reduce vision loss by increasing awareness of glaucoma, diabetic eye disease, and low vision amongst selected high-risk target audiences in the USA. These goals include 'early detection of glaucoma, diabetic eye disease, as well as the utilization of low-vision services, with the ultimate outcome of effecting appropriate behaviour change'. Other major objectives include increasing the number of healthcare providers, enhancing awareness of the need for regular, comprehensive eye examinations with dilated pupils for those at risk for glaucoma and diabetic eye disease, and the need for referrals to low-vision services, with the ultimate goal of effecting appropriate behaviour change.

An increase in ageing brings not only a huge upswing in vision loss, but also serious medical conditions including coronary artery disease, hypertension, diabetes, stroke, and cancers. The modifiable risk factors such as diet and smoking will gain increasing importance in disease prevention. An additional consideration that will impact every national economy throughout the world is the spectre of global warming. Climate change will impact upon the allocation of financial resources that will both directly and indirectly affect the well-being of the elderly. Already underway is a trend that will result in a dramatic reduction of valuable natural global resources, such as clean water and air, as well as the impact of population migrations due to climate change.

An increase in longevity will lead to an increase in those major eye conditions associated with ageing including AMD, diabetic retinopathy, glaucoma, cataract (**Table 31.3**) as well as those associated with stroke and brain tumours. But basic conditions such as uncorrected refractive errors continue to remain a worldwide issue, and account for more than 5 million cases of blindness according to Vision 2020: The Right to Sight.

Table 31.3 Eye disease prevalence and projections. (Number of adults 40 years and older in the USA)

	Current estimates (in millions)	2020 projections (in millions)
Advanced AMD (with associated vision loss)	1.8*	2.9
Glaucoma	2.2	3.3
Diabetic retinopathy	4.1	7.2
Cataract	20.5	30.1

* Another 7.3 million people are at substantial risk for vision loss from AMD
Data from: http://www.census.gov/ipc/prod/wp02/tabA-07b.xls

This rise in the ageing population will also lead to an increase in the prevalence of co-morbid conditions such as coronary arterial disease, Alzheimer's, atherosclerosis, cancers, diabetes, stroke, psychiatric disorders, arthritis and frailty.

Vision and ageing

The proportion of adults reporting some form of visual impairment increases dramatically with age. Seventeen per cent of Americans aged 65 to 74 years and 26% of Americans 75 years of age and older self-report some form of vision loss according to The Lighthouse National Survey on Vision Loss (The Lighthouse Inc. 1995). Even moderate vision loss can result in difficulty performing activities such as managing personal affairs, driving, watching television, independent travel or reading. This will translate into a greater need for specialist geriatric optometric practitioners, as well as low-vision practices devoted to the problems of the elderly. However, primary care optometric practices will also witness a greater influx of older patients who will present with common eye problems as well as pathological changes including cataracts, AMD, diabetic retinopathy, corneal changes, glaucoma, visual field loss from stroke, reduced tear film and dry eye and lid anomalies including ptosis, entropian, and ectropian.

Age is the greatest risk factor for AMD (Hyman 1992; Augood et al 2004). Around 25% of people between the ages of 65 and 74 years and 33% of those above 75 years of age in the USA are likely to develop AMD (**Fig. 31.12**). The incidence of glaucoma also increases with age (Friedman et al 2004). Other risk factors include a family history of glaucoma, African or Hispanic ancestry, and diabetes. Diabetes also increases the likelihood of visual impairment. In 2005, the US Centers for Disease Control (CDC) estimated that 14.6 million people in the US had been diagnosed with diabetes, while an additional 6.2 million had diabetes that had not yet been diagnosed. Correctable visual impairment (CVI) in diabetics has been documented in several population-based studies including those of Attebo et al (1999) and Munoz et al (2002). Although the prevalence of CVI among diabetic adults aged 65 years and upwards (7.3%) was similar to that of 20–64-year-olds (7.2%), 89.2% of visual impairment cases among the younger age group were correctable, compared with only 46.4% of cases in the older age group. The age-adjusted prevalence of CVI

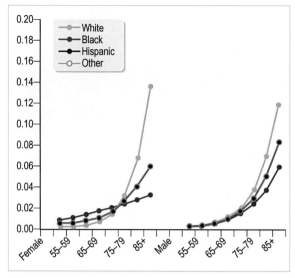

Figure 31.12 Estimated specific prevalence rate of age-related macular degeneration. (Data from: http://www.nei.nih.gov/eyedata/pdf/VPUS.pdf 7 Feb 2007)

was similar in men (7.3%) and women (7.2%). Although not statistically significant, the age-adjusted prevalence of CVI was higher amongst non-Hispanic blacks (7.9%) and Mexican-Americans (8.1%) than among non-Hispanic whites (5.6%). Zhang et al (2006) and Bresnick (2000) stated that the high prevalence of CVI amongst diabetics demonstrates a need for enhanced vision-related public health interventions (such as vision screening) in these individuals. Zhang suggested that the use of visual acuity and refractive error assessments together with recommended dilated eye examinations would contribute to improved vision outcomes for adults with diabetes. The prevalence of diabetic retinopathy amongst adults is shown in **Table 31.4**.

Falls and vision loss

Vision loss is one of the major contributing factors related to falls in the elderly, along with muscle weakness, balance and gait difficulties, a drop in blood pressure, slow heartbeat, postural hypotension, foot problems, arthritic knees, sensory problems (e.g. numbness from diabetes) and slower reflexes.

Table 31.4 Prevalence of diabetic retinopathy among adults

| Age, years | Type 1 diabetes | | | All diabetes – 40 years and older | |
	Persons	(%)		Persons	(%)
18–39	278 000	0.3%		NA	NA
40–49	172 000	0.4%		589 000	1.4%
50–64	317 000	0.4%		1 582 000	3.8%
65–74				1 068 000	5.8%
≥75				824 000	5.0%
Total	767 000	0.4%		4 063 000	3.4%

Data from: http://www.nei.nih.gov/eyedata/pbd_tables.asp

According to the CDC, the increase in fatal falls may be associated with an increased life expectancy (75.5 years in 1993 versus 77.6 years in 2003). This results in a larger proportion of older adults living with chronic diseases that render them at increased risk and vulnerability to fall-related injuries. The CDC recommends interventions to reduce the risk for falls amongst elderly individuals, which include regular exercise, a medication review to decrease contributory adverse events and interactions, annual eye examinations, and limiting fall hazards in the home.

Each year, more than 1.6 million older Americans go to the emergency room for fall-related injuries. Only half of the older adults hospitalized for a broken hip return home or live alone after the injury. Falls are the number one cause of fractures, hospital admissions for trauma, loss of independence and injury-related deaths in older adults, but these need not be inevitable, even as one ages.

Creuss et al (2006) noted that vision loss may be one of the greatest contributors to falls, with patients having AMD being twice as likely to fall as those with normal vision. Contributing factors may also include high anisometropia, significant differences in visual acuity or contrast sensitivity between the two eyes, visual field losses, spatial neglect, difficulty adapting to changes in light intensity, significant uncompensated retinal disparity, and the development of cataracts or glaucoma. De Boer et al (2004) also reported that impaired vision is an independent risk factor for falling and fractures, but indicated that various aspects of visual function may contribute differently to falls and fractures. Lord and Dayhew (2001) found that falls can contribute to the placement of an older person into institutional care.

Examination frequency

One of the most commonly asked questions, which may cause profound disagreement amongst eye care practitioners, is the recommended frequency of examinations for the elderly. The American Optometric Association (2005) recommends an annual examination after the age of 61. More frequent monitoring is advised for patients with diabetes or hypertension, a family history of glaucoma, AMD or cataracts, persons taking systemic medications with ocular side effects or those with other significant health concerns. Prevent Blindness America recommends an eye examination every one to two years after the age of 65. Those at higher risk as a result of co-morbid conditions such as high blood pressure, high cholesterol, diabetes, obesity, cardiac abnormalities, or having risk factors such as previous or current smoking should be examined more frequently.

Special accommodations for the elderly

The Americans with Disabilities Act (2002) has developed standards for small business accessibility that should be considered when setting up an optometric practice. Accommodations include wheelchair accessibility to the office entrance, waiting room area, lavatories, the examination and special testing rooms and the dispensary. Staff should be trained to be sensitive to other sensory deficits such as hearing impairment or known visual field loss.

Telephone interviews can both save time and minimize frustration for patients with decreased visual function. A detailed task analysis can be done over the telephone, or via mail, fax, or even e-mail. Indeed, many elderly patients and especially the new 'baby boomer' cohort feel very comfortable using a computer to transmit much of the necessary information, especially if it is set in a large, clear font (e.g. 16–18 point and bold faced).

Amplifiers for the hard of hearing should be available to facilitate communication. Ethnic diversity may necessitate on-call translators. The Health Insurance Portability and Accountability Act (HIPAA), enacted in 1996, established national standards for efficiency and effectiveness of the healthcare system in the USA. This act requires patient permission for relatives or friends to accompany them to the examination room. However, these third parties often benefit by obtaining a greater understanding of the nature and extent of the vision loss by observing the visual difficulties experienced during the examination.

It is often easier and quicker to have the patient brought to the examination room by an assistant. However, observation of the patient by the practitioner can provide valuable information regarding visual performance. Accompanying the patient from the waiting area to the examination room helps to establish a rapport with them. It may also provide the first clue that vision loss is affecting everyday performance. Valuable observations might include problems of gait, favouring one side, noticeable head turn, being affected by indoor glare sources, or even a patient with serious vision loss who is leading a relative or friend down the hallway. Patient facility with adaptive and mobility equipment such as the use of a support cane, three-pronged cane or a walker should also be noted.

Adapting the structured eye examination for older patients

Routine eye examinations are generally straightforward in older patients, with refractive corrections for distance, intermediate, and near as the primary outcome and screening for ocular disease the secondary outcome measure. As noted previously, older patients are at greater risk for both pathological eye conditions and other co-morbid abnormalities, e.g. diabetes. Therefore, the case history of the older patient requires greater in-depth examination including task analysis as well as questions such as the fear of losing independence, history of falls, and a detailed review of systems (see Ch. 26). For some patients, questions regarding possible fear of blindness may be appropriate. The eye examination may have to be modified as well.

The examination sequence should include the history, habitual visual acuities at distance and near, external evaluation, refraction, binocular assessment, tests of visual function, e.g. contrast sensitivity, visual fields (including Amsler grid) and colour vision, and a full examination of the anterior and posterior segments. These data will allow determination of the appropriate corrective lenses for distance, intermediate, and near, including the use of absorptive lenses, low-vision aids or specialized systems such as microscopic and telescopic lenses where indicated. If necessary, additional referrals should be considered to other specialists.

Case history

The procedure for obtaining a case history was discussed in detail in Chapter 26. However, there are some specific areas that need to be emphasized for the older patient. Rosenthal and Cole (1991a) noted that the case history should not only include the patient's visual complaints but also review their distance, intermediate, and near visual activities. When patients are poor responders or poor historians, especially those with early Alzheimer's disease or cerebral vascular accidents, they should be encouraged to allow the friend, relative or caregiver to accompany them into the examination room to fill in missing details. The functionally oriented history should investigate the ocular and health history, living situation, hearing ability, employment status, social activities and other limitations including difficulty walking or tremors. Regardless of age, employment, education, and even job retraining may be areas that need to be addressed.

Visual demands

A discussion of visual demands should include activities of daily living (e.g. managing medications, cooking) and hobbies, as well as the use of a computer (which may be a desktop, laptop or hand-held) or mobile (cell) phone. A detailed task analysis might be sent home to the patient prior to the evaluation, or alternatively handed out during the examination. Questions should be included about independent travel and driving. The latter is especially important since it can affect everything from the ability to remain gainfully employed to overall independence. Currently, there are 20 million drivers in the USA over 65 years of age, and this figure is expected to double by 2020. Most of these drivers wish to maintain their autonomy. However, elderly drivers are at higher risk of injury and death following a car accident because of their reduced ability to withstand trauma (Beers et al 2005).

Questions relating to independent travel on foot should include the ability to see traffic lights and street signs, as well as the capacity to cross an intersection. In addition, the patient should be asked about their physical motility, such as whether they are able to move around people and objects easily and if they have difficulty with curbs or steps and can walk without falling. Any supplementary mobility equipment, such as the use of a support cane, walker or wheelchair should be noted.

Daily living activity questions should focus on problems with housework, cooking, seeing stove dials, food on a plate, using the phone and being able to groom themselves. Patients should also be questioned regarding identifying faces, and whether they experience any problems watching television, movies or plays. Near and intermediate visual demands are especially important since they encompass everything from reading the newspaper, labels, prices, mail and bills, to being able to sign a cheque, read medication labels or sew. Today, since the computer has become an integral part of everyday life, having adequate intermediate visual function is extremely important.

Many elderly patients accumulate multiple pairs of glasses that may no longer be appropriate, especially if they have undergone ocular procedures such as cataract surgery. It is therefore important to separate out those pair of glasses that are most useful for distance, intermediate, near, occupational or recreational use. These may be single-vision, bifocal, progressive addition or tinted/photochromic lenses. Some or all of these glasses may be appropriate under certain conditions. However, to avoid confusion, the practitioner should make recommendations as to which pair(s) to keep and which to throw out. Labelling is often helpful since patients may have similar frames for distance and near.

Ocular history

The ocular history should investigate any previous ocular disease, surgery, treatments, diagnostic tests, ocular medications and compliance with these medications. The examiner should also ask about any significant family history such as AMD or glaucoma. Medical interventions for ocular conditions such as AMD and diabetic retinopathy should be investigated for possible side effects affecting visual function. For example, thermal laser therapy is an accepted treatment for AMD and proliferative diabetic retinopathy. Stefansson et al (1981) found that such treatment, while preserving vision, may permanently damage the retina and affect visual function at the same time. In fact, both night vision and reading fluency could be seriously affected following panretinal photocoagulation. Mackie and Walsh (1998) noted that adverse effects of photocoagulation include loss of visual field and visual acuity as well as increased glare, reduced contrast sensitivity and colour contrast.

Questions should also reflect the increased incidence of ocular and systemic disease in older patients. The case history should investigate any signs and symptoms that may be indicative of serious disease including pain, headaches, blurred vision, glare, distortion, diplopia, loss of vision, bumping into objects, halos around lights, difficulty adjusting to varying lighting conditions, phantom images, night vision problems, or difficulty with depth perception. Any previous surgical procedures and postsurgical complications must be investigated.

Medical history

The medical history should include information pertaining to conditions such as diabetic retinopathy, hypertension, cardiac disease, arthritis, allergies, asthma, thyroid conditions, stroke and cancer. Visual complications from conditions such as a cerebral vascular accident may result in a visual field loss, problems in visual perception, behavioural and cognitive changes or depression. Medications should be reviewed for visual side effects.

Many hospital-based studies have found that the risk for adverse drug reactions increases with age. Nolan and O'Malley (1988), Fulton and Allen (2005) and Zarowitz et al (2005) observed that polypharmacy is often a problem for older patients as they tend to use more medications for a given condition than are clinically warranted. Both the underlying systemic condition and its treatment should be evaluated for possible ocular side effects. For example, hydroxychloroquine sulphate is indicated for the treatment of discoid and systemic lupus erythematosus and rheumatoid arthritis. However, Elder et al (2006) reported that 35 (13.4%) out of 262 patients taking hydroxychloroquine had visual field abnormalities.

A careful history should include a list of the drugs being taken, noting drug compliance, as well as any serious side effects or drug interactions that may affect vision. Over-the-counter medications may also have ocular side effects, such as therapy for allergies that may result in decreased lacrimal output and contact lens intolerance. Vitamin supplementation is common among the elderly and should be investigated. Indeed, the AREDS Study Research Group (2000) indicated that antioxidants, zinc and vitamins C and E may protect against the progression of AMD in individuals with both moderate and advanced forms of the condition. The National Eye Institute recommends that people who are at high risk for developing advanced AMD should consider taking the combination of nutrients used in that particular study. However, many older people take multiple vitamins and non-evidenced-based supplements that may be potentially harmful. For example, an increased risk of bleeding has been observed in patients who are taking supplements such as vitamin E together with blood-thinning agents such as warfarin, heparin, or aspirin according to the Merck Manual on-line library (2003). A drug reference text should be available to investigate any potential ocular side effects resulting from systemic medications.

Hearing loss

Chia et al (2006) found that hearing loss is one of the most common conditions affecting older adults, and this may be associated with vision loss. Age-related hearing loss, known as presbycusis, gradually results from ageing changes in the inner or middle ear. One in three people over 60 years of age, and half of those older than 85, have hearing loss. In fact, it has been shown by Berry et al (2004) that older persons with visual impairment are also more likely to have hearing loss. This might suggest that these sensory impairments share common risk factors or biologic ageing markers. Combined sensory impairments have a cumulative impact on health-related quality of life. Hearing problems can make it hard to understand and follow a doctor's advice, to respond to warnings and to hear doorbells and alarms. Talking with friends and family is also difficult. All of this can be frustrating, embarrassing, and even dangerous to the patient. Practitioners should be aware that dual sensory impairment, which may result in isolation as well as severe depression, may warrant referral to another healthcare professional such as a social worker, psychologist, or psychiatrist.

Visual acuity

The measurement of visual acuity (VA) is discussed in detail in Chapter 12. Clinicians specializing in the evaluation of older patients should have the facility to measure VA at multiple distances and illumination conditions. Standard instrumentation for determining distance VA should be available, as well as portable charts for patients with reduced acuity. Chart portability is especially important for wheelchair-bound patients having VA less than 6/60 (20/200)

and those with decreased contrast sensitivity. VA notations such as hand motion (HM) or counting fingers (CF) can be avoided by the use of portable charts. Light projection (LPROJ), light perception (LP), and no light perception (NLP) are acceptable methods of notation when VA cannot be recorded with optotypes.

Stimuli presented using projector charts often have insufficient contrast to be resolved by patients with pathological eye conditions such as cataracts, diabetic retinopathy, optic nerve disease, or macular degeneration. Computerized charts provide greater contrast and may be more suitable for older patients. Alternative methods are also recommended, including the use of hand-held charts such as the Designs for Vision number chart (Designs for Vision, Inc., Ronkonkoma, NY), the Colenbrander chart (e.g. Richmond Products Inc., Albuquerque, NM) and the Early Testing for Diabetic Retinopathy Study (ETDRS) logMAR chart (e.g. VectorVision, Greenville, OH). For example, the portable, high-contrast Designs for Vision number chart can be used in a variety of settings, including the examination room, alternative health facilities, residential care settings, a nursing home, or a domestic setting when examining a house-bound patient (Rosenthal & Cole 1991b). This particular chart allows VA recording down to 1/700 (equivalent to 6/4200 or 20/14 000). Another portable option is the Colenbrander logMAR chart, which is calibrated for a viewing distance of 1 m.

High-contrast ETDRS (see **Fig. 30.1**) charts also allow portability and reliability when measuring VA at distances between 6 m and 1 m. This chart allows the presentation of optotypes having Snellen equivalents between 6/3 (20/10) and 1/40. These charts, which can be mounted on rear-illuminated light boxes, are valuable for monitoring acuity over time (Ferris et al 1982).

Assessment of near VA can be accomplished with standard near-point cards. Habitual working distances often predict uncorrected refractive error, particularly myopia, which may result from pathological conditions such as cataract.

External evaluation

External evaluation of the eye is especially important in older patients. For example, the lids are susceptible to common lesions including cysts, inflammation, atopic dermatitis, infection, itching, redness and dryness. Blepharitis, a chronic inflammation of the eyelids, may be accompanied by burning, itching, photophobia and a gritty or sandy sensation, especially when arising in the morning. McCulley and Shine (2003) reported that seborrhoeic and meibomian gland dysfunction are the most common aetiologies of blepharitis in the elderly.

According to Wong et al (2003), basal cell carcinoma, which is generally found on the lower lid or the inner canthus, is the most common form of skin cancer of the lid. A common non-malignant lesion is xanthelasma, which is characterized by lipomatous yellow plaques just beneath the skin of the periorbital region. Gladstone and Myint (2000) noted that, in patients over 40 years of age, these are twice more common in females than males. The lesion may represent a localized cutaneous phenomenon, or signify a systemic hyperlipidemia associated with elevation of low density lipoprotein (Seymour 2004). Dermatochalasis is another common bilateral condition in patients over the age of 50, where there is sagging of the upper eyelids (Fay et al 2003). Patients may opt for either surgical correction of this condition or non-surgical correction with a ptosis crutch or tape.

Ectropion, and entropion, an outward or inward turning of the lower lid, respectively, are common in the elderly and may often require referral to an ophthalmic plastic surgeon. Entropion, if left untreated, may result in corneal abrasion due to the lashes rubbing the corneal epithelium.

Myasthenia gravis is another condition that affects the lids. According to the National Institute of Neurological Disorders and Strokes (2007), myasthenia gravis occurs in all ethnic groups and both genders and most commonly affects men over the age of 60. It is an *autoimmune disease* in which antibodies are directed against the body's own proteins, resulting in the loss of tonicity in the lid and producing ptosis and/or diplopia (Baets & Oosterhuis 1993; Scherer et al 2005). While leaving the ptosis untreated may be the best solution to eliminate any diplopia that is present, Cohen and Waiss (1997) found that ptosis crutches and ptosis tape are useful for raising the lid in the absence of diplopia. However, artificial tears, lubricating ointment, or hydrophilic contract lenses may be required to prevent keratitis sicca as a result of the lid being held in the elevated position for a prolonged period of time.

Slit-lamp evaluation should include careful observation of the cornea for conditions such as Fuchs' endothelial dystrophy, a dominant hereditary condition more common in females, which is often seen in the fifth or sixth decade of life. Pachymetry and a corneal cell count may be indicated to monitor this condition.

Tear production also decreases with age and may result in drying of the cornea. The Schirmer test (see Ch. 17) uses a filter paper strip placed in the lower fornix to measure the tears produced in 5 minutes. Severe forms of dry eye will result in little or no wetting of the filter paper. Decreased tear production may require supplementary artificial tears or punctual occlusion. Sjögren's syndrome, an autoimmune disease, not only results in reduced tear production, but also xerostomia (dry mouth), rheumatoid arthritis, and dental caries. In addition to Sjögren's syndrome and rheumatoid arthritis, secondary tearing deficiency can be associated with lymphoma and leukaemia. Additional tests that may be used to evaluate dry eye include tear break-up time, fluorescein and rose bengal staining, tear film osmolarity, the phenol red dye test and an evaluation of the tear lactoferrin.

Both the pupillary reflexes and pupil size should be carefully noted (Winn et al 1994). Winn et al observed that pupil size decreased linearly as a function of age at all illuminance levels. The rate of decline ranged from 0.043 mm/year at the lowest illuminance level to 0.015 mm/year at the highest. The decrease in pupil size with age often results in complaints of poor illumination and difficulties with reading, especially in the presence of a cataract or other media opacity.

It is also important to note any information that may impact prescribed low-vision devices. For example, large sector iridectomies might cause photophobia, while asymmetric pupil locations may influence the type and position of certain low-vision devices, such as spectacle-mounted telescopic lenses. As noted previously, partial ptosis of the eyelid may obscure the pupil, leading to functional difficulties in poor lighting, especially in the presence of a cataract.

Keratometric measurements with either automated or manual instruments provide valuable objective information (see Ch. 17), especially if cataract or corneal surgery is anticipated. Keratometry can also be used as a non-invasive test for dry eye, by observing break-up of the tear film. It may be used as an objective technique for estimating the astigmatism in non-verbal patients, including aphasic stroke patients and individuals with Alzheimer's disease, as well as those who may have undergone brain surgery and are unable to communicate verbally.

Refraction

Refraction remains one of the primary responsibilities, as well as being one of the strengths, of the profession of optometry, especially with regards to the elderly. Changes in refractive error may correlate with other age-related changes such as cataract formation. Brown and Hill (1987) found that cortical cataracts produce a change in the astigmatic correction whereas nuclear cataracts lead to a myopic shift. The latter appears to be the most likely cause of uncorrected refractive error in the elderly (Wormald et al 1992). Okamoto et al (2000) showed that co-morbid conditions such as diabetes may also lead to a change in refractive error. Haegerstrom-Portnoy et al (2002) found large amounts of astigmatism in the oldest patients studied in a cohort of 569 patients in which the mean age was 75.2 years with a range from 59 to 106 years. They concluded that the 'prevalence of large amounts of astigmatism (as well as anisometropia) emphasize the importance of regular refractive evaluations in the oldest of the old'.

Older patients are often wearing an old and inappropriate correction or may be using incorrect, non-prescribed, over-the-counter reading lenses. Most patients will benefit from a traditional subjective refraction utilizing a phoropter or trial frame (see Ch. 14). However, over-refraction is useful in patients with high astigmatic correction, high refractive error, eccentric viewing and those with poor best-corrected VA. Over-refractions can be done with Halberg/Janelli clips over the existing spectacles.

In addition to the standard retinoscopy techniques, the examiner should consider either radical or off-axis retinoscopy. Radical retinoscopy is recommended when either the reflex is very dim or no reflex is seen. This involves moving the retinoscope towards the patient, until some motion is detected, to estimate the refractive error. In off-axis retinoscopy, the retinoscope is moved away from the line of sight to determine whether a reflex can be obtained. This is especially useful in the presence of media opacities.

Techniques such as the 'just noticeable difference' (JND) will often provide better information on the refractive error than traditional procedures. Weber's law states that the difference threshold or JND is the minimum amount by which stimulus intensity must be changed in order to produce a noticeable variation in sensory experience. For VA, the JND is the minimum angle of resolution (MAR) divided by 5. As noted in Chapter 12, the MAR is the reciprocal of the Snellen fraction. Thus, for a patient with best corrected VA in the better eye of 2/40 (MAR = 20'), JND = 20/5 = 4 D. Similarly, the JND for best corrected VA of 6/60 (20/200) or 6/15 (20/50) is 2 D and 0.50 D, respectively.

Subjective evaluation utilizing a trial frame is preferred when there is a substantial decrease in the VA. Bracketing may enable the examiner to find the most appropriate lens quickly. For example, the bracketing lenses used with an incoming acuity of 4/40 (MAR = 10; JND = 2.00) are ±1.00. The bracketing lenses for acuity of 2/40 would be ±2.00 D, while the lenses used for 1/40 would be ±4.00 D. If the acuity improves during refinement, for example, from 4/40 to 4/20, the bracketing lens should be changed to ±0.50 because the sensitivity is increased to smaller lens changes.

Contrast sensitivity testing

Contrast sensitivity testing was discussed in detail in Chapter 12. Waiss and Cohen (1991) noted that the contrast sensitivity function reflects the integrity of the entire visual system and problems anywhere in the system will impact negatively upon the final curve. In the past 25 years, contrast sensitivity testing (see Ch.12) has become an established method to monitor the progression of eye disease including cataracts, AMD, corneal dystrophies, media opacities, optic nerve disease, and glaucoma as well as uncorrected refractive errors.

The Mars Letter Contrast Sensitivity Test (**Fig. 31.13**) is a quick, easy to use, portable way to assess contrast sensitivity. It consists of a 23 cm by 36 cm. (9 in by 14 in) chart with eight rows of Sloan optotypes, each containing six letters. There is a 0.04 log unit decrease in contrast from letter to letter. Three charts are included, to be used for the right and left eyes and binocular testing. Both Dougherty et al (2005) and Haymes and Roberts (2006) found the Mars Test to have excellent agreement with the Pelli–Robson test, with superior repeatability.

Arden (1978) demonstrated that sensitivity to higher spatial frequencies exhibits an age-related decline beginning around 40 to 50 years of age. Rubin et al (1997) also noted that visual function decreased linearly with age for VA, contrast sensitivity, glare performance and visual fields. Guirao et al (1999) found that the average optical performance of the human eye progressively declines with age. Cognitive

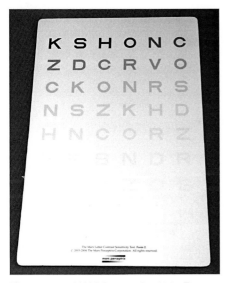

Figure 31.13 MARS Contrast Sensitivity Test. (Reproduced with permission from MARS Perceptrix.)

function may be affected in patients having a history of a cerebral vascular accident as well as individuals diagnosed with conditions such as Alzheimer's disease.

Other testing

As noted previously, early detection of eye disease will help to maintain the patient's quality of life, and can also translate into significant savings for the healthcare system. Accordingly, other screening tests should be considered essential, as well as best care practice, for older patients. Visual field testing (see Ch. 20) is indicated, especially for those at risk of glaucoma, ischaemic conditions or diabetes. Either automated or Goldmann perimetry is recommended for the evaluation of peripheral fields while home monitoring of central fields can be done with the Amsler grid (see p 325) for patients with a family history of AMD.

All of the evaluative skills come into play when dealing with an elderly population. Essential procedures for every examination include a thorough slit-lamp evaluation of the anterior segment of the eye including angle estimation, applanation tonometry, slit-lamp and head-set binocular indirect ophthalmoscopy. Gonioscopy should be added when indicated (see Chs 17 and 18).

Prescriptive devices

Older patients, even those wearing bifocals or progressive addition lenses, should be offered the option of a single-vision lens for distance, intermediate or near use as well as an absorptive lens for outdoor wear. Lord et al (2002) found that bifocals may represent a significant problem for older people, as they are more likely to fall over a hazardous object. In a prospective cohort study of 156 subjects between 63 and 90 years of age, about half (56%) were regular wearers of multifocal glasses (Lord et al 2002). Older patients with neck or spine problems may find it difficult to hold their head up while looking through a small bifocal segment for long periods of time.

Anti-reflective coatings are recommended for all lenses, to reduce glare as well as increasing light transmission. Particular attention should be paid to incorporating a UV filter into the lenses, especially for those patients who have undergone cataract extraction (even if a UV-absorbing intraocular lens has been implanted). Absorptive lenses should be considered for all patients with early cataracts, AMD, reduced contrast sensitivity, or if they are involved in outdoor activities or complaining of glare difficulties.

Prescribing habits have conventionally set the upper limit of the near addition for most practitioners at +2.50 to +3.00 D. But +4.00 and +5.00 D adds in the form of a single-vision or bifocal lens can be very beneficial for those with reduced vision. Even clinicians not specializing in low vision may find binocular prism half-eye spectacles helpful for patients with best corrected VA around 6/60 (20/200) or worse. These lenses are available for binocular use from +4.00 D with 6Δ base-in to +12.00 D with 14Δ base-in for each eye. Practitioners should refer the patient to a low-vision specialist if they feel uncomfortable prescribing very high adds, microscopic or telescopic lenses, or hand-held or stand magnifiers.

Lighting

One area that should not be overlooked is the use of task lighting for reading and close work as well as enhancing colour contrast. Eye disorders in older individuals often result in reduced transparency of the ocular media, thereby reducing the amount of light reaching the retina. These losses are greater for short rather than long wavelengths of light. Arditi and Knoblauch (1996) noted that colour deficits associated with visual impairment may affect the ability to distinguish nearby wavelengths of monochromatic light. They suggested that effective colour contrast may be enhanced by increasing the lightness differences between the foreground and background colours, and avoiding using colours of similar lightness against one another, even if they differ in chroma or hue. Haymes et al (2006) found that task lighting improved visual function in AMD. They suggested that this finding supports the provision of additional task illuminance as an important part of low-vision rehabilitation for patients with AMD. Brunnström et al (2004) noted that it is possible to increase quality of life by improving the lighting conditions. In addition, Boyce (2003) found that improved lighting can be used to compensate for some age-related changes in the visual system, and to support the independence and quality of life of the elderly.

Case disposition

It is beneficial to have a relative or friend of the patient (with their permission) listen to any recommendations and advice given. All recommendations, including instructions for the use of the various spectacles, appliances or treatments, should be given in writing to improve compliance. Additionally, return visits should be scheduled to determine progress and monitor eye pathology, if necessary.

Co-management of patients and treatment

Optometry's role in eye care has changed dramatically with the use of diagnostic and pharmaceutical agents. As the scope of practice continues to expand, the role of the optometrist in the management of elderly populations is likely to increase. Co-management of patients undergoing cataract extraction by optometrists and ophthalmologists is becoming the norm in the United States, as is the treatment of patients with glaucoma by optometrists.

Clinicians will have to re-evaluate their professional equipment for the future cohort of elderly patients. Offices should be equipped with the most modern devices for visual field analysis and assessment of the anterior and posterior segments of the eye (see Chs 17 and 18).

F C Donders (1818–1889), a pioneer in the physiology of vision, was the first investigator of age-related vision changes over 150 years ago. There is still a huge amount of work to be done to improve disease prevention and detection, the quality of clinical care, containment of healthcare costs and access to eye care. Hopefully, society will realize the extent of these problems and invest for our future generations.

References

Age-Related Eye Disease Study Research Group 2000 Risk factors associated with age-related macular degeneration. A case-control study in the age-related eye disease study: Age-Related Eye Disease Study Report Number 3. Ophthalmology 107(12):2224–2232

American Optometric Clinical Guideline Comprehensive Adult Eye and Vision Examination 2005 Clinical Practice Guideline 1, 2nd edn

Americans with Disabilities Act ADA Guide for Small Businesses 2002 U.S. small business administration office of entrepreneurial development, U.S. Department of Justice Civil Rights Division

Arden G B 1978 The importance of measuring contrast sensitivity in cases of visual disturbances. British Journal of Ophthalmology 65:198–209

Arditi A, Knoblauch K 1996 Effective color contrast and low vision. In: Rosenthal B P, Cole R G (eds) Functional assessment of low vision. Mosby-Year Book, St Louis, pp 129–158

Attebo K, Ivers R Q, Mitchell P 1999 Refractive errors in an older population: the Blue Mountains Eye Study. Ophthalmology 106:1066–1072

Augood C, Fletcher A, Bentham G et al 2004 Methods for a population-based study of the prevalence of and risk factors for age-related maculopathy and macular degeneration in elderly European populations: the EUREYE study. Ophthalmic Epidemiology 11:117–129

Baets M H, de, Oosterhuis H J 1993 Myasthenia gravis. DRD Press, Boca Raton

Beers M H, John T V, Berkwits M et al 2005 Section II, Falls, fractures, and injury, Chapter 23, The Elderly Driver, The Merck Manual of Geriatrics, 3rd ed., Online. Available: http://www.merck.com/mrkshared/mmg/sec2/ch23/ch23a.jsp July, 2005

Berry P, Mascia J, Steinman B A 2004 Vision and hearing loss in older adults: Double trouble. Care Management Journals Spring 5 (1):35–40

Boyce P 2003 Lighting for the elderly. Technology and Disability 15:3

Branch L G, Horowitz A, Carr C 1989 The implications for everyday life of incident self-reported visual decline among people over age 65 living in the community. Gerontologist 29:359–365

Bresnick G A 2000 Screening approach to the surveillance of patients with diabetes for the presence of vision-threatening retinopathy. Ophthalmology 107(1):19–24

Brown N A P, Hill A R 1987 Cataract, the relation between myopia and cataract morphology. British Journal of Ophthalmology 71:405–414

Brunnström G, Sörensen S, Alsterstad K et al 2004 Quality of light and quality of life – the effect of lighting adaptation among people with low vision. Ophthalmic and Physiological Optics 24(4):274–280

Campbell V A, Crews J E, Moriarty D G et al 1999 Surveillance for sensory impairment, activity limitation, and health-related quality of life among older adults – United States, 1993–1997. Morbidity and Mortality Weekly Report 48(SS-8):131–157

Caraballese C, Appollonio I, Rozzini R et al 1993 Sensory impairment and quality of life in a community elderly population. Journal of the American Geriatrics Society 41(4):401–407

Centers for Disease Control 2005 National diabetes fact sheet: general information and national estimates on diabetes in the United States. US Department of Health and Human Services, CDC, Online. Atlanta, GA. Online. Available: http://www.cdc.gov/diabetes/pubs/pdf/ndfs_2005.pdf

Chia E, Mitchell P, Rochtchina E et al 2006 Association between vision and hearing impairments and their combined effects on quality of life. Archives of Ophthalmology 124:1465–1470

Cohen J M, Waiss B 1997 Combination ptosis crutch and moisture chamber for management of progressive external ophthalmoplegia. Journal of American Optometric Association 68(10):663–667

Crews J E, Campbell V A 2004 Vision impairment and hearing loss among community-dwelling older Americans: implications for health and functioning. American Journal of Public Health 94:823–829

Cruess A, Xu X, Mones J et al 2006 Humanistic burden and health resource utilization among neovascular age-related macular degeneration patients: results from a multi-country cross-sectional study.

Investigative Ophthalmology and Visual Science 47: ARVO e-abstract 2199

De Boer M R, Pluijm S M, Lips P et al 2004 Different aspects of visual impairment as risk factors for falls and fractures in older men and women. Journal of Bone and Mineral Research 19(9):1539–1547

Dougherty B, Flom R, Bullimore M 2005 An evaluation of the Mars Letter Contrast Sensitivity Test. Optometry and Vision Science 82 (11):970–975

Elder M, Anmar M, Rahman A et al 2006 Early paracentral visual field loss in patients taking hydroxychloroquine. Archives of Ophthalmology 124:1729–1733

Fay A, Lee L C, Pasquale L R. 2003 Dermatochalasis causing apparent bitemporal hemianopsia. Ophthalmologic Plastic Reconstructive Surgery 19(2):151–153

Ferris F, Kassoff A, Bresnick G et al 1982 New visual acuity charts for clinical research. American Journal of Ophthalmology 94:91–96

Friedman D S, Wolfs R C, O'Colmain B J et al 2004 Prevalence of open-angle glaucoma among adults in the United States. Archives of Ophthalmology 122:532–538

Fulton M M, Allen E R 2005 Polypharmacy in the elderly: a literature review. Journal of the American Academy of Nurse Practitioners 17:123–132

Gingrich N, Gill J T 2006 Prodigal state. The Wall Street Journal. Online. Available: http://www.opinionjournal.com/cc/? id=110008328

Gladstone G J, Myint S 2000 Xanthelasma. In: Fraunfelder F T, Roy F H (eds) Current ocular therapy, 5th edn. W B Saunders, Philadelphia, pp 452–453

Guirao A, Gonzalez C, Redondo M et al 1999 Average optical performance of the human eye as a function of age in a normal population. Investigative Ophthalmology and Visual Science 40:203–213

Haegerstrom-Portnoy G, Schneck M E, Brabyn J A et al 2002 Eye development of refractive errors into old age. Optometry and Vision Science 79:643–649

Haymes S A, Roberts K F 2006 The letter contrast sensitivity test: clinical evaluation of a new design. Investigative Ophthalmology and Visual Science 47:2739–2745

Horowitz A, Reinhardt J P 2000 Mental health issues in visual impairment: Research in depression, disability, and rehabilitation. In: Silverstone B, Lang M, Rosenthal B et al (eds) The lighthouse handbooks on vision impairment and vision rehabilitation Oxford University Press, New York, pp 1089–1109

Hyman L 1992 The epidemiology of AMD. In: Hampton R G, Nelson P T (eds) Age-related macular degeneration: principles and practice. Raven Press, New York, pp 1–35

The Lighthouse Inc. 1995 The Lighthouse National Survey on Vision Loss: the experience, attitudes, and knowledge of middle-aged and older Americans. The Lighthouse, New York

Lord S R, Dayhew J 2001 Visual risk factors for falls in older people. Journal of the American Geriatric Society 49:508–515

Lord S R, Dayhew J, Howland A 2002 Multifocal glasses impair edge-contrast sensitivity and depth perception and increase the risk of falls in older people. Journal of the American Geriatric Society 50 (11):1760–1766

McCulley, J P, Shine, W E 2003 Eyelid disorders: the meibomian gland, blepharitis, and contact lenses. Eye and Contact Lens: Science and Clinical Practice 29(1) Supplement 1:S93–S95

Mackie S W, Walsh G 1998 Contrast and glare sensitivity in diabetic patients with and without pan-retinal photocoagulation. Ophthalmic and Physiological Optometry 18:173–181

Merck on-line Manual 2003 Online. Available: http://www.merck.com/ mmhe/sec12/ch154/ch154d.html

Munoz B, West S K, Rodriguez J et al 2002 Blindness, visual impairment, and the problem of uncorrected refractive error in a Mexican-American population: Proyecto VER. Investigative Ophthalmology and Visual Science 43:608–614

National Institute of Neurological Disorders and Strokes (2007) http:// www.ninds.nih.gov/disorders/myasthenia_gravis/ detail_myasthenia_gravis

Nolan L, O'Malley K 1988 Prescribing for the elderly. Part I: Sensitivity of the elderly to adverse drug reactions. Journal of the American Geriatric Society 36:142–149

Ojha R P, Thertulien R A 2005 Health care policy issues as a result of the genetic revolution: implications for public health. American Journal of Public Health 95(3):385–388

Okamoto F, Sone H, Nonoyama T et al 2000 Refractive changes in diabetic patients during intensive glycaemic control. British Journal of Ophthalmology 84(10):1097–1102

Rein D B, Zhang P, Wirth K E et al 2006 The economic burden of major adult visual disorders in the United States. Archives of Ophthalmology 124:1754–1760

Rizzo M, Kellison I L 2004 Eyes, brains, and autos. Archives of Ophthalmology 122:641–647

Rosenthal B P, Cole R G 1991a The low vision history. In: Eskridge J B, Amos J, Bartlett I (eds) Clinical procedures in optometry. J B Lippincott, Philadelphia, pp 749–761

Rosenthal B P, Cole R G 1991b Problems in Optometry 3(3):385–407

Rubin G S, West S K, Munoz B et al 1997 A comprehensive assessment of visual impairment in a population of older Americans. The SEE Study. Salisbury Eye Evaluation Project. Investigative Ophthalmology and Visual Science 38:557–568

Saaddine J, Benjamin S, Pan L et al 2005 Visual impairment and eye care among older adults – five states, Div of Diabetes Translation, National Center for Chronic Disease. Morbidity and Mortality Weekly Report 55:1321–1327

Scherer K, Bedlack R S, Simel D L 2005 Does this patient have myasthenia gravis? Journal of the American Medical Association 293:1906–1914

Seymour C A 2004 Xanthomas and abnormalities of lipid metabolism and storage. In: Champion R H, Burton J L, Burns D A et al (eds) Rook/Wilkinson/Ebling textbook of dermatology, 7th edn. Blackwell Science, Oxford, pp 57–65

Stefansson E, Landers M B, Wolbarsht M L 1981 Increased retinal oxygen supply following pan-retinal photocoagulation and vitrectomy and lensectomy. Transactions of the American Ophthalmological Society 79:307–334

Waiss B, Cohen J M 1991 Glare and contrast sensitivity for low vision practitioners. Problems in Optometry 3(3):433–448

Winn B, Whitaker D, Elliott D B 1994 Factors affecting light-adapted pupil size in normal human subjects. Investigative Ophthalmology and Visual Science 35:1132–1137

Wong C S M, Strange R C, Lear J T 2003 Basal cell carcinoma. British Medical Journal 327:794–798

Wormald R P, Wright L A, Courtney P et al 1992 Visual problems in the elderly population and implications for services. British Medical Journal 304:1226–1229

Zarowitz B J, Stebelshky L A, Muma B K et al 2005 Reduction of high-risk polypharmacy drug combinations in patients in a managed care setting. Pharmacotherapy 25:1636–1645

Zhang X, Gregg E W, Cheng Y J et al 2006 Mental health issues in visual impairment. Morbidity and Mortality Weekly Report 55:1221–1242

CHAPTER 32

Optometric assessment and management of patients with developmental disability

Kathryn J Saunders

'I like my glasses. My coach looks nice with my glasses on,' is a quotation from an athlete with Down's syndrome participating at the Special Olympics, Glasgow, 2005 after being given glasses for the first time.

'Since my son got his glasses he is like a new child, we didn't realize what a difference seeing better could make to him,' is a quotation from the mother of a 6-year-old boy with severe developmental disability and previously uncorrected high hyperopia.

Terminology

The present chapter will address the optometric needs of patients who have intellectual and/or physical disabilities for whom a modified approach to testing and management may be appropriate. There are many terms used to describe such patients and the terminology changes as society seeks descriptions that neither patronize individuals nor define them by their physical or intellectual abilities or limitations. Doubtless, the terms used today will seem clumsy and inappropriate in the future. For the purposes of this chapter the term 'developmental disability' has been chosen in an attempt to provide a meaningful description, across a wide geographical readership, of conditions that impair intellectual and/or physical function in such a way that the standard eye examination and its environment may need to be modified to optimize vision care.

A developmental disability is defined as a severe, chronic disability that begins any time from birth through the first 22 years of life and is expected to last for a lifetime. Developmental disabilities may be intellectual, physical or a combination of both. The terms intellectual disability (Australia, Europe, UK), or mental retardation (USA) are often used when describing this group. However, these terms describe conditions that impair cognitive function and do not strictly encompass physical limitations. In the UK the term 'learning disability' is often used, but in North America a person with a 'learning disability' is generally thought of as one who has normal intellect but has specific difficulties with certain aspects of learning.

It should be noted that while the term developmental disability applies strictly only to those with disabilities beginning during childhood and early adulthood, disabilities acquired later in life may also impact on optometric assessment and management. The issues addressed in the present chapter are likely to be applicable to such patients.

Developmental disabilities may be classified as severe, profound, moderate or mild, and the classification is usually assigned in relation to the individual's need for external support. A person with a developmental disability is likely to have problems functioning in several of the following areas; learning, mobility, language (receptive and expressive), economic self-sufficiency, independent living, and self-care. The British Institute of Learning Disabilities (BILD) states that such a person 'will have difficulties understanding and learning new things, and in generalising any learning to new situations, as well as having difficulties with social tasks, for example, communication, self-care, awareness of health and safety' (Northfield 2001).

Terminology is important; misuse can upset patients, families and carers and reduce the rapport the optometrist aims to establish with the patient and accompanying persons. When referring to the patient, put them first in relation to their disability, i.e. 'the patient with Down's syndrome' rather than the 'Down's syndrome patient'. The patient has many facets and should not be defined by their disability.

It is never wise to generalize about people and patients and this is a particularly dangerous practice when applied to people with a disability. A 'one size fits all' approach is unsatisfactory and each patient will present different challenges, rewards and insights. The aim of the present chapter is not to provide a prescriptive approach to the optometric management of patients with developmental disability, but to outline briefly some of the vision problems reported amongst this patient group, to describe modifications in approach that might be appropriate when testing and managing those with a developmental disability and to encourage practitioners to clearly communicate the results of their work with patients, families and other professionals.

Prevalence of developmental disability and visual impairment

The number of individuals in the population with developmental disability is growing (Foundation for People with Learning Disability, UK 2004). It is estimated that in the UK there are 3–4 people with a severe developmental disability for every 1000 people in the population and about 6 per 1000 people with a mild developmental disability. The rise in prevalence is due, in part, to advances in medical science which impact on the survival rate of those born too early, too small or with birth- and development-related complications, and those for whom function is impaired in later life by trauma, disease or degenerative conditions. There is a large body of literature which describes the increased incidence of visual anomalies amongst individuals with developmental disability (Warburg 1994, 2001a,b; Evenhuis 1995; Evenhuis et al 1997, 2001; Woodhouse et al 2000a; van Splunder et al 2003; Lindsay et al 2004) and many people with developmental disability have some difficulty with vision. This is perhaps unsurprising. Many areas of the brain are involved in the processing of visual information. Neurological damage to the brain often has implications for vision and visual processing. In particular, the immature infant brain, which requires normal visual experience to develop normal visual processing, is particularly susceptible to influence from environmental and internal factors. Evenhuis et al (2001) describes a large percentage (23%) of people with developmental disability as having a visual impairment, and reports that the risk of visual impairment increases in association with Down's syndrome, an age of 50 years or greater and with severe or profound developmental disability. In addition to long-term visual difficulties arising in early life, treatable conditions such as uncorrected refractive errors and ocular pathologies such as glaucoma and cataract account for a sizeable proportion of visual impairment in older people with

developmental disability (Evenhuis 1995; Evenhuis et al 2001; Warburg 2001a). Warburg (2001a) examined visual function in 837 Danish adults with developmental disabilities. He reports that 256 had a visual impairment and the primary source of this impairment is described in **Table 32.1**.

Visual difficulties may be unrecognized by families and carers of those with developmental disability (Haire et al 1991; Warburg 1994; Kerr et al 2003), with behaviour attributed to the disability and not identified as a symptom of visual impairment. Deterioration in behaviour may be interpreted as a sign of the onset of dementia rather than a consequence of deteriorating vision. An individual may be thought to be developing dementia because they have become disorientated, anxious or confused. These signs, which are indicative of dementia, may be more simply attributed to reducing vision due to undiagnosed, but treatable, ocular pathology such as cataract. Other scenarios that are not uncommon include adults with a developmental disability who become disinterested in near tasks which they previously enjoyed due to the onset of presbyopia or adults who begin to avoid going outside as lenticular opacities develop and result in uncomfortable glare. Relatively simple ocular changes can markedly reduce quality of life but, once identified, can be managed with straightforward optometric intervention and/or advice.

According to the UK College of Optometrists, children account for a significant proportion of those with developmental disability (approximately 30%) and it is important that visual difficulties are identified at an early stage so that a visual problem does not further exacerbate or complicate an underlying impairment. Whilst the visual requirements of those with complex needs and profound developmental disability might seem less pressing than other acute health problems, early intervention can improve quality of life and maximize visual and general potential (Sonksen & Dale 2002). Developmental setback has been demonstrated in children with visual impairment in the absence of coexisting developmental

Table 32.1 The primary source of visual impairment found amongst adults with a developmental disability surveyed in Denmark (Warburg 2001a)

Primary cause of visual impairment	Number of cases (%)
Cortical visual impairment	51 (6.1)
Optic atrophy	42 (5.0)
Myopia ≥ 5 DS	40 (4.8)
Cataract	36 (4.3)
No attributable cause	24 (2.9)
Keratoconus	18 (2.2)
Nystagmus	12 (1.4)
Retinitis pigmentosa	6 (0.7)
Age-related macular degeneration	6 (0.7)
Glaucoma	5 (0.6)
Diabetic retinopathy (4 with glaucoma)	5 (0.6)
Malformations	6 (0.7)
Other acquired disorders	5 (0.6)

disability (Cass et al 1994). Visual impairment is likely to be even more detrimental to development when a developmental disability is also present. Optometric practitioners should be aware that children with developmental disability are at an increased risk for vision problems and should either have the tools to investigate and manage such patients or be prepared to refer them to others with this expertise.

Common developmental disabilities

For many patients, a clear diagnosis relating to the origin of their developmental disability may not be available. However, some of the common conditions that can impair development are discussed below.

Down's syndrome

Down's syndrome is the most common form of diagnosed developmental disability, affecting approximately 1 in 1000 live births. It is essentially a chromosomal abnormality and, in addition to the characteristic facial features and intellectual disability, Down's syndrome is associated with a greater risk of hearing impairment, heart defects, leukaemia, epilepsy, Alzheimer's disease, digestive problems, hypothyroidism and a reduced ability to combat infection.

It has long been recognized that Down's syndrome affects the eyes and vision. Visible ocular differences, such as epicanthal folds, slanting palpebral apertures, nystagmus, blepharitis and strabismus have been noted for many decades (Sutherland 1899; Ormond 1912; Brushfield 1924; Gifford 1928; Benda 1947; Catalano 1990). More recently, reports have described an increase in the incidence of keratoconus, thinner, steeper corneas, and early-onset cataract (Shapiro & France 1985; Catalano 1990; Doyle et al 1998; Haugen et al 2001a; Evereklioglu et al 2002; Vincent et al 2005). The optometrist must be aware of the increased incidence of these physical anomalies and be prepared to manage them, through referral for surgery or treatment, or with advice on lid hygiene as appropriate.

In addition to these physical differences, there is clear evidence of a reduction in visual performance amongst individuals with Down's syndrome. Infant visual acuity and contrast sensitivity measures fall within normal age limits in Down's syndrome, but beyond 2 years of age, while typically developing children continue to show an improvement in function, visual acuity and contrast sensitivity measures for children with Down's syndrome begin to fall outside normal ranges for age (Woodhouse et al 1996; Woodhouse 1998). Older children and adults with Down's syndrome who have no clinically significant pathology do not typically achieve visual acuities better than about 6/9 Snellen equivalent (Woodhouse et al 1996) and contrast sensitivity is also poorer than their peers (Perez-Carpinell et al 1994).

Refractive error development is similarly atypical. High refractive errors, which can be considered normal in early infancy, fail to reduce and in some cases increase with age (Cregg et al 2001, 2003). The pattern of refractive development in typically developing infants and children is contrasted with the failure of emmetropization in Down's syndrome in **Figures 32.1** and **32.2**. The graphs demonstrate the broadening distribution of refractive error found with increasing age from 6 months to 6 years in Down's

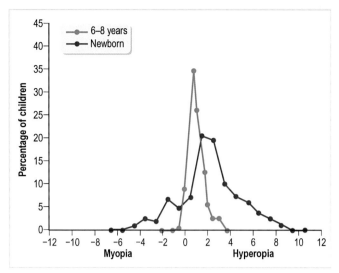

Figure 32.1 Distribution of refractive errors for typically developing newborn infants (Cook & Glasscock 1951) and 6–8-year-old children. (Sorsby et al 1961).

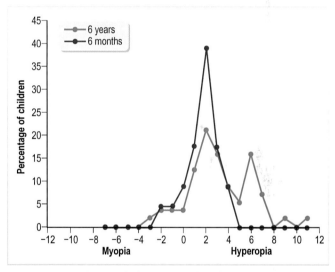

Figure 32.2 Distribution of refractive errors for infants and children with Down's syndrome at 6 months and 6 years (Woodhouse 2006, personal communication).

syndrome. The distribution of errors amongst children with Down's syndrome at 6 years more closely resembles the infant data from typically developing children, rather than that of their peers. At school age approximately 60% of children with Down's syndrome can be expected to require spectacle correction (Woodhouse, personal communication, 2006) compared to about 6% of typically developing children (Sorsby et al 1961). The most common form of refractive error in Down's syndrome is hyperopia, not myopia, as is often believed. Bronham et al (2002) demonstrate that myopia in Down's syndrome is more likely to develop in the presence of heart defect.

In addition to increased levels of ametropia, approximately 75% of children with Down's syndrome have been shown to have anomalies of accommodation (Woodhouse et al 1993; Cregg et al 2001; Haugen & Høvding 2001; Haugen et al 2001b). Normally developing children demonstrate accurate accommodation and high amplitudes from the early months of life (Duane 1922; Banks 1980; Chen & O'Leary 2000). Most children with Down's syndrome, while they are able to produce an accommodative response, fail to produce sufficient accommodation to focus near targets accurately even when wearing appropriate distance correction. They appear to have a 'tolerance' for blur which makes them consistently underaccommodate for near targets. Accommodation must be assessed objectively in all patients with Down's syndrome (see Ch. 15). This is done with the distance refractive correction in place, and when accommodative lags outside normal limits are detected, bifocal correction must be considered. This strategy has been shown to be highly successful (Stewart et al 2005).

In addition to the physical and functional differences in ocular structures and vision described above, there is evidence for cognitive visual problems and perceptual difficulties amongst people with Down's syndrome. Clinical experience suggests that children with Down's syndrome have difficulties characteristic of dorsal stream dysfunction and find going down steps and stairs problematical and changes in surface texture hard to navigate.

Cerebral palsy

Cerebral palsy is defined as a disorder of movement and posture resulting from damage to the brain (Bax 1964). Cerebral palsy is non-progressive and most commonly exists from birth, but may be acquired postnatally through infection or traumatic injury. Cerebral palsy is classified into three subtypes; ataxic, spastic and dyskinetic, based on the type of motor characteristics displayed. Spastic cerebral palsy, in which muscles are tight and stiff, is by far the most common subtype, making up approximately 75–94% of the population. Dyskinetic cerebral palsy affects 3–5% of the cerebral palsy population and is characterized by uncontrolled, slow writhing movements affecting hands, feet, legs, face and tongue. The least common form, affecting 1–4% of the population, is ataxic cerebral palsy, in which balance and coordination are the primary difficulties. It is currently estimated that the incidence of cerebral palsy, in the general population is approximately 1.9–2.5 cases per 1000 live births and this figure is increasing due to the improved survival rates of extremely preterm babies with advances in medical technology (Parkes et al 2001; Doyle 2004).

Cerebral palsy is essentially a problem with the production and coordination of movement, affecting muscles and their actions. Whilst intellectual function may also be impaired as a consequence of brain injury, between 56% and 77% of people with cerebral palsy have little or no intellectual impairment (SCPE 2000). The optometrist should not assume when talking to a person with cerebral palsy whose communication is impaired that their understanding is similarly affected. They may simply have difficulty in controlling the muscles required for clear speech.

Visual problems such as nystagmus, strabismus, cataracts, visual field loss, eye movement disorders and visual perceptual difficulties are all present at an increased rate in cerebral palsy when compared with the general population (Bax 1964; Altman et al 1966; Landau & Berson 1971; Lo Cascio 1977; Black 1982; Scheiman 1984; Schenk-Rootlieb et al 1992; McClelland et al 2005). Many of these conditions arise directly from the damage sustained to the brain early

in development and the pattern of visual impairment can often be related to the type and area of injury if this information is available. For the general optometric practitioner, formal brain imaging data are unlikely to be available, but obvious associations such as reduced physical function on a patient's left-hand side and the increased likelihood of a left visual field defect should be considered.

In a population-based study of school-aged children with cerebral palsy, visual acuity was reduced (less than 6/9 Snellen equivalent) in 22.3% of children (McClelland 2004). Those children with the most profound physical and intellectual impairment were found to have the poorest visual acuities. Visual acuity may be reduced in cerebral palsy due to various factors including strabismus, nystagmus, cataract and cortical visual impairment. Reduced visual acuity, in the form of bilateral amblyopia, may also result from high, uncorrected refractive errors in childhood. Poor control of eye movements may make obtaining visual acuity estimates and interpreting them more challenging. An increased incidence of ocular motor apraxia can disguise relatively good vision through an inability to control eye movements. In such cases, patients may seem visually unresponsive and, indeed, people with ocular motor apraxia have a significant visual impairment because eye movements are an integral part of normal visual function. However, strategies may be developed to help such patients make the best use of their vision, which may be near normal when viewing appropriately sited, stationary objects.

No prospective studies have been conducted in children with cerebral palsy to examine whether a failure to emmetropize, like that postulated for Down's syndrome, occurs. However, high refractive errors are common and present across all types and severities of cerebral palsy, suggesting that emmetropization is impaired or erroneous (Altman et al 1966; Lo Casio 1977; Duckman 1979; Black 1982).

People with cerebral palsy, including children, have also been shown by various authors to have an increased incidence of reduced accommodative function, even when distance refractive errors are fully corrected (Duckman 1984; Leat 1996; McClelland et al 2006). Successful use of near vision additions has been recorded (Ross et al 1996; Saunders & McClelland 2004). Like visual acuity performance, poorer accommodative function is associated with more severe physical and intellectual problems. However, McClelland et al (2006) demonstrated that accommodative deficits requiring a near addition were also present in 17.9% of children with cerebral palsy attending mainstream schools (i.e. with little or no intellectual impairment), highlighting the importance of investigating accommodative function in all eye examinations.

Extreme preterm birth

There are an increasing number of children surviving after extreme preterm birth or extremely low birth weight (Doyle 2004). These children often have complex difficulties, frequently including a visual component (Flanagan et al 2003). High refractive errors and retinopathy of prematurity are well-recognized associations, while cortical visual impairment and associated perceptual difficulties often feature (Robinson 1987; Rogers 1996; Rosenberg et al 1996; Repka 2002; Doyle 2004; O'Connor et al 2004; Hack et al 2005). Children with complex difficulties resulting from preterm birth are likely to require a multidisciplinary approach to vision care involving paediatric and education professionals in conjunction with eye care practitioners (Matsuba & Jan 2006). Hospital centres are increasingly adopting this approach and it is likely that hospital optometrists, rather than those working in general practice, will be involved in the assessment of such patients. However, professionals in general practice may be required to provide dispensing services.

Fragile X syndrome

Fragile X syndrome is a recessive X-linked disorder that affects males more severely than females and is the most common inherited cause of developmental disability. Other problems associated with fragile X syndrome are autistic-like behaviours affecting social interactions and attention, connective tissue anomalies such as hypotonia (lack of tone in the muscles), epilepsy, cardiovascular problems, and hearing difficulties. Fragile X is estimated to affect 1 in 4000 to 5530 males in the UK (Pembrey et al 2001). Affected males are more severely learning disabled than females, who may be unaffected carriers of the genetic defect. Patients with fragile X syndrome have been reported to have an increased incidence of moderate to high refractive errors, strabismus, nystagmus, ptosis, blepharitis, epicanthal folds, and visual perceptual difficulties (Storm et al 1987; Maino et al 1990a,b, 1991; Martinez & Maino 1993; Hatton et al 1998; Maino 2001; Hagerman & Hagerman 2002; Scheiman & Rouse 2006).

Autistic spectrum disorders

Much attention has been directed towards autistic spectrum disorders over recent years, but understanding of the conditions and behaviours that are encompassed by this term is limited. Autism is a developmental disability that affects the way a person communicates and relates to people around them. It is often, but not always, accompanied by an intellectual disability. The recorded prevalence of autism is increasing, and it is estimated that about half a million people in the UK have autistic spectrum disorders (The National Autistic Society, UK 2008). These disorders are more common in males than females by a ratio of approximately four to one (Volkmar & Pauls 2003; Taub et al 2006; The National Autistic Society, UK 2008) but, when affected, females demonstrate more severe difficulties (Volkmar & Pauls 2003). Many of the commonly reported difficulties displayed by people with autistic spectrum disorders are related to social interaction and communication, which may make the experience of an eye examination challenging for the patient. Some of the visual characteristics noted in autistic spectrum disorders include an increased incidence of strabismus and ocular motor dysfunction (Rosenhall et al 1988; Scharre & Creedon 1992; Kemner et al 1998). Limited data related to refractive error suggest the practitioner should anticipate moderate ametropia (Scharre & Creedon 1992).

Fetal alcohol syndrome

The central nervous system of the developing fetus is susceptible to damage by maternal alcohol consumption. Children born subsequent to such damage are described as having fetal alcohol syndrome, the most common non-genetic cause of developmental disability in the Western world (Abel and Sokel 1987), with a prevalence of 1.9 per 1000 live births in the USA.

Children born with fetal alcohol syndrome have distinctive facial characteristics and developmental disability which can range from mild to profound. Fetal alcohol syndrome is known to impact on the eyes and visual system, and children with the syndrome often have physical anomalies such as reduced palpebral apertures, micro-ophthalmus, bilateral ptosis and telecanthus that are easily appreciated (Strömland 1985, 1987, 2004). Ophthalmoscopic examination of children with fetal alcohol syndrome also reveals structural anomalies, the most consistently reported being optic nerve hypoplasia (Miller et al 1981; Chan et al 1991; Carones et al 1992; Hug et al 2000). In addition to these structural aspects, functional differences have been reported including reduced visual acuity, increased incidence of refractive errors (particularly myopia), nystagmus and strabismus (usually convergent) (Altman 1976; Miller et al 1981, 1984; Strömland 1985; Chan et al 1991; Carones et al 1992; Edward et al 1993; Hug et al 2000). In a study of 30 children with fetal alcohol syndrome, Strömland reported that 19% had visual acuities of 6/30 or worse. Reported success rates of occlusion therapy for treatment of amblyopia are poor in fetal alcohol syndrome, but this is generally attributed to poor compliance due to the complex social situations and behavioural difficulties often associated with the syndrome (Strömland & Hellström 1996). Nonetheless, early detection of visual anomalies is important so that appropriate treatment or intervention may be attempted and advice given to families.

Spina bifida

Spina bifida is a defect in embryonic development in which the developing neural tube fails to close. Babies born with spina bifida usually have a part of the meninges or spinal cord protruding from their back. In the most common form of spina bifida (meningomyelocele), which has a prevalence in the USA of approximately 0.37 per 1000 live births (Cauldfield et al 2006), the protrusion results in damage to the spinal cord. Spina bifida is often, but not always, accompanied by hydrocephalus (Stein & Schut 1979). It characteristically results in impairment in motor function, but intellectual function may also be affected. Dietary intervention in the form of increased folic acid consumption by women planning pregnancy or during its early stages has reduced the incidence of this condition in developed countries (Milunsky et al 1989).

Biglan (1990) discussed the evidence for ophthalmological defects in spina bifida, citing previous studies and his own prospective investigation of 304 patients with the condition. He described an increased prevalence of ophthalmic disorders associated with spina bifida (particularly when accompanied by hydrocephalus). Optic atrophy, nystagmus, strabismus (particularly paralytic), amblyopia, and cortical blindness are present more often than would be anticipated from the general population (Goddard 1965; Harcourt 1968, 1974; Keen 1973; Goodner 1974; Rabinowicz 1974; Houtman et al 1981; Biglan 1990). The few studies that report visual acuity measures in spina bifida demonstrate some vision loss, with most children having visual acuities better than 6/12 in their preferred eye (Rabinowicz 1974; Biglan 1990).

Data relating to refractive development and status in the presence of spina bifida are limited, but suggest that refractive errors are essentially normal in childhood, although oblique astigmatism may be slightly more prevalent (Biglan 1990). Biglan demonstrated that amblyopia treatment is successful in this group, and recommended early vision testing and close monitoring of visual development for optimal visual outcome and quality of life.

Cognitive visual dysfunction and perceptual difficulties

Damage to the brain, whether in infancy or adulthood, may lead to overt intellectual impairment and physical restrictions. It may also result in more subtle cognitive visual disorders, with or without associated physical and intellectual disability. When dealing with people with a developmental disability, when there is known damage to specific areas of the brain, it may be beneficial for optometrists to be aware of the cognitive visual impairments that may co-exist, even if the patient cannot describe them clearly. Structured history taking has been advocated in the identification of cognitive visual dysfunction (Dutton et al 1996; Dutton 2003). Whilst a full discussion is beyond the scope of the present chapter, some of the symptoms and signs related to cognitive visual dysfunction are described below. Simple strategies aimed at reducing their impact on daily living are discussed in the management section.

Dorsal stream dysfunction

Damage to the brain's parietal and occipital lobes and the connections between the two areas is known as dorsal stream dysfunction. This can be found in a range of conditions but Dutton (2003) highlighted a particular association with periventricular leucomalacia, a form of brain injury found following preterm birth and in patients with cerebral palsy. Patients with dorsal stream dysfunction may have difficulty in identifying objects in a crowded scene because processing of visual information is reduced and performance falls when too much information is present. Such a patient might demonstrate high levels of visual acuity when tested with single letters or an isolated grating or picture. However, they may struggle to 'see' a bus across the road which, despite its large size, is competing with all the other visual information in the wider scene. 'Seeing' a toy on a patterned carpet or a pair of trousers on a patterned bedspread can also be challenging. Logically, visual performance and attention are likely to improve when less information is present. For similar reasons, people with dorsal stream dysfunction are likely to be more comfortable in open spaces rather than in cluttered, noisy, visually diverse places. Behaviour may improve in an open park, and become challenging or disturbed in a noisy, busy supermarket. People with dorsal stream dysfunction are likely to respond best to one-on-one communication in a quiet environment.

Another aspect of dorsal stream dysfunction is a reduced appreciation of moving scenes. Many people with dorsal stream dysfunction will be most interested in TV programmes and films which have little movement, e.g. static cartoons and news programmes in which images are fairly static. They may also find moving through three-dimensional space problematic and can be regarded as clumsy. People with dorsal stream dysfunction often have problems with changes in surface texture, kerbs and stairs, particularly when going down. Visual fields should be checked to determine whether a lower visual field defect is present.

Ventral stream dysfunction

The ventral stream is the processing pathway between the occipital and temporal lobes of the brain, mediating the links between seeing, recognizing and remembering objects, people and places. Damage to the temporal lobes, responsible for visual memory and recognition processes, will impair these functions. This is likely to impinge on the ability to recognize words, places, shapes and faces and reduce visual memory that is important for tasks such as copying from the black- or white-board at school. In particular, right-sided damage is more likely to cause difficulty with face recognition and orientation in new environments.

Communication

Many people with a developmental disability also have other impairments. Hearing impairments are common; approximately 40% of those with developmental disability have significant hearing problems and practitioners must take this into account (Levy 2004). In addition, 50–90% of people with developmental disability have communication difficulties (Emerson et al 2001). About 80% of people with a severe developmental disability fail to acquire effective speech, which means that for a successful assessment optometrists will have to modify the way in which they gather information prior to and during optometric assessment. It is important to establish the best mode of communication prior to testing: whether it is slow, clear, speech; a form of sign language such as Makaton; or communication through touch (**Fig. 32.3**). It is also important to learn from the patient and accompanying persons how the patient can best communicate with you. Many patients can communicate their needs and feelings very well using unconventional or unique methods and it is important to ask accompanying persons about this at the start of the test.

Whatever the form of communication most appropriate for the patient, it is important to treat all patients with respect and without a patronizing manner. Treat adults as

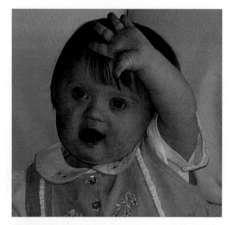

Figure 32.3 An infant with Down's syndrome learns to say 'hello' in Makaton.

adults, don't shout, and speak directly to the patient rather than to carers or family members over the top of the patient's head. Many people with developmental disability have difficulty in processing a lot of information at one time. Questions directed to patients should be simple and short. Do not string a list of questions together, but ask them individually so that the patient is not confused. Some patients may take time to respond to questions. Allow them time to answer, and if one does not understand their response ask them to repeat it or include the family/carer in the discussion to clarify what is meant.

Consent

Issues surrounding consent have become an area for great debate in recent years. Optometrists assume consent during an eye examination, as most 'normal' patients make and willingly attend their appointments. A person with a developmental disability may not have initiated their visit to the optometrist but their consent to participate in the eye examination should, when possible, be ascertained. This is usually done by explaining the procedures as the test proceeds and ensuring the patient is happy to continue. When a patient has a profound developmental disability, explicit consent may not be possible to obtain, but the optometrist and the patient's family/carer should be sensitive to the patient's responses and cease testing if it becomes clear that the patient is not happy with the process. At all times, as with all patients, optometrists must ensure they are acting in the patient's best interests.

History and symptoms

In order to address the patient's needs, optometrists routinely gather a full case history at the start of an eye examination (see Ch. 26). It is important to know the following before examining a patient with a developmental disability (adapted from John & Woodhouse 2004):

- What prompted the examination (pain? changes in behaviour?)?
- What do family/carers know about the patient's vision and past ocular history?
- What is the patient's general health? Are they taking any medications?
- Are there visual problems in the family?
- What behaviours do the family/carer observe (symptoms e.g. eye rubbing, behaviour changes)?
- What are their concerns?
- What are the patient's likes, dislikes?
- What are the patient's hobbies and preferred activities?

It is much easier to obtain this information from an accompanying person who actually knows and has spent time with the patient. If it is known that such a person cannot accompany the patient to the eye examination and that a 'stand-in' care worker will be sent instead, it may be possible to send out a questionnaire to the patient's residence prior to the test to elicit this information from someone who can give useful responses.

A visit to the optometrist might be challenging for a patient with a developmental disability who does not like new environments or new experiences. It is helpful if the patient's family/carers can talk through what might happen at the examination. Many families are happy to practise turning room lights off and looking at penlights, or covering up one eye at a time, and practising matching pictures if it improves the value that they and their family member get from the visit. The optometrist should make sure that the testing environment is as calm as possible and explain what is going to happen, giving the patient time to understand and consent to new procedures. Familiarization with test procedures may increase test times, but it will also increase the quality of the results obtained. In collaboration with speech and language therapists, optometrists providing visual assessment for adults with developmental disabilities within care homes and day centres in Northern Ireland have developed pre-testing information packs which care workers and families can use to familiarize patients with eye examination procedures. Familiarity with and reassurance about what is going to take place during the eye examination improves cooperation and the quality of test results.

A discussion about whether the patient is averse to physical contact is also valuable. Some people with a developmental disability will find physical contact highly disturbing. Others may feel threatened or upset by being touched about the face and head by a 'stranger', and consent should be sought and an explanation given of what will happen before such contact.

Optometric assessment

In order to provide a service for patients with developmental disabilities who may have physical, communication or hearing difficulties optometrists require a flexible approach. However, some core skills and techniques are valuable and these will be discussed.

The most useful vision tests for the majority of patients with developmental disability are arguably objective tests that require limited input from the patient. Such tests have been developed by vision researchers primarily to assess visual function in infancy and early childhood. However, due to their objective nature they can be applied, across the age range, to non-verbal patients and those with limited cooperation skills. These techniques are fully described and discussed in Chapter 13.

Refractive error assessment

High refractive errors are a common feature amongst patients with developmental disability. Uncorrected refractive errors are likely to be responsible for a significant proportion of visual difficulties amongst those with developmental disability, and accurate retinoscopy is essential as it may be difficult or impossible to refine prescriptions subjectively.

Distance static retinoscopy is often successful if an interesting enough distance target is available. This could be a family member making faces or showing the patient items of interest. The Thomson Test Chart 2000 software also has an excellent range of fixation targets including cartoons, images of wildlife, and space pictures. These can be changed throughout the test to maintain interest. TV or video/DVDs can also be used as fixation targets.

Mohindra or near retinoscopy is a very valuable technique for assessing refractive error (Mohindra 1977; Mohindra & Molinari 1979; Saunders & Westall 1992). The patient views a dimmed retinoscope light in a totally darkened room. It is generally easy to maintain fixation under these conditions as long as the patient is comfortable in the dark. Trial lenses can be used in sphere/cylinder combinations to neutralize the retinoscope reflex. This technique is discussed further in Chapter 28.

Cycloplegic refraction may be appropriate, particularly when fixation patterns are unusual and cooperation is limited. It is also very useful when patients are not happy in darkened conditions as it can be done with room lights on. Standard procedures apply and are discussed elsewhere (Ch. 7). This technique has obvious disadvantages. Firstly, the discomfort experienced by the patient on instillation of the cycloplegic agent can be unsettling for the patient and may reduce further cooperation. Secondly, even if the patient is compliant with further testing, cycloplegia renders further functional assessment redundant. The value of using a non-cycloplegic retinoscopy technique is that knowledge about refractive error can then be used during subsequent assessment of accommodative function and visual acuity. A cycloplegic agent may then be instilled if necessary to confirm non-cycloplegic findings and aid prescribing decisions.

Assessment of accommodative function

Even when appropriately corrected for distance refractive error many patients with cerebral palsy and Down's syndrome fail to accommodate fully for near targets *regardless of age*. Older patients entering presbyopia are likely to have issues relating to diminishing accommodative function. An objective assessment of accommodative function in all patients with developmental disability is essential. Subjective appreciation of blur and comparison of distance and near acuities to imply accommodative function is not sufficient. The former is often unsuccessful and the latter often misleading. The modified Cross–Nott dynamic retinoscopy technique has been validated for use in paediatric populations and those with developmental disabilities (Leat 1996; Woodhouse et al 2000b; Cregg et al 2001; McClelland & Saunders 2003, 2004; McClelland et al 2006) and was described in Chapter 15. Dynamic retinoscopy provides an objective assessment of whether accommodation is accurate for a target at a given distance, whether there is an accommodative lag (under-accommodation) or lead (over-accommodation). The patient does not need to respond other than fixing an appropriately detailed near vision target (**Fig. 32.4**).

McClelland and Saunders (2004) describe the normal range of accommodative lags for children aged 4 to 15 years when using dynamic retinoscopy at three test distances (**Table 32.2**). These normal ranges can be used to identify children failing to accommodate normally for their age. Another, less formal method for deciding when a patient is under-accommodating is based on the data of Brookman (1981, 1983), which suggest a normal lag for a target at 25 cm does not exceed 0.75 D. Accommodative lags greater than this may be considered significant. Clinical experience suggests that most children who fail to accommodate do not fall just outside the normal ranges or have lags which are slightly more than 0.75 D at 25 cm but demonstrate large lags and gross under-accommodation.

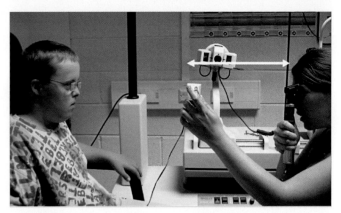

Figure 32.4 Dynamic retinoscopy through distance prescription on a teenager with Down's syndrome. The white arrow indicates the lag of accommodation demonstrated.

Table 32.2 Mean accommodative response and 95% confidence limits for visually and developmentally normal children aged 4–15 years

	4 D demand (target at 25 cm)	6 D demand (target at 16.7 cm)	10 D demand (target at 10 cm)
Normal range (D) (mean response ±2SD)	2.94–4.46	4.12–6.40	5.02–10.00
Mean response (D) (±SD)	3.70±0.39	5.26±0.58	7.51±1.27
Mean lag (D) (±SD)	0.30±0.39	0.74±0.58	2.49±1.27

n = 125
SD = standard deviation

Visual acuity measures

Many families and carers are keen to discover what the person they are caring for can see. Many patients cannot explain this for themselves and an assessment of both distance and near visual acuity and/or vision is central to the eye examination. Most of the visual acuity tests that are suitable for people with a developmental disability are those used to assess paediatric populations and are fully described in Chapter 28. These include preferential looking tests such as the Cardiff Acuity Test and the Keeler acuity cards, picture naming and matching tests such as the Kay picture test and the Lea symbols, or the use of visual evoked potentials (see p 315). It is important that both distant and near visual acuity are assessed. Near vision charts include the Near Kay picture test and the Lea symbols near test (**Fig. 32.5**).

When applying tests originally designed for younger children to older patients with a developmental disability, the tests may seem 'babyish' or patronizing. For example, the Cardiff Acuity Test is a very useful way of assessing visual acuity from a patient who has limited communication skills but can demonstrate their ability to resolve a visual target by making eye movements. The pictures used in the test are

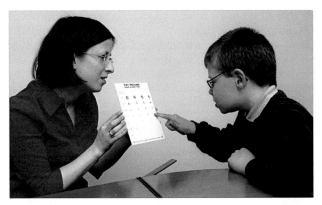

Figure 32.5 Measuring near visual acuity with the Near Kay picture test.

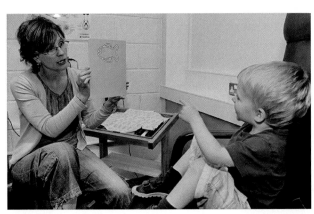

Figure 32.6 The Cardiff Acuity Test can be used to assess preferential-looking visual acuity across all age groups where communication is limited. Eye movement responses are used to judge where the target is positioned.

simple outlines of a house, car, duck, etc. (**Fig. 32.6**) that an older patient may find childish. For this reason an alternative version of the Cardiff Acuity Test has been developed with pictures that are less child-centred.

A common characteristic of a person with a developmental disability is that he or she may not be motivated to try when a task becomes difficult. When assessing acuity, the optometrist deliberately makes the task harder and harder until the patient 'fails'. People with a developmental disability may not be willing to 'fail' and may give up, resulting in falsely poor acuity measures. With this in mind, it is important to use plenty of praise and it can be helpful to intersperse 'hard' tasks with easier ones to keep up motivation and obtain more accurate acuity scores.

Electrophysiological assessment of visual acuity using the visual evoked potential (VEP) is not widely available to optometric practitioners, but is a valuable addition to the test battery in hospitals or academic environments. An example of the utility of the VEP in assessing visual function is in Rett's syndrome (Saunders et al 1995; McCulloch et al 2000). This condition, which affects only females, manifests over the first years of life as developmental milestones are gained and then subsequently lost. Girls with Rett's syndrome may learn to walk and talk, but subsequently lose these skills, and are usually severely developmentally disabled and non-verbally communicative. When using preferential looking tests to assess visual acuity, practitioners are likely to find a poor visual response, but reports from families and carers often indicate good vision

when such girls are motivated. In particular, the author was given reports by families that the girls used eye and facial movements to choose between offered foods, but when preferential looking was applied to assess vision no eye movement responses were observed. However, electrophysiological testing of responses to pattern stimuli demonstrated excellent, reproducible VEP responses to relatively detailed stimuli, suggesting normal levels of pattern vision (Saunders et al 1995). It is thought that whilst vision remains good in these children, behavioural methods of acuity testing, such as preferential looking, fail to interest sufficiently to elicit eye movement responses. Parental reports of good vision were accurate, but only an objective VEP assessment of acuity was able to confirm this.

Contrast sensitivity assessment

Most optometrists do not routinely measure contrast sensitivity (see Ch. 12). While it provides useful information about visual function, optometrists rely on the fact that most patients are able to describe quite well the nature and extent of their visual difficulties. Formal measures of contrast sensitivity are put aside and the evidence of reduced contrast sensitivity gleaned from reports of new difficulties with recognizing faces, navigating steps, etc., in addition to physical evidence of, for example, media opacities. The patient with a developmental disability may not be able to describe their symptoms clearly and a formal assessment of contrast sensitivity can be useful. Some patients may be able to complete contrast sensitivity testing with the Pelli–Robson chart, but for many a less challenging test is appropriate. The Cardiff Contrast Test provides measures of contrast sensitivity using a preferential looking method which can be applied across all levels of intellectual ability (see **Fig. 28.6**). Reduced contrast sensitivity may signal pathology and indicate that environmental adaptations would be beneficial.

Non-standard assessment of vision

In addition to formal methods of visual acuity assessment, less formal methods may be appropriate for the most impaired individuals. When patients are non-responsive to formal methods of visual assessment such as preferential looking, and VEP testing is not available, some information regarding the level of visual functioning and responsiveness can be gained from non-formal methods. Large, silent objects such as flashlights, tinsel balls or bright, coloured balls can be presented to severely impaired patients, and their reaction gauged. These may be presented very close to the patient, in different sectors of the visual field, to gain information regarding the type of visual stimuli that elicit a reaction and the preferred position of presentation. Such evidence can be used to inform family, carers and therapists working with the patient on the best ways to stimulate vision and maximize visual potential.

Visual field assessment

Damage to the brain that has led to a developmental disability may also have implications for the visual field. In particular, when there has been a vascular accident, such as cases of hydrocephalus, cerebral palsy or following pre-term birth, there is an increased risk of gross visual field restriction. Altitudinal defects reducing the extent of the lower visual field are reported in periventricular leucomalacia (a relatively common consequence of extreme preterm birth) (Jacobson & Dutton 2000). Identification of visual field defects and explanation of their impact on everyday activities can be a revelation for patients, families and carers.

For many patients with a developmental disability, automated visual field testing may not be appropriate. However, when time and sufficient energy is given to explanation and familiarization with the equipment, automated central field screening may be possible. For many patients, a gross assessment of visual fields may be more practical and informative. A common technique is arc perimetry, in which the examiner brings silent, appropriately sized targets from non-seeing to seeing areas of the visual field to estimate its extent (see Ch. 20). This technique usually works best in people with developmental disability (and young children) if the examiner stands behind the patient. The target used to assess the gross visual field may be the examiner's hands, a silent toy or a Stycar ball (**Fig. 32.7**). To provide information on day-to-day activities it is generally acceptable to make these measures binocularly.

Assessment of eye movements

Patients with developmental disabilities have an increased incidence of strabismus, nystagmus and other ocular motor disorders. Distance and near cover test and assessment of fixing and following must be carried out. Some patients may respond better to a face being used as a distance fixation target for cover test and the examiner's face at near.

Note should be made of any strabismus present and which eye is dominant, as this will have functional implications for the patient. People with cerebral palsy and other more complex neurological disorders may have abnormal eye movements and information about this must be incorporated into the picture being formed by the optometrist of the patient's visual status.

Ocular health

The increase in visual impairment in populations with developmental disability and aged over 50 years (Evenhuis et al 2001) is likely to be in part attributable to unidentified ocular pathology. Treatable conditions such as cataract have been reported as causes of visual impairment in studies of groups with developmental disability (Woodhouse et al 2000a; Evenhuis et al 2001; Warburg 2001a). It is important that appropriate referral is made in the presence of pathology, and treatment applied when necessary. Traditional reluctance to treat patients with developmental disabilities for conditions such as cataract should not be a barrier to surgery. Cooke et al (2006) demonstrated that cataract removal surgery and outcomes are as successful for patients with moderate to severe developmental disability as for their peers.

Indirect ophthalmoscopy may be the most appropriate method for internal eye examination of patients who are averse to close contact (see Ch. 18), but direct ophthalmoscopy is often highly successful if time is taken to familiarize the patient with the procedure and its purpose. Intraocular pressures can be measured with non-contact methods, particularly with hand-held apparatus such as the Pulsair and the Tiolat. Familiarization and explanation is, once again, pivotal to success.

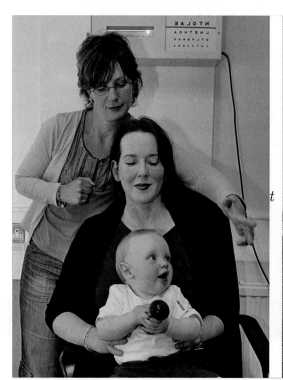
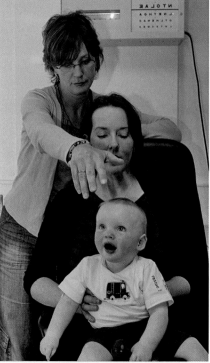

Figure 32.7 A modification of arc perimetry can provide gross information on the extent of the visual field.

Management

At the conclusion of an eye examination the optometrist generally sums up what has been done, what results have been found, how these relate to the patient's pre-test concerns and what the future plan is. The same procedure should apply for the patient with a developmental disability. It is important to address the reason why the patient initially attended for an eye examination in addition to any additional concerns that testing may have highlighted.

Refractive error

Many patients with developmental disability will need a prescription for spectacles. This will be an important part of the management plan, and prescribing decisions depend on factors such as age, unaided and aided visual acuity, as well as considerations relating to binocular function.

When testing children with developmental disability it is appropriate to start with the guidelines available for typically developing children (see Ch. 28). Practitioners generally 'hold off' prescribing for typically developing young children without strabismus or amblyopia to ensure that emmetropization, if it is going to occur, has a chance to proceed (Leat 1988; American Academy of Ophthalmology 2002). However, because it is known that children with all types of developmental disability are likely to retain high refractive errors beyond infancy and the failure of emmetropization in children with Down's syndrome has been shown empirically (Cregg et al 2001, 2003), it may be useful to prescribe earlier for children with developmental disability. This is particularly true when hyperopia is present alongside reduced accommodation, a relatively common feature in conditions that affect development. A child's sphere of interest is essentially relatively close and if significant hyperopia exists in conjunction with reduced accommodative facility then near objects will be blurred. This is likely to affect both general and visual development.

To summarize, when a child has a developmental disability, hyperopic prescriptions should be applied earlier than for typically developing children, particularly when there is evidence of reduced accommodation. These hyperopic prescriptions should not be reduced routinely as advised for typically developing children, and 'full plus' may be appropriate. Frequent review (e.g. 2–3 months after spectacle correction and regularly thereafter) is important and monitoring of visual acuity, accommodation and binocular status are essential.

Adults with extremely high, previously uncorrected refractive errors are not uncommon (Warburg 1994, 2001a; van Splunder et al 2003) and when prescribing for older children and adults it may be necessary to introduce the full correction slowly, through successive visits to the optometrist. Instant full spectacle correction of refractive errors is likely to be neither safe nor comfortable for the patient. A gradual approach to the introduction of high-powered spectacle lenses may to be sensible, allowing patients to adapt visually to changes such as the sudden appearance of previously unseen detail and the introduction of spectacle lens aberrations, and spatially to minification, magnification and the implications of these effects on tasks such as judging distances.

It is vital to monitor the impact of refractive correction on visual acuity and visual functioning. Review appointments are necessary not only to assess visual performance but to find out how the patient is getting on with their glasses, to check compliance and fit.

Near vision correction

When near function is impaired by poor accommodation as a result of either presbyopia or accommodative dysfunction in childhood, the optometrist must consult with the patient and family or carers to decide on the most appropriate management. For many this will mean the provision of a near addition in a separate pair of reading glasses, bifocals or progressive addition lenses (PALs). The choice will depend on the patient's preference, prescription, head posture and any physical limitations they may have, including difficulties controlling eye movements. Cost implications must also be discussed. Stewart et al (2005) have demonstrated great success with bifocal correction in children with Down's syndrome. Dutton described a case when PALs provided excellent results for a child with dyskinetic cerebral palsy (Ross et al 1996).

The power of the near addition prescribed will depend on the level of accommodative deficit found and the visual needs of the patient, taking into consideration their hobbies, the type of educational material they are using and their habitual working distance. Saunders and McClelland (2004), when prescribing near additions for children with cerebral palsy, measured the size of the accommodative lag at the preferred working distance and calculated the amount of near addition required to bring the accommodative response into the normal range for the child's age. Using this method they prescribed near additions which varied between patients. A more straightforward method was utilized by Stewart et al (2005) when prescribing near additions for children with Down's syndrome. Stewart et al used a standard +2.50 DS addition for all children with accommodative dysfunction and demonstrated excellent results in terms of compliance, visual performance and improvement in attention to educational and other near material. This successful strategy may be generally recommended for children with accommodative deficits.

There are no published guidelines available describing the correct age at which to commence near vision correction for a child with a developmental disability and reduced accommodative function. However, the practitioner should bear in mind the type and size of educational and play material the patient is using. Books and toys suitable for infants and young children tend not to require a high level of detailed vision, offering large, bright, uncomplicated visual targets. However, with progression through the education system and with increasing age, appropriate toy and educational material becomes more detailed and visually challenging. School-aged children should be encouraged to bring school or hobby material to the eye examination in order that the practitioner can see whether near vision correction is beneficial. Clinical experience suggests that school entry is an appropriate age for the introduction of a near vision correction. This decision must be made in consultation with the child and their family and with other visual and general factors being taken into consideration.

For some patients the most appropriate solution may not be a near vision spectacle correction. For myopic individuals, removal of distance glasses and advice about optimal near viewing distance may be more appropriate. A −10.00 D myope with poor vision may benefit from the magnification gained by removing spectacles and working at 10 cm for close tasks. However, it is important that the usefulness of this close working distance is stressed to the patient and to family and carers, as such near working distances may otherwise be discouraged or thought to 'damage the eyes'.

For some patients, non-optical methods of achieving better near vision may be optimal. If this is the case, or if spectacles have been tried and rejected, information on non-optical modifications must be included in the discussion with the patient and family/carers. In particular, the production of suitably enlarged, high-contrast images and the availability of other large-print formats including increasing text size on computer screens can be discussed, and advice regarding localized lighting and modifications to the home such as might be suitable for any person with reduced vision should be offered (see Ch. 30). It may also be appropriate to demonstrate simple magnifying aids or to refer patients to a low-vision specialist if vision cannot be improved with spectacles.

The management options described above may also be supplemented by vision therapy and/or orthoptic treatment where appropriate expertise exists. The popularity of such treatment modalities varies across regions and evidence supporting the efficacy of vision therapy is limited.

Dispensing

Finding spectacles to fit patients with developmental disabilities may require the optometrist or dispensing optician to modify and adjust frames more often than for other patients. Some patients with developmental disability may have unusual features. For example, people with Down's syndrome have smaller interpupillary distances but wider than average faces. Their heads tend also to be shorter antero-posteriorly than average, requiring the sides of frames to be shortened for a good fit. Frames may need to be sourced specifically for the patient with developmental disability who has particularly unusual facial features. However, on the whole, drastic measures are not required, and stock frames can usually be adapted. The practitioner has a duty to ensure that frames fit well, are comfortable, that the patient is happy with them and they are cosmetically acceptable.

Many families/carers are concerned that patients will not wear their glasses. On the contrary, excellent compliance with bifocal correction has been demonstrated for children with Down's syndrome (Stewart et al 2005). Clinical experience supports this and suggests that success rates increase if time is taken to ensure a good fit and encouragement and support from the practitioner and family/carers is sustained. For this to happen it is essential that everyone understands why the spectacles are important. Clear information should be given verbally and in a written report describing why glasses are needed, how they will help the patient and when they should be worn. In this way the patient and everyone working with them appreciates the importance of the glasses. If more than two pairs are necessary it will also clarify when each pair is to be worn. It may be necessary to introduce spectacle wear slowly and the best method for doing this will depend on the individual patient. However, it is often helpful to begin wearing the glasses during a favourite activity, which the clear vision the spectacles provide will enhance, for example, reading a book with a child or watching a favourite television programme.

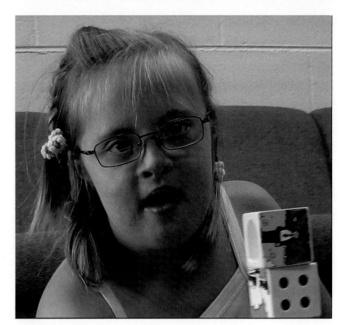

Figure 32.8 Bifocal segments should be fitted high when prescribing to children.

It is important when fitting bifocals to children that segment heights are fitted high, to pupil centre, rather than lid margin (**Fig. 32.8**). This must be made clear on prescriptions issued for children requiring near additions.

When more than one pair of spectacles is required for different uses, it is sensible to chose frames which are sufficiently different to allow easy distinction and identification.

Reporting

Following a 'routine' eye examination, a verbal summary for the patient and a written note on the record card is the usual format for reporting findings. Formal reports are generally only generated when onward referral is required. For the patient with a developmental disability it is important to provide a written report routinely summarizing findings and clearly stating management decisions. This report should be provided for the patient and, with their consent (or their family/carers), disseminated to their family/carers, their school, day centre or place of work and to other health, social and education professionals who are working with them. It may be important to send a report to the educational support services and to request visual support for children in education or for such support to be re-evaluated. A good relationship between stakeholders such as the rehabilitation services, teachers of the visually impaired and other therapists can be built up through sharing of information.

When writing a report it may be useful to start with a brief description of the patient and why they attended for an eye examination, followed by a summary in lay language of their visual strengths and difficulties, strategies for improving and maximizing visual potential, information on spectacle wear and the plan for future follow-up or onward referral. This is supplemented with a technical report on the details of the optometric findings such as the refractive error, accommodative function, ocular motor posture, extent of visual field and visual acuity. The value of 'plain English' reporting of findings and management cannot be underestimated. Kerr et al (2003) investigated visual impairment in a residential setting and fed back visual information to the institution in a 'plain English' report. These reports were so well received that they became standard procedure in the local service.

When vision is irreversibly, severely reduced this should be acknowledged in the report and it may be appropriate to refer the patient for registration as sight-impaired if this has not already been done. Onward referral to low-vision services may also be valuable.

Translating visual acuity measures

For a report to be in 'plain English' it is useful to translate visual acuity measures into a form which lay people find meaningful. Many families/carers ask, 'What can this person see?' It is useful if eye care professionals can provide clear information regarding the level of detail that is appreciable to the patient and what size and type of material should be used in educational and recreational material. This must also be related to the distance at which the material is being viewed. A measure of visual acuity related in terms of Snellen fraction or logMAR decimal, e.g. 6/60 or 1.0 logMAR, is unlikely to be helpful in isolation. The members of a multidisciplinary team providing visual assessment for children with complex difficulties in Northern Ireland have developed a website from which images of appropriate sizes for people with a range of acuities can be downloaded (http://www.science.ulst.ac.uk/visionsci/links.htm). A visual acuity of 6/60, for example, can be translated into images of appropriate size and detail for a child or adult to work with at a range of distances from 30 cm to 3 m. The recommended size of visual material is given as double the estimated visual acuity level, so that letters and images are well within the visual potential of the patient rather than at their limit.

Another way of describing visual acuity in a meaningful way is to indicate how much bigger or closer an object will need to be for the patient to see it, compared to a 'normally' sighted individual. Therefore, if visual acuity is measured as 6/60, the person with such acuity is likely to need to have objects 10 times closer or 10 times larger than others before they are seen. This may be a more useful approach when vision is relatively good, i.e. 6/18 (three times bigger, three times closer) because larger multiples can seem alarming for carers. Another difficulty with this method of relating acuity measures to real life is that it deals with the limits of vision. If a person with 6/18 visual acuity has reading material made three times larger than 6/6 they are still likely to be working near the threshold of their visual ability, which is stressful and tiring.

Strategies for maximizing vision and visual potential

Reports should clearly state what spectacles, if any, are needed and why, and when they should be worn. If more than one pair is appropriate, then their different usage must be clarified.

The report may include strategies for maximizing vision and visual potential. For example, if a patient is found to have a right visual field deficit they are likely to respond best to being approached from their left and to educational, recreational or edible material being placed on their left. Care will need to be taken with road crossing and navigation in unfamiliar places. A different seat in the classroom or social group may make participation and inclusion easier. Recognition and understanding of the implications of visual field deficits can make a big difference to the day-to-day practicalities of working with a person with a developmental disability. Spoon-feeding a child (or older person with a physical impairment) with an unidentified hemianopia can be a frustrating and messy business if the spoon is presented from the 'unseeing' side. The patient may willingly open their mouth when they see the spoon coming from their sighted side whereas if it is brought towards them from their non-sighted side they may only 'open up' when they feel the spoon on their lips. Such modifications sound trivial, but feedback from families and carers support their utility.

When nystagmus exists it is important to acknowledge and describe this in the report. Most patients with nystagmus have a 'null point', a position in which their eyes achieve the least amount of movement. The null point is likely to provide the best vision and it should be described, encouraged and supported in reports. Physiotherapists and occupational therapists need this information when working with the person so that they can take into account visually useful head postures. These head postures may also be present with incomitant deviations of the extraocular muscles and these should also be identified and their utility in reducing diplopia discussed.

Ocular motor apraxia is significantly visually disabling. The ability to initiate eye movements and move fixation to new objects or follow moving objects is key for our appreciation of visual material. Children with developmental disability and ocular motor apraxia may appear visually unresponsive and be wrongly thought to have severely reduced vision. A clear description of their eye movement difficulties and advice relating to appropriate placement of visual targets (toys, food, books) directly in the line of sight and limiting the speed at which visual material is presented can be useful.

Dutton (2003) suggested that even if cognitive visual disorders are masked by intellectual and communication difficulties, one should assume they are present and simplify the visual world, limiting the amount and complexity of visual information presented. Straightforward advice such as presenting educational or toy material as isolated single objects on a plain background may be appropriate when cognitive visual problems are suspected. Reduction of visual clutter in the home environment can help a person with cognitive visual dysfunction (and others with poor vision) find important objects more easily. By minimizing patterns (e.g. in carpets and bed coverings) and other visual distractions (e.g. unnecessary ornaments, superfluous clutter) visual performance can improve. Children with cognitive visual dysfunction can become more independent in finding their own toys and clothes following reorganization and simplification of their home environment.

For many patients with reduced vision, poor contrast sensitivity or a combination of visual difficulties, advice regarding modification to the visual environment is likely to be beneficial. The sort of advice that is given commonly to patients with visual impairment is often suitable for patients with a developmental disability, even when visual acuity is relatively good, because these modifications help to simplify visual information and maximize visual potential. Such modifications might include the use of high-contrast plates and cutlery (e.g. white utensils on a plain, dark cloth) and the use of black felt-tip pens rather than pencils or ballpoint pens to draw and write.

Case reports

Below are examples of reports written for patients with developmental disabilities attending an optometric clinic and sent to families, carers, health and education professionals. Reports should include patient details such as date of birth and address and identify all those to whom the report has been sent.

1. Thirteen-year-old girl with Down's syndrome and accommodative dysfunction

N (aged 13 years) is a shy young lady with Down's syndrome and hypothyroidism. She attended for an eye examination as her mother was concerned about her progress at school and whether her glasses needed to be changed. Her current glasses were 3 years old and had been prescribed by the local hospital eye service (R +3.50 DS L +3.75 DS). They were in poor condition and required replacement. N was very cooperative during testing and my results are described below.

Summary of findings

N is moderately long-sighted and her right eye tends to turn in. When she wears her glasses her eyes are straighter, work together better and her vision is better. However, in addition to these previously identified issues N also has difficulty with focusing (ocular accommodation). This is a common problem amongst people with Down's syndrome. It means that when N looks at objects close to her they are blurred, even with her ordinary glasses on. This will make it particularly difficult for her when doing schoolwork. To overcome this problem N needs to have a stronger prescription for near vision and, after discussion with her and her mother, she has been issued with a prescription for bifocals as follows:

R + 3.50/− 0.50 × 180 L + 3.50 DS ADD + 2.50 DS

These glasses should be worn at all times and this has been explained to N. Wearing these glasses should give N excellent vision for distance and close-up and she should be able to see all standard school material.

I will review N again in 3 months to see how she is managing with her bifocals and assess her vision and focusing through them.

Technical details

Refractive error (distant static): R +3.50/−0.50×180 L +3.50 DS

Ocular posture: right accommodative esotropia, well controlled with glasses

Ocular motility: grossly full

Stereopsis (Frisby stereotest with glasses): at least 300 sec arc

Visual acuity (Crowded Kay pictures @ 3 m) with glasses: R 6/24 (0.6 logMAR) L 6/6 part (0.02 logMAR)

Near acuity (Near Kay pictures @ 20 cm) with glasses: R 6/19 (0.5 logMAR) L 6/6 with difficulty (0.0 logMAR)

Accommodation (dynamic retinoscopy through distance Rx): reduced

Ophthalmoscopy: media clear, fundi and discs healthy and normal as seen (right and left)

2. Twenty-year-old man with physical/intellectual impairment, visual field loss and myopia

M is a 20-year-old man who was involved in a road traffic accident 5 years ago. He now uses a wheelchair, has impaired understanding and difficulty communicating. His mother reports that M's vision, which was significantly impaired immediately following the accident, has improved remarkably over the past few years. M is short-sighted (myopic) and wears his spectacles most of the time. He tends to remove them for close work. M's current glasses were prescribed 1 year ago and are in good condition. His mother attended with M today. She was interested to make sure that M's glasses were correct, to find out how well he sees and how he can make the most of his vision.

Summary of findings

M is short-sighted but when wearing his glasses he has good distance vision (better in his right eye than in his left) and should wear them for the television and general use. His glasses do not need to be changed; they are in good condition and of an appropriate strength. M's vision for reading and other close work is better when he takes his glasses off and holds things close (about 20 cm from his eyes). He should be encouraged to do this and when he does his near vision is excellent. After M's accident it was noted that he had difficulty seeing objects to his right side. This problem persists and he failed to respond to targets presented on his right side during testing. When sitting at a table or in a room, M is likely to feel more comfortable and included if he sits so that others are on his left side. It is important when showing M objects that they are presented on his left side. M should continue to have regular eye examinations and we will recall him in 2 years time.

Technical details

Current prescription: R −5.00 DS L −5.00 DS

Ocular posture: no manifest deviation

Visual acuity with glasses (LogMAR Crowded – matching): R 6/9.5(0.2 logMAR), L 6/19 (0.5 logMAR)

Near visual acuity with glasses (Kay near crowded test at 33 cm): Binoc 6/12 (0.3 logMAR)

Near visual acuity *without* glasses (Kay near crowded test at 20 cm): Binoc 6/7.5 (0.1 logMAR)

Accommodation (dynamic retinoscopy): normal

Visual fields to confrontation: marked restriction of right field

Ophthalmoscopy: unremarkable

3. Ten-year-old girl with cerebral palsy, high myopia, visual field restriction and ocular motor apraxia

P is a very engaging 10-year-old girl with quadriplegic cerebral palsy (affecting her right side more than her left) and significant intellectual impairment. She is considerably short-sighted (myopic) and has been successfully wearing glasses for some years. Her mother feels that it might be useful to provide P's school with some guidance regarding her visual status.

Summary of findings

P is significantly short-sighted and her glasses need to be updated as she has become more myopic. A prescription for new glasses was issued today (R −12.00/−3.00 × 10, L −10.00/−2.00 × 10) and her mother was advised to retain the current spectacles as a spare pair.

P's glasses allow her to see much better than she does without spectacles, but even when wearing them her vision is reduced (by the same amount in each eye). In addition, P has difficulty in controlling her eye movements and moving her eyes smoothly and quickly from one object to the next. From what we have seen today and from what we know about her condition it is also likely that P processes visual information rather slowly and has difficulty seeing moving objects. For these reasons P attends best to stationary objects presented straight in front of her and will probably find it difficult to see objects presented alongside others or in a complex scene. The more complicated the picture the less able she may be to see the detail within it. In order to help P see and understand visual information more clearly it would be useful if educational and play material are presented:

- slowly
- straight ahead or slightly to the left of centre
- in a non-crowded format (e.g. simple, isolated images on a plain background)
- at high contrast (e.g. black on white).

P may find it easier to locate objects or toys with her eyes if she is also holding or touching them. In this way her other senses may be useful to help direct her eyes. We have enclosed some examples of images that are of an appropriate size and complexity for P's vision.

Additionally, P has a problem noticing objects positioned on her right-hand side. When speaking to P, feeding P and when working with P she will find it easier if people and objects are positioned straight ahead or to her left-hand side. To compensate for the loss of vision to the right side P may turn her head to the right. This is visually useful for her and ought not to be discouraged.

Partial sight registration has been discussed with P's mother and onward referral has been initiated to the low-vision service of her local hospital. P should have a further eye examination in 2 years time.

Technical details

Current prescription (18 months old, poor condition):
R −10.00/−2.75×10 L −9.00/−2.25×10

Refractive error (distance static): R −12.00/−3.00×10
L −10.00/−2.00×10

Ocular posture: no manifest strabismus

Eye movements: Motility grossly full but intermittent tonic deviation to extreme left gaze and difficulty in re-fixating to new target (ocular motor apraxia)

Visual acuity with glasses (Cardiff Acuity Test @ 1m): R 6/19, L 6/19

Accommodation (dynamic retinoscopy): delayed response but within normal range

Visual fields to confrontation: gross restriction/neglect on right side

Summary

Following the 1995 Disability Discrimination Act in the UK, eye care professionals must not refuse to accept a patient on the grounds that they have a developmental disability. Some practitioners may feel less comfortable or qualified to examine patients with developmental disability and where another local practitioner specializes in this field it might be appropriate to mention them to families/carers. The practitioner who agrees to perform an optometric assessment on a patient with a developmental disability has a professional and ethical duty to ensure that this assessment is of high quality. Small modifications in the eye examination and modest amounts of additional equipment are required to meet these commitments. Extra time for testing and completing written reports must also be considered to ensure best practice. Just as importantly, the practitioner must be empathetic to the patient's needs and difficulties and flexible in the way they approach each eye examination. As with any area of expertise, there is no substitute for experience and this is readily gained the more patients are examined.

Providing high-quality optometric care for patients with developmental disabilities can be challenging but when done properly is very rewarding and can make a significant difference to the quality of a patient's life.

References

Abel E L, Sokel R J 1987 Incidence of fetal alcohol syndrome and economic impact of FAS-related anomalies. Drug and Alcohol Dependency 19(1):51–70

Altman B 1976 Fetal alcohol syndrome. Journal of Pediatric Ophthalmology 13:255–258

Altman H E, Hiatt R L, Deweese M W 1966 Ocular findings in cerebral palsy. Southern Medical Journal 59:1015–1018

The American Academy of Ophthalmology 2002 Preferred Practice Patterns: paediatric eye evaluations. Online. Available: www.aao.org

Banks M S 1980 The development of visual accommodation during early infancy. Child Development 51:646–666

Bax M C 1964 Terminology and classification of cerebral palsy. Developmental Medicine and Child Neurology 6:295–307

Benda C 1947 Mongolism and cretinism. Grune & Stratton, New York

Biglan A W 1990 Ophthalmologic complications of meningomyelocele: a longitudinal study. Transactions of the American Ophthalmological Society 88:389–462

Black P 1982 Visual disorders associated with cerebral palsy. British Journal of Ophthalmology 66:46–52

Bronham N R, Woodhouse J M, Cregg M et al 2002 Heart defects and ocular anomalies in children with Down's syndrome. British Journal of Ophthalmology 86:1367–1368

Brookman K E 1981 A retinoscopic method of assessing accommodative performance of young human infants. Journal of the American Optometric Association 52:865–869

Brookman K E 1983 Ocular accommodation in human infants. American Journal of Optometry and Physiological Optics 60:91–99

Brushfield T 1924 Mongolism. British Journal of Childhood Diseases 21:241–258

Carones F, Brancato R, Venturi E et al 1992 Corneal endothelial anomalies in the fetal alcohol syndrome. Archives of Ophthalmology 110:1128–1131

Cass H D, Sonksen P M, McConachie H R 1994 Developmental setback in severe visual impairment. Archives of Disease in Childhood 70:192–196

Catalano R A 1990 Down syndrome. Survey of Ophthalmology 34(5): 385–398

Cauldfield M A, Honein M A, Yuskiv N et al 2006 National estimates and race/ethnic-specific variation of selected birth defects in the United States, 1999–2001. Birth Defects Research (Part A) 76:747–756

Chan T, Bowell R, O'Keefe M et al 1991 Ocular manifestations in fetal alcohol syndrome. British Journal of Ophthalmology 75: 524–526

Chen A H, O'Leary D J 2000 Free-space accommodative response and minus lens-induced accommodative response in pre-school children. Optometry 71(7):454–458

Cook R C, Glasscock R E 1951 Refractive and ocular findings in the newborn. American Journal of Ophthalmology 34(10):1407–1413

Cooke C A, Frazer D G, Jackson A J 2006 Corneal graft and cataract surgery in patients with moderate to severe intellectual disability. Journal of Applied Research in Intellectual Disabilities 19(4): 383–390

Cregg M, Woodhouse J M, Pakeman V H et al 2001 Accommodation and refractive error in children with Down's syndrome: cross-sectional and longitudinal studies. Investigative Ophthalmology and Visual Science 42(1):55–63

Cregg M, Woodhouse J M, Stewart R E et al 2003 Development of refractive error and strabismus in children with Down's syndrome. Investigative Ophthalmology and Visual Science 44(3):1023–1030

Doyle L W 2004 Victorian Infant Collaborative Study Group. Evaluation of neonatal intensive care for extremely low birth weight infants in Victoria over two decades: 1. Effectiveness. Pediatrics 113(3 Pt1): 505–509

Doyle S, Bullock J, Gray C et al 1998 Emmetropisation, axial length and corneal topography in teenagers with Down's syndrome. The British Journal of Ophthalmology 82(7):793–796

Duane A 1922 Studies in monocular and binocular accommodation with their clinical applications. American Journal of Ophthalmology 20:132–157

Duckman R H 1979 The incidence of visual anomalies in a population of cerebral palsied children. Journal of the American Optometric Association 50:1013–1016

Duckman R H 1984 Accommodation in cerebral palsy: function and remediation. Journal of the American Optometric Association 55:281–283

Dutton G N 2003 Cognitive vision, its disorders and differential diagnosis in adults and children: knowing where and what things are. Eye 17(3):289–304

Dutton G, Ballantyne J, Boyd G et al 1996 Cortical visual dysfunction in children: a clinical study. Eye 10:302–309

Edward D, Li J, Sawaguchi S et al 1993 Diffuse corneal clouding in siblings with fetal alcohol syndrome. American Journal of Ophthalmology 111:484–493

Emerson E, Hatton C, Felce D et al 2001 Learning disabilities – the fundamental facts. The Foundation for People with Learning Disabilities, London

Evenhuis H M 1995 Medical aspects of ageing in a population with intellectual disability: 1. Visual impairment. Journal of Intellectual Disability Research 39(1):19–25

Evenhuis H M, Mul M, Lemaire E K G et al 1997 Diagnosis of sensory impairment in people with intellectual disability in general practice. Journal of Intellectual Disability Research 41(5):422–429

Evenhuis H M, Theunissen M, Denker I et al 2001 Prevalence of visual and hearing impairment in a Dutch institutionalized population with intellectual disability. Journal of Intellectual Disability Research 45(5):457–464

Evereklioglu C, Yilmaz K, Bekir N A 2002 Decreased central corneal thickness in children with Down syndrome. Journal of Pediatric Ophthalmology and Strabismus 39(5):274–277

Flanagan N M, Jackson A J, Hill A E 2003 Visual impairment in childhood: insights from a community-based survey. Child Care, Health and Development 29:493–499

The Foundation for People with Learning Disabilities 2004 Online. Available: www.learningdisabilities.org.uk

Gifford H 1928 The Mongolian eye. American Journal of Ophthalmology 11:887–893

Goddard U K 1965 Ocular changes in hydrocephalus. British Orthoptic Journal 22:72–80

Goodner E K 1974 Myelomeningocele: Part II. Ophthalmologic problems. The Western Journal of Medicine 121:291–292

Hack M, Taylor H G, Drotar D et al 2005 Chronic conditions, functional limitations and special health care needs of school-aged children born with extremely low-birth-weight in the 1990s. Journal of the American Medical Association 2994:318–325

Hagerman R J, Hagerman P H 2002 Fragile X syndrome diagnosis, treatment and research, 3rd edn. The Johns Hopkins University Press 1:3–109

Haire A R, Vernon S A, Rubinstein M P 1991 Levels of visual impairment in a day centre for people with a mental handicap. Journal of the Royal Society of Medicine 84:542–544

Harcourt R B 1968 Ophthalmic complication of meningomyelocele and hydrocephalus in children. British Journal of Ophthalmology 52:670–676

Harcourt B 1974 Strabismus affecting children with multiple handicaps. British Journal of Ophthalmology 58:272–280

Hatton D D, Buckley E, Lachiewicz A et al 1998 Ocular status of boys with fragile X syndrome: a prospective study. Journal of the American Association for Pediatric Ophthalmology and Strabismus 2:298–301

Haugen O H, Høvding G 2001 Strabismus and binocular function in children with Down syndrome: a population-based, longitudinal study. Acta Ophthalmologica Scandinavica 79(2):133–139

Haugen O H, Høvding G, Eide G E 2001a Biometric measurements of the eyes of teenagers and young adults with Down syndrome. Acta Ophthalmologica Scandinavia 79(6):616–625

Haugen O H, Høvding G, Lundstrom I 2001b Refractive development in children with Downs syndrome: a population based, longitudinal study. The British Journal of Ophthalmology 85(6):714–719

Houtman W A, Meihuizen-De Regt M J, Rutgers C H 1981 Strabismus and meningomyelocele. Documenta Ophthalmologica 50:255–261

Hug T, Fitzgerald K, Cibis G 2000 Clinical and electroretinographic findings in fetal alcohol syndrome. Journal of the American Association for Pediatric Ophthalmology and Strabismus 4:200–204

Jacobson L K, Dutton G N 2000 Periventricular leukomalacia: an important cause of visual and ocular motility dysfunction in children. Survey of Ophthalmology 45:1–13

John F M, Woodhouse J M 2004 Optometric assessment and management of children with learning disability. Optometry 7(2):57–62

Keen J H 1973 Blindness in children with myelomeningocele and hydrocephalus. Developmental Medicine and Child Neurology 15:112

Kemner C, Verbaten M N, Cuperus J M et al 1998 Abnormal saccadic eye movements in autistic children. Journal of Autism and Developmental Disorders 28(1):61–67

Kerr A M, McCulloch D, Oliver K et al 2003 Medical needs of people with intellectual disability require regular reassessment, and the provision of client- and carer-held reports. Journal of Intellectual Disability Research 47(2):134–145

Landau L, Berson D 1971 Cerebral palsy and mental retardation: ocular findings. Journal of Pediatric Ophthalmology 8:245–248

Leat S J 1988 Taking action. In: Leat S J, Shute R H, Westall C A (eds) Assessing children's vision: a handbook. Butterworth-Heinemann, Oxford, pp 344–386

Leat S J 1996 Reduced accommodation in children with cerebral palsy. Ophthalmic and Physiology Optics 16:375–384

Levy G 2004 People with learning disabilities – labels, language and health needs. Optometry 7(2):48–51

Lindsay J, McGlade A, Jackson A J 2004 Visual impairment and learning disability in adults. Optometry 7(2):63–67

Lo Casio G P 1977 A study of vision in cerebral palsy. American Journal of Optometry and Physiology Optics 54:332–337

McClelland J F 2004 Accommodative dysfunction and refractive anomalies in children with cerebral palsy. PhD thesis, University of Ulster

McClelland J F, Saunders K J 2003 Dynamic retinoscopy: a valid method for objectively assessing accommodative function? Ophthalmic and Physiological Optics 23:243–250

McClelland J F, Saunders K J 2004 Accommodative lag using Nott dynamic retinoscopy: age norms for school age children. Optometry and Vision Science 81(12):929–933

McClelland J F, Saunders K J, Jackson A J et al May 2005 Visual acuity and disorders of ocular posture in children with cerebral palsy. Investigative Ophthalmology and Visual Science Abstract No. 1395

McClelland J F, Parkes J, Hill N et al 2006 Accommodative dysfunction in children with cerebral palsy; a population based study. Investigative Ophthalmology and Visual Science 47:1824–1830

McCulloch D L, Henderson R M, Saunders K J et al 2000 Vision in Rett syndrome: studies using evoked potentials and event-related potentials. In: Kerr A, Witt Engerströn I (eds) Rett disorder and the developing brain. Oxford University Press, Inc., New York, pp 343–348

Maino D M 2001 Diagnosis and management of special populations, 1st edn. Mosby Inc. Ch. 7 pp 189–205

Maino D M, Maino J H, Maino S A 1990a Mental retardation syndromes with associated ocular defects. Journal of the American Optometric Association 61:707–716

Maino D M, Schlange D, Maino J H et al 1990b Ocular anomalies in fragile syndrome. Journal of the American Optometric Association 61:316–323

Maino D M, Wesson M, Schlange D et al 1991 Optometric findings in fragile X syndrome. Optometry and Vision Science 68(8):634–640

Martinez S, Maino D M 1993 Fragile X syndrome: oculo-visual, developmental and physical characteristics. Journal of Behavioral Optometry 4(3):59–63

Matsuba C A, Jan J E 2006 Long-term outcome of children with cortical visual impairment. Developmental Medicine and Child Neurology 48:508–512

Miller M, Israel J, Cuttone J 1981 Fetal alcohol syndrome. Journal Paediatric Ophthalmology and Strabismus 18:6–15

Miller M, Epstein R, Sugar J et al 1984 Anterior segment anomalies associated with the fetal alcohol syndrome. Journal Pediatric Ophthalmology and Strabismus 21:8–18

Milunsky A, Jick H, Jick S et al 1989 Multivitamin folic acid supplementation in early pregnancy reduces the prevalence of neural tube defects. Journal of the American Medical Association 262:2847–2852

Mohindra I 1977 Comparison of near retinoscopy and subjective refraction in adults. American Journal of Optometry and Physiological Optics 54:319–322

Mohindra I, Molinari J F 1979 Near retinoscopy and cycloplegic retinoscopy in early primary grade school children. American Journal of Optometry and Physiological Optics 56:34–38

The National Autistic Society UK 2008 Online. Available: www.nas.org.uk

Northfield J 2001 What is learning disability? British Journal of Learning Disabilities Factsheets number 001:2

O'Connor A R, Stephenson T J, Johnson A et al 2004 Visual function in low birth weight children. British Journal of Ophthalmology 88:1149–1153

Ormond A W 1912 Notes on the ophthalmic condition of forty-two Mongolian imbeciles. Transactions of the American Ophthalmological Society 32:69–76

Parkes J, Dolk H, Hill N et al 2001 Cerebral palsy in Northern Ireland: 1981–93. Paediatric Perinatal Epidemiology 15:278–286

Pembrey M E, Barnicoat A J, Carmichael B et al 2001 An assessment of screening strategies for fragile X syndrome in the UK. Health Technology Assessment (Winchester, England) 5(7):1–95

Perez-Carpinell J, de Fez M D, Climent V 1994 Visual evaluation in people with Down's syndrome. Ophthalmic and Physiological Optics 14(2):115–121

Rabinowicz I M 1974 Visual function in children with hydrocephalus. Transactions of the Ophthalmological Society of the United Kingdom 94:353–365

Repka M X 2002 Ophthalmological problems of the premature infant. Mental Retardation Developmental and Disabilities Research Reviews 8:249–257

Robinson G C 1987 Congenital ocular blindness in children, 1945–1984. American Journal of Diseases of Children 141:1321–1324

Rogers M 1996 Vision impairment in Liverpool: prevalence and morbidity. Archives of Disease in Childhood 74:299–303

Rosenberg T, Flage T, Hansen E et al 1996 Incidence of registered visual impairment in the Nordic child population. British Journal of Ophthalmology 80:49–53

Rosenhall U, Johansson E, Gillberg C 1988 Oculomotor findings in autistic children. Journal of Laryngology and Otology 102:435–439

Ross L M, Heron G, Mackie R et al 1996 Reduced accommodative function in dyskinetic cerebral palsy: a novel management strategy. Developmental Medicine and Child Neurology 42(10):701–703

Saunders K J, McClelland J F 2004 Spectacle intervention in children with cerebral palsy. Investigative Ophthalmology and Visual Science Abstract No. 1394

Saunders K J, Westall C A 1992 A comparison between near and cycloplegic retinoscopy in the refraction of infants and young children. Optometry and Vision Science 69(8):615–622

Saunders K J, McCulloch D L, Kerr A 1995 Visual function in Rett syndrome. Developmental Medicine and Child Neurology 37:496–504

Scharre J, Creedon M 1992 Assessment of visual function in autistic children. Optometry and Vision Science 69(6):433–439

Scheiman M M 1984 Optometric findings in children with cerebral palsy. American Journal of Optometry and Physiology Optics 61:321–323

Scheiman M M, Rouse M W 2006 Optometric management of learning-related vision problems, 2nd edn. Mosby Inc. Ch 4: pp 85–106

Schenk-Rootlieb A J F, van Nieuwenhuizen O, van der Graaf Y et al 1992 The prevalence of cerebral visual disturbance in children with cerebral palsy. Developmental Medicine and Child Neurology 34:473–480

SCPE Collaborative Group 2000 Surveillance of Cerebral Palsy in Europe (SCPE): a collaboration of cerebral palsy surveys and registers. Developmental Medicine and Child Neurology 42:816–824

Shapiro M B, France T D 1985 The ocular features of Downs syndrome. American Journal of Ophthalmology 99(6):659–663

Sonksen P, Dale N 2002 Visual impairment in infancy: impact on neurodevelopmental and neurobiological processes. Developmental Medicine and Child Neurology 44:782–791

Sorsby A, Benjamin B, Sheridan M et al 1961 In: Refraction and its components during growth of the eye from the age of three. Medical Research Council Special Report Series No. 301. London HMSO

Stein S C, Schut L 1979 Hydrocephalus in myelomeningocele. Childs Brain 4:413–419

Stewart R E, Woodhouse J M, Trojanowska L D 2005 In focus: the use of bifocal spectacles with children with Down's syndrome. Ophthalmic and Physiological Optics 25(6):514–522

Storm R L, PeBenito R, Ferretti C 1987 Ophthalmologic findings in the fragile X syndrome. Archives of Ophthalmology 105:1099–1102

Strömland K 1985 Ocular abnormalities in the fetal alcohol syndrome. Acta Ophthalmologica 63(suppl 171):1–50

Strömland K 1987 Ocular involvement in the fetal alcohol syndrome. Survey of Ophthalmology 31:277–284

Strömland K 2004 Visual impairment and ocular abnormalities in children with fetal alcohol syndrome. Addiction Biology 9:153–157

Strömland K, Hellström A 1996 Fetal alcohol syndrome – an ophthalmological and socioeducational prospective study. Pediatrics 97:845–850

Sutherland G A 1899 Mongolian imbecility in infants. Practitioner 63:632

Taub M B, Rowe S, Bartuccio M 2006 Examining special populations, Part 2: Fragile X syndrome and autism spectrum disorders. Optometry Today February:31–34

van Splunder J, Stilma J S, Bernsen R M D et al 2003 Refractive error and visual impairment in 900 adults with intellectual disabilities in the Netherlands. Acta Ophthalmologica Scandinavica 81:123–129

Vincent A L, Weiser B A, Crupryn M et al 2005 Computerized corneal topography in a paediatric population with Down syndrome. Clinical and Experimental Ophthalmology 33(1):47–52

Volkmar F R, Pauls D 2003 Autism. Lancet 342:1133–1141

Warburg M 1994 Visual impairment among people with developmental delay. Journal of Intellectual Disability Research 38:423–432

Warburg M 2001a Visual impairment in adult people with moderate, severe, and profound intellectual disability. Acta Ophthalmologica Scandinavica 79(5):450–454

Warburg M 2001b Visual impairment in adult people with intellectual disability: Literature review. Journal of Intellectual Disability Research 45(5):421–438

Woodhouse J M 1998 Investigating and managing the child with special needs. Ophthalmic and Physiological Optics 18(2):147–152

Woodhouse J M, Meades J S, Leat S J et al 1993 Reduced accommodation in children with Downs syndrome. Investigative Ophthalmology and Visual Science 34(7):2382–2387

Woodhouse J M, Pakeman V H, Saunders K J et al 1996 Visual acuity and accommodation in infants and young children with Down's syndrome. Journal of Intellectual Disability Research 40:49–55

Woodhouse J M, Griffiths C, Gedling A 2000a The prevalence of ocular defects and the provision of eye care in adults with learning disabilities living in the community. Ophthalmic and Physiological Optics 20(2):79–89

Woodhouse J M, Cregg M, Gunter H L et al 2000b The effect of age, size of target, and cognitive factors on accommodative responses of children with Down's syndrome. Investigative Ophthalmology and Visual Science 41(9):2479–2485

Index